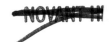

Litt's
DRUG ERUPTION &
REACTION MANUAL

24th
EDITION

Jerome Z. Litt
Neil H. Shear

CRC Press
Taylor & Francis Group
Boca Raton London New York

CRC Press is an imprint of the
Taylor & Francis Group, an **informa** business

CRC Press
Taylor & Francis Group
6000 Broken Sound Parkway NW, Suite 300
Boca Raton, FL 33487-2742

© 2018 by Taylor & Francis Group, LLC
CRC Press is an imprint of Taylor & Francis Group, an Informa business

No claim to original U.S. Government works

Printed in Canada on acid-free paper

International Standard Book Number-13: 978-0-8153-6699-7 (Pack – Paperback and eBook)
International Standard Book Number-13: 978-1-138-49097-0 (Hardback)

Visit the Taylor & Francis Web site at
http://www.taylorandfrancis.com

and the CRC Press Web site at
http://www.crcpress.com

CONTENTS

To Vel – my Muse

JZL

Editors' introductory notes

Any drug has the potential to cause an adverse reaction. An adverse drug reaction (ADR) is an unwanted, unpleasant, noxious, or harmful consequence associated with the use of a medication that has been administered in a standard dose by the proper route, for the purpose of prophylaxis, diagnosis, or treatment. Death is the ultimate adverse drug event.

ADRs are a major problem in drug therapy. They are the most common of all iatrogenic illnesses that complicate up to 15% of therapeutic drug courses, and are a leading cause of morbidity and mortality in healthcare. ADRs should therefore be considered in the differential diagnosis of a wide variety of medical disorders. Many more people – particularly the elderly – are taking more and more prescription and over-the-counter medications. In addition, new drugs are appearing in the medical marketplace on an almost daily basis. It is unsurprising, then, that more and more drug reactions and cutaneous eruptions are emerging.

Prevention, diagnosis and treatment of adverse drug events are becoming increasingly complex, and it is to be expected that physicians in all specialties are often perplexed by the nature of ADRs. To this end, I now offer a new and improved edition that has evolved from the treasured Drug Eruption Reference Manual of previous editions. I hope that you will find this new edition informative and valuable.

Enjoy!

Jerome Z. Litt, M.D.

"Is it safe?"

I am frequently asked that big question from a patient: "Is it safe?" This text is meant to help all prescribers, dispensers and patients understand what the risk of harm might be; whether it is from a drug reaction or interaction, Litt's is the go-to information source. How does this information help answer the unanswerable? Simply put, safety is a process, not a question. With the right information at hand a safe environment can thrive; the most up-to-date relevant data help peel away background noise from a seemingly infinite number of sources. This new edition adds additional support to a risk management environment, and we will continue to provide the most up-to-date and relevant information. I look forward to feedback and suggestions. I thank Jerry Litt for this great opportunity and the awesome work of the team at T&F to keep on top of all new medications that are making the landscape even more complex.

Neil H. Shear, M.D., F.R.C.P.C., F.A.C.P.

Litt's Drug Eruption & Reaction Manual – at a glance

This 24th edition has been revised and updated throughout to present a quick clinical reference guide to adverse drug reactions (ADRs), side effects, drug interactions and other safety information for prescription and over-the-counter medications. There is also material on reactions caused by classes of drugs, enabling you to see at a glance whether a reaction is common to all the drugs in that particular class, or to a majority of them, or only to a significant few.

The aims of this edition remain:
1. To help medical practitioners make informed and safe decisions when diagnosing and prescribing, and also when generally seeking information.
2. To help healthcare professionals remain pharmacovigilant.
3. To provide all physicians, lecturers, educators and pharmacists with an easy-to-use and reliable quick reference tool.

The full and comprehensive picture for all drugs – from which our information derives – can be found at our website database (www.drugeruptiondata.com), which is updated continually. Space in the manual is, unfortunately, constrained, so full profiles for various generic drugs have been eliminated from this print manual because either they have been withdrawn from the marketplace or they are rarely, if ever, prescribed today; new to this edition are links to their basic profiles in the website database. Important new drugs added to this edition of the manual are noted with an asterisk.

A note on ADRs

The incidence and severity of ADRs are influenced by a number of factors:

1. Patient-related factors:

- Age – geriatric, pediatric, adolescent . . . older patients are taking more medications—hence more of a possibility of developing reactions; pediatric patients have more delicate skins; hormonal changes occur in adolescents . . . All these factors play roles in the development of possible adverse reactions.

- Gender – male or female – and if the latter, then pregnant/breast-feeding/menopausal . . .

- Disease – not only the disease being treated, but also other pre-existing health conditions and comorbid diseases. For example, atopic patients are at increased risk for serious allergic reactions. Also, there would be an increased risk for hypersensitivity drug reactions if the patient has asthma or lupus erythematosus.

- Genetics – a patient could have abnormal drug metabolism by cytochrome P450 due to inheriting abnormal alleles.

- Geography – patients living in sunny climes could develop photoxicities from photosensitizing drugs more readily than those who inhabit cooler, less sunny climates.

2. Drug-related factors:

- Type/class of drug – for example, there is a heightened risk of hypersensitivity with the use of beta-blockers (see further the tables on class reactions).

- Duration of therapy – the longer a patient maintains the therapy, the greater the possibility that he/she could develop a reaction.

- Dosage – the greater the dosage, the more likely an adverse side effect.

- Bioavailability – the extent to and rate at which the drug enters systemic circulation, thereby accessing the site of action.

- Interactions with other drugs – for example, synergistic QT prolongation can occur when two QT prolonging agents, such as erythromycin + ritonavir, are used together.

- Route of administration – intramuscular, intravenous, subcutaneous, and topical administrations are more likely to cause hypersensitivity reactions; oral medications are less likely to result in drug hypersensitivity.

The terms "drug allergy," "drug hypersensitivity," and "drug reaction" are often used interchangeably. Drug allergy specifically refers to a reaction mediated by IgE; drug hypersensitivity is an immune-mediated response to a drug agent in a sensitized patient; and drug reactions comprise all adverse events related to drug administration, regardless of etiology.

Vigilance at point of care:

While the possibilities for adverse drug reactions seem endless, we must be on the lookout for any new medication(s) the patient might be taking. A thorough, detailed history of all medications must be made in order to elicit any remote possibility that the drug in question might be the culprit for the side effect. People do not often realize that the common over-the-counter analgesics – aspirin, Tylenol, Advil, Motrin, Naprosyn, and others – are actually medications. Herbals and supplements such as St. John's wort, ginkgo biloba, and echinacea can be responsible for various hypersensitivity reactions. For example, St. John's wort, in particular, interacts adversely with SSRIs and tricyclic antidepressants.

Contents of the book, and how to use them

1. **The A–Z**

    The major portion of the manual lists in alphabetical order the 900+ generic drugs, biologics, and supplements, and the adverse reactions that can arise from their use. An asterisk against the entry title indicates this drug is new to this edition. If you do not find a drug in the main A–Z listing under the name you know it by, you can turn to the concordance of synonyms and trade names to find the generic name it will be listed under. Occasionally a drug has been omitted from the listing but a cross-reference will link to the profile found in our website database (www.drugeruptiondata.com).

Trade (Brand) name(s) are then listed alphabetically. When there are many trade names, the ten (or so) most commonly recognized ones are listed.

Following the trade names is – in parentheses – the latest name of the pharmaceutical company that markets the drug. Many of the names of the companies have changed from earlier editions of this manual because of acquisitions, mergers, and other factors in the pharmaceutical industry.

Next appear the Indication(s), the Class in which the drug belongs, and the Half-life of each drug, where known.

Drug interactions: many severe, hazardous drug–drug interactions are recorded. Only clinically significant drug interactions that have been reported to trigger potential harm and that could be life threatening have been included here in the profile. These interactions are predictable and well documented in controlled studies; they should be avoided.

Pregnancy category: for new drugs approved on or after 30 June, 2015 this field gives (where available) a brief summary of the full statement reflecting the risk for pregnant women as given in the prescribing guidelines; health care providers are advised to check the individual label where necessary.

An explanation of the categories for older drugs (A, B, C, D and X) can be found on our website www.drugeruptiondata.com.

Adverse Drug Reactions: under each drug profile is a list of related ADRs. These adverse events have been classified under the following categories: **Skin**, **Hair**, **Nails**, **Mucosal**, **Cardiovascular**, **Central Nervous System**, **Neuromuscular/Skeletal**, **Gastrointestinal/Hepatic**, **Respiratory**, **Endocrine/Metabolic**, **Genitourinary**, **Renal**, **Hematologic**, **Otic**, **Ocular**, **Local**, **Other**.

Within each category, the reactions are listed alphabetically. Thus, the order of listing does not reflect severity or frequency in any way.

The terminology used to list reaction patterns has been simplified as far as possible by eliminating, for the most part, tags such as "like" (as in "-Psoriasis-like"), "-reactivation," "-syndrome," "-dissemination," "-iform," etc.

The number of reports is given for each reaction in square brackets. The incidence of the most important reactions is given in parentheses where indicated (usually from the full prescribing information for the relevant drug). For example, the profile for Amoxicillin begins:

Skin
> AGEP [28]
> Anaphylactoid reactions/Anaphylaxis [15]
> Angioedema (<10%) [5]

This means that we have 28 journal articles referring to occurrence of AGEP (acute generalized exanthematous pustulosis); 15 articles mentioning the occurrence of anaphylaxis; and 5 articles discussing angioedema, as reactions to Amoxicillin within the Skin category. All these articles appear on the website www.drugeruptiondata.com together with links to the article abstracts on PubMed®. Additionally, the incidence of angioedema as a reaction has been reported as up to 10%.

On some occasions, there are very few adverse reactions to a specific drug. These drugs are still included in the manual as there is a positive significance in negative findings.

2. **Important eruptions / reactions**
i) This section of the manual includes a listing of descriptions of important eruption and reaction patterns. Over 40 eruptions/reactions are described here in alphabetical order, from Acanthosis nigricans to Xerostomia.
ii) Following this section are lists of all drugs that have been found to cause these important eruptions/reactions. This section is a quick look-up tool for drugs that cause important reaction patterns.
    (Descriptions of several other reactions, and lists of drugs associated with these reactions, can be found on our website – www.drugeruptiondata.com.)
iii) We then have a list of the main classes of drugs, from 5-HT1 agonists to Xanthine alkaloids, as a quick reference guide.
iv) There follow lists of the classes of drugs most likely to cause important interactions with other drugs, with the drugs in those classes.
v) We then have an enlarged section of tables of class reactions, enabling you to see at a glance whether a reaction is common to all the drugs in that particular class, or to a majority of them, or only to a significant few.

3. The Concordance

The final part of the manual is a concordance to match synonyms (noted in italic) and trade names with the generic drug name. If you know only the synonym or trade name, you can use this list to find the corresponding generic name to look up in the main A–Z listing section of the book.

ABACAVIR

Trade names: Epzicom (ViiV), Triumeq (ViiV), Trizivir (ViiV), Ziagen (ViiV)
Indications: HIV infections in combination with other antiretrovirals
Class: Nucleoside analog reverse transcriptase inhibitor
Half-life: 1.5 hours
Clinically important, potentially hazardous interactions with: alcohol, arbutamine, argatroban, arsenic, darunavir, ganciclovir, lopinavir, methadone, phenobarbital, phenytoin, protease inhibitors, ribavirin, rifampin, tipranavir, valganciclovir
Pregnancy category: C
Important contra-indications noted in the prescribing guidelines for: nursing mothers
Note: Epzicom is abacavir and lamivudine; Triumeq is abacavir, dolutegravir and lamivudine; Trizivir is abacavir, lamivudine and zidovudine.
Warning: HYPERSENSITIVITY REACTIONS, LACTIC ACIDOSIS and SEVERE HEPATOMEGALY, and EXACERBATIONS OF HEPATITIS B

Skin
Anaphylactoid reactions/Anaphylaxis (3%) [3]
Exanthems [2]
Hypersensitivity (8–9%) [69]
Lipoatrophy [2]
Rash (5–7%) [17]
Stevens-Johnson syndrome [2]
Toxic epidermal necrolysis [2]

Cardiovascular
Myocardial infarction [9]

Central Nervous System
Abnormal dreams (10%) [2]
Anxiety (5%)
Chills (6%)
Depression (6%)
Fever (6%) [2]
Headache (7–13%) [4]
Insomnia [2]
Migraine (7%)
Neuropsychiatric disturbances [3]
Sleep related disorder (10%)
Vertigo (dizziness) (6%) [3]

Neuromuscular/Skeletal
Asthenia (fatigue) (7–12%) [2]
Bone or joint pain (5–6%)
Myalgia/Myopathy (5–6%) [2]

Gastrointestinal/Hepatic
Abdominal pain (6%)
Diarrhea (7%) [2]
Gastritis (6%)
Hepatotoxicity [4]
Nausea (7–19%) [5]
Vomiting (2–10%)

Respiratory
Bronchitis (4%)
Cough [2]
Pneumonia (4%)

Endocrine/Metabolic
ALT increased (6%)
AST increased (6%)
Hyperamylasemia (2–4%)
Hypertriglyceridemia (2–6%)

Renal
Fanconi syndrome [2]

Hematologic
Agranulocytosis [3]
Neutropenia (2–5%)

Other
Adverse effects [4]
Infection (5%)

ABALOPARATIDE *

Trade name: Tymlos (Radius Health)
Indications: Osteoporosis in postmenopausal women
Class: Parathyroid hormone analog
Half-life: <2 hours
Clinically important, potentially hazardous interactions with: none known
Pregnancy category: N/A (Not indicated for use in females of reproductive potential)
Important contra-indications noted in the prescribing guidelines for: pediatric patients
Warning: RISK OF OSTEOSARCOMA

Cardiovascular
Orthostatic hypotension (<4%)
Palpitation (5%)
Tachycardia (2%)

Central Nervous System
Headache (8%)
Vertigo (dizziness) (2–10%)

Neuromuscular/Skeletal
Asthenia (fatigue) (3%)

Gastrointestinal/Hepatic
Abdominal pain (3%)
Nausea (8%)

Endocrine/Metabolic
Hypercalcemia (3%) [2]
Hyperuricemia (25%)

Genitourinary
Hypercalciuria (11%)
Urolithiasis (2%)

Local
Injection-site edema (10%)
Injection-site erythema (58%)
Injection-site pain (9%)

ABARELIX

See: www.drugeruptiondata.com/drug/id/1011

ABATACEPT

Trade name: Orencia (Bristol-Myers Squibb)
Indications: Rheumatoid arthritis, juvenile idiopathic arthritis in pediatric patients 6 years of age and older
Class: Disease-modifying antirheumatic drug (DMARD), T-cell co-stimulation modulator
Half-life: 12–23 days
Clinically important, potentially hazardous interactions with: adalimumab, anakinra, certolizumab, denosumab, echinacea, etanercept, golimumab, infliximab, lenalidomide, live vaccines, natalizumab, pimecrolimus, sipuleucel-T, tacrolimus, TNF antagonists, trastuzumab
Pregnancy category: C
Important contra-indications noted in the prescribing guidelines for: nursing mothers; pediatric patients

Skin
Basal cell carcinoma [3]
Eczema [2]
Herpes simplex (<5%) [3]
Herpes zoster [3]
Hypersensitivity [2]
Malignancies [10]
Psoriasis [13]
Rash (4%) [6]
Sjögren's syndrome [4]
Squamous cell carcinoma [5]
Vasculitis [2]

Mucosal
Stomatitis [3]

Cardiovascular
Hypertension (7%) [4]
Hypotension [2]

Central Nervous System
Fever (5%) [2]
Headache (5–18%) [6]
Vertigo (dizziness) (9%) [3]

Neuromuscular/Skeletal
Asthenia (fatigue) [2]
Back pain (7%) [2]
Pain in extremities (3%)

Gastrointestinal/Hepatic
Abdominal pain (5%)
Diarrhea (5%) [3]
Dyspepsia (6%)
Gastroenteritis [5]
Nausea (5%) [2]
Vomiting [2]

Respiratory
Bronchitis (<13%) [4]
Cough (5–8%)
Influenza (5–13%) [2]
Nasopharyngitis (12%) [6]
Pharyngitis [3]
Pneumonia (<5%) [7]
Pulmonary toxicity [2]
Rhinitis (<5%) [2]
Sinusitis (5–13%) [3]
Tuberculosis [2]
Upper respiratory tract infection (>10%) [9]

Genitourinary
Urinary tract infection (5–13%) [10]

Local
Infusion-related reactions [4]
Infusion-site reactions (9%) [5]
Injection-site erythema [3]
Injection-site hematoma [2]
Injection-site pain [3]
Injection-site pruritus [2]
Injection-site reactions (3%) [8]

Other
Adverse effects [24]
Death [2]
Infection (36–54%) [25]

ABCIXIMAB

See: www.drugeruptiondata.com/drug/id/2

ABEMACICLIB *

Trade name: Verzenio (Lilly)
Indications: Hormone receptor-positive, human epidermal growth factor 2-negative advanced or metastatic breast cancer, either as monotherapy or in combination with fulvestrant
Class: Kinase inhibitor
Half-life: 18 hours
Clinically important, potentially hazardous interactions with: grapefruit juice, ketoconazole, strong CYP3A4 inducers and inhibitors
Pregnancy category: N/A (Can cause fetal harm)
Important contra-indications noted in the prescribing guidelines for: nursing mothers; pediatric patients

Hair
Alopecia (12%)
Mucosal
Stomatitis (14%)
Xerostomia (17%)
Central Nervous System
Anorexia [3]
Dysgeusia (taste perversion) (12%)
Fever (11%)
Headache (20%)
Vertigo (dizziness) (11%)
Neuromuscular/Skeletal
Arthralgia (15%)
Asthenia (fatigue) (65%) [7]
Gastrointestinal/Hepatic
Abdominal pain (39%) [2]
Constipation (17%)
Diarrhea (90%) [7]
Nausea (64%) [7]
Vomiting (35%) [4]
Respiratory
Cough (19%)
Endocrine/Metabolic
ALT increased (31%)
Appetite decreased (45%) [2]
AST increased (30%)
Dehydration (10%)
Serum creatinine increased (13%) [3]
Weight loss (14%) [2]

Hematologic
Anemia (25%) [3]
Leukopenia (17%) [4]
Neutropenia (37%) [5]
Thrombocytopenia (20%) [3]
Other
Infection (31%)

ABIRATERONE

Trade name: Zytiga (Janssen Biotech)
Indications: Metastatic castration-resistant prostate cancer (in combination with prednisone)
Class: CYP17 inhibitor, Enzyme inhibitor
Half-life: 12 hours
Clinically important, potentially hazardous interactions with: atazanavir, carbamazepine, clarithromycin, CYP3A4 inhibitors or inducers, indinavir, itraconazole, ketoconazole, nefazodone, nelfinavir, phenobarbital, phenytoin, rifabutin, rifampin, rifapentine, ritonavir, saquinavir, telithromycin, thioridazine, voriconazole
Pregnancy category: X
Important contra-indications noted in the prescribing guidelines for: nursing mothers; pediatric patients
Note: Contra-indicated in women who are or may become pregnant.

Skin
Edema (27%) [19]
Hot flashes (19%) [3]
Cardiovascular
Arrhythmias (7%)
Atrial fibrillation [3]
Cardiac failure (2%)
Cardiotoxicity [4]
Chest pain (4%)
Hypertension (9%) [23]
Tachycardia [3]
Central Nervous System
Headache [2]
Neuromuscular/Skeletal
Arthralgia [5]
Asthenia (fatigue) [11]
Back pain [4]
Bone or joint pain (30%) [8]
Myalgia/Myopathy (26%)
Pain in extremities [2]
Rhabdomyolysis [2]
Gastrointestinal/Hepatic
Constipation [7]
Diarrhea (18%) [5]
Dyspepsia (6%)
Hepatotoxicity (2%) [12]
Nausea [8]
Respiratory
Cough (11%)
Dyspnea [2]
Upper respiratory tract infection (5%) [2]
Endocrine/Metabolic
ALT increased (11%) [5]
AST increased (31%) [3]
Hypercholesterolemia [2]
Hypertriglyceridemia (63%)
Hypokalemia [21]

Genitourinary
Nocturia (6%)
Urinary frequency (7%)
Urinary tract infection (12%) [2]
Hematologic
Anemia [5]
Thrombocytopenia [2]
Other
Adverse effects [7]

ACAMPROSATE

See: www.drugeruptiondata.com/drug/id/1047

ACARBOSE

Trade names: Glucobay (Bayer), Precose (Bayer)
Indications: Non-insulin dependent diabetes Type II
Class: Alpha-glucosidase inhibitor, Antidiabetic
Half-life: 2 hours
Clinically important, potentially hazardous interactions with: alcohol, anabolic steroids, beta blockers, cholestyramine, corticosteroids, diazoxide, digoxin, diuretics, estrogens, hypoglycemic agents, MAO inhibitors, neomycin, orlistat, pancreatin, pegvisomant, pramlintide, progestogens, somatropin, testosterone
Pregnancy category: B
Important contra-indications noted in the prescribing guidelines for: nursing mothers; pediatric patients
Note: Contra-indicated in patients with diabetic ketoacidosis or cirrhosis; also in patients with inflammatory bowel disease, colonic ulceration, partial intestinal obstruction or in patients predisposed to intestinal obstruction.

Skin
AGEP [2]
Gastrointestinal/Hepatic
Abdominal distension [2]
Abdominal pain (19%)
Diarrhea (31%)
Flatulence (74%) [3]
Hepatitis [2]
Hepatotoxicity [3]
Pneumatosis intestinalis [8]
Other
Adverse effects [5]

ACEBUTOLOL

See: www.drugeruptiondata.com/drug/id/4

ACECLOFENAC

See: www.drugeruptiondata.com/drug/id/1261

ACEMETACIN

See: www.drugeruptiondata.com/drug/id/1691

ACENOCOUMAROL

See: www.drugeruptiondata.com/drug/id/1276

ACETAMINOPHEN

Synonyms: APAP; paracetamol
Trade names: Anacin-3 (Wyeth), Darvocet-N (aaiPharma), Excedrin (Bristol-Myers Squibb), Lorcet (Forest), Panadol (GSK), Percocet (Endo), Tylenol (Ortho-McNeil), Vicodin (AbbVie)
Indications: Pain, fever
Class: Analgesic, non-narcotic
Half-life: <3 hours
Clinically important, potentially hazardous interactions with: alcohol, anticonvulsants, barbiturates, busulfan, carbamazepine, cholestyramine, conivaptan, coumarins, didanosine, dong quai, exenatide, imatinib, isoniazid, liraglutide, melatonin, metoclopramide, metyrapone, PEG-interferon, pramlintide, probenecid, St John's wort
Pregnancy category: C
Important contra-indications noted in the prescribing guidelines for: nursing mothers
Note: Acetaminophen is the active metabolite of phenacetin. [IV] = intravenous. As a general point most reactions listed are those that have developed following the normal prescribing doses for acetaminophen and the overdosing, poisoning, and other toxicities that have been reported have been excluded.

Skin
AGEP [10]
Anaphylactoid reactions/Anaphylaxis [19]
Angioedema [8]
Dermatitis [3]
Erythema [3]
Erythema multiforme [3]
Exanthems [7]
Exfoliative dermatitis [2]
Fixed eruption [41]
Hyperhidrosis [2]
Hypersensitivity [12]
Neutrophilic eccrine hidradenitis [2]
Pemphigus [2]
Pruritus [5]
Purpura [6]
Rash [IV] [2]
Stevens-Johnson syndrome [10]
Toxic epidermal necrolysis [13]
Urticaria [17]
Vasculitis [4]

Mucosal
Xerostomia [3]

Cardiovascular
Hypertension [IV] [3]
Hypotension [2]

Central Nervous System
Agitation [IV] (>5%)
Fever [IV] (5%)
Headache [IV] (10%) [5]
Insomnia [IV] (7%)
Somnolence (drowsiness) [8]
Vertigo (dizziness) [15]

Neuromuscular/Skeletal
Rhabdomyolysis [4]

Gastrointestinal/Hepatic
Abdominal distension [2]
Abdominal pain [IV] [3]
Constipation [IV] (>5%) [7]
Diarrhea [IV] [2]
Hepatotoxicity [70]
Nausea [IV] (34%) [18]
Pancreatitis [6]
Vomiting (15%) [16]

Respiratory
Asthma [3]
Pulmonary toxicity [IV] (>5%)

Endocrine/Metabolic
Acidosis [3]

Renal
Nephrotoxicity [9]
Renal failure [3]

Hematologic
Thrombocytopenia [2]

Other
Adverse effects [16]
Death [6]

ACETAZOLAMIDE

Trade name: Diamox (Duramed)
Indications: Epilepsy, glaucoma
Class: Carbonic anhydrase inhibitor, Diuretic
Half-life: 2–6 hours
Clinically important, potentially hazardous interactions with: arsenic, aspirin, ephedra, indacaterol, lisdexamfetamine, lithium, metformin, mivacurium, triamcinolone
Pregnancy category: C
Important contra-indications noted in the prescribing guidelines for: the elderly; nursing mothers; pediatric patients
Note: Acetazolamide is a sulfonamide and can be absorbed systemically. Sulfonamides can produce severe, possibly fatal, reactions such as toxic epidermal necrolysis and Stevens-Johnson syndrome.

Skin
AGEP [2]
Anaphylactoid reactions/Anaphylaxis [3]
Exanthems [2]
Pemphigus [2]
Stevens-Johnson syndrome [6]
Toxic epidermal necrolysis [2]

Central Nervous System
Depression [2]
Dysgeusia (taste perversion) (>10%) [8]
Paresthesias [6]

Neuromuscular/Skeletal
Asthenia (fatigue) [4]

Gastrointestinal/Hepatic
Diarrhea [2]
Dyspepsia [2]
Nausea [2]
Vomiting [2]

Endocrine/Metabolic
Acidosis [3]
Libido decreased [2]
Weight loss [2]

Renal
Nephrolithiasis [3]

Ocular
Choroidal detachment [2]
Corneal edema [2]
Glaucoma [3]
Myopia [2]

ACETOHEXAMIDE

See: www.drugeruptiondata.com/drug/id/7

ACETYLCHOLINE

See: www.drugeruptiondata.com/drug/id/2445

ACETYLCYSTEINE

Synonyms: N-acetylcysteine; L-Cysteine; NAC
Indications: Emphysema, bronchitis, tuberculosis, bronchiectasis, tracheostomy care, antidote for acetaminophen toxicity
Class: Antidote, Antioxidant
Half-life: N/A
Clinically important, potentially hazardous interactions with: carbamazepine, nitroglycerin
Pregnancy category: B
Note: As an antidote, it is difficult to differentiate side effects due to the drug from those due to the effects of the poison.

Skin
Anaphylactoid reactions/Anaphylaxis (8–18%) [13]
Angioedema [6]
Pruritus (<4%) [3]
Rash (2–4%) [4]
Urticaria (6–8%)

Cardiovascular
Flushing (<8%) [2]
Tachycardia (<4%)

Central Nervous System
Seizures [2]

Gastrointestinal/Hepatic
Diarrhea [2]
Nausea (<6%) [3]
Vomiting (2–10%) [2]

Other
Adverse effects [2]
Death [2]

ACIPIMOX

See: www.drugeruptiondata.com/drug/id/1343

ACITRETIN

Trade names: Neotigason (Actavis), Soriatane (Stiefel)
Indications: Psoriasis
Class: Retinoid
Half-life: 49 hours
Clinically important, potentially hazardous interactions with: alcohol, bexarotene, chloroquine, cholestyramine, corticosteroids, coumarins, danazol, demeclocycline, doxycycline, ethanolamine, isotretinoin, lithium, lymecycline, medroxyprogesterone, methotrexate, minocycline, oxytetracycline, phenytoin, progestins, St John's wort, tetracycline, tigecycline, vitamin A
Pregnancy category: X
Important contra-indications noted in the prescribing guidelines for: nursing mothers; pediatric patients
Note: Oral retinoids can cause birth defects, and women should avoid acitretin when pregnant or trying to conceive.
Warning: PREGNANCY

Skin
Angioedema [2]
Atrophy (10–25%)
Bromhidrosis (<10%)
Bullous dermatitis (<10%)
Clammy skin (<10%)
Dermatitis (<10%)
Diaphoresis (<10%) [2]
Edema (<10%)
Erythema (18%)
Erythroderma [3]
Exanthems (10–25%) [2]
Exfoliative dermatitis (25–50%) [3]
Fissures (<10%)
Hot flashes (<10%)
Hyperhidrosis (<10%) [2]
Palmar–plantar desquamation (20–80%) [7]
Photosensitivity [3]
Pigmentation [3]
Pruritus (10–50%) [10]
Psoriasis (aggravated) (<10%)
Purpura (<10%)
Rash (>10%)
Seborrhea (<10%)
Stickiness (3–50%) [7]
Sunburn (<10%)
Toxicity [3]
Ulcerations (<10%)
Xerosis (25–50%) [14]

Hair
Alopecia (10–75%) [21]
Curly hair [3]
Hair changes (<10%)
Hair pigmentation [2]

Nails
Brittle nails [3]
Nail changes (25–50%)
Paronychia (10–25%) [6]
Pyogenic granuloma (<10%) [4]

Mucosal
Cheilitis (>75%) [14]
Dry mucous membranes [4]
Epistaxis (nosebleed) (10–25%) [2]
Gingival bleeding (<10%)
Gingivitis (<10%)
Mucocutaneous reactions [3]
Sialorrhea (<10%)
Stomatitis (<10%) [2]
Tongue disorder (<10%)
Ulcerative stomatitis (<10%)
Xerostomia (10–60%) [7]

Cardiovascular
Capillary leak syndrome [2]

Central Nervous System
Anorexia (<10%)
Depression (<10%) [4]
Dysgeusia (taste perversion) (<10%)
Headache (<10%) [2]
Hyperesthesia (10–25%)
Insomnia (<10%)
Neurotoxicity [3]
Pain (<10%)
Paralysis (facial) (<10%)
Paresthesias (10–25%) [2]
Pseudotumor cerebri [5]
Rigors (10–25%) [2]
Somnolence (drowsiness) (<10%)
Stroke [2]
Suicidal ideation [2]

Neuromuscular/Skeletal
Arthralgia (10–25%) [2]
Asthenia (fatigue) (<10%) [3]
Back pain (<10%)
Bone or joint pain [2]
Hyperostosis [10]
Myalgia/Myopathy [4]
Osteoporosis [2]

Gastrointestinal/Hepatic
Abdominal pain (<10%)
Diarrhea (<10%) [2]
Hepatitis [5]
Hepatotoxicity [8]
Nausea (<10%) [2]
Pancreatitis [3]
Vomiting [2]

Respiratory
Laryngitis [2]
Rhinitis (25–50%) [2]
Sinusitis (<10%)

Endocrine/Metabolic
GGT increased [2]
Hyperbilirubinemia [2]
Hypercholesterolemia (25–50%) [3]
Hyperlipidemia [5]
Hypertriglyceridemia (50–75%) [4]

Genitourinary
Vulvovaginal candidiasis [2]

Otic
Ear pain (<10%)
Tinnitus (<10%)

Ocular
Blepharitis (<10%)
Cataract (<10%)
Conjunctivitis (<10%) [2]
Diplopia (<10%)
Night blindness (<10%) [2]
Ocular adverse effects [2]
Ocular itching [2]
Ocular pain (<10%)
Photophobia (<10%) [2]
Vision blurred (<10%)
Xerophthalmia (10–25%) [3]

Other
Adverse effects [9]
Dipsia (thirst) (<10%)
Infection [2]
Side effects [4]
Teratogenicity [7]

ACLIDINIUM

See: www.drugeruptiondata.com/drug/id/3007

ACYCLOVIR

Synonyms: aciclovir; ACV; acycloguanosine
Trade names: Sitavig (Cipher), Zovirax (GSK)
Indications: Herpes simplex, herpes zoster
Class: Antiviral, Antiviral, topical, Guanine nucleoside analog
Half-life: 3 hours (adults)
Clinically important, potentially hazardous interactions with: cobicistat/elvitegravir/ emtricitabine/tenofovir alafenamide, cobicistat/ elvitegravir/emtricitabine/tenofovir disoproxil, meperidine, tenofovir disoproxil
Pregnancy category: B
Important contra-indications noted in the prescribing guidelines for: nursing mothers

Skin
Acneform eruption (<3%)
Dermatitis [12]
Exanthems (<5%) [5]
Facial edema (3–5%)
Peripheral edema [2]
Pruritus (<10%)
Radiation recall dermatitis [2]
Rash (<3%) [3]
Urticaria (<5%) [4]

Hair
Alopecia (<3%)

Central Nervous System
Headache (2%) [4]
Neurotoxicity [8]

Neuromuscular/Skeletal
Asthenia (fatigue) (12%)

Gastrointestinal/Hepatic
Diarrhea (2–3%)
Nausea (2–5%) [3]
Vomiting (3%)

Renal
Nephrotoxicity [12]
Renal failure [4]

Ocular
Hallucinations, visual [2]
Periorbital edema (3–5%)

Local
Injection-site inflammation (>10%)
Injection-site thrombophlebitis (9%)

Other
Adverse effects [2]

ADALIMUMAB

Trade names: Amjevita (Amgen), Humira (AbbVie)
Indications: Rheumatoid arthritis, polyarticular juvenile idiopathic arthritis, psoriatic arthritis, ankylosing spondylitis, Crohn's disease, ulcerative colitis, psoriasis
Class: Cytokine inhibitor, Disease-modifying antirheumatic drug (DMARD), Monoclonal antibody, TNF inhibitor
Half-life: 10–20 days
Clinically important, potentially hazardous interactions with: abatacept, anakinra, live vaccines
Pregnancy category: B
Important contra-indications noted in the prescribing guidelines for: nursing mothers
Note: TNF inhibitors should be used in patients with heart failure only after consideration of other treatment options. TNF inhibitors are contra-indicated in patients with a personal or family history of multiple sclerosis or demyelinating disease. TNF inhibitors should not be administered to patients with moderate to severe heart failure (New York Heart Association Functional Class III/IV).
Warning: SERIOUS INFECTIONS AND MALIGNANCY

Skin
Acneform eruption [3]
Angioedema [3]
Carcinoma [2]
Cellulitis (<5%) [2]
Dermatomyositis [5]
Eczema [2]
Erysipelas (<5%)
Granulomatous reaction [5]
Henoch–Schönlein purpura [2]
Herpes zoster [10]
Hidradenitis [2]
Hypersensitivity [3]
Lesions [2]
Lichenoid eruption [5]
Lupus erythematosus [16]
Lupus syndrome [3]
Lymphoma [8]
Malignancies [4]
Melanoma [6]
Neoplasms [2]
Palmoplantar pustulosis [3]
Peripheral edema (<5%)
Pruritus [6]
Psoriasis [39]
Rash (12%) [4]
Sarcoidosis [8]
Squamous cell carcinoma [5]
Stevens-Johnson syndrome [2]
Urticaria [3]
Vasculitis [9]
Vitiligo [2]

Hair
Alopecia [5]
Alopecia areata [7]
Alopecia universalis [2]

Cardiovascular
Arrhythmias (<5%)
Cardiac arrest (<5%)
Chest pain (<5%)
Congestive heart failure (<5%)
Hypertension (<5%)
Myocardial infarction (<5%)
Palpitation [2]
Pericarditis (<5%)
Tachycardia (<5%)
Thromboembolism [2]

Central Nervous System
Aseptic meningitis [2]
Confusion (<5%)
Encephalitis [2]
Fever (<5%) [3]
Guillain–Barré syndrome [5]
Headache (12%) [6]
Leukoencephalopathy [3]
Multiple sclerosis (<5%) [3]
Neurotoxicity [3]
Paresthesias (<5%) [2]
Syncope (<5%)
Tremor (<5%)
Vertigo (dizziness) [2]

Neuromuscular/Skeletal
Arthralgia (<5%) [6]
Asthenia (fatigue) [2]
Back pain (6%) [3]
Tuberculous arthritis [2]

Gastrointestinal/Hepatic
Abdominal pain (7%) [2]
Cholecystitis (<5%)
Colitis [2]
Esophagitis (<5%)
Gastroenteritis (<5%)
Hepatitis [7]
Hepatotoxicity [10]
Nausea (9%) [2]
Vomiting (<5%)

Respiratory
Asthma (<5%)
Bronchitis [2]
Bronchospasm (<5%)
Dyspnea (<5%)
Flu-like syndrome (7%)
Nasopharyngitis [4]
Pleural effusion (<5%)
Pneumonia (<5%) [6]
Pneumonitis [3]
Pulmonary fibrosis [3]
Pulmonary toxicity [7]
Sinusitis (11%) [2]
Tuberculosis [9]
Upper respiratory tract infection (17%) [8]

Endocrine/Metabolic
Creatine phosphokinase increased (<5%)
Hypercholesterolemia (6%)

Genitourinary
Cystitis (<5%)
Hematuria (5%)
Pelvic pain (<5%)
Urinary tract infection (8%)

Renal
Nephrotoxicity [2]

Hematologic
Agranulocytosis (<5%)
Eosinophilia [3]
Hemolytic anemia [2]
Leukopenia (<5%)
Pancytopenia [2]
Sepsis [2]

Ocular
Cataract (<5%)
Optic neuritis [5]
Uveitis [4]

Local
Injection-site edema (15%) [2]
Injection-site erythema (15%) [3]
Injection-site pain (12%)
Injection-site reactions [26]

Other
Adverse effects [45]
Death [8]
Infection (5%) [70]
Side effects [2]

ADAPALENE

Trade names: Differin (Galderma), Epiduo (Galderma)
Indications: Acne vulgaris
Class: Retinoid
Half-life: N/A
Clinically important, potentially hazardous interactions with: resorcinol, salicylates
Pregnancy category: C
Important contra-indications noted in the prescribing guidelines for: nursing mothers; pediatric patients
Note: Epiduo is adapalene and benzoyl peroxide.

Skin
Burning (38%) [7]
Erythema (38%) [9]
Pruritus (>10%) [11]
Scaling (44%) [6]
Stinging (38%) [3]
Xerosis (45%) [10]

Other
Adverse effects [3]

ADEFOVIR

Trade name: Hepsera (Gilead)
Indications: HIV infection, hepatitis B infection
Class: Antiretroviral, Nucleotide analog reverse transcriptase inhibitor
Half-life: 16–18 hours
Clinically important, potentially hazardous interactions with: amikacin, amphotericin B, cobicistat/elvitegravir/emtricitabine/tenofovir disoproxil, delavirdine, drugs causing kidney toxicity, foscarnet, gentamicin, hydroxyurea, pentamidine, tenofovir disoproxil, tobramycin
Pregnancy category: C
Important contra-indications noted in the prescribing guidelines for: the elderly; nursing mothers; pediatric patients
Warning: SEVERE ACUTE EXACERBATIONS OF HEPATITIS, NEPHROTOXICITY, HIV RESISTANCE, LACTIC ACIDOSIS AND SEVERE HEPATOMEGALY WITH STEATOSIS

Skin
Pruritus (<10%)
Rash (<10%)

Central Nervous System
Headache (9%) [2]
Pain [2]

Neuromuscular/Skeletal
Asthenia (fatigue) (13%) [3]
Back pain (<10%)
Osteomalacia [6]

Gastrointestinal/Hepatic
Abdominal pain (9%)
Diarrhea (3%)
Dyspepsia (3%)
Flatulence (4%)
Hepatotoxicity (<25%)
Nausea (5%)
Vomiting (<10%)

Respiratory
Cough (6–8%)
Rhinitis (<5%)

Endocrine/Metabolic
Hypophosphatemia [5]

Genitourinary
Hematuria (11%)

Renal
Fanconi syndrome [11]
Nephrotoxicity [14]

ADENOSINE

Synonym: ATP
Trade names: Adenocard (Astellas), Adenocur (Sanofi-Aventis)
Indications: Paroxysmal supraventricular tachycardia, varicose vein complications with stasis dermatitis
Class: Antiarrhythmic class IV, Neurotransmitter
Half-life: <10 seconds
Clinically important, potentially hazardous interactions with: aminophylline, antiarrhythmics, beta blockers, bupivacaine, carbamazepine, dipyridamole, levobupivacaine, nicotine, prilocaine, QT prolonging agents, ropivacaine
Pregnancy category: C
Important contra-indications noted in the prescribing guidelines for: pediatric patients

Cardiovascular
Arrhythmias [2]
Atrial fibrillation [6]
Chest pain [5]
Coronary vasospasm [2]
Flushing (18–44%)
Torsades de pointes [2]

Central Nervous System
Headache (2–18%) [2]
Vertigo (dizziness) (2–12%)

Neuromuscular/Skeletal
Jaw pain (<15%)

Gastrointestinal/Hepatic
Abdominal pain (13%)

Respiratory
Cough (6–8%)
Dyspnea [3]
Respiratory distress (11%)

Other
Adverse effects [2]

ADO-TRASTUZUMAB EMTANSINE

Synonym: T-DM1
Trade name: Kadcyla (Genentech)
Indications: HER2-positive, metastatic breast cancer in patients who previously received trastuzumab and a taxane, separately or in combination
Class: Antibody drug conjugate (ADC), HER2-targeted antibody-drug conjugate
Half-life: 4 days
Clinically important, potentially hazardous interactions with: none known
Pregnancy category: D
Important contra-indications noted in the prescribing guidelines for: nursing mothers; pediatric patients
Warning: HEPATOTOXICITY, CARDIAC TOXICITY, EMBRYO-FETAL TOXICITY

Skin
Hypersensitivity (2%)
Peripheral edema (7%)
Pruritus (6%)
Rash (12%)
Telangiectasia [2]

Mucosal
Epistaxis (nosebleed) (23%)
Stomatitis (14%)
Xerostomia (17%)

Cardiovascular
Cardiotoxicity [2]
Hypertension (5%)

Central Nervous System
Chills (8%)
Dysgeusia (taste perversion) (8%)
Fever (19%) [2]
Headache (28%) [4]
Insomnia (12%)
Peripheral neuropathy (21%)
Vertigo (dizziness) (10%)

Neuromuscular/Skeletal
Arthralgia (19%) [3]
Asthenia (fatigue) (18–36%) [12]
Bone or joint pain (36%)
Myalgia/Myopathy (14%)

Gastrointestinal/Hepatic
Abdominal pain (19%)
Constipation (27%) [3]
Diarrhea (24%) [5]
Dyspepsia (9%)
Hepatotoxicity [14]
Nausea (40%) [9]
Vomiting (19%)

Respiratory
Cough (18%)
Dyspnea (12%)
Pneumonia [3]

Endocrine/Metabolic
ALP increased (5%)
ALT increased (82%) [3]
AST increased (98%) [6]

Hypokalemia (10%) [3]

Genitourinary
Urinary tract infection (9%)

Hematologic
Anemia (14%) [6]
Febrile neutropenia [3]
Hemorrhage (32%) [2]
Neutropenia (7%) [4]
Thrombocytopenia (31%) [23]

Ocular
Conjunctivitis (4%)
Lacrimation (3%)
Vision blurred (5%)
Xerophthalmia (4%)

Other
Adverse effects [5]
Death [3]

AFAMELANOTIDE

See: www.drugeruptiondata.com/drug/id/1315

AFATINIB

Trade name: Gilotrif (Boehringer Ingelheim)
Indications: Metastatic non-small cell lung cancer in patients whose tumors have epidermal growth factor receptor exon 19 deletions or exon 21 (L858R) substitution mutations, metastatic squamous non-small cell lung cancer progressing following platinium-based chemotherapy
Class: Tyrosine kinase inhibitor
Half-life: 37 hours
Clinically important, potentially hazardous interactions with: amiodarone, carbamazepine, cyclosporine, erythromycin, itraconazole, ketoconazole, nelfinavir, P-glycoprotein inhibitors, phenobarbital, phenytoin, quinidine, rifampin, ritonavir, saquinavir, St John's wort, tacrolimus, verapamil
Pregnancy category: D
Important contra-indications noted in the prescribing guidelines for: nursing mothers; pediatric patients

Skin
Acneform eruption [25]
Fissures [2]
Hand–foot syndrome [2]
Pruritus [2]
Rash [49]
Toxicity [3]
Xerosis [6]

Nails
Nail changes [2]
Paronychia (58%) [10]

Mucosal
Epistaxis (nosebleed) [3]
Mucosal inflammation [7]
Mucositis [10]
Rhinorrhea (11%)
Stomatitis (71%) [19]

Central Nervous System
Anorexia [3]
Fever (12%)

Neuromuscular/Skeletal
Asthenia (fatigue) [17]
Gastrointestinal/Hepatic
Diarrhea (96%) [65]
Dysphagia [2]
Hepatotoxicity (10%) [5]
Nausea [15]
Vomiting [10]
Respiratory
Dyspnea [3]
Pneumonitis [2]
Pulmonary toxicity [5]
Endocrine/Metabolic
ALT increased [2]
Appetite decreased (29%) [5]
Dehydration [3]
Hypokalemia [2]
Hematologic
Anemia [3]
Febrile neutropenia [2]
Leukopenia [2]
Neutropenia [6]
Thrombocytopenia [2]
Other
Adverse effects [7]
Death [4]

AFLIBERCEPT

Synonym: ziv-aflibercept
Trade names: Eylea (Regeneron), Zaltrap (Sanofi-Aventis)
Indications: Neovascular (wet) age-related macular degeneration (Eylea), metastatic colorectal cancer (Zaltrap) in combination with FOLFIRI (fluorouracil, leucovorin and irinotecan)
Class: Fusion protein
Half-life: terminal 5–6 days
Clinically important, potentially hazardous interactions with: none known
Pregnancy category: C
Important contra-indications noted in the prescribing guidelines for: nursing mothers; pediatric patients
Note: Eylea: Contra-indicated in patients with ocular or periocular infection or active intraocular inflammation.
Warning: Zaltrap: HEMORRHAGE, GASTROINTESTINAL PERFORATION, COMPROMISED WOUND HEALING

Mucosal
Epistaxis (nosebleed) [3]
Stomatitis [6]
Cardiovascular
Hypertension [12]
Myocardial infarction (<2%)
Venous thromboembolism [2]
Central Nervous System
Anorexia [2]
Headache [2]
Stroke (<2%)
Neuromuscular/Skeletal
Asthenia (fatigue) [6]
Gastrointestinal/Hepatic
Diarrhea [5]

Gastrointestinal perforation [4]
Respiratory
Dysphonia [5]
Dyspnea [2]
Pulmonary embolism [2]
Endocrine/Metabolic
Weight loss [2]
Renal
Proteinuria [8]
Hematologic
Hemorrhage [3]
Neutropenia [10]
Ocular
Cataract (7%) [2]
Conjunctival hemorrhage (25%) [2]
Conjunctival hyperemia (4%)
Corneal erosion (4%)
Intraocular pressure increased (5%) [2]
Lacrimation (3%)
Ocular adverse effects [3]
Ocular pain (3–9%)
Vision blurred (2%)
Vitreous detachment (6%)
Vitreous floaters (6%)
Local
Injection-site pain (3%)
Other
Adverse effects [2]
Death [2]
Infection [2]

AGALSIDASE

See: www.drugeruptiondata.com/drug/id/993

ALBENDAZOLE

Trade name: Albenza (GSK)
Indications: Nematode infections, hydatid cyst disease
Class: Anthelmintic
Half-life: 8–12 hours
Clinically important, potentially hazardous interactions with: antimalarials, conivaptan, dexamethasone, high fat foods
Pregnancy category: C
Important contra-indications noted in the prescribing guidelines for: nursing mothers

Skin
Fixed eruption [2]
Pruritus [4]
Urticaria [2]
Hair
Alopecia (reversible) (<2%) [4]
Central Nervous System
Fever (<2%)
Headache (<11%) [5]
Intracranial pressure increased (<2%)
Psychosis [2]
Vertigo (dizziness) (<2%) [2]
Neuromuscular/Skeletal
Dystonia [3]

Gastrointestinal/Hepatic
Abdominal pain (<7%) [7]
Hepatitis [4]
Nausea (4–6%) [3]
Vomiting (4–6%) [2]
Other
Adverse effects [5]

ALBIGLUTIDE

Trade name: Tanzeum (GSK)
Indications: To improve glycemic control in adults with Type II diabetes mellitus
Class: Glucagon-like peptide-1 (GLP-1) receptor agonist
Half-life: 5 days
Clinically important, potentially hazardous interactions with: none known
Pregnancy category: C
Important contra-indications noted in the prescribing guidelines for: nursing mothers; pediatric patients
Note: Contra-indicated in patients with a personal or family history of medullary thyroid carcinoma or in patients with multiple endocrine neoplasia syndrome Type 2.
Warning: RISK OF THYROID C-CELL TUMORS

Central Nervous System
Headache [4]
Vertigo (dizziness) [2]
Neuromuscular/Skeletal
Arthralgia (7%)
Back pain (7%) [2]
Gastrointestinal/Hepatic
Constipation [2]
Diarrhea (13%) [15]
Dyspepsia (3%)
Gastroesophageal reflux (4%)
Nausea (11%) [20]
Pancreatitis [4]
Vomiting (4%) [15]
Respiratory
Cough (7%)
Influenza (5%)
Nasopharyngitis [3]
Pneumonia (2%)
Sinusitis (6%)
Upper respiratory tract infection (14%) [4]
Endocrine/Metabolic
GGT increased (2%)
Hypoglycemia (2%) [5]
Local
Injection-site hematoma (2%)
Injection-site reactions (11%) [15]
Other
Adverse effects [4]

ALBUTEROL

Synonym: salbutamol
Trade names: AccuNeb (Mylan Specialty), Combivent (Boehringer Ingelheim), Duoneb (Mylan Specialty), Proventil (Schering), Ventolin (GSK), Volmax (Muro)
Indications: Bronchospasm associated with asthma
Class: Beta-2 adrenergic agonist, Bronchodilator, Tocolytic
Half-life: 3–6 hours
Clinically important, potentially hazardous interactions with: atomoxetine, epinephrine, insulin degludec, insulin detemir, insulin glargine, insulin glulisine
Pregnancy category: C
Important contra-indications noted in the prescribing guidelines for: nursing mothers
Note: Combivent is albuterol and ipratropium.

Skin
Dermatitis [2]
Diaphoresis (<10%)
Erythema (palmar) (with infusion) [2]
Mucosal
Xerostomia (<10%)
Cardiovascular
Flushing (<10%)
Hypertension [2]
Myocardial infarction [2]
Palpitation [2]
Tachyarrhythmia [2]
Tachycardia [2]
Central Nervous System
Dysgeusia (taste perversion) (<10%)
Tremor [2]
Respiratory
Dyspnea [2]
Endocrine/Metabolic
Acidosis [3]
Other
Adverse effects [2]

ALCAFTADINE

See: www.drugeruptiondata.com/drug/id/1851

ALCLOMETASONE

See: www.drugeruptiondata.com/drug/id/1082

ALDESLEUKIN

Synonyms: IL-2; interleukin-2
Trade name: Proleukin (Chiron)
Indications: Metastatic renal cell carcinoma and metastatic melanoma
Class: Biologic, Immunomodulator, Interleukin-2
Half-life: 6–85 minutes
Clinically important, potentially hazardous interactions with: acebutolol, alfuzosin, altretamine, amikacin, aminoglycosides, antineoplastics, betamethasone, bleomycin, busulfan, captopril, carboplatin, carmustine, chlorambucil, ciclesonide, cilazapril, cisplatin, corticosteroids, cyclophosphamide, cytarabine, dacarbazine, dactinomycin, daunorubicin, docetaxel, doxorubicin, enalapril, estramustine, etoposide, fludarabine, fluorouracil, fosinopril, gemcitabine, gentamicin, hydroxyurea, idarubicin, ifosfamide, indomethacin, interferon alfa, irbesartan, kanamycin, levamisole, lisinopril, lomustine, mechlorethamine, melphalan, mercaptopurine, methotrexate, mitomycin, mitotane, mitoxantrone, neomycin, olmesartan, PEG-interferon, pentostatin, plicamycin, procarbazine, quinapril, ramipril, streptomycin, streptozocin, thioguanine, thiotepa, tobramycin, trandolapril, tretinoin, triamcinolone, uracil, vinblastine, vincristine, vinorelbine
Pregnancy category: C
Important contra-indications noted in the prescribing guidelines for: nursing mothers; pediatric patients
Note: Contra-indicated in patients with significant cardiac, pulmonary, renal, hepatic, or CNS impairment.
Warning: CAPILLARY LEAK SYNDROME

Skin
Angioedema [2]
Dermatitis [2]
Edema (47%) [3]
Erythema (41%) [5]
Erythema nodosum [3]
Erythroderma [4]
Exanthems [5]
Exfoliative dermatitis (18%)
Linear IgA bullous dermatosis [4]
Necrosis [2]
Pemphigus [2]
Peripheral edema (28%)
Petechiae (4%)
Pruritus (24%) [7]
Psoriasis [4]
Purpura (4%)
Rash (42%) [2]
Scleroderma [2]
Toxic epidermal necrolysis [2]
Toxicity [6]
Urticaria (2%) [3]
Vitiligo [3]
Xerosis (15%)
Hair
Alopecia [2]
Mucosal
Oral mucosal eruption [2]
Stomatitis (22%)
Cardiovascular
Arrhythmias (10%)
Capillary leak syndrome [12]
Cardiotoxicity (11%) [2]
Hypotension (71%) [6]
Supraventricular tachycardia (12%)
Tachycardia (23%)
Vascular leak syndrome [6]
Vasodilation (13%)
Central Nervous System
Anorexia (20%)
Anxiety (12%)
Chills (52%)
Confusion (34%)
Depression [3]
Dysgeusia (taste perversion) (7%)
Fever (29%) [8]
Neurotoxicity [3]
Pain (12%)
Rigors [3]
Somnolence (drowsiness) (22%)
Vertigo (dizziness) (11%)
Neuromuscular/Skeletal
Asthenia (fatigue) (23–27%)
Myalgia/Myopathy (6%)
Myasthenia gravis [2]
Gastrointestinal/Hepatic
Abdominal pain (11%)
Diarrhea (67%) [3]
Hepatotoxicity [2]
Nausea (35%) [9]
Vomiting (50%) [6]
Respiratory
Cough (11%)
Dyspnea (43%)
Pulmonary toxicity (11–24%) [2]
Rhinitis (10%)
Endocrine/Metabolic
Acidosis (12%)
ALP increased (10%)
AST increased (23%)
Creatine phosphokinase increased (33%) [2]
Hypocalcemia (11%)
Hypomagnesemia [2]
Hypophosphatemia [2]
Weight gain (16%)
Weight loss [2]
Genitourinary
Oliguria (63%)
Renal
Nephrotoxicity [4]
Hematologic
Anemia (29%)
Leukopenia (16%) [2]
Sepsis [3]
Thrombocytopenia (37%) [2]
Local
Injection-site inflammation [2]
Injection-site nodules [2]
Injection-site reactions (3%) [2]
Other
Adverse effects [3]
Death [5]
Infection (13%) [2]

ALECTINIB

Trade name: Alecensa (Genentech)
Indications: Anaplastic lymphoma kinase-positive, metastatic non-small cell lung cancer in patients who have progressed on, or are intolerant to, crizotinib
Class: Kinase inhibitor
Half-life: 33 hours
Clinically important, potentially hazardous interactions with: none known

Pregnancy category: N/A (Can cause fetal harm)
Important contra-indications noted in the prescribing guidelines for: nursing mothers; pediatric patients

Skin
Edema (30%)
Peripheral edema [5]
Photosensitivity (10%) [2]
Rash (18%) [2]

Hair
Alopecia [2]

Central Nervous System
Dysgeusia (taste perversion) [2]
Headache (17%) [2]

Neuromuscular/Skeletal
Asthenia (fatigue) (41%) [5]
Back pain (12%)
Myalgia/Myopathy (29%) [6]

Gastrointestinal/Hepatic
Constipation (34%) [7]
Diarrhea (16%) [2]
Nausea (18%) [3]
Vomiting (12%) [2]

Respiratory
Cough (19%)
Dyspnea (16%)
Pulmonary toxicity [3]

Endocrine/Metabolic
ALP increased (47%) [3]
ALT increased (34%) [5]
AST increased (51%) [6]
Creatine phosphokinase increased (43%) [6]
GGT increased [2]
Hyperbilirubinemia (39%) [5]
Hyperglycemia (36%)
Hypocalcemia (32%)
Hypokalemia (29%)
Hyponatremia (20%)
Hypophosphatemia (21%)
Serum creatinine increased (28%)
Weight gain (11%)

Hematologic
Anemia (56%) [2]
Lymphopenia (22%)
Neutropenia [5]

Ocular
Visual disturbances (10%)

Other
Adverse effects [2]

ALEFACEPT

See: www.drugeruptiondata.com/drug/id/939

ALEMTUZUMAB

Trade names: Campath (Bayer), MabCampath (Schering)
Indications: B-cell chronic lymphcyotic leukemia, non-Hodgkin's lymphoma
Class: Biologic, Immunosuppressant, Monoclonal antibody
Half-life: 12 days
Clinically important, potentially hazardous interactions with: none known
Pregnancy category: C
Note: Prophylactic therapy against PCP pneumonia and herpes viral infections is recommended upon initiation of therapy and for at least 2 months following last dose.
Warning: CYTOPENIAS, INFUSION REACTIONS, and INFECTIONS

Skin
Carcinoma [2]
Erythema (4%)
Herpes [2]
Herpes simplex [2]
Herpes zoster [3]
Lymphoma [2]
Lymphoproliferative disease (64–70%)
Peripheral edema (13%)
Pruritus (14–24%)
Purpura (8%)
Rash (13–40%) [5]
Thrombocytopenic purpura [10]
Urticaria (16–30%) [2]

Mucosal
Stomatitis (14%)

Cardiovascular
Flushing [2]
Hypertension (11–15%)
Hypotension (15–32%) [2]
Tachycardia (10%)

Central Nervous System
Anorexia (20%)
Anxiety (8%)
Chills (53%)
Depression (7%)
Dysesthesia (15%)
Fever (69–85%) [6]
Guillain–Barré syndrome [2]
Headache (13–24%) [3]
Insomnia (10%)
Intracranial hemorrhage [2]
Leukoencephalopathy [5]
Rigors (87%)
Tremor (3%)
Vertigo (dizziness) (12%)

Neuromuscular/Skeletal
Asthenia (fatigue) (22–34%)
Bone or joint pain (24%)
Myalgia/Myopathy (11%)

Gastrointestinal/Hepatic
Abdominal pain (11%)
Diarrhea (10–22%) [2]
Nausea (47–54%) [4]
Vomiting (33–41%) [2]

Respiratory
Dyspnea (14–26%)
Flu-like syndrome [2]
Pharyngitis (12%)

Pneumonia (16%) [3]
Pneumonitis [2]
Respiratory tract infection [2]
Tuberculosis [2]

Endocrine/Metabolic
Hyperthyroidism [2]
Hypothyroidism [2]
Thyroid dysfunction [14]

Renal
Nephrotoxicity [2]

Hematologic
Anemia (76%) [4]
Cytopenia [2]
Hemolytic anemia [2]
Hemotoxicity [4]
Leukopenia [4]
Lymphopenia (97%) [2]
Neutropenia (77%) [7]
Sepsis [2]
Thrombocytopenia (71%) [10]

Local
Application-site reactions [2]
Infusion-related reactions [10]
Infusion-site reactions [6]
Injection-site pruritus (30–40%)
Injection-site reactions (90%) [5]

Other
Adverse effects [6]
Death [13]
Infection (43–74%) [51]

ALENDRONATE

Trade names: Binosto (Mission), Fosamax (Merck)
Indications: Osteoporosis in postmenopausal women, Paget's disease
Class: Bisphosphonate
Half-life: >10 years
Clinically important, potentially hazardous interactions with: none known
Pregnancy category: C
Important contra-indications noted in the prescribing guidelines for: nursing mothers; pediatric patients

Skin
Angioedema [2]
Erythema multiforme [2]
Hypersensitivity [3]
Rash [5]

Mucosal
Oral ulceration [9]

Central Nervous System
Headache [2]

Neuromuscular/Skeletal
Arthralgia [6]
Bone or joint pain (<6%) [5]
Fractures [20]
Osteonecrosis [12]

Gastrointestinal/Hepatic
Abdominal pain (<7%) [8]
Dyspepsia [8]
Dysphagia [4]
Esophageal perforation [2]
Esophagitis [12]

Hepatotoxicity [7]
Nausea [7]
Vomiting [4]
Endocrine/Metabolic
Hypocalcemia (18%) [5]
Renal
Nephrotoxicity [2]
Renal failure [2]
Ocular
Conjunctivitis [2]
Ocular adverse effects [2]
Ocular inflammation [2]
Scleritis [3]
Uveitis [6]
Other
Adverse effects [5]

ALFENTANIL

See: www.drugeruptiondata.com/drug/id/15

ALFUZOSIN

Trade names: Uroxatral (Concordia), Xatral
(Sanofi-Aventis)
Indications: Benign prostatic hyperplasia
Class: Adrenergic alpha-receptor antagonist
Half-life: 10 hours
**Clinically important, potentially hazardous
interactions with:** ACE inhibitors, adrenergic
neurone blockers, alcohol, aldesleukin,
alprostadil, amitriptyline, angiotensin II receptor
antagonists, antipsychotics, anxiolytics and
hypnotics, arsenic, atazanavir, atenolol, baclofen,
beta blockers, boceprevir, calcium channel
blockers, cimetidine, citalopram, clonidine,
conivaptan, corticosteroids, CYP3A4 inhibitors or
inducers, darunavir, dasabuvir/ombitasvir/
paritaprevir/ritonavir, dasatinib, deferasirox,
degarelix, delavirdine, diazoxide, diltiazem,
diuretics, estrogens, food, general anesthetics,
hydralazine, indinavir, itraconazole, ketoconazole,
lapatinib, levodopa, levofloxacin, lopinavir, MAO
inhibitors, methyldopa, minoxidil, moxifloxacin,
moxisylyte, moxonidine, nelfinavir, nitrates,
nitroprusside, NSAIDs, pazopanib,
phosphodiesterase 5 inhibitors, protease
inhibitors, QT prolonging agents, ritonavir,
sildenafil, St John's wort, tadalafil, telaprevir,
telavancin, telithromycin, tipranavir, tizanidine,
vardenafil, voriconazole, vorinostat, ziprasidone
Pregnancy category: B
**Important contra-indications noted in the
prescribing guidelines for:** pediatric patients

Cardiovascular
Hypotension [2]
Orthostatic hypotension [3]
QT prolongation [2]
Central Nervous System
Headache (3%)
Pain (<2%)
Vertigo (dizziness) (6%) [19]
Neuromuscular/Skeletal
Asthenia (fatigue) (3%)

Gastrointestinal/Hepatic
Abdominal pain (<2%)
Hepatotoxicity [2]
Respiratory
Bronchitis (<2%)
Pharyngitis (<2%)
Sinusitis (<2%)
Upper respiratory tract infection (3%)
Genitourinary
Ejaculatory dysfunction [3]
Erectile dysfunction [2]
Ocular
Floppy iris syndrome [4]
Other
Adverse effects [2]

ALGLUCERASE

See: www.drugeruptiondata.com/drug/id/1054

ALGLUCOSIDASE ALFA

See: www.drugeruptiondata.com/drug/id/1164

ALIROCUMAB

Trade name: Praluent (Regeneron)
Indications: Adjunct to diet and statin therapy in
hypercholesterolemia or clinical atherosclerotic
cardiovascular disease where additional lowering
of low density lipoprotein cholesterol is required
Class: Monoclonal antibody, Proprotein
convertase subtilisin kexin type 9 (PCSK9)
inhibitor
Half-life: 17–20 days
**Clinically important, potentially hazardous
interactions with:** none known
Pregnancy category: N/A (No data available but
likely to cross the placenta in second and third
trimester)
**Important contra-indications noted in the
prescribing guidelines for:** pediatric patients

Skin
Hematoma (2%)
Cardiovascular
Cardiotoxicity [3]
Myocardial infarction [3]
Central Nervous System
Cognitive impairment [2]
Headache [4]
Neurotoxicity [4]
Stroke [2]
Vertigo (dizziness) [6]
Neuromuscular/Skeletal
Arthralgia [6]
Asthenia (fatigue) [2]
Back pain [5]
Bone or joint pain (2%) [2]
Muscle spasm (3%)
Myalgia/Myopathy (4%) [7]
Gastrointestinal/Hepatic
Diarrhea (5%) [3]
Hepatotoxicity (3%)

Nausea [2]
Respiratory
Bronchitis (4%)
Cough (3%)
Influenza (6%) [4]
Nasopharyngitis (11%) [8]
Sinusitis (3%) [2]
Upper respiratory tract infection [7]
Endocrine/Metabolic
ALT increased [3]
Creatine phosphokinase increased [3]
Genitourinary
Urinary tract infection (5%)
Ocular
Ocular adverse effects [2]
Local
Injection-site pain [2]
Injection-site reactions (7%) [16]
Other
Adverse effects [4]
Allergic reactions (9%)
Death [2]

ALISKIREN

See: www.drugeruptiondata.com/drug/id/1225

ALITRETINOIN

Trade name: Panretin (Ligand)
Indications: Kaposi's sarcoma cutaneous lesions
Class: Retinoid
Half-life: N/A
**Clinically important, potentially hazardous
interactions with:** ketoconazole, simvastatin,
vitamin A
Pregnancy category: D
**Important contra-indications noted in the
prescribing guidelines for:** the elderly; pediatric
patients
Note: Oral alitretinoin (Toctino) is not available in
the USA.

Skin
Edema (3–8%)
Erythema [2]
Exfoliative dermatitis (3–9%)
Pigmentation (3%)
Pruritus (8–11%)
Rash (25–77%)
Ulcerations (2%)
Xerosis (10%)
Hair
Curly hair [2]
Mucosal
Mucocutaneous reactions [2]
Cardiovascular
Flushing [2]
Central Nervous System
Depression [2]
Headache [7]
Paresthesias (3–22%)
Gastrointestinal/Hepatic
Nausea [2]

Endocrine/Metabolic
Creatine phosphokinase increased [2]
Hypertriglyceridemia [2]

ALLOPURINOL

Trade names: Duzallo (AstraZeneca), Zyloprim (Prometheus)
Indications: Gouty arthritis
Class: Purine analog, Xanthine oxidase inhibitor
Half-life: <3 hours
Clinically important, potentially hazardous interactions with: acenocoumarol, amoxicillin, ampicillin, ampicillin/sulbactam, azathioprine, benazepril, capecitabine, captopril, cilazapril, cyclopenthiazide, dicumarol, enalapril, fosinopril, imidapril, lisinopril, mercaptopurine, pantoprazole, quinapril, ramipril, trandolapril, uracil/tegafur, vidarabine, zofenopril
Pregnancy category: C
Note: HLA-B*5801 confers a risk of allopurinol-induced serious skin reactions like SJS/TEN and DRESS.
Duzallo is allopurinol and lesinurad (see separate entry).

Skin
AGEP [6]
DRESS syndrome [45]
Eosinophilic pustular folliculitis [2]
Erythema multiforme [7]
Exanthems (<5%) [20]
Exfoliative dermatitis (>10%) [15]
Fixed eruption [11]
Granuloma annulare (disseminated) [2]
Hypersensitivity [49]
Lupus erythematosus [3]
Pityriasis rosea [2]
Pruritus [7]
Purpura (>10%) [2]
Rash (>10%) [11]
Stevens-Johnson syndrome (>10%) [53]
Toxic epidermal necrolysis [72]
Toxic pustuloderma [3]
Toxicity [2]
Urticaria (>10%) [6]
Vasculitis [7]

Hair
Alopecia (<10%) [2]

Mucosal
Oral ulceration [3]
Stomatitis [2]

Cardiovascular
Polyarteritis nodosa [3]

Central Nervous System
Chills (<10%)
Fever [2]
Headache [3]
Vertigo (dizziness) [3]

Neuromuscular/Skeletal
Arthralgia [3]
Asthenia (fatigue) [2]
Back pain [2]
Bone or joint pain [2]
Joint disorder [2]
Myalgia/Myopathy [3]

Gastrointestinal/Hepatic
Diarrhea [5]
Hepatotoxicity [7]
Nausea [3]

Respiratory
Nasopharyngitis [2]
Upper respiratory tract infection [4]

Endocrine/Metabolic
ALT increased [2]
AST increased [3]

Renal
Nephrotoxicity [3]

Other
Adverse effects [13]
Allergic reactions (severe) [2]
Death [9]

ALMOTRIPTAN

Trade names: Almogran (Almirall), Axert (Ortho-McNeil)
Indications: Migraine headaches
Class: 5-HT1 agonist, Serotonin receptor agonist, Triptan
Half-life: 3–4 hours
Clinically important, potentially hazardous interactions with: conivaptan, darunavir, delavirdine, dihydroergotamine, ergotamine, indinavir, ketoconazole, methysergide, SNRIs, SSRIs, telithromycin, triptans, voriconazole
Pregnancy category: C
Important contra-indications noted in the prescribing guidelines for: pediatric patients
Note: Contra-indicated in patients with history, symptoms, or signs of ischemic cardiac, cerebrovascular, or peripheral vascular syndromes, or with uncontrolled hypertension.

Cardiovascular
Chest pain [3]

Central Nervous System
Headache [2]
Neurotoxicity [2]
Paresthesias [4]
Somnolence (drowsiness) [5]
Vertigo (dizziness) [6]

Neuromuscular/Skeletal
Asthenia (fatigue) [4]

Gastrointestinal/Hepatic
Nausea [6]
Vomiting [3]

Respiratory
Flu-like syndrome (12%)
Upper respiratory tract infection (20%)

Other
Adverse effects [10]

ALOGLIPTIN

Trade name: Nesina (Takeda)
Indications: Type II diabetes mellitus
Class: Antidiabetic, Dipeptidyl peptidase-4 (DPP-4) inhibitor
Half-life: 21 hours
Clinically important, potentially hazardous interactions with: none known
Pregnancy category: B
Important contra-indications noted in the prescribing guidelines for: nursing mothers; pediatric patients

Skin
Hypersensitivity [2]
Pruritus [2]

Central Nervous System
Headache (4%) [8]
Vertigo (dizziness) [3]

Neuromuscular/Skeletal
Arthralgia [2]

Gastrointestinal/Hepatic
Constipation [2]
Diarrhea [2]
Pancreatitis [3]

Respiratory
Nasopharyngitis (4%) [8]
Upper respiratory tract infection (4%) [6]

Endocrine/Metabolic
Hypoglycemia [14]

Other
Adverse effects [6]
Infection [3]

ALOSETRON

See: www.drugeruptiondata.com/drug/id/18

ALPHA-LIPOIC ACID

See: www.drugeruptiondata.com/drug/id/1224

ALPRAZOLAM

Trade name: Xanax (Pfizer)
Indications: Anxiety, depression, panic attacks
Class: Benzodiazepine
Half-life: 11–16 hours
Clinically important, potentially hazardous interactions with: alcohol, amprenavir, aprepitant, boceprevir, clarithromycin, CNS depressants, darunavir, delavirdine, digoxin, efavirenz, fluconazole, fluoxetine, fluvoxamine, grapefruit juice, indinavir, itraconazole, ivermectin, kava, ketoconazole, posaconazole, propoxyphene, ritonavir, saquinavir, St John's wort, telaprevir, tipranavir
Pregnancy category: D
Important contra-indications noted in the prescribing guidelines for: the elderly; nursing mothers; pediatric patients

Skin
 Dermatitis (4%) [5]
 Diaphoresis (16%)
 Edema (5%)
 Photosensitivity [4]
 Pruritus (<10%) [2]
 Rash (11%) [4]
Mucosal
 Sialopenia (33%)
 Sialorrhea (4%)
 Xerostomia (15%) [6]
Cardiovascular
 Hypotension (<10%)
Central Nervous System
 Cognitive impairment (>10%)
 Coma [2]
 Depression (>10%)
 Dysarthria (>10%)
 Incoordination (<10%)
 Memory loss [2]
 Neurotoxicity [2]
 Paresthesias (2%)
 Restlessness [2]
 Sedation [2]
 Seizures (<10%) [2]
 Somnolence (drowsiness) (>10%)
Neuromuscular/Skeletal
 Asthenia (fatigue) (>10%) [2]
Endocrine/Metabolic
 Galactorrhea [2]
Genitourinary
 Micturition difficulty (>10%)

ALPROSTADIL

Synonyms: PGE; prostaglandin E₁
Trade names: Caverject (Pfizer), Edex (Schwarz), Muse (Vivus), Prostin VR (Pfizer)
Indications: Impotence, to maintain patent ductus arteriosus
Class: Prostaglandin
Half-life: 5–10 minutes
Clinically important, potentially hazardous interactions with: acebutolol, alfuzosin, captopril, cilazapril, enalapril, fosinopril, irbesartan, lisinopril, olmesartan, quinapril, ramipril
Pregnancy category: D (not indicated for use in women)
Important contra-indications noted in the prescribing guidelines for: pediatric patients
Warning: APNEA (in neonates with congenital heart defects)

Skin
 Edema (<10%)
 Penile rash (<10%)
Mucosal
 Nasal congestion (<10%)
Cardiovascular
 Bradycardia (<10%)
 Flushing (>10%)
 Hypertension (<10%)
 Hypotension (<10%)
 Tachycardia (<10%)

Central Nervous System
 Fever (>10%)
 Headache (>10%)
 Pain (>10%)
 Vertigo (dizziness) (>10%)
Neuromuscular/Skeletal
 Back pain (<10%)
Gastrointestinal/Hepatic
 Diarrhea (<10%)
Respiratory
 Apnea (>10%)
 Cough (<10%)
 Flu-like syndrome (<10%)
 Sinusitis (<10%)
Genitourinary
 Erectile dysfunction (prolonged erection / >4 hours) (4%)
 Penile pain (>10%)
 Priapism (4%) [8]
 Urethral burning (>10%) [2]
Local
 Application-site burning [3]
 Application-site erythema [3]
 Application-site pain [2]
 Application-site pruritus [2]
 Injection-site ecchymoses (<10%)
 Injection-site hematoma (3%)
 Injection-site pain (2%)

ALTEPLASE

Synonym: tPA
Trade name: Activase (Genentech)
Indications: Acute myocardial infarction, acute pulmonary embolism
Class: Fibrinolytic, Plasminogen activator
Half-life: 30–45 minutes
Clinically important, potentially hazardous interactions with: defibrotide, nitroglycerin, ticlopidine
Pregnancy category: C
Important contra-indications noted in the prescribing guidelines for: the elderly; nursing mothers

Skin
 Anaphylactoid reactions/Anaphylaxis [5]
 Angioedema [12]
 Ecchymoses (<10%)
 Purpura (<10%)
Central Nervous System
 Fever (<10%)
 Intracranial hemorrhage [8]
Gastrointestinal/Hepatic
 Hemorrhagic colitis (5%)
Hematologic
 Bleeding [2]
 Hemorrhage (4%)
Other
 Death [4]

ALTRETAMINE

See: www.drugeruptiondata.com/drug/id/22

ALVIMOPAN

See: www.drugeruptiondata.com/drug/id/1292

AMANTADINE

See: www.drugeruptiondata.com/drug/id/23

AMBRISENTAN

Trade names: Letairis (Gilead), Volibris (GSK)
Indications: Pulmonary arterial hypertension
Class: Antihypertensive, Endothelin receptor (ETR) antagonist, Vasodilator
Half-life: 9 hours
Clinically important, potentially hazardous interactions with: conivaptan, cyclosporine, CYP2C19 inhibitors and inducers, CYP3A4 inhibitors and inducers, dasatinib, deferasirox, grapefruit juice, St John's wort
Pregnancy category: X
Important contra-indications noted in the prescribing guidelines for: nursing mothers; pediatric patients
Note: Also contra-indicated in patients with idiopathic pulmonary fibrosis.
Warning: CONTRA-INDICATED IN PREGNANCY

Skin
 Edema [3]
 Peripheral edema (17%) [8]
Mucosal
 Nasal congestion (6%) [2]
Cardiovascular
 Flushing (4%)
 Palpitation (5%)
Central Nervous System
 Headache (15%) [3]
Gastrointestinal/Hepatic
 Abdominal pain (3%)
 Constipation (4%)
 Hepatotoxicity [3]
Respiratory
 Dyspnea (4%)
 Nasopharyngitis (3%)
 Sinusitis (3%)
Hematologic
 Anemia [4]

AMCINONIDE

See: www.drugeruptiondata.com/drug/id/1096

AMIFOSTINE

See: www.drugeruptiondata.com/drug/id/24

AMIKACIN

Trade name: Amikacin sulfate (Bedford)
Indications: Short-term treatment of serious infections due to gram-negative bacteria
Class: Antibiotic, aminoglycoside
Half-life: 1.5–2.5 hours (adults)
Clinically important, potentially hazardous interactions with: adefovir, aldesleukin, aminoglycosides, atracurium, bumetanide, cephalexin, doxacurium, ethacrynic acid, furosemide, succinylcholine, teicoplanin, torsemide
Pregnancy category: D
Important contra-indications noted in the prescribing guidelines for: nursing mothers; pediatric patients
Note: Aminoglycosides may cause neurotoxicity and/or nephrotoxicity.

Skin
 Dermatitis [2]
 Exanthems [2]

Central Nervous System
 Neurotoxicity (<10%)

Renal
 Nephrotoxicity (<10%) [11]

Otic
 Hearing loss [5]
 Ototoxicity (<10%) [8]
 Tinnitus [3]

Ocular
 Macular infarction [3]

AMILORIDE

Trade names: Midamor (Merck), Moduretic (Merck)
Indications: Prevention of hypokalemia associated with kaliuretic diuretics, management of edema in hypertension
Class: Diuretic, potassium-sparing
Half-life: 6–9 hours
Clinically important, potentially hazardous interactions with: ACE inhibitors, benazepril, captopril, cyclosporine, enalapril, fosinopril, lisinopril, magnesium, metformin, moexipril, potassium salts, quinapril, quinidine, ramipril, spironolactone, trandolapril, zofenopril
Pregnancy category: B
Note: Moduretic is amiloride and hydrochlorothiazide. Hydrochlorothiazide is a sulfonamide and can be absorbed systemically. Sulfonamides can produce severe, possibly fatal, reactions such as toxic epidermal necrolysis and Stevens-Johnson syndrome.

Skin
 Photosensitivity [4]

Central Nervous System
 Headache (<10%)
 Vertigo (dizziness) (<10%)

Neuromuscular/Skeletal
 Asthenia (fatigue) (<10%)
 Myalgia/Myopathy (<10%)

Respiratory
 Cough (<10%)
 Dyspnea (<10%)

Endocrine/Metabolic
 Gynecomastia (<10%)
 Hyperkalemia [2]

Genitourinary
 Impotence (<10%)

AMINOCAPROIC ACID

See: www.drugeruptiondata.com/drug/id/27

AMINO-GLUTETHIMIDE

See: www.drugeruptiondata.com/drug/id/28

AMINOLEVULINIC ACID

Trade names: Ameluz (Biofrontera), Levulan Kerastick (Dusa)
Indications: Non-hyperkeratotic actinic keratoses of face and scalp
Class: Photosensitizer, Protoporphyrin IX (PpIX) (wakefulness promoting agent)
Half-life: 20–40 hours
Clinically important, potentially hazardous interactions with: none known
Pregnancy category: C
Important contra-indications noted in the prescribing guidelines for: nursing mothers; pediatric patients
Note: In photodynamic therapy: to be used in conjunction with the relevant illuminator as approved by the manufacturer.

Skin
 Burning (>50%) [6]
 Crusting (64–71%) [2]
 Dermatitis [2]
 Desquamation [2]
 Edema (35%) [9]
 Erosions (14%) [2]
 Erythema (99%) [13]
 Exfoliative dermatitis (from topical
  treatment) [3]
 Hypomelanosis (22%)
 Photosensitivity [3]
 Pigmentation (from topical treatment) (22%)
  [7]
 Pruritus (25%) [2]
 Pustules (<4%)
 Scaling (64–71%)
 Stinging (>50%) [2]
 Ulcerations (4%)
 Vesiculation (4%) [2]

Central Nervous System
 Dysesthesia (2%)
 Pain [12]

AMINOPHYLLINE

Synonym: theophylline ethylenediamine
Trade names: Elixophyllin (Forest), Phyllocontin (Napp), Quibron (Monarch)
Indications: Prevention or treatment of reversible bronchospasm
Class: Xanthine alkaloid
Half-life: 3–15 hours (in adult nonsmokers)
Clinically important, potentially hazardous interactions with: adenosine, anagrelide, arformoterol, azithromycin, BCG vaccine, caffeine, capsicum, carbimazole, cimetidine, ciprofloxacin, clorazepate, cocoa, erythromycin, eucalyptus, febuxostat, fluvoxamine, halothane, indacaterol, influenza vaccine, levofloxacin, mebendazole, methylprednisolone, moxifloxacin, nilutamide, norfloxacin, obeticholic acid, ofloxacin, oral contraceptives, prednisolone, prednisone, propranolol, rasagiline, raspberry leaf, roflumilast, ropivacaine, roxithromycin, St John's wort, torasemide, torsemide, triamcinolone, zafirlukast
Pregnancy category: C
Important contra-indications noted in the prescribing guidelines for: the elderly; nursing mothers

Skin
 Dermatitis [7]
 Exanthems [5]
 Exfoliative dermatitis [6]
 Hypersensitivity [6]
 Pruritus [3]
 Stevens-Johnson syndrome [3]
 Urticaria [6]

Cardiovascular
 Arrhythmias [2]
 Palpitation [3]
 Tachycardia [2]

Central Nervous System
 Insomnia [2]
 Seizures [11]
 Tremor [2]

Neuromuscular/Skeletal
 Rhabdomyolysis [5]

Gastrointestinal/Hepatic
 Abdominal pain [2]
 Nausea [5]
 Vomiting [2]

Endocrine/Metabolic
 SIADH [2]

Other
 Adverse effects [3]
 Allergic reactions [5]
 Death [2]

AMINOSALICYLATE SODIUM

See: www.drugeruptiondata.com/drug/id/30

NOVANT HEALTH LIBRARY SERVICES

AMIODARONE

Trade names: Cordarone (Wyeth), Pacerone (Upsher-Smith)
Indications: Ventricular fibrillation, ventricular tachycardia
Class: Antiarrhythmic, Antiarrhythmic class III, CYP1A2 inhibitor, CYP3A4 inhibitor
Half-life: 26–107 days
Clinically important, potentially hazardous interactions with: abarelix, acebutolol, acenocoumarol, afatinib, amisulpride, amitriptyline, amprenavir, anisindione, anticoagulants, arsenic, artemether/lumefantrine, asenapine, astemizole, atazanavir, atorvastatin, azoles, betrixaban, boceprevir, bosentan, carbimazole, celiprolol, cholestyramine, cimetidine, ciprofloxacin, clopidogrel, cobicistat/elvitegravir/emtricitabine/tenofovir alafenamide, cobicistat/elvitegravir/emtricitabine/tenofovir disoproxil, colchicine, cyclosporine, dabigatran, daclatasvir, darunavir, degarelix, delavirdine, dextromethorphan, dicumarol, digoxin, diltiazem, disopyramide, dronedarone, droperidol, echinacea, enoxacin, fentanyl, flecainide, fosamprenavir, gatifloxacin, grapefruit juice, indinavir, ledipasvir & sofosbuvir, lesinurad, levofloxacin, levomepromazine, lidocaine, lomefloxacin, lopinavir, loratadine, macrolide antibiotics, methotrexate, moxifloxacin, naldemedine, nelfinavir, nevirapine, nilotinib, norfloxacin, ofloxacin, orlistat, oxprenolol, pentamidine, phenytoin, pimavanserin, procainamide, propranolol, quinidine, quinine, quinolones, ribociclib, rifabutin, rifampin, rifapentine, ritonavir, ropivacaine, rosuvastatin, simvastatin, sofosbuvir & velpatasvir, sofosbuvir/velpatasvir/voxilaprevir, sotalol, sparfloxacin, St John's wort, sulpiride, tacrolimus, telaprevir, tetrabenazine, thalidomide, tipranavir, trazodone, vandetanib, venetoclax, verapamil, warfarin, zuclopenthixol
Pregnancy category: D
Important contra-indications noted in the prescribing guidelines for: the elderly; nursing mothers; pediatric patients
Warning: PULMONARY TOXICITY

Skin
Anaphylactoid reactions/Anaphylaxis [2]
Angioedema [2]
Diaphoresis [2]
Edema (<10%)
Erythema nodosum [2]
Exanthems [5]
Facial erythema (3%) [2]
Iododerma [2]
Linear IgA bullous dermatosis [6]
Lupus erythematosus [5]
Myxedema [3]
Photosensitivity (10–75%) [41]
Phototoxicity [3]
Pigmentation (blue) (<10%) [68]
Pruritus (<5%) [2]
Psoriasis [2]
Purpura (2%)
Toxic epidermal necrolysis [2]
Toxicity [5]
Vasculitis [6]

Hair
Alopecia [5]
Mucosal
Sialorrhea (<10%)
Cardiovascular
Arrhythmias (<3%) [3]
Atrial fibrillation (paroxysmal) [3]
Atrioventricular block [3]
Bradycardia [18]
Cardiotoxicity [3]
Flushing (<10%)
Hypotension (16%) [4]
QT prolongation [24]
Tachycardia [2]
Thrombophlebitis [2]
Torsades de pointes [35]
Ventricular arrhythmia [2]
Central Nervous System
Anorexia (10–33%)
Coma [2]
Dysgeusia (taste perversion) (<10%)
Headache (3–40%)
Insomnia (3–40%)
Neurotoxicity [5]
Paresthesias (4–9%)
Parkinsonism [4]
Parosmia (<10%)
Peripheral neuropathy [4]
Syncope [2]
Tremor (3–40%) [4]
Vertigo (dizziness) (3–40%)
Neuromuscular/Skeletal
Ataxia [4]
Myoclonus [2]
Rhabdomyolysis [7]
Gastrointestinal/Hepatic
Abdominal pain (<10%)
Constipation (10–33%)
Hepatic failure [2]
Hepatic steatosis [2]
Hepatitis (<3%) [3]
Hepatotoxicity [27]
Nausea (10–33%)
Pancreatitis [4]
Vomiting (10–33%)
Respiratory
Cough [2]
Eosinophilic pneumonia [2]
Pneumonia [4]
Pneumonitis [5]
Pulmonary toxicity [24]
Endocrine/Metabolic
Hyperthyroidism (<3%) [10]
Hyponatremia [2]
Hypothyroidism (<3%) [18]
SIADH [10]
Thyroid dysfunction [25]
Thyrotoxicosis [19]
Genitourinary
Epididymitis [2]
Ocular
Corneal deposits (>90%) [2]
Keratopathy [6]
Ocular adverse effects [4]
Ocular toxicity [2]
Optic neuropathy [7]
Visual disturbances (2–9%)

Other
Adverse effects [5]
Death [8]
Side effects (12%) [4]

AMISULPRIDE

See: www.drugeruptiondata.com/drug/id/1281

AMITRIPTYLINE

Trade names: Elavil (AstraZeneca), Limbitrol (Valeant)
Indications: Depression
Class: Antidepressant, tricyclic, Muscarinic antagonist
Half-life: 10–25 hours
Clinically important, potentially hazardous interactions with: adrenergic neurone blockers, alcohol, alfuzosin, altretamine, amiodarone, amphetamines, amprenavir, anticholinergics, antiepileptics, antihistamines, antimuscarinics, antipsychotics, apraclonidine, arsenic, artemether/lumefantrine, aspirin, atomoxetine, baclofen, barbiturates, brimonidine, bupropion, cannabis extract, carbamazepine, cimetidine, cinacalcet, ciprofloxacin, cisapride, clonidine, clozapine, cobicistat/elvitegravir/emtricitabine/tenofovir alafenamide, cobicistat/elvitegravir/emtricitabine/tenofovir disoproxil, conivaptan, coumarins, CYP2D6 inhibitors, desmopressin, dexmethylphenidate, diltiazem, disopyramide, disulfiram, diuretics, dronedarone, droperidol, duloxetine, entacapone, ephedra, epinephrine, estrogens, eucalyptus, flecainide, gadobutrol, general anesthetics, gotu kola, grapefruit juice, guanethidine, histamine, interferon alfa, iobenguane, isocarboxazid, isoproterenol, kava, linezolid, lithium, MAO inhibitors, methylphenidate, metoclopramide, moclobemide, moxifloxacin, moxonidine, nefopam, nicorandil, nilotinib, nitrates, NSAIDs, opioid analgesics, paroxetine hydrochloride, pentamidine, phenelzine, phenothiazines, phenytoin, pimozide, pramlintide, primidone, propafenone, propoxyphene, protease inhibitors, QT interval prolonging agents, quinidine, quinine, quinolones, rasagiline, ritonavir, saquinavir, selegiline, sibutramine, sodium oxybate, sotalol, sparfloxacin, SSRIs, St John's wort, sulfonylureas, terbinafine, tetrabenazine, thioridazine, thyroid hormones, tramadol, tranylcypromine, valerian, valproic acid, verapamil, vitamin K antagonists, yohimbine, ziprasidone
Pregnancy category: C
Important contra-indications noted in the prescribing guidelines for: the elderly; nursing mothers; pediatric patients
Note: Limbitrol is amitriptyline and chlordiazepoxide.
Warning: SUICIDALITY AND ANTIDEPRESSANT DRUGS

Skin
Diaphoresis (<10%)
DRESS syndrome [2]
Photosensitivity [3]
Pigmentation [4]

Pruritus [3]
Pseudolymphoma [2]
Purpura [2]

Mucosal
Xerostomia (>10%) [16]

Cardiovascular
Brugada syndrome [4]
Myocardial infarction [2]
Postural hypotension [2]
QT prolongation [2]

Central Nervous System
Delirium [2]
Depression [2]
Dysgeusia (taste perversion) (>10%) [2]
Hallucinations [3]
Headache [2]
Restless legs syndrome [2]
Sedation [3]
Seizures [7]
Serotonin syndrome [4]
Somnolence (drowsiness) [6]
Vertigo (dizziness) [6]

Neuromuscular/Skeletal
Asthenia (fatigue) [3]
Rhabdomyolysis [2]

Gastrointestinal/Hepatic
Cholestasis [2]
Constipation [4]
Nausea [2]

Endocrine/Metabolic
SIADH [5]
Weight gain [7]

Otic
Tinnitus [3]

Ocular
Hallucinations, visual [2]
Vision blurred [2]

Other
Adverse effects [5]
Death [3]

AMLEXANOX

See: www.drugeruptiondata.com/drug/id/1200

AMLODIPINE

Trade names: Caduet (Pfizer), Exforge (Novartis), Istin (Pfizer), Lotrel (Novartis), Norvasc (Pfizer), Prestalia (Symplmed), Tekamlo (Novartis)
Indications: Hypertension, angina
Class: Antiarrhythmic class IV, Calcium channel blocker
Half-life: 30–50 hours
Clinically important, potentially hazardous interactions with: amprenavir, carbamazepine, cobicistat/elvitegravir/emtricitabine/tenofovir alafenamide, cobicistat/elvitegravir/emtricitabine/tenofovir disoproxil, conivaptan, delavirdine, epirubicin, imatinib, phenytoin, primidone, sildenafil, simvastatin, St John's wort, tadalafil, telaprevir

Pregnancy category: C
Important contra-indications noted in the prescribing guidelines for: the elderly; nursing mothers; pediatric patients
Note: Caduet is amlodipine and atorvastatin; Exforge is amlodipine and valsartan; Lotrel is amlodipine and benazepril; Prestalia is amlodipine and perindopril; Tekamlo is amlodipine and aliskiren.

Skin
Angioedema [6]
Dermatitis (<10%)
Edema (5–14%) [20]
Erythema multiforme [2]
Exanthems (2–4%) [2]
Peripheral edema (>10%) [44]
Pigmentation [2]
Pruritus (2–4%) [3]
Rash (<10%)
Telangiectasia (facial) [5]
Toxic epidermal necrolysis [2]
Toxicity [2]
Vasculitis [2]

Mucosal
Gingival hyperplasia/hypertrophy [29]

Cardiovascular
Flushing (<10%) [5]
Hypotension [7]

Central Nervous System
Headache [12]
Parkinsonism [2]
Syncope [2]
Vertigo (dizziness) [13]

Neuromuscular/Skeletal
Asthenia (fatigue) [5]
Rhabdomyolysis [2]

Gastrointestinal/Hepatic
Diarrhea [3]
Gastritis [2]
Hepatotoxicity [3]
Nausea [5]
Vomiting [2]

Respiratory
Bronchitis [2]
Cough [2]
Upper respiratory tract infection [4]

Other
Adverse effects [8]

AMOBARBITAL

See: www.drugeruptiondata.com/drug/id/34

AMODIAQUINE

Trade names: Camoquin (Pfizer), Flavoquin (Sanofi-Aventis)
Indications: Malaria
Class: Anti-inflammatory, Antimalarial
Half-life: 15.7–19.5 hours
Clinically important, potentially hazardous interactions with: none known

Pregnancy category: N/A
Important contra-indications noted in the prescribing guidelines for: pediatric patients

Skin
Pruritus [3]

Central Nervous System
Extrapyramidal symptoms [3]

Neuromuscular/Skeletal
Asthenia (fatigue) [4]

Gastrointestinal/Hepatic
Abdominal pain [3]
Diarrhea [3]
Vomiting [7]

Hematologic
Neutropenia [2]

Other
Adverse effects [2]
Death [2]

AMOXAPINE

Trade name: Amoxapine (Watson)
Indications: Depression
Class: Antidepressant, tricyclic, Muscarinic antagonist
Half-life: 11–30 hours
Clinically important, potentially hazardous interactions with: amprenavir, artemether/lumefantrine, clonidine, dronedarone, epinephrine, fluoxetine, guanethidine, iobenguane, isocarboxazid, linezolid, MAO inhibitors, nilotinib, phenelzine, pimozide, quetiapine, quinine, quinolones, sparfloxacin, tetrabenazine, thioridazine, toremifene, tranylcypromine, vandetanib, vemurafenib, ziprasidone
Pregnancy category: C
Important contra-indications noted in the prescribing guidelines for: the elderly; nursing mothers; pediatric patients
Warning: SUICIDALITY AND ANTIDEPRESSANT DRUGS

Skin
AGEP [3]
Diaphoresis (<10%)
Edema (<10%)
Exanthems [2]
Rash (<10%)
Toxic epidermal necrolysis [2]

Mucosal
Xerostomia (14%)

Central Nervous System
Dysgeusia (taste perversion) (>10%)
Headache (<10%)
Insomnia (<10%)
Neuroleptic malignant syndrome [2]
Somnolence (drowsiness) (14%)
Vertigo (dizziness) (<10%)

Neuromuscular/Skeletal
Asthenia (fatigue) (<10%)

Gastrointestinal/Hepatic
Constipation (12%)
Nausea (<10%)

Endocrine/Metabolic
Galactorrhea [2]
Ocular
Vision blurred (7%)
Other
Side effects (5%)

AMOXICILLIN

Synonym: amoxycillin
Trade names: Amoxil (GSK), Augmentin (GSK),
Prevpac (TAP), Trimox (Bristol-Myers Squibb)
Indications: Infections of the respiratory tract,
skin and urinary tract
Class: Antibiotic, penicillin
Half-life: 0.7–1.4 hours
**Clinically important, potentially hazardous
interactions with:** allopurinol, bromelain,
chloramphenicol, demeclocycline, doxycycline,
erythromycin, imipenem/cilastatin, methotrexate,
minocycline, omeprazole, oxytetracycline,
sulfonamides, tetracycline
Pregnancy category: B
Note: Augmentin is amoxicillin and clavulanic
acid.

Skin
AGEP [28]
Anaphylactoid reactions/Anaphylaxis [15]
Angioedema (<10%) [5]
Baboon syndrome (SDRIFE) [11]
Bullous pemphigoid [2]
Dermatitis [4]
DRESS syndrome [6]
Edema [2]
Erythema multiforme [18]
Exanthems (>5%) [33]
Fixed eruption [10]
Hypersensitivity [5]
Jarisch–Herxheimer reaction [2]
Linear IgA bullous dermatosis [3]
Pemphigus [4]
Pruritus [7]
Pustules [8]
Rash (<10%) [14]
Serum sickness-like reaction (<10%) [6]
Stevens-Johnson syndrome [11]
Toxic epidermal necrolysis [13]
Toxic pustuloderma [2]
Urticaria (<5%) [16]
Mucosal
Stomatitis [2]
Central Nervous System
Anorexia [2]
Dysgeusia (taste perversion) [6]
Hallucinations [3]
Headache [5]
Somnolence (drowsiness) [3]
Vertigo (dizziness) [5]
Neuromuscular/Skeletal
Asthenia (fatigue) [3]
Rhabdomyolysis [2]
Gastrointestinal/Hepatic
Abdominal distension [2]
Abdominal pain [7]
Diarrhea [18]
Dyspepsia [2]

Hepatotoxicity [36]
Nausea [13]
Vomiting [9]
Genitourinary
Vaginitis [3]
Renal
Nephrotoxicity [2]
Other
Adverse effects [20]
Kounis syndrome [6]
Side effects [4]
Tooth fluorosis [2]

AMPHOTERICIN B

Trade names: Abelcet (Sigma-Tau), AmBisome
(Astellas), Amphocin (Pfizer), Amphotec
(Alkopharma)
Indications: Potentially life-threatening fungal
infections
Class: Antifungal
Half-life: initial: 15–48 hours; terminal: 15 days
**Clinically important, potentially hazardous
interactions with:** adefovir, aminoglycosides,
arsenic, astemizole, betamethasone, cephalothin,
cidofovir, cyclosporine, digoxin, ethoxzolamide,
fluconazole, flucytosine, ganciclovir, griseofulvin,
hydrocortisone, itraconazole, ketoconazole,
micafungin, pentamidine, probenecid, sulpiride,
terbinafine, triamcinolone, voriconazole
Pregnancy category: B
**Important contra-indications noted in the
prescribing guidelines for:** nursing mothers

Skin
Anaphylactoid reactions/Anaphylaxis [4]
Diaphoresis (7%)
Exanthems [4]
Peripheral edema (15%)
Pruritus (11%) [2]
Purpura [3]
Rash (25%)
Toxicity [2]
Urticaria [2]
Mucosal
Epistaxis (nosebleed) (15%)
Cardiovascular
Chest pain (12%)
Flushing (<10%) [2]
Hypertension (8%) [4]
Hypotension (14%)
Tachycardia (13%)
Thrombophlebitis (<10%)
Central Nervous System
Anorexia (>10%)
Anxiety (14%)
Chills (48%) [5]
Confusion (11%)
Delirium (>10%)
Fever (>10%) [5]
Headache (20%)
Insomnia (17%)
Leukoencephalopathy [4]
Pain (14%)
Paresthesias (<10%)
Parkinsonism [2]

Neuromuscular/Skeletal
Asthenia (fatigue) (13%)
Back pain (12%)
Gastrointestinal/Hepatic
Abdominal pain (20%)
Diarrhea (30%)
Gastrointestinal bleeding (10%)
Hepatotoxicity [5]
Nausea (40%)
Vomiting (32%)
Respiratory
Bronchospasm [2]
Cough (18%)
Dyspnea (23%)
Hypoxia (8%)
Pleural effusion (13%)
Pulmonary toxicity (18%)
Rhinitis (11%)
Tachypnea (>10%)
Endocrine/Metabolic
ALP increased (22%)
ALT increased (15%)
AST increased (13%)
Creatine phosphokinase increased (22%)
Hyperglycemia (23%)
Hypernatremia (4%)
Hypervolemia (12%)
Hypocalcemia (18%)
Hypokalemia [2]
Hypomagnesemia (20%)
Genitourinary
Hematuria (14%)
Urinary retention (<10%)
Renal
Nephrotoxicity [50]
Hematologic
Anemia (>10%) [4]
Leukocytosis (<10%)
Sepsis (14%)
Local
Infusion-related reactions [5]
Injection-site pain (>10%)
Injection-site reactions [5]
Other
Adverse effects [5]
Death [4]
Infection (11%)

AMPICILLIN

Trade name: Totacillin (GSK)
Indications: Susceptible strains of gram-negative
and gram-positive bacterial infections
Class: Antibiotic, penicillin
Half-life: 1–1.5 hours
**Clinically important, potentially hazardous
interactions with:** allopurinol, anticoagulants,
chloramphenicol, cyclosporine, demeclocycline,
doxycycline, erythromycin, levodopa,
methotrexate, minocycline, oxytetracycline,
sulfonamides, tetracycline
Pregnancy category: B
**Important contra-indications noted in the
prescribing guidelines for:** nursing mothers
Note: Five to 10% of people taking ampicillin
develop eruptions between the 5th and 14th day
following initiation of therapy. Also, there is a

95% incidence of exanthematous eruptions in patients who are treated for infectious mononucleosis with ampicillin. The allergenicity of ampicillin appears to be enhanced by allopurinol or by hyperuricemia. Ampicillin is clearly the more allergenic of the two drugs when given alone.

Skin
AGEP [9]
Anaphylactoid reactions/Anaphylaxis [10]
Angioedema [2]
Baboon syndrome (SDRIFE) [3]
Dermatitis [8]
Erythema multiforme [11]
Exanthems (>10%) [84]
Exfoliative dermatitis [3]
Fixed eruption [10]
Hypersensitivity [5]
Linear IgA bullous dermatosis [4]
Pemphigus [6]
Pruritus (<5%) [5]
Psoriasis [5]
Purpura [6]
Pustules [4]
Rash (<10%)
Stevens-Johnson syndrome [10]
Toxic epidermal necrolysis [15]
Urticaria [16]
Vasculitis [4]

Hematologic
Thrombocytopenia [2]

Local
Injection-site pain (>10%)

Other
Allergic reactions (<10%) [3]

AMPICILLIN/ SULBACTAM

Trade name: Unasyn (Pfizer)
Indications: Various infections caused by susceptible organisms
Class: Antibiotic, beta-lactam, Antibiotic, penicillin
Half-life: 1 hour
Clinically important, potentially hazardous interactions with: allopurinol, probenecid
Pregnancy category: B
Important contra-indications noted in the prescribing guidelines for: nursing mothers
Note: Serious and occasionally fatal hypersensitivity (anaphylactic) reactions have been reported in patients on penicillin therapy. Contra-indicated in patients with a history of hypersensitivity reactions to any of the penicillins.

Skin
Anaphylactoid reactions/Anaphylaxis [2]
Linear IgA bullous dermatosis [3]
Rash (<10%)

Gastrointestinal/Hepatic
Diarrhea (<10%)

Local
Injection-site pain (16%)

AMPRENAVIR

See: www.drugeruptiondata.com/drug/id/39

AMYL NITRITE

See: www.drugeruptiondata.com/drug/id/40

ANAGRELIDE

See: www.drugeruptiondata.com/drug/id/896

ANAKINRA

Trade name: Kineret (Amgen)
Indications: Rheumatoid arthritis, neonatal-onset multisystem inflammatory disease
Class: Disease-modulating antirheumatoid drug, Interleukin-1 receptor antagonist (IL-1Ra)
Half-life: 4–6 hours
Clinically important, potentially hazardous interactions with: abatacept, adalimumab, certolizumab, etanercept, golimumab, infliximab, lenalidomide, live vaccines
Pregnancy category: B
Important contra-indications noted in the prescribing guidelines for: nursing mothers

Central Nervous System
Fever (12%)
Headache (12–14%) [2]

Neuromuscular/Skeletal
Arthralgia (6–12%)

Gastrointestinal/Hepatic
Abdominal pain (5%)
Diarrhea (8%)
Nausea (8%)
Vomiting (14%)

Respiratory
Flu-like syndrome (6%)
Nasopharyngitis (12%)
Sinusitis (7%)
Upper respiratory tract infection (4%) [2]

Local
Injection-site edema [2]
Injection-site erythema [3]
Injection-site inflammation [2]
Injection-site pain [4]
Injection-site reactions (71%) [31]

Other
Adverse effects [5]
Infection (40%) [11]

ANASTROZOLE

Trade name: Arimidex (AstraZeneca)
Indications: Breast carcinoma (localized – advanced or metastatic)
Class: Antineoplastic, Aromatase inhibitor
Half-life: 50 hours
Clinically important, potentially hazardous interactions with: estradiol, estrogens, tamoxifen

Pregnancy category: N/A (Contra-indicated in women of premenopausal endocrine status, including pregnant women)
Important contra-indications noted in the prescribing guidelines for: nursing mothers
Note: The efficacy of anastrozole in the treatment of pubertal gynecomastia in adolescent boys and in the treatment of precocious puberty in girls with McCune-Albright syndrome has not been demonstrated.

Skin
Hot flashes (12–36%) [12]
Lupus erythematosus [3]
Peripheral edema (10%)
Pruritus (2–5%)
Rash (6–11%) [2]

Hair
Alopecia (2–5%)

Cardiovascular
Angina (2%)
Flushing (>5%)
Hypertension (2–13%)
Thrombophlebitis (2–5%)

Central Nervous System
Carpal tunnel syndrome [2]
Depression (5–13%)
Headache (9–13%) [2]
Pain (14%)
Tumor pain (>5%)

Neuromuscular/Skeletal
Arthralgia (2–5%) [8]
Asthenia (fatigue) (19%) [7]
Back pain (12%) [2]
Bone or joint pain (6–11%) [2]
Joint disorder [3]
Myalgia/Myopathy (2–5%) [2]
Osteoporosis (11%)

Gastrointestinal/Hepatic
Diarrhea [2]
Hepatitis [2]
Hepatotoxicity [5]
Nausea (11–19%)
Vomiting (8–13%)

Respiratory
Cough (11%)
Flu-like syndrome (7%)
Pharyngitis (6–14%)

Endocrine/Metabolic
Mastodynia (2–5%)

Genitourinary
Vaginal dryness (2%) [2]

Other
Infection (2–5%)

ANDROSTENEDIONE

See: www.drugeruptiondata.com/drug/id/801

ANIDULAFUNGIN

Trade names: Ecalta (Pfizer), Eraxis (Pfizer)
Indications: Candidemia, candidal esophagitis
Class: Antimycobacterial, echinocandin
Half-life: 40–50 hours
Clinically important, potentially hazardous interactions with: none known
Pregnancy category: C
Important contra-indications noted in the prescribing guidelines for: nursing mothers; pediatric patients

Skin
Angioedema (<2%)
Erythema (<2%)
Hot flashes (<2%)
Hyperhidrosis (<2%)
Peripheral edema (11%)
Pruritus (<2%)
Ulcerations (5%)
Urticaria (<2%)

Mucosal
Oral candidiasis (5%)

Cardiovascular
Atrial fibrillation (<2%)
Bundle branch block (<2%)
Chest pain (5%)
Flushing (<2%) [2]
Hypertension (12%)
Hypotension (15%)
Phlebitis [2]
Thrombophlebitis (<2%)
Venous thromboembolism (10%)

Central Nervous System
Confusion (8%)
Depression (6%)
Fever (9–18%) [3]
Headache (8%) [5]
Insomnia (15%)
Rigors (<2%)
Seizures (<2%)
Vertigo (dizziness) (<2%)

Neuromuscular/Skeletal
Back pain (5%)

Gastrointestinal/Hepatic
Abdominal pain (6%)
Cholestasis (<2%)
Constipation (8%)
Diarrhea (9–18%)
Dyspepsia (aggravated) (7%)
Hepatotoxicity [4]
Nausea (7–24%) [4]
Vomiting (7–18%) [4]

Respiratory
Cough (7%)
Dyspnea (12%)
Pleural effusion (10%)
Pneumonia (6%)
Respiratory distress (6%)

Endocrine/Metabolic
ALP increased (12%)
ALT increased (2%)
Creatine phosphokinase increased (5%)
Dehydration (6%)
Hyperglycemia (6%)
Hyperkalemia (6%)
Hypoglycemia (7%)
Hypokalemia (5–15%)
Hypomagnesemia (12%)

Genitourinary
Urinary tract infection (15%)

Hematologic
Anemia (8–9%)
Coagulopathy (<2%)
Leukocytosis (5%)
Sepsis (7%)
Thrombocythemia (6%)
Thrombocytopenia (<2%)

Ocular
Ocular pain (<2%)
Vision blurred (<2%)
Visual disturbances (<2%)

Local
Infusion-related reactions [2]

Other
Adverse effects [3]
Infection (63%)

ANISINDIONE

See: www.drugeruptiondata.com/drug/id/898

ANISTREPLASE

See: www.drugeruptiondata.com/drug/id/41

ANTHRAX VACCINE

Trade name: BioThrax (Emergent BioSolutions)
Indications: Anthrax prophylaxis
Class: Vaccine
Half-life: Requires 1 month to achieve immunity (92.5% efficient)
Clinically important, potentially hazardous interactions with: corticosteroids, immunosuppressive therapies, other vaccines
Pregnancy category: D
Important contra-indications noted in the prescribing guidelines for: the elderly; nursing mothers; pediatric patients
Note: Dr. Sue Bailey, Assistant Secretary for Health Affairs, released a statement on June 29, 1999 that 'almost one million shots given, the anthrax immunization is proving to be one of the safest vaccination programs on record.' The ADRs reported occurred for '50 service members at one installation alone.' Note that no number of military personnel was mentioned at this installation, nor did it give any percentages for the reactions reported.

Skin
Diaphoresis [2]
Edema (3%) [2]
Hypersensitivity [5]
Lupus erythematosus [2]
Pruritus (<10%) [2]
Rash [2]
Stevens-Johnson syndrome [2]
Urticaria [2]

Central Nervous System
Chills [2]
Fever [3]
Guillain–Barré syndrome [2]
Headache (4–64%) [2]

Neuromuscular/Skeletal
Arthralgia [3]
Asthenia (fatigue) (5–62%)
Myalgia/Myopathy (2–72%) [3]

Gastrointestinal/Hepatic
Diarrhea (6–8%)
Nausea (6%)

Respiratory
Flu-like syndrome [3]
Nasopharyngitis (12–15%)

Genitourinary
Dysmenorrhea (7%)

Local
Injection-site edema [4]
Injection-site nodules [2]
Injection-site pain [4]
Injection-site pruritus [2]
Injection-site reactions [6]

Other
Allergic reactions [2]

ANTI-THYMOCYTE GLOBULIN (EQUINE)

See: www.drugeruptiondata.com/drug/id/2587

ANTI-THYMOCYTE IMMUNOGLOBULIN (RABBIT)

See: www.drugeruptiondata.com/drug/id/1415

ANTIHEMOPHILIC FACTOR

Synonym: rFVIIIFc
Trade names: Afstyla (CSL Behring), Eloctate (Biogen Idec), Kovaltry (Bayer)
Indications: Control and prevention of bleeding episodes in Hemophilia A
Class: Antihemorrhagic, Recombinant fusion protein
Half-life: 20 hours (adults)
Clinically important, potentially hazardous interactions with: none known

Pregnancy category: C
Important contra-indications noted in the prescribing guidelines for: nursing mothers

APIXABAN

Trade name: Eliquis (Bristol-Myers Squibb)
Indications: Reduce the risk of stroke and systemic embolism in patients with nonvalvular atrial fibrillation
Class: Anticoagulant, Direct factor Xa inhibitor
Half-life: 5–12 hours
Clinically important, potentially hazardous interactions with: carbamazepine, darunavir, phenytoin, rifampin, St John's wort, tipranavir, voriconazole
Pregnancy category: B
Important contra-indications noted in the prescribing guidelines for: nursing mothers; pediatric patients
Note: Contra-indicated in patients with active pathological bleeding.
Warning: DISCONTINUING ELIQUIS IN PATIENTS WITHOUT ADEQUATE CONTINUOUS ANTICOAGULATION INCREASES RISK OF STROKE

Gastrointestinal/Hepatic
Hepatotoxicity [2]
Hematologic
Hemorrhage [15]
Other
Adverse effects [4]

APOMORPHINE

See: www.drugeruptiondata.com/drug/id/1055

APRACLONIDINE

Trade name: Iopidine (Alcon)
Indications: Post-surgical intraocular pressure elevation
Class: Adrenergic alpha2-receptor agonist
Half-life: 8 hours
Clinically important, potentially hazardous interactions with: amitriptyline
Pregnancy category: C
Important contra-indications noted in the prescribing guidelines for: nursing mothers; pediatric patients

Skin
Dermatitis [3]
Pruritus (10%)
Mucosal
Xerostomia (<10%)
Central Nervous System
Dysgeusia (taste perversion) (3%)
Ocular
Conjunctivitis (<5%)
Eyelid edema (<3%)
Ocular pruritus (5–15%)
Xerophthalmia (<5%)

Other
Allergic reactions [5]

APREMILAST

Trade name: Otezla (Celgene)
Indications: Psoriatic arthritis, plaque psoriasis
Class: Phosphodiesterase inhibitor, Phosphodiesterase type 4 (PDE4) inhibitor
Half-life: 6–9 hours
Clinically important, potentially hazardous interactions with: carbamazepine, phenobarbital, phenytoin, rifampin
Pregnancy category: C
Important contra-indications noted in the prescribing guidelines for: nursing mothers; pediatric patients

Central Nervous System
Depression [3]
Headache (5–6%) [24]
Neuromuscular/Skeletal
Arthralgia [2]
Asthenia (fatigue) [5]
Gastrointestinal/Hepatic
Abdominal pain (<2%) [3]
Diarrhea (8–9%) [28]
Dyspepsia [2]
Nausea (7–9%) [29]
Vomiting (<3%) [8]
Respiratory
Nasopharyngitis (<3%) [17]
Upper respiratory tract infection (<4%) [14]
Endocrine/Metabolic
ALT increased [2]
Weight loss (10–12%) [5]
Other
Adverse effects [4]
Infection [2]

APREPITANT

Trade name: Emend (Merck)
Indications: Prevention of postoperative and chemotherapy induced nausea and vomiting
Class: Antiemetic, CYP3A4 inhibitor, Neurokinin 1 receptor antagonist
Half-life: 9–13 hours
Clinically important, potentially hazardous interactions with: alprazolam, antifungal agents, astemizole, avanafil, betamethasone, carbamazepine, cisapride, clarithromycin, colchicine, conivaptan, corticosteroids, CYP2C9 substrates, CYP3A4 inhibitors or inducers, dasatinib, deferasirox, dexamethasone, diltiazem, docetaxel, eplerenone, estrogens, everolimus, fentanyl, grapefruit juice, halofantrine, ifosfamide, imatinib, irinotecan, itraconazole, ketoconazole, methylprednisolone, midazolam, mifepristone, naldemedine, nefazodone, neratinib, olaparib, oral contraceptives, paroxetine hydrochloride, phenobarbital, phenytoin, pimecrolimus, pimozide, progestins, ranolazine, rifampin, rifamycin derivatives, rifapentine, ritonavir, salmeterol, saxagliptin, St John's wort,

telithromycin, terfenadine, tolbutamide, tolvaptan, trabectedin, triamcinolone, troleandomycin, vinblastine, vincristine, voriconazole, warfarin
Pregnancy category: N/A (Insufficient evidence to inform drug-associated risk)
Important contra-indications noted in the prescribing guidelines for: nursing mothers; pediatric patients
Note: Fosaprepitant is a prodrug of aprepitant for injection. Aprepitant treatment is given along with a 5-HT3-receptor antagonist and dexamethasone.

Skin
Pruritus (8%)
Hair
Alopecia (12%)
Mucosal
Mucocutaneous reactions (3%)
Stomatitis (3%)
Cardiovascular
Hypertension (2%)
Hypotension (6%)
Central Nervous System
Anorexia (6–10%) [2]
Encephalopathy [2]
Fever (3–6%)
Headache (5–9%) [5]
Insomnia (2–3%)
Somnolence (drowsiness) [2]
Vertigo (dizziness) (3–7%) [2]
Neuromuscular/Skeletal
Asthenia (fatigue) (5–18%) [8]
Gastrointestinal/Hepatic
Abdominal pain (5%) [3]
Constipation (9–10%) [8]
Diarrhea (<10%) [2]
Dyspepsia (5–6%)
Flatulence (4%)
Gastritis (4%)
Nausea (6–13%)
Vomiting (3–8%)
Endocrine/Metabolic
ALT increased (6%)
AST increased (3%)
Creatine phosphokinase increased (4%)
Dehydration (6%)
Genitourinary
Urinary tract infection (2%)
Renal
Proteinuria (7%)
Hematologic
Anemia (3%)
Febrile neutropenia [2]
Neutropenia (3–6%) [2]
Otic
Tinnitus (4%)
Local
Infusion-site pain [2]
Other
Hiccups (11%) [8]
Infection [3]

APROBARBITAL

See: www.drugeruptiondata.com/drug/id/44

APROTININ

See: www.drugeruptiondata.com/drug/id/45

ARBUTAMINE

See: www.drugeruptiondata.com/drug/id/873

ARFORMOTEROL

Trade name: Brovana (Sunovion)
Indications: Chronic obstructive pulmonary disease including chronic bronchitis and emphysema
Class: Beta-2 adrenergic agonist, Bronchodilator
Half-life: 26 hours
Clinically important, potentially hazardous interactions with: aminophylline, beta blockers, MAO inhibitors, tricyclic antidepressants
Pregnancy category: C
Important contra-indications noted in the prescribing guidelines for: nursing mothers; pediatric patients
Note: Studies in asthma patients showed that long-acting beta$_2$-adrenergic agonists may increase the risk of asthma-related death. Contra-indicated in patients with asthma without use of a long-term asthma control medication.
Warning: ASTHMA-RELATED DEATH

Skin
Abscess (<2%)
Edema (<2%)
Herpes simplex (<2%)
Herpes zoster (<2%)
Neoplasms (<2%)
Peripheral edema (3%)
Pigmentation (<2%)
Rash (4%)
Xerosis (<2%)

Mucosal
Oral candidiasis (<2%)

Cardiovascular
Arteriosclerosis (<2%)
Atrioventricular block (<2%)
Chest pain (7%) [2]
Digitalis intoxication (<2%)
QT prolongation (<2%)
Supraventricular tachycardia (<2%)

Central Nervous System
Agitation (<2%)
Fever (<2%)
Headache [2]
Hypokinesia (<2%)
Insomnia [2]
Nervousness [3]
Pain (8%)
Paresthesias (<2%)
Somnolence (drowsiness) (<2%)
Tremor (<2%) [3]

Neuromuscular/Skeletal
Arthralgia (<2%)
Back pain (6%)
Leg cramps (4%)
Neck rigidity (<2%)

Gastrointestinal/Hepatic
Nausea [2]

Respiratory
Bronchitis [3]
COPD (exacerbation) [3]
Dysphonia (<2%)
Dyspnea (4%)
Flu-like syndrome (3%)
Nasopharyngitis [3]
Sinusitis (4%) [2]

Genitourinary
Cystitis (<2%)
Nocturia (<2%)

Ocular
Glaucoma (<2%)
Visual disturbances (<2%)

Local
Injection-site pain (<2%)

Other
Adverse effects [2]
Allergic reactions (<2%)

ARGATROBAN

See: www.drugeruptiondata.com/drug/id/811

ARIPIPRAZOLE

Trade names: Abilify (Bristol-Myers Squibb), Aristada (Alkermes)
Indications: Schizophrenia, bipolar I disorder, major depressive disorder, irritability associated with autistic disorder
Class: Antipsychotic, Mood stabilizer
Half-life: 75–94 hours
Clinically important, potentially hazardous interactions with: alcohol, atazanavir, carbamazepine, CYP3A4 inhibitors, efavirenz, itraconazole, ketoconazole, lopinavir, nelfinavir, paroxetine hydrochloride, quinidine
Pregnancy category: C
Important contra-indications noted in the prescribing guidelines for: the elderly; pediatric patients
Warning: INCREASED MORTALITY IN ELDERLY PATIENTS WITH DEMENTIA-RELATED PSYCHOSIS
SUICIDALITY AND ANTIDEPRESSANT DRUGS

Skin
Rash (6%) [2]

Mucosal
Sialorrhea (4–9%) [5]
Xerostomia (5%) [7]

Cardiovascular
Arrhythmias [2]
Hypertension [3]
QT prolongation [2]

Central Nervous System
Agitation (19%) [4]
Akathisia (8–13%) [31]
Anxiety (17%) [11]
Compulsions [2]
Dyskinesia [3]
Extrapyramidal symptoms [9]
Fever (2%)
Headache (27%) [12]
Hypersexuality [2]
Impulse control disorder [4]
Insomnia (18%) [16]
Irritability [4]
Mania [2]
Neuroleptic malignant syndrome [14]
Neurotoxicity [2]
Parkinsonism [11]
Psychosis [2]
Restlessness [8]
Schizophrenia (exacerbation) [2]
Sedation [10]
Somnolence (drowsiness) (5–11%) [11]
Stroke [2]
Suicidal ideation [6]
Tardive dyskinesia [8]
Tic disorder [2]
Tremor (3%) [9]
Vertigo (dizziness) [5]

Neuromuscular/Skeletal
Asthenia (fatigue) [5]
Ataxia [4]
Dystonia [13]
Pisa syndrome [2]

Gastrointestinal/Hepatic
Constipation (11%) [3]
Dyspepsia (9%)
Nausea (15%) [10]
Vomiting (11%) [5]

Respiratory
Cough (3%)
Upper respiratory tract infection [3]

Endocrine/Metabolic
Appetite increased [5]
Diabetes mellitus [2]
Galactorrhea [2]
Hyperprolactinemia [2]
SIADH [2]
Weight gain (2–30%) [26]

Genitourinary
Priapism [3]
Vaginitis [2]

Hematologic
Neutropenia [2]

Ocular
Vision blurred (3–8%)

Local
Injection-site pain [5]

Other
Adverse effects [4]
Death [3]
Hiccups [3]
Toothache [2]

ARMODAFINIL

Trade name: Nuvigil (Cephalon)
Indications: Narcolepsy, obstructive sleep apnea, shift work sleep disorder
Class: Eugeroic
Half-life: 12–15 hours
Clinically important, potentially hazardous interactions with: cyclosporine
Pregnancy category: C
Important contra-indications noted in the prescribing guidelines for: the elderly; nursing mothers; pediatric patients

Central Nervous System
Anxiety [2]
Headache (14–23%) [10]
Insomnia (4–6%) [3]
Vertigo (dizziness) (5%) [2]

Gastrointestinal/Hepatic
Diarrhea [3]
Nausea [2]

Other
Adverse effects [2]

ARSENIC

See: www.drugeruptiondata.com/drug/id/46

ARTEMETHER/ LUMEFANTRINE

Trade name: Coartem (Novartis)
Indications: Acute, uncomplicated malaria infections due to *Plasmodium falciparum* in patients of 5kg bodyweight and above
Class: Antimalarial
Half-life: ~2 hours (artemether); 3–6 days (lumefantrine)
Clinically important, potentially hazardous interactions with: amiodarone, amitriptyline, amoxapine, antimalarials, antiretrovirals, arsenic, astemizole, atazanavir, atovaquone/proguanil, azithromycin, carbamazepine, ciprofloxacin, citalopram, clomipramine, conivaptan, CYP2D6 substrates, CYP3A4 inhibitors, substrates or inducers, darunavir, dasatinib, degarelix, delavirdine, disopyramide, dolasetron, duloxetine, flecainide, halofantrine, hormonal contraceptives, imipramine, indinavir, itraconazole, lapatinib, levofloxacin, levomepromazine, lopinavir, mefloquine, moxifloxacin, nelfinavir, norfloxacin, ofloxacin, paroxetine hydrochloride, pazopanib, phenytoin, pimozide, procainamide, quinidine, quinine, rifampin, risperidone, sotalol, St John's wort, telavancin, telithromycin, terfenadine, tipranavir, venlafaxine, voriconazole, vorinostat, ziprasidone, zuclopenthixol
Pregnancy category: C
Important contra-indications noted in the prescribing guidelines for: nursing mothers; pediatric patients
Note: Artemether/Lumefantrine tablets should not be used to treat severe malaria or to prevent malaria.

Skin
Abscess (<3%)
Impetigo (<3%)
Inflammation [3]
Pruritus (4%) [2]
Rash (3%) [6]
Urticaria (<3%) [2]

Cardiovascular
Palpitation (18%) [2]

Central Nervous System
Agitation (<3%)
Anorexia (40%) [6]
Chills (23%)
Fever (25–29%) [6]
Gait instability (<3%)
Headache (56%) [8]
Hypoesthesia (<3%)
Insomnia (5%) [2]
Mood changes (<3%)
Seizures [2]
Sleep disturbances (22%)
Sleep related disorder [2]
Tremor (<3%)
Vertigo (dizziness) (39%) [8]

Neuromuscular/Skeletal
Arthralgia (34%)
Asthenia (fatigue) (38%) [8]
Ataxia (<3%)
Back pain (<3%)
Myalgia/Myopathy (32%)

Gastrointestinal/Hepatic
Abdominal pain (17%) [11]
Constipation (<3%)
Diarrhea (8%) [11]
Dyspepsia (<3%)
Dysphagia (<3%)
Gastroenteritis (<3%)
Hepatomegaly (6–9%)
Nausea [8]
Peptic ulceration (<3%)
Vomiting [16]

Respiratory
Asthma (<3%)
Bronchitis (<3%)
Cough (6–23%) [2]
Influenza (<3%)
Nasopharyngitis (4%)
Pharyngolaryngeal pain (<3%)
Pneumonia (<3%)
Rhinitis (4%)
Upper respiratory tract infection (<3%)

Endocrine/Metabolic
ALT increased (<3%)
AST increased (<3%)
Hypokalemia (<3%)

Genitourinary
Hematuria (<3%)
Urinary tract infection (<3%)

Renal
Proteinuria (<3%)

Hematologic
Anemia (4–9%) [4]
Eosinophilia (<3%)
Neutropenia [2]
Platelets decreased (<3%)

Otic
Ear infection (<3%)

Hearing impairment [2]
Tinnitus (<3%)

Ocular
Conjunctivitis (<3%)
Nystagmus (<3%)

Other
Adverse effects [3]
Infection (<3%)

ARTESUNATE

Trade name: Rtsun (Wiscon)
Indications: *Plasmodium falciparum* malaria
Class: Antimalarial
Half-life: 0.5 hours
Clinically important, potentially hazardous interactions with: efavirenz
Pregnancy category: N/A (Use carefully in first three trimesters of pregnancy)
Note: Artesunate therapy should be combined with other antimalarials (e.g. mefloquine) if given for less than 5 days.

Skin
Pruritus [3]

Cardiovascular
QT prolongation [2]

Central Nervous System
Anorexia [3]
Extrapyramidal symptoms [3]
Fever [2]
Headache [8]
Insomnia [2]
Vertigo (dizziness) [12]

Neuromuscular/Skeletal
Asthenia (fatigue) [5]
Myalgia/Myopathy [2]

Gastrointestinal/Hepatic
Abdominal pain [4]
Diarrhea [5]
Nausea [6]
Vomiting [13]

Respiratory
Cough [3]

Hematologic
Anemia [4]
Hemolysis [3]
Hemolytic anemia [2]
Neutropenia [2]

Other
Adverse effects [2]

ARTICAINE

See: www.drugeruptiondata.com/drug/id/2435

ASCORBIC ACID

See: www.drugeruptiondata.com/drug/id/47

ASENAPINE

Trade name: Saphris (Merck)
Indications: Schizophrenia, bipolar disorder
Class: Antipsychotic
Half-life: 24 hours
Clinically important, potentially hazardous interactions with: alcohol, amiodarone, chlorpromazine, CYP2D6 substrates and inhibitors, fluvoxamine, gatifloxacin, moxifloxacin, paroxetine hydrochloride, procainamide, QT prolonging drugs, quinidine, sotalol, thioridazine, ziprasidone
Pregnancy category: C
Important contra-indications noted in the prescribing guidelines for: the elderly; nursing mothers; pediatric patients
Warning: INCREASED MORTALITY IN ELDERLY PATIENTS WITH DEMENTIA-RELATED PSYCHOSIS

Skin
Peripheral edema (3%)
Mucosal
Oral numbness [4]
Salivary hypersecretion (2%)
Xerostomia (2–3%)
Cardiovascular
Hypertension (2–3%) [2]
Central Nervous System
Akathisia (4–6%) [10]
Anxiety (4%)
Depression (2%) [3]
Dysgeusia (taste perversion) (3%) [4]
Extrapyramidal symptoms (6–10%) [11]
Headache (12%) [3]
Hypersomnia [2]
Hypoesthesia (4–5%) [7]
Insomnia (6–15%) [3]
Irritability (2%)
Sedation [9]
Somnolence (drowsiness) (13–24%) [15]
Tardive dyskinesia [2]
Vertigo (dizziness) (4–11%) [5]
Neuromuscular/Skeletal
Arthralgia (3%)
Asthenia (fatigue) (3–4%)
Pain in extremities (2%)
Gastrointestinal/Hepatic
Abdominal pain [2]
Constipation (5%)
Dyspepsia (3–4%)
Vomiting (5%)
Endocrine/Metabolic
Appetite increased (2–4%)
Weight gain (3–5%) [12]
Other
Adverse effects [4]

ASFOTASE ALFA

Trade name: Strensiq (Alexion)
Indications: Perinatal/infantile-and juvenile-onset hypophosphatasia
Class: Enzyme replacement
Half-life: 5 days
Clinically important, potentially hazardous interactions with: none known
Pregnancy category: N/A (No available data)
Important contra-indications noted in the prescribing guidelines for: the elderly; nursing mothers

Skin
Anaphylactoid reactions/Anaphylaxis (<10%)
Calcification (4%)
Erythema (<10%)
Cardiovascular
Flushing (<10%)
Central Nervous System
Chills (<10%)
Fever (<10%)
Headache (<10%)
Hypoesthesia (oral) (<10%)
Irritability (<10%)
Pain (<10%)
Rigors (<10%)
Gastrointestinal/Hepatic
Nausea (<10%)
Vomiting (5%)
Local
Injection-site bruising (8%)
Injection-site edema (13%)
Injection-site erythema (41%)
Injection-site hemorrhage (<17%)
Injection-site induration (13%)
Injection-site lipoatrophy/lipohypertrophy (5–8%)
Injection-site pain (14%)
Injection-site papules and nodules (3%)
Injection-site pigmentation (15%)
Injection-site pruritus (13%)
Injection-site reactions (9%)
Other
Adverse effects [2]

ASPARAGINASE

Synonym: L-asparaginase
Trade names: Elspar (Merck), Kidrolase (EUSA Pharma)
Indications: Acute lymphoblastic leukemia, lymphoma
Class: Antineoplastic, Enzyme
Half-life: 8–30 hours (intravenous); 34–49 hours (intramuscular)
Clinically important, potentially hazardous interactions with: none known
Pregnancy category: C
Important contra-indications noted in the prescribing guidelines for: nursing mothers

Skin
Anaphylactoid reactions/Anaphylaxis (3–40%) [4]
Angioedema [3]
Hypersensitivity (6–40%) [14]
Toxic epidermal necrolysis [2]
Toxicity [2]
Urticaria (<15%) [5]
Mucosal
Aphthous stomatitis (<10%)
Oral lesions (26%)
Stomatitis (<10%)
Central Nervous System
Chills (>10%)
Coma (25%)
Depression (>10%)
Encephalopathy [2]
Fever (>10%)
Leukoencephalopathy [3]
Neurotoxicity [4]
Seizures (10–60%) [2]
Somnolence (drowsiness) (>10%)
Stroke [2]
Gastrointestinal/Hepatic
Abdominal pain (70%)
Hepatotoxicity [3]
Pancreatitis (15%) [22]
Vomiting (50–60%)
Endocrine/Metabolic
Hyperglycemia [2]
Hyperlipidemia [2]
Hypertriglyceridemia [4]
Genitourinary
Azotemia (66%)
Hematologic
Sepsis [2]
Thrombosis [9]
Other
Adverse effects [2]
Allergic reactions (15–35%) [2]

ASPARAGINASE ERWINIA CHRYSANTHEMI

See: www.drugeruptiondata.com/drug/id/2697

ASPARTAME

See: www.drugeruptiondata.com/drug/id/49

ASPIRIN

Synonyms: acetylsalicylic acid; ASA
Trade names: Aggrenox (Boehringer Ingelheim), Anacin (Wyeth), Ascriptin (Novartis) (Wallace), Darvon Compound (aaiPharma), Durlaza (New Haven), Ecotrin (GSK), Equagesic (Women First), Excedrin (Bristol-Myers Squibb), Fiorinal (Watson), Norgesic (3M), Soma Compound (MedPointe), Talwin Compound (Sanofi-Aventis), Yosprala (Aralez)
Indications: Pain, fever, inflammation
Class: Antiplatelet, Non-steroidal anti-inflammatory (NSAID), Salicylate
Half-life: 15–20 minutes
Clinically important, potentially hazardous interactions with: acemetacin, acenocoumarol, amitriptyline, anagrelide, anticoagulants, azficel-t, bismuth, calcium hydroxylapatite, capsicum, celecoxib, cholestyramine, cilazapril, citalopram, desvenlafaxine, devil's claw, dexamethasone, dexibuprofen, dichlorphenamide, diclofenac, dicumarol, duloxetine, enoxaparin, etodolac, evening primrose, flunisolide, flurbiprofen, ginkgo biloba, ginseng, heparin, ibuprofen, iloprost, indomethacin, ketoprofen, ketorolac, lumiracoxib, meloxicam, methotrexate, methyl salicylate, methylprednisolone, milnacipran, nilutamide, NSAIDs, paroxetine hydrochloride, phellodendron, piroxicam, prednisone, resveratrol, reteplase, rivaroxaban, sermorelin, sulfites, tinzaparin, tirofiban, tolmetin, triamcinolone, urokinase, valdecoxib, valproic acid, venlafaxine, verapamil, vilazodone, warfarin, zafirlukast
Pregnancy category: D
Important contra-indications noted in the prescribing guidelines for: nursing mothers; pediatric patients
Note: NSAIDs may cause an increased risk of serious cardiovascular and gastrointestinal adverse events, which can be fatal. This risk may increase with duration of use.
Aggrenox is aspirin and dipyridamole; Yosprala is aspirin and omeprazole.

Skin
Anaphylactoid reactions/Anaphylaxis (<10%) [8]
Angioedema (<5%) [32]
Bullous dermatitis [4]
Erythema multiforme [9]
Erythema nodosum [9]
Erythroderma [2]
Exanthems [11]
Fixed eruption [22]
Hypersensitivity [5]
Lichenoid eruption [2]
Pityriasis rosea [3]
Pruritus [6]
Psoriasis [3]
Purpura [8]
Rash (<10%)
Stevens-Johnson syndrome [6]
Toxic epidermal necrolysis [9]
Urticaria (<10%) [72]
Vasculitis [2]

Mucosal
Aphthous stomatitis [3]
Nasal polyp [4]
Oral mucosal eruption [3]
Oral ulceration [4]

Central Nervous System
Stroke [2]

Gastrointestinal/Hepatic
Black stools [3]
Gastritis [2]
Gastrointestinal bleeding [8]
Gastrointestinal ulceration [7]
Hepatotoxicity [4]
Pancreatitis [2]

Respiratory
Asthma [10]
Pulmonary toxicity [2]
Rhinitis [3]
Sinusitis [2]

Renal
Fanconi syndrome [2]

Hematologic
Bleeding [12]

Otic
Tinnitus [17]

Ocular
Periorbital edema [3]

Other
Adverse effects [9]
Allergic reactions [2]

ASTEMIZOLE

See: www.drugeruptiondata.com/drug/id/1308

ATAZANAVIR

Trade names: Evotaz (Bristol-Myers Squibb), Reyataz (Bristol-Myers Squibb)
Indications: HIV infection
Class: Antiretroviral, HIV-1 protease inhibitor
Half-life: 7 hours
Clinically important, potentially hazardous interactions with: abiraterone, alfuzosin, amiodarone, antacids, aripiprazole, artemether/lumefantrine, atorvastatin, avanafil, bepridil, bosentan, buprenorphine, cabazitaxel, cabozantinib, calcifediol, cisapride, clarithromycin, colchicine, crizotinib, cyclosporine, darifenacin, dasatinib, dexlansoprazole, diltiazem, dofetilide, efavirenz, elbasvir & grazoprevir, eluxadoline, ergot derivatives, erlotinib, estrogens, etravirine, everolimus, famotidine, felodipine, fentanyl, fesoterodine, flibanserin, fluticasone propionate, garlic, glecaprevir & pibrentasvir, indinavir, irinotecan, itraconazole, ixabepilone, ketoconazole, lapatinib, lidocaine, lopinavir, lovastatin, maraviroc, marihuana, midazolam, mifepristone, naldemedine, nevirapine, nicardipine, nifedipine, olaparib, ombitasvir/paritaprevir/ritonavir, omeprazole, oral contraceptives, paclitaxel, pantoprazole, pazopanib, pimozide, posaconazole, proton-pump inhibitors, quetiapine, quinidine, quinine, rabeprazole, raltegravir, ranolazine, rifabutin, rifampin, rilpivirine, ritonavir, rivaroxaban, romidepsin, rosuvastatin, salmeterol, saquinavir, sildenafil, simeprevir, simvastatin, sirolimus, sofosbuvir/velpatasvir/voxilaprevir, solifenacin, sonidegib, St John's wort, sunitinib, tacrolimus, tadalafil, telaprevir, telithromycin, temsirolimus, tenofovir disoproxil, ticagrelor, tipranavir, trazodone, triazolam, tricyclic antidepressants, vardenafil, vemurafenib, verapamil, voriconazole, warfarin
Pregnancy category: B
Important contra-indications noted in the prescribing guidelines for: the elderly; nursing mothers; pediatric patients
Note: Evotaz is atazanavir and cobicistat.

Skin
Jaundice (5–7%) [11]
Rash (3–20%) [7]

Cardiovascular
QT prolongation [2]
Torsades de pointes [2]

Central Nervous System
Depression (2%)
Fever (2%)
Headache (<6%) [3]
Insomnia (3%)
Neurotoxicity [2]
Pain (3%)
Vertigo (dizziness) (3%)

Neuromuscular/Skeletal
Asthenia (fatigue) (2%)
Back pain (2%)
Myalgia/Myopathy (4%)

Gastrointestinal/Hepatic
Abdominal pain (4%)
Cholelithiasis (gallstones) [4]
Diarrhea (2%) [3]
Hepatotoxicity [3]
Nausea (6–14%) [4]
Vomiting (3–4%)

Respiratory
Upper respiratory tract infection [2]

Endocrine/Metabolic
ALT increased (3%)
AST increased (3%)
Creatine phosphokinase increased (8%)
Hyperbilirubinemia [6]

Genitourinary
Urolithiasis [4]

Renal
Nephrolithiasis [5]
Nephrotoxicity [6]

Hematologic
Neutropenia (5%)

Other
Adverse effects [5]
Infection (~50%)

ATENOLOL

Trade names: Beta-Adalat (Bayer), Kalten (BPC), Tenif (AstraZeneca), Tenoret 50 (AstraZeneca), Tenoretic (AstraZeneca), Tenormin (AstraZeneca)
Indications: Angina, hypertension, acute myocardial infarction
Class: Antiarrhythmic class II, Beta adrenergic blocker, Beta blocker
Half-life: 6–7 hours (adults)
Clinically important, potentially hazardous interactions with: alfuzosin, calcium channel blockers, cisplatin, clonidine, digitalis glycosides, diltiazem, disopyramide, epinephrine, indomethacin, reserpine, verapamil
Pregnancy category: D
Important contra-indications noted in the prescribing guidelines for: the elderly; nursing mothers; pediatric patients
Note: Contra-indicated in patients with sinus bradycardia, heart block greater than first degree, cardiogenic shock, or overt cardiac failure. Beta-Adalat and Tenif are atenolol and nifedipine. Kalten, Tenoret 50 and Tenoretic are atenolol and chlorthalidone. Chlorthalidone is a sulfonamide and can be absorbed systemically. Sulfonamides can produce severe, possibly fatal, reactions such as toxic epidermal necrolysis and Stevens-Johnson syndrome.
Warning: CESSATION OF THERAPY

Skin
Anaphylactoid reactions/Anaphylaxis [2]
Lupus erythematosus [2]
Necrosis [3]
Pruritus (<5%)
Psoriasis [7]
Raynaud's phenomenon [2]
Urticaria [2]

Cardiovascular
Atrial fibrillation (5%) [2]
Atrial flutter (2%)
Bradycardia (3–18%) [8]
Cardiac arrest (2%)
Cardiac failure (19%)
Heart block (5%)
Hypotension (25%) [2]
Postural hypotension (12%)
Supraventricular tachycardia (12%)
Ventricular tachycardia (16%)

Central Nervous System
Depression (12%)
Somnolence (drowsiness) (2%)
Stroke [2]
Syncope [2]
Vertigo (dizziness) (15%)

Neuromuscular/Skeletal
Asthenia (fatigue) (26%)
Leg pain (3%)

Gastrointestinal/Hepatic
Diarrhea (3%)
Nausea (3%)

Respiratory
Dyspnea (6%)
Wheezing (3%)

Other
Adverse effects [5]

ATEZOLIZUMAB

Trade name: Tecentriq (Genentech)
Indications: Locally advanced or metastatic urothelial carcinoma in patients having disease progression following platinum-containing chemotherapy
Class: Monoclonal antibody, Programmed death-ligand (PD-L1) inhibitor
Half-life: 27 days
Clinically important, potentially hazardous interactions with: none known
Pregnancy category: N/A (Can cause fetal harm)
Important contra-indications noted in the prescribing guidelines for: nursing mothers; pediatric patients

Skin
Peripheral edema (18%)
Pruritus (13%) [2]
Rash (15%) [3]

Cardiovascular
Venous thromboembolism (>2%)

Central Nervous System
Fever (21%)

Neuromuscular/Skeletal
Arthralgia (14%)
Asthenia (fatigue) (52%) [3]
Back pain (15%)
Neck pain (15%)

Gastrointestinal/Hepatic
Abdominal pain (17%)
Colitis [2]
Constipation (21%)
Diarrhea (18%)
Gastric obstruction (>2%)
Nausea (25%)
Vomiting (17%)

Respiratory
Cough (14%)
Dyspnea (16%)
Pneumonia (>2%)
Pneumonitis (3%)

Endocrine/Metabolic
ALP increased (4%)
ALT increased (2%) [2]
Appetite decreased (26%)
AST increased (2%) [3]
Dehydration (>2%)
Diabetes mellitus [2]
Hyperglycemia (5%)
Hyperthyroidism (2%)
Hyponatremia (10%)
Hypothyroidism (6%)
Serum creatinine increased (3%)

Genitourinary
Hematuria (14%)
Urinary tract infection (22%)

Renal
Nephrotoxicity (>2%)

Hematologic
Anemia (8%)
Lymphopenia (10%)
Sepsis (>2%)

Local
Infusion-related reactions (3%)

Other
Adverse effects [3]
Infection (38%)

ATOMOXETINE

Trade name: Strattera (Lilly)
Indications: Attention deficit hyperactivity disorder
Class: Norepinephrine reuptake inhibitor
Half-life: 5 hours
Clinically important, potentially hazardous interactions with: albuterol, amitriptyline, cinacalcet, citalopram, delavirdine, droperidol, duloxetine, levalbuterol, levomepromazine, linezolid, lisdexamfetamine, MAO inhibitors, moxifloxacin, paroxetine hydrochloride, sotalol, terbinafine, terbutaline, tipranavir, venlafaxine, zuclopenthixol
Pregnancy category: C
Important contra-indications noted in the prescribing guidelines for: nursing mothers; pediatric patients
Warning: SUICIDAL IDEATION IN CHILDREN AND ADOLESCENTS

Skin
Pruritus (>2%)

Mucosal
Xerostomia (>5%) [9]

Cardiovascular
Cardiotoxicity [2]
Tachycardia [2]

Central Nervous System
Aggression [3]
Anorexia [5]
Depression (>2%) [3]
Headache [9]
Hypomania [2]
Insomnia [7]
Irritability [8]
Mania [2]
Mood changes [5]
Nervousness [3]
Somnolence (drowsiness) [11]
Suicidal ideation [6]
Tic disorder [7]
Tremor (>2%) [2]
Vertigo (dizziness) (>5%) [10]

Neuromuscular/Skeletal
Asthenia (fatigue) [11]

Gastrointestinal/Hepatic
Abdominal pain [12]
Constipation [2]
Dyspepsia [3]
Hepatotoxicity [12]
Nausea [18]
Vomiting [10]

Endocrine/Metabolic
Appetite decreased [27]
Weight loss [5]

Genitourinary
Erectile dysfunction [4]
Urinary hesitancy [2]

Other
Adverse effects [10]
Bruxism [2]

ATORVASTATIN

Trade names: Caduet (Pfizer), Lipitor (Pfizer), Liptruzet (Merck Sharpe & Dohme)
Indications: Hypercholesterolemia
Class: HMG-CoA reductase inhibitor, Statin
Half-life: 14 hours
Clinically important, potentially hazardous interactions with: alcohol, aliskiren, amiodarone, amprenavir, antifungals, atazanavir, azithromycin, bexarotene, boceprevir, bosentan, ciprofibrate, clarithromycin, clopidogrel, cobicistat/elvitegravir/emtricitabine/tenofovir alafenamide, cobicistat/elvitegravir/emtricitabine/tenofovir disoproxil, colchicine, conivaptan, cyclosporine, CYP3A4 inhibitors, dabigatran, danazol, daptomycin, darunavir, dasatinib, delavirdine, digoxin, diltiazem, dronedarone, efavirenz, elbasvir & grazoprevir, eltrombopag, erythromycin, estradiol, etravirine, everolimus, fenofibrate, fenofibric acid, fibrates, fluconazole, fosamprenavir, fusidic acid, gemfibrozil, glecaprevir & pibrentasvir, grapefruit juice, imatinib, imidazoles, indinavir, itraconazole, liraglutide, lopinavir, macrolide antibiotics, midazolam, nefazodone, nelfinavir, niacin, niacinamide, norethisterone, oral contraceptives, P-glycoprotein inhibitors, posaconazole, protease inhibitors, quinine, red rice yeast, rifampin, ritonavir, rivaroxaban, saquinavir, silodosin, St John's wort, telaprevir, telithromycin, tipranavir, topotecan, trabectedin, verapamil, voriconazole, warfarin
Pregnancy category: X
Important contra-indications noted in the prescribing guidelines for: the elderly; nursing mothers; pediatric patients
Note: Caduet is atorvastatin and amlodipine; Liptruzet is atorvastatin and ezetimibe.

Skin
Acneform eruption (<2%)
Angioedema [2]
Dermatitis (<2%)
Dermatomyositis [4]
Diaphoresis (<2%)
Ecchymoses (<2%)
Eczema (<2%)
Edema (<2%)
Facial edema (<2%)
Jaundice [2]
Lupus erythematosus [2]
Petechiae (<2%)
Photosensitivity (<2%)
Pruritus (<2%)
Rash (>3%) [2]
Seborrhea (<2%)
Toxic epidermal necrolysis [2]
Toxicity [2]
Ulcerations (<2%)
Urticaria (<2%)
Xerosis (<2%)

Hair
Alopecia (<2%)

Mucosal
Cheilitis (<2%)
Glossitis (<2%)
Oral ulceration (<2%)
Stomatitis (<2%)

Cardiovascular
Hypotension [2]

Central Nervous System
Ageusia (taste loss) (<2%)
Cognitive impairment [2]
Depression [3]
Dysgeusia (taste perversion) (<2%)
Headache [4]
Neurotoxicity [2]
Paresthesias (<2%)
Parosmia (<2%)

Neuromuscular/Skeletal
Arthralgia (4–12%)
Asthenia (fatigue) [5]
Back pain [2]
Muscle spasm [2]
Myalgia/Myopathy (3–8%) [30]
Pain in extremities (6%)
Rhabdomyolysis [41]
Tendinopathy/Tendon rupture [2]

Gastrointestinal/Hepatic
Cholelithiasis (gallstones) [2]
Diarrhea (5–14%)
Hepatitis [2]
Hepatotoxicity [11]
Nausea (4–7%)
Pancreatitis [8]

Respiratory
Nasopharyngitis (4–13%)

Endocrine/Metabolic
ALT increased [3]
Creatine phosphokinase increased [5]
Diabetes mellitus [2]
Gynecomastia (<2%)

Genitourinary
Urinary tract infection (4–8%)

Renal
Nephrotoxicity [3]

Otic
Hearing loss [2]

Other
Adverse effects [10]
Allergic reactions (<2%)
Death [6]
Multiorgan failure [2]

ATOVAQUONE

See: www.drugeruptiondata.com/drug/id/54

ATOVAQUONE/ PROGUANIL

Trade name: Malarone (GSK)
Indications: Malaria prophylaxis and treatment
Class: Antimalarial
Half-life: 24 hours
Clinically important, potentially hazardous interactions with: artemether/lumefantrine, dapsone, etoposide, hypoglycemic agents, indinavir, metoclopramide, phenothiazines, rifabutin, rifampin, ritonavir, tetracycline, typhoid vaccine
Pregnancy category: C
Important contra-indications noted in the prescribing guidelines for: the elderly; nursing mothers

Skin
Erythema multiforme [2]
Pruritus (<10%)

Mucosal
Oral ulceration (6%) [3]

Central Nervous System
Abnormal dreams (7%)
Anorexia (5%)
Headache (10%) [4]
Insomnia (3%)
Vertigo (dizziness) (5%) [3]

Neuromuscular/Skeletal
Asthenia (fatigue) (8%)

Gastrointestinal/Hepatic
Abdominal pain (17%) [5]
Diarrhea (8%)
Dyspepsia (2%)
Gastritis (3%)
Hepatotoxicity [2]
Nausea (12%)
Vomiting (12%) [2]

Respiratory
Cough [3]

Ocular
Vision impaired (2%)

Other
Adverse effects [3]

ATRACURIUM

See: www.drugeruptiondata.com/drug/id/55

ATROPINE SULFATE

Trade name: Lomotil (Pfizer)
Indications: Salivation, sinus bradycardia, uveitis, peptic ulcer
Class: Muscarinic antagonist
Half-life: 2–3 hours
Clinically important, potentially hazardous interactions with: anticholinergics, zuclopenthixol
Pregnancy category: C
Note: Many of the trade name drugs for atropine sulfate contain phenobarbital, scopolamine, hyoscyamine, hydrocodone, methenamine, etc.

Skin
Anaphylactoid reactions/Anaphylaxis [3]
Dermatitis [3]
Erythema multiforme [2]
Photosensitivity (<10%)

Mucosal
Xerostomia (>10%) [4]

Cardiovascular
Arrhythmias [2]
Atrial fibrillation [2]
Bradycardia [3]
Tachycardia [5]

Central Nervous System
Confusion [2]

Ocular
Amblyopia [5]
Hallucinations, visual [3]
Periocular dermatitis [3]

Local
Injection-site irritation (>10%)

Other
Allergic reactions [2]
Central anticholinergic syndrome [2]

AVANAFIL

Trade name: Stendra (Vivus)
Indications: Erectile dysfunction
Class: Phosphodiesterase type 5 (PDE5) inhibitor
Half-life: 5 hours
Clinically important, potentially hazardous interactions with: alcohol, alpha blockers, amprenavir, antihypertensives, aprepitant, atazanavir, clarithromycin, diltiazem, erythromycin, fluconazole, fosamprenavir, indinavir, itraconazole, ketoconazole, nefazodone, nelfinavir, nitrates, ritonavir, saquinavir, strong CYP3A4 inhibitors, telithromycin, verapamil
Pregnancy category: C (Not indicated for use in women)
Important contra-indications noted in the prescribing guidelines for: pediatric patients
Note: Contra-indicated in patients using any form of nitrates.

Skin
Facial flushing [2]
Rash (<2%)

Mucosal
Nasal congestion (<3%) [7]

Cardiovascular
Flushing (3–10%) [10]
Hypertension (<2%)

Central Nervous System
Headache (5–12%) [9]
Vertigo (dizziness) (<2%) [2]

Neuromuscular/Skeletal
Arthralgia (<2%)
Asthenia (fatigue) [2]
Back pain (<3%) [3]

Gastrointestinal/Hepatic
Constipation (<2%)
Diarrhea (<2%)
Dyspepsia (<2%) [4]
Nausea (<2%)

Respiratory
Bronchitis (<2%)
Influenza (<2%)
Nasopharyngitis (<5%) [5]
Sinusitis (<2%) [2]
Upper respiratory tract infection (<3%)

Other
Adverse effects [4]

AVELUMAB *

Trade name: Bavencio (Merck Serono)
Indications: Metastatic Merkel cell carcinoma
Class: Monoclonal antibody, Programmed death-ligand (PD-L1) inhibitor
Half-life: 6 days
Clinically important, potentially hazardous interactions with: none known
Pregnancy category: N/A (Can cause fetal harm)
Important contra-indications noted in the prescribing guidelines for: nursing mothers; pediatric patients

Skin
Peripheral edema (20%)
Pruritus (10%)
Rash (22%)

Cardiovascular
Hypertension (13%)

Central Nervous System
Headache (10%)
Vertigo (dizziness) (14%)

Neuromuscular/Skeletal
Arthralgia (16%)
Asthenia (fatigue) (50%) [3]
Bone or joint pain (32%)

Gastrointestinal/Hepatic
Abdominal pain (16%)
Colitis (2%)
Constipation (17%)
Diarrhea (23%)
Nausea (22%) [2]
Vomiting (13%)

Respiratory
Cough (18%)
Dyspnea (11%)

Endocrine/Metabolic
ALT increased (20%)
Appetite decreased (20%)
AST increased (34%) [2]
Creatine phosphokinase increased [3]
Hyperamylasemia (8%)
Hyperbilirubinemia (6%)
Hyperglycemia (>10%)
Thyroid dysfunction (6%)
Weight loss (15%)

Hematologic
Anemia (35%)
Hyperlipasemia (14%)
Lymphopenia (49%)
Neutropenia (6%)
Thrombocytopenia (27%)

Local
Infusion-related reactions (22%) [3]

AXITINIB

Trade name: Inlyta (Pfizer)
Indications: Advanced renal cell carcinoma (after failure of one prior systemic therapy)
Class: Tyrosine kinase inhibitor
Half-life: 2–6 hours
Clinically important, potentially hazardous interactions with: ketoconazole, rifampin
Pregnancy category: D
Important contra-indications noted in the prescribing guidelines for: nursing mothers; pediatric patients

Skin
Erythema (2%)
Hand–foot syndrome (27%) [15]
Pruritus (7%)
Rash (13%) [3]
Xerosis (10%)

Hair
Alopecia (4%) [2]

Mucosal
Mucosal inflammation (15%) [2]
Stomatitis (15%)

Cardiovascular
Hypertension (40%) [34]

Central Nervous System
Anorexia [5]
Dysgeusia (taste perversion) (11%)
Headache (14%) [4]
Leukoencephalopathy [2]

Neuromuscular/Skeletal
Arthralgia (15%) [2]
Asthenia (fatigue) (39%) [26]
Pain in extremities (13%)

Gastrointestinal/Hepatic
Abdominal pain (14%)
Constipation (20%) [2]
Diarrhea (55%) [25]
Dyspepsia (10%)
Nausea (32%) [10]
Vomiting (24%) [6]

Respiratory
Cough (15%) [2]
Dysphonia (>20%) [12]
Dyspnea (15%) [4]

Endocrine/Metabolic
ALT increased (22%) [2]
Appetite decreased (34%) [7]
AST increased [2]
Dehydration [2]
Hyperthyroidism [2]
Hyponatremia [2]
Hypothyroidism (19%) [8]
Serum creatinine increased [2]
Thyroid dysfunction [2]
Weight loss (25%) [3]

Renal
Proteinuria (11%) [5]

Hematologic
Anemia [2]
Hemorrhage (16%)
Neutropenia [2]
Thrombotic complications (3%)

Other
    Adverse effects [4]

AZACITIDINE

Trade name: Vidaza (Celgene)
Indications: Myelodysplastic syndromes, refractory anemia
Class: Antimetabolite, Antineoplastic, Cytosine analog
Half-life: 40–56 minutes
Clinically important, potentially hazardous interactions with: BCG vaccine, denosumab, echinacea, leflunomide, natalizumab, pimecrolimus, sipuleucel-T, tacrolimus, trastuzumab, vaccines
Pregnancy category: D
Important contra-indications noted in the prescribing guidelines for: nursing mothers; pediatric patients
Note: Contra-indicated in patients with advanced malignant hepatic tumors.

Skin
    Anaphylactoid reactions/Anaphylaxis (<5%)
    Cellulitis (8%)
    Diaphoresis (11%)
    Ecchymoses (31%)
    Edema (14%)
    Erythema (7–17%)
    Hematoma (9%)
    Herpes simplex (9%)
    Hypersensitivity (<5%)
    Induration (<5%)
    Lymphoproliferative disease [2]
    Neoplasms (<5%)
    Nodular eruption (5%)
    Pallor (16%)
    Peripheral edema (19%)
    Petechiae (11–24%)
    Pruritus (12%)
    Pyoderma gangrenosum (<5%)
    Rash (10–14%) [4]
    Sweet's syndrome [4]
    Toxicity [2]
    Urticaria (6%)
    Xerosis (5%)

Mucosal
    Gingival bleeding (10%)
    Oral bleeding (5%)
    Stomatitis (8%)
    Tongue ulceration (5%)

Cardiovascular
    Arrhythmias [2]
    Atrial fibrillation (<5%)
    Cardiac failure (<5%)
    Cardiomyopathy (<5%)
    Cardiotoxicity [3]
    Chest pain (5–16%) [4]
    Congestive heart failure (<5%)
    Hypertension (9%)
    Hypotension (7%) [2]
    Orthostatic hypotension (<5%)
    QT prolongation [2]
    Tachycardia [3]

Central Nervous System
    Anorexia (21%)
    Anxiety (5–13%)

Cerebral hemorrhage (<5%)
    Depression (12%)
    Fever (30–52%) [4]
    Headache (22%)
    Insomnia (9–11%)
    Intracranial hemorrhage (<5%)
    Pain (11%)
    Seizures (<5%)
    Syncope [2]
    Vertigo (dizziness) (19%)

Neuromuscular/Skeletal
    Arthralgia (22%) [2]
    Asthenia (fatigue) (7–36%) [4]
    Back pain (19%)
    Bone or joint pain (<5%)
    Myalgia/Myopathy (16%)
    Neck pain (<5%)

Gastrointestinal/Hepatic
    Abdominal pain (12–13%)
    Black stools (<5%)
    Cholecystitis (<5%)
    Constipation (34–50%) [4]
    Diarrhea (36%) [4]
    Dyspepsia (6%)
    Dysphagia (5%)
    Gastrointestinal bleeding (<5%)
    Loose stools (6%)
    Nausea (48–71%) [6]
    Vomiting (27–54%) [4]

Respiratory
    Cough (30%)
    Dyspnea (14–29%) [2]
    Hemoptysis (<5%)
    Nasopharyngitis (15%)
    Pharyngolaryngeal pain (6%)
    Pneumonia (11%) [2]
    Pneumonitis (<5%) [2]
    Pulmonary toxicity [2]
    Respiratory distress (<5%)
    Rhinitis (6%)
    Upper respiratory tract infection (9–13%)

Endocrine/Metabolic
    Dehydration (<5%)
    Hypokalemia (6%)
    Weight loss (8%)

Genitourinary
    Hematuria (6%)
    Urinary tract infection (9%)

Renal
    Renal failure (<5%)

Hematologic
    Agranulocytosis (<5%)
    Anemia (51–70%) [4]
    Bleeding [3]
    Bone marrow suppression (<5%)
    Cytopenia [4]
    Febrile neutropenia (14–16%) [6]
    Leukopenia (18–48%)
    Myelosuppression [3]
    Neutropenia (32–66%) [7]
    Pancytopenia (<5%)
    Splenomegaly (<5%)
    Thrombocytopenia (66–70%) [4]

Ocular
    Ocular hemorrhage (<5%)

Local
    Injection-site bruising (5–14%)
    Injection-site edema (5%)

Injection-site erythema (35–43%)
    Injection-site hematoma (6%)
    Injection-site pain (19–23%)
    Injection-site pigmentation (5%)
    Injection-site pruritus (7%)
    Injection-site purpura (14%)
    Injection-site reactions (14–29%) [7]

Other
    Adverse effects [5]
    Death [4]
    Infection (<5%) [9]

AZATADINE

See: www.drugeruptiondata.com/drug/id/59

AZATHIOPRINE

Trade names: Azasan (aaiPharma), Imuran (Prometheus)
Indications: Lupus nephritis, psoriatic arthritis, rheumatoid arthritis, autoimmune diseases, as an adjunct for the prevention of rejection in kidney transplant patients
Class: Antimetabolite, Disease-modifying antirheumatic drug (DMARD), Immunosuppressant, Purine anaolog
Half-life: 12 minutes
Clinically important, potentially hazardous interactions with: allopurinol, aminosalicylates, balsalazide, benazepril, captopril, chlorambucil, co-trimoxazole, cyclophosphamide, cyclosporine, enalapril, febuxostat, fosinopril, Hemophilus B vaccine, imidapril, lisinopril, mesalamine, mycophenolate, natalizumab, olsalazine, quinapril, ramipril, ribavirin, sulfamethoxazole, tofacitinib, trimethoprim, typhoid vaccine, vaccines, warfarin, yellow fever vaccine
Pregnancy category: D
Important contra-indications noted in the prescribing guidelines for: nursing mothers; pediatric patients
Note: Patients receiving immunosuppressants, including azathioprine, are at increased risk of developing lymphoma and other malignancies, particularly of the skin.
Warning: MALIGNANCY

Skin
    Acanthosis nigricans [2]
    Acneform eruption [2]
    AGEP [2]
    Angioedema [2]
    Basal cell carcinoma [2]
    Carcinoma [3]
    Dermatitis [4]
    Erythema gyratum repens [2]
    Erythema multiforme [2]
    Erythema nodosum [4]
    Exanthems [10]
    Herpes simplex [3]
    Herpes zoster [8]
    Hypersensitivity [28]
    Kaposi's sarcoma [14]
    Lymphoproliferative disease [4]
    Neoplasms [2]
    Neutrophilic dermatosis [4]

Nevi [3]
Porokeratosis [4]
Rash (<10%) [10]
Scabies [5]
Squamous cell carcinoma [11]
Sweet's syndrome [12]
Tinea [3]
Toxicity [3]
Tumors [8]
Urticaria [5]
Vasculitis [5]
Verrucae [3]

Hair
Alopecia [9]

Nails
Onychomycosis [2]

Mucosal
Oral ulceration [2]

Cardiovascular
Atrial fibrillation [3]

Central Nervous System
Chills (>10%)
Fever [7]
Headache [3]
Leukoencephalopathy [2]

Neuromuscular/Skeletal
Arthralgia [4]
Asthenia (fatigue) [7]

Gastrointestinal/Hepatic
Abdominal pain [2]
Hepatitis [5]
Hepatotoxicity [27]
Nausea [8]
Pancreatitis [44]
Vomiting [4]

Respiratory
Flu-like syndrome [2]
Pneumonitis [2]
Pulmonary toxicity [3]

Hematologic
Bone marrow suppression [5]
Leukopenia [12]
Myelosuppression [2]
Myelotoxicity [5]
Neutropenia [2]
Pancytopenia [4]
Thrombocytopenia [5]

Other
Adverse effects [7]

Allergic reactions [5]
Death [2]
Infection [9]

AZELASTINE

See: www.drugeruptiondata.com/drug/id/61

AZFICEL-T

See: www.drugeruptiondata.com/drug/id/2617

AZILSARTAN

See: www.drugeruptiondata.com/drug/id/2275

AZITHROMYCIN

Trade names: AzaSite (Merck), Zithromax (Pfizer)
Indications: Infections of the upper and lower respiratory tract, skin infections, sexually transmitted diseases, conjunctivitis (ophthalmic preparations only)
Class: Antibacterial, Antibiotic, macrolide
Half-life: 68 hours
Clinically important, potentially hazardous interactions with: aminophylline, antacids, artemether/lumefantrine, astemizole, atorvastatin, betrixaban, bromocriptine, cabergoline, colchicine, coumarins, cyclosporine, digoxin, droperidol, ergotamine, fluvastatin, lovastatin, methysergide, mizolastine, oral typhoid vaccine, pimozide, pravastatin, quetiapine, reboxetine, rifabutin, ritonavir, simvastatin, venetoclax, warfarin
Pregnancy category: B
Important contra-indications noted in the prescribing guidelines for: nursing mothers; pediatric patients
Note: AzaSite is for topical ophthalmic use only (for reactions see [Ophth] below).

Skin
AGEP [3]
Anaphylactoid reactions/Anaphylaxis [2]

Churg-Strauss syndrome [2]
DRESS syndrome [4]
Erythema [2]
Exanthems [3]
Hypersensitivity [3]
Jarisch–Herxheimer reaction [2]
Pruritus [3]
Rash [Ophth] (2–10%) [6]
Stevens-Johnson syndrome [6]
Urticaria [Ophth] [2]

Cardiovascular
Bradycardia [2]
Cardiotoxicity [8]
QT prolongation [11]
Torsades de pointes [4]

Central Nervous System
Anorexia (2–10%)
Headache [3]
Vertigo (dizziness) [2]

Gastrointestinal/Hepatic
Abdominal pain (2–10%) [4]
Diarrhea (4–9%) [17]
Gastrointestinal disorder [2]
Hepatotoxicity [7]
Nausea (7%) [8]
Vanishing bile duct syndrome [2]
Vomiting (2–10%) [5]

Genitourinary
Vaginitis (2–10%)

Otic
Hearing loss [3]
Tinnitus [2]

Ocular
Keratitis [2]

Local
Injection-site erythema (2–10%)
Injection-site pain (2–10%) [3]

Other
Adverse effects [14]
Death [2]
Hiccups [2]
Side effects [2]

AZTREONAM

See: www.drugeruptiondata.com/drug/id/63

BACAMPICILLIN

See: www.drugeruptiondata.com/drug/id/64

BACITRACIN

See: www.drugeruptiondata.com/drug/id/1199

BACLOFEN

Trade names: Baclofen (Watson), Gablofen (Mallinckrodt), Lioresal (Medtronic)
Indications: Spasticity resulting from multiple sclerosis
Class: GABA receptor agonist, Skeletal muscle relaxant
Half-life: 2.5–4 hours
Clinically important, potentially hazardous interactions with: acebutolol, alcohol, alfuzosin, amitriptyline, captopril, cilazapril, diclofenac, enalapril, fosinopril, irbesartan, levodopa, lisinopril, meloxicam, olmesartan, quinapril, ramipril, trandolapril
Pregnancy category: C
Important contra-indications noted in the prescribing guidelines for: pediatric patients
Note: Children appear to be at higher risk for complications than adults when using intrathecal baclofen (ITB). ITB therapy is a safe and effective treatment for severe spasticity in the pediatric population, but does have a 31% rate of complications requiring surgical management over a 3-year treatment period.
Warning: DO NOT DISCONTINUE ABRUPTLY

Skin
Exanthems [2]
Rash (<10%)
Toxicity [2]

Cardiovascular
Bradycardia [2]
Hypertension [2]
Hypotension [3]

Central Nervous System
Coma [3]
Confusion (<10%)
Dyskinesia [2]
Encephalopathy [2]
Hallucinations [4]
Headache (<10%)
Insomnia (>10%)
Seizures [9]
Slurred speech (>10%)
Somnolence (drowsiness) (>10%) [6]
Vertigo (dizziness) (>10%) [5]

Neuromuscular/Skeletal
Asthenia (fatigue) (>10%) [6]

Gastrointestinal/Hepatic
Constipation (<10%)
Nausea (<10%)

Genitourinary
Polyuria (<10%)

Other
Infection [2]
Side effects (<2%)

BALSALAZIDE

Trade names: Colazal (Salix), Colazide (Almirall)
Indications: Mild to moderately active ulcerative colitis
Class: Aminosalicylate
Half-life: N/A
Clinically important, potentially hazardous interactions with: azathioprine, cardiac glycosides, folic acid, heparin, low molecular weight heparins, mercaptopurine, thiopurine analogs, varicella virus-containing vaccines
Pregnancy category: B
Important contra-indications noted in the prescribing guidelines for: nursing mothers; pediatric patients

Skin
Hypersensitivity [2]

Mucosal
Stomatitis (3%)

Central Nervous System
Anorexia (2%)
Fever (2–6%)
Headache (15%)
Insomnia (2%)

Neuromuscular/Skeletal
Arthralgia (4%)
Asthenia (fatigue) (2%)

Gastrointestinal/Hepatic
Abdominal pain (6–13%)
Colitis (ulcerative, exacerbation) (6%)
Diarrhea (5–9%)
Dyspepsia (2%)
Flatulence (2%)
Nausea (4%)
Vomiting (10%)

Respiratory
Cough (2–3%)
Flu-like syndrome (<4%)
Nasopharyngitis (6%)
Pharyngitis (2%)
Pharyngolaryngeal pain (3%)
Rhinitis (2%)

Genitourinary
Dysmenorrhea (3%)

BASILIXIMAB

Trade name: Simulect (Novartis)
Indications: Prophylaxis of organ rejection in renal transplantation
Class: Interleukin-2 receptor antagonist, Monoclonal antibody
Half-life: 7.2 days
Clinically important, potentially hazardous interactions with: cyclosporine, Hemophilus B vaccine, mycophenolate
Pregnancy category: B
Important contra-indications noted in the prescribing guidelines for: nursing mothers

Skin
Acneform eruption (>10%)
Candidiasis (3–10%)
Cyst (3–10%)
Edema (generalized) (3–10%)
Facial edema (3–10%)
Genital edema (3–10%)
Hematoma (3–10%)
Herpes simplex (3–10%)
Herpes zoster (3–10%)
Peripheral edema (>10%)
Pruritus (3–10%)
Rash (3–10%)
Ulcerations (3–10%)
Wound complications (>10%)

Hair
Hypertrichosis (3–10%)

Mucosal
Gingival hyperplasia/hypertrophy (3–10%)
Stomatitis (3–10%)
Ulcerative stomatitis (3–10%)

Cardiovascular
Angina (3–10%)
Arrhythmias (3–10%)
Atrial fibrillation (3–10%)
Cardiac failure (3–10%)
Chest pain (3–10%)
Hypertension (>10%)
Hypotension (3–10%)
Pulmonary edema (3–10%)
Tachycardia (3–10%)

Central Nervous System
Agitation (3–10%)
Anxiety (3–10%)
Depression (3–10%)
Fever (>10%)
Headache (>10%)
Hypoesthesia (3–10%)
Insomnia (>10%)
Pain (>10%)
Paresthesias (3–10%)
Rigors (3–10%)
Tremor (>10%)
Vertigo (dizziness) (3–10%)

Neuromuscular/Skeletal
Arthralgia (3–10%)
Asthenia (fatigue) (3–10%)
Back pain (3–10%)
Cramps (3–10%)
Fractures (3–10%)
Leg pain (3–10%)
Myalgia/Myopathy (3–10%)

Gastrointestinal/Hepatic
Abdominal distension (3–10%)
Abdominal pain (>10%)
Black stools (3–10%)
Constipation (>10%)
Diarrhea (>10%)
Dyspepsia (>10%)
Esophagitis (3–10%)
Flatulence (3–10%)
Gastroenteritis (3–10%)
Gastrointestinal bleeding (3–10%)
Gastrointestinal disorder (69%)
Hernia (3–10%)
Nausea (>10%)
Vomiting (>10%)

Respiratory
Bronchitis (3–10%)
Bronchospasm (3–10%)
Cough (3–10%)
Dyspnea (>10%)
Pharyngitis (3–10%)
Pneumonia (3–10%)
Rhinitis (3–10%)
Sinusitis (3–10%)
Upper respiratory tract infection (>10%)

Endocrine/Metabolic
Acidosis (3–10%)
Dehydration (3–10%)
Diabetes mellitus (3–10%)
Hypercalcemia (3–10%)
Hypercholesterolemia (>10%)
Hyperglycemia (>10%)
Hyperkalemia (>10%)
Hyperlipidemia (3–10%)
Hypertriglyceridemia (3–10%)
Hyperuricemia (>10%)
Hypocalcemia (3–10%)
Hypoglycemia (3–10%)
Hypokalemia (>10%)
Hypophosphatemia (>10%)
Weight gain (3–10%)

Genitourinary
Albuminuria (3–10%)
Dysuria (3–10%)
Hematuria (3–10%)
Impotence (3–10%)
Oliguria (3–10%)
Urinary frequency (3–10%)
Urinary retention (3–10%)
Urinary tract infection (>10%)

Renal
Renal tubular necrosis (3–10%)

Hematologic
Anemia (>10%)
Hemorrhage (3–10%)
Leukopenia (3–10%)
Polycythemia (3–10%)
Sepsis (3–10%)
Thrombocytopenia (3–10%)
Thrombosis (3–10%)

Ocular
Abnormal vision (3–10%)
Cataract (3–10%)
Conjunctivitis (3–10%)

Other
Infection (viral) (>10%)

BCG VACCINE

Synonym: Bacille Calmette-Guerin
Trade names: Mycobax (Sanofi-Aventis), TICE BCG (Organon)
Indications: Immunization against tuberculosis
Class: Vaccine
Half-life: N/A
Clinically important, potentially hazardous interactions with: alefacept, aminophylline, azacitidine, betamethasone, cabazitaxel, cefazolin, cefixime, ceftaroline fosamil, ceftobiprole, ciprofloxacin, demeclocycline, denileukin, docetaxel, doripenem, doxycycline, fingolimod, gefitinib, gemifloxacin, leflunomide, levofloxacin, monosodium glutamate, moxifloxacin, ofloxacin, oxaliplatin, pazopanib, sulfadiazine, telavancin, telithromycin, temsirolimus
Pregnancy category: C

Skin
Abscess [16]
Anaphylactoid reactions/Anaphylaxis [5]
Churg-Strauss syndrome [15]
Dermatitis [2]
Erythema [3]
Fixed eruption [2]
Hypersensitivity [2]
Keloid [4]
Lupus vulgaris [22]
Lymphadenitis [8]
Lymphadenopathy [92]
Papular lesions [6]
Sarcoidosis [4]
Scar [8]
Scrofuloderma [5]
Sweet's syndrome [2]
Ulcerations [6]
Vasculitis [2]

Mucosal
Mucocutaneous lymph node syndrome (Kawaski syndrom) [2]

Central Nervous System
Fever [6]
Neurotoxicity [2]

Neuromuscular/Skeletal
Arthralgia [7]
Asthenia (fatigue) [4]
Osteomyelitis [33]

Gastrointestinal/Hepatic
Hepatitis [3]
Hepatotoxicity [2]

Genitourinary
Balanitis [3]
Bladder disorder [2]
Hematuria [2]

Hematologic
Sepsis [3]

Ocular
Optic neuritis [2]
Uveitis [4]

Local
Injection-site abscess [3]
Injection-site reactions [3]
Injection-site ulceration [3]

Other
Adverse effects [3]
Cancer [3]
Death [14]
Infection [2]
Systemic reactions [2]

BECAPLERMIN

See: www.drugeruptiondata.com/drug/id/1325

BECLOMETHASONE

Trade names: Beconase AQ (GSK), Qnasl (Teva), Qvar (3M), Vanceril (Schering)
Indications: Allergic rhinitis, asthma
Class: Corticosteroid, inhaled
Half-life: N/A
Clinically important, potentially hazardous interactions with: diuretics, estrogens, ketoconazole, live vaccines, oral contraceptives, phenytoin, rifampin, warfarin
Pregnancy category: C
Important contra-indications noted in the prescribing guidelines for: nursing mothers; pediatric patients

Skin
Bruising [3]
Candidiasis [2]

Mucosal
Epistaxis (nosebleed) (with nasally-inhaled formulation) (2%)
Nasal discomfort (5%)
Oral candidiasis [4]

Central Nervous System
Headache (2%) [2]

Neuromuscular/Skeletal
Osteoporosis [5]

Respiratory
Upper respiratory tract infection [2]

Ocular
Cataract [4]
Glaucoma [3]

Other
Adverse effects [10]

BEDAQUILINE

Trade name: Sirturo (Janssen)
Indications: Pulmonary multi-drug resistant tuberculosis
Class: Antimycobacterial, Diarylquinoline
Half-life: 5.5 months
Clinically important, potentially hazardous interactions with: ketoconazole, rifabutin, rifampin, rifapentine, stong CYP3A4 inhibitors and inducers
Pregnancy category: B
Important contra-indications noted in the prescribing guidelines for: nursing mothers; pediatric patients
Warning: INCREASED RISK OF DEATH / QT PROLONGATION

Skin
Rash (8%)

Cardiovascular
Chest pain (11%) [2]
QT prolongation [2]

Central Nervous System
Anorexia (9%)
Headache (28%) [3]
Vertigo (dizziness) [2]

Neuromuscular/Skeletal
Arthralgia (33%) [2]

Pain in extremities [2]
Gastrointestinal/Hepatic
Hepatotoxicity [2]
Nausea (38%) [4]
Vomiting [2]
Respiratory
Hemoptysis (18%)
Endocrine/Metabolic
ALT increased (<10%)
AST increased (<10%)
Hyperuricemia [2]
Otic
Hearing loss [2]
Other
Infection [3]

BELATACEPT

Trade name: Nulojix (Bristol-Myers Squibb)
Indications: Prophylaxis of organ rejection in kidney transplantation
Class: Immunosuppressant, T-cell co-stimulation blocker
Half-life: 7–10 days
Clinically important, potentially hazardous interactions with: live vaccines, mycophenolate
Pregnancy category: C
Important contra-indications noted in the prescribing guidelines for: nursing mothers; pediatric patients
Note: Contra-indicated in patients without immunity to Epstein-Barr virus.
Warning: POST-TRANSPLANT LYMPHOPROLIFERATIVE DISORDER, OTHER MALIGNANCIES, AND SERIOUS INFECTIONS

Skin
Acneform eruption (8%)
Hematoma (<10%)
Hyperhidrosis (<10%)
Lymphoproliferative disease (post-transplant) [7]
Malignancies [3]
Peripheral edema (34%)
Hair
Alopecia (<10%)
Mucosal
Aphthous stomatitis (<10%)
Stomatitis (<10%)
Cardiovascular
Atrial fibrillation (<10%)
Hypertension (32%)
Hypotension (18%)
Central Nervous System
Anxiety (10%)
Fever (28%)
Guillain–Barré syndrome (<10%)
Headache (21%)
Insomnia (15%)
Tremor (8%)
Vertigo (dizziness) (9%)
Neuromuscular/Skeletal
Arthralgia (17%)
Back pain (13%)
Bone or joint pain (<10%)

Gastrointestinal/Hepatic
Abdominal pain (9–19%)
Constipation (33%)
Diarrhea (39%)
Nausea (24%)
Vomiting (22%)
Respiratory
Bronchitis (10%)
Cough (24%)
Dyspnea (12%)
Influenza (11%)
Nasopharyngitis (13%)
Upper respiratory tract infection (15%)
Endocrine/Metabolic
Creatine phosphokinase increased (15%)
Hypercholesterolemia (11%)
Hyperglycemia (19%)
Hyperkalemia (20%)
Hyperuricemia (5%)
Hypocalcemia (13%)
Hypokalemia (21%)
Hypomagnesemia (7%)
Hypophosphatemia (19%)
Genitourinary
Dysuria (11%)
Hematuria (16%)
Urinary incontinence (<10%)
Urinary tract infection (37%) [2]
Renal
Proteinuria (16%)
Renal failure (<10%)
Renal tubular necrosis (9%)
Hematologic
Anemia (45%)
Dyslipidemia (19%)
Leukopenia (20%)
Neutropenia (<10%) [2]
Other
Graft dysfunction (25%)
Infection (<10%) [7]

BELIMUMAB

See: www.drugeruptiondata.com/drug/id/2285

BELINOSTAT

Trade name: Beleodaq (Spectrum)
Indications: Peripheral T-cell lymphoma
Class: Histone deacetylase (HDAC) inhibitor
Half-life: 1 hour
Clinically important, potentially hazardous interactions with: strong UGT1A1 inhibitors
Pregnancy category: D
Important contra-indications noted in the prescribing guidelines for: nursing mothers; pediatric patients

Skin
Peripheral edema (20%) [2]
Pruritus (16%)
Rash (20%)
Hair
Alopecia [2]

Cardiovascular
Hypotension (10%)
Phlebitis (10%)
QT prolongation (11%) [2]
Central Nervous System
Anorexia [2]
Chills (16%)
Fever (35%) [2]
Headache (15%) [3]
Peripheral neuropathy [2]
Vertigo (dizziness) (10%) [2]
Neuromuscular/Skeletal
Asthenia (fatigue) (37%) [11]
Myalgia/Myopathy [2]
Gastrointestinal/Hepatic
Abdominal pain (11%)
Constipation (23%) [5]
Diarrhea (23%) [6]
Nausea (42%) [10]
Vomiting (29%) [10]
Respiratory
Cough (19%)
Dyspnea (22%) [4]
Pneumonia (>2%)
Pneumonitis [2]
Endocrine/Metabolic
Appetite decreased (15%)
Creatine phosphokinase increased (>2%)
Hypokalemia (12%)
Hematologic
Anemia (32%) [5]
Leukopenia [2]
Lymphopenia [2]
Neutropenia [4]
Thrombocytopenia (16%) [3]
Thrombosis [2]
Local
Infusion-site pain (14%)
Injection-site reactions [2]
Other
Allergic reactions [2]
Hiccups [2]
Multiorgan failure (>2%)

BENACTYZINE

See: www.drugeruptiondata.com/drug/id/66

BENAZEPRIL

Trade names: Lotensin (Novartis), Lotensin HCT (Novartis), Lotrel (Novartis)
Indications: Hypertension
Class: Angiotensin-converting enzyme (ACE) inhibitor, Antihypertensive, Vasodilator
Half-life: 10–11 hours
Clinically important, potentially hazardous interactions with: allopurinol, amifostine, amiloride, angiotensin II receptor blockers, antacids, antidiabetics, antihypertensives, azathioprine, cyclosporine, diazoxide, diuretics, eplerenone, everolimus, gold & gold compounds, herbals, lithium, MAO inhibitors, methylphenidate, NSAIDs, pentoxifylline, phosphodiesterase 5 inhibitors, potassium salts,

prostacyclin analogues, rituximab, sirolimus, spironolactone, temsirolimus, tizanidine, tolvaptan, triamterene, trimethoprim, yohimbine
Pregnancy category: D
Important contra-indications noted in the prescribing guidelines for: pediatric patients
Note: Lotrel is benazepril and amlodipine. Lotensin-HCT is benazepril and hydrochlorothiazide. Hydrochlorothiazide is a sulfonamide and can be absorbed systemically. Sulfonamides can produce severe, possibly fatal, reactions such as toxic epidermal necrolysis and Stevens-Johnson syndrome.
Contra-indicated in patients with a history of angioedema with or without previous ACE inhibitor treatment.
Warning: FETAL TOXICITY

Skin
  Angioedema [8]
  Peripheral edema [3]
Central Nervous System
  Headache (6%)
  Vertigo (dizziness) (4%)
Respiratory
  Cough [10]

BENDAMUSTINE

See: www.drugeruptiondata.com/drug/id/1282

BENDROFLUME-THIAZIDE

See: www.drugeruptiondata.com/drug/id/68

BENZALKONIUM

See: www.drugeruptiondata.com/drug/id/1041

BENZNIDAZOLE *

Indications: Chagas disease (trypanosomiasis) in pediatric patients aged 2–12 years
Class: Antibiotic, nitroimidazole
Half-life: 13 hours
Clinically important, potentially hazardous interactions with: disulfiram
Pregnancy category: N/A (Can cause fetal harm)
Important contra-indications noted in the prescribing guidelines for: nursing mothers
Note: Has the potential for genotoxicity and carcinogenicity.

Skin
  Edema [4]
  Hypersensitivity [3]
  Pigmentation [2]
  Pruritus [5]
  Rash [7]
  Stevens-Johnson syndrome [2]
  Urticaria [2]

Central Nervous System
  Anorexia (<5%)
  Fever [6]
  Headache (<5%) [5]
  Neurotoxicity [2]
  Peripheral neuropathy (2%)
  Tremor (2%)
  Vertigo (dizziness) (4%)
Neuromuscular/Skeletal
  Arthralgia (<5%) [4]
  Asthenia (fatigue) [5]
  Myalgia/Myopathy [3]
Gastrointestinal/Hepatic
  Abdominal distension [2]
  Abdominal pain (25%) [4]
  Diarrhea [2]
  Dyspepsia [2]
  Hepatotoxicity (5%) [2]
  Nausea [4]
  Vomiting [2]
Hematologic
  Eosinophilia [2]
  Neutropenia [2]
Other
  Adverse effects [7]
  Allergic reactions [2]

BENZONATATE

See: www.drugeruptiondata.com/drug/id/917

BENZPHETAMINE

See: www.drugeruptiondata.com/drug/id/959

BENZTHIAZIDE

See: www.drugeruptiondata.com/drug/id/69

BENZTROPINE

See: www.drugeruptiondata.com/drug/id/70

BENZYDAMINE

See: www.drugeruptiondata.com/drug/id/1332

BENZYL ALCOHOL

See: www.drugeruptiondata.com/drug/id/1721

BEPOTASTINE

See: www.drugeruptiondata.com/drug/id/1731

BEPRIDIL

See: www.drugeruptiondata.com/drug/id/71

BERACTANT

See: www.drugeruptiondata.com/drug/id/1166

BESIFLOXACIN

See: www.drugeruptiondata.com/drug/id/1422

BETA-CAROTENE

See: www.drugeruptiondata.com/drug/id/72

BETAMETHASONE

See: www.drugeruptiondata.com/drug/id/1101

BETAXOLOL

Trade names: Betoptic [Ophthalmic] (Alcon), Kerlone (Pfizer)
Indications: Open-angle glaucoma, hypertension
Class: Adrenergic beta-receptor antagonist
Half-life: 14–22 hours
Clinically important, potentially hazardous interactions with: clonidine, verapamil
Pregnancy category: C
Important contra-indications noted in the prescribing guidelines for: nursing mothers; pediatric patients
Note: Cutaneous side effects of beta-receptor blockers are clinically polymorphous. They apparently appear after several months of continuous therapy.

Skin
  Cold extremities (2%)
  Dermatitis [3]
  Diaphoresis (<2%)
  Eczema (<2%)
  Edema (<2%)
  Erythema (<2%)
  Lymphadenopathy (<2%)
  Pruritus (<2%)
  Purpura (<2%)
  Rash (<2%) [3]
Hair
  Alopecia (<2%)
  Hypertrichosis (<2%)
Mucosal
  Epistaxis (nosebleed) (<2%)
  Oral ulceration (<2%)
  Sialorrhea (<2%)
  Xerostomia (<2%)
Cardiovascular
  Angina (<2%)
  Arrhythmias (<2%)
  Atrioventricular block (<2%)
  Bradycardia (6–8%)
  Cardiac failure (<2%)
  Chest pain (2–7%)
  Flushing (<2%)
  Hypertension (<2%)
  Hypotension (<2%)

Myocardial infarction (<2%)
Palpitation (2%)
Peripheral ischemia (<2%)

Central Nervous System
Ageusia (taste loss) (<2%)
Amnesia (<2%)
Anorexia (<2%)
Confusion (<2%)
Dysgeusia (taste perversion) (<2%)
Emotional lability (<2%)
Fever (<2%)
Hallucinations (<2%)
Headache (7–15%)
Insomnia (<5%)
Pain (<2%)
Paresthesias (2%)
Rigors (<2%)
Stupor (<2%)
Syncope (<2%)
Tremor (<2%)
Twitching (<2%)
Vertigo (dizziness) (5–15%)

Neuromuscular/Skeletal
Arthralgia (3%)
Asthenia (fatigue) (3–10%)
Ataxia (<2%)
Bone or joint pain (5%)
Leg cramps (<2%)
Myalgia/Myopathy (3%)
Neck pain (<2%)
Tendinitis (<2%)

Gastrointestinal/Hepatic
Constipation (<2%)
Diarrhea (2%)
Dyspepsia (4–5%)
Dysphagia (<2%)
Nausea (2–6%)
Vomiting (<2%)

Respiratory
Bronchitis (<2%)
Bronchospasm (<2%)
Cough (<2%)
Dysphonia (<2%)
Dyspnea (2%)
Influenza (<2%)
Pharyngitis (2%)
Pneumonia (<2%)
Sinusitis (<2%)
Upper respiratory tract infection (3%)

Endocrine/Metabolic
Acidosis (<2%)
ALT increased (<2%)
Appetite increased (<2%)
AST increased (<2%)
Diabetes mellitus (<2%)
Gynecomastia (<2%)
Hypercholesterolemia (<2%)
Hyperglycemia (<2%)
Hyperkalemia (<2%)
Hyperuricemia (<2%)
Hypokalemia (<2%)
Libido decreased (<2%)
Mastodynia (<2%)
Menstrual irregularities (<2%)
Weight gain (<2%)
Weight loss (<2%)

Genitourinary
Cystitis (<2%)
Dysuria (<2%)

Oliguria (<2%)
Peyronie's disease (<2%)
Prostatitis (<2%)

Renal
Proteinuria (<2%)
Renal function abnormal (<2%)

Hematologic
Anemia (<2%)
Lymphocytosis (<2%)
Thrombocytopenia (<2%)
Thrombosis (<2%)

Otic
Ear pain (<2%)
Hearing loss (<2%)
Tinnitus (<2%)

Ocular
Abnormal vision (<2%)
Blepharitis (<2%)
Cataract (<2%)
Conjunctivitis (<2%)
Iritis (<2%)
Lacrimation (<2%)
Ocular hemorrhage (<2%)
Scotoma (<2%)
Xerophthalmia (<2%)

Other
Allergic reactions (<2%)
Dipsia (thirst) (<2%)

BETHANECHOL

See: www.drugeruptiondata.com/drug/id/74

BETRIXABAN *

Trade name: Bevyxxa (Portola)
Indications: Prophylaxis of venous thromboembolism in adult patients hospitalized for an acute medical illness who are at risk for thromboembolic complications
Class: Direct factor Xa inhibitor
Half-life: 19–27 hours
Clinically important, potentially hazardous interactions with: amiodarone, anticoagulants, antiplatelet drugs and thrombolytics, azithromycin, clarithromycin, ketoconazole, verapamil
Pregnancy category: N/A (Likely to increase the risk of hemorrhage during pregnancy and delivery)
Important contra-indications noted in the prescribing guidelines for: nursing mothers; pediatric patients
Note: Contra-indicated in patients with active pathological bleeding.
Warning: SPINAL/EPIDURAL HEMATOMA

Mucosal
Epistaxis (nosebleed) (2%)

Cardiovascular
Hypertension (2%)

Central Nervous System
Headache (2%)

Gastrointestinal/Hepatic
Constipation (3%)

Diarrhea (2%)
Nausea (2%)

Endocrine/Metabolic
Hypokalemia (3%)

Genitourinary
Hematuria (2%)
Urinary tract infection (3%)

Hematologic
Bleeding (<2%) [2]

BEVACIZUMAB

Trade name: Avastin (Genentech)
Indications: Colon cancer
Class: Biologic, Monoclonal antibody, Vascular endothelial growth factor antagonist
Half-life: 20 days
Clinically important, potentially hazardous interactions with: antineoplastics, irinotecan, sorafenib, sunitinib
Pregnancy category: C
Important contra-indications noted in the prescribing guidelines for: the elderly; nursing mothers; pediatric patients
Warning: GASTROINTESTINAL PERFORATIONS, SURGERY AND WOUND HEALING COMPLICATIONS, and HEMORRHAGE

Skin
Acneform eruption [6]
Hand–foot syndrome [12]
Necrosis [2]
Rash [16]
Toxicity [9]
Ulcerations [3]
Wound complications [8]

Hair
Alopecia [5]

Mucosal
Epistaxis (nosebleed) [5]
Mucosal inflammation [2]
Mucositis [11]
Oral ulceration [2]
Stomatitis [8]

Cardiovascular
Cardiac failure [2]
Cardiotoxicity [6]
Hypertension (23–67%) [79]
Hypotension (7–15%)
Thromboembolism (<21%) [14]
Venous thromboembolism [5]

Central Nervous System
Anorexia [14]
Cerebral hemorrhage [5]
Headache [6]
Intracranial hemorrhage [2]
Leukoencephalopathy [19]
Neurotoxicity [13]
Peripheral neuropathy [9]
Seizures [2]

Neuromuscular/Skeletal
Arthralgia [2]
Asthenia (fatigue) [35]
Osteonecrosis [5]

Gastrointestinal/Hepatic
Abdominal pain [4]
Colitis [3]
Diarrhea [42]
Gastrointestinal bleeding [5]
Gastrointestinal fistula [2]
Gastrointestinal perforation [25]
Hepatotoxicity [4]
Nausea [11]
Vomiting [9]

Respiratory
Hemoptysis [4]
Pulmonary embolism [4]
Pulmonary toxicity [2]

Endocrine/Metabolic
ALT increased [3]
Creatine phosphokinase increased [2]
Hyperglycemia [2]
Hypokalemia [3]
Hypomagnesemia [2]

Renal
Proteinuria [32]

Hematologic
Anemia [12]
Bleeding [9]
Febrile neutropenia [13]
Hemorrhage [13]
Leukocytopenia [2]
Leukopenia [13]
Lymphopenia [4]
Neutropenia [41]
Thrombocytopenia [22]
Thrombosis [16]
Thrombotic complications [3]
Thrombotic microangiopathy [2]

Ocular
Hallucinations, visual [2]
Intraocular pressure increased [3]
Iritis [2]
Ocular adverse effects [2]
Uveitis [2]

Other
Adverse effects [22]
Allergic reactions [3]
Death [16]
Hiccups [2]
Infection [9]

BEXAROTENE

Trade name: Targretin (Eisai)
Indications: Cutaneous T-cell lymphoma, mycosis fungoides
Class: Antineoplastic, Retinoid
Half-life: 7 hours
Clinically important, potentially hazardous interactions with: acitretin, atorvastatin, beta-carotene, carboplatin, conivaptan, dexamethasone, dong quai, gemfibrozil, grapefruit juice, isotretinoin, oral contraceptives, paclitaxel, saxagliptin, St John's wort, tamoxifen, tetracyclines, tretinoin, vitamin A

Pregnancy category: X
Important contra-indications noted in the prescribing guidelines for: nursing mothers; pediatric patients
Note: Retinoids can cause birth defects, and women should avoid bexarotene when pregnant or trying to conceive.
Warning: AVOID IN PREGNANCY

Skin
Acneform eruption (<10%)
Bacterial infection (<13%)
Dermatitis [2]
Erythema [2]
Exanthems (<10%)
Exfoliative dermatitis (10–28%)
Necrosis [2]
Nodular eruption (<10%)
Peripheral edema (13%)
Pruritus (20–30%) [5]
Rash (17%) [2]
Ulcerations (<10%)
Vesiculobullous eruption (<10%)
Xerosis (11%) [2]

Hair
Alopecia (4–11%)

Mucosal
Cheilitis (<10%)
Gingivitis (<10%)
Mucositis [2]
Xerostomia (<10%)

Central Nervous System
Chills (10%)
Hyperesthesia (<10%)

Neuromuscular/Skeletal
Arthralgia [2]
Asthenia (fatigue) [2]
Myalgia/Myopathy (<10%) [2]

Respiratory
Flu-like syndrome (4–13%)

Endocrine/Metabolic
Hypercholesterolemia [4]
Hyperlipidemia [4]
Hypertriglyceridemia [6]
Hypothyroidism [6]
Mastodynia (<10%)

Hematologic
Anemia [4]
Leukopenia [4]
Lymphopenia [2]
Neutropenia [6]

Other
Adverse effects [2]

BEZAFIBRATE

See: www.drugeruptiondata.com/drug/id/1318

BEZLOTOXUMAB

Trade name: Zinplava (Merck)
Indications: To reduce the recurrence of *Clostridium difficile* infection (CDI) in patients who are receiving antibacterial treatment of CDI and are at high risk for CDI recurrence
Class: C. difficile toxin inhibitor, Monoclonal antibody
Half-life: ~19 days
Clinically important, potentially hazardous interactions with: none known
Pregnancy category: N/A (No data available)
Important contra-indications noted in the prescribing guidelines for: nursing mothers; pediatric patients

Cardiovascular
Cardiac failure (2%)

Central Nervous System
Fever (5%)
Headache (4%)

Gastrointestinal/Hepatic
Diarrhea [2]
Nausea (7%) [2]

Local
Infusion-related reactions (10%)

BICALUTAMIDE

Trade name: Casodex (AstraZeneca)
Indications: Metastatic prostatic carcinoma
Class: Androgen antagonist
Half-life: up to 10 days
Clinically important, potentially hazardous interactions with: CYP3A4 substrates
Pregnancy category: X (not indicated for use in women)
Important contra-indications noted in the prescribing guidelines for: pediatric patients

Skin
Diaphoresis (6%)
Edema (2–5%)
Hot flashes (49%) [9]
Peripheral edema (8%)
Pruritus (2–5%)
Rash (6%)
Xerosis (2–5%)

Hair
Alopecia (2–5%)

Mucosal
Xerostomia (2–5%)

Central Nervous System
Paresthesias (6%)

Neuromuscular/Skeletal
Asthenia (fatigue) [4]
Myalgia/Myopathy (2–5%)

Gastrointestinal/Hepatic
Constipation [2]
Hepatotoxicity [4]

Endocrine/Metabolic
Gynecomastia (38%) [34]
Mastodynia (39%) [16]

Local
  Injection-site reactions (2–5%)

BIMATOPROST

Trade names: Latisse (Allergan), Lumigan (Allergan)
Indications: Reduction of elevated intraocular pressure in open-angle glaucoma or ocular hypertension, hypotrichosis of the eyelashes
Class: Prostaglandin analog
Half-life: 45 minutes
Clinically important, potentially hazardous interactions with: none known
Pregnancy category: C
Important contra-indications noted in the prescribing guidelines for: nursing mothers; pediatric patients

Skin
  Pigmentation [2]

Hair
  Hirsutism (<5%)
  Hypertrichosis [2]

Central Nervous System
  Headache (<5%)

Neuromuscular/Skeletal
  Asthenia (fatigue) (<5%)

Respiratory
  Nasopharyngitis [2]
  Upper respiratory tract infection (10%)

Ocular
  Asthenopia (<10%)
  Blepharitis (<10%)
  Cataract (<10%)
  Choroidal detachment [2]
  Conjunctival edema (<10%)
  Conjunctival hemorrhage (<10%)
  Conjunctival hyperemia (25–45%) [42]
  Conjunctivitis (<10%)
  Deepening of upper lid sulcus [9]
  Eyelashes – hypertrichosis (>10%) [13]
  Eyelashes – pigmentation (<10%) [3]
  Eyelid erythema (3–10%) [2]
  Eyelid irritation (3–10%)
  Eyelid pain (3–10%)
  Eyelid pigmentation (3–10%) [6]
  Eyelid xerosis (3–10%)
  Eyes – adverse effects [2]
  Foreign body sensation (<10%)
  Iris pigmentation (<10%) [4]
  Keratitis [2]
  Lacrimation (<10%)
  Macular edema [2]
  Ocular adverse effects [10]
  Ocular burning (<10%)
  Ocular discharge (<10%)
  Ocular hyperemia [4]
  Ocular itching (<10%)
  Ocular pain [2]
  Ocular pigmentation (<3%) [5]
  Ocular pruritus (>10%) [5]
  Periorbital pigmentation (<10%) [3]
  Photophobia (<10%)
  Punctate keratitis (<10%) [2]
  Uveitis [3]

BIPERIDEN

See: www.drugeruptiondata.com/drug/id/77

BISACODYL

See: www.drugeruptiondata.com/drug/id/78

BISMUTH

Trade names: Helidac (Prometheus), Pepto-Bismol (Procter & Gamble)
Indications: As part of 'triple therapy' (antibiotics + bismuth) for eradication of *H. pylori*. Bismuth subgallate initiates clotting via activation of factor XII, and is used for bleeding during tonsillectomy and adenoidectomy. BIPP impregnated ribbon gauze is used for packing following ear surgery. Bismuth subsalicylate is in OTC products for gastrointestinal complaints and peptic ulcer disease
Class: Disinfectant, Heavy metal
Half-life: 21–72 days
Clinically important, potentially hazardous interactions with: aspirin, ciprofloxacin, demeclocycline, doxycycline, hypoglycemics, lomefloxacin, lymecycline, methotrexate, minocycline, tetracycline, warfarin
Pregnancy category: D (category C in first and second trimesters; category D in third trimester)

Skin
  Dermatitis [2]
  Hypersensitivity [2]
  Pigmentation [5]
  Pruritus (triple therapy) [2]
  Rash [4]

Mucosal
  Oral pigmentation [3]
  Stomatitis [4]
  Tongue pigmentation (>10%) [3]
  Xerostomia (triple therapy) (41%)

Central Nervous System
  Dysgeusia (taste perversion) (triple therapy) (46%) [9]
  Encephalopathy [4]
  Pain (triple therapy) (10%)
  Tremor [2]
  Vertigo (dizziness) [2]

Neuromuscular/Skeletal
  Arthralgia [10]
  Asthenia (fatigue) [2]

Gastrointestinal/Hepatic
  Diarrhea [5]
  Nausea [4]
  Vomiting [2]

Other
  Adverse effects (triple therapy) [52]
  Allergic reactions [2]
  Death [10]

BISOPROLOL

Trade names: Cardicor (Merck Serono), Concor (Merck Serono), Emcor (Merck Serono), Zebeta (Barr), Ziac (Barr)
Indications: Hypertension
Class: Beta adrenergic blocker, Beta blocker
Half-life: 9–12 hours
Clinically important, potentially hazardous interactions with: diltiazem, disopyramide, guanethidine, reserpine, rifampin, verapamil
Pregnancy category: C
Important contra-indications noted in the prescribing guidelines for: nursing mothers; pediatric patients
Note: Ziac is bisoprolol and hydrochlorothiazide. Hydrochlorothiazide is a sulfonamide and can be absorbed systemically. Sulfonamides can produce severe, possibly fatal, reactions such as toxic epidermal necrolysis and Stevens-Johnson syndrome.
Contra-indicated in patients with cardiogenic shock, overt cardiac failure, second or third degree AV block, and marked sinus bradycardia.

Skin
  Edema (3%)
  Peripheral edema (<10%)
  Rash (<10%)
  Raynaud's phenomenon (<10%)

Cardiovascular
  Bradycardia [6]
  Hypotension [3]

Central Nervous System
  Headache [2]
  Hyperesthesia (2%)
  Vertigo (dizziness) [3]

Neuromuscular/Skeletal
  Myalgia/Myopathy (<10%)

Other
  Adverse effects [4]

BIVALIRUDIN

Trade name: Angiomax (The Medicines Company)
Indications: Angioplasty adjunct
Class: Thrombin inhibitor
Half-life: 25 minutes
Clinically important, potentially hazardous interactions with: anisindione, dicumarol, heparin, reteplase, streptokinase, tenecteplase, urokinase, warfarin
Pregnancy category: B

Central Nervous System
  Pain (15%)

Neuromuscular/Skeletal
  Back pain (42%)

Hematologic
  Bleeding [5]
  Thrombosis [3]

Local
  Injection-site pain (8%)

BLEOMYCIN

Synonyms: bleo; BLM
Trade name: Blenoxane (Mead Johnson)
Indications: Melanomas, sarcomas, lymphomas, testicular carcinoma
Class: Antibiotic, anthracycline
Half-life: 1.3–9 hours
Clinically important, potentially hazardous interactions with: aldesleukin, brentuximab vedotin
Pregnancy category: D
Important contra-indications noted in the prescribing guidelines for: nursing mothers; pediatric patients

Skin
Acral erythema [2]
Acral necrosis [2]
Bullous dermatitis (<5%)
Calcification [2]
Erythema [6]
Exanthems [3]
Flagellate dermatitis [8]
Flagellate erythema/pigmentation [44]
Gangrene (digital) [3]
Hyperkeratosis (palms and soles) [2]
Hypersensitivity (<10%) [5]
Linear streaking [4]
Lipodystrophy [2]
Neutrophilic eccrine hidradenitis [2]
Pigmentation (~50%) [21]
Pruritus (>5%) [7]
Raynaud's phenomenon (>10%) [34]
Scleroderma [16]
Stevens-Johnson syndrome [2]
Toxicity [2]

Hair
Alopecia (~50%) [7]

Nails
Nail growth reduced [2]
Nail loss [3]
Onychodystrophy [2]
Onycholysis [3]

Mucosal
Oral ulceration [2]
Stomatitis (>10%) [8]

Central Nervous System
Chills (>10%)

Neuromuscular/Skeletal
Digital necrosis [3]

Respiratory
Pneumonitis [3]
Pulmonary fibrosis [3]
Pulmonary toxicity [7]

Endocrine/Metabolic
SIADH [2]

Hematologic
Hemolytic uremic syndrome [8]

Local
Injection-site phlebitis (<10%)

Other
Adverse effects [2]
Allergic reactions [2]

BLINATUMOMAB

Trade name: Blincyto (Amgen)
Indications: Precursor B-cell acute lymphoblastic leukemia
Class: Bispecific CD19-directed CD3 T-cell engager, Monoclonal antibody
Half-life: 1.4 hours
Clinically important, potentially hazardous interactions with: none known
Pregnancy category: C
Important contra-indications noted in the prescribing guidelines for: nursing mothers
Warning: CYTOKINE RELEASE SYNDROME and NEUROLOGICAL TOXICITIES

Skin
Edema (5%) [4]
Peripheral edema (25%) [2]
Rash (21%) [2]
Tumor lysis syndrome (4%)

Cardiovascular
Chest pain (11%)
Hypertension (8%)
Hypotension (11%)
Tachycardia (8%)

Central Nervous System
Aphasia (4%) [5]
Chills (15%)
Confusion (7%) [4]
Cytokine release syndrome (11%) [12]
Disorientation (3%) [3]
Encephalopathy (5%) [6]
Fever (62%) [9]
Headache (36%) [7]
Insomnia (15%)
Memory loss (2%)
Neurotoxicity [8]
Paresthesias (5%) [2]
Seizures (2%) [7]
Somnolence (drowsiness) [2]
Speech disorder [3]
Tremor (20%) [7]
Vertigo (dizziness) (14%) [2]

Neuromuscular/Skeletal
Arthralgia (10%)
Asthenia (fatigue) (17%) [4]
Ataxia [2]
Back pain (14%) [2]
Bone or joint pain (11%)
Pain in extremities (12%)

Gastrointestinal/Hepatic
Abdominal pain (15%)
Constipation (20%) [2]
Diarrhea (20%) [3]
Hepatotoxicity [2]
Nausea (25%) [4]
Vomiting (13%)

Respiratory
Cough (19%) [2]
Dyspnea (15%)
Pneumonia (9%) [4]

Endocrine/Metabolic
ALT increased (12%) [2]
Appetite decreased (10%)
AST increased (11%)
GGT increased (6%) [2]
Hyperbilirubinemia (8%)
Hyperglycemia (11%) [2]
Hypoalbuminemia (4%)
Hypokalemia (23%) [5]
Hypomagnesemia (12%)
Hypophosphatemia (6%)
Weight gain (11%)

Hematologic
Anemia (18%) [5]
Febrile neutropenia (25%) [8]
Leukocytosis (2%)
Leukopenia (9%) [5]
Lymphopenia [3]
Neutropenia (16%) [4]
Sepsis (7%) [3]
Thrombocytopenia (11%) [6]

Local
Catheter-related infection [2]

BOCEPREVIR

Trade name: Victrelis (Merck)
Indications: Chronic hepatitis C
Class: CYP3A4 inhibitor, Direct-acting antiviral, Hepatitis C virus NS3/4A protease inhibitor
Half-life: 3 hours
Clinically important, potentially hazardous interactions with: alfuzosin, alprazolam, amiodarone, atorvastatin, bepridil, bosentan, brigatinib, budesonide, buprenorphine, cabozantinib, carbamazepine, cisapride, clarithromycin, colchicine, copanlisib, cyclosporine, dasatinib, desipramine, dexamethasone, digoxin, dihydroergotamine, drospirenone, efavirenz, ergonovine, ergotamine, estradiol, felodipine, flecainide, flibanserin, fluticasone propionate, gefitinib, itraconazole, ketoconazole, lomitapide, lovastatin, methadone, methylergonovine, midazolam, midostaurin, mifepristone, neratinib, nicardipine, nifedipine, olaparib, pazopanib, phenobarbital, phenytoin, pimozide, ponatinib, posaconazole, propafenone, quinidine, ribociclib, rifabutin, rifampin, ritonavir, ruxolitinib, salmeterol, sildenafil, simvastatin, sirolimus, St John's wort, tacrolimus, tadalafil, trazodone, triazolam, vardenafil, vorapaxar, voriconazole, warfarin
Pregnancy category: X (boceprevir is pregnancy category B but must not be used in monotherapy)
Important contra-indications noted in the prescribing guidelines for: nursing mothers; pediatric patients
Note: Must be used in combination with PEG-interferon and ribavirin (see separate entries) Combination treatment is contra-indicated in pregnant women and men whose female partners are pregnant because of the risks for birth defects and fetal death associated with ribavirin, or in coadministration with drugs that are highly dependent on CYP3A4/5 for clearance, or with potent CYP3A4/5 inducers.

Skin
Pruritus [3]
Rash [3]

Central Nervous System
Dysgeusia (taste perversion) [6]

Gastrointestinal/Hepatic
Hepatotoxicity [2]

Hematologic
Anemia [24]
Neutropenia [8]
Thrombocytopenia [8]

Other
Adverse effects [6]
Infection [2]

BORTEZOMIB

Trade name: Velcade (Millennium)
Indications: Multiple myeloma, mantle cell lymphoma
Class: Biologic, Proteasome inhibitor
Half-life: 9–15 hours
Clinically important, potentially hazardous interactions with: conivaptan, darunavir, delavirdine, efavirenz, indinavir, strong CYP3A4 inhibitors or inducers, telithromycin, thalidomide, voriconazole
Pregnancy category: D
Important contra-indications noted in the prescribing guidelines for: nursing mothers; pediatric patients
Note: Contra-indicated in patients with hypersensitivity to boron or mannitol.

Skin
Edema (23%)
Erythema [2]
Folliculitis [2]
Herpes zoster (12%) [13]
Peripheral edema [5]
Pruritus (11%)
Purpura [2]
Rash (18%) [9]
Sweet's syndrome [7]
Toxicity [4]
Tumor lysis syndrome [2]
Vasculitis [4]

Mucosal
Mucositis [2]

Cardiovascular
Arrhythmias [2]
Cardiac failure [3]
Cardiotoxicity [4]
Congestive heart failure [3]
Hypertension [3]
Hypotension (13%) [4]
QT prolongation [2]

Central Nervous System
Anxiety (10%)
Dysesthesia (23%)
Dysgeusia (taste perversion) (13%)
Encephalopathy [3]
Fever (34%) [7]
Guillain–Barré syndrome [2]
Headache [3]
Hypoesthesia [2]
Insomnia (20%) [2]
Neurotoxicity [26]
Pain [2]
Paresthesias (22%) [3]
Peripheral neuropathy (39%) [58]
Vertigo (dizziness) (17%)

Neuromuscular/Skeletal
Arthralgia (17%) [2]
Asthenia (fatigue) (64%) [35]
Back pain (13%)
Bone or joint pain (14%) [2]
Cramps (11%)
Myalgia/Myopathy (12%)

Gastrointestinal/Hepatic
Abdominal distension [2]
Abdominal pain [3]
Colitis [2]
Constipation (41%) [7]
Diarrhea (52%) [22]
Gastrointestinal disorder [2]
Hepatotoxicity [4]
Nausea (55%) [10]
Pancreatitis [2]
Vomiting (33%) [4]

Respiratory
Cough (20%) [2]
Dyspnea (21%) [6]
Nasopharyngitis (12%)
Pneumonia (12%) [8]
Pneumonitis [4]
Pulmonary toxicity [3]
Upper respiratory tract infection (12%) [3]

Endocrine/Metabolic
Appetite decreased (36%)
Dehydration (10%)
Hypocalcemia [2]
Hypokalemia [3]
Serum creatinine increased [2]
Weight loss [2]

Renal
Nephrotoxicity [2]

Hematologic
Anemia (29%) [16]
Febrile neutropenia [5]
Hemotoxicity [5]
Leukopenia [8]
Lymphopenia [11]
Myelosuppression [2]
Neutropenia (17%) [35]
Sepsis [4]
Thrombocytopenia (36%) [51]

Local
Infusion-related reactions [2]
Injection-site irritation (5%)
Injection-site reactions [4]

Other
Adverse effects [13]
Death [6]
Infection [11]

BOSENTAN

Trade name: Tracleer (Actelion)
Indications: Pulmonary arterial hypertension
Class: Antihypertensive, Endothelin receptor (ETR) antagonist, Vasodilator
Half-life: ~5 hours
Clinically important, potentially hazardous interactions with: amiodarone, amprenavir, astemizole, atazanavir, atorvastatin, boceprevir, cobicistat/elvitegravir/emtricitabine/tenofovir alafenamide, cobicistat/elvitegravir/emtricitabine/tenofovir disoproxil, cyclosporine, diltiazem,

elbasvir & grazoprevir, enzalutamide, erythromycin, fluconazole, fluvastatin, glibenclamide, glyburide, indinavir, itraconazole, ketoconazole, levonorgestrel, lopinavir, lovastatin, neratinib, olaparib, oral contraceptives, palbociclib, progestogens, reboxetine, rifampin, ritonavir, sildenafil, simvastatin, St John's wort, tacrolimus, tadalafil, telaprevir, tipranavir, ulipristal, vardenafil, venetoclax, voriconazole, warfarin
Pregnancy category: X
Important contra-indications noted in the prescribing guidelines for: nursing mothers; pediatric patients
Warning: RISKS OF HEPATOTOXICITY and TERATOGENICITY

Skin
Edema (8%) [2]
Peripheral edema (8%) [5]
Pruritus (4%)

Cardiovascular
Flushing (9%) [2]

Central Nervous System
Headache [2]
Syncope [2]

Gastrointestinal/Hepatic
Hepatotoxicity [17]

Respiratory
Bronchitis [2]

Endocrine/Metabolic
AST increased [2]

Hematologic
Anemia [4]

Other
Adverse effects [7]

BOSUTINIB

See: www.drugeruptiondata.com/drug/id/3037

BOTULINUM TOXIN (A & B)

Trade names: Azzalure (Galderma), Bocouture (Merz), Botox (Allergan), Dysport (Ipsen), Myobloc (Solstice), Neurobloc (Eisai), Vistabel (Allergan), Xeomin (Merz)
Indications: Blepharospasm, hemifacial spasm, spasmodic torticollis, sialorrhea, hyperhidrosis, strabismus, oromandibular dystonia, cervical dystonia, spasmodic dysphonia, chronic migraine, urinary incontinence in people with neurologic conditions such as spinal cord injury and multiple sclerosis who have overactivity of the bladder, cosmetic application for wrinkles
Class: Acetylcholine inhibitor, Neuromuscular blocker, Ophthalmic agent, toxin
Half-life: 3–6 months
Clinically important, potentially hazardous interactions with: aminoglycosides, anticholinergics, fesoterodine, tiotropium, trospium

Pregnancy category: C
Important contra-indications noted in the prescribing guidelines for: nursing mothers; pediatric patients
Note: Distant spread of toxin effect - postmarketing reports indicate that all botulinum toxin products may spread from the area of injection to produce symptoms consistent with botulinum toxin effects. These may include asthenia, generalized muscle weakness, diplopia, ptosis, dysphagia, dysphonia, dysarthria, urinary incontinence and breathing diffculties. These symptoms have been reported hours to weeks after injection.
An antitoxin is available in the event of overdose or misinjection.
Warning: DISTANT SPREAD OF TOXIN EFFECT

Skin
  Anaphylactoid reactions/Anaphylaxis [4]
  Ecchymoses [4]
  Erythema [2]
  Granulomas [2]
  Hematoma [2]
  Peripheral edema (<10%)
  Pruritus (<10%)
  Purpura (<10%)

Mucosal
  Epistaxis (nosebleed) [2]
  Stomatitis (<10%)
  Xerostomia (3–34%) [13]

Central Nervous System
  Dysgeusia (taste perversion) (<10%)
  Gait instability [2]
  Headache [7]
  Hyperesthesia (<10%)
  Neurotoxicity [3]
  Pain (6–13%) [4]
  Seizures [2]
  Tremor (<10%)
  Vertigo (dizziness) [2]

Neuromuscular/Skeletal
  Arthralgia (<7%)
  Asthenia (fatigue) [16]
  Myasthenia gravis [2]
  Neck pain [2]

Gastrointestinal/Hepatic
  Constipation [2]
  Diarrhea [3]
  Dysphagia [16]

Respiratory
  Dysphonia [2]
  Dyspnea [2]
  Flu-like syndrome (2–10%) [8]
  Nasopharyngitis [2]
  Pulmonary toxicity [3]

Genitourinary
  Hematuria [4]
  Urinary incontinence [3]
  Urinary retention [12]
  Urinary tract infection [15]
  Vulvovaginal candidiasis (<10%)

Otic
  Tinnitus (<10%)

Ocular
  Blepharoptosis [2]
  Conjunctivitis [2]

  Diplopia [10]
  Eyelid edema [4]
  Ocular adverse effects [2]
  Ptosis (14–20%) [24]
  Xerophthalmia (6%) [2]

Local
  Injection-site bruising [4]
  Injection-site ecchymoses [2]
  Injection-site edema [8]
  Injection-site erythema [3]
  Injection-site pain (2–10%) [20]
  Injection-site paralysis [2]
  Injection-site reactions [6]

Other
  Adverse effects [18]
  Death [4]
  Infection (13–19%)
  Side effects [3]

BRENTUXIMAB VEDOTIN

Trade name: Adcetris (Seattle Genetics)
Indications: Hodgkin's lymphoma, systemic anaplastic large cell lymphoma
Class: Antibody drug conjugate (ADC), CD30-directed antibody-drug conjugate, Monoclonal antibody
Half-life: 4–6 days
Clinically important, potentially hazardous interactions with: bleomycin, efavirenz, ketoconazole, rifampin, strong CYP3A4 inhibitors
Pregnancy category: D
Important contra-indications noted in the prescribing guidelines for: the elderly; nursing mothers; pediatric patients
Warning: PROGRESSIVE MULTIFOCAL LEUKOENCEPHALOPATHY

Skin
  Diaphoresis (12%)
  Lymphadenopathy (11%)
  Peripheral edema (4–16%)
  Pruritus (19%)
  Rash (31%)
  Xerosis (10%)

Hair
  Alopecia (14%)

Central Nervous System
  Anxiety (11%)
  Chills (13%)
  Fever (29–38%) [3]
  Headache (19%)
  Insomnia (16%)
  Neurotoxicity [2]
  Pain (7–28%)
  Peripheral neuropathy (68%) [10]
  Vertigo (dizziness) (11–16%)

Neuromuscular/Skeletal
  Arthralgia (9–19%)
  Asthenia (fatigue) (41–49%) [4]
  Back pain (14%)
  Muscle spasm (10%)
  Myalgia/Myopathy (17%)
  Pain in extremities (10%)

Gastrointestinal/Hepatic
  Abdominal pain (9–25%)
  Constipation (19%)
  Diarrhea (36%) [3]
  Nausea (42%) [4]
  Vomiting (22%)

Respiratory
  Cough (17–25%)
  Dyspnea (13–19%)
  Pulmonary toxicity [2]
  Upper respiratory tract infection (12–47%)

Endocrine/Metabolic
  Appetite decreased (16%)
  Weight loss (6–12%)

Hematologic
  Anemia (33–52%)
  Neutropenia (55%) [6]
  Thrombocytopenia (16–28%)

Other
  Adverse effects [2]

BRETYLIUM

See: www.drugeruptiondata.com/drug/id/81

BREXPIPRAZOLE

Trade name: Rexulti (Otsuka)
Indications: Schizophrenia, major depressive disorder (with antidepressants)
Class: Antipsychotic
Half-life: 86–91 hours
Clinically important, potentially hazardous interactions with: strong or moderate CYP2D6 inhibitors, strong or moderate CYP3A4 inducers or inhibitors
Pregnancy category: N/A (Neonatal risk in third trimester exposure)
Important contra-indications noted in the prescribing guidelines for: the elderly; nursing mothers; pediatric patients
Warning: INCREASED MORTALITY IN ELDERLY PATIENTS WITH DEMENTIA-RELATED PSYCHOSIS
SUICIDAL THOUGHTS AND BEHAVIORS

Central Nervous System
  Agitation [3]
  Akathisia (6–9%) [12]
  Anxiety (3%) [2]
  Headache (7%) [6]
  Insomnia [4]
  Restlessness (3%)
  Sedation (2%) [2]
  Somnolence (drowsiness) (5%) [4]
  Tremor (3–4%)
  Vertigo (dizziness) (3%)

Neuromuscular/Skeletal
  Asthenia (fatigue) (3%) [2]

Gastrointestinal/Hepatic
  Constipation (2%)
  Diarrhea (3%) [2]
  Dyspepsia (3%)
  Nausea [4]

Respiratory
Nasopharyngitis (4%)

Endocrine/Metabolic
Appetite increased (3%)
Creatine phosphokinase increased (2%)
Weight gain (4–7%) [13]
Weight loss (10%)

Hematologic
Hemotoxicity (2%)

BRIGATINIB *

Trade name: Alunbrig (Ariad)
Indications: Anaplastic lymphoma kinase-positive metastatic non-small cell lung cancer in patients who have progressed on, or are intolerant to, crizotinib
Class: Tyrosine kinase inhibitor
Half-life: 25 hours
Clinically important, potentially hazardous interactions with: boceprevir, carbamazepine, clarithromycin, cobicistat, conivaptan, CYP3A substrates and strong CYP3A inducers or inhibitors, grapefruit juice, hormonal contraceptives, indinavir, itraconazole, ketoconazole, lopinavir, nelfinavir, phenytoin, posaconazole, rifampin, ritonavir, saquinavir, St John's wort, voriconazole
Pregnancy category: N/A (May cause fetal toxicity based on findings in animal studies)
Important contra-indications noted in the prescribing guidelines for: nursing mothers; pediatric patients

Skin
Rash (15–24%)

Cardiovascular
Bradycardia (6–8%)
Hypertension (11–21%)

Central Nervous System
Fever (6–14%)
Headache (27–28%) [2]
Insomnia (7–11%)
Peripheral neuropathy (13%)

Neuromuscular/Skeletal
Arthralgia (14%)
Asthenia (fatigue) (29–36%)
Back pain (10–15%)
Muscle spasm (12–17%)
Myalgia/Myopathy (9–15%)
Pain in extremities (4–11%)

Gastrointestinal/Hepatic
Abdominal pain (10–17%)
Constipation (15–19%)
Diarrhea (19–38%) [3]
Nausea (33–40%) [2]
Vomiting (23–24%)

Respiratory
Cough (18–34%) [2]
Dyspnea (21–27%) [3]
Hypoxia (<3%) [2]
Pneumonia (5–10%) [2]
Pneumonitis (4–9%)
Pulmonary toxicity [2]

Endocrine/Metabolic
ALT increased (34–40%)

Appetite decreased (15–22%)
AST increased (38–65%)
Creatine phosphokinase increased (27–48%)
Hyperglycemia (38–49%)
Hypophosphatemia (15–23%)

Hematologic
Anemia (23–40%)
Hyperlipasemia (21–45%)
Lymphopenia (19–27%)
Prothrombin time increased (20–22%)

Ocular
Visual disturbances (7–10%)

BRIMONIDINE

Trade names: Alphagan P (Allergan), Mirvaso (Galderma)
Indications: Open-angle glaucoma, ocular hypertension, topical application for rosacea
Class: Adrenergic alpha2-receptor agonist
Half-life: 12 hours
Clinically important, potentially hazardous interactions with: amitriptyline, MAO inhibitors, tricyclic antidepressants
Pregnancy category: B
Important contra-indications noted in the prescribing guidelines for: nursing mothers; pediatric patients
Note: [T] = Topical.

Skin
Burning [T] (2%) [4]
Contact dermatitis [T] [2]
Dermatitis [2]
Erythema [T] (4%) [7]
Hypersensitivity [3]
Irritation [3]
Pruritus [4]
Rosacea [2]
Xerosis [2]

Mucosal
Xerostomia (5–20%) [12]

Cardiovascular
Flushing [T] (3%) [3]
Hypertension (5–20%)

Central Nervous System
Dysgeusia (taste perversion) (<10%) [4]
Somnolence (drowsiness) [2]

Neuromuscular/Skeletal
Asthenia (fatigue) [4]

Respiratory
Upper respiratory tract infection (<10%)

Ocular
Blepharitis (<10%) [2]
Conjunctival hyperemia (5–20%) [5]
Conjunctivitis (5–20%) [7]
Eyelid crusting (<10%)
Eyelid edema (<10%)
Eyelid erythema (<10%)
Intraocular pressure increased [2]
Ocular adverse effects [4]
Ocular allergy (4%) [8]
Ocular burning (<10%) [7]
Ocular hyperemia [4]
Ocular itching [2]
Ocular pain [3]

Ocular pruritus (5–20%) [5]
Ocular stinging (<10%) [6]
Periocular dermatitis [2]
Uveitis [11]
Vision blurred [T] [3]
Visual disturbances (5–20%)
Xerophthalmia [3]

Other
Adverse effects [2]
Allergic reactions [2]

BRINZOLAMIDE

Trade name: Azopt (Alcon)
Indications: Open-angle glaucoma, ocular hypertension
Class: Carbonic anhydrase inhibitor, Diuretic
Half-life: 111 days
Clinically important, potentially hazardous interactions with: conivaptan, darunavir, delavirdine, indinavir, salicylates, telithromycin, voriconazole
Pregnancy category: C
Important contra-indications noted in the prescribing guidelines for: nursing mothers
Note: Brinzolamide is a sulfonamide and can be absorbed systemically. Sulfonamides can produce severe, possibly fatal, reactions such as toxic epidermal necrolysis and Stevens-Johnson syndrome.

Skin
Dermatitis (<5%)

Mucosal
Xerostomia [4]

Central Nervous System
Dysgeusia (taste perversion) (5–10%) [14]
Headache (<5%)

Neuromuscular/Skeletal
Asthenia (fatigue) [3]

Respiratory
Rhinitis (<5%)

Endocrine/Metabolic
Acidosis [2]

Ocular
Blepharitis (<5%)
Conjunctival hyperemia [8]
Conjunctivitis [3]
Corneal abnormalities [3]
Foreign body sensation (<5%)
Lacrimation [3]
Ocular adverse effects [3]
Ocular allergy [2]
Ocular burning [4]
Ocular discharge (<5%)
Ocular hyperemia [5]
Ocular itching [6]
Ocular keratitis (<5%)
Ocular pain (<5%) [6]
Ocular pruritus (<5%) [3]
Ocular stinging [4]
Vision blurred (5–10%) [15]
Xerophthalmia (<5%) [5]

Other
Adverse effects [2]

BRIVARACETAM

Trade name: Briviact (UCB)
Indications: Epilepsy adjunct therapy
Class: Anticonvulsant, Antiepileptic
Half-life: 9 hours
Clinically important, potentially hazardous interactions with: carbamazepine, phenytoin, rifampin
Pregnancy category: C
Important contra-indications noted in the prescribing guidelines for: the elderly; nursing mothers; pediatric patients

Central Nervous System
　Aggression [2]
　Balance disorder (3%)
　Depression [2]
　Dysgeusia (taste perversion) (<3%)
　Euphoria (<3%)
　Headache [11]
　Impaired concentration [2]
　Insomnia [2]
　Irritability (3%) [7]
　Neurotoxicity (13%)
　Sedation (16%)
　Seizures [3]
　Somnolence (drowsiness) (16%) [22]
　Vertigo (dizziness) (12%) [21]
Neuromuscular/Skeletal
　Asthenia (fatigue) (9%) [15]
　Back pain [2]
Gastrointestinal/Hepatic
　Constipation (2%)
　Nausea (5%) [5]
　Vomiting (5%) [3]
Respiratory
　Nasopharyngitis [6]
Genitourinary
　Urinary tract infection [2]
Hematologic
　Leukopenia (2%)
Local
　Infusion-site pain (<3%)
Other
　Adverse effects [4]

BRODALUMAB *

Trade name: Siliq (Valeant)
Indications: Moderate to severe plaque psoriasis
Class: Interleukin-17A (IL-17A) antagonist, Monoclonal antibody
Half-life: N/A
Clinically important, potentially hazardous interactions with: CYP450 substrates, live vaccines
Pregnancy category: N/A (Insufficient evidence to inform drug-associated risk)
Important contra-indications noted in the prescribing guidelines for: nursing mothers; pediatric patients
Note: Contra-indicated in patients with Crohn's disease.

Warning: SUICIDAL IDEATION AND BEHAVIOR

Skin
　Candidiasis [2]
　Contact dermatitis [2]
　Folliculitis [2]
Mucosal
　Oropharyngeal pain (2%)
Central Nervous System
　Headache (4%) [8]
　Suicidal ideation [4]
Neuromuscular/Skeletal
　Arthralgia (5%) [8]
　Asthenia (fatigue) (3%)
　Back pain [2]
　Myalgia/Myopathy (2%)
Gastrointestinal/Hepatic
　Diarrhea (2%) [4]
　Nausea (2%) [2]
Respiratory
　Nasopharyngitis [12]
　Upper respiratory tract infection [14]
Hematologic
　Neutropenia [4]
Local
　Injection-site bleeding (<2%)
　Injection-site bruising (<2%)
　Injection-site erythema (<2%) [4]
　Injection-site pain (<2%)
　Injection-site pruritus (<2%)
　Injection-site reactions (2%)
Other
　Infection (25%)

BROMFENAC

See: www.drugeruptiondata.com/drug/id/1181

BROMOCRIPTINE

Trade name: Parlodel (Novartis)
Indications: Amenorrhea, Parkinsonism, infertility, acromegaly
Class: Dopamine receptor agonist
Half-life: initial: 6–8 hours; terminal: 50 hours
Clinically important, potentially hazardous interactions with: alcohol, antipsychotics, azithromycin, domperidone, erythromycin, isometheptene, lanreotide, levomepromazine, macrolides, memantine, methyldopa, metoclopramide, octreotide, pasireotide, pseudoephedrine, risperidone, sympathomimetics, zuclopenthixol
Pregnancy category: N/A (Contra-indicated in women who become pregnant or in the postpartum period)
Important contra-indications noted in the prescribing guidelines for: nursing mothers; pediatric patients

Skin
　Livedo reticularis [3]
　Raynaud's phenomenon (<10%) [8]
　Scleroderma [2]

Hair
　Alopecia [2]
Mucosal
　Nasal congestion (3–4%)
　Xerostomia (4–10%) [3]
Cardiovascular
　Cardiotoxicity [2]
　Coronary spasm [2]
　Erythromelalgia [4]
　Flushing [2]
　Orthostatic hypotension (6%)
　Postural hypotension (6%)
Central Nervous System
　Anorexia (4%)
　Hallucinations [4]
　Headache (<19%) [3]
　Seizures (in postpartum patients) [3]
　Somnolence (drowsiness) (3%)
　Syncope (<2%)
　Vertigo (dizziness) (17%)
Neuromuscular/Skeletal
　Asthenia (fatigue) (3–7%)
Gastrointestinal/Hepatic
　Abdominal pain (4%)
　Constipation (3–14%) [2]
　Diarrhea (3%)
　Dyspepsia (4%)
　Gastrointestinal bleeding (<2%)
　Nausea (18–49%) [7]
　Vomiting (2–5%) [4]
Respiratory
　Pleural effusion [2]
　Pulmonary fibrosis [2]
Other
　Adverse effects [2]

BROMPHENIRAMINE

See: www.drugeruptiondata.com/drug/id/84

BUCILLAMINE

See: www.drugeruptiondata.com/drug/id/1079

BUCLIZINE

See: www.drugeruptiondata.com/drug/id/85

BUDESONIDE

Trade names: Pulmicort Turbuhaler (AstraZeneca), Rhinocort (AstraZeneca), Symbicort (AstraZeneca)
Indications: Asthma, rhinitis
Class: Corticosteroid, inhaled
Half-life: N/A
Clinically important, potentially hazardous interactions with: boceprevir, efavirenz, itraconazole, ketoconazole, live vaccines, oral contraceptives, telaprevir

Pregnancy category: C
Important contra-indications noted in the prescribing guidelines for: nursing mothers; pediatric patients
Note: Symbicort is budesonide and formoterol.

Skin
Acneform eruption [2]
Dermatitis [8]
Exanthems [2]
Pruritus [2]
Rash [2]

Mucosal
Oral candidiasis [2]

Respiratory
Asthma (exacerbation) [4]
Cough [2]

Endocrine/Metabolic
Adrenal insufficiency [3]
Cushing's syndrome [2]

Ocular
Cataract [2]

Other
Adverse effects [11]
Allergic reactions [3]
Infection [2]
Systemic reactions [2]

BUMETANIDE

See: www.drugeruptiondata.com/drug/id/86

BUPIVACAINE

See: www.drugeruptiondata.com/drug/id/1192

BUPRENORPHINE

Trade names: Probuphine (Braeburn), Suboxone (Reckitt Benckiser), Subutex (Reckitt Benckiser), Transtec (Napp)
Indications: Opioid dependence, moderate to severe pain
Class: Analgesic, Mixed opioid agonist/antagonist, Narcotic
Half-life: 37 hours
Clinically important, potentially hazardous interactions with: antihistamines, atazanavir, azole antifungals, benzodiazepines, boceprevir, carbamazepine, cimetidine, cobicistat/elvitegravir/emtricitabine/tenofovir alafenamide, cobicistat/elvitegravir/emtricitabine/tenofovir disoproxil, delavirdine, diazepam, efavirenz, erythromycin, HIV protease inhibitors, hydrocodone, hydromorphone, ketoconazole, ketorolac, linezolid, macrolide antibiotics, morphine, neuroleptics, oxymorphone, phenobarbital, phenytoin, rifampin, ritonavir, tapentadol, tipranavir
Pregnancy category: C
Important contra-indications noted in the prescribing guidelines for: nursing mothers; pediatric patients
Note: Suboxone contains naloxone; Probuphine is an implant for subdermal administration.

Warning: ABUSE POTENTIAL, LIFE-THREATENING RESPIRATORY DEPRESSION, and ACCIDENTAL EXPOSURE
Probuphine: IMPLANT MIGRATION, PROTRUSION, EXPULSION, and NERVE DAMAGE ASSOCIATED WITH INSERTION and REMOVAL

Skin
Abscess (2%)
Dermatitis [2]
Diaphoresis (12–14%)
Erythema [4]
Hyperhidrosis [4]
Pruritus [11]

Mucosal
Xerostomia [3]

Cardiovascular
Bradycardia [3]
Hypotension [4]
Pulmonary edema [2]
QT prolongation [2]
Vasodilation (9%)

Central Nervous System
Anxiety (12%)
Chills (6–8%)
Depression (11%)
Fever (3%)
Headache (30–36%) [6]
Insomnia (14–25%)
Nervousness (6%)
Neurotoxicity [2]
Pain (22–24%)
Seizures [3]
Somnolence (drowsiness) (5%) [4]
Vertigo (dizziness) (4%) [14]

Neuromuscular/Skeletal
Asthenia (fatigue) (7–14%) [4]
Back pain (4–14%)
Myalgia/Myopathy [2]

Gastrointestinal/Hepatic
Abdominal pain (11%) [2]
Constipation (11–12%) [12]
Diarrhea (4–5%) [2]
Dyspepsia (3%)
Hepatotoxicity [6]
Nausea (10–15%) [15]
Vomiting (5–8%) [12]

Respiratory
Cough (4%)
Flu-like syndrome (6%)
Pharyngitis (4%)
Respiratory depression [3]
Rhinitis (5–11%)

Ocular
Lacrimation (5%)

Local
Application-site reactions [3]

Other
Adverse effects [4]
Death [9]
Infection (6–20%)

BUPROPION

Trade names: Wellbutrin (GSK), Zyban (GSK)
Indications: Depression, aid to smoking cessation
Class: Antidepressant, Dopamine reuptake inhibitor
Half-life: 14 hours
Clinically important, potentially hazardous interactions with: amitriptyline, citalopram, cobicistat/elvitegravir/emtricitabine/tenofovir alafenamide, cobicistat/elvitegravir/emtricitabine/tenofovir disoproxil, cyclosporine, deutetrabenazine, efavirenz, eluxadoline, erythromycin, escitalopram, isocarboxazid, levodopa, linezolid, lopinavir, lorcaserin, methylphenidate, mifepristone, phenelzine, ritonavir, tranylcypromine, trimipramine, vortioxetine
Pregnancy category: C
Important contra-indications noted in the prescribing guidelines for: nursing mothers; pediatric patients
Warning: NEUROPSYCHIATRIC REACTIONS; AND SUICIDAL THOUGHTS AND BEHAVIORS

Skin
Acneform eruption (<10%)
AGEP [3]
Anaphylactoid reactions/Anaphylaxis [2]
Angioedema [3]
Diaphoresis (5%) [4]
Erythema multiforme [4]
Exanthems [2]
Hypersensitivity [6]
Lupus erythematosus [2]
Peripheral edema [2]
Pruritus (4%) [3]
Psoriasis [2]
Rash (4%) [3]
Serum sickness [3]
Serum sickness-like reaction [9]
Stevens-Johnson syndrome [2]
Thrombocytopenic purpura [2]
Urticaria [9]
Xerosis (<10%)

Hair
Hirsutism (<10%)

Mucosal
Tongue edema [2]
Xerostomia (<64%) [18]

Cardiovascular
Arrhythmias [2]
Flushing (4%)
Hypertension [2]
Myocardial ischemia [2]
Tachycardia [3]

Central Nervous System
Agitation [4]
Anxiety [4]
Delirium [2]
Depression [3]
Dysgeusia (taste perversion) (4%)
Hallucinations [6]
Headache [5]
Insomnia [7]
Nightmares [2]
Paresthesias (2%)

Parkinsonism [2]
Psychosis [6]
Seizures [40]
Serotonin syndrome [2]
Sleep related disorder [2]
Somnolence (drowsiness) [4]
Suicidal ideation [5]
Tremor (>10%) [7]
Twitching (2%)
Vertigo (dizziness) [5]

Neuromuscular/Skeletal
Arthralgia [3]
Asthenia (fatigue) [3]
Dystonia [3]
Myalgia/Myopathy (6%) [2]
Rhabdomyolysis [3]

Gastrointestinal/Hepatic
Constipation [4]
Hepatotoxicity [2]
Nausea [13]
Vomiting [5]

Respiratory
Upper respiratory tract infection [2]

Genitourinary
Priapism [2]

Ocular
Hallucinations, visual [3]

Other
Adverse effects [2]
Congenital malformations [2]
Death [5]

BUSERELIN

See: www.drugeruptiondata.com/drug/id/1326

BUSPIRONE

Trade name: BuSpar (Bristol-Myers Squibb)
Indications: Anxiety
Class: Anxiolytic, Serotonin antagonist
Half-life: 2–3 hours
Clinically important, potentially hazardous interactions with: citalopram, cobicistat/elvitegravir/emtricitabine/tenofovir alafenamide, cobicistat/elvitegravir/emtricitabine/tenofovir disoproxil, grapefruit juice, itraconazole, linezolid, nefazodone, paclitaxel, rifapentine, ritonavir, St John's wort, telithromycin, vilazodone, voriconazole
Pregnancy category: B

Hair
Alopecia [2]

Mucosal
Xerostomia (3%)

Central Nervous System
Serotonin syndrome [4]

BUSULFAN

Trade name: Myleran (GSK)
Indications: Chronic myelogenous leukemia, bone marrow disorders
Class: Alkylating agent
Half-life: 3.4 hours (after first dose)
Clinically important, potentially hazardous interactions with: acetaminophen, aldesleukin, itraconazole, metronidazole, voriconazole
Pregnancy category: D
Warning: LEUKEMOGENESIS and PANCYTOPENIA

Skin
Erythema (macular) (>10%)
Erythema multiforme [5]
Erythema nodosum [3]

Exanthems [2]
Pigmentation ('busulfan tan') (<10%) [13]
Urticaria (>10%) [5]
Vasculitis [3]

Hair
Alopecia (>10%) [7]

Mucosal
Mucositis [4]
Oral mucositis [2]
Stomatitis [2]

Central Nervous System
Neurotoxicity [3]
Seizures [3]

Gastrointestinal/Hepatic
Hepatotoxicity [4]

Respiratory
Pulmonary toxicity [3]

Endocrine/Metabolic
Gynecomastia [3]
Porphyria cutanea tarda [2]

Hematologic
Febrile neutropenia [3]

Other
Death [4]
Infection [3]

BUTABARBITAL

See: www.drugeruptiondata.com/drug/id/90

BUTALBITAL

See: www.drugeruptiondata.com/drug/id/91

BUTORPHANOL

See: www.drugeruptiondata.com/drug/id/92

C1-ESTERASE INHIBITOR

See: www.drugeruptiondata.com/drug/id/1352

CABAZITAXEL

See: www.drugeruptiondata.com/drug/id/1701

CABERGOLINE

Trade name: Dostinex (Pfizer)
Indications: Hyperprolactinemia, Parkinsonism
Class: Dopamine receptor agonist
Half-life: 63–69 hours
Clinically important, potentially hazardous interactions with: azithromycin, levomepromazine, risperidone, zuclopenthixol
Pregnancy category: B
Important contra-indications noted in the prescribing guidelines for: the elderly; nursing mothers; pediatric patients

Skin
 Edema [2]
 Hot flashes (3%)

Mucosal
 Xerostomia (2%)

Cardiovascular
 Cardiac failure [2]
 Hypotension [5]
 Myocardial toxicity [3]
 Pericarditis [4]
 Valve regurgitation [2]
 Valvulopathy [9]

Central Nervous System
 Dyskinesia [2]
 Headache (26%) [6]
 Mania [3]
 Neurotoxicity [3]
 Paresthesias (5%) [2]
 Psychosis [3]
 Somnolence (drowsiness) (<5%)
 Vertigo (dizziness) (15–17%) [6]

Neuromuscular/Skeletal
 Asthenia (fatigue) (6%) [5]

Gastrointestinal/Hepatic
 Abdominal pain (5%)
 Constipation (7–10%)
 Nausea (28%) [3]

Endocrine/Metabolic
 Mastodynia (2%)

CABOZANTINIB

Trade names: Carbometyx (Exelixis), Cometriq (Exelixis)
Indications: Metastatic medullary thyroid cancer (Cometriq), advanced renal cell carcinoma (Cabometyx)
Class: Tyrosine kinase inhibitor
Half-life: 55 hours (Cometriq); 99 hours (Cabometyx)
Clinically important, potentially hazardous interactions with: atazanavir, boceprevir, carbamazepine, clarithromycin, conivaptan, grapefruit juice, indinavir, itraconazole, ketoconazole, lopinavir, nefazodone, nelfinavir, phenobarbital, phenytoin, posaconazole, rifabutin, rifampin, rifapentine, ritonavir, saquinavir, St John's wort, telithromycin, voriconazole
Pregnancy category: D
Important contra-indications noted in the prescribing guidelines for: the elderly; nursing mothers; pediatric patients
Warning: PERFORATIONS AND FISTULAS, and HEMORRHAGE

Skin
 Erythema (11%)
 Hand–foot syndrome (50%) [16]
 Hyperkeratosis (7%)
 Jaundice (25%)
 Rash (19%)
 Toxicity [2]
 Xerosis (19%)

Hair
 Alopecia (16%)
 Hair changes (34%)
 Hair pigmentation (34%) [2]

Mucosal
 Mucosal inflammation [2]
 Stomatitis (51%)

Cardiovascular
 Chest pain (9%)
 Hypertension (33%) [13]
 Hypotension (7%)

Central Nervous System
 Anorexia [2]
 Anxiety (9%)
 Dysgeusia (taste perversion) (34%)
 Headache (18%)
 Paresthesias (7%)
 Peripheral neuropathy (5%)
 Vertigo (dizziness) (14%)

Neuromuscular/Skeletal
 Arthralgia (14%)
 Asthenia (fatigue) (21–41%) [17]
 Muscle spasm (12%)
 Pain in extremities (14%)

Gastrointestinal/Hepatic
 Abdominal pain (27%)
 Constipation (27%) [2]
 Diarrhea (63%) [15]
 Dyspepsia (11%)
 Dysphagia (13%)
 Gastrointestinal perforation (3%)
 Hemorrhoids (9%)
 Nausea (43%) [7]
 Vomiting (24%) [4]

Respiratory
 Cough (18%)
 Dysphonia (20%)
 Dyspnea (19%)
 Pulmonary embolism [2]

Endocrine/Metabolic
 ALP increased (52%)
 ALT increased (86%) [2]
 Appetite decreased (46%) [4]
 AST increased (86%) [2]
 Dehydration (7%)
 GGT increased (27%)
 Hypoalbuminemia (36%)
 Hypocalcemia (52%)
 Hypokalemia (18%)
 Hypomagnesemia (19%)
 Hyponatremia (10%)
 Hypophosphatemia (28%)
 Serum creatinine increased (58%)
 Weight loss (48%) [7]

Renal
 Proteinuria (2%)

Hematologic
 Anemia [2]
 Lymphopenia (53%)
 Neutropenia (35%) [2]
 Thrombocytopenia (35%) [2]
 Thrombosis [2]

Other
 Adverse effects [4]
 Death (6%) [5]

CALCIFEDIOL

Synonym: calcidiol
Trade name: Rayaldee (Opko)
Indications: Hyperparathyroidism in stage 3 or 4 chronic kidney disease
Class: Vitamin D analog
Half-life: 11 days
Clinically important, potentially hazardous interactions with: anticonvulsants, atazanavir, cholestyramine, clarithromycin, indinavir, itraconazole, ketoconazole, nefazodone, nelfinavir, phenobarbital, ritonavir, saquinavir, telithromycin, thiazides, voriconazole
Pregnancy category: C
Important contra-indications noted in the prescribing guidelines for: nursing mothers; pediatric patients

Skin
 Hematoma (2%)

Cardiovascular
 Congestive heart failure (4%)

Neuromuscular/Skeletal
 Arthralgia (2%)

Gastrointestinal/Hepatic
 Constipation (3%)

Respiratory
 Bronchitis (3%)
 Cough (4%)
 Dyspnea (4%)
 Nasopharyngitis (5%)

Endocrine/Metabolic
 Hyperkalemia (3%)

Hyperuricemia (2%)
Serum creatinine increased (5%)
Hematologic
Anemia (5%)

CALCIPOTRIOL

Synonym: calcipotriene
Trade name: Dovonex (Leo Pharma)
Indications: Psoriasis
Class: Antipsoriatic agent, Vitamin D analog
Half-life: ~30 minutes
Clinically important, potentially hazardous interactions with: none known
Pregnancy category: C
Important contra-indications noted in the prescribing guidelines for: nursing mothers; pediatric patients
Note: Contra-indicated in patients with acute psoriatic eruptions, hypercalcemia or vitamin D toxicity.

Skin
Burning (23%)
Contact dermatitis [8]
Erythema (<10%)
Pigmentation [3]
Pruritus (>10%) [6]
Psoriasis (<10%) [3]
Rash (11%)
Xerosis (<5%)
Respiratory
Nasopharyngitis [3]
Endocrine/Metabolic
Hypercalcemia [3]
Local
Application-site pain [3]
Application-site pruritus [2]
Application-site reactions [2]
Other
Adverse effects [3]

CALCITONIN

Trade names: Calcimar (Sanofi-Aventis), Miacalcin (Novartis)
Indications: Paget's disease of bone
Class: Parathyroid hormone antagonist
Half-life: 70–90 minutes
Clinically important, potentially hazardous interactions with: none known
Pregnancy category: C

Cardiovascular
Flushing (>10%) [5]
Gastrointestinal/Hepatic
Diarrhea [2]
Nausea [2]
Respiratory
Rhinitis (12%)
Local
Injection-site edema (>10%)
Injection-site inflammation (>10%) [2]
Injection-site reactions (10%)

CALCIUM HYDROXYLAPATITE

Trade name: Radiesse (Merz)
Indications: Correction of facial wrinkles and folds
Class: Dermal filler
Half-life: N/A
Clinically important, potentially hazardous interactions with: anticoagulants, antiplatelet drugs, aspirin

Skin
Ecchymoses [2]
Granulomas [5]
Necrosis [2]
Nodular eruption [3]
Mucosal
Oral lesions [3]

CALFACTANT

See: www.drugeruptiondata.com/drug/id/95

CANAGLIFLOZIN

Trade names: Invokamet (Janssen), Invokana (Janssen)
Indications: Type II diabetes mellitus
Class: Sodium-glucose co-transporter 2 (SGLT2) inhibitor
Half-life: 11–13 hours
Clinically important, potentially hazardous interactions with: digoxin, rifampin
Pregnancy category: C
Important contra-indications noted in the prescribing guidelines for: nursing mothers; pediatric patients
Note: Contra-indicated in patients with severe renal impairment, end stage renal disease, or on dialysis. Invokamet is canagliflozin and metformin.

Cardiovascular
Postural hypotension [2]
Central Nervous System
Headache [3]
Neuromuscular/Skeletal
Arthralgia [2]
Asthenia (fatigue) (2%)
Back pain [2]
Gastrointestinal/Hepatic
Abdominal pain (2%) [3]
Constipation (2%) [2]
Diarrhea [2]
Nausea (2%) [4]
Respiratory
Nasopharyngitis [2]
Upper respiratory tract infection [2]
Endocrine/Metabolic
Hypoglycemia [7]
Genitourinary
Genital mycotic infections (4–11%) [27]
Pollakiuria [6]

Polyuria [2]
Urinary frequency (5%) [6]
Urinary tract infection (4–6%) [20]
Vulvovaginal pruritus (2–3%) [2]
Renal
Nephrotoxicity [2]
Other
Adverse effects [3]
Dipsia (thirst) (2–3%) [3]

CANAKINUMAB

Trade name: Ilaris (Novartis)
Indications: Periodic fever syndromes, systemic juvenile idiopathic arthritis
Class: Interleukin-1 inhibitor, Monoclonal antibody
Half-life: 26 days
Clinically important, potentially hazardous interactions with: cytochrome P450, IL-1 blockers, lenalidomide, TNF-blockers
Pregnancy category: C
Important contra-indications noted in the prescribing guidelines for: nursing mothers; pediatric patients
Note: Interleukin-1 blockade may interfere with immune response to infections. Treatment with medications that work through inhibition of IL-1 has been associated with an increased risk of serious infections.

Central Nervous System
Headache [2]
Vertigo (dizziness) (11%) [2]
Neuromuscular/Skeletal
Myalgia/Myopathy (11%)
Gastrointestinal/Hepatic
Gastroenteritis (11%) [2]
Nausea (14%)
Respiratory
Bronchitis (11%)
Flu-like syndrome (20%)
Nasopharyngitis (34%) [3]
Pharyngitis (11%)
Rhinitis (17%)
Upper respiratory tract infection [4]
Endocrine/Metabolic
Weight gain (11%)
Hematologic
Macrophage activation syndrome [2]
Neutropenia [2]
Local
Injection-site reactions [4]
Other
Adverse effects [4]
Infection [11]

CANDESARTAN

Trade name: Atacand (AstraZeneca)
Indications: Hypertension and heart failure
Class: Angiotensin II receptor antagonist (blocker), Antihypertensive
Half-life: 9 hours
Clinically important, potentially hazardous interactions with: aliskiren
Pregnancy category: D
Important contra-indications noted in the prescribing guidelines for: nursing mothers; pediatric patients
Warning: FETAL TOXICITY

Skin
Angioedema [3]

Cardiovascular
Hypotension [5]

Central Nervous System
Dysgeusia (taste perversion) [2]
Headache [5]
Vertigo (dizziness) (4%) [6]

Neuromuscular/Skeletal
Back pain (3%) [3]

Gastrointestinal/Hepatic
Gastroenteritis [2]

Respiratory
Pharyngitis (2%)
Rhinitis (2%)
Upper respiratory tract infection (6%) [3]

Endocrine/Metabolic
Hyperkalemia (2%)

Renal
Renal failure [3]

Hematologic
Neutropenia [2]

Other
Adverse effects [4]
Fetotoxicity [2]

CANGRELOR

Trade name: Kengreal (Medicines Co)
Indications: Adjunct to percutaneous coronary intervention for reducing the risk of periprocedural myocardial infarction, repeat coronary revascularization and stent thrombosis
Class: Antiplatelet, Antiplatelet, cyclopentyl triazolo-pyrimidine (CPTP)
Half-life: 3–6 minutes
Clinically important, potentially hazardous interactions with: clopidogrel, prasugrel
Pregnancy category: C
Important contra-indications noted in the prescribing guidelines for: nursing mothers; pediatric patients
Note: Contra-indicated in patients with significant active bleeding.

Respiratory
Dyspnea [5]

Renal
Nephrotoxicity (3%)

Hematologic
Bleeding (<15%) [7]

CAPECITABINE

Trade name: Xeloda (Roche)
Indications: Metastatic breast or colorectal cancer, adjuvant colon cancer
Class: Antimetabolite, Antineoplastic
Half-life: 0.5–1 hour
Clinically important, potentially hazardous interactions with: allopurinol, anticoagulants, CYP2C9 substrates, erlotinib, leucovorin, phenprocoumon, phenytoin, warfarin
Pregnancy category: D
Important contra-indications noted in the prescribing guidelines for: nursing mothers
Note: Patients receiving concomitant capecitabine and oral coumarin-derivative anticoagulants such as warfarin and phenprocoumon should have their anticoagulant response (INR or prothrombin time) monitored frequently in order to adjust the anticoagulant dose accordingly. Altered coagulation parameters and/or bleeding, including death, have been reported during concomitant use.
Contra-indicated in patients with severe renal impairment or with known hypersensitivity to fluorouracil.
Warning: XELODA - WARFARIN INTERACTION

Skin
Acneform eruption [3]
Actinic keratoses [3]
Dermatitis (37%) [10]
Edema (9%) [3]
Exfoliative dermatitis (31–37%)
Hand–foot syndrome (7–58%) [167]
Jaundice [3]
Lupus erythematosus [4]
Photosensitivity [2]
Pigmentation [10]
Pruritus [2]
Radiation recall dermatitis [6]
Rash [14]
Toxicity [4]
Vitiligo [2]
Xerosis [2]

Hair
Alopecia [10]

Nails
Nail changes (7%)
Onycholysis [3]
Onychomadesis [2]
Paronychia [2]
Pyogenic granuloma [2]

Mucosal
Mucosal inflammation [2]
Mucositis [16]
Stomatitis (24%) [19]

Cardiovascular
Angina [4]
Cardiotoxicity [4]
Chest pain [3]
Coronary vasospasm [4]
Hypertension [6]
Myocardial infarction [4]
QT prolongation [2]
Thromboembolism [2]
Ventricular fibrillation [2]

Central Nervous System
Anorexia [12]
Fever [2]
Headache [2]
Leukoencephalopathy [5]
Neurotoxicity [14]
Pain [4]
Paresthesias (21%)
Peripheral neuropathy [11]
Vertigo (dizziness) [3]

Neuromuscular/Skeletal
Asthenia (fatigue) [50]
Ataxia [2]
Myalgia/Myopathy (9%) [3]
Pain in extremities [2]

Gastrointestinal/Hepatic
Abdominal pain [9]
Constipation [3]
Diarrhea [72]
Hepatotoxicity [6]
Ileus [2]
Nausea [36]
Vomiting [29]

Respiratory
Nasopharyngitis [2]

Endocrine/Metabolic
ALT increased [5]
Appetite decreased [2]
AST increased [5]
Hyperammonemia [2]
Hyperbilirubinemia [4]
Hyperglycemia [3]
Hypertriglyceridemia [2]
Hypophosphatemia [2]

Hematologic
Anemia [24]
Febrile neutropenia [4]
Hemotoxicity [2]
Leukocytopenia [3]
Leukopenia [14]
Neutropenia [44]
Thrombocytopenia [20]

Other
Adverse effects [6]
Allergic reactions [2]
Death [7]
Infection [2]

CAPREOMYCIN

See: www.drugeruptiondata.com/drug/id/1025

CAPTOPRIL

Trade names: Capoten (Par), Capozide (Par)
Indications: Hypertension, congestive heart failure, to improve survival following myocardial infarction in clinically stable patients with left ventricular dysfunction, diabetic nephropathy in patients with Type I insulin-dependent diabetes mellitus and retinopathy
Class: Angiotensin-converting enzyme (ACE) inhibitor, Antihypertensive, Vasodilator
Half-life: <3 hours
Clinically important, potentially hazardous interactions with: alcohol, aldesleukin, allopurinol, alpha blockers, alprostadil, amifostine, amiloride, angiotensin II receptor antagonists, antacids, antidiabetics, antihypertensives, antipsychotics, anxiolytics and hypnotics, aprotinin, azathioprine, baclofen, beta blockers, calcium channel blockers, clonidine, cyclosporine, CYP2D6 inhibitors, darunavir, diazoxide, digoxin, diuretics, eplerenone, estrogens, everolimus, general anesthetics, gold & gold compounds, heparins, herbals, hydralazine, hypotensives, insulin, interferon alfa, levodopa, lithium, MAO inhibitors, metformin, methyldopa, methylphenidate, minoxidil, moxisylyte, moxonidine, naldemedine, nitrates, nitroprusside, NSAIDs, pentoxifylline, phosphodiesterase 5 inhibitors, potassium salts, probenecid, prostacyclin analogues, rituximab, salicylates, sirolimus, spironolactone, sulfonylureas, temsirolimus, tizanidine, tolvaptan, triamterene, trimethoprim, venetoclax, yohimbine
Pregnancy category: D (category C in first trimester; category D in second and third trimesters)
Important contra-indications noted in the prescribing guidelines for: nursing mothers; pediatric patients
Note: Capozide is captopril and hydrochlorothiazide. Hydrochlorothiazide is a sulfonamide and can be absorbed systemically. Sulfonamides can produce severe, possibly fatal, reactions such as toxic epidermal necrolysis and Stevens-Johnson syndrome.
Warning: FETAL TOXICITY

Skin

Angioedema (<15%) [45]
Bullous pemphigoid [2]
Dermatitis [3]
DRESS syndrome [2]
Erythroderma [2]
Exanthems (4–7%) [19]
Exfoliative dermatitis (<2%) [4]
Kaposi's sarcoma [2]
Lichen planus pemphigoides [2]
Lichenoid eruption [12]
Linear IgA bullous dermatosis [5]
Lupus erythematosus [8]
Mycosis fungoides [2]
Pemphigus (<2%) [23]
Pemphigus foliaceus [2]
Penile ulceration [2]
Photosensitivity [3]
Phototoxicity (<2%)
Pigmentation [2]
Pityriasis rosea (<2%) [6]
Pruritus (<7%) [8]
Pseudolymphoma [2]
Psoriasis [8]
Rash (4–7%) [12]
Toxic epidermal necrolysis [3]
Urticaria [9]
Vasculitis [7]

Hair

Alopecia (<2%) [4]

Nails

Nail dystrophy [2]
Onycholysis [2]

Mucosal

Aphthous stomatitis (<2%) [5]
Glossitis [3]
Oral mucosal eruption [3]
Oral ulceration [4]
Sialadenitis [2]
Tongue ulceration [3]
Xerostomia (<2%)

Cardiovascular

Flushing [2]

Central Nervous System

Ageusia (taste loss) (2–4%) [11]
Dysgeusia (taste perversion) (metallic or salty taste) (2–4%) [14]
Hallucinations [2]
Paresthesias (<2%)

Gastrointestinal/Hepatic

Hepatotoxicity [3]
Nausea [2]

Respiratory

Cough [19]

Endocrine/Metabolic

Gynecomastia [3]

Renal

Nephrotoxicity [2]

Other

Adverse effects [4]
Allergic reactions [2]

CARBACHOL

See: www.drugeruptiondata.com/drug/id/1042

CARBAMAZEPINE

Trade names: Epitol (Teva), Tegretol (Novartis)
Indications: Epilepsy, pain or trigeminal neuralgia
Class: Anticonvulsant, Antipsychotic, CYP1A2 inducer, CYP3A4 inducer, Mood stabilizer
Half-life: 18–55 hours
Clinically important, potentially hazardous interactions with: abiraterone, acetaminophen, acetylcysteine, adenosine, afatinib, amitriptyline, amlodipine, amprenavir, apixaban, apremilast, aprepitant, aripiprazole, artemether/lumefantrine, boceprevir, brigatinib, brivaracetam, buprenorphine, cabazitaxel, cabozantinib, caffeine, caspofungin, cefixime, ceritinib, charcoal, citalopram, clarithromycin, clobazam, clopidogrel, clorazepate, clozapine, cobicistat/elvitegravir/emtricitabine/tenofovir disoproxil, cobimetinib, copanlisib, crizotinib, dabigatran, daclatasvir, darunavir, dasabuvir/ombitasvir/paritaprevir/ritonavir, dasatinib, deflazacort, delavirdine, dexamethasone, diltiazem, doxacurium, doxycycline, dronedarone, efavirenz, elbasvir & grazoprevir, eliglustat, emtricitabine/rilpivirine/tenofovir alafenamide, enzalutamide, erythromycin, eslicarbazepine, estradiol, ethosuximide, etravirine, ezogabine, felodipine, fesoterodine, flibanserin, fosamprenavir, gefitinib, glecaprevir & pibrentasvir, ibrutinib, idelalisib, imatinib, indinavir, influenza vaccine, isavuconazonium sulfate, isotretinoin, itraconazole, ixabepilone, ixazomib, lacosamide, lapatinib, ledipasvir & sofosbuvir, lesinurad, levetiracetam, levomepromazine, levonorgestrel, linezolid, lopinavir, methylprednisolone, midazolam, midostaurin, mifepristone, naldemedine, nelfinavir, neratinib, nevirapine, nifedipine, nilotinib, nintedanib, olanzapine, olaparib, ombitasvir/paritaprevir/ritonavir, ondansetron, osimertinib, oxcarbazepine, oxtriphylline, paclitaxel, palbociclib, paliperidone, perampanel, pimavanserin, piracetam, ponatinib, prednisolone, propoxyphene, regorafenib, rilpivirine, riociguat, risperidone, ritonavir, rivaroxaban, roflumilast, romidepsin, rufinamide, simeprevir, simvastatin, sodium picosulfate, sofosbuvir, sofosbuvir & velpatasvir, sofosbuvir/velpatasvir/voxilaprevir, solifenacin, sonidegib, sorafenib, St John's wort, sunitinib, telaprevir, telithromycin, temsirolimus, tenofovir alafenamide, terbinafine, thalidomide, tiagabine, ticagrelor, tipranavir, tolvaptan, tramadol, triamcinolone, troleandomycin, ulipristal, valbenazine, vandetanib, vemurafenib, venetoclax, verapamil, vorapaxar, voriconazole, vortioxetine, ziprasidone, zuclopenthixol
Pregnancy category: D
Note: Carbamazepine is the main cause of Stevens-Johnson syndrome (SJS), toxic epidermal necrolysis (TEN), and the hypersensitivity syndrome in Han Chinese, and in peoples of other Southeast Asian countries, as a result of a strong pharmacogenetic association that has been reported in these patients between the human leukocyte antigen (HLA)-B*1502 and carbamazepine.
Warning: SERIOUS DERMATOLOGIC REACTIONS AND HLA-B*1502 ALLELE; APLASTIC ANEMIA AND AGRANULOCYTOSIS

Skin

AGEP [5]
Angioedema [5]
Anticonvulsant hypersensitivity syndrome [19]
Bullous dermatitis [4]
Dermatitis [7]
Diaphoresis (<10%)
DRESS syndrome [48]
Eczema [2]
Erythema multiforme [16]
Erythroderma [12]
Exanthems (>5%) [35]
Exfoliative dermatitis [24]
Facial edema [2]
Fixed eruption [10]
Hypersensitivity [71]
Lichen planus [2]
Lichenoid eruption [8]
Lupus erythematosus [35]
Lymphoma [2]

Lymphoproliferative disease [5]
Mycosis fungoides [3]
Pemphigus [3]
Photosensitivity [9]
Pruritus [7]
Pseudolymphoma [17]
Purpura [8]
Pustules [5]
Rash (>10%) [30]
Serum sickness [2]
Stevens-Johnson syndrome (<10%) [98]
Toxic epidermal necrolysis (<10%) [88]
Toxic pustuloderma [3]
Toxicity [2]
Urticaria [14]
Vasculitis [7]

Hair
Alopecia [7]

Mucosal
Mucocutaneous eruption [4]
Mucocutaneous lymph node syndrome
  (Kawasaki syndrome) [2]
Oral ulceration [2]
Tongue ulceration [2]

Cardiovascular
Bradycardia [3]
Myocarditis [2]

Central Nervous System
Ageusia (taste loss) [3]
Coma [2]
Dysgeusia (taste perversion) [2]
Headache [5]
Memory loss [2]
Seizures [12]
Somnolence (drowsiness) [8]
Tic disorder [4]
Vertigo (dizziness) [8]

Neuromuscular/Skeletal
Asthenia (fatigue) [3]
Ataxia [5]
Myasthenia gravis [2]
Osteoporosis [2]

Gastrointestinal/Hepatic
Diarrhea [2]
Hepatotoxicity [11]
Nausea [5]
Pancreatitis [3]
Vanishing bile duct syndrome [4]
Vomiting [3]

Endocrine/Metabolic
Acute intermittent porphyria [5]
Hyponatremia [4]
SIADH [17]
Weight gain [5]

Renal
Nephrotoxicity [2]

Hematologic
Agranulocytosis [2]
Leukopenia [3]
Thrombocytopenia [3]

Otic
Hallucinations, auditory [2]

Ocular
Diplopia [2]

Other
Adverse effects [8]
Allergic reactions [9]

Death [6]
Side effects [3]
Teratogenicity [12]

CARBENICILLIN

See: www.drugeruptiondata.com/drug/id/100

CARBETOCIN

See: www.drugeruptiondata.com/drug/id/1372

CARBIMAZOLE

See: www.drugeruptiondata.com/drug/id/1277

CARBINOXAMINE

See: www.drugeruptiondata.com/drug/id/1026

CARBOPLATIN

Trade name: Paraplatin (Bristol-Myers Squibb)
Indications: Various carcinomas and sarcomas
Class: Alkylating agent, Antineoplastic
Half-life: terminal: 22–40 hours
**Clinically important, potentially hazardous
interactions with:** aldesleukin, bexarotene
Pregnancy category: D
**Important contra-indications noted in the
prescribing guidelines for:** the elderly; nursing
mothers; pediatric patients

Skin
Anaphylactoid reactions/Anaphylaxis [5]
Erythema (2%) [2]
Exanthems [3]
Hand–foot syndrome [4]
Hypersensitivity (2%) [27]
Pigmentation [2]
Pruritus (2%) [2]
Radiation recall dermatitis [2]
Rash (2%) [9]
Scleroderma [2]
Toxicity [5]
Urticaria (2%) [4]

Hair
Alopecia (3%) [16]
Alopecia areata [2]

Mucosal
Epistaxis (nosebleed) [2]
Mucositis [4]
Stomatitis (>10%) [2]

Cardiovascular
Flushing [3]
Hypertension [7]

Central Nervous System
Anorexia [7]
Headache [2]
Leukoencephalopathy [2]
Neurotoxicity [15]
Pain [2]

Paresthesias [2]
Peripheral neuropathy [8]
Vertigo (dizziness) [2]

Neuromuscular/Skeletal
Asthenia (fatigue) [22]
Myalgia/Myopathy [2]

Gastrointestinal/Hepatic
Constipation [3]
Diarrhea [13]
Dyspepsia [2]
Gastrointestinal perforation [2]
Hepatotoxicity [4]
Nausea [15]
Pancreatitis [2]
Vomiting [16]

Respiratory
Cough [2]
Hemoptysis [2]
Pneumonia [2]
Pulmonary toxicity [3]

Endocrine/Metabolic
ALT increased [3]
AST increased [2]
Hyperglycemia [5]
Hyponatremia [3]
SIADH [3]

Renal
Nephrotoxicity [9]

Hematologic
Anemia [25]
Febrile neutropenia [18]
Hemorrhage [2]
Hemotoxicity [8]
Leukopenia [11]
Lymphopenia [2]
Myelosuppression [2]
Myelotoxicity [2]
Neutropenia [48]
Pancytopenia [2]
Thrombocytopenia [35]

Otic
Ototoxicity [7]
Tinnitus [3]

Local
Injection-site pain (>10%)

Other
Adverse effects [2]
Allergic reactions [3]
Death [4]
Infection [5]

CARFILZOMIB

Trade name: Kyprolis (Onyx)
Indications: Multiple myeloma
Class: Proteasome inhibitor
Half-life: ~1 hour
**Clinically important, potentially hazardous
interactions with:** none known
Pregnancy category: D
**Important contra-indications noted in the
prescribing guidelines for:** nursing mothers;
pediatric patients

Skin
Herpes zoster (reactivation) (2%) [2]

Peripheral edema (24%) [3]
Tumor lysis syndrome [2]

Cardiovascular
Cardiac failure (7%) [2]
Cardiotoxicity [6]
Chest pain (11%)
Hypertension (14%) [6]

Central Nervous System
Anorexia (12%)
Chills (16%)
Fever (30%) [7]
Headache (28%) [3]
Hypoesthesia (12%)
Insomnia (18%) [2]
Pain (12%)
Peripheral neuropathy (14%) [14]
Vertigo (dizziness) (13%)

Neuromuscular/Skeletal
Arthralgia (16%)
Asthenia (fatigue) (13–56%) [16]
Back pain (20%)
Muscle spasm (14%) [2]
Pain in extremities (13%)

Gastrointestinal/Hepatic
Constipation (21%) [3]
Diarrhea (33%) [6]
Nausea (45%) [14]
Vomiting (22%) [4]

Respiratory
Cough (26%) [5]
Dyspnea (35%) [10]
Pneumonia (13%) [6]
Pulmonary hypertension (2%)
Upper respiratory tract infection (28%) [5]

Endocrine/Metabolic
AST increased (13%)
Hypercalcemia (11%)
Hyperglycemia (12%) [3]
Hypokalemia (14%) [3]
Hypomagnesemia (14%)
Hyponatremia (10%) [2]
Hypophosphatemia (11%) [3]
Serum creatinine increased [5]

Renal
Nephrotoxicity [3]

Hematologic
Anemia (47%) [20]
Hemotoxicity [2]
Leukopenia (14%) [4]
Lymphopenia (24%) [7]
Neutropenia (21%) [10]
Thrombocytopenia (36%) [18]

Other
Adverse effects [3]

CARGLUMIC ACID

See: www.drugeruptiondata.com/drug/id/1671

CARIPRAZINE

Trade name: Vraylar (Forest)
Indications: Schizophrenia, manic or mixed episodes associated with bipolar I disorder
Class: Antipsychotic
Half-life: 2–4 days
Clinically important, potentially hazardous interactions with: CYP3A4 inducers
Pregnancy category: N/A (Neonatal risk in third trimester exposure)
Important contra-indications noted in the prescribing guidelines for: the elderly; nursing mothers; pediatric patients
Warning: INCREASED MORTALITY IN ELDERLY PATIENTS WITH DEMENTIA-RELATED PSYCHOSIS

Skin
Rash (<2%)

Mucosal
Oropharyngeal pain (<3%)
Xerostomia (<3%)

Cardiovascular
Hypertension (2–6%)
Tachycardia (<3%)

Central Nervous System
Agitation (3–5%)
Akathisia (20–21%) [23]
Anxiety (3–6%) [3]
Extrapyramidal symptoms (15–29%) [18]
Fever (<4%) [4]
Headache (9–18%) [10]
Insomnia (8–13%) [13]
Mania (worsening) [2]
Parkinsonism (13–26%) [4]
Restlessness (4–7%) [8]
Schizophrenia (worsening) [3]
Sedation [7]
Somnolence (drowsiness) (5–10%) [4]
Tremor [10]
Vertigo (dizziness) (3–7%) [8]

Neuromuscular/Skeletal
Arthralgia (<2%)
Asthenia (fatigue) (<5%)
Back pain (<3%)
Dystonia (2–5%) [2]
Pain in extremities [2]

Gastrointestinal/Hepatic
Abdominal pain (3–8%) [2]
Constipation (6–11%) [11]
Diarrhea (<5%) [5]
Dyspepsia (4–9%) [6]
Hepatotoxicity (<3%)
Nausea (5–13%) [11]
Vomiting (4–10%) [9]

Respiratory
Cough (<4%)
Nasopharyngitis (<2%)

Endocrine/Metabolic
Appetite decreased (<4%)
Creatine phosphokinase increased (<3%)
Weight gain (2–3%) [7]

Genitourinary
Urinary tract infection (<2%)

Ocular
Vision blurred (4%) [3]

Other
Adverse effects [3]
Toothache (3–6%) [2]

CARISOPRODOL

Trade name: Soma (MedPointe)
Indications: Painful musculoskeletal disorders
Class: Central muscle relaxant
Half-life: 4–6 hours
Clinically important, potentially hazardous interactions with: CNS depressants, eucalyptus, meprobamate
Pregnancy category: C
Important contra-indications noted in the prescribing guidelines for: the elderly; nursing mothers; pediatric patients
Note: Contra-indicated in patients with acute intermittent porphyria.

Skin
Angioedema (<10%)
Fixed eruption [2]
Urticaria [2]

Cardiovascular
Flushing (<10%)

Central Nervous System
Amnesia [2]
Trembling (<10%)

Other
Death [2]

CARMUSTINE

Trade names: BiCNU (Bristol-Myers Squibb), Gliadel Wafer (Guilford)
Indications: Brain tumors, Hodgkin's disease, multiple myeloma
Class: Alkylating agent, Nitrosourea
Half-life: initial: 1.4 minutes; secondary: 20 minutes
Clinically important, potentially hazardous interactions with: aldesleukin, cimetidine, clorazepate
Pregnancy category: D
Important contra-indications noted in the prescribing guidelines for: nursing mothers; pediatric patients

Skin
Dermatitis [3]
Pigmentation (on accidental contact) [2]
Telangiectasia [2]

Hair
Alopecia (<10%)

Mucosal
Stomatitis (<10%)

Cardiovascular
Flushing (<10%) [2]

Central Nervous System
Intracranial hemorrhage [2]
Meningococcal infection [2]
Seizures [2]

Neuromuscular/Skeletal
Asthenia (fatigue) [2]

Gastrointestinal/Hepatic
Nausea [2]
Vomiting [2]

Hematologic
Leukopenia [2]
Thrombocytopenia [2]

Local
Injection-site burning (>10%)

CARTEOLOL

See: www.drugeruptiondata.com/drug/id/105

CARVEDILOL

Trade name: Coreg (GSK)
Indications: Hypertension
Class: Adrenergic beta-receptor antagonist
Half-life: 7–10 hours
Clinically important, potentially hazardous interactions with: cinacalcet, delavirdine, efavirenz, irbesartan, leflunomide, propafenone, trimethoprim, venetoclax, voriconazole, zafirlukast
Pregnancy category: C
Important contra-indications noted in the prescribing guidelines for: nursing mothers; pediatric patients

Skin
Diaphoresis (3%)
Edema (generalized) (5–6%) [2]
Peripheral edema (<7%)
Purpura (<3%)

Cardiovascular
Angina (2–6%)
Atrial fibrillation [2]
Atrioventricular block (<3%)
Bradycardia (2–10%) [7]
Cardiac failure [2]
Congestive heart failure [2]
Extrasystoles [2]
Hypertension (<3%)
Hypotension (9–14%) [8]
Palpitation (<3%)
Postural hypotension (<3%)

Central Nervous System
Fever (<3%)
Headache (5–8%) [2]
Pain (9%)
Paresthesias (2%)
Somnolence (drowsiness) (<3%)
Syncope (3–8%)
Vertigo (dizziness) (24–32%) [5]

Neuromuscular/Skeletal
Arthralgia (<6%)
Asthenia (fatigue) (7–24%) [2]
Muscle spasm (<3%)
Myalgia/Myopathy (3%)

Gastrointestinal/Hepatic
Black stools (<3%)
Diarrhea (2–12%)
Nausea (4–9%)
Vomiting (<6%)

Respiratory
Cough (5–8%)
Dyspnea [4]
Stridor [2]

Endocrine/Metabolic
ALP increased (<3%) [2]
Creatine phosphokinase increased (<3%) [3]
Diabetes mellitus (<3%)
GGT increased (<3%)
Hypercholesterolemia (<4%)
Hyperglycemia (5–12%)
Hyperkalemia (<3%) [2]
Hyperuricemia (<3%)
Hypervolemia (<3%)
Hypoglycemia (<3%)
Hyponatremia (<3%)
Hypovolemia (<3%)
Weight gain (10–12%)
Weight loss (<3%)

Genitourinary
Albuminuria (<3%)
Hematuria (<3%)
Impotence (<3%)

Hematologic
Anemia [2]
Prothrombin time decreased (<3%)
Thrombocytopenia (<3%)

Ocular
Abnormal vision (5%)
Vision blurred (<3%)

Other
Adverse effects [8]
Infection (2%)

CASPOFUNGIN

Trade name: Cancidas (Merck)
Indications: Invasive *Aspergillus* and *Candida* infections
Class: Antifungal
Half-life: beta phase: 9–11 hours; terminal: 40–50 hours
Clinically important, potentially hazardous interactions with: carbamazepine, cyclosporine, dexamethasone, efavirenz, nevirapine, phenytoin, rifampin, tacrolimus
Pregnancy category: C
Important contra-indications noted in the prescribing guidelines for: nursing mothers; pediatric patients

Skin
Anaphylactoid reactions/Anaphylaxis (<2%)
Edema (~3%)
Erythema (<4%)
Facial edema (3%)
Jaundice (<5%)
Peripheral edema (11%)
Petechiae (<5%)
Pruritus (2–7%)
Rash (4–16%) [5]
Septic–toxic shock (11–13%)
Ulcerations (3%)
Urticaria (<5%)
Vasculitis (2%)

Mucosal
Epistaxis (nosebleed) (<5%)
Mucosal inflammation (6–10%)

Cardiovascular
Arrhythmias (<5%)
Atrial fibrillation (<5%)
Bradycardia (<5%)
Cardiac arrest (<5%)
Flushing (3%)
Hypertension (5–10%)
Hypotension (6–12%)
Myocardial infarction (<5%)
Phlebitis (18%) [3]
Tachycardia (4–7%)
Thrombophlebitis [2]

Central Nervous System
Anxiety (<5%)
Chills (9–23%)
Confusion (<5%)
Depression (<5%)
Fever (6–29%) [8]
Headache (5–15%) [3]
Insomnia (<5%)
Pain (<5%)
Paresthesias (<3%)
Seizures (<5%)
Tremor (<2%)
Vertigo (dizziness) (<5%)

Neuromuscular/Skeletal
Arthralgia (<5%)
Asthenia (fatigue) (<5%)
Back pain (<5%)
Myalgia/Myopathy (~3%)
Pain in extremities (<5%)

Gastrointestinal/Hepatic
Abdominal distension (<5%)
Abdominal pain (7–9%)
Constipation (<5%)
Diarrhea (6–27%)
Dyspepsia (<5%)
Hepatic failure (<5%)
Hepatotoxicity (<5%) [8]
Nausea (5–15%) [2]
Vomiting (9–17%) [2]

Respiratory
Cough (6–11%)
Dyspnea (9%)
Flu-like syndrome (3%)
Hypoxia (<5%)
Pleural effusion (9%)
Pneumonia (4–11%)
Respiratory distress (8%)
Respiratory failure (6–11%)
Tachypnea (8%)

Endocrine/Metabolic
ALP increased (12–23%) [4]
ALT increased (4–18%) [4]
Appetite decreased (<5%)
AST increased (6–16%) [5]
Hypercalcemia (<5%)
Hyperglycemia (<5%)
Hypokalemia (6–8%) [3]
Hypomagnesemia (<5%)

Genitourinary
Hematuria (<5%)
Urinary tract infection (<5%)

Renal
Nephrotoxicity [5]

Renal failure (<5%)
Hematologic
Anemia (2–11%)
Coagulopathy (<5%)
Eosinophilia [2]
Febrile neutropenia (<5%)
Neutropenia (<5%)
Sepsis (5%)
Thrombocytopenia (<5%) [2]
Local
Infusion-related reactions [4]
Infusion-site pain (<5%)
Infusion-site reactions (<5%) [2]
Injection-site induration (~3%)
Injection-site reactions (2–12%) [4]
Other
Adverse effects [8]

CEFACLOR

Trade name: Ceclor (Lilly)
Indications: Various infections caused by susceptible organisms
Class: Cephalosporin, 2nd generation
Half-life: 0.6–0.9 hours
Clinically important, potentially hazardous interactions with: none known
Pregnancy category: B
Important contra-indications noted in the prescribing guidelines for: the elderly; nursing mothers; pediatric patients
Note: Penicillin and cephalosporins share a common beta-lactam structure. People who are allergic to penicillin are approximately 4 times more likely to develop an allergic reaction to a cephalosporin than those people who have no penicillin allergy (from 5–16% of patients allergic to penicillin develop reactions to cephalosporins).

Skin
AGEP [2]
Anaphylactoid reactions/Anaphylaxis [4]
Erythema multiforme [6]
Exanthems [9]
Fixed eruption [2]
Pruritus [4]
Purpura [2]
Rash (<2%) [2]
Serum sickness [7]
Serum sickness-like reaction [23]
Urticaria [5]
Gastrointestinal/Hepatic
Diarrhea [2]
Other
Adverse effects [3]

CEFADROXIL

Trade name: Duricef (Warner Chilcott)
Indications: Various infections caused by susceptible organisms
Class: Cephalosporin, 1st generation
Half-life: 1.2–1.5 hours
Clinically important, potentially hazardous interactions with: none known

Pregnancy category: B
Important contra-indications noted in the prescribing guidelines for: nursing mothers
Note: Penicillin and cephalosporins share a common beta-lactam structure. People who are allergic to penicillin are approximately 4 times more likely to develop an allergic reaction to a cephalosporin than those people who have no penicillin allergy (from 5–16% of patients allergic to penicillin develop reactions to cephalosporins).

Skin
Urticaria [2]
Gastrointestinal/Hepatic
Diarrhea [2]
Nausea [2]
Other
Adverse effects [3]

CEFAMANDOLE

See: www.drugeruptiondata.com/drug/id/109

CEFAZOLIN

See: www.drugeruptiondata.com/drug/id/110

CEFDINIR

Trade name: Omnicef (Medicis)
Indications: Community-acquired pneumonia and various infections caused by susceptible organisms
Class: Cephalosporin, 3rd generation
Half-life: 1–2 hours
Clinically important, potentially hazardous interactions with: none known
Pregnancy category: B
Important contra-indications noted in the prescribing guidelines for: pediatric patients
Note: Penicillin and cephalosporins share a common beta-lactam structure. People who are allergic to penicillin are approximately 4 times more likely to develop an allergic reaction to a cephalosporin than those people who have no penicillin allergy (from 5–16% of patients allergic to penicillin develop reactions to cephalosporins).

Skin
Rash (3%)
Gastrointestinal/Hepatic
Red stools [2]
Genitourinary
Vulvovaginal candidiasis (5%)
Other
Adverse effects [2]

CEFDITOREN

See: www.drugeruptiondata.com/drug/id/903

CEFEPIME

Trade name: Maxipime (Elan)
Indications: Various infections caused by susceptible organisms
Class: Cephalosporin, 4th generation
Half-life: 2–2.3 hours
Clinically important, potentially hazardous interactions with: none known
Pregnancy category: B
Important contra-indications noted in the prescribing guidelines for: the elderly; nursing mothers
Note: Penicillin and cephalosporins share a common beta-lactam structure. People who are allergic to penicillin are approximately 4 times more likely to develop an allergic reaction to a cephalosporin than those people who have no penicillin allergy (from 5–16% of patients allergic to penicillin develop reactions to cephalosporins).

Skin
Exanthems (2%)
Hypersensitivity [2]
Lupus erythematosus [2]
Pruritus [3]
Rash (51%) [12]
Central Nervous System
Encephalopathy [10]
Headache [3]
Neurotoxicity [14]
Seizures [16]
Status epilepticus [5]
Neuromuscular/Skeletal
Myoclonus [2]
Local
Injection-site reactions (3%) [2]
Other
Adverse effects [2]

CEFIXIME

Trade name: Suprax (Lupin)
Indications: Various infections caused by susceptible organisms
Class: Cephalosporin, 3rd generation
Half-life: 3–4 hours
Clinically important, potentially hazardous interactions with: aminoglycosides, anticoagulants, BCG vaccine, carbamazepine, probenecid, typhoid vaccine, warfarin
Pregnancy category: B
Important contra-indications noted in the prescribing guidelines for: nursing mothers; pediatric patients
Note: Penicillin and cephalosporins share a common beta-lactam structure. People who are allergic to penicillin are approximately 4 times more likely to develop an allergic reaction to a cephalosporin than those people who have no penicillin allergy (from 5–16% of patients allergic to penicillin develop reactions to cephalosporins).

Skin
Anaphylactoid reactions/Anaphylaxis (<2%)
Angioedema (<2%)
Erythema multiforme (<2%)

Facial edema (<2%)
Jaundice (<2%)
Pruritus (<2%)
Pruritus ani et vulvae (<2%)
Rash (<2%) [2]
Serum sickness-like reaction (<2%)
Stevens-Johnson syndrome (<2%)
Toxic epidermal necrolysis (<2%)
Urticaria (<2%) [2]

Central Nervous System
Fever (<2%)

Gastrointestinal/Hepatic
Abdominal pain (3%)
Diarrhea (16%)
Dyspepsia (3%)
Flatulence (4%)
Hepatitis (<2%)
Loose stools (6%)
Nausea (7%)
Pseudomembranous colitis (<2%)

Endocrine/Metabolic
ALP increased (<2%)
Creatine phosphokinase increased (<2%)

Genitourinary
Vaginitis (<2%)
Vulvovaginal candidiasis (<2%)

Renal
Renal failure (<2%)

CEFMETAZOLE

See: www.drugeruptiondata.com/drug/id/114

CEFONICID

See: www.drugeruptiondata.com/drug/id/115

CEFOPERAZONE

See: www.drugeruptiondata.com/drug/id/116

CEFOTAXIME

Trade name: Claforan (Sanofi-Aventis)
Indications: Various infections caused by
susceptible organisms
Class: Cephalosporin, 3rd generation
Half-life: 1 hour (adults)
**Clinically important, potentially hazardous
interactions with:** none known
Pregnancy category: B
**Important contra-indications noted in the
prescribing guidelines for:** nursing mothers
Note: Penicillin and cephalosporins share a
common beta-lactam structure. People who are
allergic to penicillin are approximately 4 times
more likely to develop an allergic reaction to a
cephalosporin than those people who have no
penicillin allergy (from 5–16% of patients allergic
to penicillin develop reactions to cephalosporins).

Skin
Anaphylactoid reactions/Anaphylaxis (2%)

DRESS syndrome [4]
Erythema multiforme [2]
Exanthems [3]
Hypersensitivity [2]
Pruritus (2%) [3]
Rash (2%) [3]
Urticaria (2%)

Local
Injection-site inflammation (4%)
Injection-site pain (<10%)

Other
Adverse effects [2]

CEFOTETAN

Indications: Various infections caused by
susceptible organisms
Class: Cephalosporin, 2nd generation
Half-life: 3–5 hours
**Clinically important, potentially hazardous
interactions with:** none known
Pregnancy category: B
**Important contra-indications noted in the
prescribing guidelines for:** nursing mothers;
pediatric patients
Note: Penicillin and cephalosporins share a
common beta-lactam structure. People who are
allergic to penicillin are approximately 4 times
more likely to develop an allergic reaction to a
cephalosporin than those people who have no
penicillin allergy (from 5–16% of patients allergic
to penicillin develop reactions to cephalosporins).

Skin
Anaphylactoid reactions/Anaphylaxis [3]
Rash [2]

Hematologic
Hemolytic anemia [12]

Other
Death [5]

CEFOXITIN

See: www.drugeruptiondata.com/drug/id/119

CEFPODOXIME

See: www.drugeruptiondata.com/drug/id/120

CEFPROZIL

See: www.drugeruptiondata.com/drug/id/121

CEFTAROLINE FOSAMIL

Trade name: Teflaro (Forest)
Indications: Acute bacterial skin and skin
structure infections, community-acquired
bacterial pneumonia
Class: Antibacterial, Cephalosporin, 5th
generation
Half-life: 3 hours
**Clinically important, potentially hazardous
interactions with:** BCG vaccine, probenecid,
typhoid vaccine
Pregnancy category: B
**Important contra-indications noted in the
prescribing guidelines for:** the elderly; nursing
mothers; pediatric patients
Note: Penicillin and cephalosporins share a
common beta-lactam structure. People who are
allergic to penicillin are approximately 4 times
more likely to develop an allergic reaction to a
cephalosporin than those people who have no
penicillin allergy (from 5–16% of patients allergic
to penicillin develop reactions to cephalosporins).

Skin
Anaphylactoid reactions/Anaphylaxis (<2%)
Hypersensitivity (<2%) [2]
Pruritus [7]
Rash (3%) [9]
Urticaria (<2%)

Cardiovascular
Bradycardia (<2%)
Hypertension [2]
Palpitation (<2%)
Phlebitis (2%) [3]

Central Nervous System
Fever (<2%)
Headache [9]
Insomnia [5]
Seizures (<2%)
Vertigo (dizziness) (<2%)

Gastrointestinal/Hepatic
Abdominal pain (<2%)
Colitis (<2%)
Constipation (2%)
Diarrhea (5%) [10]
Hepatotoxicity (<2%)
Nausea (4%) [9]
Vomiting (2%)

Respiratory
Eosinophilic pneumonia [3]

Endocrine/Metabolic
ALT increased (2%)
Hyperglycemia (<2%)
Hyperkalemia (<2%)
Hypokalemia (2%) [2]

Renal
Renal failure (<2%)

Hematologic
Anemia (<2%)
Eosinophilia (<2%) [2]
Neutropenia (<2%) [3]
Thrombocytopenia (<2%)

Other
Adverse effects [4]
Infection [2]

CEFTAZIDIME

Trade names: Ceptaz (GSK), Fortaz (Concordia), Tazicef (Hospira)
Indications: Various infections caused by susceptible organisms
Class: Cephalosporin, 3rd generation
Half-life: 1–2 hours
Clinically important, potentially hazardous interactions with: none known
Pregnancy category: B
Important contra-indications noted in the prescribing guidelines for: the elderly; nursing mothers
Note: Penicillin and cephalosporins share a common beta-lactam structure. People who are allergic to penicillin are approximately 4 times more likely to develop an allergic reaction to a cephalosporin than those people who have no penicillin allergy (from 5–16% of patients allergic to penicillin develop reactions to cephalosporins). See also separate profile for Ceftazidime & Avibactam.

Skin
Anaphylactoid reactions/Anaphylaxis (2%) [3]
Angioedema (2%)
Erythema multiforme (2%)
Hypersensitivity (2%)
Pemphigus erythematodes [2]
Pruritus (2%) [3]
Rash (2%) [5]
Stevens-Johnson syndrome (2%)
Toxic epidermal necrolysis (2%)
Central Nervous System
Encephalopathy [2]
Seizures [3]
Local
Injection-site inflammation (2%)
Injection-site reactions [2]
Injection-site thrombophlebitis (2%)
Other
Adverse effects [3]
Death [2]

CEFTAZIDIME & AVIBACTAM

Trade name: Avycaz (Cerexa)
Indications: Various infections caused by susceptible organisms
Class: Antibiotic, beta-lactam (avibactam), Cephalosporin, 3rd generation (ceftazidime)
Half-life: <3 hours
Clinically important, potentially hazardous interactions with: probenecid
Pregnancy category: B
Important contra-indications noted in the prescribing guidelines for: the elderly; nursing mothers; pediatric patients
Note: See also separate entry for ceftazidime.

Skin
Rash (<5%)
Central Nervous System
Anxiety (10%) [3]
Fever [4]
Headache [3]
Vertigo (dizziness) (6%)
Gastrointestinal/Hepatic
Abdominal pain (7%) [5]
Constipation (10%) [2]
Diarrhea [5]
Hepatotoxicity [4]
Nausea (2%) [5]
Vomiting [5]
Endocrine/Metabolic
ALP increased (3%)
ALT increased (3%) [3]
AST increased [3]
GGT increased (<5%)
Renal
Nephrotoxicity (<5%)
Renal failure (<5%) [4]
Hematologic
Eosinophilia (<5%)
Prothrombin time increased (<5%)
Thrombocytopenia (<5%)
Local
Injection-site reactions [4]
Other
Adverse effects [2]

CEFTIBUTEN

See: www.drugeruptiondata.com/drug/id/123

CEFTIZOXIME

See: www.drugeruptiondata.com/drug/id/124

CEFTOBIPROLE

Trade names: BAL5788 (Basilea) (Cilag AG), Zeftera (Janssen)
Indications: Bacterial infections, MRSA
Class: Cephalosporin, 5th generation
Half-life: 3 hours
Clinically important, potentially hazardous interactions with: alcohol, anticoagulants, BCG vaccine, carbenicillin, dipyridamole, heparin, pentoxifylline, plicamycin, sulfinpyrazone, ticarcillin, typhoid vaccine, valproic acid
Pregnancy category: N/A (not recommended in pregnancy)
Important contra-indications noted in the prescribing guidelines for: nursing mothers; pediatric patients
Note: Penicillin and cephalosporins share a common beta-lactam structure. People who are allergic to penicillin are approximately 4 times more likely to develop an allergic reaction to a cephalosporin than those people who have no penicillin allergy (from 5–16% of patients allergic to penicillin develop reactions to cephalosporins).

Skin
Erythema (9%)
Pruritus (9%)
Central Nervous System
Dysgeusia (taste perversion) (8%) [3]
Headache [2]
Gastrointestinal/Hepatic
Abdominal pain [2]
Diarrhea [4]
Nausea [6]
Vomiting [4]
Endocrine/Metabolic
Hyponatremia [2]
Local
Infusion-site reactions [2]
Other
Adverse effects [3]

CEFTOLOZANE & TAZOBACTAM

Trade name: Zerbaxa (Cubist)
Indications: Various infections caused by susceptible organisms
Class: Antibacterial, Antibiotic, beta-lactam, Cephalosporin, 5th generation
Half-life: <3 hours
Clinically important, potentially hazardous interactions with: none known
Pregnancy category: B
Important contra-indications noted in the prescribing guidelines for: the elderly; nursing mothers; pediatric patients

Cardiovascular
Hypertension [3]
Central Nervous System
Fever (2%) [5]
Headache (3%) [8]
Insomnia [2]
Somnolence (drowsiness) [2]
Neuromuscular/Skeletal
Myalgia/Myopathy [2]
Gastrointestinal/Hepatic
Constipation (4%) [4]
Diarrhea (2%) [10]
Nausea (3%) [11]
Vomiting [3]
Endocrine/Metabolic
ALT increased (2%)
AST increased (2%)
Hematologic
Anemia [2]
Local
Infusion-site reactions [2]

CEFTRIAXONE

Trade name: Rocephin (Roche)
Indications: Various infections caused by susceptible organisms
Class: Antibiotic, Cephalosporin, 3rd generation
Half-life: 5–9 hours
Clinically important, potentially hazardous interactions with: aminoglycosides, coumarins, histamine H$_2$ antagonists, oral typhoid vaccine, probenecid
Pregnancy category: B
Important contra-indications noted in the prescribing guidelines for: nursing mothers; pediatric patients
Note: Penicillin and cephalosporins share a common beta-lactam structure. People who are allergic to penicillin are approximately 4 times more likely to develop an allergic reaction to a cephalosporin than those people who have no penicillin allergy (from 5–16% of patients allergic to penicillin develop reactions to cephalosporins).

Skin
AGEP [4]
Anaphylactoid reactions/Anaphylaxis [15]
Angioedema [3]
Candidiasis (5%) [3]
Dermatitis [2]
DRESS syndrome [2]
Erythroderma [2]
Exanthems [7]
Hypersensitivity [4]
Linear IgA bullous dermatosis [2]
Pruritus [2]
Rash (2%) [5]
Serum sickness-like reaction [2]
Urticaria [4]

Mucosal
Glossitis [2]

Cardiovascular
Flushing [2]
Hypotension [2]
Phlebitis [2]

Central Nervous System
Fever [2]

Gastrointestinal/Hepatic
Cholelithiasis (gallstones) [4]
Diarrhea [6]
Hepatotoxicity [7]
Nausea [4]
Vomiting [2]

Respiratory
Dyspnea [2]

Renal
Biliary pseudolithiasis [7]
Nephrolithiasis [2]
Nephrotoxicity [6]
Renal failure [3]

Hematologic
Eosinophilia [2]
Hemolysis [9]
Hemolytic anemia [15]
Thrombocytopenia [4]

Local
Injection-site pain (<10%) [3]
Injection-site phlebitis [2]

Other
Adverse effects [7]
Death [9]
Side effects (3%) [2]

CEFUROXIME

Trade names: Ceftin (GSK), Zinacef (Concordia)
Indications: Various infections caused by susceptible organisms
Class: Cephalosporin, 2nd generation
Half-life: 1–2 hours
Clinically important, potentially hazardous interactions with: none known
Pregnancy category: B
Important contra-indications noted in the prescribing guidelines for: nursing mothers
Note: Penicillin and cephalosporins share a common beta-lactam structure. People who are allergic to penicillin are approximately 4 times more likely to develop an allergic reaction to a cephalosporin than those people who have no penicillin allergy (from 5–16% of patients allergic to penicillin develop reactions to cephalosporins).

Skin
AGEP [2]
Anaphylactoid reactions/Anaphylaxis [7]
Exanthems [2]
Hypersensitivity [4]
Serum sickness-like reaction [2]
Toxic epidermal necrolysis [2]
Urticaria [2]

Cardiovascular
Thrombophlebitis (<10%)

Gastrointestinal/Hepatic
Nausea [2]

Ocular
Ocular toxicity [2]

Other
Kounis syndrome [3]

CELECOXIB

Trade name: Celebrex (Pfizer)
Indications: Osteoarthritis, rheumatoid arthritis (adults and juveniles aged 2 years and over), ankylosing spondylitis, acute pain, primary dysmenorrhea
Class: COX-2 inhibitor, Non-steroidal anti-inflammatory (NSAID), Sulfonamide
Half-life: 11 hours
Clinically important, potentially hazardous interactions with: ACE inhibitors, aliskiren, angiotensin II receptor antagonists, aspirin, dexibuprofen, fluconazole, furosemide, lithium, NSAIDs, warfarin
Pregnancy category: D (pregnancy category C prior to 30 weeks gestation; category D starting at 30 weeks gestation)
Important contra-indications noted in the prescribing guidelines for: the elderly; nursing mothers; pediatric patients
Note: Celecoxib is a sulfonamide and can be absorbed systemically. Sulfonamides can produce severe, possibly fatal, reactions such as toxic epidermal necrolysis and Stevens-Johnson syndrome. NSAIDs may cause an increased risk of serious cardiovascular and gastrointestinal adverse events, which can be fatal. This risk may increase with duration of use.
Contra-indicated in patients with known hypersensitivity to celecoxib, aspirin, or other NSAIDs; in patients who have demonstrated allergic-type reactions to sulfonamides; in patients who have experienced asthma, urticaria, or allergic-type reactions after taking aspirin or other NSAIDs; and for the treatment of peri-operative pain in the setting of coronary artery bypass graft surgery.
Warning: CARDIOVASCULAR AND GASTROINTESTINAL RISKS

Skin
AGEP [7]
Anaphylactoid reactions/Anaphylaxis [8]
Angioedema [9]
Bacterial infection (<2%)
Candidiasis (<2%)
Dermatitis (<2%) [2]
Diaphoresis (<2%)
Edema (<2%) [5]
Erythema [2]
Erythema multiforme [3]
Exanthems (<2%) [7]
Facial edema (<2%)
Fixed eruption [2]
Herpes simplex (<2%)
Herpes zoster (<2%)
Hot flashes (<2%)
Hypersensitivity [8]
Nodular eruption (<2%)
Peripheral edema (2%) [2]
Photosensitivity (<2%)
Pruritus (<2%) [6]
Rash (2%) [11]
Stevens-Johnson syndrome [2]
Sweet's syndrome [3]
Toxic epidermal necrolysis [5]
Urticaria (<2%) [11]
Vasculitis [4]
Xerosis (<2%)

Hair
Alopecia (<2%) [3]

Nails
Nail changes (<2%)

Mucosal
Stomatitis (<2%) [4]
Xerostomia (<2%)

Cardiovascular
Cardiotoxicity [2]
Hypertension [2]
Myocardial infarction [4]

Central Nervous System
Anorexia [3]
Depression [2]
Dysgeusia (taste perversion) (<2%)
Headache [3]
Paresthesias (<2%)
Stroke [3]
Vertigo (dizziness) [3]

Neuromuscular/Skeletal
Asthenia (fatigue) [6]
Myalgia/Myopathy (<2%)

Tendinopathy/Tendon rupture (<2%)

Gastrointestinal/Hepatic
Abdominal pain [10]
Constipation [5]
Diarrhea [11]
Dyspepsia [10]
Flatulence [2]
Gastrointestinal bleeding [4]
Hepatotoxicity [3]
Nausea [14]
Vomiting [9]

Endocrine/Metabolic
Dehydration [2]
Mastodynia (<2%)

Genitourinary
Vaginitis (<2%)
Vulvovaginal candidiasis (<2%)

Renal
Nephrotoxicity [4]

Hematologic
Anemia [2]
Neutropenia [4]

Ocular
Visual disturbances [3]

Local
Application-site cellulitis (<2%)
Application-site reactions (<2%)

Other
Adverse effects [16]
Allergic reactions (<2%) [2]
Death [4]
Infection (<2%)
Tooth disorder (<2%)

CELIPROLOL

Trade names: Celectol (Winthrop), Celol
(Pacific), Selectol (Sanofi-Aventis)
Indications: Hypertension, angina pectoris
Class: Beta blocker
Half-life: 5–6 hours
**Clinically important, potentially hazardous
interactions with:** amiodarone, bepridil,
diltiazem, disopyramide, floctafenine, quinidine,
theophylline, verapamil
Pregnancy category: N/A
**Important contra-indications noted in the
prescribing guidelines for:** nursing mothers

Central Nervous System
Headache [2]
Vertigo (dizziness) [2]

Neuromuscular/Skeletal
Asthenia (fatigue) [3]

CEPHALEXIN

Synonym: cefalexin
Trade names: Keflex (Advancis), Keftab (Biovail)
Indications: Various infections caused by
susceptible organisms
Class: Cephalosporin, 1st generation
Half-life: 0.9–1.2 hours
**Clinically important, potentially hazardous
interactions with:** amikacin, gentamicin,
metformin
Pregnancy category: B
**Important contra-indications noted in the
prescribing guidelines for:** the elderly; nursing
mothers
Note: Penicillin and cephalosporins share a
common beta-lactam structure. People who are
allergic to penicillin are approximately 4 times
more likely to develop an allergic reaction to a
cephalosporin than those people who have no
penicillin allergy (from 5–16% of patients allergic
to penicillin develop reactions to cephalosporins).

Skin
AGEP [4]
Anaphylactoid reactions/Anaphylaxis [4]
Angioedema [2]
Bullous pemphigoid [2]
Erythema multiforme [3]
Exanthems [3]
Pemphigus [2]
Pruritus [3]
Pustules [2]
Stevens-Johnson syndrome [3]
Toxic epidermal necrolysis [4]
Urticaria [2]

Other
Adverse effects [2]
Side effects (2%) [2]

CEPHALOTHIN

See: www.drugeruptiondata.com/drug/id/129

CEPHAPIRIN

See: www.drugeruptiondata.com/drug/id/130

CEPHRADINE

See: www.drugeruptiondata.com/drug/id/131

CERITINIB

See: www.drugeruptiondata.com/drug/id/3527

CERTOLIZUMAB

Trade name: Cimzia (Celltech) (UCB)
Indications: Crohn's disease, rheumatoid
arthritis
Class: Disease-modifying antirheumatic drug
(DMARD), Monoclonal antibody, TNF inhibitor
Half-life: 14 days
**Clinically important, potentially hazardous
interactions with:** abatacept, anakinra,
lenalidomide, live vaccines, natalizumab,
rituximab
Pregnancy category: N/A (Limited evidence
insufficient to inform drug-associated risk)
**Important contra-indications noted in the
prescribing guidelines for:** nursing mothers;
pediatric patients
Note: TNF inhibitors should be used in patients
with heart failure only after consideration of other
treatment options. TNF inhibitors are contra-
indicated in patients with a personal or family
history of multiple sclerosis or demyelinating
disease. TNF inhibitors should not be
administered to patients with moderate to severe
heart failure (New York Heart Association
Functional Class III/IV).
Warning: SERIOUS INFECTIONS AND
MALIGNANCY

Skin
Herpes zoster [3]
Neoplasms [2]
Psoriasis [6]
Rash [2]

Cardiovascular
Hypertension [2]

Central Nervous System
Fever (5%) [2]
Headache (7–18%) [5]
Vertigo (dizziness) (~6%)

Neuromuscular/Skeletal
Arthralgia (6–7%) [4]
Back pain [3]

Gastrointestinal/Hepatic
Nausea [2]

Respiratory
Nasopharyngitis (4–13%) [8]
Pneumonia [2]
Pulmonary toxicity [4]
Sinusitis [2]
Upper respiratory tract infection (20%) [11]

Endocrine/Metabolic
Creatine phosphokinase increased [2]

Genitourinary
Urinary tract infection (~8%) [8]

Local
Injection-site pain [3]
Injection-site reactions (~7%) [4]

Other
Adverse effects [14]
Death [2]
Infection (14–38%) [14]

CETIRIZINE

Trade name: Zyrtec (Pfizer)
Indications: Allergic rhinitis, urticaria
Class: Histamine H1 receptor antagonist
Half-life: 8–11 hours
Clinically important, potentially hazardous interactions with: alcohol, CNS depressants, pilsicainide
Pregnancy category: B
Important contra-indications noted in the prescribing guidelines for: nursing mothers

Skin
Acneform eruption (<2%)
Anaphylactoid reactions/Anaphylaxis (<2%) [2]
Angioedema (<2%)
Bullous dermatitis (<2%)
Dermatitis (<2%)
Diaphoresis (<2%)
Exanthems (<2%)
Fixed eruption [6]
Furunculosis (<2%)
Hyperkeratosis (<2%)
Photosensitivity (<2%)
Phototoxicity (<2%)
Pruritus (<2%)
Purpura (<2%)
Rash (<2%)
Seborrhea (<2%)
Urticaria (<2%) [9]
Xerosis (<2%)

Hair
Alopecia (<2%)
Hypertrichosis (<2%)

Mucosal
Sialorrhea (<2%)
Stomatitis (<2%)
Tongue edema (<2%)
Tongue pigmentation (<2%)
Xerostomia (6%) [2]

Cardiovascular
Flushing (<2%)
QT prolongation [2]

Central Nervous System
Ageusia (taste loss) (<2%)
Dysgeusia (taste perversion) (<2%)
Headache [2]
Hyperesthesia (<2%)
Insomnia [2]
Paresthesias (<2%)
Parosmia (<2%)
Somnolence (drowsiness) [5]

Neuromuscular/Skeletal
Asthenia (fatigue) [3]
Dystonia [6]
Myalgia/Myopathy (<2%)

Endocrine/Metabolic
Mastodynia (<2%)

Genitourinary
Vaginitis (<2%)

Other
Adverse effects [4]

CETRORELIX

Trade name: Cetrotide (Merck)
Indications: Inhibition of premature luteinizing hormone surges in women undergoing controlled ovarian stimulation
Class: Gonadotropin-releasing hormone (GnRH) antagonist
Half-life: 5 hours
Clinically important, potentially hazardous interactions with: none known
Pregnancy category: X
Important contra-indications noted in the prescribing guidelines for: nursing mothers

Skin
Hot flashes [2]

Central Nervous System
Headache [2]

CETUXIMAB

Trade name: Erbitux (Bristol-Myers Squibb)
Indications: Metastatic colorectal cancer, squamous cell carcinoma of the head and neck
Class: Antineoplastic, Biologic, Epidermal growth factor receptor (EGFR) inhibitor, Monoclonal antibody
Half-life: 75–188 hours
Clinically important, potentially hazardous interactions with: none known
Pregnancy category: C
Important contra-indications noted in the prescribing guidelines for: nursing mothers; pediatric patients
Warning: SERIOUS INFUSION REACTIONS and CARDIOPULMONARY ARREST

Skin
Acneform eruption (88%) [62]
Anaphylactoid reactions/Anaphylaxis [5]
Dermatitis [4]
Desquamation (89%) [3]
Erythema [3]
Exanthems [5]
Fissures [4]
Folliculitis [13]
Hand–foot syndrome [5]
Hypersensitivity [8]
Papulopustular eruption [7]
Peripheral edema (10%)
Pruritus (40%) [9]
Radiation recall dermatitis [2]
Rash (89%) [47]
Toxic epidermal necrolysis [2]
Toxicity [18]
Xerosis (49%) [14]

Hair
Abnormal hair growth [2]
Alopecia (5%)
Hair changes [3]
Hypertrichosis [3]

Nails
Nail changes (21%)
Nail disorder [2]
Paronychia [15]

Mucosal
Mucositis [10]
Oral mucositis [2]
Stomatitis (25%) [3]
Xerostomia (11%)

Cardiovascular
Cardiotoxicity [2]
Flushing [2]
Thromboembolism [2]

Central Nervous System
Anorexia [2]
Anxiety (14%)
Aseptic meningitis [6]
Chills (13%) [2]
Confusion (15%)
Depression (13%)
Fever (30%) [4]
Headache (33%)
Insomnia (30%)
Pain (51%)
Peripheral neuropathy [3]
Rigors (13%)
Seizures [2]

Neuromuscular/Skeletal
Asthenia (fatigue) (89%) [24]
Back pain (11%)
Bone or joint pain (15%)

Gastrointestinal/Hepatic
Abdominal pain (59%)
Constipation (46%)
Diarrhea (39%) [19]
Dysphagia [2]
Hepatotoxicity [4]
Nausea [11]
Vomiting (37%) [7]

Respiratory
Cough (29%)
Dyspnea (48%) [5]
Pneumonia [2]
Pneumonitis [3]
Pulmonary toxicity [6]

Endocrine/Metabolic
Hypokalemia [6]
Hypomagnesemia [16]
Hyponatremia [5]

Hematologic
Anemia [6]
Febrile neutropenia [5]
Leukopenia [9]
Neutropenia [22]
Sepsis (<4%)
Thrombocytopenia [5]
Thrombosis [3]

Ocular
Blepharitis [3]
Conjunctivitis (7%) [2]
Ectropion [2]
Eyelashes – hypertrichosis [3]
Trichomegaly [11]

Local
Application-site reactions (~3%)
Infusion-related reactions [7]
Infusion-site reactions (15–21%) [10]

Other
Adverse effects [8]
Allergic reactions [3]

Death [6]
Infection (13–35%) [3]

CEVIMELINE

Trade name: Evoxac (Daiichi Sankyo)
Indications: Sicca syndrome in patients with Sjøgren's syndrome
Class: Muscarinic cholinergic agonist
Half-life: 3–4 hours
Clinically important, potentially hazardous interactions with: none known
Pregnancy category: C
Important contra-indications noted in the prescribing guidelines for: nursing mothers; pediatric patients
Note: Contra-indicated in patients with uncontrolled asthma, acute iritis or narrow-angle glaucoma.

Skin
Abscess (<3%)
Candidiasis (<3%)
Diaphoresis (20%)
Edema (<3%)
Erythema (<3%)
Exanthems (<10%)
Fungal dermatitis (<10%)
Hot flashes (2%)
Hyperhidrosis (19%) [5]
Peripheral edema (<3%)
Pruritus (<3%)
Rash (4%)

Mucosal
Epistaxis (nosebleed) (<3%)
Sialadenitis (<3%)
Sialorrhea (2%)
Ulcerative stomatitis (<3%)
Xerostomia (<3%)

Cardiovascular
Chest pain (<3%)
Palpitation (<3%)

Central Nervous System
Anorexia (<3%)
Depression (<3%)
Fever (<3%)
Headache (14%)
Hypoesthesia (<3%)
Hyporeflexia (<3%)
Insomnia (2%)
Migraine (<3%)
Pain (3%)
Tremor (<3%)
Vertigo (dizziness) (4%)

Neuromuscular/Skeletal
Arthralgia (4%)
Back pain (5%)
Bone or joint pain (3%)
Hypertonia (<3%)
Leg cramps (<3%)
Myalgia/Myopathy (<3%)

Gastrointestinal/Hepatic
Abdominal pain (8%)
Constipation (<3%)
Diarrhea (10%)
Dyspepsia (8%)
Eructation (belching) (<3%)

Gastroesophageal reflux (<3%)
Nausea (14%) [3]
Vomiting (5%)

Respiratory
Bronchitis (4%)
Cough (6%)
Flu-like syndrome (<3%)
Pharyngitis (5%)
Pneumonia (<3%)
Rhinitis (11%)
Sinusitis (12%)
Upper respiratory tract infection (11%)

Genitourinary
Urinary tract infection (6%)
Vaginitis (<3%)

Hematologic
Anemia (<3%)

Otic
Ear pain (<3%)
Otitis media (<3%)

Ocular
Abnormal vision (<3%)
Conjunctivitis (4%)
Ocular pain (<3%)
Xerophthalmia (<3%)

Other
Allergic reactions (<3%)
Infection (<3%)
Tooth disorder (<3%)

CHARCOAL

See: www.drugeruptiondata.com/drug/id/1158

CHLORAL HYDRATE

Indications: Insomnia, sedation
Class: Anesthetic, general, Hypnotic
Half-life: 8–11 hours
Clinically important, potentially hazardous interactions with: antihistamines, azatadine, brompheniramine, buclizine, chlorpheniramine, clemastine, dexchlorpheniramine, diphenhydramine, meclizine, tripelennamine
Pregnancy category: C
Important contra-indications noted in the prescribing guidelines for: nursing mothers

Skin
Acneform eruption [2]
Angioedema [2]
Dermatitis [2]
Erythema multiforme [2]
Exanthems [3]
Fixed eruption [5]
Pruritus [2]
Purpura [2]
Rash (<10%)
Urticaria (<10%) [2]

Mucosal
Oral lesions [2]

Cardiovascular
Hypotension [2]

Central Nervous System
Agitation [2]

Sedation (prolonged) [2]

Gastrointestinal/Hepatic
Vomiting [4]

Respiratory
Apnea [2]

Other
Adverse effects [3]
Death [3]

CHLORAMBUCIL

See: www.drugeruptiondata.com/drug/id/136

CHLORAMPHENICOL

Indications: Various infections caused by susceptible organisms
Class: Antibiotic, CYP3A4 inhibitor
Half-life: 1.5–3.5 hours
Clinically important, potentially hazardous interactions with: amoxicillin, ampicillin, clopidogrel, clozapine, ethotoin, fosphenytoin, gliclazide, levodopa, mephenytoin, phenytoin, propyphenazone, voriconazole
Pregnancy category: C
Important contra-indications noted in the prescribing guidelines for: nursing mothers

Skin
AGEP [2]
Dermatitis [18]
Erythema multiforme [6]
Exanthems (<5%) [5]
Hypersensitivity [2]
Purpura [2]
Pustules [2]
Sensitization [2]
Toxic epidermal necrolysis [2]
Urticaria [3]

Nails
Photo-onycholysis [2]

CHLORDIAZEPOXIDE

Trade names: Libritabs (Valeant), Librium (Valeant), Limbitrol (Valeant)
Indications: Anxiety
Class: Benzodiazepine
Half-life: 6–25 hours
Clinically important, potentially hazardous interactions with: chlorpheniramine, clarithromycin, efavirenz, esomeprazole, imatinib, indinavir, ketoconazole, nelfinavir, nilutamide, ritonavir
Pregnancy category: D
Important contra-indications noted in the prescribing guidelines for: the elderly; nursing mothers; pediatric patients
Note: Limbitrol is chlordiazepoxide and amitriptyline.

Skin
Angioedema [3]
Dermatitis (<10%)
Diaphoresis (>10%)

Edema (<10%)
Erythema multiforme [5]
Erythema nodosum [2]
Exanthems [3]
Fixed eruption [7]
Lupus erythematosus [3]
Photosensitivity [6]
Purpura [5]
Rash (>10%)
Urticaria [4]
Vasculitis [2]

Hair
Alopecia [3]

Mucosal
Sialopenia (>10%)
Sialorrhea (<10%)
Xerostomia (>10%)

Endocrine/Metabolic
Galactorrhea [3]

CHLORHEXIDINE

Trade name: Hibiclens (SSL)
Indications: Skin antisepsis, gingivitis
Class: Antiseptic
Half-life: N/A
Clinically important, potentially hazardous interactions with: none known
Pregnancy category: B
Important contra-indications noted in the prescribing guidelines for: nursing mothers; pediatric patients

Skin
Anaphylactoid reactions/Anaphylaxis [29]
Dermatitis [16]
Hypersensitivity [9]
Rash [2]
Urticaria [4]

Mucosal
Gingival pigmentation [2]
Gingivitis [3]
Glossitis (<10%)
Mucosal ulceration [2]
Oral mucosal irritation [2]
Stomatitis (<10%)
Tongue irritation (<10%)
Tongue pigmentation (>10%)

Central Nervous System
Dysgeusia (taste perversion) (>10%) [7]

Other
Allergic reactions [6]
Tooth pigmentation [4]

CHLORMEZANONE

See: www.drugeruptiondata.com/drug/id/140

CHLOROQUINE

Trade name: Aralen (Sanofi-Aventis)
Indications: Malaria, rheumatoid arthritis, lupus erythematosus
Class: Antimalarial, Antiprotozoal, Disease-modifying antirheumatic drug (DMARD)
Half-life: 3–5 days
Clinically important, potentially hazardous interactions with: acitretin, antacids, arsenic, cholera vaccine, cholestyramine, citalopram, dapsone, dasatinib, degarelix, droperidol, ethosuximide, furazolidone, halofantrine, hydroxychloroquine, lacosamide, lanthanum, lapatinib, levofloxacin, methotrexate, methoxsalen, mivacurium, moxifloxacin, neostigmine, nilotinib, oxcarbazepine, pazopanib, penicillamine, ribociclib, sulfonamides, telavancin, telithromycin, tiagabine, typhoid vaccine, vandetanib, vigabatrin, voriconazole, vorinostat, ziprasidone
Pregnancy category: D
Important contra-indications noted in the prescribing guidelines for: nursing mothers

Skin
Dermatitis [2]
Erythema annulare centrifugum [2]
Erythroderma [3]
Exanthems (<5%) [3]
Exfoliative dermatitis [4]
Lichenoid eruption [6]
Photosensitivity [8]
Pigmentation [15]
Pruritus [36]
Psoriasis [18]
Stevens-Johnson syndrome [4]
Toxic epidermal necrolysis [5]
Toxicity [2]
Urticaria [4]
Vitiligo [7]

Hair
Hair pigmentation [10]
Poliosis [3]

Nails
Nail pigmentation [2]

Mucosal
Mucosal membrane pigmentation [2]
Oral pigmentation [12]

Cardiovascular
Atrioventricular block [2]
Cardiac failure [2]
Cardiomyopathy [8]
Cardiotoxicity [3]
Congestive heart failure [2]
Myocardial toxicity [2]
QT prolongation [3]
Torsades de pointes [2]

Central Nervous System
Headache [4]
Psychosis [4]
Seizures [2]
Vertigo (dizziness) [4]

Neuromuscular/Skeletal
Myalgia/Myopathy [8]
Myasthenia gravis [7]

Gastrointestinal/Hepatic
Diarrhea [2]
Nausea [3]
Vomiting [5]

Endocrine/Metabolic
Porphyria [7]

Ocular
Corneal deposits [2]
Keratopathy [2]
Maculopathy [3]
Ocular adverse effects [2]
Ocular toxicity [4]
Retinopathy [10]
Vision blurred [2]

Other
Adverse effects [2]
Death [3]

CHLOROTHIAZIDE

See: www.drugeruptiondata.com/drug/id/142

CHLOROTRIANISENE

See: www.drugeruptiondata.com/drug/id/143

CHLORPHENIRAMINE

Synonym: chlorphenamine
Trade names: Chlor-Trimeton (Schering), Triaminic (Novartis)
Indications: Allergic rhinitis, urticaria
Class: Histamine H1 receptor antagonist, Muscarinic antagonist
Half-life: 20–40 hours
Clinically important, potentially hazardous interactions with: alcohol, anticholinergics, barbiturates, benzodiazepines, butabarbital, chloral hydrate, chlordiazepoxide, chlorpromazine, clonazepam, clorazepate, diazepam, ethchlorvynol, fluphenazine, flurazepam, hypnotics, lopinavir, lorazepam, MAO inhibitors, mephobarbital, mesoridazine, midazolam, narcotics, oxazepam, pentobarbital, phenobarbital, phenothiazines, phenylbutazone, primidone, prochlorperazine, promethazine, quazepam, secobarbital, sedatives, temazepam, thioridazine, tranquilizers, trifluoperazine, zolpidem
Pregnancy category: B
Important contra-indications noted in the prescribing guidelines for: the elderly; nursing mothers; pediatric patients

Skin
Angioedema (<10%)
Dermatitis (<10%) [4]
Photosensitivity (<10%)

Mucosal
Xerostomia (<10%)

Central Nervous System
Seizures [2]

CHLORPROMAZINE

Trade name: Thorazine (GSK)
Indications: Psychosis, manic-depressive disorders
Class: Antiemetic, Antipsychotic, Muscarinic antagonist, Phenothiazine
Half-life: initial: 2 hours; terminal: 30 hours
Clinically important, potentially hazardous interactions with: alcohol, antihistamines, arsenic, asenapine, chlorpheniramine, dofetilide, epinephrine, evening primrose, guanethidine, lisdexamfetamine, mivacurium, pimavanserin, propranolol, quinolones, sodium picosulfate, sparfloxacin, tetrabenazine, zolpidem
Pregnancy category: N/A
Important contra-indications noted in the prescribing guidelines for: the elderly; nursing mothers; pediatric patients
Note: The prolonged use of chlorpromazine can produce a gray-blue or purplish pigmentation over light-exposed areas. This is a result of either dermal deposits of melanin, a chlorpromazine metabolite, or to a combination of both. Chlorpromazine melanosis is seen more often in women.
Warning: INCREASED MORTALITY IN ELDERLY PATIENTS WITH DEMENTIA-RELATED PSYCHOSIS

Skin
Exanthems (>5%) [8]
Lupus erythematosus [12]
Photosensitivity (<10%) [22]
Phototoxicity [6]
Pigmentation [16]
Pruritus (<10%) [2]
Purpura [6]
Rash (<10%)
Seborrheic dermatitis [4]
Toxic epidermal necrolysis [2]
Urticaria [4]
Vasculitis [3]

Nails
Nail pigmentation [4]

Mucosal
Xerostomia (<10%)

Cardiovascular
Hypotension [4]
QT prolongation [4]
Tachycardia [2]
Torsades de pointes [2]

Central Nervous System
Neuroleptic malignant syndrome [7]
Sedation [3]
Seizures [2]

Endocrine/Metabolic
Galactorrhea (<10%)
Gynecomastia (<10%)
Mastodynia (<10%)
Weight gain [2]

Genitourinary
Priapism [7]

Otic
Tinnitus [2]

Ocular
Cataract [2]
Corneal opacity [2]
Eyelid edema [2]
Retinopathy [2]

Other
Adverse effects [3]

CHLORPROPAMIDE

See: www.drugeruptiondata.com/drug/id/146

CHLORTETRACYCLINE

See: www.drugeruptiondata.com/drug/id/147

CHLORTHALIDONE

See: www.drugeruptiondata.com/drug/id/148

CHLORZOXAZONE

See: www.drugeruptiondata.com/drug/id/149

CHOLERA VACCINE

Trade name: Vaxchora (PaxVax)
Indications: Immunization against cholera for adults traveling to cholera-affected areas
Class: Vaccine
Half-life: N/A
Clinically important, potentially hazardous interactions with: antibiotics, chloroquine
Pregnancy category: N/A (Not expected to cause fetal risk)
Important contra-indications noted in the prescribing guidelines for: the elderly; pediatric patients

Central Nervous System
Headache (29%)

Neuromuscular/Skeletal
Asthenia (fatigue) (31%)

Gastrointestinal/Hepatic
Abdominal pain (19%)
Diarrhea (4%)
Nausea (18%)
Vomiting (18%)

Endocrine/Metabolic
Appetite decreased (17%)

CHOLESTYRAMINE

Trade name: Questran (Par)
Indications: Pruritus associated with biliary obstruction, primary hypercholesterolemia
Class: Bile acid sequestrant
Half-life: N/A
Clinically important, potentially hazardous interactions with: acarbose, acetaminophen, acitretin, amiodarone, aspirin, bezafibrate, calcifediol, chloroquine, cyclopenthiazide, cyclosporine, deferasirox, digoxin, doxepin, doxercalciferol, ergocalciferol, hydroxychloroquine, isotretinoin, leflunomide, levodopa, lovastatin, meloxicam, mycophenolate, phytonadione, propranolol, raloxifene, sulfasalazine, sulfonylureas, tetracycline, tricyclic antidepressants, troglitazone, ursodiol, valproic acid, vitamin A, vitamin E
Pregnancy category: C
Important contra-indications noted in the prescribing guidelines for: nursing mothers; pediatric patients
Note: Contra-indicated in patients with complete biliary obstruction.

Skin
Pruritus [2]

Neuromuscular/Skeletal
Osteomalacia [2]

Hematologic
Hemorrhage [2]

CHOLIC ACID

Trade name: Cholbam (Asklepion Pharmaceuticals)
Indications: Bile acid synthesis disorders, adjunctive treatment of peroxisomal disorders
Class: Bile acid
Half-life: N/A
Clinically important, potentially hazardous interactions with: cyclosporine
Pregnancy category: N/A
Important contra-indications noted in the prescribing guidelines for: the elderly; nursing mothers

Gastrointestinal/Hepatic
Diarrhea (2%)

CHOLINE C11

See: www.drugeruptiondata.com/drug/id/3057

CHOLINE FENOFIBRATE

See: www.drugeruptiondata.com/drug/id/2095

CICLESONIDE

See: www.drugeruptiondata.com/drug/id/1263

CICLOPIROX

See: www.drugeruptiondata.com/drug/id/2335

CIDOFOVIR

Trade name: Vistide (Gilead)
Indications: Cytomegalovirus (CMV) retinitis in patients with acquired immunodeficiency syndrome (AIDS)
Class: Antiviral, nucleotide analog
Half-life: ~2.6 hours
Clinically important, potentially hazardous interactions with: amphotericin B, cobicistat/elvitegravir/emtricitabine/tenofovir alafenamide, cobicistat/elvitegravir/emtricitabine/tenofovir disoproxil, tenofovir disoproxil
Pregnancy category: C
Important contra-indications noted in the prescribing guidelines for: the elderly; nursing mothers; pediatric patients
Warning: RENAL TOXICITY and NEUTROPENIA

Skin
Acneform eruption (>10%)
Diaphoresis (<10%)
DRESS syndrome [2]
Pallor (<10%)
Pigmentation (>10%)
Pruritus (<10%) [2]
Rash (27%) [2]
Toxicity [3]
Ulcerations [2]
Urticaria (<10%)

Hair
Alopecia (22%) [2]

Mucosal
Stomatitis (<10%)

Central Nervous System
Chills (24%)
Dysgeusia (taste perversion) (<10%)
Headache [4]
Paresthesias (>10%)

Neuromuscular/Skeletal
Asthenia (fatigue) [2]
Myalgia/Myopathy [2]

Renal
Fanconi syndrome [2]
Nephrotoxicity [5]

Ocular
Intraocular inflammation [2]
Iritis [6]
Ocular hypotension [2]
Retinal detachment [3]
Uveitis [18]
Vision impaired [3]
Vision loss [3]

Local
Application-site reactions (39%) [3]

Other
Allergic reactions (<10%)

CILAZAPRIL

See: www.drugeruptiondata.com/drug/id/1241

CILOSTAZOL

Trade name: Pletal (Otsuka)
Indications: Peripheral vascular disease, intermittent claudication
Class: Antiplatelet, Phosphodiesterase inhibitor, Vasodilator, peripheral
Half-life: 11–13 hours
Clinically important, potentially hazardous interactions with: anagrelide, anticoagulants, antifungals, antiplatelet agents, clarithromycin, collagenase, conivaptan, CYP2C19 inhibitors, CYP3A4 inhibitors and inducers, dasatinib, deferasirox, diltiazem, drotrecogin alfa, erythromycin, esomeprazole, fondaparinux, glucosamine, grapefruit juice, high-fat foods, ibritumomab, itraconazole, ketoconazole, macrolide antibiotics, NSAIDs, omeprazole, PEG-interferon, pentosan, pentoxifylline, prostacyclin analogues, salicylates, St John's wort, telithromycin, thrombolytic agents, tositumomab & iodine[131], voriconazole
Pregnancy category: C
Important contra-indications noted in the prescribing guidelines for: nursing mothers; pediatric patients
Note: Contra-indicated in patients with congestive heart failure or active pathological bleeding.
Warning: CONTRA-INDICATED IN HEART FAILURE PATIENTS

Skin
Ecchymoses (<2%)
Edema (<2%)
Facial edema (<2%)
Furunculosis (<2%)
Hypertrophy (<2%)
Peripheral edema (7–9%)
Purpura (<2%)
Rash (2%) [2]
Urticaria (<2%)
Varicosities (<2%)
Xerosis (<2%)

Mucosal
Epistaxis (nosebleed) (<2%)
Gingival bleeding (<2%)
Perioral abscess (<2%)
Rectal hemorrhage (<2%)
Tongue edema (<2%)

Cardiovascular
Arrhythmias (<2%)
Atrial fibrillation (<2%)
Atrial flutter (<2%)
Cardiac arrest (<2%)
Cardiotoxicity [4]
Congestive heart failure (<2%)
Extrasystoles (<2%)
Hypotension (<2%)
Myocardial infarction (<2%) [4]
Myocardial ischemia (<2%)
Palpitation (5–10%) [7]
Postural hypotension (<2%)
Supraventricular tachycardia (<2%)
Tachycardia (4%) [4]
Vasodilation (<2%)
Ventricular tachycardia (<2%)

Central Nervous System
Anorexia (<2%)

Anxiety (<2%)
Cerebral ischemia (<2%)
Chills (<2%)
Headache (27–34%) [19]
Hyperesthesia (2%)
Insomnia (<2%)
Neurotoxicity (<2%)
Paresthesias (2%)
Syncope (<2%)
Vertigo (dizziness) (<10%) [4]

Neuromuscular/Skeletal
Arthralgia (<2%)
Asthenia (fatigue) (<2%)
Back pain (6–7%)
Bone or joint pain (<2%)
Gouty tophi (<2%)
Myalgia/Myopathy (2–3%)

Gastrointestinal/Hepatic
Abdominal pain (4–5%)
Black stools (<2%)
Cholelithiasis (gallstones) (<2%)
Colitis (<2%)
Diarrhea (12–19%) [7]
Dyspepsia (6%)
Esophagitis (<2%)
Flatulence (2–3%)
Gastritis (<2%)
Gastroenteritis (<2%)
Gastrointestinal ulceration (<2%)
Hematemesis (<2%)
Nausea (6–7%) [4]
Peptic ulceration (<2%)
Vomiting (>2%)

Respiratory
Asthma (<2%)
Cough (3–4%) [2]
Hemoptysis (<2%)
Pharyngitis (7–10%)
Pneumonia (<2%)
Rhinitis (7–12%)
Sinusitis (<2%)

Endocrine/Metabolic
Creatine phosphokinase increased (<2%)
Diabetes mellitus (<2%)
GGT increased (<2%)
Hyperlipidemia (<2%)
Hyperuricemia (<2%)

Genitourinary
Albuminuria (<2%)
Cystitis (<2%)
Urinary frequency (<2%)
Vaginal bleeding (<2%)
Vaginitis (<2%)

Renal
Retroperitoneal bleeding (<2%)

Hematologic
Anemia (<2%)
Hemorrhage (<2%)
Polycythemia (<2%)
Thrombosis [3]

Otic
Ear pain (<2%)
Tinnitus (<2%)

Ocular
Amblyopia (<2%)
Blindness (<2%)
Conjunctivitis (<2%)
Diplopia (<2%)

Ocular hemorrhage (<2%)
Other
Adverse effects [4]
Death [3]
Infection (10–14%)

CIMETIDINE

Trade name: Tagamet (GSK)
Indications: Duodenal ulcer
Class: CYP1A2 inhibitor, CYP3A4 inhibitor, Histamine H2 receptor antagonist
Half-life: 2 hours
Clinically important, potentially hazardous interactions with: acenocoumarol, alfuzosin, aminophylline, amiodarone, amitriptyline, anisindione, anticoagulants, buprenorphine, butorphanol, caffeine, carmustine, citalopram, clobazam, clopidogrel, clozapine, cocoa, delavirdine, dicumarol, dofetilide, duloxetine, dutasteride, epirubicin, eszopiclone, fentanyl, ferrous sulfate, floxuridine, fluorouracil, galantamine, gliclazide, hydromorphone, itraconazole, ketoconazole, labetalol, levomepromazine, lidocaine, lomustine, meptazinol, metformin, metronidazole, midazolam, mizolastine, moclobemide, morphine, narcotic analgesics, neratinib, oxprenolol, oxtriphylline, oxycodone, oxymorphone, pentazocine, phenytoin, pimecrolimus, posaconazole, prednisone, propranolol, quinine, rilpivirine, risperidone, roflumilast, sertindole, sildenafil, sufentanil, tamsulosin, terbinafine, thalidomide, tolazoline, warfarin, xanthines, zaleplon, zofenopril, zolmitriptan, zolpidem
Pregnancy category: B
Important contra-indications noted in the prescribing guidelines for: nursing mothers; pediatric patients

Skin
Angioedema [3]
Erythema annulare centrifugum [2]
Erythema multiforme [5]
Exanthems [3]
Exfoliative dermatitis [2]
Fixed eruption [2]
Hypersensitivity [4]
Lupus erythematosus [3]
Pruritus [6]
Pseudolymphoma [2]
Psoriasis [6]
Rash (<2%)
Stevens-Johnson syndrome [3]
Toxic epidermal necrolysis [2]
Urticaria [6]
Vasculitis [3]
Hair
Alopecia [4]
Central Nervous System
Hallucinations [3]
Neuromuscular/Skeletal
Myalgia/Myopathy [2]
Endocrine/Metabolic
Gynecomastia [12]

Renal
Nephrotoxicity [3]

CINACALCET

See: www.drugeruptiondata.com/drug/id/1021

CINNARIZINE

See: www.drugeruptiondata.com/drug/id/1076

CINOXACIN

See: www.drugeruptiondata.com/drug/id/154

CIPROFIBRATE

See: www.drugeruptiondata.com/drug/id/1140

CIPROFLOXACIN

Trade names: Ciloxan Ophthalmic (Alcon), Cipro (Bayer), Ciproxin (Bayer)
Indications: Various infections caused by susceptible organisms, inhalational anthrax (post exposure)
Class: Antibiotic, fluoroquinolone, CYP1A2 inhibitor, CYP3A4 inhibitor
Half-life: 4 hours
Clinically important, potentially hazardous interactions with: agomelatine, aminophylline, amiodarone, amitriptyline, antacids, antineoplastics, arsenic, artemether/lumefantrine, BCG vaccine, bendamustine, bepridil, bismuth, bismuth subsalicylate, bretylium, calcium salts, citalopram, clopidogrel, clozapine, corticosteroids, cyclosporine, dairy products, dasatinib, degarelix, didanosine, disopyramide, dolasetron, duloxetine, dutasteride, eluxadoline, erlotinib, erythromycin, flibanserin, insulin, lanthanum, lapatinib, levofloxacin, magnesium salts, meptazinol, methotrexate, methylxanthines, mifepristone, moxifloxacin, mycophenolate, neratinib, NSAIDs, olanzapine, olaparib, opiod analgesics, oral iron, oxtriphylline, P-glycoprotein inhibitors, pazopanib, pentoxifylline, phenothiazines, phenytoin, pirfenidone, probenecid, procainamide, propranolol, QT prolonging agents, quinapril, quinidine, rasagiline, ropinirole, ropivacaine, sevelamer, sotalol, St John's wort, strontium ranelate, sucralfate, sulfonylureas, telavancin, telithromycin, tizanidine, tricyclic antidepressants, typhoid vaccine, venetoclax, vitamin K antagonists, voriconazole, vorinostat, warfarin, zinc, ziprasidone, zolmitriptan
Pregnancy category: C
Important contra-indications noted in the prescribing guidelines for: the elderly; nursing mothers
Note: Fluoroquinolones are associated with an increased risk of tendinitis and tendon rupture in all ages. This risk is further increased in older patients usually over 60 years of age, in patients

taking corticosteroid drugs, and in patients with kidney, heart or lung transplants. Fluoroquinolones may exacerbate muscle weakness in persons with myasthenia gravis. Ciprofloxacin is chemically related to nalidixic acid.
Warning: SERIOUS ADVERSE REACTIONS INCLUDING TENDINITIS, TENDON RUPTURE, PERIPHERAL NEUROPATHY, CENTRAL NERVOUS SYSTEM EFFECTS and EXACERBATION OF MYASTHENIA GRAVIS

Skin
Acneform eruption [3]
AGEP [4]
Anaphylactoid reactions/Anaphylaxis [15]
Angioedema [8]
Candidiasis [2]
Diaphoresis [5]
Erythema multiforme [5]
Exanthems [4]
Facial edema [2]
Fixed eruption [13]
Hypersensitivity [5]
Jaundice [2]
Linear IgA bullous dermatosis [2]
Photosensitivity [19]
Phototoxicity [5]
Pruritus [11]
Purpura [4]
Rash (<10%) [13]
Serum sickness-like reaction [3]
Stevens-Johnson syndrome [9]
Toxic epidermal necrolysis [11]
Toxicity [3]
Urticaria [9]
Vasculitis [11]
Mucosal
Stomatitis [4]
Xerostomia [3]
Cardiovascular
Palpitation [2]
QT prolongation [11]
Torsades de pointes [8]
Central Nervous System
Dysgeusia (taste perversion) [3]
Fever [3]
Headache [6]
Mania [4]
Peripheral neuropathy [2]
Psychosis [5]
Seizures [5]
Syncope [2]
Tremor [2]
Vertigo (dizziness) [2]
Neuromuscular/Skeletal
Arthralgia [2]
Asthenia (fatigue) [3]
Myalgia/Myopathy [2]
Myasthenia gravis (exacerbation) [2]
Myoclonus [4]
Rhabdomyolysis [4]
Tendinitis [4]
Tendinopathy/Tendon rupture [31]
Gastrointestinal/Hepatic
Abdominal pain [2]
Constipation [2]
Flatulence [2]
Hepatitis [4]

Hepatotoxicity [7]
Nausea (3%) [4]
Pancreatitis [2]
Vomiting [2]

Genitourinary
Vaginitis [2]

Renal
Nephrotoxicity [9]
Renal failure [3]

Hematologic
Bone marrow suppression [2]
Hemolytic anemia [2]
Thrombocytopenia [4]

Otic
Hearing loss [2]

Ocular
Hallucinations, visual [6]
Vision blurred [2]

Local
Injection-site pain [2]

Other
Adverse effects [8]
Death [4]

CISATRACURIUM

See: www.drugeruptiondata.com/drug/id/897

CISPLATIN

Synonym: CDDP
Trade name: Platinol (Bristol-Myers Squibb)
Indications: Carcinomas, lymphomas
Class: Alkylating agent, Antineoplastic
Half-life: alpha phase: 25–49 minutes; beta phase: 58–73 hours
Clinically important, potentially hazardous interactions with: aldesleukin, atenolol, chlorothiazide, gadobenate, methotrexate, paclitaxel, pentamidine, rituximab, selenium, thalidomide, zinc
Pregnancy category: D
Important contra-indications noted in the prescribing guidelines for: the elderly; nursing mothers

Skin
Acneform eruption [6]
Anaphylactoid reactions/Anaphylaxis [10]
Angioedema [4]
Edema [3]
Erythema [3]
Exanthems [4]
Hand–foot syndrome [9]
Hypersensitivity [5]
Necrosis [2]
Peripheral edema [2]
Pigmentation [5]
Pruritus [7]
Rash [21]
Raynaud's phenomenon [14]
Thrombocytopenic purpura [2]
Toxic epidermal necrolysis [2]
Toxicity [7]
Urticaria [7]

Hair
Alopecia (>10%) [24]

Mucosal
Epistaxis (nosebleed) [3]
Mucositis [16]
Oral lesions [2]
Stomatitis [16]

Cardiovascular
Cardiotoxicity [2]
Flushing [5]
Hypertension [7]
Thromboembolism [6]
Venous thromboembolism [4]

Central Nervous System
Anorexia [23]
Dysgeusia (taste perversion) [3]
Fever [5]
Headache [4]
Insomnia [4]
Leukoencephalopathy [10]
Neurotoxicity [14]
Pain [3]
Peripheral neuropathy [8]
Seizures [4]
Vertigo (dizziness) [2]

Neuromuscular/Skeletal
Asthenia (fatigue) [34]
Ataxia [2]
Myalgia/Myopathy [3]

Gastrointestinal/Hepatic
Abdominal pain [4]
Constipation [4]
Diarrhea [34]
Esophagitis [2]
Gastrointestinal bleeding [2]
Hepatotoxicity [6]
Nausea [48]
Pancreatitis [2]
Vomiting [35]

Respiratory
Cough [4]
Dysphonia [4]
Dyspnea [4]
Pneumonia [4]
Pneumonitis [3]
Pulmonary toxicity [5]

Endocrine/Metabolic
ALP increased [2]
ALT increased [5]
Appetite decreased [7]
AST increased [5]
Dehydration [3]
Hyperglycemia [3]
Hyperkalemia [2]
Hypocalcemia [2]
Hypokalemia [5]
Hypomagnesemia [13]
Hyponatremia [18]
Serum creatinine increased [8]
SIADH [18]
Weight loss [4]

Renal
Nephrotoxicity [65]
Proteinuria [2]
Renal failure [3]
Renal function abnormal [2]

Hematologic
Anemia [48]

Febrile neutropenia [36]
Hemolytic uremic syndrome [12]
Hemotoxicity [3]
Leukopenia [30]
Lymphopenia [5]
Myelosuppression [7]
Myelotoxicity [3]
Neutropenia [88]
Thrombocytopenia [48]
Thrombosis [2]

Otic
Hearing loss [14]
Ototoxicity [39]
Tinnitus [27]

Local
Injection-site cellulitis [4]

Other
Adverse effects [15]
Death [16]
Hiccups [6]
Infection [9]

CITALOPRAM

Trade names: Celexa (Forest), Cipramil (Lundbeck)
Indications: Depression, obsessive-compulsive disorder, panic disorder
Class: Antidepressant, Selective serotonin reuptake inhibitor (SSRI)
Half-life: ~35 hours
Clinically important, potentially hazardous interactions with: alcohol, alfuzosin, alpha or beta blockers, antidepressants, antiepileptics, antiplatelet agents, artemether/lumefantrine, aspirin, atomoxetine, barbiturates, bupropion, buspirone, carbamazepine, chloroquine, cimetidine, ciprofloxacin, clozapine, CNS depressants, collagenase, conivaptan, coumarins/anticoagulants, CYP2C19 inhibitors, CYP3A4 inhibitors, cyproheptadine, desmopressin, dexibuprofen, dextromethorphan, dronedarone, drotrecogin alfa, duloxetine, efavirenz, fluconazole, gadobutrol, glucosamine, haloperidol, ibritumomab, iobenguane, isocarboxazid, lithium, macrolide antibiotics, MAO inhibitors, methadone, methylphenidate, metoclopramide, mexiletine, moclobemide, nilotinib, NSAIDs, opioid anagesics, pentoxifylline, phenelzine, phenytoin, pimozide, QT prolonging agents, quinine, rasagiline, risperidone, ritonavir, salicylates, selegiline, serotonin modulators, sibutramine, SSRIs, St John's wort, sumatriptan, tetrabenazine, thioridazine, thrombolytic agents, tositumomab & iodine[131], tramadol, tranylcypromine, trazodone, tricyclic antidepressants, tryptophan, vitamin K antagonists, ziprasidone
Pregnancy category: C
Important contra-indications noted in the prescribing guidelines for: nursing mothers; pediatric patients
Warning: SUICIDALITY AND ANTIDEPRESSANT DRUGS

Skin
Diaphoresis (11%) [3]
Hyperhidrosis (11%) [2]

Pigmentation [2]
Pruritus (<10%) [2]
Rash (<10%)

Mucosal
Xerostomia (20%) [4]

Cardiovascular
Bradycardia [2]
Cardiotoxicity [4]
Chest pain [2]
Palpitation [2]
QT prolongation [22]
Tachycardia [3]
Torsades de pointes [9]

Central Nervous System
Agitation (3%)
Akathisia [2]
Anorexia (4%)
Anxiety (4%) [2]
Fever (2%)
Headache [5]
Incoordination [2]
Insomnia (15%) [3]
Nightmares [2]
Restless legs syndrome [4]
Seizures (overdose) [5]
Serotonin syndrome [19]
Somnolence (drowsiness) (18%) [6]
Suicidal ideation [3]
Tremor (8%) [5]
Vertigo (dizziness) [5]
Yawning (2%)

Neuromuscular/Skeletal
Arthralgia (2%)
Asthenia (fatigue) (5%) [4]
Dystonia [2]
Myalgia/Myopathy (2%)

Gastrointestinal/Hepatic
Abdominal pain (3%)
Constipation [2]
Diarrhea (8%) [2]
Dyspepsia (5%)
Nausea (21%) [3]
Vomiting (4%) [2]

Respiratory
Rhinitis (5%)
Sinusitis (3%)
Upper respiratory tract infection (5%)

Endocrine/Metabolic
Galactorrhea [4]
Hyponatremia [2]
Libido decreased (2%)
SIADH [18]
Weight gain [2]

Genitourinary
Dysmenorrhea (3%)
Ejaculatory dysfunction (6%) [2]
Impotence (3%)
Priapism [4]
Sexual dysfunction [4]
Urinary frequency [2]

Otic
Hallucinations, auditory [2]

Ocular
Diplopia [2]
Glaucoma [2]
Hallucinations, visual [3]

Other
Adverse effects [2]
Death [8]

CLADRIBINE

Trade name: Leustatin (Janssen Biotech)
Indications: Leukemias
Class: Antimetabolite, Antineoplastic
Half-life: alpha phase: 25 minutes; beta phase: 7 hours
Clinically important, potentially hazardous interactions with: none known
Pregnancy category: D
Important contra-indications noted in the prescribing guidelines for: the elderly; nursing mothers

Skin
Diaphoresis (<10%)
Edema (6%)
Erythema (6%)
Exanthems (27–50%) [2]
Herpes zoster [5]
Petechiae (8%)
Pruritus (6%)
Purpura (10%)
Rash (27%) [3]

Mucosal
Mucositis [2]

Neuromuscular/Skeletal
Myalgia/Myopathy (7%)

Hematologic
Lymphocytopenia [4]
Lymphopenia [3]
Neutropenia [8]
Thrombocytopenia [2]

Local
Injection-site edema (9%)
Injection-site erythema (9%)
Injection-site pain (9%)
Injection-site phlebitis (2%)
Injection-site thrombosis (2%)

Other
Adverse effects [2]
Death [3]
Infection [7]

CLARITHROMYCIN

Trade name: Biaxin (AbbVie)
Indications: Various infections caused by susceptible organisms
Class: Antibiotic, macrolide, CYP3A4 inhibitor
Half-life: 5–7 hours
Clinically important, potentially hazardous interactions with: abiraterone, alprazolam, aprepitant, astemizole, atazanavir, atorvastatin, avanafil, benzodiazepines, betrixaban, boceprevir, brigatinib, cabazitaxel, cabozantinib, calcifediol, carbamazepine, chlordiazepoxide, cilostazol, clonazepam, clorazepate, cobicistat/elvitegravir/emtricitabine/tenofovir alafenamide, cobicistat/elvitegravir/emtricitabine/tenofovir disoproxil, colchicine, conivaptan, copanlisib, crizotinib, cyclosporine, dabigatran, darunavir, dasatinib,

deflazacort, delavirdine, diazepam, digoxin, dihydroergotamine, disopyramide, dronedarone, efavirenz, eletriptan, eluxadoline, ergot alkaloids, estradiol, etravirine, everolimus, fesoterodine, flibanserin, fluoxetine, flurazepam, fluticasone propionate, fluvastatin, HMG-CoA reductase inhibitors, ibrutinib, imatinib, indinavir, itraconazole, ixabepilone, lapatinib, lomitapide, lopinavir, lorazepam, lovastatin, maraviroc, methylergonovine, methylprednisolone, methysergide, midazolam, midostaurin, mifepristone, naldemedine, neratinib, nevirapine, nilotinib, olaparib, omeprazole, oxazepam, oxtriphylline, paclitaxel, palbociclib, paroxetine hydrochloride, pazopanib, pimavanserin, pimozide, ponatinib, pravastatin, prednisone, quazepam, ranolazine, regorafenib, repaglinide, ribociclib, rilpivirine, rimonabant, rivaroxaban, romidepsin, ruxolitinib, sertraline, sildenafil, silodosin, simeprevir, simvastatin, solifenacin, sunitinib, tadalafil, temazepam, temsirolimus, ticagrelor, tipranavir, tolvaptan, trabectedin, triazolam, ulipristal, valbenazine, vandetanib, vemurafenib, venetoclax, vorapaxar, warfarin, zidovudine
Pregnancy category: C
Important contra-indications noted in the prescribing guidelines for: the elderly; nursing mothers; pediatric patients

Skin
Anaphylactoid reactions/Anaphylaxis [2]
Exanthems [2]
Fixed eruption [3]
Hypersensitivity [3]
Psoriasis [2]
Purpura [3]
Rash (3%) [2]
Serum sickness-like reaction [2]
Toxic epidermal necrolysis [4]
Vasculitis [3]

Mucosal
Stomatitis [2]

Cardiovascular
QT prolongation [7]
Torsades de pointes [9]

Central Nervous System
Anorexia [2]
Dysgeusia (taste perversion) (3%) [9]
Mania [4]
Neurotoxicity [4]
Psychosis [3]

Neuromuscular/Skeletal
Arthralgia [2]
Rhabdomyolysis [14]

Gastrointestinal/Hepatic
Abdominal distension [2]
Abdominal pain [5]
Diarrhea [10]
Dyspepsia [2]
Hepatotoxicity [4]
Nausea [5]
Vomiting [3]

Endocrine/Metabolic
Hypoglycemia [3]

Renal
Nephrotoxicity [2]

Ocular
Hallucinations, visual [4]
Local
Injection-site pain [2]
Other
Adverse effects [11]

CLEMASTINE

See: www.drugeruptiondata.com/drug/id/161

CLEVIDIPINE

See: www.drugeruptiondata.com/drug/id/1295

CLIDINIUM

See: www.drugeruptiondata.com/drug/id/162

CLINDAMYCIN

Trade names: Benzaclin (Dermik), Cleocin (Pfizer), Cleocin-T (Pfizer), Clindagel (Galderma), Clindets (Stiefel)
Indications: Various serious infections caused by susceptible organisms
Class: Antibiotic, lincosamide
Half-life: 2–3 hours
Clinically important, potentially hazardous interactions with: cisatracurium, erythromycin, kaolin, mivacurium, neostigmine, pyridostigmine, rocuronium, saquinavir
Pregnancy category: B
Note: See also separate entry for the combination product clindamycin/tretinoin.

Skin
AGEP [8]
Anaphylactoid reactions/Anaphylaxis [5]
Dermatitis (from topical preparations) [7]
DRESS syndrome [2]
Erythema multiforme [2]
Erythroderma [2]
Exanthems [5]
Hypersensitivity [4]
Rash (<10%) [3]
Stevens-Johnson syndrome [3]
Sweet's syndrome [2]
Toxic epidermal necrolysis [3]
Urticaria [3]
Vasculitis [2]
Mucosal
Burning mouth syndrome [2]
Xerostomia [2]
Central Nervous System
Ageusia (taste loss) [2]
Gastrointestinal/Hepatic
Colitis [2]
Diarrhea [4]
Esophagitis [2]
Hepatotoxicity [3]
Pseudomembranous colitis [5]

Hematologic
Neutropenia [2]
Otic
Tinnitus [2]
Local
Application-site erythema [3]
Other
Adverse effects [6]
Death [3]

CLINDAMYCIN/ TRETINOIN

See: www.drugeruptiondata.com/drug/id/1841

CLIOQUINOL

See: www.drugeruptiondata.com/drug/id/1250

CLOBAZAM

See: www.drugeruptiondata.com/drug/id/1128

CLOBETASOL

See: www.drugeruptiondata.com/drug/id/1102

CLOFARABINE

See: www.drugeruptiondata.com/drug/id/1066

CLOFAZIMINE

See: www.drugeruptiondata.com/drug/id/164

CLOFIBRATE

See: www.drugeruptiondata.com/drug/id/165

CLOMIPHENE

See: www.drugeruptiondata.com/drug/id/166

CLOMIPRAMINE

Trade name: Anafranil (Mallinckrodt)
Indications: Obsessive-compulsive disorder
Class: Antidepressant, tricyclic, Muscarinic antagonist
Half-life: 21–31 hours
Clinically important, potentially hazardous interactions with: amprenavir, arbutamine, arsenic, artemether/lumefantrine, clonidine, duloxetine, epinephrine, formoterol, guanethidine, isocarboxazid, linezolid, MAO inhibitors, milnacipran, moclobemide, phenelzine, quinolones, sparfloxacin, tranylcypromine

Pregnancy category: C
Important contra-indications noted in the prescribing guidelines for: the elderly; nursing mothers; pediatric patients
Warning: SUICIDALITY AND ANTIDEPRESSANT DRUGS

Skin
Acneform eruption (2%)
Cellulitis (2%)
Dermatitis (2%)
Diaphoresis (29%) [2]
Edema (2%)
Hypersensitivity [2]
Photosensitivity [3]
Pruritus (6%)
Purpura (3%)
Rash (8%)
Xerosis (2%)
Mucosal
Xerostomia (84%) [6]
Cardiovascular
Flushing (8%)
QT prolongation [4]
Torsades de pointes [2]
Central Nervous System
Dysgeusia (taste perversion) (8%)
Seizures [4]
Serotonin syndrome [3]
Neuromuscular/Skeletal
Myalgia/Myopathy (13%)
Endocrine/Metabolic
Gynecomastia (2%)
SIADH [3]
Genitourinary
Vaginitis (2%)
Other
Adverse effects [3]
Allergic reactions (<3%)

CLONAZEPAM

Trade name: Klonopin (Roche)
Indications: Petit mal and myoclonic seizures
Class: Benzodiazepine
Half-life: 18–50 hours
Clinically important, potentially hazardous interactions with: amprenavir, chlorpheniramine, clarithromycin, cobicistat/elvitegravir/emtricitabine/tenofovir disoproxil, efavirenz, esomeprazole, imatinib, indinavir, nelfinavir, nevirapine, oxycodone, piracetam
Pregnancy category: D
Important contra-indications noted in the prescribing guidelines for: the elderly; nursing mothers; pediatric patients

Skin
Bullous dermatitis [2]
Dermatitis (<10%)
Diaphoresis (>10%)
Pseudolymphoma [2]
Rash (>10%)
Hair
Alopecia [2]

Mucosal
Sialopenia (>10%)
Sialorrhea (<10%)
Xerostomia (>10%)

Central Nervous System
Psychosis [2]
Seizures [2]

Other
Adverse effects [2]
Allergic reactions (<10%)

CLONIDINE

Trade name: Catapres (Boehringer Ingelheim)
Indications: Hypertension
Class: Adrenergic alpha-receptor agonist
Half-life: 6–24 hours
Clinically important, potentially hazardous interactions with: acebutolol, alfuzosin, amitriptyline, amoxapine, atenolol, betaxolol, captopril, carteolol, cilazapril, clomipramine, desipramine, dexmethylphenidate, diclofenac, doxepin, enalapril, esmolol, fosinopril, imipramine, insulin aspart, insulin degludec, insulin detemir, insulin glargine, insulin glulisine, irbesartan, levodopa, levomepromazine, lisinopril, meloxicam, metoprolol, milnacipran, nadolol, nebivolol, nortriptyline, olmesartan, oxprenolol, penbutolol, pericyazine, pindolol, propranolol, protriptyline, quinapril, ramipril, sotalol, sulpiride, timolol, trandolapril, triamcinolone, tricyclic antidepressants, trimipramine, verapamil
Pregnancy category: C
Important contra-indications noted in the prescribing guidelines for: nursing mothers; pediatric patients

Skin
Depigmentation [2]
Dermatitis (from patch) (20%) [23]
Eczema [2]
Erythema [2]
Lupus erythematosus [5]
Pigmentation [2]
Pityriasis rosea [2]
Pruritus (>5%) [6]
Psoriasis [2]
Rash (<10%) [4]
Ulcerations (<10%)

Mucosal
Xerostomia (40%) [13]

Cardiovascular
Bradycardia [8]
Hypotension [18]

Central Nervous System
Fever [2]
Hallucinations [3]
Headache [4]
Hyperesthesia (<10%)
Sedation [2]
Seizures [2]
Somnolence (drowsiness) [4]
Vertigo (dizziness) [4]

Neuromuscular/Skeletal
Asthenia (fatigue) [2]

Gastrointestinal/Hepatic
Nausea [2]

Other
Adverse effects [3]

CLOPIDOGREL

Trade name: Plavix (Bristol-Myers Squibb) (Sanofi-Aventis)
Indications: Acute coronary syndrome, recent myocardial infarction, recent stroke, or established peripheral arterial disease
Class: Antiplatelet, Antiplatelet, thienopyridine
Half-life: 6 hours
Clinically important, potentially hazardous interactions with: amiodarone, anisindione, anticoagulants, atorvastatin, calcium channel blockers, cangrelor, carbamazepine, chloramphenicol, cimetidine, ciprofloxacin, collagenase, dabigatran, dasatinib, delavirdine, dexlansoprazole, diclofenac, dicumarol, dipyridamole, drotrecogin alfa, efavirenz, enoxaparin, erythromycin, esomeprazole, etravirine, fluconazole, fluoxetine, fluvoxamine, fondaparinux, glucosamine, herbals with anticoagulant properties, ibritumomab, iloprost, itraconazole, ketoconazole, lansoprazole, lepirudin, macrolide antibiotics, meloxicam, miconazole, moclobemide, NSAIDs, omega-3 fatty acids, omeprazole, oxcarbazepine, pantoprazole, pentosan, pentoxifylline, polysulfate sodium, prasugrel, rabeprazole, rifapentine, rivaroxaban, salicylates, simvastatin, telithromycin, thrombolytic agents, tinzaparin, tositumomab & iodine[131], voriconazole, warfarin
Pregnancy category: B
Important contra-indications noted in the prescribing guidelines for: nursing mothers; pediatric patients
Note: Contra-indicated in patients with active pathological bleeding.
Warning: DIMINISHED EFFECTIVENESS IN POOR METABOLIZERS

Skin
AGEP [2]
Angioedema [4]
Bullous dermatitis (<3%)
Eczema (<3%)
Edema (3–5%)
Exanthems (<3%) [2]
Hypersensitivity [9]
Pruritus (3%) [2]
Psoriasis [2]
Purpura [18]
Rash (4%) [5]
Stevens-Johnson syndrome [2]
Thrombocytopenic purpura [9]
Ulcerations (<3%)
Urticaria (<3%) [3]

Cardiovascular
Acute coronary syndrome [2]
Myocardial infarction [2]

Central Nervous System
Ageusia (taste loss) [3]
Fever [3]
Hyperesthesia (<3%)
Intracranial hemorrhage [2]
Paresthesias (<3%)

Neuromuscular/Skeletal
Arthralgia [5]
Rhabdomyolysis [3]

Gastrointestinal/Hepatic
Gastrointestinal bleeding [3]
Hepatotoxicity [6]

Respiratory
Dyspnea [3]
Flu-like syndrome (8%)

Hematologic
Bleeding [16]
Hemolytic uremic syndrome [2]
Neutropenia [4]
Thrombocytopenia [3]
Thrombosis [2]

Other
Adverse effects [2]
Allergic reactions (<3%) [2]

CLORAZEPATE

Trade name: Tranxene (Recordati)
Indications: Anxiety and panic disorders
Class: Benzodiazepine
Half-life: 48–96 hours
Clinically important, potentially hazardous interactions with: aminophylline, amprenavir, antacids, carbamazepine, carmustine, chlorpheniramine, clarithromycin, cobicistat/elvitegravir/emtricitabine/tenofovir alafenamide, cobicistat/elvitegravir/emtricitabine/tenofovir disoproxil, efavirenz, esomeprazole, imatinib, indinavir, itraconazole, ketoconazole, MAO inhibitors, midazolam, moclobemide, nelfinavir, phenytoin, sucralfate, warfarin
Pregnancy category: D
Important contra-indications noted in the prescribing guidelines for: nursing mothers; pediatric patients

Skin
Dermatitis (<10%)
Diaphoresis (>10%)
Rash (>10%)

Mucosal
Sialopenia (>10%)
Sialorrhea (<10%)
Xerostomia (>10%)

CLOTRIMAZOLE

See: www.drugeruptiondata.com/drug/id/827

CLOXACILLIN

See: www.drugeruptiondata.com/drug/id/172

CLOZAPINE

Trade names: Clozaril (Novartis), Denzapine (Merz), Leponex (Novartis), Zaponex (Teva)
Indications: Treatment-resistant schizophrenia
Class: Antipsychotic
Half-life: 4–12 hours
Clinically important, potentially hazardous interactions with: alcohol, amitriptyline, antimuscarinics, arsenic, benzodiazepines, cabazitaxel, caffeine, carbamazepine, chloramphenicol, cimetidine, ciprofloxacin, citalopram, cocoa, cyclophosphamide, cytotoxics, darifenacin, dasatinib, encainide, epinephrine, erythromycin, everolimus, flecainide, fluoxetine, flupentixol, fluphenazine, fluvoxamine, gefitinib, guarana, haloperidol, insulin degludec, insulin detemir, insulin glargine, insulin glulisine, lapatinib, lithium, lomustine, lorazepam, MAO inhibitors, nilotinib, norfloxacin, ofloxacin, omeprazole, oxaliplatin, oxybutynin, paroxetine hydrochloride, pazopanib, pemetrexed, penicillamine, pipotiazine, propafenone, quinidine, rifampin, risperidone, ritonavir, saquinavir, selenium, sertraline, sorafenib, sulfonamides, sunitinib, telithromycin, temozolomide, temsirolimus, tetrazepam, tricyclic antidepressants, trospium, uracil/tegafur, valproic acid, venlafaxine, zuclopenthixol
Pregnancy category: B
Important contra-indications noted in the prescribing guidelines for: the elderly; nursing mothers; pediatric patients
Note: Contra-indicated in patients with myeloproliferative disorders, uncontrolled epilepsy, paralytic ileus, or a history of clozapine-induced agranulocytosis or severe granulocytopenia.
Warning: AGRANULOCYTOSIS / SEIZURES / MYOCARDITIS / OTHER ADVERSE CARDIOVASCULAR AND RESPIRATORY EFFECTS
INCREASED MORTALITY IN ELDERLY PATIENTS WITH DEMENTIA-RELATED PSYCHOSIS

Skin
Angioedema [2]
Diaphoresis (6%) [4]
Exanthems [2]
Lupus erythematosus [4]
Pityriasis rosea [2]
Rash (2%) [2]
Toxicity [5]

Mucosal
Parotitis [3]
Sialorrhea (31%) [75]
Xerostomia [3]

Cardiovascular
Atrial fibrillation [2]
Cardiomyopathy [13]
Cardiotoxicity [2]
Hypertension (4%) [4]
Hypotension (9%) [4]
Myocarditis [38]
Orthostatic hypotension [3]
Pericardial effusion [3]
Pericarditis [8]
QT prolongation [5]
Tachycardia (25%) [11]
Venous thromboembolism [5]

Central Nervous System
Akathisia [3]
Anxiety [2]
Compulsions [9]
Fever [8]
Headache (7%)
Neuroleptic malignant syndrome [30]
Neurotoxicity [2]
Pain [2]
Restless legs syndrome [2]
Sedation (39%) [11]
Seizures [25]
Somnolence (drowsiness) [10]
Syncope [2]
Tardive dyskinesia [6]
Tic disorder [2]
Tremor (<10%) [2]
Vertigo (dizziness) (19%) [2]

Neuromuscular/Skeletal
Myoclonus [2]
Rhabdomyolysis [8]

Gastrointestinal/Hepatic
Colitis [2]
Constipation (14%) [6]
Gastric obstruction [3]
Gastrointestinal hypomotility [4]
Hepatotoxicity [6]
Ileus [6]
Pancreatitis [6]

Respiratory
Pleural effusion [4]
Pneumonia [3]
Pulmonary embolism [2]

Endocrine/Metabolic
Diabetes mellitus [7]
Diabetic ketoacidosis [2]
Galactorrhea [2]
Hyperglycemia [6]
Hyperlipidemia [3]
Metabolic syndrome [13]
Weight gain [28]

Genitourinary
Priapism [14]

Renal
Enuresis [4]

Hematologic
Agranulocytosis [31]
Dyslipidemia [3]
Eosinophilia [9]
Granulocytopenia [2]
Hemotoxicity [2]
Leukopenia [10]
Neutropenia [16]
Pancytopenia [2]
Thrombosis [2]

Ocular
Maculopathy [2]

Other
Adverse effects [10]
Death [15]
Serositis [6]

CO-TRIMOXAZOLE

Synonyms: sulfamethoxazole-trimethoprim; SMX-TMP; SMZ-TMP; TMP-SMX; TMP-SMZ
Trade names: Bactrim (GSK), Septra (Monarch)
Indications: Various infections caused by susceptible organisms
Class: Antibiotic, sulfonamide
Half-life: 6–10 hours
Clinically important, potentially hazardous interactions with: anticoagulants, azathioprine, cyclosporine, dofetilide, isotretinoin, methotrexate, prilocaine, repaglinide, warfarin
Pregnancy category: C
Important contra-indications noted in the prescribing guidelines for: the elderly; nursing mothers; pediatric patients
Note: Co-trimoxazole is a sulfonamide and can be absorbed systemically. Sulfonamides can produce severe, possibly fatal, reactions such as toxic epidermal necrolysis and Stevens-Johnson syndrome.
Co-trimoxazole is sulfamethoxazole and trimethoprim.

Skin
AGEP [4]
Anaphylactoid reactions/Anaphylaxis [6]
Angioedema [3]
Bullous dermatitis [2]
Dermatitis [4]
DRESS syndrome [9]
Erythema multiforme [19]
Erythema nodosum [2]
Exanthems [35]
Exfoliative dermatitis [5]
Fixed eruption [50]
Hypersensitivity [18]
Jarisch–Herxheimer reaction [2]
Linear IgA bullous dermatosis [4]
Lupus erythematosus [4]
Photosensitivity [4]
Pruritus [10]
Purpura [3]
Pustules [6]
Radiation recall dermatitis [3]
Rash (>10%) [14]
Stevens-Johnson syndrome (<10%) [40]
Sweet's syndrome [9]
Toxic epidermal necrolysis (<10%) [51]
Toxicity [2]
Urticaria [12]
Vasculitis [11]

Mucosal
Oral mucosal eruption [2]
Oral ulceration [2]

Cardiovascular
QT prolongation [2]
Torsades de pointes [3]

Central Nervous System
Aseptic meningitis [5]
Fever [4]
Psychosis [4]
Tremor [4]
Vertigo (dizziness) [2]

Neuromuscular/Skeletal
Asthenia (fatigue) [2]
Myalgia/Myopathy [2]

Rhabdomyolysis [7]

Gastrointestinal/Hepatic
Hepatotoxicity [7]
Nausea [2]
Pancreatitis [4]
Vomiting [4]

Endocrine/Metabolic
ALT increased [2]
Hyperkalemia [4]
Hypoglycemia [5]
Hyponatremia [2]
Serum creatinine increased [4]

Hematologic
Agranulocytosis [2]
Anemia [3]
Methemoglobinemia [2]
Neutropenia [5]
Thrombocytopenia [9]

Ocular
Glaucoma [2]
Myopia [2]

Other
Adverse effects [14]
Allergic reactions [2]
Death [4]
Side effects [2]

COAGULATION FACTOR IX (RECOMBINANT)

See: www.drugeruptiondata.com/drug/id/1366

COBICISTAT/ ELVITEGRAVIR/ EMTRICITABINE/ TENOFOVIR ALAFENAMIDE

Trade name: Genvoya (Gilead)
Indications: HIV-1 infection
Class: Antiretroviral, CYP3A inhibitor (cobicistat), Hepatitis B virus necleoside analog reverse transcriptase inhibitor (tenofovir alafenamide), Integrase strand transfer inhibitor (elvitegravir), Nucleoside analog reverse transcriptase inhibitor (emtricitabine)
Half-life: 3.5 hours (cobicistat); 13 hours (elvitegravir); 10 hours (emtricitabine); <1 hour (tenofovir alafenamide)
Clinically important, potentially hazardous interactions with: acyclovir, aminoglycosides, amiodarone, amitriptyline, amlodipine, antacids, antiarrhythmics, atorvastatin, benzodiazepines, bepridil, beta blockers, bosentan, buprenorphine, bupropion, buspirone, calcium channel blockers, cidofovir, clarithromycin, clorazepate, colchicine, desipramine, dexamethasone, diazepam, digoxin, diltiazem, disopyramide, drugs affecting renal function, estazolam, ethosuximide, felodipine, flecainide, flurazepam, fluticasone furoate, fluticasone propionate, ganciclovir, gentamicin,

hormonal contraceptives, imipramine, immunosuppressants, itraconazole, ketoconazole, lidocaine, lorazepam, metoprolol, mexiletine, midazolam, naloxone, neuroleptics, nicardipine, nifedipine, nortriptyline, oxcarbazepine, paroxetine hydrochloride, perphenazine, propafenone, quinidine, rifabutin, rifapentine, risperidone, salmeterol, sildenafil, SSRIs, tadalafil, telithromycin, thioridazine, timolol, trazodone, tricyclic antidepressants, valacyclovir, valganciclovir, vardenafil, verapamil, voriconazole, warfarin, zolpidem
Pregnancy category: B
Important contra-indications noted in the prescribing guidelines for: nursing mothers
Note: See also separate profiles for emtricitabine and tenofovir alafenamide.
Warning: LACTIC ACIDOSIS/SEVERE HEPATOMEGALY WITH STEATOSIS and POST TREATMENT ACUTE EXACERBATION OF HEPATITIS B

Central Nervous System
Headache (6%)

Neuromuscular/Skeletal
Asthenia (fatigue) (5%)

Gastrointestinal/Hepatic
Diarrhea (7%)
Nausea (5%) [2]

Other
Adverse effects [2]

COBICISTAT/ ELVITEGRAVIR/ EMTRICITABINE/ TENOFOVIR DISOPROXIL

Trade name: Stribild (Gilead)
Indications: HIV-1 infection
Class: Antiretroviral, CYP3A inhibitor (cobicistat), Integrase strand transfer inhibitor (elvitegravir), Nucleoside analog reverse transcriptase inhibitor (emtricitabine and tenofovir disoproxil)
Half-life: 3.5 hours (cobicistat); 13 hours (elvitegravir); 10 hours (emtricitabine); 12–18 hours (tenofovir disoproxil)
Clinically important, potentially hazardous interactions with: acyclovir, adefovir, amiodarone, amitriptyline, amlodipine, antacids, antiarrhythmics, antiretrovirals, atorvastatin, benzodiazepines, bepridil, beta blockers, bosentan, buprenorphine, bupropion, buspirone, calcium channel blockers, carbamazepine, cidofovir, clarithromycin, clonazepam, clorazepate, colchicine, cyclosporine, desipramine, dexamethasone, diazepam, digoxin, diltiazem, disopyramide, drugs affecting renal function, elbasvir & grazoprevir, emtricitabine, estazolam, ethosuximide, felodipine, flecainide, flurazepam, fluticasone propionate, ganciclovir, hormonal contraceptives, imipramine, immunosuppressants, itraconazole, ketoconazole, lamivudine, ledipasvir & sofosbuvir, lidocaine,

metoprolol, mexiletine, midazolam, naloxone, neuroleptics, nicardipine, nifedipine, non-nucleoside reverse transcriptase inhibitors, nortriptyline, oxcarbazepine, paroxetine hydrochloride, perphenazine, phenobarbital, phenytoin, propafenone, protease inhibitors, quinidine, rifabutin, rifapentine, risperidone, ritonavir, salmeterol, sedatives / hypnotics, sildenafil, simeprevir, sirolimus, SSRIs, tacrolimus, tadalafil, telithromycin, tenofovir disoproxil, thioridazine, timolol, trazodone, tricyclic antidepressants, valacyclovir, valganciclovir, vardenafil, verapamil, voriconazole, warfarin, zolpidem
Pregnancy category: B
Important contra-indications noted in the prescribing guidelines for: the elderly; nursing mothers; pediatric patients
Note: See also separate profiles for emtricitabine and tenofovir disoproxil.
Warning: LACTIC ACIDOSIS/SEVERE HEPATOMEGALY WITH STEATOSIS and POST TREATMENT ACUTE EXACERBATION OF HEPATITIS B

Skin
Rash (3%) [3]

Central Nervous System
Abnormal dreams (9%) [3]
Headache (7%) [5]
Insomnia (3%) [2]
Vertigo (dizziness) (3%) [3]

Neuromuscular/Skeletal
Asthenia (fatigue) (5%) [2]

Gastrointestinal/Hepatic
Diarrhea (12%) [6]
Flatulence (2%)
Gastrointestinal disorder [2]
Hepatotoxicity [2]
Nausea (16%) [8]

Respiratory
Upper respiratory tract infection [2]

Endocrine/Metabolic
AST increased (2%)
Serum creatinine increased [2]

Genitourinary
Hematuria (3%)

Renal
Nephrotoxicity [2]
Proteinuria (39%)

Other
Adverse effects [5]

COBIMETINIB

Trade name: Cotellic (Genentech)
Indications: Melanoma (unresectable or metastatic) in patients with BRAF V600E or V600K mutations, in combination with vemurafenib
Class: MEK inhibitor
Half-life: 23–70 hours
Clinically important, potentially hazardous interactions with: carbamazepine, efavirenz, itraconazole, phenytoin, rifampin, St John's wort, strong or moderate CYP3A inhibitors or inducers

Pregnancy category: N/A (Can cause fetal harm)
Important contra-indications noted in the prescribing guidelines for: nursing mothers; pediatric patients

Skin
Acneform eruption (16%) [3]
Basal cell carcinoma (5%)
Erythema (10%) [2]
Hyperkeratosis (11%) [3]
Keratoacanthoma [3]
Photosensitivity (46%) [8]
Rash [7]
Squamous cell carcinoma (6%) [6]

Hair
Alopecia (15%) [3]

Mucosal
Stomatitis (14%)

Cardiovascular
Hypertension (15%)

Central Nervous System
Chills (10%)
Fever (28%) [3]

Neuromuscular/Skeletal
Arthralgia [3]
Asthenia (fatigue) [6]
Myalgia/Myopathy [2]

Gastrointestinal/Hepatic
Diarrhea (60%) [7]
Gastrointestinal bleeding (4%)
Hepatotoxicity [5]
Nausea (41%) [6]
Vomiting (24%) [3]

Respiratory
Pneumonitis (<10%)

Endocrine/Metabolic
ALP increased (71%) [3]
ALT increased (68%) [3]
AST increased (73%) [3]
Creatine phosphokinase increased (79%) [4]
GGT increased (65%)
Hyperkalemia (26%)
Hypoalbuminemia (42%)
Hypocalcemia (24%)
Hypokalemia (25%)
Hyponatremia (38%)
Hypophosphatemia (68%)
Serum creatinine increased (100%)

Genitourinary
Hematuria (2%)

Hematologic
Anemia (69%) [3]
Hemorrhage (13%)
Lymphopenia (73%)
Thrombocytopenia (18%)

Ocular
Chorioretinopathy (13%) [3]
Retinal detachment (12%) [2]
Vision impaired (15%)

COCAINE

Indications: Topical anesthesia
Class: Anesthetic, local, CNS stimulant
Half-life: 75 minutes
Clinically important, potentially hazardous interactions with: epinephrine, iobenguane
Pregnancy category: C (the pregnancy category is X for non-medicinal use)

Skin
Angioedema [3]
Diaphoresis [3]
Hyperkeratosis (fingers and palms) [2]
Necrosis [6]
Purpura [4]
Raynaud's phenomenon [2]
Scleroderma (reversible) [3]
Vasculitis [14]

Mucosal
Nasal septal perforation [4]
Palatal perforation [7]

Cardiovascular
Angina [2]
Brugada syndrome [3]
Chest pain [5]
Myocardial infarction [6]
Myocardial ischemia [2]

Central Nervous System
Ageusia (taste loss) (>10%)
Anosmia (>10%)
Compulsions [2]
Hallucinations [4]
Leukoencephalopathy [3]
Psychosis [2]
Seizures [6]
Suicidal ideation [2]
Tic disorder [2]
Tremor (<10%)

Neuromuscular/Skeletal
Arthralgia [2]
Rhabdomyolysis [19]

Genitourinary
Priapism [5]

Renal
Glomerulonephritis [2]
Nephrotoxicity [2]

Hematologic
Agranulocytosis [2]
Hemolytic uremic syndrome [2]
Neutropenia [6]

Otic
Hallucinations, auditory [2]

Ocular
Hallucinations, visual [3]

Other
Death [3]

CODEINE

Synonym: methylmorphine
Trade names: Halotussin (Watson), Nucofed (Monarch), Robitussin AC (Wyeth), Tussi-Organidin (MedPointe)
Indications: Pain, cough suppressant
Class: Opiate agonist
Half-life: 2.5–4 hours
Clinically important, potentially hazardous interactions with: alcohol, cinacalcet, CNS depressants, delavirdine, MAO inhibitors, mianserin, terbinafine, tipranavir
Pregnancy category: C
Important contra-indications noted in the prescribing guidelines for: the elderly; nursing mothers; pediatric patients
Warning: DEATH RELATED TO ULTRA-RAPID METABOLISM OF CODEINE TO MORPHINE

Skin
Angioedema [2]
Dermatitis [5]
Erythema multiforme [4]
Exanthems [6]
Fixed eruption [6]
Pruritus [3]
Rash (<10%)
Toxic epidermal necrolysis [2]
Urticaria (<10%) [9]

Mucosal
Xerostomia (<10%)

Central Nervous System
Somnolence (drowsiness) [2]
Vertigo (dizziness) [2]

Gastrointestinal/Hepatic
Constipation [3]
Nausea [2]
Pancreatitis [5]
Vomiting [2]

Respiratory
Respiratory depression [3]

Local
Injection-site pain (<10%)

Other
Death [5]

COLCHICINE

Indications: Gouty arthritis (in adults), gout, familial Mediterranean fever
Class: Alkaloid, Anti-inflammatory
Half-life: 27–31 hours (following multiple doses)
Clinically important, potentially hazardous interactions with: amiodarone, aprepitant, atazanavir, atorvastatin, azithromycin, boceprevir, clarithromycin, cobicistat/elvitegravir/emtricitabine/tenofovir alafenamide, cobicistat/elvitegravir/emtricitabine/tenofovir disoproxil, conivaptan, cyanocobalamin, cyclosporine, darunavir, dasatinib, delavirdine, digoxin, diltiazem, efavirenz, erythromycin, fenofibrate, fibrates, fluvastatin, gemfibrozil, grapefruit juice, HMG-CoA reductase inhibitors, indinavir, itraconazole, ketoconazole, lapatinib, lopinavir, ombitasvir/paritaprevir/ritonavir, P-glycoprotein

inhibitors or inducers, pravastatin, protease inhibitors, ritonavir, rosuvastatin, saxagliptin, simvastatin, strong CYP3A4 inhibitors, telithromycin, troleandomycin, verapamil, voriconazole
Pregnancy category: C
Important contra-indications noted in the prescribing guidelines for: the elderly
Note: Contra-indicated in patients with renal or hepatic impairment where P-glycoprotein or strong CYP3A4 inhibitors are also prescribed.

Skin
Pruritus [2]
Staphylococcal scalded skin syndrome [2]
Toxic epidermal necrolysis [3]
Vasculitis [2]

Hair
Alopecia (<10%) [6]

Central Nervous System
Headache (2%)
Neurotoxicity [3]

Neuromuscular/Skeletal
Asthenia (fatigue) (<4%)
Gouty tophi (4%)
Myalgia/Myopathy [20]
Rhabdomyolysis [18]

Gastrointestinal/Hepatic
Abdominal pain (<20%) [2]
Diarrhea (23%) [6]
Gastrointestinal disorder [2]
Hepatotoxicity [3]
Nausea (<20%) [3]
Vomiting (<20%) [4]

Respiratory
Pharyngolaryngeal pain (3%)

Other
Adverse effects [6]
Death [3]
Side effects (14%)

COLESEVELAM

Trade names: Cholestagel (Genzyme), Welchol (Sankyo)
Indications: Hypercholesterolemia, hyperlipidemia, Type II diabetes mellitus
Class: Bile acid sequestrant
Half-life: N/A
Clinically important, potentially hazardous interactions with: cyclosporine, deferasirox, estradiol, glyburide, levothyroxine, olmesartan, phenytoin, warfarin
Pregnancy category: B
Important contra-indications noted in the prescribing guidelines for: pediatric patients
Note: Contra-indicated in patients with a history of bowel obstruction, with serum triglyceride concentrations >500 mg/dL or with a history of hypertriglyceridemia-induced pancreatitis.

Cardiovascular
Hypertension (3%)

Central Nervous System
Headache [2]

Neuromuscular/Skeletal
Myalgia/Myopathy (2%)

Gastrointestinal/Hepatic
Abdominal pain (4%)
Constipation (9–10%) [3]
Diarrhea (3%)
Dyspepsia (4–6%) [3]
Flatulence (11%)
Gastrointestinal disorder [4]
Nausea (3%)

Respiratory
Nasopharyngitis (4%)

Endocrine/Metabolic
Hypoglycemia (3%) [3]

Other
Adverse effects [4]

COLESTIPOL

See: www.drugeruptiondata.com/drug/id/179

COLISTIN

See: www.drugeruptiondata.com/drug/id/1144

COLLAGEN (BOVINE)

Trade names: Bellafill (Suneva), Zyderm (Inamed), Zyplast (Inamed)
Indications: Cataract surgery (collagen shields), depressed cutaneous scars, facial lines, wrinkles, glottic insufficiency, phonosurgey, urinary incontinence
Class: Protein
Half-life: Several months to years
Clinically important, potentially hazardous interactions with: argatroban, avitene
Pregnancy category: N/A
Important contra-indications noted in the prescribing guidelines for: nursing mothers
Note: A reaction to the anesthetic, lidocaine, in liquid collagen injections may occur. Artecoll and Bellafill contain polymethyl-methacrylate microspheres.

Skin
Abscess [2]
Churg-Strauss syndrome [7]
Dermatomyositis [3]
Edema [2]
Erythema [3]
Granulomatous reaction [2]
Hypersensitivity [10]
Induration [3]
Panniculitis [2]

Neuromuscular/Skeletal
Arthralgia [2]
Polymyositis [3]

Other
Adverse effects [12]
Allergic reactions [7]

CONIVAPTAN

Trade name: Vaprisol (Astellas)
Indications: Hyponatremia, SIADH
Class: CYP3A4 inhibitor, Vasopressin receptor antagonist
Half-life: 5 hours
Clinically important, potentially hazardous interactions with: acetaminophen, albendazole, alfuzosin, almotriptan, alosetron, ambrisentan, amitriptyline, amlodipine, antifungals, aprepitant, artemether/lumefantrine, atorvastatin, bexarotene, bortezomib, brigatinib, brinzolamide, bupivacaine, cabazitaxel, cabozantinib, ciclesonide, cilostazol, cinacalcet, citalopram, clarithromycin, colchicine, copanlisib, cyclobenzaprine, CYP3A4 inhibitors or substrates, darunavir, dasatinib, deferasirox, delavirdine, dienogest, digoxin, docetaxel, dronedarone, dutasteride, efavirenz, enalapril, eplerenone, estradiol, eszopiclone, everolimus, fentanyl, fesoterodine, fingolimod, flibanserin, gefitinib, guanfacine, halofantrine, indinavir, itraconazole, ixabepilone, ketoconazole, lapatinib, lomitapide, maraviroc, meloxicam, metaxalone, methylprednisolone, micafungin, midazolam, midostaurin, mifepristone, mometasone, neratinib, nilotinib, nisoldipine, oxybutynin, pantoprazole, paricalcitol, pazopanib, pimecrolimus, pioglitazone, ponatinib, prasugrel, ramelteon, ranolazine, ribociclib, ritonavir, rivaroxaban, romidepsin, rosuvastatin, ruxolitinib, salmeterol, saxagliptin, sildenafil, silodosin, simvastatin, sorafenib, St John's wort, tadalafil, tamsulosin, telithromycin, temsirolimus, terbinafine, tiagabine, tiotropium, tipranavir, tolvaptan, trimethoprim, ulipristal, vardenafil, venetoclax, vorapaxar, voriconazole, ziprasidone
Pregnancy category: C
Important contra-indications noted in the prescribing guidelines for: nursing mothers; pediatric patients

Skin
Erythema (3%)
Peripheral edema (3–8%)
Pruritus (<5%)

Mucosal
Oral candidiasis (2%)
Xerostomia (4%)

Cardiovascular
Atrial fibrillation (2–5%)
Hypertension (6–8%)
Hypotension (5–8%) [4]
Orthostatic hypotension (6–14%)
Phlebitis (32–51%)

Central Nervous System
Confusion (<5%)
Fever (5–11%) [2]
Headache (8–10%)
Insomnia (4–5%)

Gastrointestinal/Hepatic
Constipation (6–8%)
Diarrhea (<7%)
Nausea (3–5%)
Vomiting (5–7%)

Respiratory
Pharyngolaryngeal pain (<5%)

Pneumonia (2–5%)

Endocrine/Metabolic
Hypokalemia (10–22%)
Hypomagnesemia (2–5%)
Hyponatremia (6–8%)

Genitourinary
Urinary tract infection (4–5%)

Hematologic
Anemia (5–6%)

Local
Infusion-site erythema (<6%)
Infusion-site pain (<5%)
Infusion-site reactions (63–73%) [5]

Other
Dipsia (thirst) (3–6%) [2]

COPANLISIB *

Trade name: Aliqopa (Bayer)
Indications: Relapsed follicular lymphoma in adult patients who have received at least two prior systemic therapies
Class: Kinase inhibitor
Half-life: 39 hours
Clinically important, potentially hazardous interactions with: boceprevir, carbamazepine, clarithromycin, cobicistat, conivaptan, danoprevir, dasabuvir/ombitasvir/paritaprevir/ritonavir, diltiazem, elvitegravir, enzalutamide, grapefruit juice, idelalisib, indinavir, itraconazole, ketoconazole, lopinavir, mitotane, nefazodone, nelfinavir, phenytoin, posaconazole, rifampin, ritonavir, saquinavir, St John's wort, strong CYP3A inhibitors and inducers, tipranavir, troleandomycin, voriconazole
Pregnancy category: N/A (Can cause fetal harm)
Important contra-indications noted in the prescribing guidelines for: nursing mothers; pediatric patients

Skin
Rash (15%)

Mucosal
Mucosal inflammation (8%)
Stomatitis (14%)

Cardiovascular
Hypertension (26%) [2]

Central Nervous System
Dysesthesia (7%)
Paresthesias (7%)

Neuromuscular/Skeletal
Asthenia (fatigue) (36%)

Gastrointestinal/Hepatic
Diarrhea (36%)
Nausea (26%)
Vomiting (13%)

Respiratory
Pneumonitis (9%)

Endocrine/Metabolic
Hyperglycemia (54%) [3]
Hypertriglyceridemia (58%)
Hyperuricemia (25%)
Hypophosphatemia (44%)

Hematologic
Hemoglobin decreased (78%)
Hyperlipasemia (21%)
Leukopenia (36%)
Lymphocytopenia (78%)
Neutropenia (32%)
Thrombocytopenia (22%)

Other
Infection (21%)

CORTISONE

Trade name: Cortone (Merck)
Indications: Arthralgia, dermatoses
Class: Corticosteroid
Half-life: N/A
Clinically important, potentially hazardous interactions with: chlorpropamide, diuretics, ethambutol, live vaccines, pancuronium, rifampin
Pregnancy category: C
Important contra-indications noted in the prescribing guidelines for: nursing mothers

Neuromuscular/Skeletal
Osteonecrosis [15]
Osteoporosis [10]
Tendinopathy/Tendon rupture [2]

Ocular
Cataract [5]
Glaucoma [8]

Other
Adverse effects [2]

CRISABOROLE *

Trade name: Eucrisa (Pfizer)
Indications: Atopic dermatitis
Class: Phosphodiesterase type 4 (PDE4) inhibitor
Half-life: N/A
Clinically important, potentially hazardous interactions with: none known
Pregnancy category: N/A (No available data)
Important contra-indications noted in the prescribing guidelines for: nursing mothers; pediatric patients

Local
Application-site pain (4%) [3]

CRIZOTINIB

Trade name: Xalkori (Pfizer)
Indications: Advanced or metastatic non-small cell lung cancer in ALK-positive patients
Class: Tyrosine kinase inhibitor
Half-life: 42 hours
Clinically important, potentially hazardous interactions with: alfentanil, atazanavir, carbamazepine, clarithromycin, cyclosporine, CYP3A inhibitors or inducers, CYP3A substrates, dihydroergotamine, efavirenz, ergotamine, fentanyl, grapefruit juice, indinavir, itraconazole, ketoconazole, nefazodone, nelfinavir, neratinib, olaparib, phenobarbital, phenytoin, pimozide, quinidine, rifabutin, rifampin, ritonavir, saquinavir,

sirolimus, St John's wort, tacrolimus, telithromycin, troleandomycin, voriconazole
Pregnancy category: D
Important contra-indications noted in the prescribing guidelines for: nursing mothers; pediatric patients

Skin
Edema (38%) [11]
Peripheral edema [6]
Photosensitivity [2]
Rash (16%) [4]

Mucosal
Stomatitis (11%)

Cardiovascular
Bradycardia (5%) [6]
Cardiotoxicity [2]
Chest pain (12%)
QT prolongation [6]

Central Nervous System
Dysgeusia (taste perversion) (13%) [5]
Fever (12%)
Headache (13%)
Insomnia (12%)
Neurotoxicity (23%)
Vertigo (dizziness) (24%) [5]

Neuromuscular/Skeletal
Arthralgia (11%)
Asthenia (fatigue) (31%) [8]
Back pain (11%)
Bone or joint pain [2]

Gastrointestinal/Hepatic
Abdominal pain (16%)
Constipation (38%) [13]
Diarrhea (49%) [23]
Dyspepsia [3]
Dysphagia [3]
Esophagitis [8]
Gastroesophageal reflux [2]
Hepatitis [2]
Hepatotoxicity [11]
Nausea (57%) [22]
Vomiting (45%) [22]

Respiratory
Cough (21%)
Dyspnea (22%)
Pneumonitis [6]
Pulmonary toxicity [9]
Upper respiratory tract infection (20%)

Endocrine/Metabolic
ALT increased (15%) [11]
Appetite decreased (27%) [4]
AST increased (11%) [9]
Dehydration [2]
Hypocalcemia [2]
Hypogonadism [6]
Hypophosphatemia [5]

Renal
Nephrotoxicity [8]

Hematologic
Anemia [3]
Lymphopenia (11%) [5]
Neutropenia (5%) [9]

Ocular
Diplopia [2]
Ocular adverse effects (64%) [13]
Photophobia [2]

Photopsia [3]
Reduced visual acuity [2]
Vision blurred [4]
Vision impaired [3]
Visual disturbances [15]
Vitreous floaters [2]

Other
Adverse effects [5]
Death [2]

CROFELEMER

Trade name: Fulyzaq (Salix)
Indications: Non-infectious diarrhea in adult patients with HIV/AIDS on anti-retroviral therapy
Class: Proanthocyanidin oligomer
Half-life: N/A
Clinically important, potentially hazardous interactions with: none known
Pregnancy category: C
Important contra-indications noted in the prescribing guidelines for: the elderly; nursing mothers; pediatric patients
Note: Derived from the red latex of *Croton lechleri* which is also known as Sangre de Drago or dragon's blood.

Skin
Acneform eruption (<2%)
Dermatitis (<2%)
Herpes zoster (<2%)

Mucosal
Xerostomia (<2%)

Central Nervous System
Anxiety (2%)
Depression (<2%)
Vertigo (dizziness) (<2%)

Neuromuscular/Skeletal
Arthralgia (3%)
Back pain (3%)
Bone or joint pain (2%)
Pain in extremities (<2%)

Gastrointestinal/Hepatic
Abdominal distension (2%)
Abdominal pain (<2%)
Constipation (<2%)
Dyspepsia (<2%)
Flatulence (3%)
Gastroenteritis (<2%)
Nausea (3%)

Respiratory
Bronchitis (4%)
Cough (4%)
Nasopharyngitis (2%)
Sinusitis (<2%)
Upper respiratory tract infection (6%)

Endocrine/Metabolic
ALT increased (2%)
AST increased (<2%)

Genitourinary
Pollakiuria (<2%)

Renal
Nephrolithiasis (<2%)

Hematologic
Leukopenia (<2%)

Other
Infection (giardiasis) (2%)

CROMOLYN

See: www.drugeruptiondata.com/drug/id/181

CYANOCOBALAMIN

Synonym: Vitamin B_{12}
Trade name: Nascobal (Nastech)
Indications: Vitamin B_{12} deficiency, pernicious anemia
Class: Vitamin
Half-life: 6 days
Clinically important, potentially hazardous interactions with: colchicine
Pregnancy category: C

Skin
Acneform eruption [8]
Anaphylactoid reactions/Anaphylaxis [6]
Dermatitis [2]
Exanthems [3]
Hypersensitivity [2]
Nicolau syndrome [2]
Pruritus (<10%)
Urticaria [7]

Other
Allergic reactions [3]

CYCLAMATE

See: www.drugeruptiondata.com/drug/id/183

CYCLOBENZAPRINE

Trade name: Flexeril (McNeil)
Indications: Muscle spasms
Class: Central muscle relaxant
Half-life: 8–37 hours
Clinically important, potentially hazardous interactions with: acetylcholinesterase inhibitors, anticholinergics, barbiturates, cisapride, CNS depressants, conivaptan, CYP1A2 inhibitors, droperidol, levomepromazine, linezolid, MAO inhibitors, phendimetrazine, pramlintide, safinamide
Pregnancy category: B
Important contra-indications noted in the prescribing guidelines for: the elderly; nursing mothers; pediatric patients

Mucosal
Xerostomia (7–32%) [7]

Central Nervous System
Confusion (<3%)
Dysgeusia (taste perversion) (<3%)
Headache (5%) [3]
Irritability (<3%)
Nervousness (<3%)
Serotonin syndrome [3]
Somnolence (drowsiness) (29–39%) [8]
Vertigo (dizziness) (<11%) [8]

Neuromuscular/Skeletal
Asthenia (fatigue) (6%) [3]

Gastrointestinal/Hepatic
Abdominal pain (<3%)
Constipation (<3%) [3]
Diarrhea (<3%)
Nausea (<3%)

Respiratory
Pharyngitis (<3%)
Upper respiratory tract infection (<3%)

Ocular
Vision blurred (<3%)

Other
Adverse effects [2]

CYCLOPENTHIAZIDE

See: www.drugeruptiondata.com/drug/id/1419

CYCLOPHOSPHAMIDE

Synonyms: CPM; CTX; CYT
Trade names: Cytoxan (Mead Johnson), Neosar (Gensia)
Indications: Lymphomas, minimal change nephrotic syndrome in pediatric patients
Class: Alkylating agent
Half-life: 3–12 hours
Clinically important, potentially hazardous interactions with: aldesleukin, azathioprine, belimumab, clozapine, cyclopenthiazide, cyclosporine, dexamethasone, etanercept, itraconazole, mycophenolate, pentostatin, prednisone, vaccines
Pregnancy category: D
Important contra-indications noted in the prescribing guidelines for: nursing mothers
Note: Contra-indicated in patients with urinary outflow obstruction.

Skin
Acral erythema [3]
Anaphylactoid reactions/Anaphylaxis [3]
Edema [5]
Exanthems [4]
Graft-versus-host reaction [2]
Hand–foot syndrome [10]
Herpes zoster [4]
Hypersensitivity [6]
Kaposi's sarcoma [2]
Lupus erythematosus [2]
Lymphoma [4]
Malignancies [2]
Pemphigus [2]
Pigmentation [16]
Radiation recall dermatitis [6]
Rash (<10%) [6]
Scleroderma [2]
Squamous cell carcinoma [2]
Stevens-Johnson syndrome [2]
Toxicity [6]
Urticaria [8]
Vasculitis [2]

Hair
Alopecia [28]

Nails

Leukonychia (Mees' lines) (Muehrcke's lines) [3]
Melanonychia [2]
Nail pigmentation [16]

Mucosal

Gingival pigmentation [2]
Mucositis [3]
Oral ulceration [2]
Stomatitis (10%) [6]

Cardiovascular

Cardiotoxicity [6]
Flushing (<10%)
Hypotension [2]

Central Nervous System

Anorexia [2]
Dysgeusia (taste perversion) [2]
Fever [3]
Headache [3]
Leukoencephalopathy [6]
Neurotoxicity [7]
Peripheral neuropathy [6]

Neuromuscular/Skeletal

Arthralgia [2]
Asthenia (fatigue) [13]
Myalgia/Myopathy [7]

Gastrointestinal/Hepatic

Abdominal pain [2]
Diarrhea [8]
Hepatotoxicity [11]
Nausea [10]
Vomiting [11]

Respiratory

Pneumonia [4]

Endocrine/Metabolic

Amenorrhea [16]
Hyperglycemia [2]
Hyponatremia [3]
Menstrual irregularities [2]
SIADH [9]

Genitourinary

Cystitis [10]
Urinary tract infection [2]

Hematologic

Anemia [9]
Cytopenia [2]
Febrile neutropenia [14]
Hemorrhage [2]
Hemotoxicity [10]
Leukopenia [12]
Lymphopenia [3]
Myelosuppression [4]
Neutropenia [33]
Sepsis [2]
Thrombocytopenia [16]

Local

Infusion-related reactions [2]

Other

Adverse effects [16]
Allergic reactions [2]
Death [9]
Hiccups [4]
Infection [21]

CYCLOSERINE

Trade name: Seromycin (Lilly)
Indications: Tuberculosis
Class: Antibiotic
Half-life: 10 hours
Clinically important, potentially hazardous interactions with: none known
Pregnancy category: C
Important contra-indications noted in the prescribing guidelines for: nursing mothers; pediatric patients

Skin

Dermatitis [2]
Exanthems [4]
Lichenoid eruption [2]

Mucosal

Gingival hyperplasia/hypertrophy [3]

Central Nervous System

Depression [2]
Neurotoxicity [2]
Psychosis [7]
Seizures [4]

Renal

Nephrotoxicity [2]

Other

Adverse effects [4]

CYCLOSPORINE

Synonyms: CsA; CyA
Trade names: Neoral (Novartis), Restasis (Allergan), Sandimmune (Novartis)
Indications: Rheumatoid arthritis, prophylaxis of organ rejection in transplants, psoriasis, Restasis is indicated for patients with moderate-to-severe dry eye syndrome
Class: Calcineurin inhibitor, Disease-modifying antirheumatic drug (DMARD), Immunosuppressant
Half-life: 10–27 hours (adults)
Clinically important, potentially hazardous interactions with: afatinib, aliskiren, ambrisentan, amiloride, aminoglycosides, amiodarone, amphotericin B, ampicillin, amprenavir, anisindione, anticoagulants, armodafinil, atazanavir, atorvastatin, azathioprine, azithromycin, bacampicillin, basiliximab, benazepril, bezafibrate, boceprevir, bosentan, bupropion, captopril, carbenicillin, caspofungin, ceritinib, cholestyramine, cholic acid, choline fenofibrate, cilazapril, ciprofloxacin, clarithromycin, cloxacillin, co-trimoxazole, cobicistat/elvitegravir/emtricitabine/tenofovir disoproxil, colchicine, colesevelam, corticosteroids, crizotinib, cyclophosphamide, dabigatran, daclizumab, danazol, daptomycin, darifenacin, darunavir, dasatinib, delavirdine, dichlorphenamide, diclofenac, dicloxacillin, dicumarol, digoxin, diltiazem, disulfiram, docetaxel, doxycycline, dronedarone, echinacea, efavirenz, elbasvir & grazoprevir, eluxadoline, enalapril, enzalutamide, erythromycin, ethotoin, etoposide, etoricoxib, everolimus, ezetimibe, flunisolide, fluoxymesterone, fluvastatin, foscarnet, fosinopril, fosphenytoin, gemfibrozil,

glecaprevir & pibrentasvir, grapefruit juice, Hemophilus B vaccine, HMG-CoA reductase inhibitors, imatinib, imipenem/cilastatin, indinavir, influenza vaccine, irbesartan, itraconazole, ketoconazole, lanreotide, levofloxacin, lisinopril, lopinavir, lovastatin, meloxicam, mephenytoin, methicillin, methoxsalen, methylphenidate, methylprednisolone, methyltestosterone, mezlocillin, micafungin, mifepristone, mizolastine, moxifloxacin, mycophenolate, nafcillin, naldemedine, natalizumab, nelfinavir, neratinib, nevirapine, nifedipine, nisoldipine, norfloxacin, NSAIDs, ofloxacin, olmesartan, omeprazole, orlistat, osimertinib, oxacillin, oxcarbazepine, pasireotide, penicillins, phenytoin, pitavastatin, posaconazole, pravastatin, prednisolone, prednisone, pristinamycin, quinapril, rabeprazole, ramipril, ranolazine, ribociclib, rifabutin, rifampin, rifapentine, ritonavir, rosuvastatin, sevelamer, silodosin, simvastatin, sirolimus, sofosbuvir/velpatasvir/voxilaprevir, spironolactone, St John's wort, sulfacetamide, sulfadiazine, sulfamethoxazole, sulfisoxazole, sulfonamides, tacrolimus, telithromycin, temsirolimus, tenoxicam, terbinafine, testosterone, ticarcillin, tinidazole, tipranavir, tofacitinib, tolvaptan, trabectedin, trandolapril, triamterene, trimethoprim, troleandomycin, ursodiol, vaccines, vecuronium, venetoclax, voriconazole, warfarin, zofenopril
Pregnancy category: C
Important contra-indications noted in the prescribing guidelines for: nursing mothers; pediatric patients
Note: Restasis is an ophthalmic emulsion.

Skin

Acne keloid [2]
Acneform eruption [7]
Anaphylactoid reactions/Anaphylaxis [8]
Basal cell carcinoma [4]
Candidiasis [2]
Cyst [5]
Edema (5–14%)
Fibroadenoma [2]
Folliculitis [8]
Herpes simplex [4]
Herpes zoster [2]
Hot flashes [2]
Hypersensitivity [2]
Kaposi's sarcoma [5]
Keratoses [3]
Keratosis pilaris [2]
Linear IgA bullous dermatosis [2]
Lymphocytic infiltration [5]
Lymphoma [12]
Lymphoproliferative disease [2]
Malignancies [2]
Mycosis fungoides [2]
Peripheral edema [3]
Pruritus (<2%) [2]
Pseudolymphoma [6]
Psoriasis [2]
Purpura (3%) [4]
Rash (7–12%)
Raynaud's phenomenon [2]
Sebaceous hyperplasia [9]
Squamous cell carcinoma [12]
Thrombocytopenic purpura [5]
Toxicity [2]

Urticaria [2]
Vasculitis [3]

Hair
Alopecia (3–4%) [2]
Alopecia areata [6]
Hirsutism [10]
Hypertrichosis (5–19%) [33]
Pseudofolliculitis barbae [2]

Nails
Brittle nails (<2%)
Leukonychia (Mees' lines) [2]

Mucosal
Aphthous stomatitis [2]
Gingival hyperplasia/hypertrophy (2–6%)
[157]
Gingivitis (3–4%)
Oral ulceration [2]
Rectal hemorrhage (<3%)
Stomatitis (5–7%)

Cardiovascular
Arrhythmias (2–5%)
Capillary leak syndrome [2]
Chest pain (4–6%)
Flushing (2–5%) [5]
Hypertension (8–28%) [26]

Central Nervous System
Anorexia (3%)
Depression (<6%)
Dysesthesia [2]
Encephalopathy [4]
Fever (3–6%)
Headache (14–25%) [4]
Insomnia (<4%)
Leukoencephalopathy [17]
Migraine (2–3%)
Neurotoxicity [10]
Pain (3–13%)
Paresthesias (5–11%) [8]
Parkinsonism [6]
Pseudotumor cerebri [3]
Rigors (<3%)
Seizures [4]
Tremor (7–13%) [4]
Vertigo (dizziness) (6–8%)

Neuromuscular/Skeletal
Arthralgia (<6%)
Asthenia (fatigue) (3–6%) [4]
Myalgia/Myopathy [10]
Rhabdomyolysis [13]

Gastrointestinal/Hepatic
Abdominal pain (15%) [3]
Diarrhea (5–13%) [3]
Dyspepsia (2–12%)
Flatulence (4–5%)
Gastrointestinal disorder (2–4%) [2]
Hepatotoxicity [9]
Nausea (6–23%)
Vomiting (6–9%)

Respiratory
Bronchitis (<3%)
Bronchospasm (5%)
Cough (3–5%)
Dyspnea (<5%)
Influenza (<10%)
Pharyngitis (3–4%)
Pneumonia (<4%)
Rhinitis (<5%)
Sinusitis (3–4%)

Upper respiratory tract infection (8–15%)

Endocrine/Metabolic
Diabetes mellitus [2]
Gynecomastia (>3%) [3]
Hypertriglyceridemia [2]
Hypomagnesemia (4–6%)
Menstrual irregularities (<3%)
Serum creatinine increased (16–43%) [4]

Genitourinary
Urinary frequency (2–4%)
Urinary tract infection (3%)

Renal
Nephrotoxicity [94]
Renal function abnormal [2]

Hematologic
Anemia [3]
Dyslipidemia [4]
Hemolytic uremic syndrome [17]
Leukopenia [2]
Neutropenia [2]

Ocular
Hallucinations, visual [2]
Ocular burning (Restasis) (17%)
Papilledema [2]

Other
Adverse effects [19]
Infection [6]

CYCLOTHIAZIDE

See: www.drugeruptiondata.com/drug/id/188

CYPROHEPTADINE

See: www.drugeruptiondata.com/drug/id/189

CYPROTERONE

Trade name: Androcur (Bayer)
Indications: Control of libido in severe hypersexuality and/or sexual deviation in the adult male
Class: Androgen antagonist, Progesterone agonist
Half-life: 1.7 days
Clinically important, potentially hazardous interactions with: alcohol, clotrimazole, fingolimod, itraconazole, ketoconazole, pazopanib, phenytoin, rifampin, ritonavir, St John's wort
Pregnancy category: X (not indicated for use in women)
Important contra-indications noted in the prescribing guidelines for: pediatric patients

Skin
Tumors [3]

Cardiovascular
Venous thromboembolism [2]

Neuromuscular/Skeletal
Osteoporosis [2]

Gastrointestinal/Hepatic
Hepatotoxicity [24]

Respiratory
Dyspnea [4]

CYSTEAMINE

See: www.drugeruptiondata.com/drug/id/2637

CYTARABINE

Synonym: ara-C
Trade names: Cytosar-U (Sicor), DepoCyt (Pacira)
Indications: Leukemias
Class: Antimetabolite, Antineoplastic, Antiviral
Half-life: initial: 10–15 minutes
Clinically important, potentially hazardous interactions with: aldesleukin
Pregnancy category: D
Important contra-indications noted in the prescribing guidelines for: nursing mothers; pediatric patients
Note: DepoCyt is a liposomal formulation. Vasculitis, a part of the cytarabine syndrome, consists of fever, malaise, myalgia, conjunctivitis, arthralgia and a diffuse erythematous maculopapular eruption that occurs from 6–12 hours following the administration of the drug.
Warning: DepoCyt: CHEMICAL ARACHNOIDITIS ADVERSE REACTIONS

Skin
Acral erythema [16]
Anaphylactoid reactions/Anaphylaxis [3]
Ephelides (<10%)
Erythema [5]
Exanthems [7]
Hand–foot syndrome [21]
Herpes zoster [2]
Hypersensitivity [2]
Neutrophilic eccrine hidradenitis [11]
Pruritus (<10%)
Rash (>10%) [4]
Seborrheic keratoses (inflammation of)
(Leser–Trélat syndrome) [2]
Toxic epidermal necrolysis [2]
Toxicity [5]
Vasculitis [3]

Hair
Alopecia (<10%) [5]

Nails
Leukonychia (Mees' lines) [2]

Mucosal
Mucositis [3]
Oral lesions [5]
Oral ulceration (>10%)
Perianal ulcerations (>10%)
Stomatitis [2]

Cardiovascular
Thrombophlebitis (>10%)

Central Nervous System
Fever [3]
Headache [4]
Leukoencephalopathy [8]
Neurotoxicity [10]
Peripheral neuropathy [2]

Neuromuscular/Skeletal
Myalgia/Myopathy (<10%)
Rhabdomyolysis [3]

Gastrointestinal/Hepatic
Diarrhea [5]
Hepatotoxicity [5]
Nausea [4]
Pancreatitis [5]
Vomiting [4]

Respiratory
Pneumonia [3]

Endocrine/Metabolic
Hypokalemia [2]

Hematologic
Anemia [2]
Bleeding [2]
Febrile neutropenia [8]
Hemotoxicity [3]
Leukopenia [2]
Myelosuppression [3]
Neutropenia [7]
Sepsis [2]

Thrombocytopenia [5]

Ocular
Ocular adverse effects [2]

Local
Injection-site cellulitis (<10%)

Other
Adverse effects [5]
Death [4]
Infection [6]

DABIGATRAN

Trade name: Pradaxa (Boehringer Ingelheim)
Indications: Prevention of venous thromboembolic events, reduce stroke risk
Class: Anticoagulant, Thrombin inhibitor
Half-life: 2.5 days
Clinically important, potentially hazardous interactions with: amiodarone, antacids, anticoagulants, atorvastatin, carbamazepine, clarithromycin, clopidogrel, collagenase, cyclosporine, darunavir, dasatinib, deferasirox, desirudin, dextran, diclofenac, dronedarone, fondaparinux, heparin, ibritumomab, itraconazole, ketoconazole, ketorolac, lapatinib, meloxicam, nandrolone, neratinib, NSAIDs, P-glycoprotein inducers and inhibitors, pantoprazole, pentosan, phenytoin, polysulfate sodium, prostacyclin analogues, proton pump inhibitors, quinidine, rifampin, rivaroxaban, salicylates, St John's wort, sulfinpyrazone, tacrolimus, telaprevir, thrombolytic agents, ticlopidine, tipranavir, tositumomab & iodine[131], ulipristal, verapamil, vitamin K antagonists
Pregnancy category: C
Important contra-indications noted in the prescribing guidelines for: the elderly; nursing mothers; pediatric patients
Note: Contra-indicated in patients with active pathological bleeding or with a mechanical prosthetic heart valve.
Warning: DISCONTINUING PRADAXA IN PATIENTS WITHOUT ADEQUATE CONTINUOUS ANTICOAGULATION INCREASES RISK OF STROKE

Skin
Bruising (<10%)
Exanthems [2]
Rash [2]

Mucosal
Epistaxis (nosebleed) [2]

Cardiovascular
Myocardial infarction [5]

Central Nervous System
Headache [2]
Intracranial hemorrhage [4]
Subarachnoid hemorrhage [2]

Gastrointestinal/Hepatic
Abdominal pain [2]
Dyspepsia (11%) [7]
Esophagitis [3]
Gastritis [2]
Gastrointestinal bleeding (6%) [10]

Renal
Renal failure [4]

Hematologic
Anemia (<4%)
Anticoagulation [2]
Hemorrhage [9]
Thrombosis [3]

Other
Adverse effects [6]
Death [6]

DABRAFENIB

Trade name: Tafinlar (Novartis)
Indications: Melanoma (unresectable or metastatic) in patients with BRAF V600E mutation
Class: BRAF inhibitor, Kinase inhibitor
Half-life: 8 hours
Clinically important, potentially hazardous interactions with: strong CYP3A4 or CYP2C8 inducers or inhibitors
Pregnancy category: D
Important contra-indications noted in the prescribing guidelines for: nursing mothers; pediatric patients

Skin
Acneform eruption [4]
Actinic keratoses [3]
Basal cell carcinoma [4]
Bullae (<10%)
Erythema [2]
Exanthems [2]
Grover's disease [4]
Hand–foot syndrome (20%) [6]
Hyperkeratosis (37%) [12]
Hypersensitivity (<10%)
Keratoacanthoma (7%) [7]
Keratosis pilaris [4]
Lesions [2]
Malignant melanoma (2%)
Panniculitis [6]
Papillomas (27%) [4]
Peripheral edema [2]
Photosensitivity [7]
Pruritus [3]
Rash (17%) [5]
Seborrheic keratoses [2]
Squamous cell carcinoma (7%) [17]
Toxicity [4]
Xerosis [4]

Hair
Alopecia (22%) [7]
Hair changes [2]

Cardiovascular
Chest pain [2]
Hypertension [3]

Central Nervous System
Chills [4]
Fever (28%) [20]
Headache (32%) [7]
Intracranial hemorrhage [3]

Neuromuscular/Skeletal
Arthralgia (27%) [9]
Asthenia (fatigue) [12]
Back pain (12%)
Myalgia/Myopathy (11%) [2]

Gastrointestinal/Hepatic
Abdominal pain [2]
Constipation (11%) [2]
Diarrhea [3]
Nausea [8]
Pancreatitis (<10%)
Vomiting [6]

Respiratory
Cough (12%) [2]
Nasopharyngitis (10%)

Endocrine/Metabolic
ALP increased (19%) [2]
ALT increased [2]
Appetite decreased [3]
AST increased [3]
Hyperglycemia (50%)
Hyponatremia (8%) [2]
Hypophosphatemia (37%)

Renal
Nephrotoxicity (<10%) [2]

Hematologic
Anemia [5]
Leukopenia [2]
Neutropenia [4]

Other
Adverse effects [7]

DACARBAZINE

Synonym: DIC
Trade name: DTIC-Dome (Bayer)
Indications: Malignant melanoma, carcinomas
Class: Alkylating agent, Antineoplastic
Half-life: 5 hours
Clinically important, potentially hazardous interactions with: aldesleukin
Pregnancy category: C
Important contra-indications noted in the prescribing guidelines for: nursing mothers

Skin
Anaphylactoid reactions/Anaphylaxis (<10%)
Hypersensitivity [2]
Photosensitivity [10]
Rash (<10%) [2]
Urticaria [2]

Hair
Alopecia (<10%) [3]

Mucosal
Stomatitis (48%)

Cardiovascular
Flushing (<10%) [2]

Central Nervous System
Dysgeusia (taste perversion) (<10%)

Neuromuscular/Skeletal
Asthenia (fatigue) (75%) [4]
Myalgia/Myopathy (<10%)

Gastrointestinal/Hepatic
Hepatotoxicity [3]
Nausea [3]
Vomiting [2]

Respiratory
Flu-like syndrome [2]

Endocrine/Metabolic
ALT increased [2]
AST increased [2]

Hematologic
Neutropenia [4]
Thrombocytopenia [2]

Local
Injection-site burning (>10%)
Injection-site necrosis (>10%)
Injection-site pain (>10%)

Other
Adverse effects [7]

DACLATASVIR

Trade name: Daklinza (Bristol-Myers Squibb)
Indications: Hepatitis C (in combination with sofosbuvir)
Class: Direct-acting antiviral, Hepatitis C virus NS5A inhibitor
Half-life: 12–15 hours
Clinically important, potentially hazardous interactions with: amiodarone, carbamazepine, dabigatran, phenytoin, rifampin, St John's wort
Pregnancy category: N/A (No data available)
Important contra-indications noted in the prescribing guidelines for: nursing mothers; pediatric patients
Note: See also separate entry for sofosbuvir.

Skin
Pruritus [3]
Rash [2]

Central Nervous System
Fever [4]
Headache (14%) [17]
Insomnia [4]

Neuromuscular/Skeletal
Asthenia (fatigue) (14%) [14]

Gastrointestinal/Hepatic
Abdominal pain [2]
Diarrhea (5%) [10]
Nausea (8%) [12]

Respiratory
Nasopharyngitis [2]

Endocrine/Metabolic
ALT increased [10]
AST increased [4]

Hematologic
Anemia [6]
Lymphopenia [2]
Neutropenia [3]
Thrombocytopenia [2]

Other
Adverse effects [8]

DACLIZUMAB

Trade names: Zenapax (Roche), Zinbryta (Biogen)
Indications: Transplant rejection (Zenapax), relapsing forms of multiple sclerosis (Zinbryta)
Class: Immunosuppressant, Monoclonal antibody
Half-life: 11–38 days
Clinically important, potentially hazardous interactions with: corticosteroids, cyclosporine, Hemophilus B vaccine, methylprednisolone, mycophenolate, prednisolone

Pregnancy category: C
Important contra-indications noted in the prescribing guidelines for: the elderly; nursing mothers; pediatric patients
Warning: Zinbryta: HEPATIC INJURY INCLUDING AUTOIMMUNE HEPATITIS and OTHER IMMUNE-MEDIATED DISORDERS

Skin
Acneform eruption (>5%)
Dermatitis [2]
Eczema [6]
Edema (>5%)
Hypersensitivity [2]
Hypohidrosis (2–5%)
Lymphadenopathy [4]
Peripheral edema (>5%)
Pruritus (2–5%)
Psoriasis [2]
Rash (2–5%) [8]
Toxicity [2]
Wound complications (>5%)

Hair
Hirsutism (2–5%)

Cardiovascular
Chest pain (>5%)
Hypertension (>5%)
Hypotension (>5%)
Pulmonary edema (>5%)
Tachycardia (>5%)

Central Nervous System
Anxiety (2–5%)
Depression (2–5%)
Fever (>5%)
Headache (>5%) [3]
Insomnia (>5%)
Pain (>5%)
Tremor (>5%)
Vertigo (dizziness) (>5%)

Neuromuscular/Skeletal
Arthralgia (2–5%)
Asthenia (fatigue) (>5%)
Back pain (>5%)
Bone or joint pain (>5%)
Myalgia/Myopathy (2–5%)

Gastrointestinal/Hepatic
Abdominal distension (>5%)
Abdominal pain (>5%)
Colitis [2]
Constipation (>5%)
Diarrhea (>5%)
Flatulence (2–5%)
Gastritis (2–5%)
Hemorrhoids (2–5%)
Hepatotoxicity [5]
Nausea (>5%)
Vomiting (>5%)

Respiratory
Cough (>5%)
Dyspnea (>5%)
Hypoxia (2–5%)
Nasopharyngitis [2]
Pharyngitis (2–5%)
Pleural effusion (2–5%)
Pneumonia [2]
Rhinitis (2–5%)
Upper respiratory tract infection [3]

Endocrine/Metabolic
ALT increased [2]
AST increased [2]
Dehydration (2–5%)
Diabetes mellitus (2–5%)

Genitourinary
Urinary retention (2–5%)
Urinary tract infection [2]

Renal
Nephrotoxicity (2–5%)

Hematologic
Hemorrhage (>5%)
Thrombosis (>5%)

Ocular
Vision blurred (2–5%)

Local
Application-site reactions (2–5%)

Other
Adverse effects [4]
Infection [7]

DACTINOMYCIN

Synonyms: ACT; actinomycin-D
Trade name: Cosmegen (Merck)
Indications: Melanomas, sarcomas
Class: Antibiotic, anthracycline
Half-life: 36 hours
Clinically important, potentially hazardous interactions with: aldesleukin
Pregnancy category: D
Important contra-indications noted in the prescribing guidelines for: the elderly; nursing mothers; pediatric patients
Note: Contra-indicated in patients with chickenpox or herpes zoster infection.

Skin
Acneform eruption (>10%) [6]
Erythema [2]
Folliculitis [2]
Pigmentation [4]
Pruritus [2]
Pustules [2]
Radiation recall dermatitis (>10%) [4]

Hair
Alopecia (>10%)

Mucosal
Oral lesions [3]
Stomatitis (ulcerative) (>5%)

Hematologic
Febrile neutropenia [2]
Neutropenia [2]
Thrombocytopenia [2]

Local
Injection-site extravasation (>10%)
Injection-site necrosis (>10%)
Injection-site phlebitis (>10%)

DALBAVANCIN

See: www.drugeruptiondata.com/drug/id/1323

DALFAMPRIDINE

Synonym: 4-aminopyridine
Trade name: Ampyra (Acorda)
Indications: Multiple sclerosis (to improve walking)
Class: Potassium channel blocker
Half-life: 5–6.5 hours
Clinically important, potentially hazardous interactions with: none known
Pregnancy category: C
Important contra-indications noted in the prescribing guidelines for: nursing mothers; pediatric patients
Note: Contra-indicated in patients with a history of seizure, or with moderate or severe renal impairment.

Central Nervous System
Balance disorder (5%)
Gait instability [2]
Headache (7%) [5]
Insomnia (9%) [5]
Multiple sclerosis (relapse) (4%)
Paresthesias (4%) [2]
Seizures [5]
Vertigo (dizziness) (7%) [9]
Neuromuscular/Skeletal
Asthenia (fatigue) (7%) [3]
Back pain (5%)
Gastrointestinal/Hepatic
Constipation (3%)
Dyspepsia (2%)
Nausea (7%) [4]
Respiratory
Nasopharyngitis (4%)
Pharyngolaryngeal pain (2%)
Genitourinary
Urinary tract infection (12%) [2]
Other
Adverse effects [4]

DALTEPARIN

Trade name: Fragmin (Pfizer)
Indications: Prophylaxis of deep vein thrombosis
Class: Heparin, low molecular weight
Half-life: 4–8 hours
Clinically important, potentially hazardous interactions with: butabarbital, danaparoid
Pregnancy category: B
Important contra-indications noted in the prescribing guidelines for: nursing mothers; pediatric patients
Warning: SPINAL/EPIDURAL HEMATOMA

Skin
Anaphylactoid reactions/Anaphylaxis (<10%) [2]
Bullous dermatitis (<10%)
Pruritus (<10%)
Rash (<10%)
Hair
Alopecia [2]
Local
Injection-site hematoma (<10%)

Injection-site pain (<10%)
Other
Allergic reactions (<10%) [3]

DANAPAROID

See: www.drugeruptiondata.com/drug/id/835

DANAZOL

Indications: Endometriosis, fibrocystic breast disease
Class: Pituitary hormone inhibitor
Half-life: ~4.5 hours
Clinically important, potentially hazardous interactions with: acenocoumarol, acitretin, atorvastatin, cyclosporine, insulin aspart, insulin degludec, insulin detemir, insulin glargine, insulin glulisine, oral contraceptives, paricalcitol, simvastatin, tacrolimus, warfarin
Pregnancy category: X
Important contra-indications noted in the prescribing guidelines for: nursing mothers; pediatric patients

Skin
Acneform eruption (>10%) [6]
Diaphoresis (3%)
Edema (>10%)
Erythema multiforme [2]
Exanthems [2]
Lupus erythematosus [4]
Rash (3%)
Seborrhea [4]
Hair
Alopecia [3]
Hirsutism (<10%) [5]
Cardiovascular
Flushing [3]
Neuromuscular/Skeletal
Rhabdomyolysis [5]
Gastrointestinal/Hepatic
Hepatotoxicity [4]
Endocrine/Metabolic
Pseudomenopause [2]
Weight gain [2]
Other
Adverse effects [3]
Death [2]

DANTROLENE

Trade names: Dantrium (Par), Ryanodex (Eagle)
Indications: Spasticity, malignant hyperthermia
Class: Skeletal muscle relaxant, hydantoin
Half-life: 8.7 hours
Clinically important, potentially hazardous interactions with: verapamil
Pregnancy category: C
Important contra-indications noted in the prescribing guidelines for: the elderly; nursing mothers; pediatric patients
Warning: HEPATOTOXICITY

Skin
Acneform eruption [3]
Rash (>10%)
Cardiovascular
Pericarditis [3]
Central Nervous System
Chills (<10%)
Vertigo (dizziness) [2]
Neuromuscular/Skeletal
Asthenia (fatigue) [2]
Myalgia/Myopathy [2]
Gastrointestinal/Hepatic
Hepatotoxicity [2]
Respiratory
Eosinophillic pleural effusion [3]
Pleural effusion [5]
Other
Adverse effects [2]
Death [4]

DAPAGLIFLOZIN

Trade names: Farxiga (AstraZeneca), Qtern (AstraZeneca), Xigduo XR (AstraZeneca)
Indications: Type II diabetes mellitus
Class: Sodium-glucose co-transporter 2 (SGLT2) inhibitor
Half-life: 13 hours
Clinically important, potentially hazardous interactions with: pioglitazone
Pregnancy category: C
Important contra-indications noted in the prescribing guidelines for: the elderly; nursing mothers; pediatric patients
Note: Contra-indicated in patients with severe renal impairment, end-stage renal disease, or undergoing dialysis. Qtern is dapagliflozin and saxagliptin; Xigduo XR is dapagliflozin and metformin.

Skin
Eczema [2]
Cardiovascular
Hypertension [2]
Hypotension [3]
Central Nervous System
Headache [3]
Neuromuscular/Skeletal
Arthralgia [2]
Back pain (3–4%) [3]
Pain in extremities (2%)
Gastrointestinal/Hepatic
Constipation (2%)
Diarrhea [3]
Nausea (3%) [3]
Respiratory
Bronchitis [2]
Cough [2]
Influenza (2–3%) [2]
Nasopharyngitis (6–7%) [7]
Upper respiratory tract infection [5]
Endocrine/Metabolic
Dehydration [2]
Hypoglycemia (>10%) [13]
Hypovolemia [2]

Genitourinary
Genital mycotic infections (particularly in women) (3–8%) [32]
Pollakiuria [2]
Urinary frequency (3–4%)
Urinary tract infection (4–6%) [34]

Renal
Nephrotoxicity [2]

Hematologic
Dyslipidemia (2–3%)

Other
Adverse effects [9]
Dipsia (thirst) [2]
Infection (<10%)

DAPSONE

Trade name: Aczone (Allergan)
Indications: Leprosy, dermatitis herpetiformis, acne
Class: Antibiotic, Antimycobacterial
Half-life: 10–50 hours
Clinically important, potentially hazardous interactions with: atovaquone/proguanil, chloroquine, didanosine, furazolidone, ganciclovir, hydroxychloroquine, methotrexate, pyrimethamine, rifabutin, rifampin, rifapentine, sulfonamides, trimethoprim, ursodiol
Pregnancy category: C
Important contra-indications noted in the prescribing guidelines for: nursing mothers
Note: A hypersensitivity reaction – termed the 'sulfone syndrome' or 'dapsone syndrome' – may infrequently develop during the first six weeks of treatment. This syndrome consists of exfoliative dermatitis, fever, malaise, nausea, anorexia, hepatitis, jaundice, lymphadenopathy and hemolytic anemia.

Skin
AGEP [2]
Bullous dermatitis [2]
Cyanosis [2]
Dapsone syndrome [41]
DRESS syndrome [14]
Erythema multiforme [9]
Erythema nodosum [5]
Exanthems (<5%) [12]
Exfoliative dermatitis [10]
Fixed eruption [4]
Hypersensitivity [21]
Lupus erythematosus [6]
Photosensitivity [9]
Pigmentation [6]
Rash [6]
Stevens-Johnson syndrome [5]
Toxic epidermal necrolysis [9]
Urticaria [2]

Nails
Beau's lines (transverse nail bands) [3]

Central Nervous System
Headache (4%) [2]
Insomnia [2]
Peripheral neuropathy [2]

Neuromuscular/Skeletal
Asthenia (fatigue) [2]

Gastrointestinal/Hepatic
Hepatitis [3]
Hepatotoxicity [2]
Pancreatitis [2]

Respiratory
Cough (2%)
Eosinophilic pneumonia [2]
Nasopharyngitis (5%)
Pharyngitis (2%)
Sinusitis (2%)
Upper respiratory tract infection (3%)

Hematologic
Agranulocytosis [7]
Anemia [5]
Hemolysis [6]
Hemolytic anemia [6]
Methemoglobinemia [20]

Local
Application-site erythema (13%) [2]
Application-site reactions (18%)

Other
Adverse effects [4]
Death [5]

DAPTOMYCIN

Trade name: Cubicin (Cubist)
Indications: Complicated skin and skin structure infections, *Staphylococcus aureus* bloodstream infections
Class: Antibiotic, glycopeptide
Half-life: ~8 hours
Clinically important, potentially hazardous interactions with: atorvastatin, cyclosporine, fibrates, HMG-CoA reductase inhibitors, rosuvastatin, statins, tobramycin, typhoid vaccine, warfarin
Pregnancy category: B
Important contra-indications noted in the prescribing guidelines for: the elderly; nursing mothers; pediatric patients

Skin
AGEP [2]
Cellulitis (<2%)
Edema (<7%)
Fungal dermatitis (3%)
Hyperhidrosis (5%)
Pruritus (3–6%)
Rash (4%)

Cardiovascular
Chest pain (7%)
Hypertension (6%)
Hypotension (2%)

Central Nervous System
Fever (2%)
Headache (5%)
Insomnia (9%)
Vertigo (dizziness) (2%)

Neuromuscular/Skeletal
Back pain (<2%)
Myalgia/Myopathy [7]
Rhabdomyolysis [7]

Gastrointestinal/Hepatic
Abdominal pain (<6%)
Constipation (6%)

Diarrhea (5%) [2]
Hepatotoxicity [3]
Nausea (6%) [2]
Vomiting (3%)

Respiratory
Cough (<2%)
Dyspnea (2%)
Eosinophilic pneumonia [15]
Pharyngolaryngeal pain (8%)
Pneumonia [2]

Endocrine/Metabolic
Creatine phosphokinase increased (7%) [6]

Genitourinary
Urinary tract infection (2%)

Renal
Nephrotoxicity [2]
Renal failure [2]

Hematologic
Eosinophilia [2]
Neutropenia [2]
Thrombocytopenia [2]

Local
Injection-site reactions (6%)

Other
Adverse effects [3]

DARATUMUMAB

Trade name: Darzalex (Janssen Biotech)
Indications: Multiple myeloma in patients who have received at least three prior lines of therapy including a proteasome inhibitor (PI) and an immunomodulatory agent or who are double-refractory to a PI and an immunomodulatory agent
Class: Monoclonal antibody
Half-life: 18 days
Clinically important, potentially hazardous interactions with: none known
Pregnancy category: N/A (No data available)
Important contra-indications noted in the prescribing guidelines for: pediatric patients

Skin
Herpes zoster (3%)

Mucosal
Nasal congestion (17%)

Cardiovascular
Chest pain (12%)
Hypertension (10%)

Central Nervous System
Chills (10%)
Cytokine release syndrome [2]
Fever (21%) [3]
Headache (12%)

Neuromuscular/Skeletal
Arthralgia (17%)
Asthenia (fatigue) (39%) [4]
Back pain (23%)
Pain in extremities (15%)

Gastrointestinal/Hepatic
Constipation (15%)
Diarrhea (16%)
Nausea (27%)
Vomiting (14%)

Respiratory
Bronchospasm (<2%) [3]
Cough (21%) [3]
Dyspnea (15%) [2]
Hypoxia (<2%)
Nasopharyngitis (15%)
Pneumonia (11%) [2]
Rhinitis (>5%)
Upper respiratory tract infection (20%) [2]

Endocrine/Metabolic
Appetite decreased (15%)

Hematologic
Anemia (45%) [7]
Lymphopenia (72%) [5]
Neutropenia (60%) [4]
Thrombocytopenia (48%) [7]

Local
Infusion-related reactions (48%) [9]

DARBEPOETIN ALFA

Synonym: erythropoiesis stimulating protein
Trade name: Aranesp (Amgen)
Indications: Anemia associated with renal failure and chemotherapy
Class: Colony stimulating factor, Erythropoiesis-stimulating agent (ESA), Erythropoietin
Half-life: 21 hours
Clinically important, potentially hazardous interactions with: none known
Pregnancy category: C
Important contra-indications noted in the prescribing guidelines for: nursing mothers; pediatric patients
Note: There is an increased risk of death for patients suffering from chronic renal failure with this drug (6%).
Warning: ERYTHROPOIESIS-STIMULATING AGENTS (ESAs) INCREASE THE RISK OF DEATH, MYOCARDIAL INFARCTION, STROKE, VENOUS THROMBOEMBOLISM, THROMBOSIS OF VASCULAR ACCESS AND TUMOR PROGRESSION OR RECURRENCE

Skin
Edema (21%)
Peripheral edema (11%)
Pruritus (8%)
Rash (7%) [2]

Central Nervous System
Fever (9–19%)
Vertigo (dizziness) (8–14%)

Neuromuscular/Skeletal
Arthralgia (11–13%)
Asthenia (fatigue) (9–33%)
Back pain (8%)
Myalgia/Myopathy (21%)

Gastrointestinal/Hepatic
Abdominal pain (12%)

Respiratory
Cough (10%)
Flu-like syndrome (6%)
Upper respiratory tract infection (14%)

Hematologic
Thrombosis [2]

Local
Injection-site pain (7%)

Other
Adverse effects [3]

DARIFENACIN

Trade names: Emselex (Novartis), Enablex (Novartis)
Indications: Overactive bladder
Class: Anticholinergic, Antimuscarinic, Muscarinic antagonist
Half-life: 13–19 hours
Clinically important, potentially hazardous interactions with: anticholinergics, antihistamines, atazanavir, clozapine, cyclosporine, digoxin, disopyramide, domperidone, erythromycin, flecainide, fosamprenavir, haloperidol, imipramine, indinavir, itraconazole, ketoconazole, levodopa, lopinavir, MAO inhibitors, memantine, metoclopramide, nefopam, nelfinavir, nitrates (sublingual), parasympathomimetics, paroxetine hydrochloride, phenothiazines, potent CYP3A4 inhibitors, ritonavir, saquinavir, thioridazine, tipranavir, tricyclic antidepressants, verapamil
Pregnancy category: C
Important contra-indications noted in the prescribing guidelines for: nursing mothers; pediatric patients
Note: Contra-indicated in patients with, or at risk for, urinary retention, gastric retention or uncontrolled narrow-angle glaucoma.

Mucosal
Xerostomia (20%) [12]

Central Nervous System
Headache [2]

Gastrointestinal/Hepatic
Abdominal pain (2%)
Constipation [3]

DARUNAVIR

Trade names: Prezcobix (Janssen), Prezista (Janssen)
Indications: HIV infection (must be co-administered with ritonavir and with other antiretroviral agents)
Class: Antiretroviral, HIV-1 protease inhibitor
Half-life: 15 hours
Clinically important, potentially hazardous interactions with: abacavir, alfuzosin, almotriptan, alosetron, alprazolam, amiodarone, antifungals, apixaban, artemether/lumefantrine, astemizole, atorvastatin, bortezomib, brinzolamide, calcium channel blockers, captopril, carbamazepine, ciclesonide, cisapride, clarithromycin, colchicine, conivaptan, cyclosporine, CYP2D6 substrates, CYP3A4 inhibitors, inducers and substrates, dabigatran, dasatinib, deferasirox, delavirdine, didanosine, dienogest, digoxin, dihydroergotamine, dronedarone, duloxetine, dutasteride, efavirenz, elbasvir & grazoprevir, enfuvirtide, eplerenone, ergotamine, estrogens, etravirine, everolimus, fentanyl, fesoterodine, food, fusidic acid,

glecaprevir & pibrentasvir, guanfacine, halofantrine, HMG-CoA reductase inhibitors, indinavir, inhaled corticosteroids, ixabepilone, ketoconazole, lidocaine, lopinavir, lovastatin, maraviroc, meperidine, methadone, methylprednisolone, midazolam, mifepristone, mometasone, nefazodone, nilotinib, nisoldipine, olaparib, P-glycoprotein substrates, paricalcitol, paroxetine hydrochloride, pazopanib, phenobarbital, phenytoin, pimecrolimus, pimozide, prasugrel, pravastatin, protease inhibitors, quetiapine, quinidine, quinine, ranolazine, rifabutin, rifampin, rilpivirine, rivaroxaban, romidepsin, rosuvastatin, salmeterol, saquinavir, saxagliptin, sertraline, sildenafil, silodosin, simeprevir, simvastatin, sirolimus, sorafenib, St John's wort, tacrolimus, tadalafil, tamsulosin, telaprevir, temsirolimus, tenofovir disoproxil, terfenadine, theophylline, tolvaptan, topotecan, trazodone, triazolam, tricyclic antidepressants, vardenafil, voriconazole, warfarin, zidovudine
Pregnancy category: C
Important contra-indications noted in the prescribing guidelines for: nursing mothers; pediatric patients
Note: Darunavir is a sulfonamide and can be absorbed systemically. Sulfonamides can produce severe, possibly fatal, reactions such as toxic epidermal necrolysis and Stevens-Johnson syndrome.
Prezcobix is darunavir and cobicistat.

Skin
Angioedema (<2%)
Hypersensitivity (<2%) [2]
Pruritus (<2%)
Rash (6–10%) [9]
Stevens-Johnson syndrome (<2%)
Urticaria (<2%)

Central Nervous System
Abnormal dreams (<2%)
Anorexia (2%)
Headache (7%) [6]

Neuromuscular/Skeletal
Asthenia (fatigue) (2–3%)
Osteonecrosis (<2%)

Gastrointestinal/Hepatic
Abdominal distension (2%)
Abdominal pain (6%)
Diarrhea (9–14%) [10]
Dyspepsia (<3%)
Flatulence (<2%)
Gastrointestinal disorder [3]
Hepatotoxicity (<2%) [6]
Nausea (4–7%) [6]
Pancreatitis (<2%)
Vomiting (2–5%)

Endocrine/Metabolic
Diabetes mellitus (new onset or exacebated) (2%)

Other
Adverse effects [6]

DASABUVIR/ OMBITASVIR/PARITA-PREVIR/RITONAVIR

Trade name: Viekira XR (AbbVie)
Indications: Genotype 1a chronic hepatitis C virus with or without cirrhosis, genotype 1b chronic hepatitis C virus with or without cirrhosis in combination with ribavirin
Class: CYP3A4 inhibitor (ritonavir), Direct-acting antiviral, Hepatitis C virus non-nucleoside NS5B palm polymerase inhibitor (dasabuvir), Hepatitis C virus NS3/4A protease inhibitor (paritaprevir), Hepatitis C virus NS5A inhibitor (ombitasvir)
Half-life: 6 hours (dasabuvir); 21–25 hours (ombitasvir); 6 hours (paritaprevir); 4 hours (ritonavir)
Clinically important, potentially hazardous interactions with: alfuzosin, carbamazepine, cisapride, copanlisib, dihydroergotamine, dronedarone, efavirenz, ergotamine, ethinyl estradiol-containing medications, gemfibrozil, lovastatin, lurasidone, methylergonovine, midazolam, midostaurin, neratinib, phenobarbital, phenytoin, pimozide, ranolazine, rifampin, sildenafil, simvastatin, St John's wort, triazolam
Pregnancy category: N/A (Insufficient evidence to inform drug-associated risk; contra-indicated in pregnancy when given with ribavirin)
Important contra-indications noted in the prescribing guidelines for: nursing mothers; pediatric patients
Note: Contra-indicated in patients with moderate to severe hepatic impairment. See also separate entries for Ombitasvir/Paritaprevir/Ritonavir (co-packaged with Dasabuvir as Viekira Pak) and Ribavirin.

Skin
Pruritus (7%) [2]
Rash (7%)

Central Nervous System
Insomnia (5%) [2]

Neuromuscular/Skeletal
Asthenia (fatigue) (4%) [3]

Gastrointestinal/Hepatic
Hepatotoxicity [2]
Nausea (8%)

Endocrine/Metabolic
ALT increased [2]
Hyperbilirubinemia (2%)

DASATINIB

Trade name: Sprycel (Bristol-Myers Squibb)
Indications: Leukemia (chronic myeloid), acute lymphoblastic leukemia
Class: Antineoplastic, Biologic, Tyrosine kinase inhibitor
Half-life: 3–5 hours
Clinically important, potentially hazardous interactions with: abciximab, alfentanil, alfuzosin, ambrisentan, antacids, anticoagulants, antiplatelet agents, aprepitant, argatroban, artemether/lumefantrine, astemizole, atazanavir,

atorvastatin, boceprevir, cabazitaxel, carbamazepine, chloroquine, ciclesonide, cilostazol, cinacalcet, ciprofloxacin, cisapride, clarithromycin, clopidogrel, clozapine, colchicine, conivaptan, cyclosporine, CYP3A4 inhibitors, inducers and substrates, dabigatran, darunavir, deferasirox, dexamethasone, dihydroergotamine, docetaxel, dronedarone, efavirenz, eptifibatide, ergotamine, erythromycin, eszopiclone, famotidine, fentanyl, fesoterodine, gadobutrol, gefitinib, H$_2$ antagonists, indinavir, itraconazole, ixabepilone, ketoconazole, lopinavir, lurasidone, maraviroc, meloxicam, nefazodone, nelfinavir, nilotinib, omeprazole, pantoprazole, phenobarbital, phenytoin, pimozide, proton pump inhibitors, QT prolonging agents, quinidine, quinine, rifampin, ritonavir, saquinavir, saxagliptin, sildenafil, simvastatin, sirolimus, St John's wort, tacrolimus, tadalafil, temsirolimus, terfenadine, tetrabenazine, thioridazine, tiagabine, tinzaparin, vardenafil, ziprasidone
Pregnancy category: D
Important contra-indications noted in the prescribing guidelines for: nursing mothers; pediatric patients

Skin
Acneform eruption (<10%) [2]
Dermatitis (<10%)
Eczema (<10%)
Edema (13–18%) [6]
Erythema [2]
Herpes (<10%)
Hyperhidrosis (<10%)
Panniculitis [4]
Peripheral edema [3]
Pruritus (<10%) [4]
Rash (11–21%) [10]
Toxicity [7]
Urticaria (<10%)
Xerosis (<10%)

Hair
Alopecia (<10%) [3]
Hair pigmentation [2]

Mucosal
Mucositis (16%)

Cardiovascular
Arrhythmias (<10%)
Cardiac failure (3%)
Congestive heart failure (2%)
Flushing (<10%)
Hypertension (<10%)
Palpitation (<10%)
Pericardial effusion (2–3%) [6]
QT prolongation [3]
Tachycardia (<10%)

Central Nervous System
Anorexia (<10%) [6]
Anxiety [2]
Depression (<10%)
Dysgeusia (taste perversion) (<10%)
Fever (5–39%)
Headache (12–33%) [8]
Insomnia (<10%)
Neurotoxicity (13%)
Pain (26%) [2]
Peripheral neuropathy (<10%)
Somnolence (drowsiness) (<10%)
Subdural hemorrhage [4]

Vertigo (dizziness) (<10%)

Neuromuscular/Skeletal
Arthralgia (<19%)
Asthenia (fatigue) (8%) [15]
Bone or joint pain (12–19%) [3]
Myalgia/Myopathy (6–13%) [2]

Gastrointestinal/Hepatic
Abdominal distension (<10%)
Abdominal pain (<25%) [2]
Colitis (<10%) [3]
Constipation (<10%)
Diarrhea (18–31%) [19]
Dyspepsia (<10%)
Enterocolitis (<10%)
Gastritis (<10%)
Gastrointestinal bleeding (2–8%) [3]
Hemorrhagic colitis [2]
Hepatitis [2]
Hepatotoxicity [2]
Nausea (9–23%) [11]
Vomiting (7–15%) [6]

Respiratory
Cough (<10%)
Dyspnea (20%) [5]
Pleural effusion (12–21%) [38]
Pneumonia (<10%) [3]
Pneumonitis (<10%)
Pulmonary hypertension (<10%) [11]
Pulmonary toxicity [3]
Upper respiratory tract infection (<10%)

Endocrine/Metabolic
Weight gain (<10%)
Weight loss (<10%)

Renal
Proteinuria [2]
Renal failure [3]

Hematologic
Anemia [3]
Bleeding (6–26%)
Cytopenia [3]
Febrile neutropenia (<12%)
Hemorrhage [2]
Hemotoxicity [4]
Myelosuppression [9]
Neutropenia [7]
Pancytopenia (<10%)
Thrombocytopenia [13]

Otic
Tinnitus (<10%)

Ocular
Reduced visual acuity (<10%)
Vision blurred (<10%)
Visual disturbances (<10%)
Xerophthalmia (<10%)

Other
Adverse effects [4]
Death [2]
Infection (<14%) [2]
Side effects [2]

DAUNORUBICIN

Synonyms: daunomycin; DNR; rubidomycin
Trade name: DaunoXome (Gilead)
Indications: Acute leukemias
Class: Antibiotic, anthracycline
Half-life: 14–20 hours; 4 hours (intramuscular)
**Clinically important, potentially hazardous
interactions with:** aldesleukin, gadobenate
Pregnancy category: D
**Important contra-indications noted in the
prescribing guidelines for:** the elderly; nursing
mothers; pediatric patients
Warning: MYOCARDIAL TOXICITY /
MYELOSUPPRESSION

Skin
Angioedema [4]
Dermatitis [2]
Edema (11%)
Exanthems [2]
Folliculitis (<5%)
Hot flashes (<5%)
Hyperhidrosis (14%)
Lymphadenopathy (<5%)
Neutrophilic eccrine hidradenitis [2]
Pigmentation [3]
Pruritus (7%)
Seborrhea (<5%)
Urticaria [3]
Xerosis (<5%)

Hair
Alopecia (8%) [4]

Nails
Nail pigmentation [5]

Mucosal
Gingival bleeding (<5%)
Oral lesions [2]
Sialorrhea (<5%)
Stomatitis (10%)
Xerostomia (<5%)

Cardiovascular
Chest pain (9–14%)
Flushing (14%)
Hypertension (<5%)
Myocardial toxicity [5]
Palpitation (<5%)
Tachycardia (<5%)

Central Nervous System
Amnesia (<5%)
Anorexia (23%)
Anxiety (<5%)
Cognitive impairment (<5%)
Depression (10%)
Dysgeusia (taste perversion) (<5%)
Gait instability (<5%)
Hallucinations (<5%)
Headache (25%)
Insomnia (6%)
Meningococcal infection (<5%)
Neurotoxicity (13%)
Rigors (19%)
Seizures (<5%)
Somnolence (drowsiness) (<5%)
Syncope (<5%)
Tremor (<5%)
Vertigo (dizziness) (8%)

Neuromuscular/Skeletal
Arthralgia (7%)
Asthenia (fatigue) (10%)
Ataxia (<5%)
Back pain (16%)
Hyperkinesia (<5%)
Hypertonia (<5%)
Myalgia/Myopathy (7%)

Gastrointestinal/Hepatic
Abdominal pain (23%)
Black stools (<5%)
Constipation (7%)
Diarrhea (38%)
Dysphagia (<5%)
Gastritis (<5%)
Gastrointestinal bleeding (<5%)
Hemorrhoids (<5%)
Hepatomegaly (<5%)
Nausea (54%)
Tenesmus (5%)
Vomiting (23%)

Respiratory
Cough (28%)
Dyspnea (26%)
Flu-like syndrome (5%)
Hemoptysis (<5%)
PIE syndrome (<5%)
Rhinitis (12%)
Sinusitis (8%)

Endocrine/Metabolic
Appetite increased (<5%)
Dehydration (<5%)

Genitourinary
Dysuria (<5%)
Nocturia (<5%)
Polyuria (<5%)

Hematologic
Neutropenia (15–36%)
Splenomegaly (<5%)

Otic
Ear pain (<5%)
Hearing loss (<5%)
Tinnitus (<5%)

Ocular
Abnormal vision (5%)
Conjunctivitis (<5%)
Ocular pain (<5%)

Local
Injection-site inflammation (<5%)
Injection-site necrosis (<10%) [2]
Injection-site ulceration (<10%)

Other
Dipsia (thirst) (<5%)
Hiccups (<5%)
Infection (40%)
Tooth decay (<5%)

DECITABINE

Synonym: 5-aza-2'-deoxycytidine
Trade name: Dacogen (MGI Pharma)
Indications: Myelodysplastic syndromes,
leukemia
Class: Antineoplastic
Half-life: ~30 minutes
**Clinically important, potentially hazardous
interactions with:** none known
Pregnancy category: D
**Important contra-indications noted in the
prescribing guidelines for:** nursing mothers;
pediatric patients

Skin
Bacterial infection (5%)
Candidiasis (10%)
Cellulitis (12%)
Ecchymoses (22%)
Edema (18%)
Erythema (14%)
Facial edema (6%)
Hematoma (5%)
Lymphadenopathy (12%)
Pallor (23%)
Peripheral edema (25%)
Petechiae (39%)
Pruritus (11%)
Rash (19%) [2]
Urticaria (6%)

Mucosal
Gingival bleeding (8%)
Glossodynia (5%)
Lip ulceration (5%)
Mucositis [2]
Oral candidiasis (6%)
Stomatitis (12%)
Tongue ulceration (7%)

Cardiovascular
Chest pain (7%)
Hypotension (6%)
Pulmonary edema (6%)
QT prolongation [2]

Central Nervous System
Anorexia (16%) [2]
Anxiety (11%)
Confusion (12%)
Fever (53%) [2]
Headache (28%)
Hypoesthesia (11%)
Insomnia (28%)
Pain (13%)
Rigors (22%)
Vertigo (dizziness) (18%)

Neuromuscular/Skeletal
Arthralgia (20%)
Asthenia (fatigue) (5–12%) [6]
Back pain (17%)
Bone or joint pain (6–19%)
Myalgia/Myopathy (5%)

Gastrointestinal/Hepatic
Abdominal distension (5%)
Abdominal pain (14%)
Ascites (10%)
Constipation (35%)
Diarrhea (34%) [2]
Dyspepsia (12%)

Dysphagia (6%)
Gastroesophageal reflux (5%)
Hemorrhoids (8%)
Hepatotoxicity [2]
Loose stools (7%)
Nausea (42%) [7]
Vomiting (25%) [4]

Respiratory
Cough (40%)
Hypoxia (10%)
Pharyngitis (16%)
Pneumonia (22%) [2]
Sinusitis (5%)

Endocrine/Metabolic
ALP increased (11%)
Appetite decreased (16%)
AST increased (10%)
Dehydration (6%)
Hyperglycemia (33%)
Hyperkalemia (13%)
Hypoalbuminemia (24%)
Hypokalemia (22%)
Hypomagnesemia (24%)
Hyponatremia (19%)

Genitourinary
Dysuria (6%)
Urinary frequency (5%)
Urinary tract infection (7%)

Hematologic
Anemia (82%) [5]
Bacteremia (5%)
Febrile neutropenia (29%) [7]
Hemotoxicity [2]
Leukopenia (28%)
Lymphopenia [2]
Myelosuppression [11]
Neutropenia (90%) [12]
Thrombocytopenia (89%) [8]

Ocular
Vision blurred (6%)

Local
Injection-site edema (5%)
Injection-site erythema (5%)

Other
Adverse effects [2]
Allergic reactions [2]
Infection [3]

DEFERASIROX

Trade names: Exjade (Novartis), Jadenu (Novartis)
Indications: Chronic iron overload due to blood transfusions and in non-transfuson dependent thalassemia syndromes
Class: Chelator, iron
Half-life: 8–16 hours
Clinically important, potentially hazardous interactions with: alfuzosin, aluminum-containing antacids, ambrisentan, aprepitant, cabazitaxel, cholestyramine, cilostazol, colesevelam, colestipol, conivaptan, dabigatran, darunavir, dasatinib, delavirdine, docetaxel, efavirenz, enalapril, estradiol, eszopiclone, fesoterodine, gefitinib, indinavir, ixabepilone, lapatinib, lurasidone, maraviroc, pazopanib, phenobarbital, phenytoin, pioglitazone,

repaglinide, rifampin, ritonavir, sildenafil, telithromycin, theophylline, tiagabine, tipranavir, trimethoprim, ulipristal
Pregnancy category: C
Important contra-indications noted in the prescribing guidelines for: the elderly; nursing mothers
Warning: RENAL FAILURE, HEPATIC FAILURE, AND GASTROINTESTINAL HEMORRHAGE

Skin
Rash (2–11%) [24]
Urticaria (4%)

Central Nervous System
Headache (16%) [2]

Neuromuscular/Skeletal
Arthralgia (7%)
Asthenia (fatigue) [3]
Back pain (6%)

Gastrointestinal/Hepatic
Abdominal pain (21–28%) [12]
Diarrhea (5–20%) [18]
Gastrointestinal bleeding [3]
Gastrointestinal disorder [3]
Hepatotoxicity [8]
Nausea (2–6%) [20]
Vomiting (10–21%) [7]

Respiratory
Cough (14%)
Flu-like syndrome (11%)
Upper respiratory tract infection (9%)

Endocrine/Metabolic
ALT increased [8]
Appetite decreased [2]
AST increased [3]
Serum creatinine increased [21]

Renal
Fanconi syndrome [10]
Nephrotoxicity [7]
Proteinuria [4]
Renal failure [3]
Renal function abnormal [2]

Other
Adverse effects [15]

DEFERIPRONE

Trade name: Ferriprox (ApoPharma)
Indications: Treatment of patients with transfusional iron overload due to thalassemia syndromes when current chelation therapy is inadequate
Class: Chelator, iron
Half-life: 1.9 hours
Clinically important, potentially hazardous interactions with: antacids containing iron, aluminum, zinc, diclofenac, mineral supplements, probenecid
Pregnancy category: D
Important contra-indications noted in the prescribing guidelines for: the elderly; nursing mothers; pediatric patients
Warning: AGRANULOCYTOSIS / NEUTROPENIA

Central Nervous System
Headache (3%)

Neuromuscular/Skeletal
Arthralgia (10%) [8]
Arthropathy [5]
Back pain (2%)
Bone or joint pain [2]
Pain in extremities (2%)

Gastrointestinal/Hepatic
Abdominal pain (10%) [2]
Diarrhea (3%) [2]
Dyspepsia (2%)
Gastrointestinal disorder [5]
Hepatotoxicity [3]
Nausea (13%) [4]
Vomiting (10%)

Endocrine/Metabolic
ALT increased (8%) [5]
Appetite increased (4%)
AST increased [2]
Weight gain (2%)

Renal
Chromaturia (15%)

Hematologic
Agranulocytosis (2%) [15]
Neutropenia [12]
Thrombocytopenia [2]

Other
Adverse effects [2]
Death [2]

DEFEROXAMINE

Trade name: Desferal (Novartis)
Indications: Hemochromatosis, acute iron overload
Class: Chelator, iron
Half-life: 6.1 hours
Clinically important, potentially hazardous interactions with: ascorbic acid, ferrous sulfate, zinc
Pregnancy category: C

Skin
Anaphylactoid reactions/Anaphylaxis [3]
Hypersensitivity [2]

Central Nervous System
Neurotoxicity [2]

Neuromuscular/Skeletal
Arthralgia [6]

Endocrine/Metabolic
Serum creatinine increased [2]

Otic
Hearing loss [2]
Ototoxicity [7]

Ocular
Night blindness [2]
Retinopathy [12]

Local
Injection-site inflammation (<10%)
Injection-site pain (<10%)

Other
Death [3]

DEFIBROTIDE

Trade name: Defitelio (Jazz)
Indications: Hepatic veno-occlusive disease in patients with renal or pulmonary dysfunction following hematopoietic stem-cell transplantation
Class: Oligonucleotide
Half-life: <2 hours
Clinically important, potentially hazardous interactions with: alteplase, heparin
Pregnancy category: N/A (No data available)
Important contra-indications noted in the prescribing guidelines for: nursing mothers
Note: Contra-indicated for concomitant administration with systemic anticoagulant or fibrinolytic therapy.

Skin
Graft-versus-host reaction (6%)
Mucosal
Epistaxis (nosebleed) (14%)
Cardiovascular
Hypotension (37%) [3]
Central Nervous System
Cerebral hemorrhage (2%)
Intracranial hemorrhage (3%)
Gastrointestinal/Hepatic
Diarrhea (24%)
Gastrointestinal bleeding (9%) [3]
Nausea (16%)
Vomiting (18%)
Respiratory
Alveolar hemorrhage (pulmonary) (9%)
Pneumonia (5%)
Pulmonary hemorrhage (4%)
Pulmonary toxicity (6%)
Endocrine/Metabolic
Hyperuricemia (2%)
Hematologic
Hemorrhage [2]
Sepsis (7%)
Other
Adverse effects [3]
Infection (3%)

DEFLAZACORT *

Trade name: Emflaza (Marathon)
Indications: Duchenne muscular dystrophy
Class: Corticosteroid
Half-life: N/A
Clinically important, potentially hazardous interactions with: carbamazepine, clarithromycin, diltiazem, efavirenz, fluconazole, grapefruit juice, live vaccines, pancuronium, phenytoin, rifampin, verapamil
Pregnancy category: N/A (Should be used during pregnancy only if the potential benefit justifies the potential risk to the fetus)
Important contra-indications noted in the prescribing guidelines for: the elderly; nursing mothers; pediatric patients

Skin
Cushingoid features (33%) [2]

Erythema (8%)
Hypersensitivity [3]
Toxic epidermal necrolysis [2]
Hair
Hirsutism (10%) [2]
Mucosal
Rhinorrhea (8%)
Central Nervous System
Behavioral disturbances [2]
Irritability (8%)
Gastrointestinal/Hepatic
Abdominal pain (6%)
Respiratory
Cough (12%)
Nasopharyngitis (10%)
Upper respiratory tract infection (12%)
Endocrine/Metabolic
Appetite increased (14%) [2]
Weight gain (20%) [5]
Genitourinary
Pollakiuria (12%)
Ocular
Cataract [3]
Other
Adverse effects [2]
Side effects [2]

DEGARELIX

See: www.drugeruptiondata.com/drug/id/1362

DELAFLOXACIN *

Trade name: Baxdela (Melinta)
Indications: Acute bacterial skin and skin structure infections caused by designated susceptible bacteria
Class: Antibiotic, fluoroquinolone
Half-life: 4–9 hours
Clinically important, potentially hazardous interactions with: none known
Pregnancy category: N/A (Insufficient evidence to inform drug-associated risk)
Important contra-indications noted in the prescribing guidelines for: the elderly; nursing mothers; pediatric patients
Note: Fluoroquinolones are associated with an increased risk of tendinitis and tendon rupture in all ages. This risk is further increased in older patients usually over 60 years of age, in patients taking corticosteroid drugs, and in patients with kidney, heart or lung transplants.
Fluoroquinolones may exacerbate muscle weakness in persons with myasthenia gravis.
Warning: SERIOUS ADVERSE REACTIONS INCLUDING TENDINITIS, TENDON RUPTURE, PERIPHERAL NEUROPATHY, CENTRAL NERVOUS SYSTEM EFFECTS, and EXACERBATION OF MYASTHENIA GRAVIS

Skin
Dermatitis (<2%)
Edema (<2%)
Erythema (<2%)
Hypersensitivity (<2%)

Irritation (<2%)
Pruritus (<2%)
Rash (<2%)
Urticaria (<2%)
Mucosal
Oral candidiasis (<2%)
Cardiovascular
Bradycardia (<2%)
Flushing (<2%)
Hypertension (<2%)
Hypotension (<2%)
Palpitation (<2%)
Phlebitis (<2%)
Tachycardia (<2%)
Central Nervous System
Abnormal dreams (<2%)
Anxiety (<2%)
Dysgeusia (taste perversion) (<2%)
Headache (3%) [2]
Hypoesthesia (<2%)
Insomnia (<2%)
Paresthesias (<2%)
Presyncope (<2%)
Syncope (<2%)
Vertigo (dizziness) (<2%)
Neuromuscular/Skeletal
Myalgia/Myopathy (<2%)
Gastrointestinal/Hepatic
Abdominal pain (<2%)
Diarrhea (8%) [4]
Dyspepsia (<2%)
Nausea (8%) [3]
Vomiting (2%) [2]
Endocrine/Metabolic
ALT increased (>2%)
AST increased (>2%)
Creatine phosphokinase increased (<2%)
Hyperglycemia (<2%)
Hyperphosphatemia (<2%)
Hypoglycemia (<2%)
Serum creatinine increased (<2%)
Genitourinary
Vulvovaginal candidiasis (<2%)
Renal
Nephrotoxicity (<2%)
Renal failure (<2%)
Hematologic
Thrombosis (<2%)
Otic
Tinnitus (<2%)
Ocular
Vision blurred (<2%)
Local
Injection-site bruising (<2%)
Injection-site extravasation (<2%)
Other
Infection (<2%)

DELAVIRDINE

See: www.drugeruptiondata.com/drug/id/199

DEMECLOCYCLINE

See: www.drugeruptiondata.com/drug/id/200

DENILEUKIN

See: www.drugeruptiondata.com/drug/id/201

DENOSUMAB

Trade names: Prolia (Amgen), Xgeva (Amgen)
Indications: Osteoporosis (postmenopausal women), prevention of skeletal-related events in patients with bone metastases from solid tumors
Class: Bone resorption inhibitor, Monoclonal antibody, RANK ligand (RANKL) inhibitor
Half-life: 25–28 days
Clinically important, potentially hazardous interactions with: abatacept, alcohol, azacitidine, betamethasone, cabazitaxel, denileukin, docetaxel, fingolimod, gefitinib, immuosuppressants, leflunomide, lenalidomide, oxaliplatin, pazopanib, temsirolimus, triamcinolone
Pregnancy category: X
Important contra-indications noted in the prescribing guidelines for: nursing mothers; pediatric patients
Note: Contra-indicated in patients with hypocalcemia.

Skin
Cellulitis [9]
Dermatitis [2]
Eczema [10]
Herpes zoster (2%)
Hypersensitivity [2]
Peripheral edema (5%)
Pruritus (2%)
Rash (3%) [4]

Cardiovascular
Angina (3%)
Atrial fibrillation (2%)
Cardiotoxicity [2]

Central Nervous System
Headache [3]
Insomnia (3%)
Pain [2]
Vertigo (dizziness) (5%)

Neuromuscular/Skeletal
Arthralgia [3]
Asthenia (fatigue) (2%) [2]
Back pain (35%) [6]
Bone or joint pain (4–8%) [3]
Fractures [8]
Myalgia/Myopathy (3%)
Osteonecrosis (jaw) [25]
Pain in extremities (12%) [6]

Gastrointestinal/Hepatic
Abdominal pain (3%)
Flatulence (2%)
Gastroesophageal reflux (2%)
Pancreatitis [2]

Respiratory
Pharyngitis (2%)

Pneumonia (4%)
Upper respiratory tract infection (5%)

Endocrine/Metabolic
Hypercholerolemia (7%) [2]
Hypocalcemia (2%) [34]
Hypophosphatemia [3]

Genitourinary
Cystitis (6%)

Hematologic
Anemia (3%) [2]

Other
Adverse effects [11]
Infection [12]

DEOXYCHOLIC ACID

Trade name: Kybella (Kythera)
Indications: Improvement in the appearance of moderate to severe convexity or fullness associated with submental fat
Class: Cytolytic
Half-life: N/A
Clinically important, potentially hazardous interactions with: none known
Pregnancy category: N/A
Important contra-indications noted in the prescribing guidelines for: the elderly; pediatric patients
Note: Contra-indicated in the presence of infection at the injection sites.

Skin
Lymphadenopathy (<2%)

Mucosal
Oropharyngeal pain (3%)

Cardiovascular
Hypertension (3%)

Central Nervous System
Headache (8%)
Syncope (<2%)

Neuromuscular/Skeletal
Neck pain (<2%)

Gastrointestinal/Hepatic
Dysphagia (2%)
Nausea (2%)

Local
Injection-site bruising (72%) [2]
Injection-site edema [2]
Injection-site erythema (27%)
Injection-site hemorrhage (<2%)
Injection-site induration (23%) [2]
Injection-site nodules (13%)
Injection-site numbness (66%) [2]
Injection-site pain (70%) [2]
Injection-site pigmentation (<2%)
Injection-site pruritus (12%)
Injection-site urticaria (<2%)

Other
Adverse effects [2]

DESFLURANE

See: www.drugeruptiondata.com/drug/id/920

DESIPRAMINE

See: www.drugeruptiondata.com/drug/id/202

DESLORATADINE

Trade name: Clarinex (Schering)
Indications: Allergic rhinitis, urticaria
Class: Histamine H1 receptor antagonist
Half-life: 27 hours
Clinically important, potentially hazardous interactions with: none known
Pregnancy category: C
Important contra-indications noted in the prescribing guidelines for: nursing mothers; pediatric patients

Skin
Urticaria [2]

Mucosal
Xerostomia [5]

Central Nervous System
Headache [7]
Somnolence (drowsiness) [6]

Neuromuscular/Skeletal
Asthenia (fatigue) [7]

Gastrointestinal/Hepatic
Diarrhea [2]
Nausea [2]

Other
Adverse effects [6]

DESMOPRESSIN

Trade names: DDAVP (Sanofi-Aventis), Minirin (Ferring), Noctiva (Serenity), Stimate (CSL Behring)
Indications: Primary nocturnal enuresis, nocturia due to nocturnal polyuria (Noctiva)
Class: Antidiuretic hormone analog
Half-life: 75 minutes
Clinically important, potentially hazardous interactions with: amitriptyline, citalopram, demeclocycline, hydromorphone, meloxicam, tapentadol
Pregnancy category: B
Important contra-indications noted in the prescribing guidelines for: the elderly; nursing mothers; pediatric patients
Warning: Noctiva: HYPONATREMIA

Cardiovascular
Flushing (<10%)
Myocardial infarction [2]

Central Nervous System
Headache [6]
Seizures [5]

Endocrine/Metabolic
Hyponatremia [11]
SIADH [2]

Local
Injection-site pain (<10%)

DESONIDE

See: www.drugeruptiondata.com/drug/id/1084

DESOXIMETASONE

Trade name: Topicort (Taro)
Indications: Dermatoses
Class: Corticosteroid, topical
Half-life: N/A
Clinically important, potentially hazardous interactions with: live vaccines
Pregnancy category: C
Important contra-indications noted in the prescribing guidelines for: nursing mothers; pediatric patients

Local
Application-site irritation (3%)
Application-site pruritus (2%) [2]

Other
Adverse effects [3]

DESVENLAFAXINE

Trade name: Pristiq (Wyeth)
Indications: Major depressive disorder
Class: Antidepressant, Serotonin-norepinephrine reuptake inhibitor
Half-life: 11 hours
Clinically important, potentially hazardous interactions with: alcohol, aspirin, CNS-active agents, heparin, ketoconazole, linezolid, lithium, MAO inhibitors, NSAIDs, sibutramine, tramadol, venlafaxine, warfarin
Pregnancy category: C
Important contra-indications noted in the prescribing guidelines for: the elderly; nursing mothers; pediatric patients
Warning: SUICIDAL THOUGHTS AND BEHAVIORS

Skin
Hot flashes (<2%)
Hyperhidrosis (10–21%)
Hypersensitivity (2%)
Rash (<2%)

Mucosal
Epistaxis (nosebleed) (<2%)
Xerostomia (11–25%) [3]

Cardiovascular
Hypertension (<2%)
Hypotension (~2%)
Orthostatic hypotension (<2%)
Palpitation (<3%)
Tachycardia (<2%)

Central Nervous System
Abnormal dreams (2–4%)
Anorexia (5–8%) [2]
Anorgasmia (3–8%)
Anxiety (3–5%)
Chills (<4%)
Dysgeusia (taste perversion) (<2%)
Extrapyramidal symptoms (<2%)
Headache (20–29%) [3]

Impaired concentration (<2%)
Insomnia (9–12%) [3]
Irritability (2%)
Nervousness (<2%) [2]
Paresthesias (<3%)
Seizures (~2%)
Somnolence (drowsiness) (4–12%) [4]
Suicidal ideation [2]
Syncope (<2%)
Tremor (~3%)
Vertigo (dizziness) (10–16%) [5]
Yawning (<4%)

Neuromuscular/Skeletal
Asthenia (fatigue) (7–11%) [2]

Gastrointestinal/Hepatic
Constipation (9–14%)
Diarrhea (5–11%)
Nausea (22–41%) [6]
Vomiting (3–9%)

Endocrine/Metabolic
Appetite decreased (5–10%)
Libido decreased (3–6%)
Weight gain (<2%)
Weight loss (<2%)

Genitourinary
Ejaculatory dysfunction (<5%)
Erectile dysfunction (3–11%)
Sexual dysfunction (<2%)

Otic
Tinnitus (<2%)

Ocular
Mydriasis (2–6%)
Vision blurred (3–4%)

DEUTETRABENAZINE *

Trade name: Austedo (Teva)
Indications: Chorea associated with Huntington's disease
Class: Vesicular monoamine transporter 2 inhibitor
Half-life: 9–10 hours
Clinically important, potentially hazardous interactions with: alcohol or other sedating drugs, bupropion, dopamine antagonists or antipsychotics, fluoxetine, MAO inhibitors, paroxetine hydrochloride, quinidine, strong CYP2D6 inhibitors, tetrabenazine
Pregnancy category: N/A (Based on animal data, may cause fetal harm)
Important contra-indications noted in the prescribing guidelines for: the elderly; nursing mothers; pediatric patients
Note: Contra-indicated in suicidal or untreated/inadequately treated depression, in hepatic impairment. or in patients taking MAO inhibitors, reserpine or tetrabenazine.
Warning: DEPRESSION AND SUICIDALITY

Skin
Hematoma (4%)

Mucosal
Xerostomia (9%)

Central Nervous System
Anxiety (4%) [2]
Depression [3]

Insomnia (7%) [2]
Somnolence (drowsiness) (11%) [4]
Vertigo (dizziness) (4%)

Neuromuscular/Skeletal
Asthenia (fatigue) (9%) [3]

Gastrointestinal/Hepatic
Constipation (4%)
Diarrhea (9%) [2]

Genitourinary
Urinary tract infection (7%)

DEXAMETHASONE

Trade names: Decadron (Merck), Dexone (Solvay), Ozurdex (Allergan)
Indications: Antiemetic, arthralgias, dermatoses, diagnostic aid, macular edema following branch retinal vein occlusion (BRVO) or central retinal vein occlusion (CRVO), non-infectious uveitis affecting the posterior segment of the eye
Class: Antiemetic, Corticosteroid, systemic, Corticosteroid, topical
Half-life: N/A
Clinically important, potentially hazardous interactions with: albendazole, aminoglutethimide, amprenavir, aprepitant, aspirin, bexarotene, boceprevir, carbamazepine, caspofungin, cobicistat/elvitegravir/emtricitabine/tenofovir alafenamide, cobicistat/elvitegravir/emtricitabine/tenofovir disoproxil, cyclophosphamide, dasatinib, delavirdine, diuretics, ephedrine, imatinib, itraconazole, ixabepilone, lapatinib, lenalidomide, live vaccines, lopinavir, methotrexate, midazolam, phenobarbital, phenytoin, praziquantel, primidone, rifampin, rilpivirine, romidepsin, simeprevir, sorafenib, sunitinib, telaprevir, temsirolimus, ticagrelor, vandetanib, warfarin
Pregnancy category: C
Important contra-indications noted in the prescribing guidelines for: nursing mothers; pediatric patients

Skin
Acneform eruption [6]
AGEP [2]
Anaphylactoid reactions/Anaphylaxis [3]
Dermatitis [5]
Edema [4]
Erythema multiforme [3]
Exanthems [4]
Herpes zoster [2]
Hyperhidrosis [2]
Hypersensitivity [5]
Peripheral edema [8]
Pigmentation [2]
Pruritus [7]
Pruritus ani et vulvae [2]
Rash [10]
Striae [4]
Toxicity [5]
Tumor lysis syndrome [3]
Xerosis [2]

Mucosal
Oral candidiasis [2]

Cardiovascular
Bradycardia [8]

Litt's Drug Eruption & Reaction Manual © 2018 by Taylor & Francis Group, LLC

Flushing [5]
Hypertension [16]
Myocardial toxicity [11]
Tachycardia [2]
Thromboembolism [3]
Venous thromboembolism [5]

Central Nervous System
Anorexia [2]
Catatonia [2]
Dysgeusia (taste perversion) [3]
Fever [6]
Headache (<5%) [8]
Insomnia [9]
Leukoencephalopathy [2]
Neurotoxicity [11]
Paresthesias [2]
Peripheral neuropathy [22]
Somnolence (drowsiness) [2]
Vertigo (dizziness) [3]

Neuromuscular/Skeletal
Arthralgia [5]
Asthenia (fatigue) [38]
Back pain [5]
Bone or joint pain [4]
Muscle spasm [4]
Myalgia/Myopathy [6]
Osteonecrosis [15]
Osteoporosis [3]

Gastrointestinal/Hepatic
Abdominal distension [2]
Abdominal pain [5]
Constipation [10]
Diarrhea [17]
Dyspepsia [2]
Gastrointestinal disorder [3]
Hepatotoxicity [4]
Nausea [12]
Pancreatitis [2]
Vomiting [7]

Respiratory
Cough [3]
Dyspnea [5]
Pneumonia [14]
Pneumonitis [2]
Upper respiratory tract infection [3]

Endocrine/Metabolic
ALT increased [2]
AST increased [2]
Cushing's syndrome [2]
Dehydration [2]
Hyperglycemia [7]
Hypokalemia [5]
Hypophosphatemia [4]
Serum creatinine increased [2]

Renal
Nephrotoxicity [2]

Hematologic
Anemia [36]
Febrile neutropenia [7]
Hemoglobin decreased [2]
Hemotoxicity [7]
Leukopenia [10]
Lymphopenia [11]
Myelosuppression [5]
Neutropenia [49]
Sepsis [3]
Thrombocytopenia [49]
Thrombosis [2]

Otic
Ototoxicity [4]

Ocular
Cataract (<10%) [7]
Conjunctival hemorrhage (>10%)
Glaucoma [9]
Intraocular pressure increased (>10%) [10]
Ocular hypertension (<10%) [6]
Ocular pain (<10%) [6]
Vision blurred [3]

Local
Infusion-related reactions [2]
Infusion-site reactions [2]

Other
Adverse effects [19]
Allergic reactions [2]
Death [11]
Hiccups [17]
Infection [30]
Side effects [3]

DEXCHLOR-PHENIRAMINE

See: www.drugeruptiondata.com/drug/id/204

DEXIBUPROFEN

See: www.drugeruptiondata.com/drug/id/1284

DEXKETOPROFEN

See: www.drugeruptiondata.com/drug/id/1232

DEXLANSOPRAZOLE

Trade name: Dexilant (Takeda)
Indications: Erosive esophagitis, heartburn associated with gastroesophageal reflux disease
Class: Proton pump inhibitor (PPI)
Half-life: <2 hours
Clinically important, potentially hazardous interactions with: atazanavir, clopidogrel, digoxin, emtricitabine/rilpivirine/tenofovir alafenamide, ketoconazole, tacrolimus, warfarin
Pregnancy category: B
Important contra-indications noted in the prescribing guidelines for: nursing mothers

Skin
Acneform eruption (<2%)
Dermatitis (<2%)
Erythema (<2%)
Hot flashes (<2%)
Lesions (<2%)
Lymphadenopathy (<2%)
Pruritus (<2%)
Rash (<2%)
Urticaria (<2%)

Mucosal
Mucosal inflammation (<2%)
Oral candidiasis (<2%)
Xerostomia (<2%)

Cardiovascular
Cardiac disorder (<2%)

Central Nervous System
Headache [2]

Gastrointestinal/Hepatic
Abdominal pain (4%) [4]
Constipation [2]
Diarrhea (5%) [4]
Flatulence (<3%) [3]
Gastrointestinal disorder (<2%)
Nausea (3%) [4]
Vomiting (<2%) [2]

Respiratory
Upper respiratory tract infection (2–3%) [3]

Hematologic
Anemia (<2%)

Otic
Ear pain (<2%)
Tinnitus (<2%)

Ocular
Ocular edema (<2%)
Ocular pruritus (<2%)

Other
Adverse effects [2]

DEXMEDETOMIDINE

See: www.drugeruptiondata.com/drug/id/206

DEXMETHYL-PHENIDATE

Trade name: Focalin (Novartis)
Indications: Attention deficit disorder
Class: CNS stimulant
Half-life: 2–4.5 hours
Clinically important, potentially hazardous interactions with: amitriptyline, clonidine, linezolid, MAO inhibitors, pantoprazole
Pregnancy category: C
Important contra-indications noted in the prescribing guidelines for: nursing mothers; pediatric patients
Note: Contra-indicated in patients with marked anxiety, tension and agitation, with glaucoma, or with motor tics or history/diagnosis of Tourette's syndrome.

Central Nervous System
Fever (5%)
Headache [4]

Gastrointestinal/Hepatic
Abdominal pain (15%) [2]

Endocrine/Metabolic
Appetite decreased [2]

DEXRAZOXANE

See: www.drugeruptiondata.com/drug/id/1286

DEXTRO-AMPHETAMINE

Trade names: Adderall (Shire), Dexedrine (Alliant), Mydayis (Shire)
Indications: Narcolepsy, attention deficit disorder (ADD)
Class: Amphetamine, CNS stimulant
Half-life: 10–12 hours
Clinically important, potentially hazardous interactions with: fluoxetine, fluvoxamine, MAO inhibitors, paroxetine hydrochloride, phenelzine, sertraline, tranylcypromine
Pregnancy category: C
Important contra-indications noted in the prescribing guidelines for: nursing mothers; pediatric patients
Warning: ABUSE AND DEPENDENCE

Skin
Diaphoresis (<10%)

Mucosal
Xerostomia (<10%)

Central Nervous System
Insomnia [2]

Neuromuscular/Skeletal
Rhabdomyolysis [10]

DEXTRO-METHORPHAN

Trade names: Robitussin (Wyeth), Vicks Formula 44 (Procter & Gamble)
Indications: Nonproductive cough
Class: Analgesic, narcotic, NMDA receptor antagonist
Half-life: N/A
Clinically important, potentially hazardous interactions with: amiodarone, citalopram, iloperidone, linezolid, lorcaserin, memantine, moclobemide, phenelzine, rasagiline, safinamide, sibutramine, tranylcypromine, valdecoxib
Pregnancy category: C
Important contra-indications noted in the prescribing guidelines for: nursing mothers; pediatric patients

---

Skin
Bullous dermatitis [2]
Fixed eruption [2]

Central Nervous System
Serotonin syndrome [4]
Vertigo (dizziness) [2]

Gastrointestinal/Hepatic
Diarrhea [2]

Genitourinary
Urinary tract infection [2]

Other
Adverse effects [2]

DIATRIZOATE

See: www.drugeruptiondata.com/drug/id/1112

DIAZEPAM

Trade names: Diastat (Xcel), Valium (Roche)
Indications: Anxiety
Class: Benzodiazepine, Skeletal muscle relaxant
Half-life: 20–70 hours
Clinically important, potentially hazardous interactions with: alcohol, amprenavir, barbiturates, buprenorphine, chlorpheniramine, clarithromycin, CNS depressants, cobicistat/elvitegravir/emtricitabine/tenofovir alafenamide, cobicistat/elvitegravir/emtricitabine/tenofovir disoproxil, efavirenz, esomeprazole, eucalyptus, fluoroquinolones, imatinib, indinavir, itraconazole, ivermectin, macrolide antibiotics, MAO inhibitors, methadone, mianserin, nalbuphine, narcotics, nelfinavir, nilutamide, olanzapine, omeprazole, phenothiazines, propranolol, ritonavir, SSRIs, voriconazole
Pregnancy category: D
Important contra-indications noted in the prescribing guidelines for: nursing mothers

---

Skin
Dermatitis (<10%) [3]
Diaphoresis (>10%)
Exanthems [6]
Exfoliative dermatitis [2]
Fixed eruption [2]
Pigmentation [2]
Purpura [4]
Rash (>10%) [2]

Mucosal
Xerostomia (>10%)

Central Nervous System
Amnesia [17]
Hallucinations [2]
Sedation [3]
Somnolence (drowsiness) [6]
Vertigo (dizziness) [2]

Neuromuscular/Skeletal
Ataxia [2]

Endocrine/Metabolic
Gynecomastia [4]
Porphyria [2]

Local
Injection-site pain [2]
Injection-site phlebitis (>10%) [2]

Other
Adverse effects [3]
Allergic reactions [2]

DIAZOXIDE

See: www.drugeruptiondata.com/drug/id/211

DICHLORPHENAMIDE

See: www.drugeruptiondata.com/drug/id/1881

DICLOFENAC

Trade names: Arthrotec (Pfizer), Cataflam (Novartis), Dicolmax (Galen), Motifene (Daiichi Sankyo), Pennsaid (Mallinckrodt), Solaraze Gel (Nycomed), Voltaren (Novartis), Voltarol (Novartis), Zipsor (Depomed)
Indications: Rheumatoid and osteoarthritis, topical treatment of actinic keratosis, postoperative inflammation in patients who have undergone cataract extraction and for the temporary relief of pain and photophobia in patients undergoing corneal refractive surgery
Class: Non-steroidal anti-inflammatory (NSAID)
Half-life: 1–2 hours
Clinically important, potentially hazardous interactions with: ACE inhibitors, adrenergic neurone blockers, aldosterone antagonists, aliskiren, alpha blockers, angiotensin II receptor antagonists, anticoagulants, aspirin, baclofen, beta blockers, calcium channel blockers, cardiac glycosides, clonidine, clopidogrel, corticosteroids, coumarins, cyclosporine, dabigatran, deferiprone, diazoxide, diuretics, enoxaparin, erlotinib, furosemide, heparins, hydralazine, iloprost, ketorolac, lithium, methotrexate, methyldopa, mifamurtide, minoxidil, moxonidine, nitrates, nitroprusside, penicillamine, pentoxifylline, phenindione, potassium canrenoate, prasugrel, rifampin, ritonavir, rivaroxaban, SSRIs, sulfonylureas, tacrolimus, thiazides, tinzaparin, venlafaxine, voriconazole, warfarin, zidovudine
Pregnancy category: D (category B for topical use; category C for oral and ophthalmic use; category D in third trimester.)
Important contra-indications noted in the prescribing guidelines for: nursing mothers; pediatric patients
Note: NSAIDs may cause an increased risk of serious cardiovascular and gastrointestinal adverse events, which can be fatal. This risk may increase with duration of use.
Contra-indicated in patients who have experienced asthma, urticaria, or allergic-type reactions after taking aspirin or other NSAIDs. Severe, rarely fatal, anaphylactic-like reactions to NSAIDs have been reported in such patients. Arthrotec is diclofenac and misoprostol.
Warning: RISK OF SERIOUS CARDIOVASCULAR AND GASTROINTESTINAL EVENTS

Skin
Anaphylactoid reactions/Anaphylaxis (<3%) [16]
Angioedema (<3%) [2]
Bullous dermatitis (<3%) [2]
Dermatitis (<3%) [10]
Dermatitis herpetiformis [2]
Eczema (<3%)
Erythema [4]
Erythema multiforme [6]
Exanthems (<5%) [6]
Fixed eruption [4]
Hypersensitivity [5]
Linear IgA bullous dermatosis [6]
Nicolau syndrome [16]
Photosensitivity (<3%) [4]
Pruritus (<10%) [6]
Purpura (<3%) [2]

Purpura fulminans [2]
Rash (>10%) [4]
Stevens-Johnson syndrome [5]
Toxic epidermal necrolysis [4]
Urticaria (<3%) [7]
Vasculitis [3]
Xerosis [3]

Hair
Alopecia (<3%)

Mucosal
Tongue edema (<3%)
Xerostomia (<3%) [2]

Cardiovascular
Cardiotoxicity [2]
Myocardial infarction [4]

Central Nervous System
Dysgeusia (taste perversion) (<3%)
Headache [2]
Stroke [3]
Vertigo (dizziness) [4]

Neuromuscular/Skeletal
Rhabdomyolysis [3]

Gastrointestinal/Hepatic
Abdominal pain [7]
Constipation [3]
Diarrhea [4]
Dyspepsia [6]
Gastritis [3]
Gastrointestinal bleeding [5]
Gastrointestinal ulceration [4]
Hepatotoxicity [10]
Nausea [8]
Vomiting [4]

Renal
Nephrotoxicity [4]
Renal failure [2]

Hematologic
Agranulocytosis [3]
Bleeding [2]

Local
Application-site reactions [3]

Other
Adverse effects [11]
Allergic reactions [2]
Death [6]

DICLOXACILLIN

See: www.drugeruptiondata.com/drug/id/213

DICUMAROL

Indications: Atrial fibrillation, pulmonary embolism, venous thrombosis
Class: Coumarin
Half-life: 1–4 days
Clinically important, potentially hazardous interactions with: allopurinol, amiodarone, amobarbital, anabolic steroids, anti-thyroid agents, aprobarbital, aspirin, barbiturates, bivalirudin, butabarbital, butalbital, cimetidine, clofibrate, clopidogrel, cyclosporine, delavirdine, disulfiram, fenofibrate, fluconazole, gemfibrozil, glutethimide, imatinib, itraconazole, ketoconazole, levothyroxine, liothyronine,

mephobarbital, methimazole, metronidazole, miconazole, penicillins, pentobarbital, phenobarbital, phenylbutazones, piperacillin, prednisone, primidone, propylthiouracil, quinidine, quinine, rifabutin, rifampin, rifapentine, rofecoxib, salicylates, secobarbital, sulfinpyrazone, sulfonamides, testosterone, zileuton
Pregnancy category: D
Important contra-indications noted in the prescribing guidelines for: nursing mothers

Skin
Dermatitis [2]
Exanthems [5]
Necrosis [10]
Purplish erythema (feet and toes) [2]
Purpura [2]
Urticaria [3]

Hair
Alopecia (<10%) [5]

Hematologic
Hemorrhage [3]

DICYCLOMINE

See: www.drugeruptiondata.com/drug/id/215

DIDANOSINE

Trade name: Videx (Bristol-Myers Squibb)
Indications: Advanced HIV infection
Class: Antiretroviral, Nucleoside analog reverse transcriptase inhibitor
Half-life: 1.5 hours
Clinically important, potentially hazardous interactions with: acetaminophen, amprenavir, ciprofloxacin, corticosteroids, dapsone, darunavir, febuxostat, gemifloxacin, indinavir, itraconazole, ketoconazole, levofloxacin, lomefloxacin, lopinavir, moxifloxacin, norfloxacin, ofloxacin, sulfones, tenofovir disoproxil, tetracycline, tipranavir, voriconazole
Pregnancy category: B
Important contra-indications noted in the prescribing guidelines for: the elderly; nursing mothers
Warning: PANCREATITIS, LACTIC ACIDOSIS and HEPATOMEGALY with STEATOSIS

Skin
Erythema multiforme [2]
Lipodystrophy [2]
Pruritus (9%)
Rash (9%)
Stevens-Johnson syndrome [3]

Mucosal
Xerostomia [4]

Cardiovascular
Myocardial infarction [2]

Central Nervous System
Neurotoxicity [4]

Gastrointestinal/Hepatic
Hepatotoxicity [2]
Non-cirrhotic portal hypertension [5]

Pancreatitis [23]
Endocrine/Metabolic
Acidosis [6]
Diabetes mellitus [2]
Gynecomastia [3]

Renal
Fanconi syndrome [5]

Ocular
Retinopathy [3]

Other
Death [3]

DIETHYLPROPION

See: www.drugeruptiondata.com/drug/id/218

DIETHYLSTILBESTROL

See: www.drugeruptiondata.com/drug/id/219

DIFLUNISAL

See: www.drugeruptiondata.com/drug/id/220

DIFLUPREDNATE

See: www.drugeruptiondata.com/drug/id/1306

DIGOXIN

Trade name: Lanoxin (Concordia)
Indications: Congestive heart failure, atrial fibrillation
Class: Antiarrhythmic class IV, Cardiac glycoside, Inotrope
Half-life: 36–48 hours
Clinically important, potentially hazardous interactions with: acarbose, alprazolam, amiodarone, amphotericin B, arbutamine, atorvastatin, azithromycin, bendroflumethiazide, benzthiazide, bisacodyl, boceprevir, bosutinib, bumetanide, canagliflozin, captopril, carbimazole, chlorothiazide, chlorthalidone, cholestyramine, clarithromycin, cobicistat/elvitegravir/emtricitabine/tenofovir alafenamide, cobicistat/elvitegravir/emtricitabine/tenofovir disoproxil, colchicine, conivaptan, cyclopenthiazide, cyclosporine, cyclothiazide, darifenacin, darunavir, demeclocycline, dexlansoprazole, dexmedetomidine, doxycycline, dronedarone, erythromycin, eslicarbazepine, esomeprazole, ethacrynic acid, etravirine, everolimus, ezogabine, fingolimod, flibanserin, flunisolide, furosemide, glycopyrrolate, glycopyrronium, hydrochlorothiazide, hydroflumethiazide, indapamide, indinavir, itraconazole, lapatinib, lenalidomide, liraglutide, lomustine, lopinavir, meloxicam, mepenzolate, metformin, methylclothiazide, metolazone, milnacipran, minocycline, mirabegron, neratinib, nifedipine, nilotinib, omeprazole, oxprenolol, oxytetracycline, pantoprazole, paricalcitol, paroxetine hydrochloride, pemetrexed,

phenylbutazone, polythiazide, posaconazole, propafenone, propantheline, quinethazone, quinidine, quinine, rabeprazole, rifampin, roxithromycin, sitagliptin, sodium picosulfate, sorafenib, St John's wort, sunitinib, telaprevir, telithromycin, temozolomide, temsirolimus, teriparatide, tetracycline, thalidomide, thiazide diuretics, ticagrelor, tipranavir, tolvaptan, trichlormethiazide, trimethoprim, troglitazone, ulipristal, valbenazine, venetoclax, verapamil, zuclopenthixol

Pregnancy category: C
Important contra-indications noted in the prescribing guidelines for: the elderly; nursing mothers; pediatric patients
Note: This is the pure form of Digitalis. Contra-indicated in ventricular fibrillation.

Skin
Exanthems (2%) [2]
Psoriasis [2]
Toxicity [4]

Cardiovascular
Arrhythmias [7]
Atrial fibrillation [4]
Bradycardia [3]
Tachycardia [2]

Central Nervous System
Anorexia [2]

Neuromuscular/Skeletal
Asthenia (fatigue) [2]

Gastrointestinal/Hepatic
Nausea [4]
Vomiting [2]

Endocrine/Metabolic
Gynecomastia [2]

Ocular
Dyschromatopsia (green) [6]
Hallucinations, visual [2]

Other
Death [5]

DIHYDROCODEINE

Trade name: DHC-Continus (Napp)
Indications: Severe pain in cancer and other chronic conditions
Class: Analgesic, opioid
Half-life: 12 hours
Clinically important, potentially hazardous interactions with: CNS depressants, MAO inhibitors, phenothiazines, tranquilizers
Pregnancy category: C
Important contra-indications noted in the prescribing guidelines for: nursing mothers

Skin
AGEP [2]

Mucosal
Xerostomia [2]

Central Nervous System
Narcosis [2]
Seizures [3]
Somnolence (drowsiness) [2]

Gastrointestinal/Hepatic
Abdominal pain [2]
Constipation [2]
Nausea [2]
Vomiting [2]

Respiratory
Respiratory depression [2]

Genitourinary
Priapism [2]

Renal
Renal failure [5]

DIHYDROERGO-TAMINE

See: www.drugeruptiondata.com/drug/id/222

DIHYDROTACHYS-TEROL

See: www.drugeruptiondata.com/drug/id/223

DILTIAZEM

Trade names: Cardizem (Biovail), Dilacor XR (Watson), Teczem (Sanofi-Aventis), Tiazac (Forest)
Indications: Angina, essential hypertension
Class: Antiarrhythmic class IV, Calcium channel blocker, CYP3A4 inhibitor
Half-life: 5–8 hours (for extended-release capsules)
Clinically important, potentially hazardous interactions with: acebutolol, alfuzosin, amiodarone, amitriptyline, amprenavir, aprepitant, atazanavir, atenolol, atorvastatin, avanafil, bisoprolol, bosentan, carbamazepine, celiprolol, cilostazol, cobicistat/elvitegravir/emtricitabine/tenofovir alafenamide, cobicistat/elvitegravir/emtricitabine/tenofovir disoproxil, colchicine, copanlisib, corticosteroids, cyclosporine, deflazacort, delavirdine, dronedarone, dutasteride, efavirenz, epirubicin, erythromycin, fingolimod, flibanserin, lurasidone, midostaurin, mifepristone, moricizine, naldemedine, naloxegol, neratinib, nevirapine, nifedipine, olaparib, oxprenolol, posaconazole, ranolazine, silodosin, simvastatin, sonidegib, sulpiride, telaprevir, venetoclax
Pregnancy category: C
Important contra-indications noted in the prescribing guidelines for: the elderly; nursing mothers; pediatric patients
Note: Teczem is diltiazem and enalapril.

Skin
AGEP [21]
Angioedema [3]
Diaphoresis [2]
Edema (<10%) [4]
Erythema [2]
Erythema multiforme (<31%) [11]
Exanthems [17]
Exfoliative dermatitis [6]

Hypersensitivity [2]
Leg ulceration [2]
Lupus erythematosus [5]
Palmar–plantar desquamation [2]
Peripheral edema (5–8%)
Photosensitivity [11]
Phototoxicity [2]
Pigmentation [10]
Pruritus [6]
Psoriasis [3]
Purpura [3]
Pustules [2]
Rash [4]
Stevens-Johnson syndrome [4]
Thickening [2]
Toxic epidermal necrolysis [4]
Toxic erythema [2]
Toxicity [2]
Urticaria [5]
Vasculitis [6]

Hair
Alopecia [2]

Mucosal
Gingival hyperplasia/hypertrophy (21%) [10]
Xerostomia [2]

Cardiovascular
Atrial fibrillation [2]
Bradycardia [7]
Cardiogenic shock [2]
Flushing (<10%) [6]
Hypotension [2]

Central Nervous System
Dysgeusia (taste perversion) [2]
Parkinsonism [3]
Somnolence (drowsiness) [2]

Neuromuscular/Skeletal
Rhabdomyolysis [4]

Other
Side effects [2]

DIMENHYDRINATE

Trade name: Dramamine (Pfizer)
Indications: Motion sickness, dizziness, nausea, vomiting
Class: Antiemetic, Cholinesterase absorption inhibitor
Half-life: N/A
Clinically important, potentially hazardous interactions with: none known
Pregnancy category: B
Important contra-indications noted in the prescribing guidelines for: nursing mothers

Skin
Fixed eruption [12]

Mucosal
Xerostomia (<10%)

Central Nervous System
Somnolence (drowsiness) [5]

DIMERCAPROL

See: www.drugeruptiondata.com/drug/id/1056

DIMETHYL FUMARATE

Synonyms: dimethyl (E) butenedioate; BG-12
Trade names: Fumaderm (Biogen Idec),
Tecfidera (Biogen Idec)
Indications: Relapsing forms of multiple
sclerosis, psoriasis
Class: Fumaric acid ester
Half-life: 1 hour
**Clinically important, potentially hazardous
interactions with:** none known
Pregnancy category: C
**Important contra-indications noted in the
prescribing guidelines for:** the elderly; nursing
mothers; pediatric patients
Note: Fumaderm is mixed dimethyl fumarate and
monoethylfumarate salts.

Skin
  Contact dermatitis (from topical contact)
  [14]
  Erythema (5%) [2]
  Pruritus (8%) [4]
  Rash (8%)
Cardiovascular
  Flushing (40%) [27]
Central Nervous System
  Leukoencephalopathy [6]
Neuromuscular/Skeletal
  Asthenia (fatigue) [3]
Gastrointestinal/Hepatic
  Abdominal pain (18%) [11]
  Diarrhea (14%) [10]
  Dyspepsia (5%) [2]
  Nausea [7]
  Vomiting (9%) [3]
Endocrine/Metabolic
  AST increased (4%) [2]
Genitourinary
  Albuminuria (6%)
  Urinary tract infection [2]
Renal
  Proteinuria [2]
Hematologic
  Hemotoxicity [2]
  Lymphopenia (2%) [8]
Other
  Adverse effects (gastrointestinal) [19]
  Infection [2]

DINOPROSTONE

Trade names: Cervidel (Forest), Prepidil (Pfizer)
Indications: Pregnancy termination, uterine
content evacuation, cervical ripening
Class: Prostaglandin
Half-life: 2.5–5 minutes
**Clinically important, potentially hazardous
interactions with:** none known
Pregnancy category: C
Note: Dinoprostone is the naturally occurring
form of Prostaglandin E2 (PGE2).

DINUTUXIMAB

Trade name: Unituxin (United Therapeutics)
Indications: High-risk neuroblastoma in
combination with granulocyte-macrophage
colony-stimulating factor (GM-CSF), interleukin-2
(IL-2), and isotretinoin (13-*cis*-retinoic acid), in
pediatric patients who achieve at least a partial
response to prior first-line multiagent,
multimodality therapy
Class: GD2-binding monoclonal antibody,
Monoclonal antibody
Half-life: 10 days
**Clinically important, potentially hazardous
interactions with:** none known
Pregnancy category: N/A (May cause fetal
harm)
**Important contra-indications noted in the
prescribing guidelines for:** the elderly; nursing
mothers
Warning: SERIOUS INFUSION REACTIONS
AND NEUROTOXICITY

Skin
  Edema (17%)
  Urticaria (25–37%)
Mucosal
  Nasal congestion (20%)
Cardiovascular
  Capillary leak syndrome (22–40%)
  Hypertension (14%)
  Hypotension (60%)
  Tachycardia (19%)
Central Nervous System
  Fever (55–72%)
  Pain (61–85%) [2]
  Peripheral neuropathy (13%)
Gastrointestinal/Hepatic
  Diarrhea (31–43%)
  Nausea (10%)
  Vomiting (33–46%)
Respiratory
  Hypoxia (24%)
  Wheezing (15%)
Endocrine/Metabolic
  ALT increased (43–56%)
  AST increased (16–28%)
  Creatine phosphokinase increased (15%)
  Hyperglycemia (18%)
  Hypertriglyceridemia (16%)
  Hypoalbuminemia (29–33%)
  Hypocalcemia (20–27%)
  Hypokalemia (26–43%)
  Hypomagnesemia (12%)
  Hyponatremia (36–58%)
  Hypophosphatemia (20%)
  Weight gain (10%)
Renal
  Proteinuria (16%)
Hematologic
  Anemia (42–51%)
  Hemorrhage (17%)
  Lymphopenia (54–62%)
  Neutropenia (25–39%)
  Sepsis (18%)
  Thrombocytopenia (61–66%)

Local
  Infusion-related reactions (47–60%) [2]

DIPHENHYDRAMINE

Trade name: Benadryl (Pfizer)
Indications: Allergic rhinitis, urticaria
Class: Antiemetic, Histamine H1 receptor
antagonist, Muscarinic antagonist
Half-life: 2–8 hours
**Clinically important, potentially hazardous
interactions with:** alcohol, anticholinergics,
chloral hydrate, CNS depressants, glutethimide,
MAO inhibitors
Pregnancy category: B
**Important contra-indications noted in the
prescribing guidelines for:** nursing mothers

Skin
  Anaphylactoid reactions/Anaphylaxis [4]
  Contact dermatitis [2]
  Dermatitis [4]
  Eczema [2]
  Fixed eruption [4]
  Photosensitivity [3]
  Pruritus [2]
  Toxic epidermal necrolysis [3]
  Toxicity [2]
Mucosal
  Xerostomia (<10%)
Cardiovascular
  QT prolongation [5]
  Torsades de pointes [3]
Central Nervous System
  Delirium [2]
  Sedation [2]
  Seizures [2]
  Somnolence (drowsiness) [7]
Neuromuscular/Skeletal
  Rhabdomyolysis [5]
Ocular
  Hallucinations, visual [2]
Other
  Death [4]

DIPHENOXYLATE

Trade name: Lomotil (Pfizer)
Indications: Diarrhea
Class: Antimotility, Opioid agonist
Half-life: 2.5 hours
**Clinically important, potentially hazardous
interactions with:** oxybutynin
Pregnancy category: C
**Important contra-indications noted in the
prescribing guidelines for:** nursing mothers;
pediatric patients
Note: Diphenoxylate is almost always prescribed
with atropine sulfate.

Mucosal
  Xerostomia (3%)

DIPHTHERIA ANTITOXIN

See: www.drugeruptiondata.com/drug/id/1216

DIPYRIDAMOLE

Trade names: Aggrenox (Boehringer Ingelheim), Persantine (Boehringer Ingelheim)
Indications: Thromboembolic complications following cardiac valve replacement
Class: Adenosine reuptake inhibitor, Antiplatelet
Half-life: 10–12 hours
Clinically important, potentially hazardous interactions with: adenosine, ceftobiprole, clopidogrel, enoxaparin, fondaparinux, regadenoson, reteplase, riociguat, tinzaparin
Pregnancy category: B
Important contra-indications noted in the prescribing guidelines for: nursing mothers; pediatric patients
Note: Aggrenox is dipyridamole and aspirin.

Skin
　Rash (2%)
　Stevens-Johnson syndrome [2]
Cardiovascular
　Flushing (3%)
Central Nervous System
　Headache [3]
Other
　Adverse effects [3]

DIRITHROMYCIN

See: www.drugeruptiondata.com/drug/id/230

DISOPYRAMIDE

Trade name: Norpace (Pfizer)
Indications: Ventricular arrhythmias
Class: Antiarrhythmic, Antiarrhythmic class Ia, Muscarinic antagonist
Half-life: 4–10 hours
Clinically important, potentially hazardous interactions with: acebutolol, amiodarone, amisulpride, amitriptyline, arsenic, artemether/ lumefantrine, astemizole, atenolol, bisoprolol, celiprolol, ciprofloxacin, clarithromycin, cobicistat/elvitegravir/emtricitabine/tenofovir alafenamide, cobicistat/elvitegravir/emtricitabine/ tenofovir disoproxil, darifenacin, degarelix, dronedarone, droperidol, enoxacin, erythromycin, gatifloxacin, gliclazide, glycopyrrolate, glycopyrronium, insulin aspart, insulin degludec, insulin glargine, insulin glulisine, itraconazole, ketoconazole, levomepromazine, lomefloxacin, lurasidone, metformin, moxifloxacin, nevirapine, nilotinib, norfloxacin, ofloxacin, oxprenolol, oxybutynin, pimavanserin, quinine, quinolones, ribociclib, rifapentine, roxithromycin, sildenafil, sotalol, sparfloxacin, sulpiride, tadalafil, telithromycin, tiotropium, trospium, vandetanib, vardenafil, zuclopenthixol

Pregnancy category: C
Important contra-indications noted in the prescribing guidelines for: nursing mothers; pediatric patients

Skin
　Dermatitis (<3%)
　Edema (<3%)
　Exanthems (<5%)
　Lupus erythematosus [3]
　Pruritus (<3%)
　Rash (generalized) (<3%)
Mucosal
　Oral lesions (40%)
　Xerostomia (32%) [2]
Cardiovascular
　Chest pain (<3%)
　Hypotension (<3%)
　QT prolongation [8]
　Torsades de pointes [13]
Central Nervous System
　Anorexia (<3%)
　Headache (3–9%)
　Nervousness (<3%)
　Syncope (<3%)
　Vertigo (dizziness) (3–9%)
Neuromuscular/Skeletal
　Asthenia (fatigue) (3–9%)
Gastrointestinal/Hepatic
　Abdominal pain (3–9%)
　Constipation (11%) [2]
　Diarrhea (<3%)
　Nausea (3–9%)
　Vomiting (<3%)
Respiratory
　Dyspnea (<3%)
Endocrine/Metabolic
　Hypocalcemia [3]
　Hypoglycemia [4]
　Hypokalemia (<3%)
　Weight gain (<3%)
Genitourinary
　Impotence (<3%)
　Urinary hesitancy (14%)
　Urinary retention (3–9%)
Ocular
　Vision blurred (3–9%)
　Xerophthalmia (3–9%)

DISTIGMINE

See: www.drugeruptiondata.com/drug/id/1348

DISULFIRAM

Trade name: Antabuse (Odyssey)
Indications: Alcoholism
Class: Antialcoholism, Antioxidant
Half-life: N/A
Clinically important, potentially hazardous interactions with: acenocoumarol, alcohol, amitriptyline, anisindione, anticoagulants, benznidazole, clobazam, cyclosporine, dicumarol, dronabinol, ethanolamine, ethotoin, fosphenytoin, lopinavir, mephenytoin, metronidazole,

omeprazole, oxtriphylline, phenytoin, thalidomide, tipranavir, warfarin
Pregnancy category: C
Important contra-indications noted in the prescribing guidelines for: nursing mothers; pediatric patients

Skin
　Acneform eruption [3]
　Bullous dermatitis [2]
　Dermatitis [17]
　Eczema [2]
　Exanthems [2]
　Fixed eruption [2]
　Rash (<10%)
　Recall reaction (nickel) [4]
　Urticaria [3]
Cardiovascular
　Flushing (with alcohol) [5]
　Hypertension [2]
　Hypotension [2]
　Polyarteritis nodosa [2]
　Tachycardia [2]
Central Nervous System
　Dysgeusia (taste perversion) (metallic or
　　garlic aftertaste) (<10%)
　Neurotoxicity [6]
　Psychosis [5]
　Seizures [2]
　Somnolence (drowsiness) [2]
　Vertigo (dizziness) [2]
Neuromuscular/Skeletal
　Asthenia (fatigue) [2]
Ocular
　Optic neuropathy [2]
Other
　Adverse effects [2]

DOBUTAMINE

See: www.drugeruptiondata.com/drug/id/234

DOCETAXEL

Trade name: Taxotere (Sanofi-Aventis)
Indications: Metastatic breast cancer, non-small cell lung cancer, with prednisone in hormone refractory prostate cancer, with cisplatin and fluorouracil for gastric adenocarcinoma and squamous cell carcinoma of the head and neck
Class: Antineoplastic, Taxane
Half-life: 11–18 hours
Clinically important, potentially hazardous interactions with: alcohol, aldesleukin, anthracyclines, antifungals, aprepitant, BCG vaccine, conivaptan, cyclosporine, CYP3A4 inhibitors or inducers, dasatinib, deferasirox, denosumab, echinacea, erythromycin, itraconazole, ketoconazole, lapatinib, leflunomide, natalizumab, P-glycoprotein inhibitors or inducers, pimecrolimus, prednisone, ritonavir, sipuleucel-T, sorafenib, St John's wort, tacrolimus, thalidomide, trastuzumab, vaccines, voriconazole

Pregnancy category: D
Important contra-indications noted in the prescribing guidelines for: the elderly; nursing mothers; pediatric patients
Note: Contra-indicated in patients with hypersensitivity to docetaxel or polysorbate 80, or with neutrophil counts of <1500 cells/mm³.
Warning: TOXIC DEATHS, HEPATOTOXICITY, NEUTROPENIA, HYPERSENSITIVITY REACTIONS, and FLUID RETENTION

Skin
AGEP [2]
Anaphylactoid reactions/Anaphylaxis [3]
Edema (34%) [24]
Erythema [4]
Exanthems [3]
Facial erythema [2]
Flagellate erythema/pigmentation [2]
Hand–foot syndrome [42]
Hypersensitivity (6%) [15]
Peripheral edema [9]
Photosensitivity [6]
Pigmentation [2]
Psoriasis [3]
Radiation recall dermatitis [18]
Rash [12]
Recall reaction [2]
Scleroderma [9]
Thrombocytopenic purpura [2]
Toxicity (20–48%) [10]
Xerosis [2]

Hair
Alopecia (56–76%) [30]

Nails
Beau's lines (transverse nail bands) [2]
Discoloration [2]
Melanonychia [2]
Nail changes [17]
Nail disorder (11–41%) [2]
Nail loss [3]
Nail pigmentation [6]
Onycholysis [15]
Onychopathy [2]
Paronychia [4]
Pyogenic granuloma [2]
Subungual abscess [2]
Subungual hemorrhage [2]
Transverse superficial loss of nail plate [2]

Mucosal
Aphthous stomatitis [2]
Mucositis [15]
Oral mucositis [5]
Stomatitis (19–53%) [19]

Cardiovascular
Capillary leak syndrome [2]
Cardiotoxicity [2]
Flushing [2]
Hypertension [10]
Hypotension (3%)
Thromboembolism [2]

Central Nervous System
Anorexia [11]
Dysesthesia (4%)
Dysgeusia (taste perversion) (6%) [7]
Fever (31–35%) [6]
Headache [2]
Mood changes [2]
Neurotoxicity [20]

Pain [5]
Paresthesias (4%) [2]
Peripheral neuropathy [10]
Vertigo (dizziness) [2]

Neuromuscular/Skeletal
Arthralgia (3–9%) [3]
Asthenia (fatigue) (53–66%) [60]
Bone or joint pain [2]
Myalgia/Myopathy (3–23%) [10]

Gastrointestinal/Hepatic
Abdominal pain [4]
Constipation [3]
Diarrhea (23–43%) [48]
Dysphagia [2]
Hepatotoxicity [2]
Nausea (34–42%) [27]
Vomiting (22–23%) [20]

Respiratory
Acute respiratory distress syndrome [2]
Cough [2]
Dyspnea [5]
Pleural effusion [2]
Pneumonia [3]
Pneumonitis [10]
Pulmonary embolism [2]
Pulmonary toxicity (41%) [4]
Respiratory failure [2]
Upper respiratory tract infection [3]

Endocrine/Metabolic
ALP increased (4–7%)
ALT increased [5]
Amenorrhea [4]
Appetite decreased [3]
AST increased [4]
Dehydration [2]
Hyperglycemia [3]
Hyponatremia [4]
Hypophosphatemia [2]

Hematologic
Anemia (65–94%) [24]
Febrile neutropenia (6%) [49]
Hemolytic uremic syndrome [3]
Hemotoxicity [3]
Leukocytopenia [4]
Leukopenia (84–99%) [26]
Lymphopenia [4]
Myelosuppression [2]
Neutropenia (84–99%) [86]
Thrombocytopenia (8–14%) [12]

Ocular
Epiphora [8]

Local
Injection-site erythema [2]
Injection-site extravasation [3]
Injection-site pigmentation [3]
Injection-site reactions [2]

Other
Adverse effects [4]
Allergic reactions [2]
Death [17]
Infection (<34%) [9]

DOCOSANOL

See: www.drugeruptiondata.com/drug/id/957

DOCUSATE

See: www.drugeruptiondata.com/drug/id/236

DOFETILIDE

See: www.drugeruptiondata.com/drug/id/237

DOLASETRON

See: www.drugeruptiondata.com/drug/id/238

DOLUTEGRAVIR

Trade names: Tivicay (ViiV), Triumeq (ViiV)
Indications: HIV-1 infection
Class: Antiretroviral, Integrase strand transfer inhibitor
Half-life: ~14 hours
Clinically important, potentially hazardous interactions with: dofetilide
Pregnancy category: B
Important contra-indications noted in the prescribing guidelines for: nursing mothers; pediatric patients
Note: Triumeq is abacavir, dolutegravir and lamivudine.

Skin
Hypersensitivity [5]
Pruritus (<2%)
Rash [3]

Central Nervous System
Abnormal dreams [2]
Headache (<2%) [17]
Insomnia (<3%) [4]

Neuromuscular/Skeletal
Asthenia (fatigue) (<2%) [3]
Myalgia/Myopathy (<2%)

Gastrointestinal/Hepatic
Abdominal pain (<2%)
Diarrhea [16]
Flatulence (<2%)
Hepatitis (<2%)
Nausea [14]
Vomiting (<2%)

Respiratory
Nasopharyngitis [3]
Upper respiratory tract infection [2]

Endocrine/Metabolic
ALT increased (<2%) [3]
AST increased (<3%)
Creatine phosphokinase increased (<4%)
Hyperglycemia (5–7%)

Renal
Nephrotoxicity (<2%)

Other
Adverse effects [4]

DOMPERIDONE

See: www.drugeruptiondata.com/drug/id/843

DONEPEZIL

Trade names: Aricept (Eisai), Aricept Evess (Eisai)
Indications: Mild, moderate and severe dementia of the Alzheimer's type
Class: Acetylcholinesterase inhibitor, Cholinesterase inhibitor, Parasympathomimetic
Half-life: 50–70 hours
Clinically important, potentially hazardous interactions with: anticholinergics, cholinergic agonists, galantamine, non-depolarising muscle relaxants, ramelteon, succinylcholine
Pregnancy category: C
Important contra-indications noted in the prescribing guidelines for: nursing mothers; pediatric patients
Note: Contra-indicated in patients with known hypersensitivity to donepezil hydrochloride or to piperidine derivatives.

Skin
  Diaphoresis [2]
  Ecchymoses (4–5%)
  Eczema (3%)
  Purpura (<10%)

Cardiovascular
  Atrioventricular block [2]
  Bradycardia [7]
  Chest pain (2%)
  Hypertension [2]
  Hypotension (3%)
  QT prolongation [4]
  Torsades de pointes [2]

Central Nervous System
  Abnormal dreams (3%) [2]
  Agitation [2]
  Anorexia (4–8%) [5]
  Confusion (2%) [3]
  Delirium [2]
  Depression (2–3%) [3]
  Emotional lability (2%)
  Fever (3%)
  Gait instability [2]
  Hallucinations (3%)
  Headache (4–10%) [6]
  Hostility (3%)
  Insomnia (5–9%) [4]
  Mania [2]
  Nervousness (3%)
  Neuroleptic malignant syndrome [2]
  Pain (3–9%)
  Parkinsonism [2]
  Somnolence (drowsiness) (2%) [2]
  Syncope (2%) [5]
  Tremor [3]
  Vertigo (dizziness) (2–8%) [6]

Neuromuscular/Skeletal
  Arthralgia (2%)
  Asthenia (fatigue) (5%) [3]
  Back pain (3%)
  Dystonia [2]
  Muscle spasm [2]
  Myoclonus [2]

Gastrointestinal/Hepatic
  Constipation [3]
  Diarrhea (10%) [11]
  Hepatotoxicity [3]
  Nausea (6–11%) [14]
  Vomiting (5–8%) [8]

Endocrine/Metabolic
  Appetite decreased [4]
  Creatine phosphokinase increased (3%)
  Dehydration (2%)
  Hyperlipidemia (2%)
  Weight loss (3%)

Genitourinary
  Urinary frequency (2%) [2]
  Urinary incontinence (2%)
  Urinary tract infection [3]

Hematologic
  Hemorrhage (2%)

Other
  Adverse effects [9]
  Infection (11%)

DOPAMINE

Trade name: Intropin (Hospira)
Indications: Hemodynamic imbalances present in shock
Class: Adrenergic alpha-receptor agonist, Catecholamine, Inotropic sympathomimetic
Half-life: 2 minutes
Clinically important, potentially hazardous interactions with: ethotoin, fosphenytoin, furazolidone, lurasidone, MAO inhibitors, mephenytoin, phenelzine, phenytoin, quetiapine, tranylcypromine
Pregnancy category: C
Important contra-indications noted in the prescribing guidelines for: nursing mothers; pediatric patients

Cardiovascular
  QT prolongation [2]

Local
  Injection-site extravasation [2]
  Injection-site necrosis [3]

DOPEXAMINE

See: www.drugeruptiondata.com/drug/id/1331

DORIPENEM

See: www.drugeruptiondata.com/drug/id/1254

DORNASE ALFA

See: www.drugeruptiondata.com/drug/id/1048

DORZOLAMIDE

Trade names: Cosopt (Merck), Trusopt (Banyu)
Indications: Glaucoma, ocular hypertension
Class: Carbonic anhydrase inhibitor, Diuretic
Half-life: ~4 months
Clinically important, potentially hazardous interactions with: none known
Pregnancy category: C
Important contra-indications noted in the prescribing guidelines for: nursing mothers
Note: Dorzolamide is a sulfonamide and can be absorbed systemically. Sulfonamides can produce severe, possibly fatal, reactions such as toxic epidermal necrolysis and Stevens-Johnson syndrome.
Cosopt is dorzolamide and timolol.

Skin
  Contact dermatitis [4]

Central Nervous System
  Dysgeusia (taste perversion) (25%) [8]

Ocular
  Ocular burning (33%) [5]
  Ocular pain [2]
  Ocular pruritus [4]
  Ocular stinging [10]
  Vision blurred [3]

Other
  Adverse effects [2]

DOXACURIUM

See: www.drugeruptiondata.com/drug/id/242

DOXAPRAM

See: www.drugeruptiondata.com/drug/id/243

DOXAZOSIN

Trade name: Cardura (Pfizer)
Indications: Hypertension
Class: Adrenergic alpha-receptor antagonist
Half-life: 19–22 hours
Clinically important, potentially hazardous interactions with: tadalafil, vardenafil, zuclopenthixol
Pregnancy category: C
Important contra-indications noted in the prescribing guidelines for: the elderly; nursing mothers; pediatric patients

Skin
  Edema (4%)
  Exanthems (2%)

Mucosal
  Xerostomia (2%) [2]

Cardiovascular
  Hypotension [3]
  Orthostatic hypotension [2]
  Postural hypotension [2]

Central Nervous System
  Headache [2]
  Vertigo (dizziness) [9]

Neuromuscular/Skeletal
  Asthenia (fatigue) [4]

Gastrointestinal/Hepatic
  Abdominal pain [2]

Genitourinary
  Erectile dysfunction [3]

Ocular
Floppy iris syndrome [3]

DOXEPIN

Trade names: Adapin (LGM Pharma), Silenor (Somaxon), Sinquan (Pfizer)
Indications: Mental depression, anxiety, insomnia
Class: Antidepressant, tricyclic, Muscarinic antagonist
Half-life: 6–8 hours
Clinically important, potentially hazardous interactions with: alcohol, amprenavir, arbutamine, cholestyramine, clonidine, CNS depressants, epinephrine, formoterol, guanethidine, isocarboxazid, linezolid, MAO inhibitors, phenelzine, QT prolonging agents, quinolones, ramelteon, selegiline, sparfloxacin, sympathomimetics, tranylcypromine
Pregnancy category: C (pregnancy category is B for topical use)
Important contra-indications noted in the prescribing guidelines for: nursing mothers
Warning: SUICIDALITY AND ANTIDEPRESSANT DRUGS

Skin
Dermatitis (from topical) [9]
Diaphoresis (<10%)
Pseudolymphoma [2]

Mucosal
Xerostomia (>10%) [6]

Cardiovascular
QT prolongation [2]

Central Nervous System
Dysgeusia (taste perversion) (>10%)
Headache [4]
Somnolence (drowsiness) [7]

DOXERCALCIFEROL

See: www.drugeruptiondata.com/drug/id/246

DOXORUBICIN

Synonym: hydroxydaunomycin
Trade names: Adriamycin (Bedford), Doxil (Tibotec), Rubex (Mead Johnson)
Indications: Carcinomas, leukemias, sarcomas
Class: Antibiotic, anthracycline
Half-life: 20–48 hours
Clinically important, potentially hazardous interactions with: aldesleukin, cabazitaxel, CYP2D6 inhibitors or inducers, CYP3A4 inhibitors or inducers, gadobenate, P-glycoprotein inhibitors or inducers, paclitaxel, sorafenib, stavudine, trastuzumab, zidovudine
Pregnancy category: D
Important contra-indications noted in the prescribing guidelines for: nursing mothers
Warning: CARDIOMYOPATHY, SECONDARY MALIGNANCIES, EXTRAVASATION AND TISSUE NECROSIS, and SEVERE MYELOSUPPRESSION

Skin
Anaphylactoid reactions/Anaphylaxis [2]
Angioedema [5]
Erythema [2]
Exanthems [4]
Exfoliative dermatitis [2]
Hand–foot syndrome [60]
Hypersensitivity [2]
Intertrigo [3]
Lupus erythematosus [3]
Necrosis (local) [5]
Palmar–plantar erythema (painful) [4]
Pigmentation [15]
Pruritus [2]
Purpura [2]
Radiation recall dermatitis [8]
Rash [6]
Toxicity [12]
Urticaria [10]

Hair
Alopecia (>10%) [39]

Nails
Beau's lines [2]
Melanonychia [2]
Nail changes [2]
Nail pigmentation [16]
Onycholysis [5]

Mucosal
Aphthous stomatitis [2]
Mucositis [16]
Oral lesions [7]
Stomatitis (>10%) [19]
Tongue pigmentation [3]

Cardiovascular
Atrial fibrillation [2]
Cardiomyopathy [5]
Cardiotoxicity [18]
Chest pain [2]
Congestive heart failure [5]
Flushing (<10%) [2]
Myocardial toxicity [4]

Central Nervous System
Anorexia [3]
Dysgeusia (taste perversion) [2]
Fever [5]
Headache [3]
Leukoencephalopathy [4]
Neurotoxicity [4]
Pain [2]
Peripheral neuropathy [5]

Neuromuscular/Skeletal
Asthenia (fatigue) [17]
Bone or joint pain [2]
Myalgia/Myopathy [2]

Gastrointestinal/Hepatic
Constipation [3]
Diarrhea [5]
Gastrointestinal perforation [2]
Hepatotoxicity [6]
Nausea [11]
Pancreatitis [2]
Vomiting [10]

Respiratory
Dyspnea [3]
Pneumonia [3]
Pneumonitis [2]

Endocrine/Metabolic
ALT increased [3]

Amenorrhea [2]
Renal
Nephrotoxicity [2]
Hematologic
Anemia [12]
Febrile neutropenia [15]
Hemorrhage [2]
Hemotoxicity [2]
Leukopenia [3]
Neutropenia [31]
Thrombocytopenia [18]
Local
Injection-site erythema [7]
Injection-site extravasation (>10%) [12]
Injection-site necrosis (>10%) [5]
Injection-site reactions [2]
Injection-site ulceration (>10%) [4]
Other
Adverse effects [5]
Allergic reactions [3]
Death [10]
Infection [4]

DOXYCYCLINE

Trade names: Adoxa (Bioglan), Doryx (Warner Chilcott), Oracea (Galderma), Vibra-Tabs (Pfizer), Vibramycin-D (Pfizer)
Indications: Various infections caused by susceptible organisms
Class: Antibiotic, tetracycline
Half-life: 12–22 hours
Clinically important, potentially hazardous interactions with: acitretin, amoxicillin, ampicillin, antacids, bacampicillin, barbiturates, BCG vaccine, bismuth, calcium salts, carbamazepine, carbenicillin, cloxacillin, corticosteroids, coumarins, cyclosporine, dairy products, digoxin, ergotamine, methysergide, methotrexate, methoxyflurane, methysergide, mezlocillin, nafcillin, oral contraceptives, oral iron, oral typhoid vaccine, oxacillin, penicillins, phenindione, phenytoin, piperacillin, primidone, quinapril, retinoids, rifampin, St John's wort, strontium ranelate, sucralfate, sulfonylureas, ticarcillin, tripotassium dicitratobismuthate, zinc
Pregnancy category: D
Important contra-indications noted in the prescribing guidelines for: nursing mothers; pediatric patients

Skin
AGEP [2]
Angioedema [2]
Candidiasis [3]
Erythema multiforme [4]
Exanthems [2]
Fixed eruption [9]
Hypersensitivity [2]
Photosensitivity [20]
Phototoxicity [9]
Pigmentation [5]
Pruritus [3]
Rash [5]
Stevens-Johnson syndrome [6]
Sweet's syndrome [2]
Toxic epidermal necrolysis [2]
Urticaria [6]

Nails
Photo-onycholysis [13]

Mucosal
Black tongue [2]
Mucosal candidiasis [2]

Central Nervous System
Anosmia [2]
Fever [2]
Headache [4]
Intracranial pressure increased [2]
Paresthesias [4]
Vertigo (dizziness) [3]

Neuromuscular/Skeletal
Myalgia/Myopathy [2]

Gastrointestinal/Hepatic
Abdominal pain [3]
Diarrhea [3]
Esophagitis [3]
Hepatotoxicity [2]
Nausea [5]
Pancreatitis [3]
Ulcerative esophagitis [2]
Vomiting [3]

Endocrine/Metabolic
Hypoglycemia [2]

Genitourinary
Vaginitis [2]

Other
Adverse effects [6]
Allergic reactions [3]
Tooth pigmentation (>10%) [5]

DRONABINOL

Synonyms: tetrahydrocannabinol; THC
Trade names: Marinol (AbbVie), Syndros (Insys)
Indications: Chemotherapy-induced nausea, anorexia associated with weight loss in patients with AIDS
Class: Antiemetic, Cannabinoid
Half-life: 19–24 hours
Clinically important, potentially hazardous interactions with: disulfiram, metronidazole
Pregnancy category: C
Important contra-indications noted in the prescribing guidelines for: the elderly; nursing mothers; pediatric patients

Mucosal
Xerostomia (<10%)

Central Nervous System
Euphoria (<10%)
Paranoia (<10%)
Somnolence (drowsiness) (<10%)
Vertigo (dizziness) (<10%) [5]

Gastrointestinal/Hepatic
Abdominal pain (<10%)
Nausea (<10%) [2]
Vomiting (<10%)

Other
Adverse effects [4]

DRONEDARONE

Trade name: Multaq (Sanofi-Aventis)
Indications: Atrial fibrillation and atrial flutter
Class: Antiarrhythmic, Antiarrhythmic class III
Half-life: 13–19 hours
Clinically important, potentially hazardous interactions with: amiodarone, amitriptyline, amoxapine, antiarrhythmics, antipsychotics prolonging QT interval, arsenic, atorvastatin, beta blockers, bupivacaine, calcium channel blockers, carbamazepine, citalopram, clarithromycin, conivaptan, coumarins, cyclosporine, CYP3A inducers, dabigatran, darunavir, dasabuvir/ombitasvir/paritaprevir/ritonavir, dasatinib, degarelix, delavirdine, digoxin, diltiazem, disopyramide, dolasetron, efavirenz, erythromycin, fingolimod, grapefruit juice, indinavir, itraconazole, ketoconazole, lapatinib, levobupivacaine, levofloxacin, levomepromazine, metoprolol, moxifloxacin, nefazodone, neratinib, nifedipine, ombitasvir/paritaprevir/ritonavir, oxcarbazepine, pazopanib, phenindione, phenobarbital, phenothiazines, phenytoin, posaconazole, prilocaine, propranolol, rifampin, rifapentine, ritonavir, ropivacaine, rosuvastatin, saquinavir, simvastatin, sirolimus, sotalol, St John's wort, statins, tacrolimus, telavancin, telithromycin, tricyclic antidepressants, venetoclax, verapamil, voriconazole, vorinostat, warfarin, ziprasidone
Pregnancy category: X
Important contra-indications noted in the prescribing guidelines for: nursing mothers; pediatric patients
Warning: INCREASED RISK OF DEATH, STROKE AND HEART FAILURE IN PATIENTS WITH DECOMPENSATED HEART FAILURE OR PERMANENT ATRIAL FIBRILLATION

Skin
Anaphylactoid reactions/Anaphylaxis [2]
Dermatitis (5%)
Eczema (5%)
Erythema (5%)
Pruritus (5%)
Rash (5%) [8]

Cardiovascular
Arrhythmias [3]
Bradycardia (3%) [8]
Cardiac failure (new or worsening) [9]
Cardiotoxicity [3]
Congestive heart failure [2]
QT prolongation (28%) [10]
Torsades de pointes [3]

Central Nervous System
Vertigo (dizziness) [2]

Neuromuscular/Skeletal
Asthenia (fatigue) (7%) [3]

Gastrointestinal/Hepatic
Abdominal pain (4%) [2]
Diarrhea (9%) [14]
Dyspepsia (2%)
Gastrointestinal disorder [4]
Hepatic failure [5]
Hepatotoxicity [9]
Nausea (5%) [12]
Vomiting (2%) [6]

Respiratory
Pulmonary toxicity [9]

Endocrine/Metabolic
Serum creatinine increased (51%) [6]

Renal
Nephrotoxicity [2]
Renal failure [2]

Other
Adverse effects [2]
Death [2]
Side effects [2]

DROPERIDOL

Trade names: Inapsine (Akorn), Xomolix (ProStrakan)
Indications: Tranquilizer and antiemetic in surgical procedures
Class: Antiemetic, Antipsychotic, Butyrophenone
Half-life: 2.3 hours
Clinically important, potentially hazardous interactions with: amiodarone, amisulpride, amitriptyline, arsenic, atomoxetine, azithromycin, chloroquine, CNS depressants, cyclobenzaprine, disopyramide, duloxetine, eszopiclone, fluoxetine, fluvoxamine, hydromorphone, hydroxychloroquine, levomepromazine, lurasidone, macrolides, metaxalone, milnacipran, moxifloxacin, paliperidone, pentamidine, pimozide, QT prolonging agents, quinine, ramelteon, sertraline, sotalol, sulpiride, tamoxifen, tapentadol, thiopental, tiagabine, tricyclic antidepressants
Pregnancy category: C
Important contra-indications noted in the prescribing guidelines for: nursing mothers; pediatric patients
Note: Contra-indicated in patients with known or suspected QT prolongation.
This product is not available in the European market.
Warning: QT PROLONGATION AND TORSADE DE POINTES

Skin
Anaphylactoid reactions/Anaphylaxis [3]
Angioedema [2]

Cardiovascular
Arrhythmias [2]
QT prolongation [13]
Torsades de pointes [6]

Central Nervous System
Akathisia [5]
Extrapyramidal symptoms [2]
Neuroleptic malignant syndrome [2]
Restlessness [2]
Sedation [2]

Neuromuscular/Skeletal
Dystonia [6]

Other
Death [3]

DROTRECOGIN ALFA

See: www.drugeruptiondata.com/drug/id/918

DROXIDOPA

Synonym: L-DOPS
Trade name: Northera (Chelsea Therapeutics)
Indications: Neurogenic orthostatic hypotension
Class: Amino acid analog (synthetic)
Half-life: 2.5 hours
Clinically important, potentially hazardous interactions with: none known
Pregnancy category: C
Important contra-indications noted in the prescribing guidelines for: nursing mothers; pediatric patients
Warning: SUPINE HYPERTENSION

Cardiovascular
Hypertension (2–7%)

Central Nervous System
Gait instability (15%) [2]
Headache (6–15%) [3]
Syncope (13%)
Vertigo (dizziness) (4–10%) [2]

Gastrointestinal/Hepatic
Nausea (2–9%)

Genitourinary
Urinary tract infection (15%) [2]

DULAGLUTIDE

Trade name: Trulicity (Lilly)
Indications: To improve glycemic control in adults with Type II diabetes mellitus
Class: Glucagon-like peptide-1 (GLP-1) receptor agonist
Half-life: 5 days
Clinically important, potentially hazardous interactions with: none known
Pregnancy category: C
Important contra-indications noted in the prescribing guidelines for: nursing mothers; pediatric patients
Note: Contra-indicated in patients with a personal or family history of medullary thyroid carcinoma or in patients with multiple endocrine neoplasia syndrome Type 2.
Warning: RISK OF THYROID C-CELL TUMORS

Cardiovascular
Atrioventricular block (2%)
Tachycardia (3–6%)

Central Nervous System
Headache [3]

Neuromuscular/Skeletal
Asthenia (fatigue) (4–6%)

Gastrointestinal/Hepatic
Abdominal pain (7–9%)
Constipation [4]
Diarrhea [22]
Dyspepsia (4–6%) [3]
Nausea (12–21%) [23]
Pancreatitis [2]
Vomiting (6–13%) [16]

Respiratory
Nasopharyngitis [6]

Endocrine/Metabolic
Appetite decreased (5–9%) [2]

Local
Injection-site reactions [5]

Other
Adverse effects (gastrointestinal) [4]

DULOXETINE

Trade names: Cymbalta (Lilly), Yentreve (Lilly)
Indications: Depression
Class: Antidepressant, Noradrenaline reuptake inhibitor, Serotonin reuptake inhibitor
Half-life: 8–17 hours
Clinically important, potentially hazardous interactions with: 5HT1 agonists, alcohol, amitriptyline, artemether/lumefantrine, aspirin, atomoxetine, cimetidine, ciprofloxacin, citalopram, clomipramine, CYP1A2 inducers, CYP2D6 inhibitors and substrates, darunavir, droperidol, enoxacin, fesoterodine, fluoxetine, fluvoxamine, iobenguane, levomepromazine, MAO inhibitors, meperidine, moclobemide, naratriptan, nebivolol, NSAIDs, paroxetine hydrochloride, PEG-interferon, quinidine, sibutramine, SSRIs, St John's wort, tamoxifen, teriflunomide, thioridazine, tramadol, tricyclic antidepressants, tryptophan, venlafaxine, warfarin
Pregnancy category: C
Important contra-indications noted in the prescribing guidelines for: nursing mothers; pediatric patients
Warning: SUICIDAL THOUGHTS AND BEHAVIORS

Skin
Diaphoresis (6%) [2]
Hot flashes (>2%)
Hyperhidrosis (7%) [8]

Mucosal
Oropharyngeal pain (>2%)
Xerostomia (13%) [23]

Cardiovascular
Flushing (3%)
Palpitation (>2%)

Central Nervous System
Agitation (5%)
Anxiety (3%)
Headache (14%) [11]
Insomnia (10%) [13]
Paresthesias (>2%)
Restless legs syndrome [2]
Serotonin syndrome [4]
Somnolence (drowsiness) (10%) [15]
Suicidal ideation [4]
Tardive dyskinesia [3]
Tremor (3%)
Vertigo (dizziness) (10%) [15]
Yawning (>2%) [2]

Neuromuscular/Skeletal
Arthralgia (>2%)
Asthenia (fatigue) (10%) [14]
Back pain (>2%)
Bone or joint pain (4%)
Muscle spasm (3%)

Gastrointestinal/Hepatic
Abdominal pain (>2%)
Colitis [2]
Constipation (10%) [8]
Diarrhea (9%) [6]
Hepatotoxicity (rare) [4]
Nausea (24%) [24]
Vomiting (>2%) [3]

Respiratory
Cough (>2%)
Influenza (3%)
Nasopharyngitis (5%)
Upper respiratory tract infection (4%)

Endocrine/Metabolic
ALT increased [2]
Appetite decreased (8–9%) [2]
Hyponatremia [2]
Libido decreased (4%)
SIADH [6]
Weight loss (>2%)

Genitourinary
Ejaculatory dysfunction (2–5%)
Sexual dysfunction [6]

Ocular
Vision blurred (>2%)

Other
Adverse effects [11]
Bruxism [3]
Death [2]

DUPILUMAB *

Trade name: Dupixent (Regeneron)
Indications: Moderate-to-severe atopic dermatitis
Class: Interleukin-4 receptor alpha antagonist, Monoclonal antibody
Half-life: N/A
Clinically important, potentially hazardous interactions with: none known
Pregnancy category: N/A (Insufficient evidence to inform drug-associated risk)
Important contra-indications noted in the prescribing guidelines for: pediatric patients

Skin
Herpes simplex (2%)

Mucosal
Oral candidiasis (4%)

Central Nervous System
Headache [2]

Respiratory
Nasopharyngitis [3]

Ocular
Conjunctivitis (10%) [3]

Local
Injection-site reactions (10%) [3]

DURVALUMAB *

Trade name: Imfinzi (AstraZeneca)
Indications: Locally advanced or metastatic urothelial carcinoma in patients having disease progression following platinum-containing chemotherapy
Class: Monoclonal antibody, Programmed death-ligand (PD-L1) inhibitor
Half-life: 17 days
Clinically important, potentially hazardous interactions with: none known
Pregnancy category: N/A (Can cause fetal harm)
Important contra-indications noted in the prescribing guidelines for: the elderly; nursing mothers; pediatric patients

Skin
 Peripheral edema (15%)
 Rash (11%)
Central Nervous System
 Fever (14%)
Neuromuscular/Skeletal
 Asthenia (fatigue) (39%)
 Bone or joint pain (24%)
Gastrointestinal/Hepatic
 Abdominal pain (14%)
 Colitis (13%)
 Constipation (21%)
 Diarrhea (13%) [3]
 Nausea (16%)
Respiratory
 Cough (10%)
 Dyspnea (13%)
 Pneumonitis (2%)
Endocrine/Metabolic
 ALP increased (4%)
 Appetite decreased (19%)
 AST increased (2%)
 Hypercalcemia (3%)
 Hyperglycemia (3%)
 Hypermagnesemia (4%)
 Hyperthyroidism (5–6%)
 Hyponatremia (12%)
 Hypothyroidism (6–10%)
Genitourinary
 Urinary tract infection (15%)
Hematologic
 Anemia (8%)
 Lymphopenia (11%)
Local
 Infusion-related reactions (2%)
Other
 Death [2]
 Infection (30–38%)

DUTASTERIDE

Trade names: Avodart (GSK), Jalyn (GSK)
Indications: Benign prostatic hyperplasia, male pattern baldness (anecdotal)
Class: 5-alpha reductase inhibitor, Androgen antagonist
Half-life: 3–5 weeks
Clinically important, potentially hazardous interactions with: cimetidine, ciprofloxacin, conivaptan, darunavir, delavirdine, diltiazem, indinavir, ketoconazole, ritonavir, telithromycin, troleandomycin, verapamil, voriconazole
Pregnancy category: X
Important contra-indications noted in the prescribing guidelines for: nursing mothers; pediatric patients
Note: Jalyn is dutasteride and tamsulosin.

Endocrine/Metabolic
 Gynecomastia [2]
 Libido decreased (<3%) [3]
Genitourinary
 Ejaculatory dysfunction [3]
 Erectile dysfunction [8]
 Impotence (<5%)
 Sexual dysfunction [6]
Other
 Adverse effects [2]

ECALLANTIDE

See: www.drugeruptiondata.com/drug/id/1425

ECONAZOLE

See: www.drugeruptiondata.com/drug/id/1342

ECULIZUMAB

Trade name: Soliris (Alexion)
Indications: Paroxysmal nocturnal hemoglobinuria, atypical hemolytic uremic syndrome
Class: Complement inhibitor, Monoclonal antibody
Half-life: ~12 days
Clinically important, potentially hazardous interactions with: none known
Pregnancy category: C
Important contra-indications noted in the prescribing guidelines for: nursing mothers; pediatric patients
Warning: SERIOUS MENINGOCOCCAL INFECTIONS

Skin
Peripheral edema [2]
Pruritus [2]

Mucosal
Nasal congestion [2]

Cardiovascular
Hypertension [2]

Central Nervous System
Fever [3]
Headache (44%) [5]
Insomnia [2]
Meningococcal infection [4]
Vertigo (dizziness) [3]

Neuromuscular/Skeletal
Asthenia (fatigue) (12%) [4]
Back pain (19%) [3]
Pain in extremities [2]

Gastrointestinal/Hepatic
Abdominal pain [2]
Diarrhea [3]
Nausea [4]
Vomiting [3]

Respiratory
Cough (12%) [4]
Nasopharyngitis (23%) [5]
Pharyngolaryngeal pain [2]
Upper respiratory tract infection [2]

Genitourinary
Urinary tract infection [3]

Hematologic
Anemia [2]
Leukopenia [2]

EDARAVONE *

Trade name: Radicava (Mitsubishi Tanabe Pharma)
Indications: Amyotrophic lateral sclerosis
Class: Antioxidant
Half-life: 4–6 hours
Clinically important, potentially hazardous interactions with: none known
Pregnancy category: N/A (May cause fetal toxicity based on findings in animal studies)
Important contra-indications noted in the prescribing guidelines for: nursing mothers; pediatric patients
Note: Radicava contains sodium bisulfite which may cause allergic type reactions.

Skin
Dermatitis (8%)
Eczema (7%) [2]
Hematoma (15%) [2]
Tinea (4%)

Central Nervous System
Gait instability (13%) [2]
Headache (10%) [2]
Insomnia [2]

Gastrointestinal/Hepatic
Constipation [2]
Diarrhea [2]
Dysphagia [3]
Hepatotoxicity [2]

Respiratory
Hypoxia (6%)
Nasopharyngitis [2]
Respiratory failure (6%) [2]

Genitourinary
Glycosuria (4%) [2]

Renal
Nephrotoxicity [2]

Other
Adverse effects [2]

EDOXABAN

Trade name: Savaysa (Daiichi Sankyo)
Indications: Reduce the risk of stroke and systemic embolism in patients with nonvalvular atrial fibrillation, treatment of deep vein thrombosis and pulmonary embolism
Class: Direct factor Xa inhibitor
Half-life: 10–14 hours
Clinically important, potentially hazardous interactions with: anticoagulants, rifampin
Pregnancy category: C
Important contra-indications noted in the prescribing guidelines for: nursing mothers; pediatric patients
Note: Contra-indicated in patients with active pathological bleeding.
Warning: REDUCED EFFICACY IN NONVALVULAR ATRIAL FIBRILLATION PATIENTS WITH CRCL>95ml/min
ISCHEMIC EVENTS ON PREMATURE DISCONTINUATION
SPINAL/EDPIDURAL HEMATOMA

Skin
Rash (4%)

Mucosal
Epistaxis (nosebleed) (5%)
Gingival bleeding [2]
Oral bleeding (3%)

Gastrointestinal/Hepatic
Diarrhea [2]
Gastrointestinal bleeding (4%)
Hepatotoxicity (5–8%) [2]

Genitourinary
Hematuria (2%) [2]

Hematologic
Anemia (2–10%)
Bleeding (>5%) [13]

Other
Adverse effects [4]

EDROPHONIUM

See: www.drugeruptiondata.com/drug/id/251

EFALIZUMAB

See: www.drugeruptiondata.com/drug/id/1004

EFAVIRENZ

Trade names: Atripla (Gilead), Sustiva (Bristol-Myers Squibb)
Indications: HIV infection
Class: Antiretroviral, CYP1A2 inhibitor, CYP3A4 inducer, Non-nucleoside reverse transcriptase inhibitor
Half-life: 52–76 hours
Clinically important, potentially hazardous interactions with: alcohol, alprazolam, amprenavir, aripiprazole, artesunate, atazanavir, atorvastatin, atovaquone, benzodiazepines, bepridil, boceprevir, bortezomib, brentuximab vedotin, budesonide, buprenorphine, bupropion, carbamazepine, carvedilol, caspofungin, chlordiazepoxide, cisapride, citalopram, clarithromycin, clonazepam, clopidogrel, clorazepate, CNS depressants, cobimetinib, colchicine, conivaptan, crizotinib, cyclosporine, CYP2B6 inhibitors and inducers, CYP2C19 substrates, CYP2C9 substrates, CYP3A4 substrates and inducers, darunavir, dasabuvir/ombitasvir/paritaprevir/ritonavir, dasatinib, deferasirox, deflazacort, diazepam, dihydroergotamine, diltiazem, dronedarone, elbasvir & grazoprevir, enzalutamide, eplerenone, ergot, etravirine, everolimus, exemestane, fentanyl, flurazepam, fosamprenavir, fosphenytoin, gefitinib, glecaprevir & pibrentasvir, grapefruit juice, guanfacine, halofantrine, hydroxyzine, imatinib, indinavir, itraconazole, ixabepilone, lapatinib, levomepromazine, levonorgestrel, linagliptin, lopinavir, lorazepam, lovastatin, lurasidone, maraviroc, methadone, methysergide, midazolam, mifepristone, neratinib, nevirapine, nifedipine, nilotinib, nisoldipine, olaparib, ombitasvir/paritaprevir/ritonavir, oral contraceptives, oxazepam,

paclitaxel, palbociclib, pazopanib, phenytoin, pimecrolimus, pimozide, posaconazole, pravastatin, praziquantel, progestogens, propafenone, protease inhibitors, quazepam, raltegravir, ranolazine, rifabutin, rifampin, rilpivirine, ritonavir, rivaroxaban, roflumilast, romidepsin, salmeterol, saquinavir, saxagliptin, sertraline, simeprevir, simvastatin, sirolimus, sofosbuvir & velpatasvir, sofosbuvir/velpatasvir/voxilaprevir, sonidegib, sorafenib, SSRIs, St John's wort, sunitinib, tacrolimus, tadalafil, telaprevir, temazepam, ticagrelor, tipranavir, tocilizumab, tolvaptan, toremifene, triazolam, ulipristal, vandetanib, vemurafenib, venetoclax, vilazodone, vitamin K antagonists, voriconazole, warfarin, zuclopenthixol

Pregnancy category: D
Important contra-indications noted in the prescribing guidelines for: the elderly; nursing mothers; pediatric patients
Note: Atripla is efavirenz, emtricitabine and tenofovir disoproxil.

Skin
DRESS syndrome [2]
Eczema (<2%)
Erythema (11%)
Exanthems (27%) [3]
Exfoliative dermatitis (<2%)
Folliculitis (<2%)
Hot flashes (<2%)
Hypersensitivity [5]
Lipodystrophy [2]
Peripheral edema (<2%)
Photosensitivity [4]
Pruritus (11%)
Rash (26%) [16]
Stevens-Johnson syndrome [3]
Toxicity [2]
Urticaria (<2%)

Hair
Alopecia (<2%)

Mucosal
Xerostomia (<2%)

Cardiovascular
Flushing (<2%)
Thrombophlebitis (<2%)

Central Nervous System
Abnormal dreams (<3%) [9]
Aggression [2]
Anorexia (<2%)
Anxiety (13%) [4]
Depression (19%) [9]
Dysgeusia (taste perversion) (<2%)
Hallucinations [2]
Headache (2–8%) [2]
Impaired concentration (3–5%) [4]
Insomnia (7%) [4]
Nervousness (7%)
Neuropsychiatric disturbances [2]
Neurotoxicity [14]
Nightmares [3]
Pain (<13%)
Paresthesias (<2%)
Parosmia (<2%)
Psychosis [6]
Sleep related disorder [2]
Somnolence (drowsiness) (2%) [3]
Suicidal ideation [5]

Tremor (<2%)
Vertigo (dizziness) (2–9%) [15]

Neuromuscular/Skeletal
Asthenia (fatigue) (2–8%) [3]
Myalgia/Myopathy (<2%)

Gastrointestinal/Hepatic
Abdominal pain (2–3%)
Diarrhea (3–14%) [2]
Dyspepsia (4%)
Hepatic failure [2]
Hepatotoxicity [13]
Nausea (2–10%) [3]
Vomiting (3–6%)

Endocrine/Metabolic
ALT increased [2]
Gynecomastia [14]

Genitourinary
Urolithiasis [3]

Hematologic
Dyslipidemia [2]

Other
Adverse effects [10]
Teratogenicity [4]

EFINACONAZOLE

Trade name: Jublia (Valeant)
Indications: Onychomycosis
Class: Antifungal
Half-life: 30 hours
Clinically important, potentially hazardous interactions with: none known
Pregnancy category: C
Important contra-indications noted in the prescribing guidelines for: nursing mothers; pediatric patients

---

Nails
Onychocryptosis (2%)

Local
Application-site dermatitis (2%)
Application-site reactions [4]
Application-site vesicles (2%)

EFLORNITHINE

Trade name: Vaniqa (Women First)
Indications: Sleeping sickness, hypertrichosis
Class: Ornithine decarboxylase inhibitor
Half-life: 3–3.5 hours (intravenous); 8 hours (topical)
Clinically important, potentially hazardous interactions with: none known
Pregnancy category: C
Important contra-indications noted in the prescribing guidelines for: nursing mothers; pediatric patients

---

Skin
Acneform eruption (24%)
Burning (4%)
Facial edema (3%)
Pruritus (4%) [2]
Rash (3%)
Stinging (8%)

Xerosis (2%)

Hair
Alopecia (5–10%)
Ingrown (2%)
Pseudofolliculitis barbae (5–15%)

Central Nervous System
Headache (5%)
Paresthesias (4%)
Seizures (7%) [2]
Vertigo (dizziness) (<10%)

Gastrointestinal/Hepatic
Diarrhea (<10%)
Vomiting (<10%)

Hematologic
Eosinophilia (<10%)

Otic
Hearing impairment (<10%)

ELBASVIR & GRAZOPREVIR

Trade name: Zepatier (Merck)
Indications: Chronic hepatitis C virus genotypes 1 or 4 (with or without ribavirin)
Class: Direct-acting antiviral, Hepatitis C virus NS3/4A protease inhibitor (grazoprevir), Hepatitis C virus NS5A inhibitor (elbasvir)
Half-life: 24 hours (elbasvir); 31 hours (grazoprevir)
Clinically important, potentially hazardous interactions with: atazanavir, atorvastatin, bosentan, carbamazepine, cobicistat/elvitegravir/emtricitabine/tenofovir disoproxil, cyclosporine, darunavir, efavirenz, fluvastatin, ketoconazole, lopinavir, lovastatin, modafinil, moderate CYP3A inducers, nafcillin, OATP1B1/3 inhibitors, phenytoin, rifampin, rosuvastatin, saquinavir, simvastatin, strong CYP3A inducers, tacrolimus, tipranavir
Pregnancy category: N/A (No available data; contra-indicated in pregnant women and in men with pregnant partners when administered with ribavirin)
Important contra-indications noted in the prescribing guidelines for: pediatric patients
Note: Contra-indicated in patients with moderate or severe hepatic impairment (Child-Pugh B or C).

Central Nervous System
Headache (10–11%) [8]

Neuromuscular/Skeletal
Asthenia (fatigue) (5–11%) [8]

Gastrointestinal/Hepatic
Abdominal pain (2%)
Diarrhea (2%) [2]
Nausea (11%) [7]

ELETRIPTAN

Trade name: Relpax (Pfizer)
Indications: Migraine headaches
Class: 5-HT1 agonist, Serotonin receptor agonist, Triptan
Half-life: 4–5 hours
Clinically important, potentially hazardous interactions with: clarithromycin, dihydroergotamine, itraconazole, ketoconazole, methysergide, nefazodone, nelfinavir, paclitaxel, ritonavir, SNRIs, SSRIs, telithromycin, triptans, troleandomycin, voriconazole
Pregnancy category: C
Important contra-indications noted in the prescribing guidelines for: nursing mothers; pediatric patients
Note: Contra-indicated in patients with history, symptoms, or signs of ischemic cardiac, cerebrovascular, or peripheral vascular syndromes, or in patients with uncontrolled hypertension.

Mucosal
Xerostomia (2–4%)
Cardiovascular
Chest pain (<4%) [3]
Flushing (2%)
Central Nervous System
Headache (3–4%)
Neurotoxicity [2]
Paresthesias (3–4%)
Somnolence (drowsiness) (3–7%) [2]
Vertigo (dizziness) (3–7%)
Warm feeling (2%)
Neuromuscular/Skeletal
Asthenia (fatigue) (4–10%) [4]
Gastrointestinal/Hepatic
Abdominal pain (<2%)
Dyspepsia (<2%)
Dysphagia (<2%)
Nausea (3–7%) [5]
Vomiting [2]
Other
Adverse effects [2]

ELIGLUSTAT

Trade name: Cerdelga (Genzyme)
Indications: Gaucher disease
Class: Glucosylceramide synthase inhibitor
Half-life: 7–9 hours
Clinically important, potentially hazardous interactions with: carbamazepine, grapefruit juice, phenobarbital, phenytoin, rifampin, St John's wort, strong or moderate CYP2D6 inhibitors
Pregnancy category: C
Important contra-indications noted in the prescribing guidelines for: nursing mothers; pediatric patients

Skin
Rash (5%)
Mucosal
Oropharyngeal pain (10%)

Cardiovascular
Palpitation (5%) [3]
Central Nervous System
Headache (13–40%) [2]
Migraine (10%)
Vertigo (dizziness) (8%)
Neuromuscular/Skeletal
Asthenia (fatigue) (8–14%)
Back pain (12%)
Pain in extremities (11%)
Gastrointestinal/Hepatic
Abdominal pain (10%) [2]
Constipation (5%)
Diarrhea (12%) [2]
Dyspepsia (7%)
Flatulence (10%)
Gastroesophageal reflux (7%)
Nausea (10–12%)
Respiratory
Cough (7%)
Other
Adverse effects [2]

ELOSULFASE ALFA

Trade name: Vimizim (BioMarin)
Indications: Mucopolysaccharidosis IVA (Morquio A syndrome)
Class: Enzyme
Half-life: 8–36 minutes
Clinically important, potentially hazardous interactions with: none known
Pregnancy category: C
Important contra-indications noted in the prescribing guidelines for: nursing mothers; pediatric patients
Warning: RISK OF ANAPHYLAXIS

Skin
Anaphylactoid reactions/Anaphylaxis (8%)
Hypersensitivity (19%)
Central Nervous System
Chills (10%)
Fever (33%)
Headache (26%)
Neuromuscular/Skeletal
Asthenia (fatigue) (10%)
Gastrointestinal/Hepatic
Abdominal pain (21%)
Nausea (24%)
Vomiting (31%) [2]
Local
Infusion-related reactions [2]

ELOTUZUMAB

Trade name: Empliciti (Bristol-Myers Squibb)
Indications: Multiple myeloma (in combination with lenalidomide and dexamethasone) in patients who have received one to three prior therapies
Class: Monoclonal antibody
Half-life: N/A
Clinically important, potentially hazardous interactions with: none known

Pregnancy category: N/A (Embryo-fetal toxicity with combination dosage)
Important contra-indications noted in the prescribing guidelines for: nursing mothers; pediatric patients
Note: See separate entries for dexamethasone and lenalidomide.

Skin
Herpes zoster (14%)
Hyperhidrosis (>5%)
Hypersensitivity (>5%) [2]
Peripheral edema [5]
Rash [2]
Mucosal
Oropharyngeal pain (10%)
Cardiovascular
Chest pain (>5%) [3]
Flushing [2]
Tachycardia [2]
Central Nervous System
Anorexia [3]
Chills [4]
Fever (37%) [6]
Headache (15%) [5]
Hypoesthesia (>5%)
Insomnia [4]
Mood changes (>5%)
Neurotoxicity [2]
Peripheral neuropathy (27%) [3]
Neuromuscular/Skeletal
Arthralgia [2]
Asthenia (fatigue) (62%) [10]
Back pain [3]
Muscle spasm [3]
Pain in extremities (16%)
Gastrointestinal/Hepatic
Constipation (36%) [4]
Diarrhea (47%) [6]
Nausea [5]
Vomiting (15%) [4]
Respiratory
Cough [3]
Dyspnea [5]
Nasopharyngitis (25%)
Pneumonia (20%) [5]
Upper respiratory tract infection (23%) [2]
Endocrine/Metabolic
ALP increased (39%)
Appetite decreased (21%)
Hyperglycemia (89%) [2]
Hyperkalemia (32%)
Hypocalcemia (78%)
Hypokalemia [4]
Serum creatinine increased [3]
Weight loss (14%) [2]
Hematologic
Anemia [4]
Leukopenia (91%) [3]
Lymphocytopenia [3]
Lymphopenia (13–99%) [4]
Neutropenia [8]
Thrombocytopenia (84%) [5]
Ocular
Cataract (12%)
Local
Infusion-related reactions (10%) [10]

ELTROMBOPAG

Trade names: Promacta (Novartis), Revolade (Novartis)
Indications: Thrombocytopenic purpura, severe aplastic anemia in patients with insufficient response to immunosuppressive therapy
Class: Thrombopoietin receptor (TPO) agonist
Half-life: 21–32 hours
Clinically important, potentially hazardous interactions with: antacids, atorvastatin, dairy products, eluxadoline, lopinavir, mineral supplements, olmesartan, rosuvastatin, selenium, zinc
Pregnancy category: C
Important contra-indications noted in the prescribing guidelines for: nursing mothers; pediatric patients
Warning: RISK FOR HEPATIC DECOMPENSATION IN PATIENTS WITH CHRONIC HEPATITIS C

Skin
Peripheral edema (3–4%)
Pigmentation [2]
Rash (3–7%)

Hair
Alopecia (2%)

Mucosal
Oropharyngeal pain (4%)
Xerostomia (2%)

Cardiovascular
Thromboembolism [5]
Venous thromboembolism [2]

Central Nervous System
Dysgeusia (taste perversion) (4%)
Headache (10–21%) [10]
Paresthesias (3%)

Neuromuscular/Skeletal
Arthralgia (3%) [2]
Asthenia (fatigue) (3–4%) [4]
Back pain (3%)
Myalgia/Myopathy (5%)
Pain in extremities (7%)

Gastrointestinal/Hepatic
Abdominal pain [2]
Constipation [2]
Diarrhea (9%)
Hepatotoxicity [3]
Nausea (4–9%) [5]
Vomiting (6%)

Respiratory
Cough (5%)
Nasopharyngitis [2]
Pharyngitis (4%)
Upper respiratory tract infection (7%)

Endocrine/Metabolic
ALP increased (2%)
ALT increased (5–6%) [4]
AST increased (4%)

Genitourinary
Urinary tract infection (5%)

Renal
Renal failure [3]

Hematologic
Bleeding [3]
Neutropenia [2]
Thrombocytopenia [2]
Thrombosis [5]

Ocular
Cataract (5%) [2]

Other
Adverse effects [8]

ELUXADOLINE

Trade name: Viberzi (Forest)
Indications: Irritable bowel syndrome with diarrhea
Class: Opioid mu receptor agonist
Half-life: 4–6 hours
Clinically important, potentially hazardous interactions with: alfentanil, alosetron, anticholinergics, atazanavir, bupropion, ciprofloxacin, clarithromycin, cyclosporine, dihydroergotamine, eltrombopag, ergotamine, fentanyl, fluconazole, gemfibrozil, lopinavir, opioids, paroxetine hydrochloride, paroxetine mesylate, pimozide, quinidine, rifampin, ritonavir, rosuvastatin, saquinavir, sirolimus, tacrolimus, tipranavir
Pregnancy category: N/A (Insufficient evidence to inform drug-associated risk)
Important contra-indications noted in the prescribing guidelines for: pediatric patients
Note: Contra-indicated in patients with known or suspected biliary duct obstruction, or sphincter of Oddi disease or dysfunction; alcoholism, alcohol abuse, alcohol addiction, or drink more than 3 alcoholic beverages/day; a history of pancreatitis; structural diseases of the pancreas, including known or suspected pancreatic duct obstruction; severe hepatic impairment (Child-Pugh Class C); severe constipation or sequelae from constipation, or known or suspected mechanical gastrointestinal obstruction.

Skin
Rash (3%)

Central Nervous System
Euphoria (<2%)
Sedation (<2%)
Somnolence (drowsiness) (<2%)
Vertigo (dizziness) (3%) [2]

Gastrointestinal/Hepatic
Abdominal distension (3%) [2]
Abdominal pain (6–7%) [4]
Constipation (7–8%) [7]
Flatulence (3%)
Gastroenteritis (<3%) [2]
Gastroesophageal reflux (<2%)
Nausea (7–8%) [5]
Pancreatitis [5]
Vomiting (4%) [3]

Respiratory
Asthma (<2%)
Bronchitis (3%)
Bronchospasm (<2%)
Nasopharyngitis (3–4%) [2]
Respiratory failure (<2%)
Wheezing (<2%)

Endocrine/Metabolic
ALT increased (2–3%)
AST increased (<2%)

Other
Adverse effects [2]

EMPAGLIFLOZIN

Trade names: Glyxambi (Boehringer Ingelheim), Jardiance (Boehringer Ingelheim), Synjardy (Boehringer Ingelheim)
Indications: Type II diabetes mellitus
Class: Sodium-glucose co-transporter 2 (SGLT2) inhibitor
Half-life: 12 hours
Clinically important, potentially hazardous interactions with: none known
Pregnancy category: C
Important contra-indications noted in the prescribing guidelines for: nursing mothers; pediatric patients
Note: Contra-indicated in patients with severe renal impairment, end stage renal disease, or on dialysis. Glyxambi is empagliflozin and linagliptin; Synjardy is empagliflozin and metformin.

Central Nervous System
Headache [2]

Gastrointestinal/Hepatic
Constipation [2]

Respiratory
Nasopharyngitis [4]

Endocrine/Metabolic
Hypoglycemia [3]

Genitourinary
Genital mycotic infections (2–6%) [7]
Pollakiuria [3]
Urinary frequency (3%)
Urinary tract infection (8–9%) [7]

Other
Adverse effects [7]
Dipsia (thirst) (2%)

EMTRICITABINE

Trade names: Atripla (Gilead), Complera (Gilead), Descovy (Gilead), Emtriva (Gilead), Truvada (Gilead)
Indications: HIV-1 infection
Class: Antiretroviral, Nucleoside analog reverse transcriptase inhibitor
Half-life: ~10 hours
Clinically important, potentially hazardous interactions with: cobicistat/elvitegravir/emtricitabine/tenofovir disoproxil, ganciclovir, lamivudine, ribavirin, valganciclovir
Pregnancy category: B
Important contra-indications noted in the prescribing guidelines for: nursing mothers
Note: Emtricitabine is a fluorinated derivative of lamivudine. Atripla is emtricitabine, efavirenz and tenofovir disoproxil; Complera is emtricitabine, rilpivirine and tenofovir disoproxil; Descovy is emtricitabine and tenofovir alafenamide; Truvada is emtricitabine and tenofovir disoproxil. See also separate profiles for emtricitabine in combination with cobicistat, elvitegravir and tenofovir disoproxil or tenofovir alafenamide.

Warning: LACTIC ACIDOSIS / SEVERE HEPATOMEGALY WITH STEATOSIS and POST TREATMENT EXACERBATION OF HEPATITIS B

Skin
Exanthems (17%)
Pigmentation (palms and soles) (32%)
Pruritus (17–30%)
Pustules (17–30%)
Rash (17–30%) [5]
Urticaria (17–30%)
Vesiculobullous eruption (17–30%)

Central Nervous System
Abnormal dreams (2–11%) [3]
Anxiety [2]
Depression (6–9%)
Fever (18%)
Headache (13–22%) [5]
Insomnia (7–16%)
Neurotoxicity [5]
Paresthesias (6%)
Peripheral neuropathy (4%)
Somnolence (drowsiness) [2]
Vertigo (dizziness) (4–25%) [4]

Neuromuscular/Skeletal
Arthralgia (3–5%)
Asthenia (fatigue) (12–16%) [4]
Myalgia/Myopathy (4–6%) [2]

Gastrointestinal/Hepatic
Abdominal pain (8–14%) [2]
Diarrhea (20–23%) [6]
Dyspepsia (4–8%)
Gastroenteritis (11%)
Hepatic failure [2]
Hepatotoxicity [2]
Nausea (13–18%) [7]
Vomiting (9–23%) [4]

Respiratory
Cough (14–28%)
Pneumonia (15%)
Rhinitis (12–20%)

Hematologic
Anemia (7%)

Otic
Otitis media (23%)

Other
Adverse effects [5]
Allergic reactions (17–30%)
Infection (44%)

EMTRICITABINE/ RILPIVIRINE/ TENOFOVIR ALAFENAMIDE

Trade name: Odefsey (Gilead)
Indications: HIV-1 infection
Class: Hepatitis B virus necleoside analog reverse transcriptase inhibitor (tenofovir alafenamide), Non-nucleoside reverse transcriptase inhibitor (rilpivirine), Nucleoside analog reverse transcriptase inhibitor (emtricitabine)
Half-life: 10 hours (emtricitabine); 50 hours (rilpivirine); <1 hour (tenofovir alafenamide)
Clinically important, potentially hazardous interactions with: carbamazepine, dexamethasone, dexlansoprazole, esomeprazole, lansoprazole, omeprazole, oxcarbazepine, pantoprazole, phenobarbital, phenytoin, rabeprazole, rifampin, rifapentine, St John's wort
Pregnancy category: N/A (Insufficient evidence to inform drug-associated risk)
Important contra-indications noted in the prescribing guidelines for: nursing mothers; pediatric patients
Warning: LACTIC ACIDOSIS/SEVERE HEPATOMEGALY WITH STEATOSIS and POST TREATMENT ACUTE EXACERBATION OF HEPATITIS B

Central Nervous System
Depression (<2%)
Headache (<2%)
Insomnia (<2%)

ENALAPRIL

Trade names: Innovace (Merck Sharpe & Dohme), Lexxel (AstraZeneca), Teczem (Sanofi-Aventis), Vaseretic (Valeant), Vasotec (Valeant)
Indications: Hypertension, symptomatic congestive heart failure, asymptomatic left ventricular dysfunction
Class: Angiotensin-converting enzyme (ACE) inhibitor, Antihypertensive, Vasodilator
Half-life: 11 hours
Clinically important, potentially hazardous interactions with: alcohol, aldesleukin, allopurinol, alpha blockers, alprostadil, amifostine, amiloride, angiotensin II receptor antagonists, antacids, antidiabetics, antihypertensives, antipsychotics, anxiolytics and hypnotics, aprotinin, azathioprine, baclofen, beta blockers, calcium channel blockers, clonidine, conivaptan, corticosteroids, cyclosporine, CYP3A4 inducers, deferasirox, diazoxide, diuretics, eplerenone, estrogens, everolimus, general anesthetics, gold & gold compounds, grapefruit juice, heparins, hydralazine, hypotensives, insulin, levodopa, lithium, MAO inhibitors, metformin, methyldopa, methylphenidate, minoxidil, moxisylyte, moxonidine, nitrates, nitroprusside, NSAIDs, pentoxifylline, phosphodiesterase 5 inhibitors, potassium salts, prostacyclin analogues, quinine, rituximab, salicylates, sirolimus, spironolactone, sulfonylureas, tadalafil, temsirolimus, tizanidine, tolvaptan, triamterene, trimethoprim
Pregnancy category: D (category C in first trimester; category D in second and third trimesters)
Important contra-indications noted in the prescribing guidelines for: nursing mothers
Note: Lexxel is enalapril and felodipine; Teczem is enalapril and diltiazem; Vaseretic is enalapril and hydrochlorothiazide. Hydrochlorothiazide is a sulfonamide and can be absorbed systemically. Sulfonamides can produce severe, possibly fatal, reactions such as toxic epidermal necrolysis and Stevens-Johnson syndrome.
Contra-indicated in patients with a history of angioedema with or without previous ACE inhibitor treatment.
Warning: FETAL TOXICITY

Skin
Angioedema [73]
Bullous pemphigoid [2]
Exanthems [9]
Lichenoid eruption [2]
Lupus erythematosus [2]
Pemphigus [10]
Pemphigus foliaceus [2]
Peripheral edema [2]
Photosensitivity [2]
Pruritus [3]
Psoriasis [3]
Rash [5]
Urticaria [5]
Vasculitis [2]

Mucosal
Oral lesions [4]
Oral ulceration [2]
Tongue edema [2]

Cardiovascular
Flushing [4]
Hypotension [2]

Central Nervous System
Ageusia (taste loss) [4]
Dysgeusia (taste perversion) (<10%) [7]
Headache (5%)
Vertigo (dizziness) (4–8%) [2]

Neuromuscular/Skeletal
Asthenia (fatigue) (<3%)
Pseudopolymyalgia [2]

Gastrointestinal/Hepatic
Hepatotoxicity [3]
Pancreatitis [2]

Respiratory
Cough (8–23%) [40]

Endocrine/Metabolic
Hyperkalemia [4]
SIADH [3]

Renal
Nephrotoxicity [2]

Other
Adverse effects [9]
Death [4]

ENASIDENIB *

Trade name: Idhifa (Celgene)
Indications: Relapsed or refractory acute myeloid leukemia
Class: Isocitrate dehydrogenase-2 inhibitor
Half-life: 137 hours
Clinically important, potentially hazardous interactions with: none known
Pregnancy category: N/A (Can cause fetal harm)
Important contra-indications noted in the prescribing guidelines for: nursing mothers; pediatric patients
Warning: DIFFERENTIATION SYNDROME

Skin
   Differentiation syndrome (14%)
   Tumor lysis syndrome (6%)
Cardiovascular
   Pulmonary edema (<10%)
Central Nervous System
   Dysgeusia (taste perversion) (12%)
Gastrointestinal/Hepatic
   Diarrhea (43%)
   Nausea (50%)
   Vomiting (34%)
Respiratory
   Acute respiratory distress syndrome (<10%)
Endocrine/Metabolic
   Appetite decreased (34%)
   Hyperbilirubinemia (81%)
   Hypocalcemia (74%)
   Hypokalemia (41%)
   Hypophosphatemia (27%)
Hematologic
   Leukocytosis (12%)

ENFLURANE

See: www.drugeruptiondata.com/drug/id/879

ENFUVIRTIDE

Trade name: Fuzeon (Roche)
Indications: HIV-1 infection (in combination with other antiretroviral agents)
Class: Antiretroviral, HIV cell fusion inhibitor
Half-life: 3.8 hours
Clinically important, potentially hazardous interactions with: darunavir, indinavir, tipranavir
Pregnancy category: B
Important contra-indications noted in the prescribing guidelines for: the elderly; nursing mothers

Skin
   Folliculitis (2%)
   Herpes simplex (4%)
   Hypersensitivity [3]
   Papillomas (4%)
   Pruritus (62%)

Mucosal
   Xerostomia (2%)
Central Nervous System
   Anorexia (2%)
   Depression (9%)
Neuromuscular/Skeletal
   Asthenia (fatigue) (16%) [2]
   Myalgia/Myopathy (3%)
   Pain in extremities (3%)
Gastrointestinal/Hepatic
   Abdominal pain (4%)
   Pancreatitis (3%)
Respiratory
   Cough (4%)
   Flu-like syndrome (2%)
   Pneumonia (3%)
   Sinusitis (6%)
Endocrine/Metabolic
   ALT increased (<4%)
   Appetite decreased (3%)
   Creatine phosphokinase increased (3–7%)
   Weight loss (7%)
Hematologic
   Eosinophilia (2–9%)
Ocular
   Conjunctivitis (2%)
Local
   Injection-site bruising (52%)
   Injection-site erythema (91%)
   Injection-site induration (90%)
   Injection-site nodules (80%) [4]
   Injection-site pain (96%)
   Injection-site pruritus (65%)
   Injection-site reactions (98%) [27]
   Injection-site scleroderma [2]
Other
   Infection [3]

ENOXACIN

See: www.drugeruptiondata.com/drug/id/255

ENOXAPARIN

Trade names: Clexane (Sanofi-Aventis), Lovenox (Sanofi-Aventis)
Indications: Prevention of deep vein thrombosis, ischemic complications of unstable angina and non-Q wave myocardial infarction, treatment of acute ST-segment elevation myocardial infarction
Class: Heparin, low molecular weight
Half-life: 4.5 hours
Clinically important, potentially hazardous interactions with: ACE inhibitors, angiotensin II receptor antagonists, anticoagulants, aspirin, butabarbital, clopidogrel, danaparoid, diclofenac, dipyridamole, drotrecogin alfa, iloprost, infused nitrates, ketorolac, NSAIDs, platelet inhibitors, rivaroxaban, salicylates, sulfinpyrazone
Pregnancy category: B
Important contra-indications noted in the prescribing guidelines for: nursing mothers; pediatric patients
Note: Epidural or spinal hematomas may occur in patients who are anticoagulated with low

molecular weight heparins or heparinoids and are receiving neuraxial anesthesia or undergoing spinal puncture.
Contra-indicated in patients with active major bleeding; thrombocytopenia with a positive *in vitro* test for anti-platelet antibody in the presence of enoxaparin; hypersensitivity to heparin or pork products; hypersensitivity to benzyl alcohol (multi-dose formulation only).
Warning: SPINAL/EPIDURAL HEMATOMA

Skin
   Anaphylactoid reactions/Anaphylaxis [3]
   Angioedema [2]
   Bullous dermatitis [7]
   Ecchymoses (2%)
   Edema (3%)
   Erythema (<10%) [2]
   Exanthems [2]
   Hematoma [11]
   Hypersensitivity [7]
   Necrosis [4]
   Peripheral edema (3%)
   Pruritus [2]
   Purpura (<10%)
Cardiovascular
   Venous thromboembolism [2]
Gastrointestinal/Hepatic
   Hepatotoxicity [5]
Endocrine/Metabolic
   ALT increased [4]
   AST increased [3]
Genitourinary
   Hematuria [2]
Hematologic
   Bleeding [8]
   Hemorrhage [4]
   Thrombocytopenia [5]
Local
   Injection-site necrosis [4]
   Injection-site plaques [2]
Other
   Adverse effects [4]
   Death [2]

ENTACAPONE

Trade names: Comtan (Orion), Comtess (Orion), Stalevo (Orion)
Indications: Parkinsonism
Class: Catechol-O-methyl transferase inhibitor
Half-life: 2.4 hours
Clinically important, potentially hazardous interactions with: amitriptyline, MAO inhibitors, paroxetine hydrochloride, phenelzine, rasagiline, tranylcypromine, venlafaxine
Pregnancy category: C
Important contra-indications noted in the prescribing guidelines for: nursing mothers; pediatric patients

Skin
   Diaphoresis (2%)
   Purpura (2%)
Mucosal
   Xerostomia (3%)

Central Nervous System
Anxiety (2%)
Dyskinesia (25%) [3]
Hyperactivity (10%)
Hypokinesia (9%)
Parkinsonism (17%)
Somnolence (drowsiness) (2%)
Vertigo (dizziness) (8%) [2]

Neuromuscular/Skeletal
Asthenia (fatigue) (8%)
Back pain (4%)

Gastrointestinal/Hepatic
Abdominal pain (8%)
Constipation (6%)
Diarrhea (10%) [3]
Dyspepsia (2%)
Flatulence (2%)
Nausea (14%) [3]
Vomiting (4%)

Respiratory
Dyspnea (3%)

Genitourinary
Melanuria (10%) [2]

ENTECAVIR

Trade name: Baraclude (Bristol-Myers Squibb)
Indications: Chronic hepatitis B virus infection
Class: Antiviral, Guanosine nucleoside analog
Half-life: ~24 hours
Clinically important, potentially hazardous interactions with: none known
Pregnancy category: C
Important contra-indications noted in the prescribing guidelines for: nursing mothers; pediatric patients
Warning: SEVERE ACUTE EXACERBATIONS OF HEPATITIS B, PATIENTS CO-INFECTED WITH HIV AND HBV, and LACTIC ACIDOSIS AND HEPATOMEGALY

Skin
Rash [2]

Hair
Alopecia [2]

Central Nervous System
Headache (2–4%) [3]
Neurotoxicity [3]
Peripheral neuropathy [2]

Neuromuscular/Skeletal
Asthenia (fatigue) (<3%) [6]
Myalgia/Myopathy [3]

Gastrointestinal/Hepatic
Abdominal pain [2]
Diarrhea [2]
Pancreatitis [3]

Respiratory
Cough [2]
Upper respiratory tract infection [2]

Endocrine/Metabolic
Acidosis [6]
ALT increased (2–12%) [2]
Creatine phosphokinase increased (<2%)
Hypophosphatemia [2]

Genitourinary
Hematuria (9%)

Other
Adverse effects [4]

ENZALUTAMIDE

Trade name: Xtandi (Medivation)
Indications: Metastatic castration-resistant prostate cancer in patients who have previously received docetaxel
Class: Androgen antagonist
Half-life: 8–9 days
Clinically important, potentially hazardous interactions with: alfentanil, bosentan, carbamazepine, copanlisib, cyclosporine, dihydroergotamine, efavirenz, ergotamine, fentanyl, gemfibrozil, itraconazole, midazolam, midostaurin, modafinil, nafcillin, neratinib, omeprazole, phenobarbital, phenytoin, pimozide, quinidine, rifabutin, rifampin, rifapentine, sirolimus, St John's wort, tacrolimus, warfarin
Pregnancy category: X (not indicated for use in women)
Important contra-indications noted in the prescribing guidelines for: nursing mothers; pediatric patients

Skin
Hot flashes (20%) [11]
Peripheral edema (15%) [3]
Pruritus (4%)
Xerosis (4%)

Mucosal
Epistaxis (nosebleed) (3%)

Cardiovascular
Hypertension (6%) [5]

Central Nervous System
Amnesia (>2%)
Anxiety (7%)
Cognitive impairment (4%)
Gait instability [3]
Hallucinations (2%)
Headache (12%) [4]
Hypoesthesia (4%)
Insomnia (9%)
Paresthesias (7%) [2]
Seizures [12]
Spinal cord compression (7%)
Vertigo (dizziness) (10%) [2]

Neuromuscular/Skeletal
Arthralgia (21%) [4]
Asthenia (fatigue) (51%) [22]
Back pain (26%) [5]
Bone or joint pain (15%) [7]
Fractures (4%) [2]

Gastrointestinal/Hepatic
Constipation [3]
Diarrhea (22%) [9]
Nausea [4]

Respiratory
Bronchitis (>2%)
Laryngitis (>2%)
Nasopharyngitis (>2%)
Pharyngitis (>2%)
Pneumonia (>2%)
Sinusitis (>2%)

Upper respiratory tract infection (11%) [3]

Endocrine/Metabolic
ALT increased (10%)
Appetite decreased [5]
Gynecomastia [2]
Weight loss [3]

Genitourinary
Hematuria (7%)
Pollakiuria (5%)

Hematologic
Anemia [2]
Neutropenia (15%)

Other
Adverse effects [4]

EPHEDRINE

Trade names: Rynatuss (MedPointe), Vicks Vatronol (Procter & Gamble)
Indications: Nasal congestion, acute hypotensive states, asthma
Class: Adrenergic alpha-receptor agonist, Sympathomimetic
Half-life: 3–6 hours
Clinically important, potentially hazardous interactions with: antihypertensives, dexamethasone, furazolidone, guanethidine, iobenguane, levomepromazine, MAO inhibitors, methyldopa, oxprenolol, phenelzine, phenylpropanolamine, selegiline, tranylcypromine, tricyclic antidepressants
Pregnancy category: C
Important contra-indications noted in the prescribing guidelines for: nursing mothers

Skin
Dermatitis [5]
Diaphoresis (<10%)
Fixed eruption [6]
Pallor (<10%)
Urticaria [2]

Mucosal
Xerostomia (<10%)

Central Nervous System
Trembling (<10%)
Tremor (<10%)

EPINASTINE

See: www.drugeruptiondata.com/drug/id/1013

EPINEPHRINE

Synonym: adrenaline
Trade names: Adrenaclick (Amedra), Adrenalin (JHP Pharmaceuticals), Auvi-Q (Sanofi-Aventis), Epipen (Mylan)
Indications: Cardiac arrest, hay fever, asthma, anaphylaxis
Class: Catecholamine, Sympathomimetic
Half-life: N/A
Clinically important, potentially hazardous interactions with: albuterol, alpha blockers, amitriptyline, amoxapine, atenolol, beta blockers,

carteolol, chlorpromazine, clomipramine, clozapine, cocaine, desipramine, doxepin, ergotamine, furazolidone, halothane, imipramine, insulin aspart, insulin degludec, insulin detemir, insulin glargine, insulin glulisine, levalbuterol, lisdexamfetamine, lurasidone, MAO inhibitors, metoprolol, milnacipran, nadolol, nortriptyline, oxprenolol, penbutolol, phenelzine, phenoxybenzamine, phenylephrine, pindolol, prazosin, propranolol, protriptyline, sympathomimetics, terbutaline, thioridazine, timolol, tranylcypromine, tricyclic antidepressants, trimipramine, vasopressors
Pregnancy category: C
Important contra-indications noted in the prescribing guidelines for: the elderly

Skin
Dermatitis [4]
Diaphoresis (<10%)
Necrosis [3]
Pemphigus (cicatricial) [2]

Cardiovascular
Arrhythmias [3]
Chest pain [2]
Flushing (<10%)
Hypertension [3]
Hypotension [3]
Myocardial infarction [5]
Palpitation [2]
QT prolongation [2]
Ventricular tachycardia [2]

Central Nervous System
Anxiety [2]
Trembling (<10%)
Tremor [3]

EPIRUBICIN

Trade name: Ellence (Pfizer)
Indications: Adjuvant therapy in primary breast cancer
Class: Antibiotic, anthracycline
Half-life: 33 hours
Clinically important, potentially hazardous interactions with: amlodipine, bepridil, cimetidine, diltiazem, felodipine, isradipine, nicardipine, nifedipine, nimodipine, nisoldipine, verapamil
Pregnancy category: D
Important contra-indications noted in the prescribing guidelines for: nursing mothers
Warning: SEVERE OR LIFE-THREATENING HEMATOLOGICAL AND OTHER ADVERSE REACTIONS

Skin
Erythroderma (5%)
Hand–foot syndrome [5]
Hot flashes (5–39%)
Pruritus (9%)
Rash (<9%) [2]
Vasculitis [2]

Hair
Alopecia (69–95%) [17]

Mucosal
Mucositis [5]

Stomatitis [9]

Cardiovascular
Cardiotoxicity [3]
QT prolongation [3]

Central Nervous System
Anorexia [5]
Dysgeusia (taste perversion) [2]
Fever [2]
Headache [2]
Neurotoxicity [2]
Peripheral neuropathy [3]

Neuromuscular/Skeletal
Arthralgia [2]
Asthenia (fatigue) (6%) [9]
Myalgia/Myopathy (55%) [5]

Gastrointestinal/Hepatic
Abdominal pain [2]
Constipation [2]
Diarrhea [7]
Hepatotoxicity [2]
Nausea [12]
Vomiting [11]

Endocrine/Metabolic
ALT increased [2]
Amenorrhea [2]
AST increased [2]

Hematologic
Anemia [9]
Febrile neutropenia [5]
Leukopenia [4]
Neutropenia [12]
Thrombocytopenia [5]

Local
Injection-site reactions (3–20%)

Other
Allergic reactions [2]

EPLERENONE

See: www.drugeruptiondata.com/drug/id/944

EPOETIN ALFA

Synonyms: erythropoietin; EPO
Trade names: Epogen (Amgen), Eprex (Janssen-Cilag), Procrit (Ortho)
Indications: Anemia
Class: Erythropoiesis-stimulating agent (ESA), Erythropoietin
Half-life: 4–13 hours (in patients with chronic renal failure)
Clinically important, potentially hazardous interactions with: none known
Pregnancy category: C
Important contra-indications noted in the prescribing guidelines for: nursing mothers
Warning: ERYTHROPOIESIS-STIMULATING AGENTS (ESAs) INCREASE THE RISK OF DEATH, MYOCARDIAL INFARCTION, STROKE, VENOUS THROMBOEMBOLISM, THROMBOSIS OF VASCULAR ACCESS AND TUMOR PROGRESSION OR RECURRENCE

Skin
Angioedema (<5%)

Edema (17%)
Pruritus (12–21%) [2]
Rash (2–19%)

Cardiovascular
Hypertension (3–28%)

Central Nervous System
Fever (10–42%) [2]
Headache (5–18%)
Paresthesias (11%)

Neuromuscular/Skeletal
Arthralgia (10–16%)

Gastrointestinal/Hepatic
Constipation [2]
Nausea (35–56%)

Respiratory
Cough (4–26%)
Dyspnea [2]

Hematologic
Thrombocytopenia [2]

Ocular
Hallucinations, visual [2]

Local
Injection-site reactions (7%)

EPOPROSTENOL

Trade names: Flolan (GSK), Veletri (Actelion)
Indications: Pulmonary arterial hypertension
Class: Peripheral vasodilator
Half-life: 6 minutes
Clinically important, potentially hazardous interactions with: anticoagulants, antihypertensives, diuretics, vasodilators
Pregnancy category: B
Important contra-indications noted in the prescribing guidelines for: the elderly; nursing mothers; pediatric patients
Note: Contra-indicated in patients with heart failure induced by reduced left ventricular ejection fraction.

Skin
Diaphoresis (41%)
Pruritus (4%)
Rash (10%) [2]

Cardiovascular
Bradycardia (5%) [2]
Cardiac failure (31%)
Chest pain (11%) [2]
Flushing [6]
Hypotension (16%) [5]
Tachycardia (35%) [2]

Central Nervous System
Agitation (11%)
Anxiety (21%) [2]
Chills (25%)
Fever (25%)
Headache (83%) [13]
Insomnia (9%)
Paresthesias (12%)
Seizures (4%)
Somnolence (drowsiness) (4%)
Syncope (13%)
Tremor (21%)

Neuromuscular/Skeletal
  Back pain (13%)
  Jaw pain (54%) [6]
  Myalgia/Myopathy (44%)
Gastrointestinal/Hepatic
  Abdominal pain (14%)
  Diarrhea [2]
  Nausea [4]
Respiratory
  Alveolar hemorrhage (pulmonary) [2]
  Dyspnea (2%)
  Flu-like syndrome (25%)
  Pneumonia [2]
Endocrine/Metabolic
  Weight loss (27%)
Hematologic
  Sepsis (25%)
Local
  Injection-site infection (21%)
  Injection-site pain (13%)
Other
  Adverse effects [3]

EPROSARTAN

Trade name: Teveten (AbbVie)
Indications: Hypertension
Class: Angiotensin II receptor antagonist (blocker), Antihypertensive
Half-life: 5–9 hours
Clinically important, potentially hazardous interactions with: none known
Pregnancy category: D (category C in first trimester; category D in second and third trimesters)
Important contra-indications noted in the prescribing guidelines for: nursing mothers; pediatric patients
Warning: FETAL TOXICITY

Central Nervous System
  Dysgeusia (taste perversion) [2]
  Vertigo (dizziness) [2]
Neuromuscular/Skeletal
  Arthralgia (2%)
  Asthenia (fatigue) (2%)
Gastrointestinal/Hepatic
  Abdominal pain (2%)
Respiratory
  Cough (4%) [3]
  Pharyngitis (4%)
  Rhinitis (4%)
  Upper respiratory tract infection (8%) [2]
Other
  Adverse effects [3]

EPTIFIBATIDE

Trade name: Integrilin (Merck)
Indications: Acute coronary syndrome, unstable angina
Class: Antiplatelet, Glycoprotein IIb/IIIa inhibitor
Half-life: 2.5 hours
Clinically important, potentially hazardous interactions with: anticoagulants, antiplatelet agents, collagenase, dasatinib, drotrecogin alfa, fondaparinux, glucosamine, ibritumomab, iloprost, lepirudin, NSAIDs, pentoxifylline, salicylates, thrombolytic agents, tositumomab & iodine[131]
Pregnancy category: B
Important contra-indications noted in the prescribing guidelines for: nursing mothers; pediatric patients
Note: Contra-indicated in patients with a history of bleeding diathesis, or evidence of active abnormal bleeding within the previous 30 days; severe hypertension not adequately controlled on antihypertensive therapy; major surgery within the preceding 6 weeks; history of stroke within 30 days or any history of hemorrhagic stroke; current or planned administration of another parenteral GP IIb/IIIa inhibitor; or dependency on renal dialysis.

Cardiovascular
  Hypotension (7%)
Hematologic
  Bleeding [3]
  Hemorrhage (<10%)
  Thrombocytopenia [16]
  Thrombosis [3]
Other
  Death [2]

ERDOSTEINE

See: www.drugeruptiondata.com/drug/id/1258

ERGOCALCIFEROL

See: www.drugeruptiondata.com/drug/id/264

ERGOMETRINE

Trade name: Ergometrine (Hameln)
Indications: Management of the third stage of labor and in the treatment of postpartum hemorrhage
Class: Amine alkaloid
Half-life: N/A
Clinically important, potentially hazardous interactions with: halothane, sympathomimetic agents
Important contra-indications noted in the prescribing guidelines for: nursing mothers

Cardiovascular
  Myocardial infarction [4]
  Myocardial ischemia [3]

ERGOTAMINE

Trade name: Wigrettes (Organon)
Indications: Migraine, migraine variants
Class: Ergot alkaloid
Half-life: 2 hours
Clinically important, potentially hazardous interactions with: acebutolol, almotriptan, amprenavir, azithromycin, boceprevir, ceritinib, chlortetracycline, crizotinib, darunavir, dasabuvir/ombitasvir/paritaprevir/ritonavir, dasatinib, delavirdine, demeclocycline, doxycycline, eluxadoline, enzalutamide, epinephrine, erythromycin, indinavir, itraconazole, lopinavir, lymecycline, methylergonovine, mifepristone, minocycline, naratriptan, nelfinavir, nilotinib, ombitasvir/paritaprevir/ritonavir, oxytetracycline, posaconazole, propyphenazone, ribociclib, ritonavir, telaprevir, telithromycin, tetracycline, tigecycline, tipranavir, troleandomycin, voriconazole, warfarin
Pregnancy category: X
Important contra-indications noted in the prescribing guidelines for: nursing mothers
Note: Ergotamine is excreted in breast milk and may cause symptoms of vomiting, diarrhea, weak pulse and unstable blood pressure in nursing infants.

Skin
  Toxicity [4]
Cardiovascular
  Valvulopathy [3]
Respiratory
  Pleural effusion [2]

ERIBULIN

Trade name: Halaven (Eisai)
Indications: Metastatic breast cancer in patients who have previously received at least two chemotherapeutic regimens (prior therapy should have included an anthracycline and a taxane in either the adjuvant or metastatic setting), unresectable or metastatic liposarcoma in patients who have received a prior anthracycline-containing regimen
Class: Antineoplastic, Microtubule inhibitor
Half-life: 40 hours
Clinically important, potentially hazardous interactions with: none known
Pregnancy category: N/A (No available data but caused embryo-fetal toxicity in animal studies)
Important contra-indications noted in the prescribing guidelines for: nursing mothers; pediatric patients

Skin
  Peripheral edema (5–10%)
  Rash (5–10%)
Hair
  Alopecia (45%) [10]
Mucosal
  Mucosal inflammation (9%)
  Stomatitis (5–10%)
  Xerostomia (5–10%)

Central Nervous System
Anorexia (20%) [3]
Depression (5–10%)
Dysgeusia (taste perversion) (5–10%)
Fever (21%)
Headache (19%)
Insomnia (5–10%)
Neurotoxicity [6]
Peripheral neuropathy (35%) [25]
Vertigo (dizziness) (5–10%)

Neuromuscular/Skeletal
Arthralgia (22%)
Asthenia (fatigue) (54%) [29]
Back pain (16%)
Muscle spasm (5–10%)
Myalgia/Myopathy (22%)
Pain in extremities (11%)

Gastrointestinal/Hepatic
Abdominal pain (5–10%)
Constipation (25%) [2]
Diarrhea (18%) [3]
Dyspepsia (5–10%)
Hepatotoxicity [2]
Nausea (35%) [9]
Vomiting (18%)

Respiratory
Cough (14%)
Dyspnea (16%) [2]
Upper respiratory tract infection (5–10%)

Endocrine/Metabolic
Appetite decreased [2]
Hypokalemia (5–10%)
Weight loss (21%)

Genitourinary
Urinary tract infection (10%)

Hematologic
Anemia (58%) [11]
Febrile neutropenia (5%) [14]
Leukopenia [16]
Lymphopenia [3]
Neutropenia (82%) [47]

Ocular
Lacrimation (increased) (5–10%)

Other
Adverse effects [3]
Death [2]

ERLOTINIB

Trade name: Tarceva (OSI)
Indications: Non-small cell lung cancer, pancreatic cancer (with gemcitabine)
Class: Antineoplastic, Biologic, Epidermal growth factor receptor (EGFR) inhibitor, Tyrosine kinase inhibitor
Half-life: ~36 hours
Clinically important, potentially hazardous interactions with: atazanavir, capecitabine, carbamazepine, ciprofloxacin, clarithromycin, diclofenac, itraconazole, ketoconazole, meloxicam, nefazodone, nelfinavir, omeprazole, pantoprazole, phenobarbital, phenytoin, rifabutin, rifampin, rifapentine, ritonavir, saquinavir, St John's wort, troleandomycin, voriconazole, warfarin

Pregnancy category: D
Important contra-indications noted in the prescribing guidelines for: nursing mothers; pediatric patients

Skin
Acne keloid [2]
Acneform eruption [27]
Dermatitis [4]
DRESS syndrome [2]
Erythema (18%)
Exanthems [3]
Folliculitis [9]
Hand–foot syndrome [3]
Papulopustular eruption [9]
Pruritus (13%) [8]
Purpura [3]
Rash (75%) [112]
Rosacea [2]
Toxicity [9]
Xerosis (12%) [12]

Hair
Alopecia [10]
Hair changes [4]
Hypertrichosis [4]

Nails
Nail changes [3]
Paronychia [11]

Mucosal
Mucositis [10]
Stomatitis (17%) [10]

Cardiovascular
Hypertension [2]

Central Nervous System
Anorexia [9]
Fever [2]

Neuromuscular/Skeletal
Asthenia (fatigue) (52%) [31]
Rhabdomyolysis [2]

Gastrointestinal/Hepatic
Abdominal pain (11%)
Cholangitis [2]
Diarrhea [67]
Gastrointestinal bleeding [3]
Hepatotoxicity [13]
Nausea [16]
Vomiting [8]

Respiratory
Cough (33%)
Dyspnea [4]
Pneumonia [2]
Pneumonitis [7]
Pneumothorax [2]
Pulmonary toxicity [15]

Endocrine/Metabolic
ALT increased [3]
Appetite decreased [4]
AST increased [3]
Dehydration [3]
Hyperglycemia [3]

Hematologic
Anemia [12]
Febrile neutropenia [2]
Hemotoxicity [2]
Leukopenia [4]
Neutropenia [14]
Thrombocytopenia [10]

Ocular
Conjunctivitis (12%) [3]
Corneal perforation [2]
Ectropion [4]
Ocular adverse effects [3]
Periorbital rash [2]
Trichomegaly [13]

Other
Adverse effects [12]
Death [10]
Infection (24%) [7]

ERTAPENEM

Trade name: Invanz (Merck)
Indications: Severe resistant bacterial infections caused by susceptible organisms
Class: Antibiotic, carbapenem
Half-life: 4 hours
Clinically important, potentially hazardous interactions with: probenecid
Pregnancy category: B
Important contra-indications noted in the prescribing guidelines for: the elderly; nursing mothers

Skin
Edema (3%)
Erythema (<2%)
Pruritus (<2%)
Rash (2–3%)
Wound complications [2]

Cardiovascular
Phlebitis (2%)
Thrombophlebitis (2%)

Central Nervous System
Delirium [2]
Hallucinations [2]
Seizures [7]

Gastrointestinal/Hepatic
Nausea [2]

Respiratory
Cough (<2%)

Genitourinary
Vaginitis (<3%)

Local
Injection-site extravasation (2%)

Other
Death (2%)

ERYTHROMYCIN

Trade names: Eryc (Warner Chilcott), PCE (AbbVie)
Indications: Various infections caused by susceptible organisms
Class: Antibiotic, macrolide, CYP3A4 inhibitor
Half-life: 1.4–2 hours
Clinically important, potentially hazardous interactions with: afatinib, alfentanil, aminophylline, amisulpride, amoxicillin, ampicillin, anticonvulsants, arsenic, astemizole, atorvastatin, avanafil, benzodiazepines, bosentan, bromocriptine, buprenorphine, bupropion, carbamazepine, cilostazol, ciprofloxacin,

cisapride, clindamycin, clindamycin/tretinoin, clopidogrel, clozapine, colchicine, cyclosporine, CYP3A inhibitors, darifenacin, dasatinib, digoxin, dihydroergotamine, diltiazem, disopyramide, docetaxel, doxercalciferol, dronedarone, enoxacin, eplerenone, ergotamine, estradiol, eszopiclone, everolimus, flibanserin, fluconazole, fluoxetine, fluvastatin, gatifloxacin, HMG-CoA reductase inhibitors, imatinib, indacaterol, itraconazole, ketoconazole, levodopa, lomefloxacin, lorazepam, lovastatin, methadone, methylergonovine, methylprednisolone, methysergide, midazolam, mifepristone, mizolastine, moxifloxacin, naldemedine, naloxegol, neratinib, nintedanib, nitrazepam, norfloxacin, ofloxacin, olaparib, oxtriphylline, paroxetine hydrochloride, pentamidine, pimecrolimus, pimozide, pitavastatin, pravastatin, quetiapine, quinolones, ranolazine, repaglinide, rilpivirine, rivaroxaban, roflumilast, rosuvastatin, rupatadine, sertraline, sildenafil, silodosin, simeprevir, simvastatin, sparfloxacin, sulpiride, tacrolimus, tadalafil, tamsulosin, terfenadine, tramadol, triamcinolone, triazolam, troleandomycin, vardenafil, venetoclax, verapamil, vilazodone, vinblastine, warfarin, zafirlukast, zaleplon, zolpidem, zuclopenthixol

Pregnancy category: B
Important contra-indications noted in the prescribing guidelines for: the elderly; nursing mothers

Skin
AGEP [2]
Anaphylactoid reactions/Anaphylaxis [2]
Baboon syndrome (SDRIFE) [2]
Dermatitis (systemic) [4]
Exanthems (<5%) [4]
Fixed eruption [6]
Hypersensitivity (<10%) [3]
Rash [3]
Stevens-Johnson syndrome [7]
Toxic epidermal necrolysis [7]
Urticaria [4]

Mucosal
Oral candidiasis (<10%)

Cardiovascular
QT prolongation [5]
Torsades de pointes [8]

Neuromuscular/Skeletal
Rhabdomyolysis [4]

Gastrointestinal/Hepatic
Abdominal pain [3]
Diarrhea [4]
Nausea [4]

Otic
Tinnitus [3]

Local
Injection-site phlebitis (<10%) [2]

Other
Allergic reactions (<2%) [3]

ESCITALOPRAM

Trade name: Lexapro (Forest)
Indications: Major depressive disorders, anxiety
Class: Antidepressant, Selective serotonin reuptake inhibitor (SSRI)
Half-life: 27–32 hours
Clinically important, potentially hazardous interactions with: alcohol, bupropion, MAO inhibitors, methylphenidate, omeprazole, selegiline, St John's wort, sumatriptan, telaprevir, valerian
Pregnancy category: C
Important contra-indications noted in the prescribing guidelines for: the elderly; nursing mothers; pediatric patients
Warning: SUICIDALITY AND ANTIDEPRESSANT DRUGS

Skin
Diaphoresis (5%)
Hot flashes (<10%)
Rash (<10%)

Mucosal
Oral vesiculation (<19%)
Xerostomia (6%) [6]

Cardiovascular
QT prolongation [9]
Torsades de pointes [2]

Central Nervous System
Anxiety [2]
Headache (24%) [5]
Insomnia (9–12%) [4]
Paresthesias (<10%)
Restless legs syndrome [5]
Serotonin syndrome [5]
Somnolence (drowsiness) (6–13%) [7]
Tremor (<10%)
Vertigo (dizziness) (5%) [6]

Neuromuscular/Skeletal
Asthenia (fatigue) [4]
Myalgia/Myopathy (<10%)

Gastrointestinal/Hepatic
Abdominal pain [3]
Constipation [2]
Diarrhea [3]
Dyspepsia [2]
Nausea [9]
Vomiting [3]

Respiratory
Cough (<10%)
Flu-like syndrome (5%)

Endocrine/Metabolic
Galactorrhea [2]
Hyponatremia [3]
SIADH [6]
Weight gain [3]

Genitourinary
Ejaculatory dysfunction (9–14%)
Sexual dysfunction [4]

Otic
Tinnitus (<10%)

Ocular
Glaucoma [3]

Other
Adverse effects [2]

Allergic reactions (<10%)
Toothache (<10%)

ESLICARBAZEPINE

Trade names: Aptiom (Sunovion), Zebinix (Eisai)
Indications: Partial-onset seizures
Class: Antiepileptic
Half-life: 13–20 hours
Clinically important, potentially hazardous interactions with: carbamazepine, digoxin, lamotrigine, levetiracetam, MAO inhibitors, oral contraceptives, oxcarbazepine, phenytoin, topiramate, valproic acid, warfarin
Pregnancy category: C
Important contra-indications noted in the prescribing guidelines for: nursing mothers; pediatric patients

Skin
Peripheral edema (<2%)
Rash (<3%) [2]

Cardiovascular
Hypertension (<2%)

Central Nervous System
Balance disorder (3%)
Depression (<3%)
Dysarthria (<2%)
Gait instability (2%)
Headache (13–15%) [12]
Incoordination [3]
Insomnia (2%)
Somnolence (drowsiness) (11–18%) [15]
Tremor (2–4%)
Vertigo (dizziness) (20–28%) [20]

Neuromuscular/Skeletal
Asthenia (fatigue) (4–7%) [7]
Ataxia (4–6%)

Gastrointestinal/Hepatic
Constipation (2%)
Diarrhea (2–4%)
Nausea (10–16%) [10]
Vomiting (6–10%) [4]

Respiratory
Cough (<2%)
Nasopharyngitis [2]

Endocrine/Metabolic
Hyponatremia (2%) [3]

Genitourinary
Urinary tract infection (2%)

Ocular
Diplopia (9–11%) [8]
Nystagmus (<2%)
Vision blurred (5–6%) [3]
Vision impaired (<2%)

ESMOLOL

Trade name: Brevibloc (Baxter)
Indications: Tachyarrhythmias, tachycardia
Class: Adrenergic beta-receptor antagonist, Antiarrhythmic class II
Half-life: 9 minutes
Clinically important, potentially hazardous interactions with: clonidine, verapamil

Pregnancy category: C
Important contra-indications noted in the prescribing guidelines for: nursing mothers; pediatric patients

Skin
Diaphoresis (>10%)
Cardiovascular
Bradycardia [5]
Hypotension [12]
Local
Injection-site pain (8%)
Injection-site reactions (<10%)
Other
Death [2]

ESOMEPRAZOLE

Trade name: Nexium (AstraZeneca)
Indications: Gastroesophageal reflux disease
Class: Proton pump inhibitor (PPI)
Half-life: 1.5 hours
Clinically important, potentially hazardous interactions with: benzodiazepines, chlordiazepoxide, cilostazol, clonazepam, clopidogrel, clorazepate, diazepam, digoxin, flurazepam, lorazepam, midazolam, oxazepam, posaconazole, quazepam, rifampin, rilpivirine, St John's wort, temazepam, tipranavir, voriconazole
Pregnancy category: C
Important contra-indications noted in the prescribing guidelines for: nursing mothers; pediatric patients

Skin
DRESS syndrome [2]
Fixed eruption [2]
Lupus erythematosus [2]
Central Nervous System
Dysgeusia (taste perversion) [3]
Fever [2]
Headache (8–11%) [6]
Somnolence (drowsiness) [2]
Vertigo (dizziness) [3]
Neuromuscular/Skeletal
Rhabdomyolysis [2]
Gastrointestinal/Hepatic
Abdominal pain [3]
Constipation [3]
Diarrhea [7]
Nausea [5]
Vomiting [4]
Respiratory
Bronchitis (4%)
Endocrine/Metabolic
Hypomagnesemia [2]
Other
Adverse effects [6]

ESTAZOLAM

See: www.drugeruptiondata.com/drug/id/267

ESTRADIOL

Trade names: Alora (Watson), Climara (Bayer), Divigel (Upsher-Smith), Elestrin (Azur Pharma), Esclim (Women First), Estrace (Bristol-Myers Squibb) (Warner Chilcott), Estraderm (Novartis), Estring (Pharmacia & Upjohn), Estrogel (Ascend), Evamist (KV Pharm), Fempatch (Pfizer), Gynodiol (Barr), Innofem (Novo Nordisk), Menostar (Bayer), Vagifem (Novo Nordisk), Vivelle (Novartis), Vivelle-Dot (Novartis)
Indications: Menopausal symptoms, hypoestrogenism due to hypogonadism, castration or primary ovarian failure, postmenopausal osteoporosis
Class: Estrogen, Hormone
Half-life: 1.75±2.87 hours
Clinically important, potentially hazardous interactions with: alcohol, amprenavir, anastrozole, ascorbic acid, atorvastatin, boceprevir, carbamazepine, chenodiol, clarithromycin, colesevelam, conivaptan, corticosteroids, CYP1A2 inducers, CYP3A4 inducers, deferasirox, delavirdine, erythromycin, folic acid, grapefruit juice, itraconazole, ketoconazole, lopinavir, minocycline, oxtriphylline, P-glycoprotein inhibitors or inducers, PEG-interferon, phenobarbital, rifampin, ritonavir, ropinirole, saxagliptin, somatropin, St John's wort, telaprevir, thyroid products, tipranavir, ursodiol
Pregnancy category: X
Important contra-indications noted in the prescribing guidelines for: the elderly; nursing mothers; pediatric patients
Note: See also separate entry for estrogens.
Warning: ENDOMETRIAL CANCER, CARDIOVASCULAR DISORDERS, BREAST CANCER and PROBABLE DEMENTIA

Central Nervous System
Headache [2]
Gastrointestinal/Hepatic
Nausea [3]
Respiratory
Nasopharyngitis (10%)
Upper respiratory tract infection (6%)
Endocrine/Metabolic
Mastodynia (7%)
Genitourinary
Metrorrhagia (4%)
Other
Adverse effects [3]

ESTRAMUSTINE

Trade name: Emcyt (Pfizer)
Indications: Prostate carcinoma
Class: Alkylating agent, Nitrosourea
Half-life: 20 hours
Clinically important, potentially hazardous interactions with: aldesleukin
Pregnancy category: X (not indicated for use in women)

Skin
Angioedema [2]
Edema (>10%) [4]
Peripheral edema [2]
Pruritus (2%) [2]
Purpura (3%)
Xerosis (2%)
Cardiovascular
Thrombophlebitis (3%)
Neuromuscular/Skeletal
Asthenia (fatigue) [3]
Gastrointestinal/Hepatic
Diarrhea [3]
Nausea [3]
Endocrine/Metabolic
Gynecomastia (>10%) [5]
Mastodynia (66%)
Hematologic
Anemia [3]
Febrile neutropenia [2]
Leukopenia [2]
Neutropenia [5]
Local
Injection-site thrombophlebitis (<10%) [3]
Other
Allergic reactions [2]
Death [2]

ESTROGENS

See: www.drugeruptiondata.com/drug/id/269

ESZOPICLONE

Trade names: Imovane (Sanofi-Aventis), Lunesta (Sunovion), Zimovane (Sanofi-Aventis)
Indications: Insomnia
Class: Hypnotic, non-benzodiazepine
Half-life: 6 hours
Clinically important, potentially hazardous interactions with: alcohol, antifungals, cimetidine, CNS depressants, conivaptan, CYP3A4 inhibitors and inducers, dasatinib, deferasirox, droperidol, erythromycin, ethanol, flumazenil, ketoconazole, levomepromazine, lorazepam, nefazodone, nelfinavir, olanzapine, rifampin, ritonavir, St John's wort, telithromycin, tricyclic antidepressants, valerian, voriconazole
Pregnancy category: C
Important contra-indications noted in the prescribing guidelines for: the elderly; nursing mothers; pediatric patients

Skin
Pruritus (<4%)
Rash (<5%)
Mucosal
Xerostomia (3–7%) [5]
Central Nervous System
Abnormal dreams (<3%)
Amnesia [3]
Anxiety (<3%)
Confusion (<3%)
Depression (<4%)
Dysgeusia (taste perversion) (8–34%) [21]

Hallucinations (<3%)
Headache (13–21%) [8]
Nervousness (<5%)
Neurotoxicity (<3%)
Pain (4–5%)
Somnolence (drowsiness) (8–10%) [2]
Vertigo (dizziness) [3]

Gastrointestinal/Hepatic
Diarrhea (2–4%)
Dyspepsia (2–6%)
Nausea (4–5%) [2]
Vomiting (<3%)

Endocrine/Metabolic
Gynecomastia (<3%)
Libido decreased (<3%)

Genitourinary
Dysmenorrhea (<3%)
Urinary tract infection (<3%)

Other
Adverse effects [4]
Infection (3–10%)

ETAMSYLATE

See: www.drugeruptiondata.com/drug/id/1374

ETANERCEPT

Trade names: Enbrel (Amgen), Erelzi (Sandoz)
Indications: Rheumatoid arthritis, polyarticular juvenile idiopathic arthritis in patients aged 2 years or older, psoriatic arthritis, ankylosing spondylitis, plaque psoriasis
Class: Cytokine inhibitor, Disease-modifying antirheumatic drug (DMARD), TNF inhibitor
Half-life: 4–13 days
Clinically important, potentially hazardous interactions with: abatacept, anakinra, cyclophosphamide, live vaccines
Pregnancy category: B
Important contra-indications noted in the prescribing guidelines for: the elderly; nursing mothers; pediatric patients
Note: TNF inhibitors should be used in patients with heart failure only after consideration of other treatment options. Contra-indicated in patients with sepsis. TNF inhibitors are contra-indicated in patients with a personal or family history of multiple sclerosis or demyelinating disease. TNF inhibitors should not be administered to patients with moderate to severe heart failure (New York Heart Association Functional Class III/IV).
Warning: SERIOUS INFECTIONS AND MALIGNANCIES

Skin
Abscess [2]
Anaphylactoid reactions/Anaphylaxis [2]
Carcinoma [2]
Cellulitis [2]
Dermatitis [3]
Dermatomyositis [4]
Exanthems [2]
Granulomas [2]
Granulomatous reaction [5]
Henoch–Schönlein purpura [3]
Herpes zoster [5]
Hidradenitis [2]
Leprosy [2]
Lichen planus [2]
Lichenoid eruption [3]
Lupus erythematosus [25]
Lupus syndrome [3]
Lymphoma [3]
Malignancies (<3%) [3]
Melanoma [2]
Neoplasms [2]
Nodular eruption [3]
Pruritus (2–5%) [2]
Psoriasis [19]
Pustules [2]
Rash (3–13%) [7]
Sarcoidosis [10]
Squamous cell carcinoma [4]
Urticaria (2%) [2]
Vasculitis [23]

Hair
Alopecia [5]

Cardiovascular
Atrial fibrillation [2]
Cardiotoxicity [2]
Hypertension [2]

Central Nervous System
Fever (2–3%)
Headache [16]
Leukoencephalopathy [3]
Multiple sclerosis [2]
Neurotoxicity [4]
Paresthesias [2]
Peripheral neuropathy [2]
Vertigo (dizziness) [2]

Neuromuscular/Skeletal
Asthenia (fatigue) [7]
Back pain [2]
Myalgia/Myopathy [2]
Myasthenia gravis [3]

Gastrointestinal/Hepatic
Abdominal pain [3]
Crohn's disease [4]
Diarrhea (8–16%) [4]
Gastroenteritis [3]
Hepatotoxicity [4]
Inflammatory bowel disease [2]
Nausea [5]

Respiratory
Asthma [2]
Bronchitis [4]
Cough [4]
Flu-like syndrome [3]
Laryngitis [2]
Nasopharyngitis [3]
Pharyngitis [4]
Pneumonia [5]
Pneumonitis [2]
Pulmonary toxicity [4]
Rhinitis [4]
Sinusitis [5]
Tuberculosis [2]
Upper respiratory tract infection (38–65%) [10]

Endocrine/Metabolic
ALT increased [3]
Hypertriglyceridemia [2]
Thyroiditis [2]

Genitourinary
Cystitis [2]
Urinary tract infection [2]

Renal
Nephrotoxicity [2]

Hematologic
Leukopenia [2]
Macrophage activation syndrome [2]
Neutropenia [2]
Pancytopenia [2]
Thrombocytopenia [2]

Otic
Otitis media [2]

Ocular
Uveitis [12]

Local
Injection-site reactions (37–43%) [56]

Other
Adverse effects [36]
Allergic reactions (<3%)
Death [6]
Infection (50–81%) [43]

ETELCALCETIDE *

Trade name: Parsabiv (Amgen)
Indications: Secondary hyperparathyroidism in adult patients with chronic kidney disease on hemodialysis
Class: Calcimimetic
Half-life: 3–4 days
Clinically important, potentially hazardous interactions with: none known
Pregnancy category: N/A (No data available)
Important contra-indications noted in the prescribing guidelines for: nursing mothers; pediatric patients

Skin
Facial edema (<4%)
Hypersensitivity (4%)
Pruritus (<4%)
Urticaria (<4%)

Cardiovascular
Cardiac failure (2%)

Central Nervous System
Headache (8%)
Paresthesias (6%)

Neuromuscular/Skeletal
Muscle spasm (12%)
Myalgia/Myopathy (2%)

Gastrointestinal/Hepatic
Diarrhea (11%)
Nausea (11%) [3]
Vomiting (9%) [3]

Endocrine/Metabolic
Hyperkalemia (4%)
Hypocalcemia (7–64%) [3]

ETHACRYNIC ACID

See: www.drugeruptiondata.com/drug/id/271

ETHAMBUTOL

Trade name: Myambutol (Stat Trade)
Indications: Tuberculosis
Class: Antimycobacterial
Half-life: 3–4 hours
Clinically important, potentially hazardous interactions with: cortisone, zinc
Pregnancy category: C
Important contra-indications noted in the prescribing guidelines for: nursing mothers; pediatric patients

Skin
  Bullous dermatitis [2]
  Dermatitis [2]
  DRESS syndrome [5]
  Erythema multiforme [2]
  Exanthems (<5%) [4]
  Hypersensitivity [3]
  Lichenoid eruption [2]
  Lupus erythematosus [2]
  Pruritus [4]
  Rash [2]
  Toxic epidermal necrolysis [2]
  Urticaria [2]
Renal
  Nephrotoxicity [2]
Ocular
  Amblyopia [2]
  Ocular toxicity [9]
  Optic neuritis [4]
  Optic neuropathy [9]
  Vision impaired [2]
Other
  Adverse effects [4]

ETHANOLAMINE

See: www.drugeruptiondata.com/drug/id/273

ETHCHLORVYNOL

See: www.drugeruptiondata.com/drug/id/274

ETHIONAMIDE

See: www.drugeruptiondata.com/drug/id/275

ETHOSUXIMIDE

Trade name: Zarontin (Pfizer)
Indications: Absence (petit mal) seizures
Class: Antiepileptic, succinimide
Half-life: 50–60 hours
Clinically important, potentially hazardous interactions with: antipsychotics, carbamazepine, chloroquine, cobicistat/elvitegravir/emtricitabine/tenofovir alafenamide, cobicistat/elvitegravir/emtricitabine/tenofovir disoproxil, hydroxychloroquine, isoniazid, levomepromazine, lisdexamfetamine, MAO inhibitors, mefloquine, nevirapine, orlistat, phenobarbital, phenytoin, primidone, risperidone, SSRIs, St John's wort, tricyclic antidepressants, valproic acid, zuclopenthixol
Pregnancy category: C
Important contra-indications noted in the prescribing guidelines for: nursing mothers
Note: Cases of birth defects have been reported with ethosuximide.

Skin
  Exanthems (<5%) [2]
  Lupus erythematosus (>10%) [22]
  Raynaud's phenomenon [3]
  Stevens-Johnson syndrome (>10%)
  Urticaria (<5%)
Hematologic
  Agranulocytosis [2]
Other
  Side effects (3%)

ETHOTOIN

See: www.drugeruptiondata.com/drug/id/277

ETHOXZOLAMIDE

See: www.drugeruptiondata.com/drug/id/1951

ETIDRONATE

Trade name: Didronel (Procter & Gamble)
Indications: Paget's disease, osteoporosis
Class: Bisphosphonate
Half-life: 6 hours
Clinically important, potentially hazardous interactions with: ferrous sulfate
Pregnancy category: C
Important contra-indications noted in the prescribing guidelines for: nursing mothers; pediatric patients

Neuromuscular/Skeletal
  Fractures [6]
  Osteomalacia [3]
  Pseudogout [2]
  Skeletal toxicity [2]
Gastrointestinal/Hepatic
  Esophagitis [2]

ETODOLAC

Trade name: Lodine (Wyeth)
Indications: Pain
Class: COX-2 inhibitor, Non-steroidal anti-inflammatory (NSAID)
Half-life: 7 hours
Clinically important, potentially hazardous interactions with: aspirin, methotrexate
Pregnancy category: C
Important contra-indications noted in the prescribing guidelines for: the elderly; nursing mothers; pediatric patients
Note: NSAIDs may cause an increased risk of serious cardiovascular and gastrointestinal adverse events, which can be fatal. This risk may increase with duration of use.

Skin
  Exanthems [2]
  Facial edema [2]
  Fixed eruption [2]
  Pruritus (<10%) [7]
  Rash (>10%) [5]
  Vasculitis [2]
Gastrointestinal/Hepatic
  Abdominal pain [2]
  Constipation [2]
  Dyspepsia [3]
  Nausea [2]
Other
  Adverse effects [2]

ETOMIDATE

See: www.drugeruptiondata.com/drug/id/1399

ETOPOSIDE

Trade name: VePesid (Bristol-Myers Squibb)
Indications: Lymphomas, carcinomas
Class: Topoisomerase 2 inhibitor
Half-life: 4–11 hours
Clinically important, potentially hazardous interactions with: aldesleukin, atovaquone, atovaquone/proguanil, cyclosporine, gadobenate, prednisolone, St John's wort
Pregnancy category: D
Important contra-indications noted in the prescribing guidelines for: the elderly; nursing mothers; pediatric patients

Skin
  Anaphylactoid reactions/Anaphylaxis (<2%) [3]
  Erythema [3]
  Exanthems [4]
  Hand–foot syndrome [4]
  Hypersensitivity [9]
  Pigmentation [2]
  Radiation recall dermatitis [3]
  Rash [2]
  Stevens-Johnson syndrome [3]
  Toxicity [2]
Hair
  Alopecia (8–66%) [8]
Mucosal
  Mucositis (>10%)
  Oral lesions (<5%) [2]
  Stomatitis (<10%) [2]
Cardiovascular
  Flushing [3]
Central Nervous System
  Anorexia [2]
  Leukoencephalopathy [2]
  Neurotoxicity [3]
Neuromuscular/Skeletal
  Asthenia (fatigue) [2]
Gastrointestinal/Hepatic
  Diarrhea [2]

Hepatotoxicity [2]
Nausea [5]
Vomiting [7]
Respiratory
Pulmonary toxicity [2]
Endocrine/Metabolic
Hyponatremia [2]
Renal
Nephrotoxicity [3]
Hematologic
Anemia [5]
Febrile neutropenia [5]
Leukopenia [3]
Neutropenia [11]
Thrombocytopenia [9]
Other
Adverse effects [3]
Allergic reactions (<2%)
Death [2]
Infection [4]

ETORICOXIB

See: www.drugeruptiondata.com/drug/id/1235

ETRAVIRINE

Trade name: Intelence (Tibotec)
Indications: HIV infection
Class: Non-nucleoside reverse transcriptase inhibitor
Half-life: 41 hours
Clinically important, potentially hazardous interactions with: atazanavir, atorvastatin, carbamazepine, clarithromycin, clopidogrel, darunavir, delavirdine, digoxin, efavirenz, fosamprenavir, indinavir, maraviroc, nelfinavir, neratinib, nevirapine, non-nucleoside reverse transcriptase inhibitors, olaparib, palbociclib, phenobarbital, phenytoin, rifabutin, rifampin, rifapentine, rilpivirine, ritonavir, sildenafil, simeprevir, St John's wort, tadalafil, telithromycin, tipranavir, vardenafil, venetoclax, voriconazole
Pregnancy category: B
Important contra-indications noted in the prescribing guidelines for: nursing mothers; pediatric patients

Skin
Facial edema (<2%)
Hyperhidrosis (<2%)
Lipohypertrophy (<2%)
Prurigo (<2%)
Rash (9%) [17]
Xerosis (<2%)
Mucosal
Stomatitis (<2%)
Xerostomia (<2%)
Cardiovascular
Angina (<2%)
Atrial fibrillation (<2%)
Hypertension (3%)
Myocardial infarction (<2%)
Central Nervous System
Abnormal dreams (<2%)

Amnesia (<2%)
Anorexia (<2%)
Anxiety (<2%)
Confusion (<2%)
Disorientation (<2%)
Headache (3%) [3]
Hypersomnia (<2%)
Hypoesthesia (<2%)
Insomnia (<2%)
Nervousness (<2%)
Neurotoxicity [3]
Nightmares (<2%)
Paresthesias (<2%)
Peripheral neuropathy (3%)
Seizures (<2%)
Sleep related disorder (<2%)
Somnolence (drowsiness) (<2%)
Syncope (<2%)
Tremor (<2%)
Vertigo (dizziness) (<2%)
Neuromuscular/Skeletal
Asthenia (fatigue) (3%)
Gastrointestinal/Hepatic
Abdominal distension (<2%)
Abdominal pain (3%)
Constipation (<2%)
Diarrhea [3]
Flatulence (<2%)
Gastritis (<2%)
Gastroesophageal reflux (<2%)
Hematemesis (<2%)
Hepatic failure (<2%)
Hepatomegaly (<2%)
Hepatotoxicity [2]
Nausea [4]
Pancreatitis (<2%)
Retching (<2%)
Respiratory
Bronchospasm (<2%)
Dyspnea (<2%)
Endocrine/Metabolic
Diabetes mellitus (<2%)
Gynecomastia (<2%)
Renal
Renal failure (<2%)
Hematologic
Dyslipidemia (<2%)
Hemolytic anemia (<2%)
Ocular
Vision blurred (<2%)
Other
Adverse effects [6]

EVEROLIMUS

Trade names: Afinitor (Novartis), Certican (Novartis), Zortress (Novartis)
Indications: Prophylaxis of organ rejection in adults following kidney or liver transplant, advanced renal cell carcinoma, neuroendocrine tumors of pancreatic, gastrointestinal or lung origin, breast cancer in post-menopausal women with advanced hormone-receptor positive, HER2-negative type cancer, renal angiomyolipoma and tuberous sclerosis complex, subependymal giant cell astrocytoma associated with tuberous sclerosis
Class: Antineoplastic, Immunosuppressant, mTOR inhibitor
Half-life: ~30 hours
Clinically important, potentially hazardous interactions with: aprepitant, atazanavir, atorvastatin, benazepril, captopril, clarithromycin, clozapine, conivaptan, cyclosporine, darunavir, delavirdine, digoxin, efavirenz, enalapril, erythromycin, grapefruit juice, indinavir, itraconazole, ketoconazole, lapatinib, lisinopril, live vaccines, nelfinavir, oxcarbazepine, phenytoin, posaconazole, quinapril, ramipril, ribociclib, rifampin, rifapentine, ritonavir, saquinavir, St John's wort, telithromycin, venetoclax, verapamil, voriconazole
Pregnancy category: D
Important contra-indications noted in the prescribing guidelines for: nursing mothers; pediatric patients
Warning: In immunosuppression therapy: MALIGNANCIES AND SERIOUS INFECTIONS, KIDNEY GRAFT THROMBOSIS; NEPHROTOXICITY
In heart transplantation: MORTALITY

Skin
Acneform eruption (3–25%) [5]
Angioedema [4]
Cellulitis (21%)
Contact dermatitis (14%)
Edema (39%) [4]
Erythema (4%)
Excoriations (14%)
Hand–foot syndrome (5%) [9]
Hypersensitivity [2]
Lymphedema [2]
Peripheral edema (4–39%) [8]
Pityriasis rosea (4%)
Pruritus (14–21%) [5]
Rash (18–59%) [47]
Tinea (18%)
Toxicity [9]
Xerosis (13–18%)
Nails
Nail disorder (4–22%) [2]
Mucosal
Aphthous stomatitis [4]
Epistaxis (nosebleed) (18–22%) [3]
Mucosal inflammation (19%) [3]
Mucositis [17]
Nasal congestion (14%)
Oral ulceration [4]
Oropharyngeal pain (11%)
Rhinorrhea (3%)
Stomatitis (44–86%) [70]

Xerostomia (8–11%)

Cardiovascular
Chest pain (5%)
Hypertension (4–13%) [14]
Tachycardia (3%)

Central Nervous System
Anorexia (25%) [12]
Anxiety (7%)
Chills (4%)
Dysgeusia (taste perversion) (10–19%) [2]
Fever (20–32%) [7]
Headache (18–30%) [4]
Insomnia (9%)
Migraine (30%)
Pain [2]
Peripheral neuropathy [2]
Seizures (29%)
Somnolence (drowsiness) (7%)
Vertigo (dizziness) (7–14%)

Neuromuscular/Skeletal
Arthralgia (15%)
Asthenia (fatigue) (7–45%) [60]
Back pain (15%)
Jaw pain (3%)
Muscle spasm (10%)
Pain in extremities (10–14%)

Gastrointestinal/Hepatic
Abdominal pain (9–36%) [4]
Constipation (11–14%)
Diarrhea (25–50%) [34]
Dysphagia (4%)
Gastritis (7%)
Gastroenteritis (18%)
Gastrointestinal bleeding [3]
Hemorrhoids (5%)
Hepatotoxicity [7]
Nausea (26–32%) [10]
Pancreatitis [2]
Vomiting (20–29%) [3]

Respiratory
Cough (21–30%) [6]
Dyspnea (20–24%) [7]
Nasopharyngitis (25%)
Pharyngitis (11%)
Pharyngolaryngeal pain (4%)
Pleural effusion (7%)
Pneumonia [10]
Pneumonitis (14–17%) [41]
Pulmonary toxicity [10]
Rhinitis (25%)
Sinusitis (39%)
Upper respiratory tract infection (25–82%)
[2]

Endocrine/Metabolic
ALT increased (21–48%) [4]
Appetite decreased (30%) [5]
AST increased (25–56%) [3]
Diabetes mellitus (2–10%) [2]
GGT increased [2]
Hypercholesterolemia [7]
Hyperglycemia [32]
Hyperlipidemia [8]
Hypertriglyceridemia [2]
Hypokalemia [4]
Hypomagnesemia [2]
Hyponatremia [3]
Hypophosphatemia [5]
Hypothyroidism [2]
Serum creatinine increased (19–50%) [4]

Weight loss (9–28%) [3]

Genitourinary
Urinary tract infection (15%)

Renal
Nephrotoxicity [5]
Proteinuria (7%) [15]
Renal failure (3%) [3]

Hematologic
Anemia [35]
Febrile neutropenia [5]
Hemoglobin decreased (86–92%) [2]
Hemolytic uremic syndrome [2]
Hemorrhage (3%) [3]
Hemotoxicity [5]
Immunosupression [2]
Leukopenia [4]
Lymphopenia [8]
Neutropenia [17]
Platelets decreased (23–45%)
Sepsis [2]
Thrombocytopenia [20]

Otic
Otitis media (36%)

Ocular
Conjunctivitis (2%)
Eyelid edema (4%) [2]
Ocular hyperemia (4%)

Other
Adverse effects [29]
Death [8]
Infection (18%) [29]
Side effects [2]

EVOLOCUMAB

Trade name: Repatha (Amgen)
Indications: Heterozygous or homozygous familial hypercholesterolemia where additional lowering of low density lipoprotein cholesterol is required
Class: Monoclonal antibody, Proprotein convertase subtilisin kexin type 9 (PCSK9) inhibitor
Half-life: 11–17 days
Clinically important, potentially hazardous interactions with: none known
Pregnancy category: N/A (No data available but likely to cross the placenta in second and third trimester)
Important contra-indications noted in the prescribing guidelines for: pediatric patients

Mucosal
Nasal congestion [2]
Oropharyngeal pain [2]

Cardiovascular
Hypertension (2%)

Central Nervous System
Headache (4%) [10]
Neurotoxicity [2]
Vertigo (dizziness) (3%)

Neuromuscular/Skeletal
Arthralgia (2%) [8]
Asthenia (fatigue) [2]
Back pain (2–6%) [10]
Bone or joint pain (3%) [3]

Muscle spasm [6]
Myalgia/Myopathy (3%) [10]
Pain in extremities [5]

Gastrointestinal/Hepatic
Diarrhea (3%) [5]
Gastroenteritis (2%) [2]
Hepatotoxicity [5]
Nausea [4]

Respiratory
Cough (<4%) [3]
Influenza (<6%) [9]
Nasopharyngitis (4–10%) [13]
Pharyngitis [2]
Sinusitis (3%) [2]
Upper respiratory tract infection (2–6%)
[10]

Endocrine/Metabolic
Creatine phosphokinase increased [9]

Genitourinary
Urinary tract infection (<4%)

Local
Injection-site bruising [4]
Injection-site edema [2]
Injection-site erythema [3]
Injection-site pain [7]
Injection-site reactions (3–5%) [9]

Other
Adverse effects [6]
Allergic reactions (5%)

EXEMESTANE

Trade name: Aromasin (Pfizer)
Indications: Advanced breast cancer
Class: Aromatase inhibitor
Half-life: 24 hours
Clinically important, potentially hazardous interactions with: efavirenz, oxcarbazepine, rifapentine
Pregnancy category: X
Important contra-indications noted in the prescribing guidelines for: nursing mothers; pediatric patients

Skin
Diaphoresis (6–12%) [2]
Edema (7%)
Hot flashes (30%) [7]
Lymphedema (2–5%)
Peripheral edema (9%) [2]
Pruritus (2–5%)
Radiation recall dermatitis [2]
Rash (2–5%) [6]

Hair
Alopecia (2–5%)

Mucosal
Stomatitis [7]

Central Nervous System
Dysgeusia (taste perversion) [2]
Headache [3]
Insomnia [2]
Paresthesias (2–5%)
Tumor pain (30%)

Neuromuscular/Skeletal
Arthralgia [4]
Asthenia (fatigue) [6]

Back pain [2]
Bone or joint pain [2]
Myalgia/Myopathy [2]

Gastrointestinal/Hepatic
Diarrhea [4]

Respiratory
Pneumonitis [5]

Endocrine/Metabolic
Hyperglycemia [4]

Hematologic
Anemia [2]

Other
Adverse effects [2]

EXENATIDE

Trade names: Bydureon (Amylin), Byetta (Amylin)
Indications: Type II diabetes mellitus
Class: Glucagon-like peptide-1 (GLP-1) receptor agonist, Incretin mimetic, Insulin secretagogue
Half-life: 2.4 hours
Clinically important, potentially hazardous interactions with: acetaminophen, alcohol, antibiotics, corticosteroids, lovastatin, oral contraceptives, pegvisomant, prandial insulin, somatropin, sulfonylureas, thiazide diuretics, vitamin K antagonists, warfarin
Pregnancy category: C
Important contra-indications noted in the prescribing guidelines for: nursing mothers; pediatric patients
Note: Risk of thyroid C-cell tumors with exenatide extended release formulations. Bydureon is contra-indicated in patients with a personal or family history of medullary thyroid carcinoma or in patients with multiple endocrine neoplasia syndrome Type 2.

Skin
Hyperhidrosis (<10%)
Urticaria [2]

Cardiovascular
Cardiotoxicity [2]

Central Nervous System
Chills (<2%)
Headache (<10%) [8]
Vertigo (dizziness) (<10%) [3]

Neuromuscular/Skeletal
Asthenia (fatigue) (<10%)

Gastrointestinal/Hepatic
Abdominal distension (<10%)
Abdominal pain (<10%) [2]
Constipation (>5%)
Diarrhea (<11%) [18]
Dyspepsia (<10%)
Flatulence (2%)
Gastroenteritis (<10%)
Gastroesophageal reflux (3%)
Nausea (<11%) [43]
Pancreatitis [10]
Vomiting (~10%) [25]

Respiratory
Nasopharyngitis [2]

Endocrine/Metabolic
Appetite decreased (<10%) [3]
Hypoglycemia (>5%) [4]

Genitourinary
Urinary tract infection [2]

Renal
Nephrotoxicity [2]
Renal failure [3]

Local
Injection-site erythema (5–7%)
Injection-site nodules (~10%) [4]
Injection-site pruritus (5–6%) [2]
Injection-site reactions [7]

Other
Adverse effects [10]
Cancer [2]

EZETIMIBE

Trade names: Ezetrol (Merck), Liptruzet (Merck Sharpe & Dohme), Vytorin (MSD), Zetia (Merck)
Indications: Hypercholesterolemia
Class: Cholesterol inhibitor
Half-life: 22 hours
Clinically important, potentially hazardous interactions with: cholestyramine, cyclosporine, fenofibrate, gemfibrozil, HMG-CoA reductase inhibitors, ritonavir
Pregnancy category: C (Pregnancy category is X when combined with a statin.)
Important contra-indications noted in the prescribing guidelines for: nursing mothers
Note: Liptruzet is ezetimibe and atorvastatin; vytorin is ezetimibe and simvastatin.

Skin
Rash [3]

Central Nervous System
Headache [5]
Vertigo (dizziness) [4]

Neuromuscular/Skeletal
Arthralgia (4%) [3]
Asthenia (fatigue) [2]
Back pain (4%) [4]
Bone or joint pain [4]
Muscle spasm [3]
Myalgia/Myopathy (5%) [16]
Pain in extremities [2]

Gastrointestinal/Hepatic
Abdominal pain (2%)
Diarrhea [4]
Hepatotoxicity [6]
Nausea [4]
Pancreatitis [3]

Respiratory
Cough (2%)
Influenza [3]
Nasopharyngitis [5]
Upper respiratory tract infection [2]

Endocrine/Metabolic
Creatine phosphokinase increased [8]

Genitourinary
Urinary tract infection [2]

Hematologic
Thrombocytopenia [2]

Local
Injection-site erythema [2]
Injection-site reactions [5]

Other
Adverse effects [6]

EZOGABINE

Synonym: retigabine
Trade names: Potiga (GSK), Trobalt (GSK)
Indications: Epilepsy
Class: Anticonvulsant, Potassium channel opener
Half-life: 7–11 hours
Clinically important, potentially hazardous interactions with: alcohol, carbamazepine, digoxin, phenytoin
Pregnancy category: C
Important contra-indications noted in the prescribing guidelines for: the elderly; nursing mothers; pediatric patients
Warning: RETINAL ABNORMALITIES AND POTENTIAL VISION LOSS

Skin
Hyperhidrosis (<2%)
Peripheral edema (<2%)
Pigmentation [2]

Mucosal
Mucosal membrane pigmentation [4]
Xerostomia (<2%)

Central Nervous System
Amnesia (2%)
Anxiety (3%)
Aphasia (4%)
Balance disorder (4%)
Confusion (9%) [6]
Disorientation (2%)
Dysarthria (4%) [3]
Dysphasia (2%)
Gait instability (4%)
Hallucinations (<2%)
Headache [6]
Hypokinesia (<2%)
Impaired concentration (6%)
Incoordination (7%)
Memory loss (6%)
Neurotoxicity [3]
Paresthesias (3%)
Somnolence (drowsiness) (22%) [14]
Speech disorder [3]
Tremor (8%) [3]
Vertigo (dizziness) (31%) [14]

Neuromuscular/Skeletal
Asthenia (fatigue) (20%) [11]
Ataxia [3]
Myoclonus (<2%)

Gastrointestinal/Hepatic
Constipation (3%)
Dyspepsia (2%)
Dysphagia (<2%)
Nausea (7%) [5]

Respiratory
Influenza (3%)

Endocrine/Metabolic
Appetite increased (<2%)
Weight gain (dose related) (3%)

Genitourinary
Dysuria (2%)
Hematuria (2%)
Urinary hesitancy (2%)
Urinary retention (<2%) [6]
Urinary tract infection [3]

Renal
Chromaturia (2%)
Ocular
Diplopia (7%) [2]
Ocular pigmentation [4]

Vision blurred (5%) [2]
Other
Adverse effects [2]

FACTOR VIII - VON WILLEBRAND FACTOR

See: www.drugeruptiondata.com/drug/id/1404

FAMCICLOVIR

Trade name: Famvir (Novartis)
Indications: Acute herpes zoster, recurrent genital herpes
Class: Antiviral, Guanine nucleoside analog
Half-life: 2–3 hours
Clinically important, potentially hazardous interactions with: none known
Pregnancy category: B
Important contra-indications noted in the prescribing guidelines for: nursing mothers; pediatric patients

Skin
 Pruritus (4%)
 Rash (<4%)
 Vasculitis [3]
Central Nervous System
 Headache (9–39%) [5]
 Paresthesias (<3%)
Neuromuscular/Skeletal
 Asthenia (fatigue) (<5%)
Gastrointestinal/Hepatic
 Abdominal pain (<8%) [2]
 Diarrhea (2–9%)
 Flatulence (<5%)
 Nausea (2–13%) [3]
 Vomiting (<5%) [2]
Genitourinary
 Dysmenorrhea (<8%)
Other
 Adverse effects [4]

FAMOTIDINE

Trade names: Duexis (Horizon), Pepcid (Valeant)
Indications: Duodenal ulcer, gastric ulcer, gastroesophageal reflux disease
Class: Histamine H2 receptor antagonist
Half-life: 2.5–3.5 hours
Clinically important, potentially hazardous interactions with: atazanavir, cefditoren, dasatinib, delavirdine, rilpivirine, thalidomide
Pregnancy category: B
Important contra-indications noted in the prescribing guidelines for: nursing mothers
Note: Duexis is famotidine and ibuprofen.

Skin
 Dermatitis [3]
 Peripheral edema [2]
 Pruritus [2]
 Rash [3]
 Urticaria [3]
 Vasculitis [2]
Cardiovascular
 Hypertension [3]

Central Nervous System
 Confusion [2]
 Delirium [3]
 Fever [2]
 Headache (5%) [4]
 Neurotoxicity [2]
 Somnolence (drowsiness) [2]
Neuromuscular/Skeletal
 Arthralgia [2]
 Back pain [2]
Gastrointestinal/Hepatic
 Abdominal pain [2]
 Diarrhea (2%) [3]
 Dyspepsia [3]
 Gastroesophageal reflux [2]
 Nausea [4]
 Vomiting [4]
Respiratory
 Influenza [2]
 Sinusitis [2]
 Upper respiratory tract infection [2]
Endocrine/Metabolic
 Hypomagnesemia [2]
 Hypophosphatemia [2]
Genitourinary
 Urinary tract infection [2]
Hematologic
 Eosinophilia [2]
 Thrombocytopenia [2]

FEBUXOSTAT

Trade name: Uloric (Takeda)
Indications: Hyperuricemia in gout
Class: Xanthine oxidase inhibitor
Half-life: 5–8 hours
Clinically important, potentially hazardous interactions with: aminophylline, azathioprine, didanosine, mercaptopurine, oxtriphylline, theophylline
Pregnancy category: C

Skin
 Rash (2%) [7]
Cardiovascular
 Cardiotoxicity [2]
Central Nervous System
 Headache [5]
 Vertigo (dizziness) [5]
Neuromuscular/Skeletal
 Arthralgia [5]
 Bone or joint pain [2]
 Gouty tophi (flare) [3]
 Joint disorder [2]
Gastrointestinal/Hepatic
 Diarrhea [9]
 Hepatotoxicity (5%) [13]
 Nausea [7]
 Vomiting [2]
Respiratory
 Upper respiratory tract infection [2]
Other
 Adverse effects [7]

FELBAMATE

See: www.drugeruptiondata.com/drug/id/283

FELBINAC

See: www.drugeruptiondata.com/drug/id/1407

FELODIPINE

See: www.drugeruptiondata.com/drug/id/284

FENBUFEN

See: www.drugeruptiondata.com/drug/id/1143

FENOFIBRATE

Trade name: Tricor (AbbVie)
Indications: Hyperlipidemia
Class: Fibrate, Lipid regulator
Half-life: 20 hours
Clinically important, potentially hazardous interactions with: atorvastatin, colchicine, dicumarol, ezetimibe, lovastatin, nicotinic acid, rosuvastatin, statins, warfarin
Pregnancy category: C
Important contra-indications noted in the prescribing guidelines for: the elderly; nursing mothers; pediatric patients

Skin
 Photosensitivity [11]
 Phototoxicity [2]
 Pruritus (4%)
 Rash (2–8%) [3]
Neuromuscular/Skeletal
 Myalgia/Myopathy [11]
 Rhabdomyolysis [18]
Gastrointestinal/Hepatic
 Hepatotoxicity [15]
 Pancreatitis [3]
Endocrine/Metabolic
 Gynecomastia [2]
Renal
 Nephrotoxicity [3]
 Renal failure [2]
Other
 Adverse effects (<10%)

FENOLDOPAM

See: www.drugeruptiondata.com/drug/id/994

FENOPROFEN

See: www.drugeruptiondata.com/drug/id/287

FENTANYL

Trade names: Actiq (Cephalon), Duragesic (Janssen)
Indications: Chronic pain
Class: Analgesic, opioid, Anesthetic
Half-life: ~7 hours
Clinically important, potentially hazardous interactions with: amiodarone, amprenavir, aprepitant, atazanavir, ceritinib, cimetidine, conivaptan, crizotinib, darunavir, dasatinib, delavirdine, efavirenz, eluxadoline, enzalutamide, indinavir, itraconazole, ketoconazole, lapatinib, lopinavir, mifepristone, nelfinavir, nevirapine, nifedipine, osimertinib, ranitidine, ribociclib, rifapentine, ritonavir, saquinavir, telithromycin, voriconazole
Pregnancy category: C
Important contra-indications noted in the prescribing guidelines for: nursing mothers; pediatric patients
Note: Contra-indicated in opioid non-tolerant patients, and for the management of acute or postoperative pain including headache/migraines and dental pain.
Warning: ADDICTION, ABUSE, and MISUSE; LIFE-THREATENING RESPIRATORY DEPRESSION; ACCIDENTAL EXPOSURE; NEONATAL OPIOID WITHDRAWAL SYNDROME; CYTOCHROME P450 3A4 INTERACTION
EXPOSURE TO HEAT (for topical patches)

Skin
Anaphylactoid reactions/Anaphylaxis [6]
Diaphoresis (>10%) [2]
Edema (>10%)
Erythema (at application site) [3]
Pruritus (3–44%) [30]
Rash [3]
Mucosal
Xerostomia (>10%) [3]
Cardiovascular
Bradycardia (>10%) [3]
Flushing (3–10%)
Hypotension [8]
Tachycardia [2]
Central Nervous System
Agitation [2]
Anorexia [2]
Confusion (>10%)
Delirium [2]
Depression (>10%)
Hallucinations [2]
Headache (>10%)
Neuroleptic malignant syndrome [2]
Sedation [2]
Serotonin syndrome [4]
Somnolence (drowsiness) [13]
Vertigo (dizziness) [12]
Neuromuscular/Skeletal
Asthenia (fatigue) (>10%) [2]
Myoclonus [3]
Gastrointestinal/Hepatic
Constipation (>10%) [11]
Nausea (>10%) [31]
Vomiting (>10%) [21]

Respiratory
Cough [15]
Respiratory depression [7]
Ocular
Miosis (>10%)
Local
Application-site erythema [2]
Other
Adverse effects [7]
Death [7]

FERRIC GLUCONATE

See: www.drugeruptiondata.com/drug/id/2817

FERROUS SULFATE

See: www.drugeruptiondata.com/drug/id/2677

FERUMOXSIL

See: www.drugeruptiondata.com/drug/id/2235

FERUMOXYTOL

Trade name: Feraheme (AMG Pharma)
Indications: Iron deficiency anemia in adults with chronic kidney disease
Class: Iron supplement
Half-life: 15 hours
Clinically important, potentially hazardous interactions with: none known
Pregnancy category: C
Important contra-indications noted in the prescribing guidelines for: the elderly; nursing mothers; pediatric patients
Note: May cause hypersensitivity reactions, hypotension and iron overload. Feraheme may transiently affect magnetic resonance (MRI) imaging for up to 3 months following dosage. Contra-indicated in patients with evidence of iron overload or anemia not caused by iron deficiency.

Skin
Anaphylactoid reactions/Anaphylaxis [3]
Hypersensitivity [3]
Pruritus [5]
Rash [2]
Urticaria [2]
Cardiovascular
Hypotension (3%) [3]
Central Nervous System
Headache [6]
Vertigo (dizziness) (3%) [3]
Neuromuscular/Skeletal
Asthenia (fatigue) [2]
Back pain [2]
Gastrointestinal/Hepatic
Abdominal pain [2]
Nausea (3%) [6]
Vomiting [2]

Respiratory
Dyspnea [3]
Local
Injection-site pain [3]
Other
Adverse effects [2]

FESOTERODINE

Trade name: Toviaz (Pfizer)
Indications: Overactive bladder syndrome, urinary incontinence, urgency and frequency
Class: Antimuscarinic, Muscarinic antagonist
Half-life: 7 hours; 4 hours (oral)
Clinically important, potentially hazardous interactions with: alcohol, amantadine, anticholinergics, antidepressants, antimuscarinics, atazanavir, botulinum toxin (A & B), carbamazepine, cinacalcet, clarithromycin, conivaptan, CYP2D6 inhibitors, CYP3A4 inhibitors, CYP3AF inhibitors, darunavir, dasatinib, deferasirox, delavirdine, duloxetine, indinavir, itraconazole, ketoconazole, nefazodone, nelfinavir, PEG-interferon, phenobarbital, phenytoin, pramlintide, rifampin, ritonavir, saquinavir, secretin, St John's wort, telithromycin, terbinafine, tipranavir, tocilizumab, voriconazole
Pregnancy category: C
Important contra-indications noted in the prescribing guidelines for: nursing mothers; pediatric patients
Note: Contra-indicated in patients with urinary retention, gastric retention, or uncontrolled narrow-angle glaucoma.

Mucosal
Xerostomia (19–35%) [28]
Central Nervous System
Headache [3]
Neuromuscular/Skeletal
Back pain (2%)
Gastrointestinal/Hepatic
Constipation (4–6%) [16]
Diarrhea (<10%)
Dyspepsia (<2%) [2]
Nausea (<2%) [2]
Respiratory
Upper respiratory tract infection (2–3%)
Genitourinary
Dysuria (<2%)
Urinary retention [2]
Urinary tract infection (3–4%) [3]
Ocular
Vision blurred [2]
Xerophthalmia (<4%) [2]
Other
Adverse effects [3]

FEXOFENADINE

Trade name: Allegra (Sanofi-Aventis)
Indications: Allergic rhinitis, pruritus, urticaria
Class: Histamine H1 receptor antagonist
Half-life: 14.4 hours
Clinically important, potentially hazardous interactions with: neratinib, St John's wort
Pregnancy category: C
Important contra-indications noted in the prescribing guidelines for: the elderly; nursing mothers; pediatric patients

Skin
Urticaria [3]

Central Nervous System
Headache (5–11%) [2]

FIDAXOMICIN

See: www.drugeruptiondata.com/drug/id/2537

FINAFLOXACIN

Trade name: Xtoro (Alcon)
Indications: Acute otitis externa caused by susceptible strains of *Pseudomonas aeruginosa* and *Staphylococcus aureus*
Class: Antibiotic, fluoroquinolone
Half-life: N/A
Clinically important, potentially hazardous interactions with: none known
Pregnancy category: C
Important contra-indications noted in the prescribing guidelines for: nursing mothers; pediatric patients

Central Nervous System
Headache [2]

Gastrointestinal/Hepatic
Diarrhea [2]
Flatulence [2]
Loose stools [2]
Nausea [2]

Respiratory
Nasopharyngitis [2]
Rhinitis [2]

FINASTERIDE

Trade names: Propecia (Merck), Proscar (Merck)
Indications: Benign prostatic hypertrophy, male-pattern baldness
Class: 5-alpha reductase inhibitor, Androgen antagonist, Enzyme inhibitor
Half-life: 5–8 hours
Clinically important, potentially hazardous interactions with: none known

Pregnancy category: N/A (Contra-indicated in women)
Important contra-indications noted in the prescribing guidelines for: nursing mothers; pediatric patients

Skin
Folliculitis [2]
Rash [3]
Urticaria [2]
Xerosis [2]

Hair
Hirsutism [3]

Cardiovascular
Postural hypotension [2]

Central Nervous System
Depression [6]
Headache [2]
Vertigo (dizziness) (7%) [3]

Neuromuscular/Skeletal
Asthenia (fatigue) (5%) [2]
Myalgia/Myopathy (severe) [2]

Endocrine/Metabolic
Gynecomastia (<2%) [15]
Libido decreased (2–10%) [8]
Mastodynia (<2%)
Menstrual irregularities [2]

Genitourinary
Ejaculatory dysfunction [9]
Erectile dysfunction [7]
Impotence (5–19%)
Sexual dysfunction [6]

Other
Adverse effects [6]

FINGOLIMOD

Trade name: Gilenya (Novartis)
Indications: Multiple sclerosis
Class: Immunosuppressant
Half-life: 6–9 days
Clinically important, potentially hazardous interactions with: BCG vaccine, beta blockers, class Ia antiarrhythmics, class III antiarrhythmics, conivaptan, cyproterone, denosumab, digoxin, diltiazem, dronedarone, ketoconazole, leflunomide, live vaccines, natalizumab, PEG-interferon, pimecrolimus, QT prolonging drugs, roflumilast, sipuleucel-T, tacrolimus, tocilizumab, trastuzumab, typhoid vaccine, verapamil, yellow fever vaccine
Pregnancy category: C
Important contra-indications noted in the prescribing guidelines for: nursing mothers; pediatric patients
Note: Contra-indicated in patients with recent (within the last 6 months) occurrence of: myocardial infarction, unstable angina, stroke, transient ischemic attack, decompensated heart failure requiring hospitalization, or Class III/IV heart failure; history or presence of Mobitz Type II 2nd degree or 3rd degree AV block or sick sinus syndrome, unless patient has a pacemaker; baseline QT interval ≥500 ms; or is receiving treatment with Class Ia or Class III anti-arrhythmic drugs.

Skin
Basal cell carcinoma [4]
Eczema (3%)
Herpes (9%) [6]
Herpes simplex [3]
Herpes zoster [3]
Kaposi's sarcoma [2]
Lymphoma [2]
Melanoma [2]
Neoplasms [2]
Pruritus (3%)
Skin cancer [3]
Tinea (4%)
Varicella zoster [5]

Hair
Alopecia (4%)

Cardiovascular
Asystole [2]
Atrial fibrillation [2]
Atrioventricular block [19]
Bradycardia (4%) [23]
Cardiac failure [2]
Cardiotoxicity [3]
Hypertension (6%) [9]

Central Nervous System
Depression (8%)
Encephalopathy [2]
Headache (25%) [10]
Leukoencephalopathy [6]
Migraine (5%)
Paresthesias (5%)
Vertigo (dizziness) (7%)

Neuromuscular/Skeletal
Asthenia (fatigue) (3%) [5]
Back pain (12%) [4]

Gastrointestinal/Hepatic
Diarrhea (12%) [3]
Gastroenteritis (5%)
Hepatotoxicity [10]

Respiratory
Bronchitis (8%)
Cough (10%) [3]
Dyspnea (8%)
Influenza (13%) [3]
Nasopharyngitis [5]
Pulmonary toxicity [4]
Respiratory tract infection [2]
Sinusitis (7%)

Endocrine/Metabolic
ALT increased (14%) [2]
AST increased (14%)
GGT increased (5%)
Weight loss (5%)

Hematologic
Leukopenia (3%)
Lymphocytopenia [3]
Lymphopenia (4%) [10]

Ocular
Macular edema [22]
Ocular pain (3%)
Vision blurred (4%)

Other
Adverse effects [11]
Death [7]
Infection [16]

FLAVOXATE

See: www.drugeruptiondata.com/drug/id/292

FLECAINIDE

Trade name: Tambocor (3M)
Indications: Atrial fibrillation
Class: Antiarrhythmic, Antiarrhythmic class Ic
Half-life: 12–16 hours
Clinically important, potentially hazardous interactions with: acebutolol, amiodarone, amisulpride, amitriptyline, artemether/lumefantrine, boceprevir, cinacalcet, clozapine, cobicistat/elvitegravir/emtricitabine/tenofovir alafenamide, cobicistat/elvitegravir/emtricitabine/tenofovir disoproxil, darifenacin, delavirdine, fosamprenavir, lopinavir, mirabegron, quinine, ritonavir, telaprevir, tipranavir
Pregnancy category: C
Important contra-indications noted in the prescribing guidelines for: nursing mothers; pediatric patients

Skin
 Diaphoresis (<3%)
 Edema (4%)
 Psoriasis [2]
 Rash (<3%)

Cardiovascular
 Arrhythmias [7]
 Atrial fibrillation [3]
 Atrial flutter [2]
 Atrioventricular block [2]
 Bradycardia [4]
 Brugada syndrome [4]
 Bundle branch block [2]
 Cardiotoxicity [3]
 Chest pain (5%)
 Congestive heart failure [2]
 Extrasystoles [2]
 Flushing (<3%)
 Hypotension [2]
 Palpitation (6%)
 QT prolongation [7]
 Supraventricular tachycardia [2]
 Tachycardia [2]
 Torsades de pointes [4]

Central Nervous System
 Headache (10%) [4]
 Hyperesthesia (<10%)
 Neurotoxicity [3]
 Seizures [2]
 Syncope [2]
 Tremor (5%)
 Vertigo (dizziness) (19%) [5]

Neuromuscular/Skeletal
 Asthenia (fatigue) (5–8%)

Gastrointestinal/Hepatic
 Abdominal pain (3%)
 Constipation (4%)
 Diarrhea (<3%) [2]
 Nausea (9%) [3]

Respiratory
 Dyspnea (10%)

Ocular
 Vision blurred [2]
 Visual disturbances (16%) [3]

Other
 Adverse effects [2]

FLIBANSERIN

Trade name: Addyi (Sprout)
Indications: Hypoactive sexual desire disorder in premenopausal women
Class: Serotonin type 1A receptor agonist, Serotonin type 2A receptor antagonist
Half-life: 11 hours
Clinically important, potentially hazardous interactions with: alcohol, amprenavir, atazanavir, boceprevir, carbamazepine, ciprofloxacin, clarithromycin, conivaptan, digoxin, diltiazem, erythromycin, fluconazole, fosamprenavir, grapefruit juice, indinavir, itraconazole, ketoconazole, nefazodone, nelfinavir, phenobarbital, phenytoin, posaconazole, rifabutin, rifampin, rifapentine, ritonavir, saquinavir, St John's wort, telaprevir, telithromycin, verapamil
Pregnancy category: N/A (No data available)
Important contra-indications noted in the prescribing guidelines for: the elderly; nursing mothers; pediatric patients
Warning: HYPOTENSION AND SYNCOPE IN CERTAIN SETTINGS

Mucosal
 Xerostomia (2%)

Central Nervous System
 Anxiety (2%)
 Insomnia (5%) [2]
 Sedation [2]
 Somnolence (drowsiness) (11%) [9]
 Vertigo (dizziness) (2%) [9]

Neuromuscular/Skeletal
 Asthenia (fatigue) (9%) [5]

Gastrointestinal/Hepatic
 Abdominal pain (2%)
 Constipation (2%)
 Nausea (10%) [6]

FLORBETAPIR F18

See: www.drugeruptiondata.com/drug/id/2897

FLOXURIDINE

See: www.drugeruptiondata.com/drug/id/960

FLUCLOXACILLIN

Trade name: Floxapen (Actavis)
Indications: Infections due to sensitive Gram-positive organisms
Class: Antibiotic, beta-lactam
Half-life: 53 minutes
Clinically important, potentially hazardous interactions with: oral contraceptives, probenecid
Pregnancy category: N/A
Important contra-indications noted in the prescribing guidelines for: nursing mothers

Skin
 AGEP [2]

Gastrointestinal/Hepatic
 Hepatotoxicity [21]

Endocrine/Metabolic
 Acidosis [2]

Renal
 Nephrotoxicity [4]

Hematologic
 Anemia [2]

FLUCONAZOLE

Trade name: Diflucan (Pfizer)
Indications: Candidiasis
Class: Antibiotic, triazole, Antifungal, azole, CYP3A4 inhibitor
Half-life: 25–30 hours
Clinically important, potentially hazardous interactions with: alprazolam, amphotericin B, anisindione, anticoagulants, atorvastatin, avanafil, betamethasone, bosentan, celecoxib, citalopram, clobazam, clopidogrel, deflazacort, dicumarol, eluxadoline, eplerenone, erythromycin, flibanserin, irbesartan, ivacaftor, lesinurad, methadone, midazolam, mifepristone, naldemedine, neratinib, nevirapine, olaparib, ospemifene, pantoprazole, phenobarbital, phenytoin, pimecrolimus, propranolol, quetiapine, ramelteon, rifapentine, rilpivirine, ruxolitinib, simeprevir, sonidegib, sulfonylureas, temsirolimus, terbinafine, tipranavir, tofacitinib, trabectedin, triamcinolone, venetoclax, vinblastine, vincristine, warfarin, zidovudine
Pregnancy category: D (fluconazole is pregnancy category C for vaginal candidiasis)
Important contra-indications noted in the prescribing guidelines for: the elderly; nursing mothers

Skin
 AGEP [3]
 Erythema multiforme [3]
 Exfoliative dermatitis [2]
 Fixed eruption [10]
 Hypersensitivity (<4%)
 Rash (2%) [4]
 Stevens-Johnson syndrome [6]
 Toxic epidermal necrolysis [4]

Hair
 Alopecia [4]

Nails
Nail changes [2]
Mucosal
Oral ulceration [2]
Cardiovascular
Hypotension [2]
QT prolongation [7]
Torsades de pointes [11]
Central Nervous System
Dysgeusia (taste perversion) [2]
Headache (2–13%) [3]
Neurotoxicity [2]
Neuromuscular/Skeletal
Rhabdomyolysis [4]
Gastrointestinal/Hepatic
Abdominal pain [2]
Diarrhea [2]
Hepatotoxicity [3]
Nausea (2–7%)
Renal
Renal failure [2]
Other
Adverse effects [5]

FLUCYTOSINE

See: www.drugeruptiondata.com/drug/id/295

FLUDARABINE

Trade names: Fludara (Genzyme), Oforta (Sanofi-Aventis)
Indications: Chronic lymphocytic leukemia (B-cell)
Class: Antimetabolite, Antineoplastic
Half-life: 9 hours
Clinically important, potentially hazardous interactions with: aldesleukin, clofazimine, live vaccines, pentostatin
Pregnancy category: D
Important contra-indications noted in the prescribing guidelines for: nursing mothers; pediatric patients
Note: Severe neurologic effects, including blindness, coma, and death were observed in dose-ranging studies in patients with acute leukemia when fludarabine phosphate was administered at high doses. Instances of life-threatening and sometimes fatal autoimmune hemolytic anemia have been reported after one or more cycles of treatment with fludarabine phosphate.
Warning: CNS TOXICITY, HEMOLYTIC ANEMIA, AND PULMONARY TOXICITY

Skin
Anaphylactoid reactions/Anaphylaxis (<3%)
Diaphoresis (14%)
Edema (8–19%)
Herpes simplex (7–8%)
Herpes zoster [2]
Paraneoplastic pemphigus [4]
Peripheral edema (7%)
Pruritus (<3%)
Rash (4–15%)

Hair
Alopecia (<10%)
Mucosal
Mucositis (2%)
Stomatitis (9%)
Cardiovascular
Angina (6%)
Arrhythmias (<4%)
Chest pain (5%)
Congestive heart failure (<4%)
Myocardial infarction (<4%)
Phlebitis (<3%)
Supraventricular tachycardia (<4%)
Central Nervous System
Aneurysm (<2%)
Anorexia (7–34%)
Cerebrovascular accident (<4%)
Chills (11–19%)
Fever (11–69%) [2]
Headache (3–9%)
Leukoencephalopathy [9]
Neurotoxicity [3]
Pain (5–22%)
Paresthesias (4–12%)
Sleep related disorder (<3%)
Neuromuscular/Skeletal
Asthenia (fatigue) (6–65%)
Back pain (4–9%)
Myalgia/Myopathy (>10%)
Gastrointestinal/Hepatic
Abdominal pain (8–10%)
Cholelithiasis (gallstones) (3%)
Constipation (<3%)
Diarrhea (5–15%)
Esophagitis (3%)
Gastrointestinal bleeding (3–13%) [2]
Hepatotoxicity [2]
Nausea (<36%)
Respiratory
Bronchitis (<9%)
Cough (6–44%)
Dyspnea (<22%)
Flu-like syndrome (5–8%)
Hemoptysis (<6%)
Pharyngitis (9%)
Pneumonia (3–22%) [3]
Pneumonitis (6%)
Pulmonary toxicity [4]
Rhinitis (3–11%)
Sinusitis (<5%)
Upper respiratory tract infection (2–14%)
Endocrine/Metabolic
Hyperglycemia (<6%)
Weight loss (<6%)
Genitourinary
Dysuria (3–4%)
Hematuria (<3%)
Urinary hesitancy (3%)
Urinary tract infection (4–15%)
Hematologic
Anemia [3]
Cytopenia [2]
Febrile neutropenia [2]
Hemolytic anemia [2]
Hemotoxicity [3]
Leukopenia [2]
Myelosuppression [3]
Myelotoxicity [2]

Neutropenia [6]
Sepsis [2]
Thrombocytopenia [4]
Thrombosis (<3%)
Otic
Hearing loss (2–6%)
Ocular
Visual disturbances (3–15%)
Other
Adverse effects [2]
Death [4]
Infection (12–44%) [6]

FLUDEOXYGLUCOSE F18

See: www.drugeruptiondata.com/drug/id/1761

FLUDROCORTISONE

See: www.drugeruptiondata.com/drug/id/1931

FLUMAZENIL

See: www.drugeruptiondata.com/drug/id/297

FLUMETASONE

See: www.drugeruptiondata.com/drug/id/1086

FLUNISOLIDE

See: www.drugeruptiondata.com/drug/id/1087

FLUOCINOLONE

See: www.drugeruptiondata.com/drug/id/1093

FLUOCINONIDE

See: www.drugeruptiondata.com/drug/id/1092

FLUORIDES

Indications: Caries prevention (topical), osteoporosis prevention (oral)
Class: Chemical
Half-life: N/A
Clinically important, potentially hazardous interactions with: caffeine
Pregnancy category: C

Skin
Acneform eruption [2]
Burning [12]
Dermatitis [4]
Edema [2]
Erythema [2]

Hypersensitivity [6]
Necrosis [2]
Pruritus [5]
Toxicity [27]
Urticaria [7]
Mucosal
Oral ulceration [2]
Stomatitis [3]
Central Nervous System
Headache [2]
Neuromuscular/Skeletal
Arthralgia [5]
Bone or joint pain [12]
Skeletal fluorosis [35]
Gastrointestinal/Hepatic
Abdominal pain [2]
Ocular
Cataract [2]
Other
Adverse effects [9]
Death [7]
Tooth fluorosis [39]

FLUOROURACIL

Trade names: 5-fluorouracil (Taj), Carac
(Valeant), Efudex (Valeant), Fluoroplex (Allergan),
Fluorouracil Injection, USP (Bioniche), Tolak (Hill
Dermac)
Indications: Palliative management of malignant
neoplasms especially of the gastrointestinal tract,
breast, liver and pancreas, topical therapy for
actinic keratoses
Class: Antimetabolite, Antineoplastic
Half-life: 8–20 minutes
**Clinically important, potentially hazardous
interactions with:** aldesleukin, bromelain,
cimetidine, granulocyte colony-stimulating factor
(G-CSF), metronidazole, tinidazole
Pregnancy category: X
**Important contra-indications noted in the
prescribing guidelines for:** nursing mothers;
pediatric patients
Note: Contra-indicated in patients with
dihydropyrimidine dehydrogenase deficiency.
Tolak cream contains peanut oil and should be
used with caution in peanut-sensitive individuals.

Skin
Acneform eruption [3]
Acral erythema [4]
Actinic keratoses [4]
Anaphylactoid reactions/Anaphylaxis [2]
Dermatitis (>10%) [4]
Eczema [2]
Edema [2]
Erythema [4]
Erythema multiforme [3]
Exanthems (<10%) [3]
Hand–foot syndrome (<38%) [54]
Lupus erythematosus [6]
Palmar–plantar pigmentation [2]
Peripheral edema [2]
Photosensitivity [3]
Pigmentation [11]
Pruritus [4]
Radiation recall dermatitis [3]

Rash [8]
Recall reaction [3]
Seborrheic dermatitis [3]
Toxicity [4]
Ulcerations [2]
Xerosis (<10%) [2]
Hair
Alopecia (>10%) [16]
Nails
Nail pigmentation [3]
Paronychia [2]
Mucosal
Epistaxis (nosebleed) [2]
Mucosal inflammation [2]
Mucositis (<79%) [15]
Oral mucositis [7]
Oral ulceration [2]
Stomatitis (>10%) [23]
Tongue pigmentation [2]
Cardiovascular
Angina [9]
Bradycardia [2]
Cardiac failure [5]
Cardiomyopathy [4]
Cardiotoxicity [13]
Hypertension [10]
Myocardial infarction [4]
QT prolongation [3]
Thromboembolism [2]
Venous thromboembolism [2]
Ventricular tachycardia [2]
Central Nervous System
Anorexia [9]
Dysgeusia (taste perversion) [2]
Encephalopathy [3]
Fever [5]
Headache [2]
Insomnia [2]
Leukoencephalopathy [27]
Neurotoxicity [12]
Peripheral neuropathy [4]
Vertigo (dizziness) [2]
Neuromuscular/Skeletal
Asthenia (fatigue) [18]
Gastrointestinal/Hepatic
Abdominal pain [4]
Constipation [3]
Diarrhea [31]
Hepatotoxicity [7]
Nausea [24]
Vomiting [19]
Respiratory
Dysphonia [2]
Pulmonary embolism [2]
Endocrine/Metabolic
Acidosis [2]
ALP increased [2]
ALT increased [2]
AST increased [2]
Hyperammonemia [3]
Hyperglycemia [2]
Hypocalcemia [2]
Hypokalemia [3]
Hypomagnesemia [3]
Hyponatremia [3]
Serum creatinine increased [2]
SIADH [4]
Weight loss [2]

Renal
Proteinuria [4]
Hematologic
Anemia [19]
Febrile neutropenia [15]
Hemolytic uremic syndrome [3]
Leukopenia [16]
Lymphopenia [2]
Myelosuppression [4]
Neutropenia [42]
Thrombocytopenia [21]
Ocular
Ectropion [2]
Epiphora [2]
Ocular inflammation [2]
Local
Application-site edema [2]
Application-site pruritus [3]
Injection-site burning [2]
Injection-site desquamation [4]
Injection-site edema [3]
Injection-site erythema [4]
Injection-site necrosis [2]
Injection-site pain [2]
Injection-site ulceration [2]
Other
Adverse effects [8]
Death [4]
Infection [6]
Side effects [2]

FLUOXETINE

Trade names: Prozac (Lilly), Sarafem (Warner
Chilcott), Symbyax (Lilly)
Indications: Depression, obsessive-compulsive
disorder
Class: Antidepressant, Selective serotonin
reuptake inhibitor (SSRI)
Half-life: 2–3 days
**Clinically important, potentially hazardous
interactions with:** alprazolam, amoxapine,
amphetamines, astemizole, clarithromycin,
clopidogrel, clozapine, desipramine,
deutetrabenazine, dexibuprofen,
dextroamphetamine, diethylpropion, droperidol,
duloxetine, erythromycin, haloperidol,
iloperidone, imipramine, insulin aspart, insulin
degludec, insulin glargine, insulin glulisine,
isocarboxazid, linezolid, lithium, MAO inhibitors,
mazindol, meperidine, methamphetamine,
midazolam, moclobemide, nifedipine,
nortriptyline, olanzapine, PEG-interferon,
phendimetrazine, phenelzine, phentermine,
phenylpropanolamine, phenytoin, pimozide,
propranolol, pseudoephedrine, rasagiline,
risperidone, selegiline, serotonin agonists,
sibutramine, St John's wort, sumatriptan,
sympathomimetics, tramadol, tranylcypromine,
trazodone, tricyclic antidepressants,
troleandomycin, tryptophan, valbenazine,
vortioxetine, zolmitriptan
Pregnancy category: C
**Important contra-indications noted in the
prescribing guidelines for:** the elderly; nursing
mothers; pediatric patients
Note: Increased risk of suicidal thinking and
behavior in children, adolescents, and young

adults taking antidepressants for Major Depressive Disorder (MDD) and other psychiatric disorders. Sarafem is not approved for use in pediatric patients with MDD and obsessive compulsive disorder. Symbyax is not approved for use in children and adolescents.

Symbyax is fluoxetine and olanzapine.

Warning: SUICIDAL THOUGHTS AND BEHAVIORS

Skin
Diaphoresis (8%) [2]
Exanthems (4%) [7]
Mycosis fungoides [2]
Phototoxicity [2]
Pruritus (2%) [4]
Pseudolymphoma [4]
Rash (6%) [3]
Raynaud's phenomenon [2]
Serum sickness-like reaction [2]
Toxic epidermal necrolysis [2]
Toxicity [2]
Urticaria (4%) [5]
Vasculitis [2]

Hair
Alopecia [7]

Mucosal
Black tongue [2]
Oral ulceration [2]
Xerostomia (12%) [7]

Cardiovascular
Flushing (<2%)
Orthostatic hypotension [2]
QT prolongation [7]
Torsades de pointes [2]

Central Nervous System
Akathisia [6]
Amnesia [2]
Delirium [3]
Depression [2]
Dysgeusia (taste perversion) (2%)
Extrapyramidal symptoms [3]
Hallucinations [3]
Headache (<27%) [3]
Neuroleptic malignant syndrome [2]
Paresthesias [2]
Restless legs syndrome [4]
Serotonin syndrome [13]
Somnolence (drowsiness) [4]
Suicidal ideation [11]
Tremor (2–10%)
Vertigo (dizziness) [3]

Neuromuscular/Skeletal
Asthenia (fatigue) [2]
Rhabdomyolysis [2]

Gastrointestinal/Hepatic
Nausea [3]

Endocrine/Metabolic
Gynecomastia [2]
SIADH [20]
Weight gain [4]

Genitourinary
Priapism [2]
Sexual dysfunction [5]

Ocular
Hallucinations, visual [4]

Other
Adverse effects [3]
Bruxism [4]
Death [3]

FLUOXYMESTERONE

See: www.drugeruptiondata.com/drug/id/300

FLUPHENAZINE

Trade name: Prolixin (Bristol-Myers Squibb)
Indications: Psychoses
Class: Antipsychotic, Phenothiazine
Half-life: 84–96 hours
Clinically important, potentially hazardous interactions with: antihistamines, arsenic, chlorpheniramine, clozapine, dofetilide, evening primrose, quinolones, sparfloxacin
Pregnancy category: C
Important contra-indications noted in the prescribing guidelines for: nursing mothers

Skin
Rash (<10%)
Vitiligo [2]

Central Nervous System
Neuroleptic malignant syndrome [14]
Parkinsonism [3]
Somnolence (drowsiness) [4]

Neuromuscular/Skeletal
Dystonia [3]

Endocrine/Metabolic
Galactorrhea (<10%)
Gynecomastia (<10%)
Mastodynia (<10%)

Genitourinary
Priapism [2]

Ocular
Maculopathy [3]

FLUPREDNISOLONE

See: www.drugeruptiondata.com/drug/id/1941

FLURAZEPAM

See: www.drugeruptiondata.com/drug/id/302

FLURBIPROFEN

Trade name: Ansaid (Pfizer)
Indications: Rheumatoid arthritis, osteoarthritis
Class: Non-steroidal anti-inflammatory (NSAID)
Half-life: 3–4 hours
Clinically important, potentially hazardous interactions with: ACE inhibitors, aspirin, furosemide, lithium, methotrexate

Pregnancy category: C
Important contra-indications noted in the prescribing guidelines for: the elderly; nursing mothers
Note: NSAIDs may cause an increased risk of serious cardiovascular and gastrointestinal adverse events, which can be fatal. This risk may increase with duration of use.
Elderly patients are at greater risk for serious gastrointestinal events.
Warning: CARDIOVASCULAR AND GASTROINTESTINAL RISKS

Skin
Eczema (3–9%)
Edema (3–9%)
Exanthems [3]
Fixed eruption [2]
Hypersensitivity [4]
Pruritus (<5%)
Rash (<3%)

Mucosal
Oral lichenoid eruption [2]

Central Nervous System
Headache [4]

Renal
Nephrotoxicity [2]

Other
Side effects (6%) [2]

FLUTAMIDE

Indications: Metastatic prostate carcinoma
Class: Androgen antagonist
Half-life: 8–10 hours
Clinically important, potentially hazardous interactions with: none known
Pregnancy category: D (not indicated for use in women)
Important contra-indications noted in the prescribing guidelines for: nursing mothers; pediatric patients
Warning: HEPATIC INJURY

Skin
Edema (4%)
Hot flashes (61%)
Photosensitivity [9]
Rash (3%)
Xerosis [2]

Central Nervous System
Paresthesias (<10%)

Gastrointestinal/Hepatic
Hepatotoxicity [13]

Endocrine/Metabolic
Gynecomastia (9%) [4]
Pseudoporphyria [3]

Local
Injection-site irritation (3%)

FLUTICASONE FUROATE

See: www.drugeruptiondata.com/drug/id/3657

FLUTICASONE PROPIONATE

See: www.drugeruptiondata.com/drug/id/1107

FLUVASTATIN

Trade name: Lescol (Novartis)
Indications: Hypercholesterolemia
Class: HMG-CoA reductase inhibitor, Statin
Half-life: 1.2 hours
Clinically important, potentially hazardous interactions with: azithromycin, bosentan, ciprofibrate, clarithromycin, colchicine, cyclosporine, delavirdine, elbasvir & grazoprevir, erythromycin, gemfibrozil, imatinib, mifepristone, red rice yeast
Pregnancy category: X
Important contra-indications noted in the prescribing guidelines for: nursing mothers

Skin
Lupus erythematosus [2]
Rash (3%)

Central Nervous System
Headache (9%)

Neuromuscular/Skeletal
Asthenia (fatigue) (3%)
Myalgia/Myopathy (5%) [4]
Rhabdomyolysis [13]

Gastrointestinal/Hepatic
Diarrhea (5%)
Dyspepsia (8%)
Hepatotoxicity [5]

Respiratory
Sinusitis (3%)
Upper respiratory tract infection (16%)

Endocrine/Metabolic
Creatine phosphokinase increased [2]

Other
Allergic reactions (3%)

FLUVOXAMINE

Trade name: Luvox (Solvay)
Indications: Obsessive-compulsive disorder, depression
Class: Antidepressant, CYP1A2 inhibitor, CYP3A4 inhibitor, Selective serotonin reuptake inhibitor (SSRI)
Half-life: 15 hours
Clinically important, potentially hazardous interactions with: alosetron, alprazolam, aminophylline, amphetamines, anagrelide, asenapine, astemizole, bendamustine, clobazam, clopidogrel, clozapine, dextroamphetamine, diethylpropion, droperidol, duloxetine, isocarboxazid, linezolid, MAO inhibitors, mazindol, methadone, methamphetamine, neratinib, olanzapine, oxtriphylline, phendimetrazine, phenelzine, phentermine, phenylpropanolamine, pirfenidone, propranolol, pseudoephedrine, ramelteon, rasagiline, roflumilast, ropivacaine, selegiline, sibutramine, St

John's wort, sumatriptan, sympathomimetics, tacrine, tasimelteon, tizanidine, tramadol, tranylcypromine, trazodone, troleandomycin, tryptophan, zolmitriptan
Pregnancy category: C
Important contra-indications noted in the prescribing guidelines for: the elderly; nursing mothers; pediatric patients
Warning: SUICIDALITY AND ANTIDEPRESSANT DRUGS

Skin
Diaphoresis (<7%)
Photosensitivity [3]

Mucosal
Oral lesions (10%)
Xerostomia (<14%) [2]

Cardiovascular
Chest pain (3%)
Palpitation (3%)
QT prolongation [3]

Central Nervous System
Anorexia (6–14%)
Anxiety (5–8%)
Dysgeusia (taste perversion) (3%)
Headache (22–35%)
Insomnia (21–35%)
Neuroleptic malignant syndrome [2]
Pain (10%)
Seizures [2]
Serotonin syndrome [6]
Somnolence (drowsiness) (22–27%)
Tremor (5–8%)
Vertigo (dizziness) (11–15%)
Yawning (2–5%)

Neuromuscular/Skeletal
Asthenia (fatigue) (14–26%) [3]
Myalgia/Myopathy (5%)

Gastrointestinal/Hepatic
Diarrhea (16–18%)
Dyspepsia (8–10%)
Nausea (34–40%)

Respiratory
Pharyngitis (6%)
Upper respiratory tract infection (9%)

Endocrine/Metabolic
Galactorrhea [2]
Libido decreased (2–10%)
SIADH [2]

Genitourinary
Ejaculatory dysfunction (8–11%)

FOLIC ACID

Synonyms: folacin; folate; vitamin B9
Indications: Anemias
Class: Vitamin
Half-life: N/A
Clinically important, potentially hazardous interactions with: balsalazide, estradiol, raltitrexed
Pregnancy category: A

Skin
Anaphylactoid reactions/Anaphylaxis [3]
Exanthems [2]

Pruritus [2]
Urticaria [2]

FOLLITROPIN ALFA/ BETA

See: www.drugeruptiondata.com/drug/id/1811

FOMEPIZOLE

See: www.drugeruptiondata.com/drug/id/941

FOMIVIRSEN

See: www.drugeruptiondata.com/drug/id/1202

FONDAPARINUX

Trade name: Arixtra (Mylan)
Indications: Prophylaxis of deep vein thrombosis
Class: Anticoagulant, Heparinoid
Half-life: 17–21 hours
Clinically important, potentially hazardous interactions with: abciximab, anagrelide, anticoagulants, cilostazol, clopidogrel, dabigatran, dipyridamole, eptifibatide, nandrolone, salicylates, ticlopidine, tirofiban
Pregnancy category: B
Important contra-indications noted in the prescribing guidelines for: the elderly; nursing mothers; pediatric patients
Warning: SPINAL/EPIDURAL HEMATOMAS

Skin
Bullous dermatitis (3%)
Edema (9%)
Hematoma [2]
Hypersensitivity [4]
Purpura (4%)
Rash (8%)

Central Nervous System
Pain (2%)

Gastrointestinal/Hepatic
Hepatotoxicity [2]

Local
Injection-site bleeding (<10%)
Injection-site pruritus (<10%)

FORMOTEROL

Trade names: Dulera (Merck Sharpe & Dohme), Foradil (Novartis), Perforomist (Mylan), Symbicort (AstraZeneca)
Indications: Asthma, bronchospasm
Class: Beta-2 adrenergic agonist, Bronchodilator
Half-life: 10–14 hours
Clinically important, potentially hazardous interactions with: beta blockers, clomipramine, desipramine, doxepin, imipramine, iobenguane, nortriptyline, protriptyline, trimipramine

Pregnancy category: C
Important contra-indications noted in the prescribing guidelines for: nursing mothers; pediatric patients
Note: Dulera is formoterol and mometasone; Symbicort is formoterol and budesonide.
Warning: ASTHMA-RELATED DEATH

Skin
Pruritus (2%)
Mucosal
Xerostomia (<3%) [3]
Cardiovascular
Chest pain (2%)
Central Nervous System
Anxiety (2%)
Fever (2%)
Headache [8]
Insomnia (2%)
Tremor (2%) [6]
Vertigo (dizziness) (2–3%) [2]
Neuromuscular/Skeletal
Back pain (4%)
Cramps (2%)
Leg cramps (2%)
Gastrointestinal/Hepatic
Diarrhea (5%) [2]
Nausea (5%)
Vomiting (2%)
Respiratory
Asthma (exacerbation) [3]
Bronchitis (5%)
Cough [5]
Dysphonia [2]
Dyspnea (2%) [2]
Nasopharyngitis [7]
Pharyngitis (4%) [2]
Pneumonia [2]
Rhinitis [2]
Upper respiratory tract infection (7%) [3]
Genitourinary
Urinary tract infection [2]
Other
Adverse effects [2]
Death [2]
Infection (17%)

FOSAMPRENAVIR

Trade name: Lexiva (ViiV)
Indications: HIV infections (in combination with other antiretrovirals)
Class: Antiretroviral, HIV-1 protease inhibitor
Half-life: 7.7 hours
Clinically important, potentially hazardous interactions with: amiodarone, atorvastatin, avanafil, bepridil, carbamazepine, darifenacin, delavirdine, dihydroergotamine, efavirenz, etravirine, flecainide, flibanserin, itraconazole, ketoconazole, lidocaine, lopinavir, lovastatin, midazolam, mifepristone, nevirapine, olaparib, phenobarbital, phenytoin, pimozide, posaconazole, propafenone, quinidine, quinine, rifabutin, rifampin, rilpivirine, ritonavir, rivaroxaban, rosuvastatin, sildenafil, simeprevir, simvastatin, St John's wort, tadalafil, telaprevir,

telithromycin, tipranavir, triazolam, vardenafil, warfarin
Pregnancy category: C
Important contra-indications noted in the prescribing guidelines for: the elderly; nursing mothers; pediatric patients
Note: Fosamprenavir is a sulfonamide and can be absorbed systemically. Sulfonamides can produce severe, possibly fatal, reactions such as toxic epidermal necrolysis and Stevens-Johnson syndrome.
Fosamprenavir is a prodrug of amprenavir (see separate entry).

Skin
Hypersensitivity [2]
Pruritus (7%)
Rash (~19%) [5]
Central Nervous System
Depression (8%)
Headache (19%)
Paresthesias (oral) (2%)
Neuromuscular/Skeletal
Asthenia (fatigue) (10%)
Gastrointestinal/Hepatic
Abdominal pain (5%)
Diarrhea [2]
Hepatotoxicity [2]
Vomiting [2]
Respiratory
Bronchitis [2]
Cough [2]
Nasopharyngitis [3]
Rhinitis [2]
Upper respiratory tract infection [2]
Other
Adverse effects [3]

FOSCARNET

See: www.drugeruptiondata.com/drug/id/308

FOSFOMYCIN

See: www.drugeruptiondata.com/drug/id/309

FOSINOPRIL

Trade name: Monopril (Bristol-Myers Squibb)
Indications: Hypertension, heart failure
Class: Angiotensin-converting enzyme (ACE) inhibitor, Antihypertensive, Vasodilator
Half-life: 12 hours
Clinically important, potentially hazardous interactions with: alcohol, aldesleukin, allopurinol, alpha blockers, alprostadil, amifostine, amiloride, angiotensin II receptor blocking agents, antacids, antidiabetics, antihypertensives, antipsychotics, anxiolytics and hypnotics, azathioprine, baclofen, beta blockers, calcium channel blockers, clonidine, corticosteroids, cyclosporine, diazoxide, diuretics, estrogens, general anesthetics, gold & gold compounds, heparins, hydralazine, hypotensives, insulin, levodopa, lithium, MAO inhibitors, metformin,

methyldopa, minoxidil, moxisylyte, moxonidine, nitrates, nitroprusside, NSAIDs, pentoxifylline, phosphodiesterase 5 inhibitors, potassium salts, prostacyclin analogues, rituximab, sirolimus, spironolactone, sulfonylureas, temsirolimus, tizanidine, tolvaptan, triamterene, trimethoprim
Pregnancy category: D (category C in first trimester; category D in second and third trimesters)
Important contra-indications noted in the prescribing guidelines for: nursing mothers
Warning: USE IN PREGNANCY

Skin
Angioedema [3]
Respiratory
Cough [3]

FOSPHENYTOIN

See: www.drugeruptiondata.com/drug/id/311

FROVATRIPTAN

See: www.drugeruptiondata.com/drug/id/856

FULVESTRANT

See: www.drugeruptiondata.com/drug/id/905

FURAZOLIDONE

See: www.drugeruptiondata.com/drug/id/312

FUROSEMIDE

Trade name: Lasix (Sanofi-Aventis)
Indications: Edema
Class: Diuretic, loop
Half-life: ~2 hours
Clinically important, potentially hazardous interactions with: acemetacin, aliskiren, amikacin, amyl nitrite, celecoxib, diclofenac, digoxin, flurbiprofen, gentamicin, hyaluronic acid, hydrocortisone, kanamycin, mivacurium, neomycin, piroxicam, probenecid, streptomycin, tobramycin, tolmetin
Pregnancy category: C
Important contra-indications noted in the prescribing guidelines for: the elderly; nursing mothers; pediatric patients
Note: Furosemide is a sulfonamide and can be absorbed systemically. Sulfonamides can produce severe, possibly fatal, reactions such as toxic epidermal necrolysis and Stevens-Johnson syndrome.

Skin
AGEP [2]
Anaphylactoid reactions/Anaphylaxis [2]
Bullous dermatitis [16]
Bullous pemphigoid [11]
Erythema multiforme [3]

Exanthems (12%) [7]
Exfoliative dermatitis [3]
Lichenoid eruption [2]
Linear IgA bullous dermatosis [2]
Photosensitivity (<10%) [2]
Phototoxicity [4]
Pruritus [2]
Purpura [3]
Pustules [3]
Stevens-Johnson syndrome [3]
Sweet's syndrome [2]
Urticaria [3]

Vasculitis [7]

Mucosal
Xerostomia [3]

Cardiovascular
Hypotension [2]

Gastrointestinal/Hepatic
Pancreatitis [3]

Endocrine/Metabolic
Porphyria cutanea tarda [3]

Otic
Hearing loss [2]
Ototoxicity [3]

Other
Adverse effects [3]
Side effects [2]

FUSIDIC ACID

See: www.drugeruptiondata.com/drug/id/1142

Litt's Drug Eruption & Reaction Manual © 2018 by Taylor & Francis Group, LLC

GABAPENTIN

Trade names: Horizant (GSK), Neurontin (Pfizer)
Indications: Postherpetic neuralgia in adults, seizures
Class: Anticonvulsant
Half-life: 5–7 hours
Clinically important, potentially hazardous interactions with: none known
Pregnancy category: C
Important contra-indications noted in the prescribing guidelines for: the elderly; nursing mothers; pediatric patients

---

Skin
 Anticonvulsant hypersensitivity syndrome [2]
 Bullous pemphigoid [2]
 Edema [5]
 Exanthems [2]
 Peripheral edema (8%) [12]
 Rash [2]
 Stevens-Johnson syndrome [2]
Hair
 Alopecia [2]
Mucosal
 Xerostomia (5%)
Central Nervous System
 Aggression [2]
 Coma [3]
 Confusion [3]
 Delirium [2]
 Fever (10%)
 Gait instability (2%) [4]
 Headache (3%) [9]
 Incoordination (2%)
 Neurotoxicity [4]
 Psychosis [2]
 Sedation [5]
 Seizures [4]
 Somnolence (drowsiness) (21%) [38]
 Tremor [3]
 Vertigo (dizziness) (17–28%) [49]
Neuromuscular/Skeletal
 Asthenia (fatigue) (6%) [13]
 Ataxia (3%) [10]
 Dystonia [2]
 Myalgia/Myopathy [4]
 Myasthenia gravis [3]
 Myoclonus [5]
 Rhabdomyolysis [4]
Gastrointestinal/Hepatic
 Abdominal pain (3%)
 Constipation (4%) [2]
 Diarrhea (6%)
 Flatulence (2%) [2]
 Nausea (4%) [5]
 Vomiting (3%) [3]
Respiratory
 Respiratory depression [2]
Endocrine/Metabolic
 Weight gain (2%) [8]
Genitourinary
 Sexual dysfunction [5]
Otic
 Hearing loss [2]

Ocular
 Diplopia [2]
 Hallucinations, visual [2]
 Nystagmus [2]
 Vision blurred (3%)
Other
 Adverse effects [7]
 Infection (5%)

GADOBENATE

See: www.drugeruptiondata.com/drug/id/3237

GADOBUTROL

See: www.drugeruptiondata.com/drug/id/1289

GADODIAMIDE

See: www.drugeruptiondata.com/drug/id/1063

GADOFOSVESET

See: www.drugeruptiondata.com/drug/id/1259

GADOPENTETATE

See: www.drugeruptiondata.com/drug/id/3207

GADOTERIDOL

See: www.drugeruptiondata.com/drug/id/3267

GADOVERSETAMIDE

See: www.drugeruptiondata.com/drug/id/3257

GADOXETATE

See: www.drugeruptiondata.com/drug/id/1390

GALANTAMINE

Trade names: Razadyne (Janssen), Reminyl (Janssen)
Indications: Alzheimer's disease
Class: Acetylcholinesterase inhibitor, Cholinesterase inhibitor
Half-life: ~7 hours
Clinically important, potentially hazardous interactions with: bethanechol, cimetidine, donepezil, edrophonium, paroxetine hydrochloride, physostigmine, pilocarpine, rivastigmine, succinylcholine, tacrine

Pregnancy category: C
Important contra-indications noted in the prescribing guidelines for: nursing mothers; pediatric patients
Note: Originally derived from snowdrop (*Galanthus* sp) bulbs.

Skin
 Peripheral edema (>2%)
 Purpura (>2%)
Cardiovascular
 Bradycardia (2%) [5]
 QT prolongation [5]
Central Nervous System
 Anorexia (7–9%) [2]
 Depression (7%)
 Headache (8%) [2]
 Insomnia (5%)
 Somnolence (drowsiness) (4%)
 Syncope (2%) [3]
 Tremor (3%)
 Vertigo (dizziness) (9%) [4]
Neuromuscular/Skeletal
 Asthenia (fatigue) (5%)
Gastrointestinal/Hepatic
 Abdominal pain (5%)
 Diarrhea (6–12%) [5]
 Dyspepsia (5%)
 Nausea (6–24%) [6]
 Vomiting (4–13%) [6]
Respiratory
 Rhinitis (4%)
 Upper respiratory tract infection (>2%)
Endocrine/Metabolic
 Weight loss (5–7%)
Genitourinary
 Hematuria (3%)
 Urinary tract infection (8%)
Hematologic
 Anemia (3%)
Other
 Adverse effects [3]

GALSULFASE

See: www.drugeruptiondata.com/drug/id/1115

GANCICLOVIR

See: www.drugeruptiondata.com/drug/id/315

GANIRELIX

See: www.drugeruptiondata.com/drug/id/316

GATIFLOXACIN

See: www.drugeruptiondata.com/drug/id/317

GEFITINIB

Trade name: Iressa (AstraZeneca)
Indications: Advanced non-small cell lung cancer
Class: Antineoplastic, Biologic, Epidermal growth factor receptor (EGFR) inhibitor, Tyrosine kinase inhibitor
Half-life: 48 hours
Clinically important, potentially hazardous interactions with: antifungals, BCG vaccine, boceprevir, carbamazepine, cardiac glycosides, clozapine, conivaptan, CYP3A4 inhibitors and inducers, dasatinib, deferasirox, denosumab, echinacea, efavirenz, grapefruit juice, itraconazole, leflunomide, natalizumab, phenobarbital, phenytoin, pimecrolimus, ranitidine, rifampin, rifapentine, sipuleucel-T, St John's wort, tacrolimus, topotecan, trastuzumab, vaccines, vitamin K antagonists, voriconazole, warfarin
Pregnancy category: D
Important contra-indications noted in the prescribing guidelines for: nursing mothers; pediatric patients

Skin
Acneform eruption (25–33%) [32]
Desquamation (39%) [2]
Exanthems [3]
Folliculitis [4]
Hand–foot syndrome [2]
Papulopustular eruption [3]
Peripheral edema (2%)
Pruritus (8–9%) [5]
Rash (43–54%) [63]
Seborrhea [2]
Toxicity [10]
Ulcerations [2]
Xerosis (13–26%) [12]

Hair
Alopecia [6]
Hypertrichosis [2]

Nails
Nail changes (17%)
Paronychia (6%) [13]
Pyogenic granuloma [2]

Mucosal
Mucositis [4]
Stomatitis [7]

Cardiovascular
Hypertension [2]

Central Nervous System
Anorexia (7–10%) [2]

Neuromuscular/Skeletal
Asthenia (fatigue) [11]

Gastrointestinal/Hepatic
Abdominal pain [3]
Diarrhea (48–67%) [37]
Gastrointestinal perforation [2]
Hepatotoxicity [26]
Nausea (13–18%) [9]
Vomiting (9–12%) [5]

Respiratory
Dyspnea (2%)
Pneumonia [2]
Pneumonitis [4]
Pulmonary toxicity [16]

Endocrine/Metabolic
ALT increased [7]
Appetite decreased [2]
AST increased [6]
Dehydration [2]
Weight loss (3–5%)

Genitourinary
Cystitis [2]

Renal
Nephrotoxicity [2]

Hematologic
Anemia [4]
Neutropenia [6]
Thrombocytopenia [3]

Ocular
Amblyopia (2%)
Blepharitis [2]
Conjunctivitis [2]

Other
Adverse effects [11]
Death [8]

GEMCITABINE

Trade name: Gemzar (Lilly)
Indications: Pancreatic carcinoma as a single agent, ovarian cancer (with carboplatin), breast cancer (with paclitaxel), non-small cell lung cancer (with cisplatin)
Class: Antimetabolite, Antineoplastic
Half-life: 42–94 minutes for short infusions; 4–11 hours for longer infusions
Clinically important, potentially hazardous interactions with: aldesleukin
Pregnancy category: D
Important contra-indications noted in the prescribing guidelines for: nursing mothers; pediatric patients

Skin
Acneform eruption [3]
Bullous dermatitis [2]
Cellulitis [5]
Dermatitis [6]
Eczema (13%)
Edema (13%) [4]
Exanthems [2]
Hand–foot syndrome [19]
Hypersensitivity [3]
Livedo reticularis [2]
Necrosis [2]
Peripheral edema (20%) [4]
Petechiae (16%)
Pruritus (13%) [2]
Radiation recall dermatitis (<74%) [17]
Rash (30%) [35]
Raynaud's phenomenon [3]
Thrombocytopenic purpura [6]
Toxic epidermal necrolysis [3]
Toxicity [5]
Vasculitis [3]

Hair
Alopecia (15%) [15]

Mucosal
Mucositis [7]
Stomatitis (11%) [13]

Cardiovascular
Arrhythmias [3]
Atrial fibrillation [4]
Capillary leak syndrome [9]
Cardiotoxicity [3]
Hypertension [3]
Hypotension [2]
Myocardial infarction [3]
Thromboembolism [2]
Venous thromboembolism [4]

Central Nervous System
Anorexia [11]
Fever (41%) [13]
Leukoencephalopathy [4]
Neurotoxicity [10]
Pain [2]
Paresthesias (10%) [2]
Peripheral neuropathy [5]
Somnolence (drowsiness) (11%)

Neuromuscular/Skeletal
Asthenia (fatigue) (18%) [44]
Myalgia/Myopathy (>10%) [6]

Gastrointestinal/Hepatic
Abdominal pain [2]
Cholangitis [2]
Constipation [3]
Diarrhea (19%) [25]
Gastrointestinal bleeding [2]
Hepatic disorder [2]
Hepatotoxicity [11]
Nausea (69%) [25]
Vomiting (69%) [20]

Respiratory
Dyspnea (10–23%) [2]
Flu-like syndrome (19%) [2]
Pneumonitis [5]
Pulmonary toxicity [11]

Endocrine/Metabolic
ALT increased [6]
Appetite decreased [2]
AST increased [6]
Dehydration [2]
Hypomagnesemia [7]
Hyponatremia [2]

Genitourinary
Hematuria (30%)

Renal
Nephrotoxicity [5]
Renal failure [2]

Hematologic
Anemia (70%) [38]
Febrile neutropenia [17]
Hemolytic uremic syndrome [32]
Hemotoxicity [6]
Leukocytopenia [3]
Leukopenia (62%) [24]
Myelosuppression [7]
Myelotoxicity [3]
Neutropenia (61%) [87]
Thrombocytopenia (30%) [63]
Thrombosis [3]
Thrombotic microangiopathy [4]

Local
Injection-site reactions (4%)

Other
Adverse effects [9]
Allergic reactions (4%)

Death [11]
Infection (16%) [9]

GEMEPROST

See: www.drugeruptiondata.com/drug/id/1375

GEMFIBROZIL

Trade name: Lopid (Pfizer)
Indications: Hyperlipidemia
Class: Fibrate, Lipid regulator
Half-life: 2 hours
Clinically important, potentially hazardous interactions with: atorvastatin, bexarotene, colchicine, cyclosporine, dasabuvir/ombitasvir/paritaprevir/ritonavir, dicumarol, eluxadoline, enzalutamide, ezetimibe, fluvastatin, interferon alfa, lovastatin, nicotinic acid, paclitaxel, pioglitazone, pitavastatin, pravastatin, repaglinide, rosiglitazone, rosuvastatin, roxithromycin, selexipag, simvastatin, treprostinil, warfarin
Pregnancy category: C
Important contra-indications noted in the prescribing guidelines for: nursing mothers; pediatric patients
Note: Contra-indicated in patients with preexisting gallbladder disease.

Skin
Eczema (2%)
Exanthems (3%) [2]
Psoriasis [3]
Rash (2%)

Central Nervous System
Headache [3]

Neuromuscular/Skeletal
Asthenia (fatigue) (2%)
Compartment syndrome [2]
Myalgia/Myopathy [5]
Rhabdomyolysis [35]

Gastrointestinal/Hepatic
Abdominal pain (10%)
Dyspepsia (20%)
Hepatotoxicity [2]
Pancreatitis [2]

Other
Death [2]

GEMIFLOXACIN

See: www.drugeruptiondata.com/drug/id/967

GEMTUZUMAB

See: www.drugeruptiondata.com/drug/id/320

GENTAMICIN

Trade names: Garamycin (Schering), Genoptic (Allergan)
Indications: Various infections caused by susceptible organisms
Class: Antibiotic, aminoglycoside
Half-life: 2–4 hours
Clinically important, potentially hazardous interactions with: adefovir, aldesleukin, aminoglycosides, atracurium, bumetanide, carbenicillin, cephalexin, cephalothin, cobicistat/elvitegravir/emtricitabine/tenofovir alafenamide, doxacurium, ethacrynic acid, furosemide, methoxyflurane, non-polarizing muscle relaxants, pancuronium, pipecuronium, polypeptide antibiotics, rocuronium, succinylcholine, teicoplanin, torsemide, tubocurarine, vecuronium
Pregnancy category: C
Important contra-indications noted in the prescribing guidelines for: the elderly; nursing mothers
Note: Aminoglycosides may cause neurotoxicity and/or nephrotoxicity.

Skin
Anaphylactoid reactions/Anaphylaxis [2]
Dermatitis [8]
Edema (<10%)
Erythema (<10%)
Exanthems [5]
Photosensitivity [2]
Pruritus (<10%)

Hair
Alopecia [2]

Renal
Fanconi syndrome [2]
Nephrotoxicity [15]

Otic
Ototoxicity [12]
Tinnitus [4]

Local
Injection-site necrosis [5]

GESTRINONE

See: www.drugeruptiondata.com/drug/id/1397

GLATIRAMER

Synonym: copolymer-1
Trade names: Copaxone (Teva), Glatopa (Novartis)
Indications: Multiple sclerosis
Class: Immunomodulator
Half-life: N/A
Clinically important, potentially hazardous interactions with: Hemophilus B vaccine
Pregnancy category: B
Important contra-indications noted in the prescribing guidelines for: the elderly; nursing mothers; pediatric patients

Skin
Acneform eruption (>2%)
Anaphylactoid reactions/Anaphylaxis [3]
Cyst (2%)
Diaphoresis (15%)
Ecchymoses (8%)
Eczema (8%)
Edema (8%)
Erythema (4%)
Facial edema (6%)
Herpes simplex (4%)
Hyperhidrosis (15%)
Hypersensitivity (3%)
Lipoatrophy [3]
Nicolau syndrome [3]
Nodular eruption (2%)
Panniculitis [2]
Peripheral edema (7%)
Pruritus (4%)
Purpura (8%)
Rash (18%)

Hair
Alopecia (>2%)

Nails
Nail changes (>2%)

Mucosal
Oral vesiculation (6%)
Xerostomia (>2%)

Cardiovascular
Chest pain (13%) [2]
Flushing [5]
Palpitation (7%) [6]
Vasodilation (20%) [2]

Central Nervous System
Anxiety (13%) [3]
Chills (4%)
Depression (>2%)
Dysgeusia (taste perversion) (>2%)
Fever (6%)
Hyperesthesia (>2%)
Migraine (4%)
Pain (28%) [2]
Paresthesias (>2%) [2]
Tremor (7%)
Vertigo (dizziness) (>2%)

Neuromuscular/Skeletal
Arthralgia (24%)
Asthenia (fatigue) (19%)
Myalgia/Myopathy (>2%)

Gastrointestinal/Hepatic
Hepatotoxicity [3]
Nausea (15%)
Vomiting (7%)

Respiratory
Cough (>2%)
Dyspnea [3]
Flu-like syndrome (26%)
Sinusitis (>2%)

Endocrine/Metabolic
Mastodynia (>2%)

Genitourinary
Urinary tract infection [2]
Vaginitis (4%)

Otic
Tinnitus (>2%)

Local
Injection-site bleeding (5%)
Injection-site ecchymoses (>2%)
Injection-site edema [2]

Injection-site erythema (66%) [4]
Injection-site induration (13%) [3]
Injection-site inflammation (49%)
Injection-site lipoatrophy/lipohypertrophy [2]
Injection-site pain (73%) [3]
Injection-site pruritus (40%) [3]
Injection-site reactions (6–67%) [15]
Injection-site urticaria (5%)

Other
Adverse effects [5]
Infection (50%) [2]

GLECAPREVIR & PIBRENTASVIR *

Trade name: Mavyret (AbbVie)
Indications: Chronic HCV genotype 1–6 infection
Class: Direct-acting antiviral, Hepatitis C virus NS3/4A protease inhibitor (glecaprevir), Hepatitis C virus NS5A inhibitor (pibrentasvir)
Half-life: 6 hours (glecaprevir); 13 hours (pibrentasvir)
Clinically important, potentially hazardous interactions with: atazanavir, atorvastatin, carbamazepine, cyclosporine, darunavir, efavirenz, lopinavir, lovastatin, oral contraceptives, rifampin, ritonavir, simvastatin, St John's wort
Pregnancy category: N/A (Insufficient evidence to inform drug-associated risk)
Important contra-indications noted in the prescribing guidelines for: nursing mothers; pediatric patients
Note: Contra-indicated in patients with severe hepatic impairment (Child-Pugh C).
Warning: RISK OF HEPATITIS B VIRUS REACTIVATION IN PATIENTS COINFECTED WITH HCV AND HBV

Central Nervous System
Headache (13%) [2]
Neuromuscular/Skeletal
Asthenia (fatigue) (11%) [2]
Gastrointestinal/Hepatic
Nausea (8%)
Endocrine/Metabolic
Hyperbilirubinemia (<4%)
Other
Adverse effects [2]

GLICLAZIDE

See: www.drugeruptiondata.com/drug/id/1329

GLIMEPIRIDE

Trade names: Amaryl (Sanofi-Aventis), Avandaryl (GSK)
Indications: Non-insulin dependent diabetes Type II
Class: Sulfonylurea
Half-life: 5–9 hours
Clinically important, potentially hazardous interactions with: none known
Pregnancy category: C
Important contra-indications noted in the prescribing guidelines for: the elderly; nursing mothers; pediatric patients
Note: Glimepiride is a sulfonamide and can be absorbed systemically. Sulfonamides can produce severe, possibly fatal, reactions such as toxic epidermal necrolysis and Stevens-Johnson syndrome
Avandaryl is glimepiride and rosiglitazone.

Central Nervous System
Headache [4]
Vertigo (dizziness) [2]
Neuromuscular/Skeletal
Arthralgia [2]
Gastrointestinal/Hepatic
Diarrhea [5]
Dyspepsia [2]
Nausea [4]
Pancreatitis [2]
Endocrine/Metabolic
Hypoglycemia [8]
Weight gain [3]
Genitourinary
Genital mycotic infections [3]
Urinary tract infection [3]
Other
Adverse effects [5]

GLIPIZIDE

Trade names: Glucotrol (Pfizer), Metaglip (Bristol-Myers Squibb)
Indications: Non-insulin dependent diabetes Type II
Class: Sulfonylurea
Half-life: 2–4 hours
Clinically important, potentially hazardous interactions with: none known
Pregnancy category: C
Important contra-indications noted in the prescribing guidelines for: the elderly; nursing mothers; pediatric patients
Note: Glipizide is a sulfonamide and can be absorbed systemically. Sulfonamides can produce severe, possibly fatal, reactions such as toxic epidermal necrolysis and Stevens-Johnson syndrome.

Skin
Photosensitivity (<10%)
Pruritus (<3%)
Rash (<10%)
Urticaria (<10%)

Central Nervous System
Hyperesthesia (<3%)
Paresthesias (<3%)
Neuromuscular/Skeletal
Myalgia/Myopathy (<3%)
Endocrine/Metabolic
Hypoglycemia [3]
Other
Adverse effects [2]

GLUCAGON

Trade name: Glucagon Emergency Kit (Lilly)
Indications: Hypoglycemic reactions
Class: Hormone, polypeptide
Half-life: 3–10 minutes
Clinically important, potentially hazardous interactions with: insulin degludec, insulin glargine, insulin glulisine, warfarin
Pregnancy category: B

Skin
Erythema necrolyticum migrans [2]
Exanthems [7]
Folliculitis [2]
Pyoderma gangrenosum [3]
Rash [2]
Sweet's syndrome [7]
Urticaria (<10%) [2]
Vasculitis [9]
Local
Injection-site reactions [3]

GLUCARPIDASE

See: www.drugeruptiondata.com/drug/id/2737

GLUCOSAMINE

Trade names: Arthro-Aid (NutraSense), Glucosamine sulfate (Rottapharm)
Indications: Arthritis, osteoarthritis, cartilage repair and maintenance, strained joints, improving joint function and range of motion, alleviating joint pain
Class: Amino sugar, Food supplement
Half-life: N/A
Clinically important, potentially hazardous interactions with: abciximab, cilostazol, citalopram, clopidogrel, eptifibatide, meloxicam
Pregnancy category: C

Mucosal
Oral vesiculation (7%)
Central Nervous System
Depression (6%)
Neuromuscular/Skeletal
Asthenia (fatigue) (9%) [2]
Gastrointestinal/Hepatic
Dyspepsia [2]
Hepatotoxicity [3]
Nausea [2]

Other
Adverse effects (6%) [4]
Allergic reactions (4%) [2]

GLYBURIDE

Synonyms: glibenclamide; glybenclamide
Trade names: Diabeta (Sanofi-Aventis),
Glucovance (Bristol-Myers Squibb), Glynase
(Pfizer), Micronase (Pfizer)
Indications: Non-insulin dependent diabetes
Type II
Class: Sulfonylurea
Half-life: 5–16 hours
**Clinically important, potentially hazardous
interactions with:** bosentan, colesevelam,
norfloxacin
Pregnancy category: C
Note: Glyburide is a sulfonamide and can be
absorbed systemically. Sulfonamides can produce
severe, possibly fatal, reactions such as toxic
epidermal necrolysis and Stevens-Johnson
syndrome.
Glucovance is glyburide and metformin.

Skin
Erythema (<5%)
Exanthems (<5%) [3]
Linear IgA bullous dermatosis [2]
Pemphigus [2]
Photosensitivity (<10%) [5]
Pruritus (<10%) [3]
Psoriasis [2]
Purpura [2]
Rash (<10%)
Urticaria (<5%) [4]
Vasculitis [5]

Cardiovascular
Flushing [2]

Endocrine/Metabolic
Hypoglycemia [2]
Weight gain [2]

Other
Adverse effects [2]

GLYCOPYRROLATE

Synonym: glycopyrronium bromide
Trade names: Cuvposa (Shionogi), Robinul
(Forte), Seebri Neohaler (Novartis), Utibron
Neohaler (Novartis)
Indications: Duodenal ulcer, irritable bowel
syndrome, hyperhidrosis
Class: Anticholinergic, Muscarinic antagonist,
Non-depolarizing muscle relaxant
Half-life: N/A
**Clinically important, potentially hazardous
interactions with:** anticholinergics, arbutamine,
belladonna alkaloids, digoxin, disopyramide,
meperidine, phenothiazines, procainamide,
quinidine, ritodrine, tricyclic antidepressants
Pregnancy category: C
**Important contra-indications noted in the
prescribing guidelines for:** the elderly; nursing
mothers; pediatric patients
Note: Utibron Neohaler is glycopyrrolate and
indacaterol.

Skin
Photosensitivity (<10%)
Xerosis (>10%)

Mucosal
Nasal congestion (30%)
Xerostomia (40%) [9]

Cardiovascular
Bradycardia [2]
Flushing (30%)

Central Nervous System
Headache (15%) [2]

Gastrointestinal/Hepatic
Constipation (35%)
Vomiting (40%)

Respiratory
Sinusitis (15%)
Upper respiratory tract infection (15%)

Genitourinary
Urinary retention (15%)

Ocular
Mydriasis [2]

Local
Injection-site irritation (>10%)

GOLD & GOLD COMPOUNDS

See: www.drugeruptiondata.com/drug/id/327

GOLIMUMAB

Trade name: Simponi (Centocor)
Indications: Rheumatoid arthritis, psoriatic
arthritis, ankylosing spondylitis, ulcerative colitis
Class: Disease-modifying antirheumatic drug
(DMARD), Monoclonal antibody, TNF inhibitor
Half-life: 2 weeks
**Clinically important, potentially hazardous
interactions with:** abatacept, anakinra, live
vaccines
Pregnancy category: B
**Important contra-indications noted in the
prescribing guidelines for:** nursing mothers;
pediatric patients
Note: TNF inhibitors should be used in patients
with heart failure only after consideration of other
treatment options. TNF inhibitors are contra-
indicated in patients with a personal or family
history of multiple sclerosis or demyelinating
disease. TNF inhibitors should not be
administered to patients with moderate to severe
heart failure (New York Heart Association
Functional Class III/IV).
Warning: SERIOUS INFECTIONS AND
MALIGNANCY

Skin
Lupus erythematosus [3]
Malignancies [5]
Psoriasis [2]
Rash [3]

Cardiovascular
Hypertension [2]

Central Nervous System
Headache [7]

Neuromuscular/Skeletal
Arthralgia [3]
Asthenia (fatigue) [2]

Gastrointestinal/Hepatic
Colitis [2]
Diarrhea [4]
Nausea [6]

Respiratory
Cough [2]
Nasopharyngitis (6%) [7]
Pneumonia [4]
Pulmonary toxicity [2]
Tuberculosis [2]
Upper respiratory tract infection (7%) [7]

Endocrine/Metabolic
ALT increased [4]
AST increased [3]

Genitourinary
Urinary tract infection [2]

Hematologic
Sepsis [4]

Local
Injection-site erythema [7]
Injection-site reactions (6%) [7]

Other
Adverse effects [12]
Death [3]
Infection (28%) [16]

GOSERELIN

See: www.drugeruptiondata.com/drug/id/328

GRANISETRON

See: www.drugeruptiondata.com/drug/id/329

GRANULOCYTE COLONY-STIMULATING FACTOR (G-CSF)

See: www.drugeruptiondata.com/drug/id/330

GREPAFLOXACIN

See: www.drugeruptiondata.com/drug/id/331

GRISEOFULVIN

Trade names: Fulvicin (Schering), Grifulvin V (Ortho), Gris-PEG (Pedinol)
Indications: Fungal infections of the skin, hair and nails
Class: Antifungal
Half-life: 9–24 hours
Clinically important, potentially hazardous interactions with: alcohol, levonorgestrel, liraglutide, midazolam, thalidomide, ulipristal
Pregnancy category: C
Important contra-indications noted in the prescribing guidelines for: nursing mothers; pediatric patients

Skin
Angioedema [3]
Bullous dermatitis [2]
Cold urticaria [2]
Erythema multiforme [6]
Exanthems [6]
Exfoliative dermatitis [2]
Fixed eruption [7]
Lichenoid eruption [2]
Lupus erythematosus [14]
Petechiae [2]
Photosensitivity (<10%) [18]
Pigmentation [2]
Pruritus [4]
Rash (>10%)
Serum sickness-like reaction [3]
Stevens-Johnson syndrome [3]
Toxic epidermal necrolysis [4]

Urticaria (>10%) [5]
Vasculitis [2]
Mucosal
Oral candidiasis (<10%)
Central Nervous System
Dysgeusia (taste perversion) [3]
Endocrine/Metabolic
Gynecomastia [2]
Porphyria [12]
Other
Adverse effects [2]
Allergic reactions (<5%)

GUANABENZ

See: www.drugeruptiondata.com/drug/id/333

GUANADREL

See: www.drugeruptiondata.com/drug/id/334

GUANETHIDINE

See: www.drugeruptiondata.com/drug/id/335

GUANFACINE

See: www.drugeruptiondata.com/drug/id/336

GUSELKUMAB *

Trade name: Tremfya (Janssen Biotech)
Indications: Plaque psoriasis
Class: Interleukin-23 inhibitor, Monoclonal antibody
Half-life: 15–18 days
Clinically important, potentially hazardous interactions with: live vaccines
Pregnancy category: N/A (Insufficient evidence to inform drug-associated risk)
Important contra-indications noted in the prescribing guidelines for: nursing mothers; pediatric patients

Central Nervous System
Headache (5%) [3]
Neuromuscular/Skeletal
Arthralgia (3%)
Back pain [2]
Gastrointestinal/Hepatic
Diarrhea (2%)
Hepatotoxicity (3%)
Respiratory
Nasopharyngitis [5]
Upper respiratory tract infection (14%) [4]
Local
Injection-site reactions (5%)
Other
Infection [3]

HALCINONIDE

See: www.drugeruptiondata.com/drug/id/1083

HALOBETASOL

See: www.drugeruptiondata.com/drug/id/1097

HALOFANTRINE

See: www.drugeruptiondata.com/drug/id/1327

HALOMETASONE

See: www.drugeruptiondata.com/drug/id/1098

HALOPERIDOL

Trade name: Haldol (Ortho-McNeil)
Indications: Schizophrenia, Tourette's disorder
Class: Antiemetic, Antipsychotic
Half-life: 20 hours
Clinically important, potentially hazardous interactions with: acemetacin, arsenic, benztropine, citalopram, clozapine, darifenacin, fluoxetine, itraconazole, lisdexamfetamine, lithium, meloxicam, methotrexate, moxifloxacin, nilotinib, oxybutynin, propranolol, quinine, ribociclib, sotalol, sulpiride, tetrabenazine, tiotropium, trospium, vandetanib, venlafaxine
Pregnancy category: C
Important contra-indications noted in the prescribing guidelines for: the elderly; pediatric patients
Warning: INCREASED MORTALITY IN ELDERLY PATIENTS WITH DEMENTIA-RELATED PSYCHOSIS

Skin
Cellulitis [2]
Diaphoresis [2]
Photosensitivity [3]
Seborrheic dermatitis [2]

Hair
Alopecia areata [2]

Mucosal
Xerostomia [4]

Cardiovascular
Arrhythmias [2]
QT prolongation [22]
Torsades de pointes [12]

Central Nervous System
Agitation [4]
Akathisia [9]
Delirium [3]
Extrapyramidal symptoms [9]
Insomnia [3]
Neuroleptic malignant syndrome [36]
Parkinsonism [8]
Sedation [3]
Somnolence (drowsiness) [5]
Tardive dyskinesia (<37%) [5]
Tremor [7]

Vertigo (dizziness) [2]

Neuromuscular/Skeletal
Dystonia [3]
Myoclonus [2]
Rhabdomyolysis [7]

Gastrointestinal/Hepatic
Constipation [2]
Pancreatitis [2]

Respiratory
Pneumonia [2]

Endocrine/Metabolic
Galactorrhea [4]
Hyperprolactinemia [2]
Hypoglycemia [2]
SIADH [3]
Weight gain [2]

Genitourinary
Priapism [3]
Urinary retention [3]

Local
Injection-site reactions [3]

Other
Adverse effects [4]
Death [7]

HALOTHANE

See: www.drugeruptiondata.com/drug/id/338

HEMOPHILUS B VACCINE

Trade names: ActHIB (Sanofi-Aventis), Comvax (Merck), HibTITER (Lederle), OmniHIB (GSK), PedivaxHIB (Merck), ProHIBIT (Connaught)
Indications: Hemophilus B immunization
Class: Vaccine
Half-life: N/A
Clinically important, potentially hazardous interactions with: azathioprine, basiliximab, corticosteroids, cyclosporine, daclizumab, glatiramer, mycophenolate, sirolimus, tacrolimus
Pregnancy category: C

Skin
Erythema [2]

HEPARIN

Trade names: Hep-Flush (Wyeth), Viaflex (Baxter)
Indications: Venous thrombosis, pulmonary embolism, intravascular coagulation, peripheral arterial embolism
Class: Anticoagulant, Heparinoid
Half-life: 2 hours
Clinically important, potentially hazardous interactions with: acenocoumarol, aliskiren, antihistamines, aspirin, balsalazide, bivalirudin, butabarbital, ceftobiprole, dabigatran, danaparoid, defibrotide, desvenlafaxine, iloprost, nandrolone, nicotine, nitroglycerin, palifermin, piperacillin/tazobactam, salicylates, tirofiban, warfarin

Pregnancy category: C
Important contra-indications noted in the prescribing guidelines for: the elderly
Note: A higher incidence of bleeding has been reported in patients over 60 years of age, especially women. Contra-indicated in patients with severe thrombocyopenia.

Skin
Anaphylactoid reactions/Anaphylaxis [4]
Bullous dermatitis [4]
Dermatitis [6]
Ecchymoses [3]
Erythema [2]
Exanthems [2]
Hypersensitivity [17]
Lesions [2]
Livedo reticularis [2]
Necrosis [56]
Petechiae [2]
Purpura (>10%)
Toxic epidermal necrolysis [2]
Urticaria [6]
Vasculitis [6]

Hair
Alopecia [2]

Mucosal
Gingivitis (>10%)

Genitourinary
Priapism [6]

Hematologic
Bleeding [2]
Hemorrhage [6]
Thrombocytopenia [97]
Thrombosis [9]

Local
Injection-site eczematous eruption [5]
Injection-site induration [4]
Injection-site necrosis [4]
Injection-site plaques [2]

Other
Allergic reactions (<10%) [3]
Death [6]

HEPATITIS A VACCINE

Trade names: Avaxim (Sanofi Pasteur), Havrix (GSK), Vaqta (Merck)
Indications: Hepatitis A immunization
Class: Vaccine
Half-life: >2 years
Clinically important, potentially hazardous interactions with: none known
Pregnancy category: C

Skin
Rash (<10%)

Central Nervous System
Anorexia (<10%)
Chills (<10%)
Fever (>10%) [2]
Guillain–Barré syndrome [2]
Headache (>10%) [3]
Somnolence (drowsiness) (>10%)

Neuromuscular/Skeletal
Arm pain (<10%)

Asthenia (fatigue) (<10%)
Back pain (<10%)
Gastrointestinal/Hepatic
Constipation (<10%)
Diarrhea (<10%)
Nausea (<10%)
Vomiting (<10%)
Respiratory
Cough (<10%)
Nasopharyngitis (<10%)
Pharyngitis (<10%)
Rhinitis (<10%)
Upper respiratory tract infection (<10%)
Otic
Otitis media (<10%)
Ocular
Conjunctivitis (<10%)
Local
Injection-site erythema [2]
Injection-site pain (<10%) [7]
Injection-site reactions [5]
Other
Adverse effects [2]

HEPATITIS B VACCINE

Trade names: Comvax (Merck), Engerix B
(GSK), Pediatrix (GSK), Recombivax HB (Merck),
Twinrix (GSK)
Other common trade names: Heptavax-B
Indications: For immunization of infection
caused by all known subtypes of hepatitis B virus
Class: Vaccine
Half-life: N/A
**Clinically important, potentially hazardous
interactions with:** none known
Pregnancy category: C

Skin
Anaphylactoid reactions/Anaphylaxis [6]
Churg-Strauss syndrome [2]
Dermatomyositis [2]
Erythema multiforme [2]
Erythema nodosum [3]
Gianotti–Crosti syndrome [2]
Granuloma annulare [2]
Lichen planus [17]
Lichenoid eruption [3]
Lupus erythematosus [9]
Pemphigus [2]
Pseudolymphoma [2]
Purpura [6]
Raynaud's phenomenon [2]
Urticaria [3]
Vasculitis [11]
Hair
Alopecia [2]
Cardiovascular
Polyarteritis nodosa [5]
Central Nervous System
Guillain–Barré syndrome [4]
Neurotoxicity [2]
Neuromuscular/Skeletal
Arthralgia [4]

Ocular
Optic neuropathy [3]
Uveitis [2]
Local
Injection-site edema [2]
Injection-site pain (22%) [3]
Other
Adverse effects [2]
Death [2]

HEROIN

Synonym: diacetylmorphine
Indications: Substance abuse drug
Class: Opiate agonist
Half-life: N/A
**Clinically important, potentially hazardous
interactions with:** none known
Pregnancy category: B (category D if used for
prolonged period or in high doses)

Skin
Abscess [7]
Acanthosis nigricans [2]
Burning (24%)
Candidiasis [3]
Cellulitis [3]
Edema [4]
Exanthems [2]
Fixed eruption [2]
Folliculitis (candidal) [4]
Necrosis [3]
Photosensitivity [2]
Pigmentation [4]
Pruritus [6]
Pustules [5]
Toxic epidermal necrolysis [2]
Ulcerations [5]
Urticaria [3]
Vasculitis [2]
Central Nervous System
Leukoencephalopathy [12]
Seizures (2%)
Neuromuscular/Skeletal
Myalgia/Myopathy [2]
Rhabdomyolysis [15]
Otic
Hearing loss [2]
Ocular
Diplopia [2]
Eyelid edema [2]
Local
Injection-site ulceration [3]
Other
Death [5]
Infection (13%)
Side effects (85%)
Teratogenicity [2]

HISTRELIN

See: www.drugeruptiondata.com/drug/id/1111

HUMAN PAPILLOMA-VIRUS (HPV) VACCINE

Synonym: HPV4
Trade names: Gardasil (Merck), Silgard (Merck)
Indications: For prevention of HPV genital
warts, cervical cancers and vulvar dysplasias
(against Types 6, 11, 16 and 18 human
papillomavirus)
Class: Vaccine
Half-life: N/A
**Clinically important, potentially hazardous
interactions with:** immunosuppressants
Pregnancy category: B
**Important contra-indications noted in the
prescribing guidelines for:** the elderly; nursing
mothers; pediatric patients

Mucosal
Oropharyngeal pain (3%)
Central Nervous System
Cognitive impairment [2]
Fever (13%) [4]
Headache (28%) [8]
Myelitis [2]
Vertigo (dizziness) (<4%) [2]
Neuromuscular/Skeletal
Asthenia (fatigue) [5]
Gastrointestinal/Hepatic
Diarrhea (3–4%)
Nausea (2–7%) [2]
Vomiting (<2%)
Respiratory
Cough (2%)
Nasopharyngitis (3%)
Upper respiratory tract infection (2%)
Local
Injection-site bruising (3%)
Injection-site edema (14–25%) [2]
Injection-site erythema (17–25%) [2]
Injection-site pain (61–84%) [4]
Injection-site pruritus (3%)
Injection-site reactions [4]
Other
Adverse effects [4]
Toothache (2%)

HUMAN PAPILLOMA-VIRUS VACCINE (BIVALENT)

Trade name: Cervarix (GSK)
Indications: Prevention of human papillomavirus
(HPV) types 16 and 18 in females aged 10–25
years old
Class: Vaccine
Half-life: N/A
**Clinically important, potentially hazardous
interactions with:** immunosuppressants
Pregnancy category: B
**Important contra-indications noted in the
prescribing guidelines for:** the elderly; nursing
mothers; pediatric patients

Skin
Anaphylactoid reactions/Anaphylaxis (3%) [2]
Erythema (<10%) [4]
Pruritus (<10%)
Rash (<10%)
Urticaria (7%)

Central Nervous System
Fever (13%) [3]
Headache (53%) [2]

Neuromuscular/Skeletal
Arthralgia (21%)
Asthenia (fatigue) (55%)
Myalgia/Myopathy (49%)

Gastrointestinal/Hepatic
Abdominal pain (28%)
Diarrhea (28%)
Nausea (28%)
Vomiting (28%)

Local
Injection-site edema (44%) [3]
Injection-site erythema (48%)
Injection-site pain (92%) [9]
Injection-site reactions [5]

Other
Adverse effects [2]

HYALURONIC ACID

Synonym: hyaluronidase
Trade names: Euflexxa (Ferring), Hyalgan (Sanofi-Aventis), Hylan G-F 20 (Synvisc), Juvederm (Allergan), Perlane (Q-Med AB), Restylane Fine Lines (Medicis), Vitrase (ISTA Pharma)
Indications: Oral: joint disorders **Injection:** adjunct in eye surgery, viscosupplementation in orthopedics, cosmetic surgery **Topical:** wounds, burns, skin ulcers, stomatitis
Class: Food supplement, Glycoaminoglycan
Half-life: 2.5–5.5 minutes
Clinically important, potentially hazardous interactions with: furosemide, local anesthetics, NSAIDs, oral anticoagulants
Pregnancy category: C
Important contra-indications noted in the prescribing guidelines for: nursing mothers; pediatric patients
Note: Most reported reactions relate to orthopedic use.

Skin
Acneform eruption (<29%)
Anaphylactoid reactions/Anaphylaxis [2]
Angioedema [6]
Churg-Strauss syndrome [12]
Dermatitis (24%)
Ecchymoses [3]
Edema [8]
Erythema [6]
Erythema multiforme [2]
Facial edema [2]
Granulomatous reaction [2]
Hematoma [2]
Herpes simplex [2]
Hypersensitivity [6]
Induration [2]

Inflammation [7]
Necrosis [3]
Nodular eruption [2]
Pruritus [4]

Cardiovascular
Arterial occlusion [2]
Hypertension (4%)

Central Nervous System
Pain [3]

Neuromuscular/Skeletal
Arthralgia [8]
Back pain (5%)
Chondritis (<11%) [2]
Gouty tophi [3]
Tendinitis (2%)

Gastrointestinal/Hepatic
Nausea (2%)

Ocular
Orbital inflammation [2]

Local
Injection-site bruising [3]
Injection-site ecchymoses [2]
Injection-site edema (20%) [12]
Injection-site erythema (47%) [8]
Injection-site granuloma [2]
Injection-site nodules [3]
Injection-site pain (8–47%) [16]
Injection-site reactions (<11%) [12]

Other
Adverse effects [14]
Infection [2]

HYDRALAZINE

Trade names: Apresazide (Novartis), Apresoline (Novartis), Ser-Ap-Es (Novartis)
Indications: Hypertension
Class: Vasodilator
Half-life: 3–7 hours
Clinically important, potentially hazardous interactions with: acebutolol, alfuzosin, captopril, cilazapril, diclofenac, enalapril, fosinopril, levodopa, levomepromazine, lisinopril, meloxicam, olmesartan, quinapril, ramipril, trandolapril, triamcinolone, trifluoperazine, zuclopenthixol
Pregnancy category: C
Note: Apresazide is hydralazine and hydrochlorothiazide; Ser-Ap-Es is hydralazine, reserpine and hydrochlorothiazide. Hydrochlorothiazide is a sulfonamide and can be absorbed systemically. Sulfonamides can produce severe, possibly fatal, reactions such as toxic epidermal necrolysis and Stevens-Johnson syndrome.

Skin
Edema [2]
Exanthems [4]
Lupus erythematosus (7%) [112]
Photosensitivity [2]
Purpura [3]
Sweet's syndrome [6]
Toxic epidermal necrolysis [2]
Ulcerations [2]
Vasculitis [13]

Mucosal
Oral ulceration [2]
Orogenital ulceration [2]

Cardiovascular
Flushing (>10%)

Gastrointestinal/Hepatic
Hepatotoxicity [2]

Respiratory
Alveolar hemorrhage (pulmonary) [2]

Renal
Glomerulonephritis [5]

HYDROCHLORO-THIAZIDE

Trade names: Accuretic (Pfizer), Aldactazide (Pfizer), Aldoril (Merck), Atacand HCT (AstraZeneca), Avalide (Bristol-Myers Squibb), Capozide (Par), Diovan HCT (Novartis), Dyazide (GSK), Hyzaar (Merck), Inderide (Wyeth), Lopressor (Novartis), Lotensin (Novartis), Lotensin HCT (Novartis), Micardis (Boehringer Ingelheim), Microzide (Watson), Moduretic (Merck), Prinzide (Merck), Tekturna HCT (Novartis), Teveten HCT (Biovail), Uniretic (Schwarz), Vaseretic (Biovail), Zestoretic (AstraZeneca), Ziac (Barr)
Indications: Edema
Class: Diuretic, thiazide
Half-life: 5.6–14.8 hours
Clinically important, potentially hazardous interactions with: digoxin, dofetilide, lithium, zinc
Pregnancy category: B
Important contra-indications noted in the prescribing guidelines for: nursing mothers; pediatric patients
Note: Hydrochlorothiazide is a sulfonamide and can be absorbed systemically. Sulfonamides can produce severe, possibly fatal, reactions such as toxic epidermal necrolysis and Stevens-Johnson syndrome.
Hydrochlorothiazide is often used in combination, e.g. with aliskiren (Tekturna HCT); amiloride (Moduretic); benazepril (Lotensin HCT); bisoprolol (Ziac); captopril (Capozide); enalapril (Vaseretic); irbesartan (Avalide); lisinopril (Prinzide and Zestoretic); losartan (Hyzaar); methyldopa (Aldoril); moexipril (Uniretic); spironolactone (Aldactazide); triamterene (Dyazide and Maxzide).

Skin
Dermatitis [2]
Diaphoresis [2]
Edema [2]
Erythema annulare centrifugum [2]
Lichenoid eruption [5]
Lupus erythematosus [16]
Peripheral edema [5]
Photosensitivity [18]
Phototoxicity [5]
Purpura [6]
Rash [2]
Toxic epidermal necrolysis [2]
Vasculitis [3]

Cardiovascular
Hypotension [5]
Central Nervous System
Headache [7]
Vertigo (dizziness) [8]
Neuromuscular/Skeletal
Asthenia (fatigue) [3]
Gastrointestinal/Hepatic
Diarrhea [2]
Nausea [2]
Pancreatitis [4]
Respiratory
Upper respiratory tract infection [3]
Endocrine/Metabolic
Hyponatremia [3]
Serum creatinine increased [2]
SIADH [4]
Ocular
Glaucoma [2]
Other
Adverse effects [5]
Death [2]

HYDROCODONE

Trade names: Duratuss (UCB), Entex HC (Andrx), Hycotuss (Endo), Hydromet (Actavis), Hysingla ER (Purdue), Lortab (UCB), Maxidone (Watson), Norco (Watson), Tussionex (Celltech), Vicodin (AbbVie), Vicoprofen (AbbVie), Zohydro ER (Pernix), Zydone (Endo)
Indications: Acute pain, coughing
Class: Opiate agonist
Half-life: 3.8 hours
Clinically important, potentially hazardous interactions with: alcohol, buprenorphine, butorphanol, CYP3A4 inhibitors or inducers, MAO inhibitors, nalbuphine, pentazocine
Pregnancy category: C
Important contra-indications noted in the prescribing guidelines for: nursing mothers; pediatric patients
Note: Hydrocodone is included in many combination drugs. Other medications that can be included in these preparations include: phenylpropanolamine, phenylephrine, pyrilamine, pseudoephedrine, acetaminophen, ibuprofen, and others. Zohydro ER is the first extended-release, single-entity hydrocodone-containing drug product approved by the FDA and reflects the newly updated labeling requirements recently announced by the FDA.
Warning: ADDICTION, ABUSE, AND MISUSE; LIFE-THREATENING RESPIRATORY DEPRESSION; ACCIDENTAL INGESTION; NEONATAL OPIOID WITHDRAWAL SYNDROME; INTERACTION WITH ALCOHOL; and CYTOCHROME P450 3A4 INTERACTION

Skin
Hot flashes (<10%)
Hyperhidrosis (<10%)
Peripheral edema (<3%)
Pruritus (3%) [2]
Rash (<10%)

Mucosal
Xerostomia (3%)
Cardiovascular
Chest pain (<10%)
Central Nervous System
Fever (<10%)
Headache [2]
Migraine (<10%)
Paresthesias (<10%)
Somnolence (drowsiness) (<5%) [3]
Tremor (3%)
Vertigo (dizziness) (2–3%) [4]
Neuromuscular/Skeletal
Arthralgia (<10%)
Asthenia (fatigue) (<4%)
Back pain (<4%) [2]
Bone or joint pain (<10%)
Muscle spasm (<3%)
Myalgia/Myopathy (<10%)
Neck pain (<10%)
Pain in extremities (<10%)
Gastrointestinal/Hepatic
Abdominal pain (2–3%)
Constipation (8–11%) [7]
Gastroesophageal reflux (<10%)
Nausea (7–10%) [9]
Vomiting [8]
Respiratory
Cough (<10%)
Dyspnea (<10%)
Upper respiratory tract infection (<3%)
Endocrine/Metabolic
Dehydration (<10%)
GGT increased (<10%)
Hypokalemia (<10%)
Genitourinary
Urinary tract infection (<5%)

HYDROCORTISONE

See: www.drugeruptiondata.com/drug/id/1103

HYDROFLU-METHIAZIDE

See: www.drugeruptiondata.com/drug/id/344

HYDROMORPHONE

Trade names: Dilaudid (AbbVie), Exalgo (Mallinckrodt), Jurnista (Janssen-Cilag), Palladone (Napp)
Indications: Pain
Class: Opiate agonist
Half-life: 1–3 hours; 2 hours (IV)
Clinically important, potentially hazardous interactions with: alcohol, alvimopan, ammonium chloride, amphetamines, anticholinergics, anxiolytics and hypnotics, buprenorphine, butorphanol, cimetidine, CNS depressants, desmopressin, domperidone, droperidol, linezolid, MAO inhibitors, metoclopramide, moclobemide, nalbuphine,

pegvisomant, pentazocine, phenothiazines, sodium oxybate, SSRIs, St John's wort, succinylcholine, thiazide diuretics
Pregnancy category: C
Important contra-indications noted in the prescribing guidelines for: nursing mothers; pediatric patients
Note: OROS hydromorphone prolonged release (Jurnista) is a once-daily formulation of hydromorphone that utilizes OROS (osmotic-controlled release oral delivery system) technology to deliver the drug at a near constant rate.
Warning: ADDICTION, ABUSE, AND MISUSE; LIFE-THREATENING RESPIRATORY DEPRESSION; ACCIDENTAL INGESTION; NEONATAL OPIOID WITHDRAWAL SYNDROME; and INTERACTION WITH ALCOHOL

Skin
Pruritus (<11%) [12]
Mucosal
Xerostomia (<10%)
Cardiovascular
Bradycardia [2]
Flushing (<10%)
Hypotension [2]
Central Nervous System
Agitation [3]
Dysgeusia (taste perversion) [3]
Headache [5]
Hyperalgesia [3]
Somnolence (drowsiness) [6]
Tremor [2]
Vertigo (dizziness) [10]
Neuromuscular/Skeletal
Asthenia (fatigue) [5]
Myoclonus [3]
Gastrointestinal/Hepatic
Constipation [10]
Nausea [17]
Vomiting [11]
Endocrine/Metabolic
Appetite decreased [2]
Other
Adverse effects [7]

HYDROQUINONE

Trade names: Ambi (Johnson & Johnson), Lustra (Taro)
Indications: Ultraviolet induced dyschromia and discoloration resulting from the use of oral contraceptives, pregnancy, hormone replacement therapy, or skin trauma
Class: Depigmentation agent
Half-life: N/A
Clinically important, potentially hazardous interactions with: none known
Pregnancy category: C
Important contra-indications noted in the prescribing guidelines for: nursing mothers; pediatric patients

Skin

Acneform eruption [2]
Burning [2]
Contact dermatitis (localized) [2]
Depigmentation [2]
Erythema [4]
Ochronosis [15]
Peeling [2]
Pigmentation [3]
Pruritus [2]
Scaling [2]
Striae [2]
Xerosis [2]

Other

Adverse effects [3]

HYDROXY-CHLOROQUINE

Trade name: Plaquenil (Sanofi-Aventis)
Indications: Malaria, lupus erythematosus, rheumatoid arthritis
Class: Antimalarial, Antiprotozoal, Disease-modifying antirheumatic drug (DMARD)
Half-life: 32–50 days
Clinically important, potentially hazardous interactions with: chloroquine, cholestyramine, dapsone, droperidol, ethosuximide, lacosamide, lanthanum, moxifloxacin, neostigmine, oxcarbazepine, penicillamine, tiagabine, typhoid vaccine, vigabatrin, yellow fever vaccine
Pregnancy category: C
Important contra-indications noted in the prescribing guidelines for: nursing mothers; pediatric patients

Skin

AGEP [22]
Bullous dermatitis [2]
DRESS syndrome [2]
Erythema annulare centrifugum [3]
Erythema multiforme [2]
Erythroderma [3]
Exanthems (<5%) [4]
Exfoliative dermatitis [3]
Lichenoid eruption [4]
Photosensitivity [6]
Phototoxicity [3]
Pigmentation (<10%) [19]
Pruritus (>10%) [13]
Psoriasis (exacerbation) [13]
Rash (<10%) [4]
Thrombocytopenic purpura [2]
Toxic epidermal necrolysis [3]
Urticaria [2]

Hair

Alopecia [2]
Hair pigmentation (bleaching) (<10%) [8]

Nails

Nail pigmentation [3]

Mucosal

Oral pigmentation [7]
Stomatitis [2]

Cardiovascular

Cardiomyopathy [8]
Cardiotoxicity [4]

QT prolongation [3]

Central Nervous System

Anorexia [2]
Dysgeusia (taste perversion) [2]
Headache [2]
Neurotoxicity [3]

Neuromuscular/Skeletal

Asthenia (fatigue) [3]
Myalgia/Myopathy [8]

Gastrointestinal/Hepatic

Diarrhea [5]
Dysphagia [2]
Nausea [6]
Vomiting [4]

Endocrine/Metabolic

Hypoglycemia [3]
Porphyria [7]
Weight loss [2]

Hematologic

Anemia [3]
Neutropenia [2]
Thrombocytopenia [4]

Otic

Hearing loss [2]

Ocular

Maculopathy [5]
Ocular adverse effects [2]
Ocular toxicity [9]
Reduced visual acuity [2]
Retinopathy [29]
Vision blurred [3]

Other

Adverse effects [8]
Death [3]

HYDROXYUREA

Synonym: hydroxycarbamide
Trade names: Droxia (Bristol-Myers Squibb), Hydrea (Bristol-Myers Squibb)
Indications: Leukemia, malignant tumors
Class: Antineoplastic, Antiretroviral
Half-life: 3–4 hours
Clinically important, potentially hazardous interactions with: adefovir, aldesleukin
Pregnancy category: D

Skin

Acral erythema [8]
Atrophy [4]
Dermatitis [3]
Dermatomyositis [28]
Exanthems (<10%)
Fixed eruption [4]
Ichthyosis [2]
Keratoses [2]
Leg ulceration (29%) [20]
Lichen planus [3]
Lichenoid eruption [3]
Lupus erythematosus [3]
Palmar–plantar desquamation [6]
Pigmentation (<58%) [17]
Poikiloderma [3]
Pruritus [3]
Purpura [2]
Radiation recall dermatitis [2]

Telangiectasia [2]
Tumors [5]
Ulcerations [27]
Vasculitis [6]
Xerosis (<10%) [7]

Hair

Alopecia (<10%) [8]

Nails

Atrophic nails [3]
Melanonychia [7]
Nail changes [4]
Nail dystrophy [2]
Nail pigmentation [18]
Onycholysis [2]

Mucosal

Oral lesions [2]
Oral pigmentation [2]
Oral squamous cell carcinoma [2]
Oral ulceration [8]
Stomatitis (>10%) [4]
Tongue pigmentation (<29%) [3]

Gastrointestinal/Hepatic

Pancreatitis [2]

Other

Adverse effects [2]
Death [2]
Side effects (7–35%) [3]

HYDROXYZINE

Trade names: Atarax (Pfizer), Vistaril (Pfizer)
Indications: Anxiety and tension, pruritus
Class: Histamine H1 receptor antagonist, Muscarinic antagonist
Half-life: 3–7 hours
Clinically important, potentially hazardous interactions with: alcohol, barbiturates, CNS depressants, efavirenz, lurasidone, narcotics, non-narcotic analgesics
Pregnancy category: C
Important contra-indications noted in the prescribing guidelines for: nursing mothers

Skin

AGEP [3]
Anaphylactoid reactions/Anaphylaxis [2]
Angioedema [3]
Erythema multiforme [2]
Exanthems [3]
Fixed eruption [3]
Urticaria [4]

Mucosal

Xerostomia (12%) [4]

Central Nervous System

Somnolence (drowsiness) [5]

Gastrointestinal/Hepatic

Vomiting [2]

HYOSCYAMINE

Trade names: IB-Stat (InKline), Levbid (Schwarz), Levsin (Schwarz), Levsin/SL (Schwarz), Levsinex (Schwarz), Nulev (Schwarz)
Indications: Treatment of gastrointestinal tract disorders caused by spasm, adjunctive therapy for peptic ulcers, cystitis, Parkinsonism, biliary and renal colic
Class: Anticholinergic, Muscarinic antagonist
Half-life: N/A
Clinically important, potentially hazardous interactions with: anticholinergics, arbutamine

Pregnancy category: C
Important contra-indications noted in the prescribing guidelines for: the elderly; nursing mothers; pediatric patients

---

Skin
  Photosensitivity (<10%)
  Xerosis (>10%)
Mucosal
  Xerostomia (>10%)
Cardiovascular
  Tachycardia [2]

Local
  Injection-site inflammation (>10%)

IBANDRONATE

Synonym: ibandronic acid
Trade names: Bondronat (Roche), Boniva (Roche)
Indications: Postmenopausal osteoporosis
Class: Bisphosphonate
Half-life: 37–157 hours
Clinically important, potentially hazardous interactions with: alcohol, aminoglycosides, antacids, calcium salts, food, magnesium salts, NSAIDs, oral iron
Pregnancy category: C
Important contra-indications noted in the prescribing guidelines for: nursing mothers; pediatric patients

Skin
Rash (<2%)

Cardiovascular
Hypertension (6–7%)

Central Nervous System
Fever (~9%) [4]
Headache (3–7%)
Vertigo (dizziness) (<4%)

Neuromuscular/Skeletal
Arthralgia (3–6%) [2]
Asthenia (fatigue) (4%) [3]
Back pain (4–14%)
Bone or joint pain [3]
Cramps (2%)
Joint disorder (4%)
Myalgia/Myopathy (<6%)
Osteonecrosis [13]
Pain in extremities (<8%)

Gastrointestinal/Hepatic
Abdominal pain (5–8%)
Constipation (3–4%)
Diarrhea (4–7%) [2]
Dyspepsia (6–12%) [4]
Gastritis (2%)
Gastrointestinal disorder [3]
Nausea (5%) [4]
Vomiting (3%) [4]

Respiratory
Bronchitis (3–10%)
Flu-like syndrome (<4%) [7]
Nasopharyngitis (4%)
Pharyngitis (3%)
Pneumonia (6%)
Upper respiratory tract infection (2–34%)

Endocrine/Metabolic
Hypercholesterolemia (5%)
Hypocalcemia [3]
Hypophosphatemia [2]

Genitourinary
Urinary tract infection (2–6%)

Other
Adverse effects [5]
Allergic reactions (3%)
Infection (4%)
Tooth disorder (4%)

IBRITUMOMAB

See: www.drugeruptiondata.com/drug/id/906

IBRUTINIB

Trade name: Imbruvica (Pharmacyclics)
Indications: Mantle cell lymphoma
Class: Bruton's tyrosine kinase (BTK) inhibitor
Half-life: 4–6 hours
Clinically important, potentially hazardous interactions with: carbamazepine, clarithromycin, grapefruit juice, itraconazole, ketoconazole, phenytoin, posaconazole, rifampin, St John's wort, strong or moderate CYP3A inhibitors or inducers, telithromycin, voriconazole
Pregnancy category: D
Important contra-indications noted in the prescribing guidelines for: nursing mothers; pediatric patients

Skin
Cellulitis [3]
Ecchymoses (30%) [4]
Panniculitis [2]
Peripheral edema (35%) [3]
Petechiae (11%)
Rash (25%) [5]
Toxicity (14%) [3]
Tumor lysis syndrome [2]

Mucosal
Epistaxis (nosebleed) (11%)
Stomatitis (17%)

Cardiovascular
Atrial fibrillation [10]
Hypertension [4]
Hypotension [2]

Central Nervous System
Fever (18%) [5]
Headache (13%) [2]
Peripheral neuropathy [2]
Vertigo (dizziness) (14%)

Neuromuscular/Skeletal
Arthralgia (11%) [3]
Asthenia (fatigue) (14–41%) [19]
Bone or joint pain (37%)
Muscle spasm (14%) [2]

Gastrointestinal/Hepatic
Abdominal pain (24%)
Constipation (25%)
Diarrhea (51%) [23]
Dyspepsia (11%)
Hepatotoxicity [2]
Nausea (31%) [14]
Vomiting (24%) [3]

Respiratory
Cough (19%) [3]
Dyspnea (27%)
Pneumonia (14%) [7]
Sinusitis (13%) [2]
Upper respiratory tract infection (34%) [6]

Endocrine/Metabolic
Appetite decreased (21%)
Dehydration (12%) [2]
Hyperuricemia (15%)
Hypokalemia [2]

Genitourinary
Urinary tract infection (14%) [2]

Hematologic
Anemia [11]
Bleeding [11]
Cytopenia [3]
Febrile neutropenia [3]
Hemorrhage [2]
Lymphocytosis [2]
Neutropenia [15]
Sepsis [2]
Thrombocytopenia [13]

Other
Adverse effects [2]
Infection [7]

IBUPROFEN

Trade names: Advil (Wyeth), Motrin (McNeil), Vicoprofen (AbbVie)
Indications: Arthritis, pain
Class: Non-steroidal anti-inflammatory (NSAID)
Half-life: 2–4 hours
Clinically important, potentially hazardous interactions with: aspirin, ciprofibrate, diuretics, methotrexate, methyl salicylate, NSAIDs, oxycodone hydrochloride, salicylates, tacrine, tacrolimus, urokinase, voriconazole
Pregnancy category: D (category C prior to 30 weeks gestation; category D starting at 30 weeks gestation)
Note: NSAIDs may cause an increased risk of serious cardiovascular and gastrointestinal adverse events, which can be fatal. This risk may increase with duration of use.

Skin
AGEP [5]
Anaphylactoid reactions/Anaphylaxis [5]
Angioedema [8]
Bullous dermatitis [3]
Bullous pemphigoid [2]
Dermatitis [5]
DRESS syndrome [4]
Erythema multiforme [11]
Erythema nodosum (<5%)
Exanthems [9]
Fixed eruption [15]
Hypersensitivity [5]
Lupus erythematosus [5]
Nicolau syndrome [2]
Peripheral edema [2]
Photosensitivity [6]
Pruritus (<5%) [5]
Psoriasis (palms) [2]
Rash (>10%) [2]
Stevens-Johnson syndrome [10]
Toxic epidermal necrolysis [8]
Urticaria (>10%) [10]
Vasculitis [8]
Vesiculobullous eruption [2]

Hair
Alopecia [2]

Cardiovascular
Cardiotoxicity [2]
Hypertension [4]

Central Nervous System
Aseptic meningitis [16]
Headache [3]

Neuromuscular/Skeletal
Arthralgia [2]
Back pain [2]

Rhabdomyolysis [3]

Gastrointestinal/Hepatic
Abdominal pain [6]
Constipation [4]
Diarrhea [4]
Dyspepsia [5]
Gastroesophageal reflux [2]
Gastrointestinal bleeding [2]
Gastrointestinal disorder [2]
Hepatotoxicity [3]
Nausea [7]
Pancreatitis [2]
Vanishing bile duct syndrome [2]
Vomiting [5]

Respiratory
Influenza [2]
Sinusitis [2]
Upper respiratory tract infection [2]

Endocrine/Metabolic
Pseudoporphyria [2]

Genitourinary
Urinary tract infection [2]

Renal
Nephrotoxicity [4]

Hematologic
Thrombocytopenia [5]

Otic
Hearing loss [2]
Tinnitus [2]

Ocular
Amblyopia [2]
Optic neuritis [2]
Periorbital edema [3]
Visual disturbances [2]

Other
Adverse effects [13]
Kounis syndrome [3]

IBUTILIDE

Trade name: Corvert (Pfizer)
Indications: Atrial fibrillation and flutter
Class: Antiarrhythmic, Antiarrhythmic class III
Half-life: 2–12 hours
Clinically important, potentially hazardous interactions with: degarelix
Pregnancy category: C
Important contra-indications noted in the prescribing guidelines for: nursing mothers; pediatric patients

Cardiovascular
Bradycardia [4]
Hypotension [2]
QT prolongation [5]
Tachycardia (3%)
Torsades de pointes [10]
Ventricular arrhythmia [4]
Ventricular tachycardia [6]

Central Nervous System
Headache (4%)

Gastrointestinal/Hepatic
Nausea (2%) [3]

ICATIBANT

See: www.drugeruptiondata.com/drug/id/1368

ICODEXTRIN

See: www.drugeruptiondata.com/drug/id/1072

IDARUBICIN

Synonyms: 4-demethoxydaunorubicin; 4-DMDR
Trade name: Idamycin (Pfizer)
Indications: Acute myeloid leukemia
Class: Antibiotic, anthracycline
Half-life: 14–35 hours (oral)
Clinically important, potentially hazardous interactions with: aldesleukin
Pregnancy category: D
Important contra-indications noted in the prescribing guidelines for: nursing mothers; pediatric patients

Skin
Rash (>10%) [4]
Urticaria (>10%)

Hair
Alopecia (77%) [8]

Mucosal
Mucositis (50%) [5]
Stomatitis (>10%)

Gastrointestinal/Hepatic
Diarrhea [3]
Hepatotoxicity [2]
Nausea [2]
Vomiting [2]

Hematologic
Febrile neutropenia [2]
Neutropenia [2]

Other
Infection [2]

IDARUCIZUMAB

Trade name: Praxbind (Boehringer Ingelheim)
Indications: Reversal of the anticoagulant effects of dabigatran in patients requiring emergency or urgent surgery or with life-threatening or uncontrolled bleeding
Class: Monoclonal antibody, Reversal agent for dabigatran
Half-life: 10 hours
Clinically important, potentially hazardous interactions with: none known
Pregnancy category: N/A (No data available)
Important contra-indications noted in the prescribing guidelines for: nursing mothers; pediatric patients
Note: Risk of serious adverse reactions in patients with hereditary fructose intolerance due to sorbitol excipient.

Skin
Irritation [2]

Central Nervous System
Delirium (7%)
Fever (6%)
Headache [2]

Neuromuscular/Skeletal
Back pain [2]

Gastrointestinal/Hepatic
Constipation (7%)

Respiratory
Nasopharyngitis [2]
Pneumonia (6%)

Endocrine/Metabolic
Hypokalemia (7%)

IDEBENONE

See: www.drugeruptiondata.com/drug/id/1062

IDELALISIB

Trade name: Zydelig (Gilead)
Indications: Relapsed chronic lymphocytic leukemia (with rituximab), follicular B-cell non-Hodgkin lymphoma, small lymphocytic lymphoma
Class: Phosphoinositide 3-kinase (PI3K) inhibitor
Half-life: 8 hours
Clinically important, potentially hazardous interactions with: carbamazepine, copanlisib, midostaurin, neratinib, phenytoin, rifampin, St John's wort, strong CYP3A inducers and substrates
Pregnancy category: D
Important contra-indications noted in the prescribing guidelines for: nursing mothers; pediatric patients
Warning: FATAL AND SERIOUS TOXICITIES: HEPATIC, SEVERE DIARRHEA, COLITIS, PNEUMONITIS, and INTESTINAL PERFORATION

Skin
Diaphoresis (12%)
Peripheral edema (10%)
Rash (21%) [7]
Toxicity [2]

Central Nervous System
Chills [5]
Fever [9]
Headache (11%)
Insomnia (12%)

Neuromuscular/Skeletal
Asthenia (fatigue) (30%) [8]

Gastrointestinal/Hepatic
Abdominal pain (26%)
Colitis [6]
Constipation [2]
Diarrhea (47%) [15]
Gastrointestinal perforation [2]
Hepatotoxicity [8]
Nausea (29%) [8]
Vomiting (15%) [3]

Respiratory
Cough (29%) [5]
Dyspnea (17%)
Pneumonia (25%) [9]

Pneumonitis [5]
Upper respiratory tract infection (12%) [3]

Endocrine/Metabolic
ALT increased (50%) [8]
Appetite decreased (16%) [2]
AST increased (41%) [8]

Hematologic
Anemia [6]
Febrile neutropenia [6]
Neutropenia [8]
Thrombocytopenia [6]

Other
Adverse effects [2]
Side effects [2]

IDURSULFASE

See: www.drugeruptiondata.com/drug/id/1185

IFOSFAMIDE

Trade name: Ifex (Bristol-Myers Squibb)
Indications: Cancers, sarcomas, leukemias, lymphomas
Class: Alkylating agent
Half-life: 4–15 hours
Clinically important, potentially hazardous interactions with: aldesleukin, aprepitant
Pregnancy category: D

Skin
Dermatitis (<10%)
Pigmentation (<10%) [2]
Toxicity [2]

Hair
Alopecia (50–100%) [4]

Nails
Ridging (<10%)

Cardiovascular
Phlebitis (2%)

Central Nervous System
Confusion [2]
Delirium [2]
Encephalopathy [10]
Neurotoxicity [11]
Seizures [2]

Neuromuscular/Skeletal
Osteomalacia [2]

Gastrointestinal/Hepatic
Hepatotoxicity [2]
Nausea [6]
Pancreatitis [2]
Vomiting [6]

Endocrine/Metabolic
SIADH [2]

Renal
Fanconi syndrome [4]
Nephrotoxicity [34]

Hematologic
Anemia [3]
Febrile neutropenia [2]
Leukopenia [2]
Myelosuppression [2]
Neutropenia [4]

Thrombocytopenia [4]
Other
Allergic reactions (<10%)
Death [2]
Infection [2]

ILOPERIDONE

Trade name: Fanapt (Vanda)
Indications: Schizophrenia
Class: Antipsychotic
Half-life: 18–33 hours
Clinically important, potentially hazardous interactions with: alcohol, dextromethorphan, fluoxetine, itraconazole, ketoconazole, paroxetine hydrochloride, QT prolonging agents
Pregnancy category: C
Important contra-indications noted in the prescribing guidelines for: the elderly; nursing mothers; pediatric patients
Warning: INCREASED MORTALITY IN ELDERLY PATIENTS WITH DEMENTIA-RELATED PSYCHOSIS

Skin
Rash (2%)

Mucosal
Nasal congestion (8%) [2]
Xerostomia (10%) [9]

Cardiovascular
Hypotension (3%)
Orthostatic hypotension (3%) [4]
QT prolongation [8]
Tachycardia (12%) [4]

Central Nervous System
Akathisia (2%) [3]
Anxiety [2]
Headache [3]
Insomnia (18%) [3]
Sedation [3]
Somnolence (drowsiness) (15%) [8]
Tremor (3%)
Vertigo (dizziness) (20%) [11]

Neuromuscular/Skeletal
Arthralgia (3%)
Asthenia (fatigue) (6%) [2]

Gastrointestinal/Hepatic
Diarrhea (7%)
Dyspepsia [3]
Nausea (10%) [2]

Respiratory
Dyspnea (2%)
Nasopharyngitis (3%)
Upper respiratory tract infection (3%)

Endocrine/Metabolic
Weight gain (9%) [10]

Genitourinary
Ejaculatory dysfunction (2%) [2]

ILOPROST

See: www.drugeruptiondata.com/drug/id/1132

IMATINIB

Trade name: Gleevec (Novartis)
Indications: Chronic myeloid leukemia
Class: Antineoplastic, Biologic, CYP3A4 inhibitor, Tyrosine kinase inhibitor
Half-life: 18 hours
Clinically important, potentially hazardous interactions with: acetaminophen, amlodipine, anisindione, anticoagulants, aprepitant, atorvastatin, barbiturates, benzodiazepines, butabarbital, carbamazepine, chlordiazepoxide, clarithromycin, clonazepam, clorazepate, corticosteroids, cyclosporine, dexamethasone, diazepam, dicumarol, efavirenz, erythromycin, ethotoin, felodipine, flurazepam, fluvastatin, fosphenytoin, isradipine, itraconazole, ketoconazole, lorazepam, lovastatin, mephenytoin, mephobarbital, midazolam, mifepristone, neratinib, nicardipine, nifedipine, nimodipine, nisoldipine, olaparib, oxazepam, oxcarbazepine, pentobarbital, phenobarbital, phenytoin, pimozide, pravastatin, primidone, quazepam, rifampin, rifapentine, safinamide, secobarbital, simvastatin, St John's wort, temazepam, voriconazole, warfarin
Pregnancy category: D
Important contra-indications noted in the prescribing guidelines for: nursing mothers

Skin
Acneform eruption [2]
AGEP [7]
Diaphoresis (13%)
DRESS syndrome [3]
Edema (<5%) [35]
Erythema (<10%) [5]
Erythema multiforme [2]
Erythroderma [3]
Exanthems [9]
Exfoliative dermatitis [4]
Facial edema (<10%) [3]
Hand–foot syndrome [3]
Hypomelanosis [5]
Lichen planus [5]
Lichenoid eruption [11]
Mycosis fungoides [2]
Neutrophilic eccrine hidradenitis [3]
Panniculitis [3]
Peripheral edema (<10%) [5]
Petechiae (<10%)
Photosensitivity (<10%) [3]
Pigmentation [12]
Pityriasis rosea [5]
Pruritus (6–10%) [3]
Pseudolymphoma [3]
Psoriasis [3]
Rash (32–39%) [26]
Squamous cell carcinoma [2]
Stevens-Johnson syndrome [13]
Sweet's syndrome [3]
Toxicity [9]
Urticaria [3]
Vasculitis [2]
Xerosis (<10%) [2]

Hair
Alopecia (10–15%) [2]
Follicular mucinosis [2]

Nails
Nail dystrophy [2]

Mucosal
Mucositis [2]
Oral lichenoid eruption [3]
Oral pigmentation [3]
Oral ulceration [3]

Cardiovascular
Cardiotoxicity [2]
Congestive heart failure [2]
QT prolongation [2]

Central Nervous System
Anorexia [4]
Chills (11%)
Depression (15%) [2]
Fever (13–41%) [2]
Headache (19–37%) [4]
Hypoesthesia (<10%)
Insomnia (10–19%)
Subdural hemorrhage [2]
Vertigo (dizziness) [2]

Neuromuscular/Skeletal
Arthralgia (21–26%) [4]
Asthenia (fatigue) (29–75%) [20]
Bone or joint pain (11–31%) [13]
Muscle spasm [9]
Myalgia/Myopathy (16–62%) [11]
Osteonecrosis [3]

Gastrointestinal/Hepatic
Abdominal pain [5]
Ascites [2]
Constipation (9–16%) [2]
Diarrhea (25–59%) [17]
Dyspepsia [2]
Gastrointestinal bleeding [5]
Hepatotoxicity (6–12%) [18]
Nausea (42–73%) [15]
Vomiting (23–58%) [13]

Respiratory
Cough (11–27%)
Dyspnea (21%)
Nasopharyngitis (10–31%)
Pharyngitis (10–15%)
Pleural effusion [3]
Pneumonitis (4–13%) [2]
Pulmonary toxicity [2]
Rhinitis (17%)
Upper respiratory tract infection (3–21%)

Endocrine/Metabolic
Creatine phosphokinase increased [2]
Gynecomastia [4]
Hypophosphatemia [2]
Hypothyroidism [2]
Porphyria cutanea tarda [3]
Pseudoporphyria [5]
Weight gain (5–32%) [3]

Renal
Fanconi syndrome [2]
Nephrotoxicity [2]
Renal failure [2]

Hematologic
Anemia [10]
Febrile neutropenia [2]
Hemotoxicity [4]
Leukopenia [3]
Myelosuppression [2]
Neutropenia [13]
Thrombocytopenia [11]

Otic
Hearing loss [4]

Ocular
Epiphora (25%)
Eyelid edema [2]
Optic edema [2]
Periorbital edema (33%) [11]

Other
Adverse effects [14]
Death [3]
Side effects [2]

IMIDAPRIL

See: www.drugeruptiondata.com/drug/id/1265

IMIGLUCERASE

See: www.drugeruptiondata.com/drug/id/1028

IMIPENEM/CILASTATIN

See: www.drugeruptiondata.com/drug/id/353

IMIPRAMINE

Trade name: Tofranil (Mallinckrodt)
Indications: Depression
Class: Antidepressant, tricyclic, Muscarinic antagonist
Half-life: 6–18 hours
Clinically important, potentially hazardous interactions with: amprenavir, arbutamine, artemether/lumefantrine, clonidine, cobicistat/elvitegravir/emtricitabine/tenofovir alafenamide, cobicistat/elvitegravir/emtricitabine/tenofovir disoproxil, darifenacin, epinephrine, fluoxetine, formoterol, guanethidine, iobenguane, isocarboxazid, labetalol, linezolid, MAO inhibitors, phenelzine, propranolol, quinolones, ropivacaine, sparfloxacin, tranylcypromine, zaleplon, zolpidem
Pregnancy category: D
Warning: SUICIDALITY AND ANTIDEPRESSANT DRUGS

Skin
Diaphoresis (<25%) [8]
Exanthems (<6%) [6]
Exfoliative dermatitis [4]
Photosensitivity [3]
Pigmentation [13]
Pruritus (3%) [6]
Purpura [3]
Urticaria [6]

Hair
Alopecia [2]

Mucosal
Glossitis [2]
Oral lesions [3]
Stomatitis [2]
Xerostomia (>10%) [16]

Cardiovascular
QT prolongation [3]
Tachycardia [2]

Central Nervous System
Dysgeusia (taste perversion) (metallic taste) (>10%) [2]
Parkinsonism (<10%)

Neuromuscular/Skeletal
Asthenia (fatigue) [2]

Endocrine/Metabolic
SIADH [4]

Otic
Tinnitus [4]

IMIQUIMOD

Trade names: Aldara (3M), Zyclara (Graceway)
Indications: External genital and perianal warts, actinic keratoses
Class: Antiviral, Immunomodulator
Half-life: N/A
Clinically important, potentially hazardous interactions with: none known
Pregnancy category: C
Important contra-indications noted in the prescribing guidelines for: nursing mothers; pediatric patients

Skin
Angioedema [2]
Burning (9–31%) [7]
Crusting [3]
Depigmentation [3]
Eczema (<10%)
Edema (12–17%) [2]
Erosions (10–32%) [5]
Erythema (33–85%) [14]
Erythema multiforme [2]
Excoriations (18–25%) [2]
Flaking (18–67%) [3]
Fungal dermatitis (<10%)
Herpes simplex (<10%)
Hypomelanosis [2]
Induration (5%)
Lichen planus [3]
Lupus erythematosus [3]
Lymphadenopathy (2%)
Pemphigus [4]
Pemphigus foliaceus [3]
Pigmentation [3]
Pruritus (22–75%) [10]
Psoriasis [3]
Scabbing (4%)
Scar [3]
Seborrheic keratoses (<10%)
Tenderness (local) (12%) [2]
Ulcerations (5–10%) [5]
Vesiculation (2–3%)
Vitiligo [7]

Hair
Alopecia (<10%)
Poliosis [2]

Cardiovascular
Chest pain (<10%)

Central Nervous System
Anorexia (<10%)
Anxiety (<10%)

Fever (<10%) [2]
Headache (<10%) [3]
Neurotoxicity [2]
Pain (2–11%) [6]
Rigors (<10%)
Vertigo (dizziness) (<10%)

Neuromuscular/Skeletal
Asthenia (fatigue) (<10%) [2]
Back pain (<10%)
Myalgia/Myopathy (<10%)

Gastrointestinal/Hepatic
Nausea (<10%) [2]
Vomiting (<10%)

Respiratory
Cough (<10%)
Flu-like syndrome (<3%)
Pharyngitis (<10%)
Rhinitis (<10%)
Sinusitis (<10%)
Upper respiratory tract infection (<10%)

Genitourinary
Urinary tract infection (<10%)

Local
Application-site burning (<10%)
Application-site edema (<10%) [4]
Application-site erythema (<10%) [3]
Application-site pruritus (<10%) [4]
Application-site reactions [9]

Other
Adverse effects [6]

IMMUNE GLOBULIN (EQUINE)

See: www.drugeruptiondata.com/drug/id/2597

IMMUNE GLOBULIN IV

Synonyms: IGIV; IVIG
Trade names: Gamimune (Bayer), Gammagard (Baxter), Gammar PIV (ZLB Behring), Gamunex (Bayer), Iveegam (Baxter), Venoglobulin (Alpha Therapeutics)
Indications: Immunodeficiency in patients unable to produce sufficient amounts of IgG antibodies
Class: Immunomodulator
Half-life: N/A
Clinically important, potentially hazardous interactions with: live vaccines
Pregnancy category: C
Important contra-indications noted in the prescribing guidelines for: nursing mothers
Warning: THROMBOSIS, RENAL DYSFUNCTION and ACUTE RENAL FAILURE

Skin
Anaphylactoid reactions/Anaphylaxis [3]
Eczema [3]
Lichenoid eruption [2]
Pompholyx [3]
Rash [2]
Vasculitis [4]

Cardiovascular
Flushing [2]
Hypertension [3]

Myocardial infarction [2]
Palpitation [2]
Thromboembolism [3]

Central Nervous System
Aseptic meningitis [6]
Chills [4]
Fever [10]
Headache [16]

Neuromuscular/Skeletal
Arthralgia [2]
Asthenia (fatigue) [3]
Myalgia/Myopathy [3]

Gastrointestinal/Hepatic
Abdominal pain [2]
Diarrhea [2]
Nausea [8]
Vomiting [2]

Respiratory
Cough [2]
Dyspnea [2]
Pulmonary embolism [2]

Renal
Nephrotoxicity [6]
Renal failure [2]

Hematologic
Anemia [2]
Hemolysis [2]
Hemolytic anemia [3]
Thrombosis [3]

Local
Application-site pain (16%)
Infusion-related reactions [4]
Injection-site edema [2]
Injection-site erythema [2]

Other
Adverse effects [9]

IMMUNE GLOBULIN SC

Synonym: SCIG
Trade names: Cuvitru (Shire), Hizentra (CSL Behring), Vivaglobin (CSL Behring)
Indications: Primary immune deficiency
Class: Immunomodulator
Half-life: N/A
Clinically important, potentially hazardous interactions with: none known
Pregnancy category: C
Warning: THROMBOSIS

Skin
Pruritus [2]
Rash (<3%)

Mucosal
Oropharyngeal pain (17%)

Cardiovascular
Tachycardia (<3%)

Central Nervous System
Fever (<3%) [2]
Headache (2–32%) [3]

Neuromuscular/Skeletal
Asthenia (fatigue) (<5%)

Gastrointestinal/Hepatic
Gastrointestinal disorder (<5%)
Nausea (<11%)

Respiratory
Bronchitis [2]
Cough (10%)
Upper respiratory tract infection [2]

Local
Injection-site reactions (49–92%) [5]

Other
Allergic reactions (11%)

INACTIVATED POLIO VACCINE

See: www.drugeruptiondata.com/drug/id/1408

INAMRINONE

See: www.drugeruptiondata.com/drug/id/355

INDACATEROL

Trade names: Arcapta Neohaler (Novartis), Onbrez Breezhaler (Novartis), Utibron Neohaler (Novartis)
Indications: Long term, once-daily maintenance bronchodilator treatment of airflow obstruction in chronic obstructive pulmonary disease (COPD), including chronic bronchitis and/or emphysema
Class: Beta-2 adrenergic agonist, Bronchodilator
Half-life: 40–56 hours
Clinically important, potentially hazardous interactions with: acetazolamide, adrenergics, aminophylline, arsenic, corticosteroids, diuretics, erythromycin, ketoconazole, MAO inhibitors, pazopanib, QT prolonging agents, ritonavir, steroids, telavancin, theophylline, tricyclic antidepressants, verapamil, xanthine derivatives
Pregnancy category: C
Important contra-indications noted in the prescribing guidelines for: nursing mothers; pediatric patients
Note: Studies in asthma patients showed that long-acting beta$_2$-adrenergic agonists may increase the risk of asthma-related death. Contra-indicated in patients with asthma without use of a long-term asthma control medication. Utibron Neohaler is indacaterol and glycopyrrolate.
Warning: ASTHMA-RELATED DEATH

Mucosal
Oropharyngeal pain [2]

Central Nervous System
Headache (5%) [3]
Pain (oropharyngeal) (2%)

Gastrointestinal/Hepatic
Nausea (2%)

Respiratory
Asthma [2]
COPD (exacerbation) [7]
Cough (7%) [9]
Dyspnea [2]
Influenza [2]
Nasopharyngitis (5%) [6]

Upper respiratory tract infection [3]
Other
Adverse effects [6]

INDAPAMIDE

Trade name: Lozol (Sanofi-Aventis)
Indications: Edema
Class: Diuretic, thiazide
Half-life: 14–18 hours
Clinically important, potentially hazardous interactions with: digoxin, lithium, zinc
Pregnancy category: B
Important contra-indications noted in the prescribing guidelines for: the elderly; nursing mothers; pediatric patients
Note: Indapamide is a sulfonamide and can be absorbed systemically. Sulfonamides can produce severe, possibly fatal, reactions such as toxic epidermal necrolysis and Stevens-Johnson syndrome.

Skin
Angioedema [3]
Erythema multiforme [2]
Pemphigus foliaceus [2]
Peripheral edema (<5%) [2]
Pruritus (<5%) [2]
Rash (<5%) [4]
Toxic epidermal necrolysis [3]
Urticaria (<5%)
Vasculitis (<5%)
Mucosal
Xerostomia (<5%) [2]
Cardiovascular
Flushing (<5%)
QT prolongation [5]
Central Nervous System
Paresthesias (<5%)
Vertigo (dizziness) [2]
Endocrine/Metabolic
Hypokalemia [2]
Hyponatremia [2]

INDINAVIR

Trade name: Crixivan (Merck)
Indications: HIV infection
Class: Antiretroviral, CYP3A4 inhibitor, HIV-1 protease inhibitor
Half-life: ~1.8 hours
Clinically important, potentially hazardous interactions with: abiraterone, alfuzosin, almotriptan, alosetron, alprazolam, amiodarone, amprenavir, antacids, antiarrhythmics, antifungal agents, artemether/lumefantrine, astemizole, atazanavir, atorvastatin, atovaquone, atovaquone/proguanil, avanafil, bepridil, bortezomib, bosentan, brigatinib, brinzolamide, cabazitaxel, cabozantinib, calcifediol, calcium channel blockers, carbamazepine, chlordiazepoxide, ciclesonide, cisapride, clarithromycin, clonazepam, clorazepate, colchicine, conivaptan, copanlisib, corticosteroids, crizotinib, cyclosporine, CYP3A4 inducers and substrates, darifenacin, darunavir, dasatinib, deferasirox,

delavirdine, diazepam, didanosine, dienogest, digoxin, dihydroergotamine, dronedarone, dutasteride, efavirenz, enfuvirtide, eplerenone, ergot derivatives, ergotamine, estazolam, estrogens, etravirine, everolimus, felodipine, fentanyl, fesoterodine, flibanserin, flurazepam, fluticasone propionate, food, fusidic acid, grapefruit juice, guanfacine, H₂-antagonists, halazepam, halofantrine, HMG-CoA reductase inhibitors, itraconazole, ixabepilone, ketoconazole, lapatinib, lidocaine, lomitapide, lopinavir, lovastatin, maraviroc, meperidine, methylergonovine, methylprednisolone, methysergide, midazolam, midostaurin, mifepristone, mometasone, nefazodone, nelfinavir, neratinib, nevirapine, nicardipine, nifedipine, nilotinib, nisoldipine, olaparib, P-glycoprotein inhibitors and inducers, paclitaxel, palbociclib, pantoprazole, paricalcitol, pazopanib, PEG-interferon, phenobarbital, phenytoin, pimavanserin, pimecrolimus, pimozide, ponatinib, prasugrel, protease inhibitors, proton pump inhibitors, quazepam, quinidine, quinine, ranolazine, ribociclib, rifabutin, rifampin, rifapentine, rilpivirine, rivaroxaban, romidepsin, rosuvastatin, ruxolitinib, salmeterol, saxagliptin, sildenafil, silodosin, simeprevir, simvastatin, sirolimus, solifenacin, sorafenib, St John's wort, sunitinib, tacrolimus, tadalafil, tamsulosin, telithromycin, temsirolimus, tenofovir disoproxil, theophylline, ticagrelor, tolvaptan, trazodone, triazolam, tricyclic antidepressants, valproic acid, vardenafil, vemurafenib, venetoclax, venlafaxine, vorapaxar, zidovudine
Pregnancy category: C
Important contra-indications noted in the prescribing guidelines for: nursing mothers; pediatric patients
Note: Protease inhibitors cause dyslipidemia which includes elevated triglycerides and cholesterol and redistribution of body fat centrally to produce the so-called 'protease paunch', breast enlargement, facial atrophy, and 'buffalo hump'.

Skin
Bromhidrosis (<2%)
Dermatitis (<2%)
Diaphoresis (<2%)
Folliculitis (<2%)
Herpes simplex (<2%)
Herpes zoster (<2%)
Jaundice (2%)
Lipodystrophy [8]
Lipomatosis [2]
Pruritus [2]
Rash [2]
Seborrhea (<2%)
Stevens-Johnson syndrome [2]
Xerosis [2]
Hair
Alopecia [5]
Nails
Onychocryptosis [2]
Paronychia [5]
Pyogenic granuloma [3]
Mucosal
Aphthous stomatitis (<2%)
Cheilitis [4]

Gingivitis (<2%)
Cardiovascular
Flushing (<2%)
Central Nervous System
Anorexia (3%)
Dysesthesia (<2%)
Dysgeusia (taste perversion) (3%)
Fever (2%)
Headache (5%)
Hyperesthesia (<2%)
Paresthesias (<2%)
Somnolence (drowsiness) (2%)
Vertigo (dizziness) (3%)
Neuromuscular/Skeletal
Asthenia (fatigue) (2%)
Back pain (8%)
Myalgia/Myopathy with lovastatin or simvastatin (<2%)
Gastrointestinal/Hepatic
Abdominal pain (17%) [2]
Diarrhea (3%)
Dyspepsia (2%)
Nausea (12%)
Vomiting (8%)
Respiratory
Cough (2%)
Endocrine/Metabolic
ALT increased (5%)
Appetite increased (2%)
AST increased (4%)
Creatine phosphokinase increased [2]
Diabetes mellitus [2]
Gynecomastia [4]
Porphyria (acute) [2]
Genitourinary
Crystalluria [2]
Dysuria (2%)
Renal
Nephrolithiasis (9%) [4]
Nephrotoxicity [13]
Ocular
Eyelid edema (<2%)
Other
Bruxism (<2%)

INDOMETHACIN

Synonym: indometacin
Indications: Arthritis
Class: Non-steroidal anti-inflammatory (NSAID)
Half-life: 4.5 hours
Clinically important, potentially hazardous interactions with: aldesleukin, aspirin, atenolol, cyclopenthiazide, diflunisal, diuretics, methotrexate, NSAIDs, prednisolone, prednisone, sermorelin, tiludronate, torsemide, triamterene, urokinase
Pregnancy category: C
Important contra-indications noted in the prescribing guidelines for: nursing mothers; pediatric patients
Note: NSAIDs may cause an increased risk of serious cardiovascular and gastrointestinal adverse events, which can be fatal. This risk may increase with duration of use.

Warning: RISK OF SERIOUS CARDIOVASCULAR AND GASTROINTESTINAL EVENTS

Skin
Angioedema [2]
Bullous dermatitis [2]
Dermatitis [5]
Dermatitis herpetiformis (exacerbation) [2]
Edema (3–9%)
Exanthems (<5%) [7]
Fixed eruption [2]
Pruritus (<10%) [3]
Psoriasis [7]
Purpura [5]
Rash (>10%)
Toxic epidermal necrolysis [6]
Urticaria [7]
Vasculitis [5]

Mucosal
Oral lesions (<7%) [2]
Oral ulceration [4]

Central Nervous System
Psychosis [3]

Gastrointestinal/Hepatic
Gastrointestinal bleeding [2]
Gastrointestinal perforation [3]
Gastrointestinal ulceration [3]
Pancreatitis [2]

Otic
Tinnitus [2]

Ocular
Periorbital edema [2]

Other
Adverse effects [8]

INDORAMIN

See: www.drugeruptiondata.com/drug/id/1341

INFLIXIMAB

Trade names: Inflectra (Celltrion) ((Remsima)), Remicade (Centocor), Renflexis (Samsung Bioepsis)
Indications: Crohn's disease, ulcerative colitis, rheumatoid arthritis, ankylosing spondylitis, psoriatic arthritis, plaque psoriasis
Class: Cytokine inhibitor, Disease-modifying antirheumatic drug (DMARD), Monoclonal antibody, TNF inhibitor
Half-life: 8–10 days
Clinically important, potentially hazardous interactions with: abatacept, anakinra, live vaccines, methotrexate, tocilizumab
Pregnancy category: B
Important contra-indications noted in the prescribing guidelines for: the elderly; nursing mothers
Note: TNF inhibitors should be used in patients with heart failure only after consideration of other treatment options.
Contra-indicated in patients with a personal or family history of multiple sclerosis or demyelinating disease. TNF inhibitors should not be administered to patients with moderate to severe heart failure (New York Heart Association Functional Class III/IV).
Warning: SERIOUS INFECTIONS and MALIGNANCY

Skin
Abscess [4]
Acneform eruption [6]
AGEP [2]
Anaphylactoid reactions/Anaphylaxis [10]
Angioedema [2]
Candidiasis (5%) [4]
Cellulitis [5]
Dermatitis [4]
Eczema [5]
Edema [3]
Erythema multiforme [2]
Exanthems [4]
Folliculitis [2]
Hand–foot syndrome [2]
Herpes [2]
Herpes simplex [4]
Herpes zoster [11]
Hypersensitivity [11]
Leukocytoclastic vasculitis [2]
Lichen planus [2]
Lichenoid eruption [3]
Lupus erythematosus [35]
Lupus syndrome [11]
Lymphoma [9]
Malignancies [2]
Molluscum contagiosum [2]
Neoplasms [2]
Nevi [2]
Palmar–plantar pustulosis [3]
Pityriasis lichenoides chronica [2]
Pruritus (7%) [8]
Pseudolymphoma [2]
Psoriasis [56]
Pustules [5]
Rash (10%) [13]
Sarcoidosis [5]
Serum sickness [2]
Serum sickness-like reaction (<3%) [5]
Toxic epidermal necrolysis [2]
Toxicity [2]
Urticaria [6]
Vasculitis [18]
Vitiligo [4]

Hair
Alopecia [6]
Alopecia areata [3]

Cardiovascular
Cardiotoxicity [2]
Chest pain [4]
Flushing [2]
Hypertension (7%) [3]
Palpitation [2]
Pericarditis [2]
Tachycardia [2]

Central Nervous System
Aseptic meningitis [2]
Chills (5–9%) [2]
Demyelination [3]
Fever (7%) [10]
Headache (18%) [11]
Leukoencephalopathy [2]
Neurotoxicity [8]
Pain (8%) [3]
Paresthesias (<4%) [2]
Peripheral neuropathy [7]
Seizures [2]
Vertigo (dizziness) [3]

Neuromuscular/Skeletal
Arthralgia (<8%) [15]
Asthenia (fatigue) (9%) [4]
Back pain (8%)
Myalgia/Myopathy (5%) [7]
Polymyositis [2]

Gastrointestinal/Hepatic
Abdominal pain (12%) [3]
Crohn's disease (26%)
Diarrhea (12%)
Dyspepsia (10%)
Hepatitis [11]
Hepatotoxicity [16]
Nausea (21%) [3]
Pancreatitis [2]

Respiratory
Bronchitis (10%)
Cough (12%) [3]
Dyspnea (6%) [3]
Pharyngitis (12%)
Pneumonia [12]
Pulmonary toxicity [6]
Rhinitis (8%)
Sinusitis (14%) [4]
Tuberculosis [13]
Upper respiratory tract infection (32%) [6]

Endocrine/Metabolic
ALT increased [2]

Genitourinary
Cystitis [2]
Urinary tract infection (8%) [2]

Renal
Nephrotoxicity [2]

Hematologic
Neutropenia [5]
Sepsis [2]
Thrombocytopenia [5]

Ocular
Optic neuritis [3]
Uveitis [2]

Local
Application-site reactions (mild) (<4%) [6]
Infusion-related reactions [20]
Infusion-site reactions (20%) [12]
Injection-site reactions (6%) [9]

Other
Adverse effects [43]
Allergic reactions [8]
Death [13]
Infection (36%) [58]
Nocardiosis [3]
Side effects [2]
Systemic reactions [2]

INFLUENZA VACCINE

Trade names: Afluria (Seqirus), Agrippal (Chiron), Comvax (Merck), Fluad (Novartis), Fluarix (GSK), FluMist (Medimmune) (Wyeth), Flurix (GSK), Fluviral (Shire), Inflexal V (Berna Biotech), Invivac (Solvay), Vaxigrip (Sanofi-Aventis)
Indications: Influenza prevention
Class: Vaccine
Half-life: N/A
Clinically important, potentially hazardous interactions with: aminophylline, carbamazepine, cyclosporine, mercaptopurine, phenobarbital, phenytoin, prednisone, vincristine, warfarin
Pregnancy category: C
Important contra-indications noted in the prescribing guidelines for: pediatric patients
Note: Inactivated influenza vaccine should not be given to persons with anaphylactic hypersensitivity to eggs or other components of the vaccine. For current data on influenza in the USA consult the Centers for Disease Control and Protection website (www.cdc.gov/flu).

Skin
Anaphylactoid reactions/Anaphylaxis (rare) [3]
Henoch–Schönlein purpura [2]
Hypersensitivity [2]
Linear IgA bullous dermatosis [2]
Purpura [2]
Rash [3]
Serum sickness-like reaction [2]
Vasculitis [10]

Central Nervous System
Fever [13]
Guillain–Barré syndrome [11]
Headache [9]
Seizures [3]

Neuromuscular/Skeletal
Arthralgia [2]
Asthenia (fatigue) [7]
Myalgia/Myopathy [11]
Polymyositis [4]

Gastrointestinal/Hepatic
Abdominal pain [2]

Respiratory
Asthma [2]
Cough [2]

Hematologic
Thrombocytopenia [2]

Ocular
Oculorespiratory syndrome [15]
Optic neuritis [2]

Local
Injection-site edema [4]
Injection-site erythema [7]
Injection-site induration [5]
Injection-site inflammation [3]
Injection-site pain (20–28%) [15]
Injection-site reactions [3]

Other
Adverse effects [7]
Side effects [4]
Systemic reactions (injection site) [5]

INGENOL MEBUTATE

Trade name: Picato (Leo Pharma)
Indications: Actinic keratosis
Class: Cell death inducer
Half-life: N/A
Clinically important, potentially hazardous interactions with: none known
Pregnancy category: C
Important contra-indications noted in the prescribing guidelines for: pediatric patients

Skin
Crusting [4]
Erythema [4]
Flaking [4]
Scaling [3]

Central Nervous System
Headache (2%) [4]

Respiratory
Nasopharyngitis (2%) [2]

Ocular
Eyelid edema [2]
Periorbital edema (3%) [2]

Local
Application-site erythema [2]
Application-site infection (3%) [2]
Application-site pain (2–15%) [6]
Application-site pruritus (8%) [4]
Application-site reactions [3]

INOSITOL

See: www.drugeruptiondata.com/drug/id/1376

INOTUZUMAB OZOGAMICIN *

Trade name: Besponsa (Wyeth)
Indications: Relapsed or refractory B-cell precursor acute lymphoblastic leukemia
Class: Antibody drug conjugate (ADC), CD22-directed antibody-drug conjugate
Half-life: 12 days
Clinically important, potentially hazardous interactions with: none known
Pregnancy category: N/A (Can cause fetal harm)
Important contra-indications noted in the prescribing guidelines for: nursing mothers; pediatric patients
Warning: HEPATOTOXICITY, INCLUDING HEPATIC VENOOCCLUSIVE DISEASE (ALSO KNOWN AS SINUSOIDAL OBSTRUCTION SYNDROME) and INCREASED RISK OF POSTHEMATOPOIETIC STEM CELL TRANSPLANT NONRELAPSE MORTALITY

Skin
Hypersensitivity (2%)
Tumor lysis syndrome (2%)

Mucosal
Stomatitis (13%)

Cardiovascular
Hypotension [2]
Veno-occlusive disease (23%) [4]

Central Nervous System
Chills (11%)
Fever (32%) [4]
Headache (28%) [2]

Neuromuscular/Skeletal
Asthenia (fatigue) (35%) [2]

Gastrointestinal/Hepatic
Abdominal distension (6%)
Abdominal pain (23%)
Ascites (4%)
Constipation (16%)
Diarrhea (17%)
Hepatotoxicity (14%) [3]
Nausea (31%) [4]
Vomiting (15%)

Respiratory
Pneumonia [2]

Endocrine/Metabolic
ALP increased (13%)
ALT increased (>10%) [2]
Appetite decreased (12%)
AST increased (>10%) [3]
GGT increased (21%)
Hyperbilirubinemia (21%) [5]
Hyperuricemia (4%)

Hematologic
Anemia (36%)
Febrile neutropenia (26%) [2]
Hemorrhage (33%)
Hyperlipasemia (9%)
Leukopenia (35%) [3]
Lymphopenia (18%) [4]
Myelosuppression (>10%)
Neutropenia (49%) [9]
Pancytopenia (2%)
Thrombocytopenia (51%) [9]

Local
Infusion-related reactions (2%)

Other
Infection (48%) [2]

INSULIN

See: www.drugeruptiondata.com/drug/id/361

INSULIN ASPART

Trade names: NovoLog (Novo Nordisk), NovoRapid (Novo Nordisk), Ryzodeg (Novo Nordisk)
Indications: Diabetes mellitus
Class: Hormone, polypeptide
Half-life: 81 minutes
Clinically important, potentially hazardous interactions with: ACE inhibitors, alcohol, atypical antipsychotics, beta blockers, clonidine, corticosteroids, danazol, disopyramide, diuretics, epinephrine, estrogens, fibrates, fluoxetine, isoniazid, isoniazid, lithium salts, MAO inhibitors, niacin, octreotide, oral contraceptives, pentamidine, phenothiazine derivatives, pramlintide, propoxyphene, salbutamol,

salicylates, somatropin, sulfonamide antibiotics, terbutaline, thyroid hormones
Pregnancy category: B
Important contra-indications noted in the prescribing guidelines for: the elderly; pediatric patients
Note: Ryzodeg is insulin aspart and insulin degludec; various forms of insulin are available - see other insulin profiles for reaction details.

___

Skin
Lipodystrophy (>5%)
Peripheral edema (>5%)

Nails
Onychomycosis (10%)

Cardiovascular
Chest pain (5%)

Central Nervous System
Headache (12%) [2]
Hyporeflexia (11%)

Gastrointestinal/Hepatic
Abdominal pain (5%)
Diarrhea (5%)
Nausea (7%)

Respiratory
Nasopharyngitis [2]
Sinusitis (5%)

Endocrine/Metabolic
Diabetic ketoacidosis [2]
Hypoglycemia (75%) [5]
Weight gain (>5%)

Genitourinary
Urinary tract infection (8%)

INSULIN DEGLUDEC

Trade names: Ryzodeg (Novo Nordisk), Tresiba (Novo Nordisk), Xultophy (Novo Nordisk)
Indications: Diabetes mellitus
Class: Human insulin analog, long-acting
Half-life: 25 hours
Clinically important, potentially hazardous interactions with: ACE inhibitors, albuterol, alcohol, angiotensin II receptor blocking agents, beta blockers, clonidine, clozapine, corticosteroids, danazol, DDP-4-inhibitors, disopyramide, diuretics, epinephrine, estrogens, fibrates, fluoxetine, GLP-1 receptor agonists, glucagon, guanethidine, isoniazid, lithium, MAO inhibitors, niacin, octreotide, olanzapine, oral contraceptives, pentamidine, pentoxifylline, phenothiazines, pramlintide, propoxyphene, protease inhibitors, reserpine, salicylates, SGLT-2 inhibitors, somatropin, sulfonamide antibiotics, terbutaline, thyroid hormones
Pregnancy category: C
Important contra-indications noted in the prescribing guidelines for: the elderly; nursing mothers; pediatric patients
Note: Contra-indicated during episodes of hypoglycemia. Ryzodeg is insulin degludec and insulin aspart; Xultophy is insulin degludec and liraglutide; various forms of insulin are available - see other insulin profiles for reaction details.

Skin
Hypersensitivity [2]
Peripheral edema (<3%)

Central Nervous System
Headache (9–12%) [10]

Gastrointestinal/Hepatic
Diarrhea (6%) [6]
Gastroenteritis (5%)
Nausea [7]
Vomiting [2]

Respiratory
Nasopharyngitis (13–24%) [11]
Sinusitis (5%)
Upper respiratory tract infection (8–12%) [3]

Endocrine/Metabolic
Diabetic ketoacidosis [2]
Hypoglycemia [9]

Ocular
Retinopathy [2]

Local
Injection-site reactions (4%) [6]

Other
Adverse effects [4]

INSULIN DETEMIR

Trade name: Levemir (Novo Nordisk)
Indications: Diabetes (Type I or II)
Class: Human insulin analog, long-acting
Half-life: 5–7 hours
Clinically important, potentially hazardous interactions with: albuterol, alcohol, antipsychotics, beta blockers, clonidine, clozapine, corticosteroids, danazol, diuretics, epinephrine, estrogens, guanethidine, isoniazid, lithium, niacin, olanzapine, oral antidiabetics, oral contraceptives, pentamidine, phenothiazines, propranolol, protease inhibitors, reserpine, somatropin, terbutaline, thiazolidinediones, thyroid hormones
Pregnancy category: B
Important contra-indications noted in the prescribing guidelines for: the elderly; nursing mothers; pediatric patients
Note: Various forms of insulin are available - see other insulin profiles for reaction details.

___

Central Nervous System
Fever (10%)
Headache (7–31%) [3]

Neuromuscular/Skeletal
Back pain (8%)

Gastrointestinal/Hepatic
Abdominal pain (6–13%)
Gastroenteritis (6–17%)
Nausea (7%)
Vomiting (7%)

Respiratory
Bronchitis (5%)
Cough (8%)
Flu-like syndrome (6–14%)
Pharyngitis (10–17%)
Rhinitis (7%)
Upper respiratory tract infection (13–36%)

Endocrine/Metabolic
Hyperglycemia [2]
Hypoglycemia [4]

Local
Injection-site reactions (3–4%) [4]

Other
Allergic reactions [3]
Infection (viral) (7%)

INSULIN GLARGINE

Trade names: Basaglar (Lilly), Lantus (Sanofi-Aventis), Soliqua (Sanofi-Aventis)
Indications: Diabetes (Type I or II)
Class: Hormone analog, polypeptide
Half-life: N/A
Clinically important, potentially hazardous interactions with: ACE inhibitors, albuterol, alcohol, beta blockers, clonidine, clozapine, corticosteroids, danazol, disopyramide, diuretics, epinephrine, estrogens, fibrates, fluoxetine, glucagon, guanethidine, isoniazid, lithium, MAO inhibitors, niacin, olanzapine, oral antidiabetic products, oral contraceptives, pentamidine, pentoxifylline, phenothiazine derivatives, pramlintide, propoxyphene, propranolol, protease inhibitors, reserpine, salicylates, somatostain analogs, somatropin, sulfonamide antibiotics, terbutaline, thyroid hormones
Pregnancy category: C
Important contra-indications noted in the prescribing guidelines for: nursing mothers; pediatric patients
Note: Soliqua is insulin glargine and lixisenatide; various forms of insulin are available - see other insulin profiles for reaction details.

___

Skin
Lipoatrophy [2]
Peripheral edema (20%)

Central Nervous System
Depression (11%)
Headache (6–10%) [4]

Neuromuscular/Skeletal
Arthralgia (14%)
Back pain (13%)
Pain in extremities (13%)

Gastrointestinal/Hepatic
Diarrhea (11%) [6]
Nausea [5]
Vomiting [4]

Respiratory
Bronchitis (15%)
Cough (12%)
Influenza (19%)
Nasopharyngitis [6]
Pharyngitis (8%)
Rhinitis (5%)
Sinusitis (19%)
Upper respiratory tract infection (11–29%) [3]

Endocrine/Metabolic
Hypoglycemia [4]

Genitourinary
Urinary tract infection (11%)

Ocular
Cataract (18%)
Retinopathy [2]

Local
Injection-site pain (3%)
Injection-site reactions [4]

Other
Adverse effects [5]
Infection (9–14%)

INSULIN GLULISINE

Trade name: Apidra (Sanofi-Aventis)
Indications: Diabetes
Class: Insulin analog
Half-life: 13–42 minutes
Clinically important, potentially hazardous interactions with: ACE inhibitors, albuterol, alcohol, anitpsychotics, beta blockers, clonidine, clozapine, corticosteroids, danazol, disopyramide, diuretics, epinephrine, fibrates, fluoxetine, glucagon, guanethidine, isoniazid, lithium, MAO inhibitors, niacin, oral antidiabetic agents, oral contraceptives, pentamidine, pentoxifylline, phenothiazine derivatives, pramlintide, propoxyphene, propranolol, protease inhibitors, reserpine, salicylates, somatostatin analogs, somatropin, sulfonamide antibiotics, terbutaline, thyroid hormones
Pregnancy category: C
Important contra-indications noted in the prescribing guidelines for: nursing mothers; pediatric patients
Note: Various forms of insulin are available - see other insulin profiles for reaction details.

Skin
Peripheral edema (8%)

Cardiovascular
Hypertension (4%)

Central Nervous System
Headache (7%)

Neuromuscular/Skeletal
Arthralgia (6%)

Respiratory
Influenza (4–6%)
Nasopharyngitis (8–11%)
Upper respiratory tract infection (7–11%)

Endocrine/Metabolic
Hypoglycemia (6–7%) [3]

Local
Injection-site reactions (10%) [2]

INTERFERON ALFA

Synonyms: IFN; INF
Trade names: Infergen (Intermune), Intron A (Schering), Rebetron (Schering), Roferon-A (Roche)
Indications: Chronic hepatitis C virus infection, hairy cell leukemia
Class: Biologic, Immunomodulator, Interferon
Half-life: 2 hours
Clinically important, potentially hazardous interactions with: aldesleukin, amitriptyline, captopril, gemfibrozil, metaxalone, methadone, ribavirin, telbivudine, theophylline, theophylline derivatives, zafirlukast, zidovudine
Pregnancy category: C (pregnancy category will be X when used in combination with ribavirin)
Important contra-indications noted in the prescribing guidelines for: nursing mothers; pediatric patients
Note: Many of the adverse reactions depend on the nature of the disease being treated. Either hairy cell leukemia [L] or AIDS-related Kaposi's sarcoma [K].

Skin
Angioedema [3]
Bullous dermatitis [4]
Dermatitis (6%)
Eczema [6]
Edema [L] (11%) [2]
Erythema [2]
Exanthems [3]
Herpes simplex [2]
Kaposi's sarcoma [2]
Lichen planus [8]
Linear IgA bullous dermatosis [3]
Livedo reticularis [2]
Lupus erythematosus [17]
Lupus syndrome [2]
Necrosis [6]
Pemphigus [2]
Photosensitivity [2]
Pigmentation [3]
Pruritus 13% [L] 5–7% [K] (13%) [4]
Psoriasis [22]
Purpura [2]
Rash 44% [L] 11% [K] [5]
Raynaud's phenomenon [11]
Sarcoidosis [47]
Seborrheic dermatitis [2]
Sjögren's syndrome [4]
Thrombocytopenic purpura [2]
Toxicity [4]
Urticaria [K] (<3%) [3]
Vasculitis [7]
Vitiligo [9]

Hair
Alopecia (23%) [16]
Hair pigmentation [3]
Hypertrichosis [3]
Straight hair [2]

Mucosal
Aphthous stomatitis [2]
Oral lichen planus [7]
Stomatitis (<10%)
Xerostomia (>10%) [4]

Cardiovascular
Cardiotoxicity [2]
Hypertension [3]
Hypotension [2]

Central Nervous System
Ageusia (taste loss) [2]
Anorexia [4]
Anosmia [4]
Anxiety [2]
Chills [4]
Depression (5–15%) [24]
Dysgeusia (taste perversion) [K] (25%) [2]
Fever (37%) [6]
Headache (54%) [5]
Insomnia (19%)
Irritability [2]
Neurotoxicity [4]
Paresthesias 8% [L] (12%)
Parkinsonism [3]
Restless legs syndrome [2]
Rigors (35%)
Seizures [2]
Suicidal ideation [6]
Tremor [2]
Vertigo (dizziness) (16%) [2]

Neuromuscular/Skeletal
Arthralgia (28%) [4]
Asthenia (fatigue) (56%) [11]
Back pain (9%)
Myalgia/Myopathy 69% [L] 71% [K] [10]
Myasthenia gravis [11]
Rhabdomyolysis [3]

Gastrointestinal/Hepatic
Abdominal pain (15%)
Constipation [2]
Diarrhea (24%) [5]
Nausea (24%) [7]
Pancreatitis [7]
Vomiting [5]

Respiratory
Cough [2]
Dyspnea (13%) [2]
Flu-like syndrome (>10%) [10]
Pulmonary hypertension [2]

Endocrine/Metabolic
ALT increased [2]
AST increased [2]
Hyperglycemia [2]
Hyperthyroidism [3]
Thyroid dysfunction [3]
Thyroiditis [2]
Weight loss (16%) [5]

Genitourinary
Impotence [2]

Renal
Nephrotoxicity [3]
Proteinuria [2]

Hematologic
Anemia (11%) [7]
Febrile neutropenia [2]
Hemolytic uremic syndrome [6]
Leukopenia [5]
Lymphopenia (14%)
Neutropenia (21%) [5]
Thrombocytopenia [7]

Otic
Tinnitus [4]

Ocular
Eyelashes – hypertrichosis [3]
Optic neuropathy [4]
Retinopathy [6]
Vision blurred (4%)

Local
Injection-site alopecia [2]
Injection-site erythema [2]
Injection-site induration [3]
Injection-site necrosis [16]

Other
Adverse effects [6]
Infection [4]
Vogt-Koyanagi-Harada syndrome [6]

INTERFERON BETA

Trade names: Avonex (Biogen), Betaferon (Bayer), Betaseron (Bayer), Plegridy (Biogen), Rebif (Merck)
Indications: Relapsing multiple sclerosis, cancers
Class: Immunomodulator, Interferon
Half-life: 10 hours
Clinically important, potentially hazardous interactions with: theophylline, theophylline derivatives, zidovudine
Pregnancy category: C
Important contra-indications noted in the prescribing guidelines for: nursing mothers; pediatric patients

Skin
Cyst (4%)
Diaphoresis (23%)
Edema (generalized) (8%)
Herpes simplex (2–3%)
Herpes zoster (3)
Hypersensitivity (3%)
Lipoatrophy [2]
Lupus erythematosus [8]
Nevi (3%)
Nicolau syndrome [2]
Rash [2]
Raynaud's phenomenon [2]
Sarcoidosis [2]
Thrombocytopenic purpura [4]
Urticaria (5%)
Vasculitis [4]

Hair
Alopecia (4%)

Mucosal
Mucosal bleeding (12–38%)

Cardiovascular
Capillary leak syndrome [3]

Central Nervous System
Chills (21%)
Depression [8]
Fever [4]
Headache [4]
Multiple sclerosis [2]
Pain (52%)
Paresthesias [2]
Psychosis [2]
Seizures (2%) [2]
Vertigo (dizziness) (35%)

Neuromuscular/Skeletal
Arthralgia [2]

Asthenia (fatigue) [2]
Myalgia/Myopathy (44%)
Rhabdomyolysis [2]

Gastrointestinal/Hepatic
Hepatotoxicity [5]

Respiratory
Flu-like syndrome (61%) [14]
Upper respiratory tract infection (31%)

Endocrine/Metabolic
Mastodynia (7%)
Thyroid dysfunction [4]

Genitourinary
Vaginitis (4%)

Renal
Nephrotoxicity [2]

Hematologic
Hemolytic uremic syndrome [3]
Thrombotic microangiopathy [4]

Ocular
Retinopathy [3]

Local
Injection-site ecchymoses (2%)
Injection-site inflammation (3%)
Injection-site necrosis [3]
Injection-site purpura (2%)
Injection-site reactions (4%) [9]

Other
Adverse effects [4]
Death [4]
Infection (11%) [3]

INTERFERON GAMMA *

Trade name: Actimmune (Horizon)
Indications: Chronic granulomatous disease, severe malignant osteopetrosis
Class: Immunomodulator, Interferon
Half-life: 6 hours
Clinically important, potentially hazardous interactions with: tasonermin, typhoid vaccine
Pregnancy category: N/A (May cause fetal toxicity based on findings in animal studies)
Important contra-indications noted in the prescribing guidelines for: nursing mothers; pediatric patients

Skin
Rash (17%)

Central Nervous System
Chills (14%) [3]
Fever (52%) [8]
Headache (33%) [3]

Neuromuscular/Skeletal
Arthralgia (2%)
Asthenia (fatigue) (14%) [3]
Myalgia/Myopathy (6%)

Gastrointestinal/Hepatic
Diarrhea (14%)
Nausea (10%)
Vomiting (13%)

Respiratory
Flu-like syndrome [4]

Local
Injection-site erythema (14%) [2]

IOBENGUANE

See: www.drugeruptiondata.com/drug/id/1324

IODIXANOL

See: www.drugeruptiondata.com/drug/id/1116

IODOQUINOL

See: www.drugeruptiondata.com/drug/id/1345

IOHEXOL

See: www.drugeruptiondata.com/drug/id/1267

IOMEPROL

See: www.drugeruptiondata.com/drug/id/1396

IOPROMIDE

See: www.drugeruptiondata.com/drug/id/1220

IOTHALAMATE

See: www.drugeruptiondata.com/drug/id/1416

IOVERSOL

See: www.drugeruptiondata.com/drug/id/1417

IPILIMUMAB

Trade name: Yervoy (Bristol-Myers Squibb)
Indications: Melanoma
Class: Biologic, CTLA-4-blocking monoclonal antibody, Monoclonal antibody
Half-life: 15 days
Clinically important, potentially hazardous interactions with: none known
Pregnancy category: C
Important contra-indications noted in the prescribing guidelines for: nursing mothers; pediatric patients
Warning: IMMUNE-MEDIATED ADVERSE REACTIONS

Skin
Dermatitis (12%) [12]
Dermatomyositis [2]
Erythema [3]
Exanthems [5]
Granulomas [3]
Lymphadenopathy [2]
Pruritus (21–31%) [22]
Rash (19–29%) [28]
Sarcoidosis [4]
Stevens-Johnson syndrome [3]

Toxic epidermal necrolysis [3]
Toxicity [3]
Urticaria (2%) [2]
Vitiligo [3]

Hair
Alopecia [3]

Cardiovascular
Atrial fibrillation [2]
Myocarditis [3]
Pericarditis [2]

Central Nervous System
Anorexia [3]
Chills [2]
Encephalitis [2]
Encephalopathy [4]
Fever [4]
Guillain–Barré syndrome [5]
Headache (14%) [3]
Neurotoxicity [5]

Neuromuscular/Skeletal
Arthralgia [4]
Asthenia (fatigue) (34–41%) [11]
Myalgia/Myopathy [3]
Myasthenia gravis [5]
Rhabdomyolysis [2]

Gastrointestinal/Hepatic
Abdominal pain [3]
Colitis (5–8%) [48]
Constipation [2]
Diarrhea (32–37%) [44]
Enterocolitis (7%) [6]
Gastrointestinal perforation [5]
Hepatitis [15]
Hepatotoxicity (<2%) [19]
Nausea [4]
Pancreatitis [4]
Vomiting [2]

Respiratory
Dyspnea [2]
Pneumonia [5]
Pneumonitis [9]

Endocrine/Metabolic
Adrenal insufficiency [3]
ALT increased [11]
AST increased [9]
Hyperthyroidism [3]
Hyponatremia [3]
Hypophysitis [34]
Hypopituitarism (<4%)
Hypothyroidism [10]
Thyroid dysfunction [4]
Thyroiditis [12]
Weight loss [2]

Renal
Nephrotoxicity [7]
Renal failure [4]

Hematologic
Anemia [3]
Hyperlipasemia [2]
Neutropenia [6]
Thrombocytopenia [6]

Ocular
Iridocyclitis [3]
Orbital inflammation [3]
Retinitis [2]
Uveitis [8]
Xerophthalmia [2]

Local
Infusion-related reactions [4]
Injection-site reactions [2]

Other
Adverse effects [28]
Death [12]

IPODATE

See: www.drugeruptiondata.com/drug/id/364

IPRATROPIUM

Trade names: Atrovent (Boehringer Ingelheim), Combivent (Boehringer Ingelheim), Duoneb (Mylan Specialty), Ipratropium Steri-Neb (Ivax), Rinatec (Boehringer Ingelheim)
Indications: Bronchospasm
Class: Anticholinergic, Muscarinic antagonist
Half-life: 2 hours
Clinically important, potentially hazardous interactions with: anticholinergics
Pregnancy category: B
Important contra-indications noted in the prescribing guidelines for: nursing mothers
Note: Combivent is ipratropium and albuterol.

Mucosal
Oral lesions (<5%)
Oral ulceration [2]
Xerostomia (3%) [3]

Central Nervous System
Dysgeusia (taste perversion) [2]
Trembling (<10%)

Ocular
Mydriasis [2]

Other
Adverse effects [2]

IRBESARTAN

Trade names: Aprovel (Bristol-Myers Squibb), Avalide (Bristol-Myers Squibb), Avapro (Sanofi-Aventis)
Indications: Hypertension, diabetic nephropathy
Class: Angiotensin II receptor antagonist (blocker), Antihypertensive
Half-life: 11–15 hours
Clinically important, potentially hazardous interactions with: ACE inhibitors, adrenergic neurone blockers, alcohol, aldesleukin, aldosterone antagonists, aliskiren, alpha blockers, alprostadil, amifostine, antihypertensives, antipsychotics, anxiolytics and hypnotics, baclofen, beta blockers, calcium channel blockers, carvedilol, clonidine, corticosteroids, cyclosporine, CYP2C8 and CYP2C9 substrates, diazoxide, diuretics, eplerenone, fluconazole, general anesthetics, heparins, hypotensives, levodopa, lithium, MAO inhibitors, methyldopa, methylphenidate, moxisylyte, moxonidine, nitrates, NSAIDs, pentoxifylline, phosphodiesterase 5 inhibitors, potassium salts, prostacyclin analogues, rifamycin derivatives, rituximab, tacrolimus, tizanidine, tolvaptan, trimethoprim
Pregnancy category: D (category C in first trimester; category D in second and third trimesters)
Important contra-indications noted in the prescribing guidelines for: nursing mothers; pediatric patients
Note: Avalide is irbesartan and hydrochlorothiazide. Hydrochlorothiazide is a sulfonamide which can be absorbed systemically. Sulfonamides can produce severe, possibly fatal, reactions such as toxic epidermal necrolysis and Stevens-Johnson syndrome.
Warning: FETAL TOXICITY

Skin
Angioedema [3]
Edema (<10%)
Peripheral edema [2]
Rash (<10%)

Gastrointestinal/Hepatic
Pancreatitis [2]

Respiratory
Cough [2]

IRINOTECAN

Trade names: Camptosar (Pfizer), Onivyde (Merrimack)
Indications: Metastatic colorectal carcinoma (Camptosar), metastatic adenocarcinoma of the pancreas (Onivyde - in combination with fluorouracil and leucovorin)
Class: Antineoplastic, Topoisomerase 1 inhibitor
Half-life: 6–10 hours
Clinically important, potentially hazardous interactions with: aprepitant, atazanavir, bevacizumab, ketoconazole, lapatinib, safinamide, sorafenib, St John's wort, strong CYP3A4 inhibitors, voriconazole
Pregnancy category: D
Important contra-indications noted in the prescribing guidelines for: the elderly; nursing mothers; pediatric patients
Warning: DIARRHEA and MYELOSUPPRESSION (Camptosar)
SEVERE NEUTROPENIA and SEVERE DIARRHEA (Onivyde)

Skin
Acneform eruption [4]
Exfoliative dermatitis (14%)
Hand–foot syndrome [6]
Pruritus [4]
Rash (46%) [7]
Toxicity [3]

Hair
Alopecia (13–61%) [24]

Mucosal
Mucositis (30%) [2]
Stomatitis (<14%) [5]

Cardiovascular
Bradycardia [2]
Flushing (11%)
Hypertension [8]

Hypotension (5%)
Thrombophlebitis (<10%)
Vasodilation (6%)

Central Nervous System
Anorexia (44%) [18]
Chills (14%)
Confusion (3%)
Dysarthria [2]
Fever (44%) [3]
Insomnia [2]
Neurotoxicity [5]
Pain (23%)
Somnolence (drowsiness) (9%)
Vertigo (dizziness) (21%)

Neuromuscular/Skeletal
Asthenia (fatigue) (69%) [19]

Gastrointestinal/Hepatic
Abdominal pain (68%) [3]
Constipation (32%) [2]
Diarrhea (83%) [41]
Hepatotoxicity [3]
Nausea (82%) [20]
Vomiting (63%) [17]

Respiratory
Cough (20%)
Dyspnea (22%)
Pneumonia (4%) [4]

Endocrine/Metabolic
Dehydration [4]

Renal
Proteinuria [4]

Hematologic
Anemia (97%) [15]
Febrile neutropenia [10]
Leukopenia (96%) [12]
Lymphopenia [2]
Neutropenia (96%) [40]
Thrombocytopenia (96%) [8]

Other
Adverse effects [3]
Allergic reactions (9%)
Death [5]
Infection (14%) [2]

ISAVUCONAZONIUM SULFATE

Trade name: Cresemba (Astellas)
Indications: Invasive aspergillosis, mucormycosis
Class: Antifungal, azole
Half-life: 130 hours
Clinically important, potentially hazardous interactions with: carbamazepine, ketoconazole, rifampin, ritonavir, St John's wort, strong CYP3A4 inducers or inhibitors
Pregnancy category: C
Important contra-indications noted in the prescribing guidelines for: nursing mothers; pediatric patients
Note: Contra-indicated in patients with familial short QT syndrome.

Skin
Dermatitis (<5%)
Erythema (<5%)

Exfoliative dermatitis (<5%)
Hypersensitivity (<5%)
Peripheral edema (15%)
Petechiae (<5%)
Pruritus (8%)
Rash (9%)
Urticaria (<5%)

Hair
Alopecia (<5%)

Mucosal
Gingivitis (<5%)
Stomatitis (<5%)

Cardiovascular
Atrial fibrillation (<5%)
Atrial flutter (<5%)
Bradycardia (<5%)
Cardiac arrest (<5%)
Chest pain (9%)
Extrasystoles (<5%)
Hypotension (8%)
Palpitation (<5%)
QT interval shortening (<5%)
Thrombophlebitis (<5%)

Central Nervous System
Anxiety (8%)
Chills (<5%)
Confusion (<5%)
Delirium (9%)
Depression (<5%)
Dysgeusia (taste perversion) (<5%)
Encephalopathy (<5%)
Gait instability (<5%)
Hallucinations (<5%)
Headache (17%)
Hypoesthesia (<5%)
Insomnia (11%)
Migraine (<5%)
Paresthesias (<5%)
Peripheral neuropathy (<5%)
Seizures (<5%)
Somnolence (drowsiness) (<5%)
Stupor (<5%)
Syncope (<5%)
Tremor (<5%)
Vertigo (dizziness) (<5%)

Neuromuscular/Skeletal
Asthenia (fatigue) (11%)
Back pain (10%)
Bone or joint pain (<5%)
Myalgia/Myopathy (<5%)
Neck pain (<5%)

Gastrointestinal/Hepatic
Abdominal distension (<5%)
Abdominal pain (17%)
Cholecystitis (<5%)
Cholelithiasis (gallstones) (<5%)
Constipation (14%)
Diarrhea (24%) [3]
Dyspepsia (6%)
Gastritis (<5%)
Hepatic failure (<5%)
Hepatomegaly (<5%)
Hepatotoxicity (17%)
Nausea (28%) [3]
Vomiting (25%)

Respiratory
Bronchospasm (<5%)
Dyspnea (17%)

Respiratory failure (7%)
Tachypnea (<5%)

Endocrine/Metabolic
Appetite decreased (9%)
Hypoalbuminemia (<5%)
Hypoglycemia (<5%)
Hypokalemia (19%)
Hypomagnesemia (5%)
Hyponatremia (<5%)

Genitourinary
Hematuria (<5%)

Renal
Proteinuria (<5%)
Renal failure (10%)

Hematologic
Agranulocytosis (<5%)
Leukopenia (<5%)
Pancytopenia (<5%)

Otic
Tinnitus (<5%)

Ocular
Optic neuropathy (<5%)

Local
Injection-site reactions (6%)

Other
Adverse effects [3]

ISOCARBOXAZID

See: www.drugeruptiondata.com/drug/id/368

ISOETHARINE

See: www.drugeruptiondata.com/drug/id/369

ISOFLURANE

See: www.drugeruptiondata.com/drug/id/950

ISONIAZID

Synonym: INH
Trade names: Rifamate (Sanofi-Aventis), Rifater (Sanofi-Aventis)
Indications: Tuberculosis
Class: Antibiotic, Antimycobacterial
Half-life: <4 hours
Clinically important, potentially hazardous interactions with: acetaminophen, betamethasone, ethosuximide, insulin aspart, insulin degludec, insulin detemir, insulin glargine, insulin glulisine, itraconazole, levodopa, metformin, phenytoin, prednisolone, propranolol, rifampin, rifapentine, safinamide, triamcinolone
Pregnancy category: C

Skin
Acneform eruption [7]
AGEP [2]
Angioedema [2]
Bullous dermatitis [2]
Dermatitis [3]

DRESS syndrome [6]
Erythema multiforme [2]
Exanthems [4]
Exfoliative dermatitis [5]
Hypersensitivity [7]
Lichenoid eruption [2]
Lupus erythematosus [58]
Peripheral edema [22]
Photosensitivity [5]
Pruritus [3]
Purpura [7]
Pustules [3]
Stevens-Johnson syndrome [5]
Toxic epidermal necrolysis [9]
Toxicity [2]
Urticaria (<5%) [4]
Vasculitis [2]

Hair
Alopecia [3]

Mucosal
Oral lesions [2]

Central Nervous System
Fever [3]
Hallucinations [3]
Neurotoxicity [2]
Psychosis [2]
Seizures [9]

Neuromuscular/Skeletal
Arthralgia [2]
Rhabdomyolysis (3%) [3]

Gastrointestinal/Hepatic
Hepatotoxicity [32]
Pancreatitis [4]

Respiratory
Pleural effusion [2]

Endocrine/Metabolic
Gynecomastia [4]

Renal
Nephrotoxicity [2]

Ocular
Hallucinations, visual [2]
Optic neuritis [2]

Other
Adverse effects [6]
Death [3]
Side effects (2%) [2]

ISOPROTERENOL

See: www.drugeruptiondata.com/drug/id/371

ISOSORBIDE

Indications: Acute angle-closure glaucoma
Class: Diuretic
Half-life: 5–9.5 hours
Clinically important, potentially hazardous interactions with: sildenafil
Pregnancy category: C
Note: Various forms of isosorbide are available – see other isosorbide profiles for reaction details.

Central Nervous System
Headache [10]

ISOSORBIDE DINITRATE

Trade names: Dilatrate-SR (Schwarz), Isordil (Wyeth), Sorbitrate (AstraZeneca)
Indications: Angina pectoris
Class: Nitrate, Vasodilator
Half-life: 4 hours (oral)
Clinically important, potentially hazardous interactions with: sildenafil
Pregnancy category: C
Important contra-indications noted in the prescribing guidelines for: the elderly; nursing mothers; pediatric patients
Note: Various forms of isosorbide are available – see other isosorbide profiles for reaction details.

Cardiovascular
Flushing (>10%)

Central Nervous System
Headache [3]

ISOSORBIDE MONO-NITRATE

Trade names: Imdur (Schering), Monoket (Schwarz)
Indications: Angina pectoris
Class: Nitrate, Vasodilator
Half-life: ~4 hours
Clinically important, potentially hazardous interactions with: sildenafil
Pregnancy category: B
Important contra-indications noted in the prescribing guidelines for: the elderly; nursing mothers; pediatric patients
Note: Various forms of isosorbide are available – see other isosorbide profiles for reaction details.

Cardiovascular
Flushing (>10%) [2]
Palpitation [2]

Central Nervous System
Headache [7]
Vertigo (dizziness) [2]

Other
Adverse effects [2]

ISOTRETINOIN

Synonym: 13-cis-retinoic acid
Trade names: Accutane (Roche), Amnesteem (Genpharm), Claravis (Barr), Roaccutane (Roche)
Indications: Cystic acne
Class: Retinoid
Half-life: 21–24 hours
Clinically important, potentially hazardous interactions with: acitretin, alcohol (ethyl), antacids, bexarotene, carbamazepine, cholestyramine, co-trimoxazole, corticosteroids, dairy products, minocycline, oral contraceptives, phenytoin, retinoids, St John's wort, tetracycline, tetracyclines, vitamin A

Pregnancy category: X
Important contra-indications noted in the prescribing guidelines for: nursing mothers; pediatric patients
Note: Oral retinoids can cause birth defects, and women should avoid isotretinoin when pregnant or trying to conceive.

Skin
Abscess [3]
Acneform eruption [19]
Angioedema [3]
Desquamation (palms and soles) (5%)
Diaphoresis [2]
Edema (subcutaneous, recurrent) [2]
Erythema nodosum [3]
Exfoliative dermatitis (<10%)
Facial edema (<10%)
Facial erythema [3]
Fragility [3]
Granulation tissue [4]
Keloid [5]
Pallor (<10%)
Photosensitivity (>10%) [7]
Pigmentation [2]
Pityriasis rosea [2]
Pruritus (<5%) [5]
Pyoderma gangrenosum [3]
Rash [3]
Sweet's syndrome [2]
Urticaria [2]
Vasculitis [4]
Xanthomas [2]
Xerosis (>10%) [12]

Hair
Alopecia (16%) [3]
Curly hair [3]

Nails
Brittle nails [2]
Elkonyxis [2]
Median canaliform dystrophy [3]
Onycholysis [3]
Paronychia [4]
Pyogenic granuloma [8]

Mucosal
Cheilitis (>90%) [16]
Epistaxis (nosebleed) [2]
Mucositis [2]
Xerostomia (>10%) [5]

Central Nervous System
Depression [7]
Headache [7]
Pseudotumor cerebri [4]

Neuromuscular/Skeletal
Arthralgia [4]
Asthenia (fatigue) [2]
Myalgia/Myopathy [8]
Rhabdomyolysis [2]
Sacroiliitis [3]
Stiff person syndrome [2]

Gastrointestinal/Hepatic
Abdominal pain [3]
Hepatotoxicity [3]
Pancreatitis [3]

Endocrine/Metabolic
Amenorrhea [2]
Gynecomastia [2]
Hypercholesterolemia [2]

Hyperlipidemia [2]
Hypertriglyceridemia [5]

Hematologic
Neutropenia [2]

Ocular
Ocular adverse effects [2]
Photophobia [2]
Xerophthalmia [2]

Other
Adverse effects [8]
Side effects [2]
Teratogenicity [8]

ISOXSUPRINE

See: www.drugeruptiondata.com/drug/id/376

ISRADIPINE

Trade name: DynaCirc (Reliant)
Indications: Hypertension
Class: Calcium channel blocker
Half-life: 8 hours
**Clinically important, potentially hazardous
interactions with:** amprenavir, delavirdine,
epirubicin, imatinib, phenytoin
Pregnancy category: C

Skin
Edema (7%) [6]
Exanthems (2%) [2]
Pruritus (<6%)
Rash (2%)

Mucosal
Oral lesions (6%)

Cardiovascular
Flushing (2–9%) [9]
QT prolongation [2]

Central Nervous System
Headache (9%)
Vertigo (dizziness) (9%)

ITRACONAZOLE

Trade names: Onmel (Merz), Sporanox
(Janssen)
Indications: Onychomycosis, deep mycoses,
oropharyngeal candidiasis (oral solution only)
Class: Antibiotic, triazole, Antifungal, azole,
CYP3A4 inhibitor
Half-life: 21 hours
**Clinically important, potentially hazardous
interactions with:** abiraterone, afatinib,
alfentanil, alfuzosin, aliskiren, alprazolam,
amphotericin B, amprenavir, anisindione, antacids,
aprepitant, aripiprazole, artemether/lumefantrine,
astemizole, atazanavir, atorvastatin, avanafil,
boceprevir, bosentan, brigatinib, budesonide,
buspirone, busulfan, cabazitaxel, cabozantinib,
calcifediol, calcium channel blockers,
carbamazepine, cerivastatin, ciclesonide,
cilostazol, cimetidine, cinacalcet, cisapride,
clarithromycin, clopidogrel, clorazepate,
cobicistat/elvitegravir/emtricitabine/tenofovir

alafenamide, cobicistat/elvitegravir/emtricitabine/
tenofovir disoproxil, cobimetinib, colchicine,
conivaptan, copanlisib, corticosteroids,
coumarins, crizotinib, cyclophosphamide,
cyclosporine, cyproterone, dabigatran,
darifenacin, dasatinib, dexamethasone, diazepam,
dicumarol, didanosine, digoxin,
dihydroergotamine, dihydropyridines,
disopyramide, docetaxel, dofetilide, dronedarone,
efavirenz, eletriptan, enzalutamide, eplerenone,
ergotamine, erlotinib, erythromycin, estradiol,
ethotoin, everolimus, felodipine, fentanyl,
fesoterodine, flibanserin, fluticasone propionate,
fosamprenavir, fosphenytoin, gefitinib, grapefruit
juice, halofantrine, haloperidol, histamine H$_2$-
antagonists, HMG-CoA reductase inhibitors,
ibrutinib, iloperidone, imatinib, indinavir,
irinotecan, isoniazid, ivabradine, ixabepilone,
lapatinib, lercanidipine, levomethadyl, lomitapide,
lopinavir, lovastatin, lurasidone, mephenytoin,
methadone, methylergonovine,
methylprednisolone, methysergide, micafungin,
midazolam(oral), midostaurin, mifepristone,
mizolastine, naldemedine, neratinib, nevirapine,
nilotinib, nisoldipine, olaparib, omeprazole, oral
hypoglycemics, osimertinib, paclitaxel,
palbociclib, paliperidone, pantoprazole,
pazopanib, phenobarbital, phenytoin,
pimavanserin, pimecrolimus, pimozide, ponatinib,
prednisolone, prednisone, proton pump
inhibitors, quetiapine, quinidine, ranolazine,
reboxetine, regorafenib, repaglinide, ribociclib,
rifabutin, rifampin, rilpivirine, rimonabant,
ritonavir, rivaroxaban, romidepsin, ruxolitinib,
saquinavir, sildenafil, silodosin, simeprevir,
simvastatin, sirolimus, solifenacin, sonidegib,
sunitinib, tacrolimus, tadalafil, telaprevir,
telithromycin, temsirolimus, terfenadine,
ticagrelor, tolterodine, tolvaptan, triamcinolone,
triazolam, trimetrexate, ulipristal, valbenazine,
vardenafil, vemurafenib, venetoclax, vinblastine,
vincristine, vinflunine, vinorelbine, vorapaxar,
warfarin
Pregnancy category: C
**Important contra-indications noted in the
prescribing guidelines for:** nursing mothers
Note: Contra-indicated in patients with evidence
of ventricular dysfunction such as congestive
heart failure (CHF) or a history of CHF except for
the treatment of life-threatening or other serious
infections.
Warning: CONGESTIVE HEART FAILURE,
CARDIAC EFFECTS AND DRUG
INTERACTIONS

Skin
AGEP [3]
Angioedema [2]
Diaphoresis (3%)
Edema (<4%) [11]
Exanthems (<3%) [7]
Peripheral edema (4%)
Phototoxicity [2]
Pruritus (<3%) [8]
Rash (8%) [10]
Urticaria [3]

Hair
Alopecia [3]

Mucosal
Xerostomia [3]

Cardiovascular
Cardiac arrest [2]
Cardiac failure [4]
Congestive heart failure [4]
Hypertension (3%) [3]
QT prolongation [5]
Torsades de pointes [2]

Central Nervous System
Fever [2]
Headache (4%) [3]
Neurotoxicity [5]
Peripheral neuropathy [4]
Seizures [2]
Tremor [2]
Vertigo (dizziness) [2]

Neuromuscular/Skeletal
Asthenia (fatigue) [3]
Back pain [2]
Rhabdomyolysis [7]

Gastrointestinal/Hepatic
Abdominal pain (2–6%) [5]
Constipation [2]
Diarrhea [4]
Hepatitis [2]
Hepatotoxicity [7]
Nausea (5–7%) [8]
Pancreatitis [2]
Vomiting [3]

Respiratory
Cough (4%)
Dyspnea (2%)
Flu-like syndrome [2]
Pneumonia (2%)

Endocrine/Metabolic
ALT increased [2]
AST increased [2]
Hyperbilirubinemia [2]
Hypertriglyceridemia [2]
Hypokalemia [6]

Renal
Renal failure [2]

Hematologic
Leukopenia [2]
Thrombocytopenia [2]

Other
Adverse effects [8]
Death [3]
Side effects [2]

IVABRADINE

Trade names: Corlanor (Amgen), Procoralan
(Servier)
Indications: Chronic stable angina pectoris
Class: Cardiotonic agent, HCN channel blocker
Half-life: 2 hours
**Clinically important, potentially hazardous
interactions with:** azole antifungals,
clarithromycin, CYP3A4 inducers, diltiazem,
grapefruit juice, itraconazole, ketoconazole,
macrolide antibiotics, nefazodone, nelfinavir,
pentamidine, phenytoin, rifampin, ritonavir,
sotalol, St John's wort, strong or moderate
CYP3A4 inhibitors, telithromycin, verapamil

Pregnancy category: N/A
Important contra-indications noted in the prescribing guidelines for: nursing mothers; pediatric patients

Cardiovascular
Atrial fibrillation (8%) [3]
Atrioventricular block (<10%)
Bradycardia (10%) [6]
Hypertension (9%)

Central Nervous System
Headache (2–5%) [2]
Vertigo (dizziness) (<10%) [3]

Neuromuscular/Skeletal
Myalgia/Myopathy (<10%)

Gastrointestinal/Hepatic
Nausea [2]

Ocular
Luminous phenomena (14%) [5]
Vision blurred (<10%) [3]
Visual disturbances [3]

IVACAFTOR

Trade name: Kalydeco (Vertex)
Indications: Cystic fibrosis in patients aged 6 years and older who have a *G551D* mutation in the *CFTR* gene
Class: CFTR potentiator
Half-life: 12 hours
Clinically important, potentially hazardous interactions with: CYP3A inducers or inhibitors, fluconazole, grapefruit juice, ketoconazole, rifampin, St John's wort
Pregnancy category: B
Important contra-indications noted in the prescribing guidelines for: nursing mothers; pediatric patients
Note: See also separate profile for lumacaftor/ivacaftor.

Skin
Acneform eruption (4–7%)
Rash (13%) [6]

Mucosal
Nasal congestion (20%) [7]
Oropharyngeal pain (22%) [7]

Cardiovascular
Chest pain (4–7%)

Central Nervous System
Fever [2]
Headache (24%) [8]
Vertigo (dizziness) (9%) [4]

Neuromuscular/Skeletal
Arthralgia (4–7%)
Myalgia/Myopathy (4–7%)

Gastrointestinal/Hepatic
Abdominal pain (16%) [4]
Diarrhea (13%) [6]
Hepatotoxicity [3]
Nausea (12%) [3]
Vomiting [2]

Respiratory
Cough [5]
Hemoptysis [2]

Nasopharyngitis (15%) [4]
Rhinitis (4–7%)
Upper respiratory tract infection (22%) [7]
Wheezing (4–7%)

Endocrine/Metabolic
AST increased (4–7%)

Otic
Otitis media [2]

Other
Adverse effects [4]

IVERMECTIN

Trade names: Sklice (Sanofi Pasteur), Soolantra (Galderma), Stromectol (Merck)
Indications: Various infections caused by susceptible helmintic organisms
Class: Anthelmintic
Half-life: 16–35 hours
Clinically important, potentially hazardous interactions with: alprazolam, barbiturates, benzodiazepines, diazepam, midazolam, valproic acid
Pregnancy category: C
Important contra-indications noted in the prescribing guidelines for: nursing mothers; pediatric patients

Skin
Edema (10–53%) [7]
Exanthems (<34%) [3]
Facial edema [3]
Pruritus (38–71%) [14]
Rash (<93%) [6]
Urticaria (23%)

Cardiovascular
Tachycardia (4%)

Central Nervous System
Fever (23%) [2]
Headache [3]
Psychosis [2]
Vertigo (dizziness) (3%) [3]

Neuromuscular/Skeletal
Arthralgia (9%)
Myalgia/Myopathy (20%) [3]

Gastrointestinal/Hepatic
Abdominal pain [3]

Other
Adverse effects [4]
Side effects (mild) [3]

IXABEPILONE

See: www.drugeruptiondata.com/drug/id/1255

IXAZOMIB

Trade name: Ninlaro (Millennium)
Indications: Multiple myeloma (in combination with lenalidomide and dexamethasone) in patients who have received at least one prior therapy
Class: Proteasome inhibitor
Half-life: 10 days
Clinically important, potentially hazardous interactions with: carbamazepine, phenytoin, rifampin, St John's wort, strong CYP3A inducers
Pregnancy category: N/A (Can cause fetal harm)
Important contra-indications noted in the prescribing guidelines for: nursing mothers; pediatric patients
Note: See separate profiles for dexamethasone and lenalidomide.

Skin
Acneform eruption [3]
Erythema [4]
Erythema multiforme [2]
Exanthems [8]
Exfoliative dermatitis [4]
Facial edema [2]
Hyperhidrosis [4]
Peripheral edema (25%) [4]
Petechiae [3]
Pigmentation [3]
Pruritus [4]
Rash (19%) [10]
Urticaria [2]
Xerosis [3]

Hair
Alopecia [2]

Central Nervous System
Chills [2]
Fever [4]
Insomnia [2]
Peripheral neuropathy (28%) [11]

Neuromuscular/Skeletal
Asthenia (fatigue) [10]
Back pain (21%)

Gastrointestinal/Hepatic
Abdominal pain [2]
Constipation (34%) [3]
Diarrhea (42%) [12]
Nausea (26%) [11]
Vomiting (22%) [10]

Respiratory
Dyspnea [2]
Pneumonia [3]
Upper respiratory tract infection (19%)

Endocrine/Metabolic
Appetite decreased [4]
Dehydration [3]
Hypokalemia [2]

Renal
Renal failure [2]

Hematologic
Anemia [8]
Leukopenia [3]
Lymphopenia [5]
Neutropenia (67%) [11]
Platelets decreased [3]
Thrombocytopenia (78%) [16]

Ocular
Conjunctivitis (6%)
Vision blurred (6%)
Xerophthalmia (5%)

Other
Adverse effects [4]

IXEKIZUMAB

Trade name: Taltz (Lilly)
Indications: Plaque psoriasis
Class: Interleukin-17A (IL-17A) antagonist,
Monoclonal antibody
Half-life: 13 days
**Clinically important, potentially hazardous
interactions with:** live vaccines

Pregnancy category: N/A (Insufficient evidence
to inform drug-associated risk)
**Important contra-indications noted in the
prescribing guidelines for:** pediatric patients

Skin
Hypersensitivity [4]
Peripheral edema [2]
Urticaria [2]

Central Nervous System
Headache [7]

Gastrointestinal/Hepatic
Crohn's disease [2]
Nausea (2%)

Respiratory
Nasopharyngitis [9]

Upper respiratory tract infection (14%) [9]

Hematologic
Neutropenia (11%) [3]
Thrombocytopenia (3%)

Otic
Ear infection (2%)

Local
Injection-site erythema [2]
Injection-site reactions (17%) [7]

Other
Infection [3]

JAPANESE ENCEPHALITIS VACCINE

Trade name: Ixiaro (Novartis)
Indications: Active immunization against Japanese encephalitis for adults
Class: Vaccine
Half-life: N/A
Clinically important, potentially hazardous interactions with: immunosuppressants

Pregnancy category: C
Important contra-indications noted in the prescribing guidelines for: nursing mothers; pediatric patients

Skin
Edema (4%)
Pruritus (4%)
Rash (<10%)

Central Nervous System
Fever [5]
Headache (28%) [5]
Seizures [2]

Neuromuscular/Skeletal
Asthenia (fatigue) (11%)
Myalgia/Myopathy (16%)

Gastrointestinal/Hepatic
Diarrhea (<10%)
Nausea (<10%)
Vomiting (<10%)

Respiratory
Flu-like syndrome (12%)

Local
Injection-site edema (<10%)
Injection-site erythema (<10%)
Injection-site induration (<10%)
Injection-site pain (33%) [3]
Injection-site pruritus (<10%)

Other
Adverse effects [5]

KANAMYCIN

Indications: Various infections caused by susceptible organisms
Class: Antibiotic, aminoglycoside
Half-life: 2–4 hours
Clinically important, potentially hazardous interactions with: aldesleukin, atracurium, bacitracin, bumetanide, doxacurium, ethacrynic acid, furosemide, methoxyflurane, neostigmine, non-depolarizing muscle relaxants, pancuronium, polypeptide antibiotics, rocuronium, succinylcholine, teicoplanin, torsemide, vecuronium
Pregnancy category: D
Important contra-indications noted in the prescribing guidelines for: nursing mothers
Note: Aminoglycosides may cause neurotoxicity and/or nephrotoxicity.

Skin
Edema (>10%)
Pruritus (<10%)
Rash (<10%)

Renal
Nephrotoxicity [2]

Otic
Ototoxicity [8]

KETAMINE

Trade name: Ketalar (Monarch)
Indications: Induction of anesthesia
Class: Anesthetic
Half-life: 2–3 hours
Clinically important, potentially hazardous interactions with: memantine, mivacurium
Pregnancy category: D

Skin
Pruritus [3]
Rash (<10%)

Mucosal
Sialorrhea [2]

Cardiovascular
Bradycardia [4]
Hypertension [5]
Hypotension [5]
Tachycardia [2]

Central Nervous System
Agitation [5]
Amnesia [2]
Hallucinations [14]
Headache [3]
Mania [2]
Nightmares [2]
Sedation [3]
Tremor (>10%)
Vertigo (dizziness) [4]

Gastrointestinal/Hepatic
Hepatotoxicity [2]
Nausea [7]
Vomiting [11]

Respiratory
Apnea [3]
Hypoxia [3]

Laryngospasm [4]

Genitourinary
Cystitis [3]

Local
Injection-site pain (<10%)

Other
Adverse effects [3]

KETOCONAZOLE

Trade name: Nizoral (Janssen)
Indications: Fungal infections
Class: Antibiotic, imidazole, Antifungal, azole, CYP3A4 inhibitor
Half-life: initial: 2 hours; terminal: 8 hours
Clinically important, potentially hazardous interactions with: abemaciclib, abiraterone, afatinib, alcohol, alfuzosin, aliskiren, alitretinoin, almotriptan, alprazolam, amphotericin B, amprenavir, anisindione, anticoagulants, aprepitant, aripiprazole, astemizole, atazanavir, avanafil, axitinib, beclomethasone, bedaquiline, benzodiazepines, betrixaban, boceprevir, bosentan, bosutinib, brentuximab vedotin, brigatinib, budesonide, buprenorphine, cabazitaxel, cabozantinib, caffeine, calcifediol, ceritinib, chlordiazepoxide, ciclesonide, cilostazol, cimetidine, cinacalcet, cisapride, clopidogrel, clorazepate, cobicistat/elvitegravir/emtricitabine/ tenofovir alafenamide, cobicistat/elvitegravir/ emtricitabine/tenofovir disoproxil, colchicine, conivaptan, copanlisib, crizotinib, cyclosporine, cyproterone, dabigatran, darifenacin, darunavir, dasatinib, desvenlafaxine, dexlansoprazole, dicumarol, didanosine, disopyramide, docetaxel, dofetilide, domperidone, doxercalciferol, dronedarone, dutasteride, echinacea, elbasvir & grazoprevir, eletriptan, eplerenone, erlotinib, erythromycin, estradiol, eszopiclone, everolimus, fentanyl, fesoterodine, fingolimod, flibanserin, flunisolide, fluticasone propionate, fosamprenavir, gastric alkanizers, halofantrine, HMG-CoA reductase inhibitors, ibrutinib, iloperidone, imatinib, indacaterol, indinavir, irinotecan, isavuconazonium sulfate, ivabradine, ivacaftor, ixabepilone, lanthanum, lapatinib, levomilnacipran, lomitapide, lopinavir, lurasidone, macitentan, maraviroc, mefloquine, methadone, methylergonovine, methylprednisolone, midazolam, midostaurin, mizolastine, mometasone, naldemedine, neratinib, nevirapine, nilotinib, nisoldipine, non-sedating antihistamines, olaparib, omeprazole, ospemifene, oxybutynin, paclitaxel, palbociclib, pantoprazole, paricalcitol, pazopanib, pimavanserin, pimecrolimus, pimozide, pomalidomide, ponatinib, prednisolone, prednisone, proton-pump inhibitors, quetiapine, quinidine, rabeprazole, ramelteon, ranolazine, reboxetine, regorafenib, ribociclib, rifampin, rilpivirine, rimonabant, ritonavir, rivaroxaban, roflumilast, romidepsin, ropivacaine, rupatadine, ruxolitinib, saquinavir, saxagliptin, sildenafil, silodosin, simeprevir, simvastatin, solifenacin, sonidegib, sucralfate, sunitinib, tacrolimus, tadalafil, tamsulosin, tasimelteon, telaprevir, telithromycin, temsirolimus, ticagrelor, tiotropium, tofacitinib, tolterodine, tolvaptan, trabectedin, tramadol,

triamcinolone, triazolam, trospium, ulipristal, valbenazine, vardenafil, vemurafenib, venetoclax, venlafaxine, vilazodone, vinblastine, vincristine, vorapaxar, warfarin, zaleplon, ziprasidone, zolpidem, zotarolimus
Pregnancy category: C
Warning: HEPATOTXICITY, QT PROLONGATION AND DRUG INTERACTIONS LEADING TO QT PROLONGATION

Skin
Anaphylactoid reactions/Anaphylaxis [3]
Angioedema [3]
Dermatitis [3]
Exanthems (<9%) [7]
Exfoliative dermatitis [2]
Fixed eruption [2]
Hypersensitivity [3]
Pigmentation [3]
Pruritus (<9%) [5]
Purpura [2]
Rash (<3%) [3]
Urticaria (<3%) [2]
Xerosis [3]

Hair
Alopecia (<4%) [4]

Mucosal
Gingivitis [2]
Oral lesions (<5%) [3]
Oral lichenoid eruption [2]
Oral pigmentation [2]

Cardiovascular
QT prolongation [4]

Central Nervous System
Chills (<3%)
Fever [2]
Neurotoxicity [3]

Neuromuscular/Skeletal
Asthenia (fatigue) [3]
Rhabdomyolysis [3]

Gastrointestinal/Hepatic
Hepatotoxicity [18]
Nausea (3–10%) [4]
Vomiting (3–10%)

Endocrine/Metabolic
Gynecomastia (<3%) [8]

Hematologic
Eosinophilia [2]

Other
Adverse effects [5]
Death [5]

KETOPROFEN

Trade names: Orudis (Sanofi-Aventis), Oruvail (Wyeth)
Indications: Arthritis
Class: Non-steroidal anti-inflammatory (NSAID)
Half-life: 1.5–4 hours
Clinically important, potentially hazardous interactions with: aspirin, caffeine, methotrexate, probenecid

Pregnancy category: C

Important contra-indications noted in the prescribing guidelines for: nursing mothers; pediatric patients

Note: NSAIDs may cause an increased risk of serious cardiovascular and gastrointestinal adverse events, which can be fatal. This risk may increase with duration of use.

Skin

Anaphylactoid reactions/Anaphylaxis [4]
Contact dermatitis [5]
Dermatitis [29]
Eczema [3]
Erythema [4]
Exanthems [3]
Peripheral edema (<3%)
Photoallergic reaction [2]
Photocontact dermatitis [5]
Photosensitivity [35]
Pruritus (<10%) [4]
Rash (>10%)
Urticaria [6]

Gastrointestinal/Hepatic

Abdominal pain (3–9%) [2]
Constipation [2]
Diarrhea (3–9%)
Dyspepsia (11%) [2]
Gastrointestinal bleeding [2]
Nausea (3–9%) [2]
Pancreatitis [3]

Endocrine/Metabolic

Pseudoporphyria [2]

Renal

Renal function abnormal (3–9%)

Local

Application-site reactions [2]

Other

Adverse effects [11]
Allergic reactions [2]

KETOROLAC

Trade names: Acular (Allergan), Toradol (Roche)
Indications: Pain, relief of inflammation following cataract surgery (ophthalmic solution)
Class: Analgesic, non-opioid, Non-steroidal anti-inflammatory (NSAID)
Half-life: 2–8 hours
Clinically important, potentially hazardous interactions with: aspirin, buprenorphine, dabigatran, diclofenac, enoxaparin, meloxicam, methotrexate, probenecid, rivaroxaban, salicylates, tiagabine, tinzaparin
Pregnancy category: C
Important contra-indications noted in the prescribing guidelines for: nursing mothers; pediatric patients
Warning: GASTROINTESTINAL, CARDIOVASCULAR, RENAL, AND BLEEDING RISK

Skin

Anaphylactoid reactions/Anaphylaxis [3]
Dermatitis (3–9%)
Diaphoresis (<10%) [2]
Edema (<10%)
Exanthems (3–9%)
Hematoma [2]
Hypersensitivity [2]
Pruritus (<10%)
Purpura (<10%)
Rash (<10%)

Mucosal

Stomatitis (<10%)
Xerostomia [2]

Cardiovascular

Hypertension (<10%)

Central Nervous System

Headache (>10%) [4]
Somnolence (drowsiness) [3]
Vertigo (dizziness) [4]

Gastrointestinal/Hepatic

Abdominal pain (>10%)
Constipation (<10%)
Diarrhea (7%) [2]
Dyspepsia (>10%)
Flatulence (<10%)
Gastrointestinal bleeding [6]
Gastrointestinal ulceration (<10%) [2]
Nausea (>10%) [12]
Vomiting (<10%) [8]

Renal

Renal function abnormal (<10%)

Hematologic

Anemia (<10%)
Prothrombin time increased (<10%)

Otic

Tinnitus (<10%)

Ocular

Corneal melting [4]
Ocular burning [2]

Local

Injection-site pain (<10%)

Other

Adverse effects [10]
Death [2]
Side effects [2]

KETOTIFEN

See: www.drugeruptiondata.com/drug/id/385

L-CARNITINE

See: www.drugeruptiondata.com/drug/id/914

L-METHYLFOLATE

See: www.drugeruptiondata.com/drug/id/1299

LABETALOL

Trade name: Trandate (Prometheus)
Indications: Hypertension
Class: Adrenergic beta-receptor antagonist, Antiarrhythmic class II
Half-life: 3–8 hours
Clinically important, potentially hazardous interactions with: cimetidine, halothane, imipramine, iobenguane, tricyclic antidepressants
Pregnancy category: C
Important contra-indications noted in the prescribing guidelines for: nursing mothers; pediatric patients
Note: Cutaneous side effects of beta-receptor blockers are clinically polymorphous. They apparently appear after several months of continuous therapy.

Skin
Anaphylactoid reactions/Anaphylaxis [2]
Edema (<2%)
Exanthems (<5%) [4]
Lichenoid eruption [4]
Lupus erythematosus [4]
Pityriasis rubra pilaris [2]
Pruritus (<10%) [3]
Psoriasis (exacerbation) [3]
Scalp tingling [3]
Cardiovascular
Flushing (19%)
Hypotension [4]
Central Nervous System
Dysgeusia (taste perversion) (<10%)
Paresthesias (7%) [2]
Neuromuscular/Skeletal
Myalgia/Myopathy [4]
Other
Side effects (6%) [2]

LACOSAMIDE

Trade name: Vimpat (UCB Pharma)
Indications: Partial-onset seizures
Class: Anticonvulsant, Antiepileptic
Half-life: 13 hours
Clinically important, potentially hazardous interactions with: alcohol, antipsychotics, carbamazepine, chloroquine, fosphenytoin, hydroxychloroquine, lamotrigine, MAO inhibitors, mefloquine, orlistat, phenobarbital, phenytoin, pregabalin, SSRIs, St John's wort, tricyclic antidepressants

Pregnancy category: C
Important contra-indications noted in the prescribing guidelines for: the elderly; nursing mothers; pediatric patients

Skin
Angioedema [2]
Pruritus (2%)
Rash [2]
Cardiovascular
Atrioventricular block [3]
Hypotension [2]
Central Nervous System
Balance disorder (4%)
Depression (2%) [2]
Gait instability (2%) [4]
Headache (13%) [14]
Incoordination [2]
Irritability [2]
Memory loss (2%)
Sedation [3]
Seizures [4]
Somnolence (drowsiness) (7%) [10]
Tremor (7%) [4]
Vertigo (dizziness) (31%) [34]
Neuromuscular/Skeletal
Asthenia (fatigue) (2–9%) [8]
Ataxia (8%) [9]
Gastrointestinal/Hepatic
Diarrhea (4%)
Nausea (11%) [17]
Pancreatitis [2]
Vomiting (9%) [8]
Respiratory
Nasopharyngitis [2]
Upper respiratory tract infection [2]
Ocular
Abnormal vision [3]
Diplopia (11%) [13]
Nystagmus (5%)
Vision blurred (8%) [4]
Local
Injection-site pain (2%)
Other
Adverse effects [8]

LACTULOSE

See: www.drugeruptiondata.com/drug/id/1360

LAMIVUDINE

Synonym: 3TC
Trade names: Combivir (ViiV), Epivir (ViiV), Epzicom (ViiV), Triumeq (ViiV), Trizivir (ViiV)
Indications: HIV progression
Class: Antiretroviral, Nucleoside analog reverse transcriptase inhibitor
Half-life: 5–7 hours
Clinically important, potentially hazardous interactions with: cobicistat/elvitegravir/emtricitabine/tenofovir disoproxil, emtricitabine, trimethoprim

Pregnancy category: C
Note: Combivir is lamivudine and zidovudine; Epzicom is lamivudine and abacavir; Triumeq is abacavir, dolutegravir and lamivudine; Trizivir is lamivudine, abacavir and zidovudine,.

Skin
Angioedema [2]
Exanthems [2]
Hypersensitivity [4]
Jaundice [2]
Pigmentation [2]
Pruritus [3]
Rash (9%) [10]
Stevens-Johnson syndrome [2]
Toxic epidermal necrolysis [2]
Hair
Alopecia [3]
Central Nervous System
Abnormal dreams [2]
Chills (<10%)
Headache [6]
Insomnia [3]
Neurotoxicity [2]
Paresthesias (>10%)
Peripheral neuropathy [3]
Vertigo (dizziness) [4]
Neuromuscular/Skeletal
Asthenia (fatigue) [5]
Myalgia/Myopathy (8%)
Rhabdomyolysis [3]
Gastrointestinal/Hepatic
Abdominal pain [4]
Diarrhea [4]
Hepatotoxicity [3]
Nausea [6]
Pancreatitis [4]
Vomiting [2]
Respiratory
Upper respiratory tract infection [2]
Endocrine/Metabolic
Acidosis [3]
Hematologic
Anemia [2]
Other
Adverse effects [9]

LAMOTRIGINE

Trade name: Lamictal (GSK)
Indications: Epilepsy
Class: Anticonvulsant, Antiepileptic, Mood stabilizer
Half-life: 24 hours
Clinically important, potentially hazardous interactions with: eslicarbazepine, lacosamide, oral contraceptives, rufinamide
Pregnancy category: C
Important contra-indications noted in the prescribing guidelines for: the elderly; nursing mothers
Warning: SERIOUS SKIN RASHES

Skin
Angioedema (<10%)

Anticonvulsant hypersensitivity syndrome [17]
DRESS syndrome [17]
Erythema (<10%) [2]
Erythema multiforme [4]
Exanthems (<10%) [18]
Hot flashes (<10%)
Hypersensitivity (<10%) [29]
Lupus erythematosus [4]
Photosensitivity [2]
Pruritus (3%) [3]
Rash (10–20%) [53]
Stevens-Johnson syndrome (<10%) [49]
Toxic epidermal necrolysis [51]

Hair
Alopecia [2]

Mucosal
Xerostomia (6%)

Central Nervous System
Agitation [2]
Aseptic meningitis [4]
Fever [2]
Hallucinations [3]
Headache [6]
Insomnia (5–10%)
Nervousness [2]
Neuroleptic malignant syndrome [2]
Pain (5%)
Seizures [9]
Somnolence (drowsiness) (9%) [7]
Suicidal ideation [2]
Tic disorder [2]
Tremor [4]
Vertigo (dizziness) [8]

Neuromuscular/Skeletal
Asthenia (fatigue) (8%) [2]
Ataxia (2–5%) [3]
Rhabdomyolysis [3]

Gastrointestinal/Hepatic
Abdominal pain (6%)
Hepatotoxicity [4]
Nausea [4]

Respiratory
Cough (5%)
Flu-like syndrome (7%)
Pharyngitis (5%)
Rhinitis (7%)

Endocrine/Metabolic
SIADH [2]

Genitourinary
Urinary frequency (<5%)
Vaginitis (4%)

Renal
Nephrotoxicity [3]

Hematologic
Agranulocytosis [3]

Ocular
Abnormal vision (2–5%)
Diplopia [5]
Hallucinations, visual [2]
Nystagmus (2–5%)

Other
Adverse effects [7]
Allergic reactions [2]
Death [6]
Multiorgan failure [2]

Side effects [2]
Teratogenicity [6]

LANREOTIDE

Trade names: Somatuline Autogel (Ipsen), Somatuline Depot (Ipsen), Somatuline LA (Ipsen)
Indications: Acromegaly, carcinoid syndrome, thyrotrophic adenoma
Class: Somatostatin analog
Half-life: 2 hours (immediate release) 5 days (sustained release).
Clinically important, potentially hazardous interactions with: antidiabetics, bromocriptine, cyclosporine, insulin, metformin, repaglinide, sulfonylureas
Pregnancy category: C
Important contra-indications noted in the prescribing guidelines for: nursing mothers; pediatric patients

Hair
Alopecia [2]

Cardiovascular
Bradycardia (5–18%)
Hypertension (5%)

Central Nervous System
Headache (7%)
Pain (7%)

Neuromuscular/Skeletal
Arthralgia (7%) [2]

Gastrointestinal/Hepatic
Abdominal pain (7–19%) [6]
Cholelithiasis (gallstones) (2–17%) [2]
Constipation (8%)
Diarrhea (31–65%) [6]
Flatulence (6–14%) [3]
Loose stools (6%)
Nausea (11%) [3]
Steatorrhea [2]
Vomiting (7%)

Endocrine/Metabolic
Diabetes mellitus (7%)
Hyperglycemia (7%)
Hypoglycemia (7%)
Weight loss (5–11%)

Hematologic
Anemia (5–14%)

Local
Injection-site induration [3]
Injection-site pain (4%) [4]
Injection-site reactions (6–22%) [2]

Other
Adverse effects [2]

LANSOPRAZOLE

Trade name: Prevacid (TAP)
Indications: Active duodenal ulcer
Class: Proton pump inhibitor (PPI)
Half-life: 2 hours
Clinically important, potentially hazardous interactions with: bosutinib, clopidogrel, delavirdine, eucalyptus, neratinib, prednisone, rilpivirine, sucralfate

Pregnancy category: C
Important contra-indications noted in the prescribing guidelines for: nursing mothers

Skin
Anaphylactoid reactions/Anaphylaxis [6]
Erythema multiforme [2]
Facial edema [2]
Hypersensitivity [3]
Lupus erythematosus [3]
Peripheral edema [2]
Pruritus (3–10%)
Rash (3–10%)
Toxic epidermal necrolysis [4]
Urticaria [3]

Mucosal
Stomatitis [2]

Central Nervous System
Dysgeusia (taste perversion) [3]
Headache (3%) [4]
Vertigo (dizziness) [2]

Gastrointestinal/Hepatic
Abdominal pain [2]
Colitis [2]
Constipation [2]
Diarrhea (<5%) [6]
Hepatitis [2]
Nausea [2]

Endocrine/Metabolic
Gynecomastia [2]

Other
Death [2]

LANTHANUM

See: www.drugeruptiondata.com/drug/id/1113

LAPATINIB

Trade name: Tykerb (Novartis)
Indications: Breast cancer
Class: Antineoplastic, Biologic, Epidermal growth factor receptor (EGFR) inhibitor, Tyrosine kinase inhibitor
Half-life: 24 hours
Clinically important, potentially hazardous interactions with: alfuzosin, artemether/lumefantrine, atazanavir, carbamazepine, chloroquine, ciprofloxacin, clarithromycin, clozapine, colchicine, conivaptan, CYP2C8 substrates, CYP3A4 inhibitors or inducers, dabigatran, deferasirox, dexamethasone, digoxin, docetaxel, dronedarone, efavirenz, eplerenone, everolimus, fentanyl, food, gadobutrol, grapefruit juice, histamine H₂-antagonists, indinavir, irinotecan, itraconazole, ketoconazole, nefazodone, nelfinavir, nilotinib, omeprazole, P-glycoprotein inducers, paclitaxel, pantoprazole, pazopanib, phenobarbital, phenytoin, pimecrolimus, pimozide, posaconazole, proton pump inhibitors, QT prolonging agents, quinine, repaglinide, rifabutin, rifampin, rifapentin, ritonavir, rivaroxaban, safinamide, salmeterol, saquinavir, saxagliptin, silodosin, St John's wort, telithromycin, tetrabenazine, thioridazine, tolvaptan, topotecan, voriconazole, ziprasidone

Pregnancy category: D
Important contra-indications noted in the prescribing guidelines for: nursing mothers; pediatric patients
Note: Lapitinib is used in conjunction with capecitabine.
Warning: HEPATOXICITY

Skin
Acneform eruption (90%) [4]
Depigmentation (21%)
Hand–foot syndrome (53%) [9]
Inflammation (15%)
Pruritus [3]
Rash (28%) [26]
Toxicity [6]
Xerosis (10%)

Hair
Alopecia [2]

Nails
Paronychia [3]

Mucosal
Mucosal inflammation (15%)
Mucositis [2]
Stomatitis (14%)

Central Nervous System
Anorexia (24%) [2]
Insomnia (10%)

Neuromuscular/Skeletal
Asthenia (fatigue) (12%) [19]
Back pain (11%)
Bone or joint pain [2]
Pain in extremities (12%)

Gastrointestinal/Hepatic
Abdominal pain (15%)
Diarrhea (65%) [44]
Dyspepsia (11%)
Hepatotoxicity [11]
Nausea (44%) [9]
Vomiting (26%) [7]

Respiratory
Dyspnea (12%) [2]

Endocrine/Metabolic
ALT increased (37%) [5]
AST increased (49%) [4]
Hyperbilirubinemia [3]

Hematologic
Anemia [5]
Febrile neutropenia [2]
Leukopenia [4]
Lymphopenia [2]
Neutropenia [8]

Otic
Tinnitus (14%)

Other
Adverse effects [11]
Death [2]

LARONIDASE

See: www.drugeruptiondata.com/drug/id/996

LATANOPROST

Trade name: Xalatan (Pfizer)
Indications: Reduction of elevated intraocular pressure in open angle glaucoma or ocular hypertension
Class: Prostaglandin analog
Half-life: 17 minutes
Clinically important, potentially hazardous interactions with: thimerosal
Pregnancy category: C
Important contra-indications noted in the prescribing guidelines for: nursing mothers; pediatric patients

Skin
Pigmentation [2]
Pruritus [2]
Rash (<10%)

Cardiovascular
Angina (<10%)
Chest pain (<10%)

Central Nervous System
Headache [3]
Vertigo (dizziness) [2]

Neuromuscular/Skeletal
Arthralgia (<10%)
Back pain (<10%)
Myalgia/Myopathy (<10%)

Respiratory
Flu-like syndrome (<10%)
Upper respiratory tract infection (<10%)

Ocular
Conjunctival hyperemia [19]
Deepening of upper lid sulcus [5]
Eyelashes – hypertrichosis [15]
Eyelashes – pigmentation [9]
Eyelid edema (<4%)
Eyelid erythema (<4%)
Eyelid pain (<10%)
Eyelid pigmentation [4]
Eyelid pruritus (2%)
Foreign body sensation [5]
Iris pigmentation [7]
Keratitis [3]
Macular edema [7]
Ocular adverse effects [7]
Ocular hyperemia [4]
Ocular itching [8]
Ocular pigmentation (5%) [12]
Periorbitopathy [2]
Uveitis [5]
Vision blurred [3]
Xerophthalmia (<10%)

Other
Allergic reactions (<10%)

LEDIPASVIR & SOFOSBUVIR

Trade name: Harvoni (Gilead)
Indications: Hepatitis C
Class: Hepatitis C virus NS5A inhibitor (ledipasvir), Hepatitis C virus nucleotide analog NS5B polymerase inhibitor (sofosbuvir)
Half-life: 47 hours (ledipasvir); <27 hours (sofosbuvir)
Clinically important, potentially hazardous interactions with: amiodarone, carbamazepine, cobicistat/elvitegravir/emtricitabine/tenofovir disoproxil, oxcarbazepine, phenobarbital, phenytoin, rifabutin, rifampin, rifapentine, ritonavir, rosuvastatin, simeprevir, St John's wort, tenofovir disoproxil
Pregnancy category: N/A (Insufficient evidence to inform drug-associated risk; contra-indicated in pregnancy when given with ribavirin)
Important contra-indications noted in the prescribing guidelines for: nursing mothers; pediatric patients
Note: See also separate entry for sofosbuvir.

Skin
Pruritus [6]
Rash [5]

Cardiovascular
Bradycardia [3]

Central Nervous System
Headache (11–17%) [32]
Insomnia (3–6%) [11]
Irritability [5]
Vertigo (dizziness) [3]

Neuromuscular/Skeletal
Arthralgia [3]
Asthenia (fatigue) (7–18%) [33]
Muscle spasm [2]
Myalgia/Myopathy [3]

Gastrointestinal/Hepatic
Diarrhea (3–7%) [12]
Hepatotoxicity [3]
Nausea (6–9%) [20]

Respiratory
Cough [3]
Dyspnea [3]
Nasopharyngitis [2]
Upper respiratory tract infection [6]

Renal
Nephrotoxicity [3]

Hematologic
Anemia [7]

Other
Adverse effects [5]
Infection [2]

LEFLUNOMIDE

See: www.drugeruptiondata.com/drug/id/391

LENALIDOMIDE

Trade name: Revlimid (Celgene)
Indications: Transfusion-dependent anemia due to myeloplastic syndromes, multiple myeloma (in combination with dexamethasone)
Class: Biologic, Immunomodulator, Thalidomide analog
Half-life: 3–5 hours
Clinically important, potentially hazardous interactions with: abatacept, anakinra, canakinumab, certolizumab, denosumab, dexamethasone, digoxin, erythropoietin stimulating agents, estrogen containing therapies, leflunomide, natalizumab, pimecrolimus, rilonacept, sipuleucel-T, tacrolimus, trastuzumab, vaccines
Pregnancy category: X
Important contra-indications noted in the prescribing guidelines for: nursing mothers; pediatric patients
Warning: FETAL RISK, HEMATOLOGIC TOXICITY, and DEEP VEIN THOMBOSIS AND PULMONARY EMBOLISM

Skin
Cellulitis (5%)
DRESS syndrome [2]
Ecchymoses (5–8%)
Edema (10%)
Erythema (5%)
Exanthems [3]
Folliculitis [2]
Graft-versus-host reaction [2]
Hyperhidrosis (7%) [2]
Malignancies (secondary) [6]
Peripheral edema (26%) [4]
Pigmentation [2]
Pruritus (42%) [3]
Rash (36%) [16]
Stevens-Johnson syndrome [5]
Sweet's syndrome [3]
Toxicity [6]
Tumor lysis syndrome [3]
Tumors [5]
Xerosis (14%) [2]

Mucosal
Epistaxis (nosebleed) (15%)
Xerostomia (7%)

Cardiovascular
Chest pain (5%)
Hypertension (6%)
Palpitation (5%)
Thromboembolism [5]
Venous thromboembolism [13]

Central Nervous System
Anorexia (10%)
Depression (5%)
Dysgeusia (taste perversion) (6%)
Fever (21%) [3]
Headache (20%)
Hypoesthesia (7%)
Insomnia (10%) [4]
Neurotoxicity (7%) [8]
Pain (7%)
Peripheral neuropathy (5%) [12]
Rigors (6%)
Somnolence (drowsiness) [2]
Tremor (21%)

Vertigo (dizziness) (20%)

Neuromuscular/Skeletal
Arthralgia (21%) [4]
Asthenia (fatigue) (15–31%) [33]
Back pain (21%) [4]
Bone or joint pain (14%)
Cramps (33%)
Muscle spasm [4]
Myalgia/Myopathy (18%) [3]
Pain in extremities (12%)

Gastrointestinal/Hepatic
Abdominal pain (8–12%)
Constipation (24%) [8]
Diarrhea (49%) [15]
Gastrointestinal disorder [4]
Hepatotoxicity [3]
Loose stools (6%)
Nausea (24%) [9]
Vomiting (10%) [5]

Respiratory
Acute respiratory distress syndrome [2]
Alveolar hemorrhage (pulmonary) [2]
Bronchitis (11%)
Cough (20%) [5]
Dyspnea (7–17%) [4]
Nasopharyngitis (23%)
Pharyngitis (16%)
Pneumonia (12%) [9]
Pneumonitis [7]
Pulmonary toxicity [3]
Rhinitis (7%)
Sinusitis (8%)
Upper respiratory tract infection (15%) [3]

Endocrine/Metabolic
ALT increased (8%) [3]
Appetite decreased (7%)
Hyperglycemia [2]
Hypocalcemia (9%)
Hypokalemia (11%) [4]
Hypomagnesemia (6%)
Hyponatremia [2]
Hypophosphatemia [3]
Hypothyroidism (7%)
Weight loss (20%)

Genitourinary
Urinary tract infection (11%)

Renal
Nephrotoxicity [3]

Hematologic
Anemia (31%) [25]
Cytopenia [3]
Febrile neutropenia (5%) [8]
Hemotoxicity [12]
Leukopenia (8%) [11]
Lymphopenia (5%) [8]
Myelosuppression [6]
Neutropenia (59%) [58]
Thrombocytopenia (62%) [50]
Thrombosis [4]

Ocular
Vision blurred (17%)

Local
Infusion-related reactions [2]
Injection-site reactions [2]

Other
Adverse effects [13]
Cancer [2]

Death [4]
Infection [20]
Teratogenicity [2]

LENVATINIB

Trade name: Lenvima (Eisai)
Indications: Differentiated thyroid cancer, renal cell cancer (in combination with everolimus)
Class: Tyrosine kinase inhibitor
Half-life: 28 hours
Clinically important, potentially hazardous interactions with: none known
Pregnancy category: N/A (Can cause fetal harm)
Important contra-indications noted in the prescribing guidelines for: nursing mothers; pediatric patients

Skin
Exanthems (21%)
Hand–foot syndrome (32%) [2]
Hyperkeratosis (7%)
Peripheral edema (21%) [3]
Rash (21%)
Toxicity [2]

Hair
Alopecia (12%)

Mucosal
Aphthous stomatitis (41%)
Epistaxis (nosebleed) (12%)
Gingivitis (10%)
Glossitis (41%)
Glossodynia (25%)
Mucosal inflammation (41%)
Oral ulceration (41%)
Oropharyngeal pain (25%)
Parotitis (10%)
Stomatitis (41%) [3]
Xerostomia (17%)

Cardiovascular
Hypertension (73%) [18]
Hypotension (9%)
QT prolongation (9%)

Central Nervous System
Anorexia [3]
Dysgeusia (taste perversion) (18%)
Headache (38%) [4]
Insomnia (12%)
Vertigo (dizziness) (15%)

Neuromuscular/Skeletal
Arthralgia (62%)
Asthenia (fatigue) (67%) [10]
Back pain (62%)
Bone or joint pain (62%)
Myalgia/Myopathy (62%)
Pain in extremities (62%)

Gastrointestinal/Hepatic
Abdominal pain (31%) [2]
Constipation (29%) [3]
Diarrhea (67%) [11]
Dyspepsia (13%)
Nausea (47%) [7]
Vomiting (36%) [5]

Respiratory
Cough (24%)
Dysphonia (31%) [2]

Nasopharyngitis [2]

Endocrine/Metabolic
ALP increased (>5%)
ALT increased (4%) [2]
Appetite decreased (54%) [6]
AST increased (5%) [2]
Creatine phosphokinase increased (3%)
Dehydration (9%)
Hyperbilirubinemia (>5%)
Hypercalcemia (>5%)
Hypercholesterolemia (>5%)
Hyperkalemia (>5%)
Hypoalbuminemia (>5%)
Hypocalcemia (9%)
Hypoglycemia (>5%)
Hypokalemia (6%)
Hypomagnesemia (>5%)
Weight loss (51%) [5]

Genitourinary
Hematuria [2]
Urinary tract infection (11%)

Renal
Proteinuria (34%) [9]

Hematologic
Leukopenia [2]
Platelets decreased (2%)
Thrombocytopenia [4]

Other
Adverse effects [3]
Death [2]
Tooth disorder (10%)

LEPIRUDIN

See: www.drugeruptiondata.com/drug/id/2145

LESINURAD

Trade names: Duzallo (AstraZeneca), Zurampic (AstraZeneca)
Indications: Gout-associated hyperuricemia (in combination with a xanthine oxidase inhibitor)
Class: URAT1 inhibitor
Half-life: 5 hours
Clinically important, potentially hazardous interactions with: amiodarone, carbamazepine, CYP2C9 inducers or inhibitors, CYP3A substrates, fluconazole, rifampin, valproic acid
Pregnancy category: N/A (No available data)
Important contra-indications noted in the prescribing guidelines for: nursing mothers; pediatric patients
Note: Contra-indicated in patients with severe renal impairment (including end stage renal disease, kidney transplant recipients or patients on dialysis), tumor lysis syndrome or Lesch-Nylan syndrome. Duzallo is lesinurad and allopurinol (see separate entry).
Warning: RISK OF ACUTE RENAL FAILURE, MORE COMMON WHEN USED WITHOUT A XANTHINE OXIDASE INHIBITOR

Cardiovascular
Cardiotoxicity (<2%)

Central Nervous System
Headache (5%) [2]

Vertigo (dizziness) [2]
Neuromuscular/Skeletal
Back pain [2]
Gastrointestinal/Hepatic
Diarrhea [2]
Gastroesophageal reflux (3%)
Respiratory
Influenza (5%)
Nasopharyngitis [2]
Endocrine/Metabolic
Serum creatinine increased (4–8%) [2]
Renal
Nephrolithiasis (<3%)
Renal failure (<4%)

LETROZOLE

Trade name: Femara (Novartis)
Indications: Breast cancer
Class: Aromatase inhibitor
Half-life: ~2 days
Clinically important, potentially hazardous interactions with: none known
Pregnancy category: X
Important contra-indications noted in the prescribing guidelines for: nursing mothers; pediatric patients

Skin
Exanthems (5%)
Hot flashes (6%) [8]
Hyperhidrosis (<5%)
Leukocytoclastic vasculitis [2]
Pruritus (2%)
Psoriasis (5%)
Rash (<10%) [5]
Vesiculation (5%)
Hair
Alopecia (<5%) [3]
Cardiovascular
Cardiac failure [2]
Hypertension [3]
Myocardial toxicity [2]
Central Nervous System
Anorexia [3]
Depression [3]
Fever [2]
Headache [3]
Insomnia [2]
Mood changes [2]
Vertigo (dizziness) [2]
Neuromuscular/Skeletal
Arthralgia [10]
Asthenia (fatigue) [9]
Back pain [3]
Bone or joint pain [3]
Myalgia/Myopathy [7]
Osteoporosis [7]
Gastrointestinal/Hepatic
Constipation [2]
Diarrhea [7]
Nausea [8]
Vomiting [4]
Respiratory
Dyspnea [3]

Endocrine/Metabolic
Hypercholesterolemia [3]
Hyperglycemia [3]
Genitourinary
Vaginal dryness [4]
Hematologic
Leukopenia [2]
Neutropenia [4]
Other
Adverse effects [2]
Infection [2]

LEUCOVORIN

Synonyms: citrovorum factor; folinic acid
Indications: Overdose of methotrexate, in combination with fluorouracil in the palliative treatment of patients with colorectal cancer
Class: Adjuvant
Half-life: 15 minutes
Clinically important, potentially hazardous interactions with: capecitabine, glucarpidase, trimethoprim
Pregnancy category: C

Skin
Hand–foot syndrome [3]
Rash [5]
Toxicity [2]
Hair
Alopecia [2]
Mucosal
Mucositis [6]
Stomatitis [5]
Cardiovascular
Hypertension [6]
Central Nervous System
Anorexia [5]
Neurotoxicity [5]
Peripheral neuropathy [4]
Neuromuscular/Skeletal
Asthenia (fatigue) [8]
Gastrointestinal/Hepatic
Abdominal pain [2]
Diarrhea [22]
Nausea [13]
Vomiting [11]
Endocrine/Metabolic
ALP increased [2]
Renal
Proteinuria [3]
Hematologic
Anemia [9]
Febrile neutropenia [3]
Leukopenia [6]
Neutropenia [24]
Thrombocytopenia [6]
Other
Adverse effects [2]
Infection [2]

LEUPROLIDE

Trade names: Eligard (Sanofi-Aventis), Lupron (TAP), Lupron Depot-Ped (AbbVie), Viadur (Bayer)
Indications: Prostate carcinoma, endometriosis
Class: Gonadotropin-releasing hormone (GnRH) agonist
Half-life: 3–4 hours
Clinically important, potentially hazardous interactions with: none known
Pregnancy category: X
Important contra-indications noted in the prescribing guidelines for: nursing mothers

Skin
Anaphylactoid reactions/Anaphylaxis [3]
Dermatitis (5%)
Dermatitis herpetiformis [2]
Ecchymoses (<5%)
Edema (<10%)
Granulomas [2]
Hot flashes (12%) [6]
Peripheral edema (4–12%)
Pigmentation (<5%)
Pruritus (<5%)
Rash (<10%)
Vasculitis [2]
Xerosis (<5%)

Hair
Alopecia (<5%)

Cardiovascular
Flushing (61%) [2]
Thrombophlebitis (2%)

Central Nervous System
Dysgeusia (taste perversion) (<5%)
Paresthesias (<5%)

Neuromuscular/Skeletal
Myalgia/Myopathy [2]

Endocrine/Metabolic
Gynecomastia (7%)
Mastodynia (7%)

Ocular
Diplopia [2]

Local
Injection-site granuloma [6]
Injection-site inflammation (2%)
Injection-site pain [2]
Injection-site reactions (24%)

LEVALBUTEROL

See: www.drugeruptiondata.com/drug/id/876

LEVAMISOLE

See: www.drugeruptiondata.com/drug/id/395

LEVETIRACETAM

Trade names: Elepsia XR (Sun Pharma), Keppra (UCB)
Indications: Partial onset seizures
Class: Anticonvulsant
Half-life: 7 hours
Clinically important, potentially hazardous interactions with: carbamazepine, eslicarbazepine
Pregnancy category: C
Important contra-indications noted in the prescribing guidelines for: nursing mothers

Skin
DRESS syndrome [7]
Erythema [2]
Erythema multiforme [2]
Rash [5]
Stevens-Johnson syndrome [3]
Toxic epidermal necrolysis [2]
Urticaria [2]

Central Nervous System
Aggression [7]
Agitation [5]
Anorexia [2]
Behavioral disturbances [4]
Compulsions [2]
Depression [8]
Encephalopathy [4]
Fever [2]
Headache (25%) [12]
Irritability [9]
Nervousness [2]
Neurotoxicity [3]
Paresthesias (2%)
Psychosis [3]
Seizures [4]
Sleep related disorder [2]
Somnolence (drowsiness) [17]
Suicidal ideation [4]
Vertigo (dizziness) (9–18%) [20]

Neuromuscular/Skeletal
Asthenia (fatigue) (<22%) [20]
Osteoporosis [2]
Rhabdomyolysis [3]

Gastrointestinal/Hepatic
Abdominal pain [2]
Diarrhea [2]
Hepatotoxicity [3]
Nausea [4]
Vomiting [4]

Respiratory
Influenza [2]
Nasopharyngitis [5]

Endocrine/Metabolic
Creatine phosphokinase increased [3]
Libido decreased [2]
Weight gain [4]

Genitourinary
Sexual dysfunction [2]

Renal
Nephrotoxicity [2]

Hematologic
Hemotoxicity [2]
Pancytopenia [2]
Thrombocytopenia [2]

Other
Adverse effects [8]
Death [2]
Infection (13–26%) [7]

LEVOBETAXOLOL

See: www.drugeruptiondata.com/drug/id/767

LEVOBUNOLOL

See: www.drugeruptiondata.com/drug/id/397

LEVOBUPIVACAINE

See: www.drugeruptiondata.com/drug/id/922

LEVOCETIRIZINE

Trade name: Xyzal (UCB Pharma)
Indications: Allergic rhinitis, chronic idiopathic urticaria
Class: Histamine H1 receptor antagonist
Half-life: 6–10 hours
Clinically important, potentially hazardous interactions with: none known
Pregnancy category: B
Important contra-indications noted in the prescribing guidelines for: the elderly; nursing mothers; pediatric patients

Skin
Fixed eruption [3]

Mucosal
Xerostomia (2–3%)

Central Nervous System
Headache [2]
Sedation [2]
Somnolence (drowsiness) (5–6%)

Neuromuscular/Skeletal
Asthenia (fatigue) (<4%)

Gastrointestinal/Hepatic
Hepatotoxicity [2]

Respiratory
Nasopharyngitis (4–6%)
Pharyngitis (<2%)

LEVODOPA

Synonyms: L-dopa; carbidopa
Trade names: Duopa (Abbvie), Rytary (Impax), Sinemet (Bristol-Myers Squibb), Stalevo (Orion)
Indications: Parkinsonism
Class: Dopamine precursor
Half-life: 1–3 hours
Clinically important, potentially hazardous interactions with: ACE inhibitors, acebutolol, alfuzosin, alpha blockers, amisulpride, ampicillin, angiotensin II receptor antagonists, anti-hypertensives, antimuscarinics, antipsychotics, baclofen, benzodiazepines, beta blockers, bupropion, calcium channel blockers, captopril,

chloramphenicol, cholestyramine, cilazapril, clobazam, clonidine, darifenacin, diazoxide, diuretics, dopamine D_2 receptor antagonists, enalapril, erythromycin, fosinopril, hydralazine, irbesartan, iron salts, isoniazid, levomepromazine, linezolid, lisinopril, MAO inhibitors, memantine, methyldopa, metoclopramide, minoxidil, moclobemide, moxonidine, nitrates, olanzapine, olmesartan, oral iron, oxybutynin, paliperidone, papaverine, pericyazine, phenelzine, phenytoin, probenecid, pyridoxine, quetiapine, quinapril, ramipril, rifampin, risperidone, sapropterin, selegiline, sodium nitroprusside, sulpiride, tetrabenazine, tiotropium, trandolapril, tranylcypromine, tricyclic antidepressants, trospium, volatile liquid general anesthetics, ziprasidone, zuclopenthixol, zuclopenthixol acetate, zuclopenthixol decanoate, zuclopenthixol dihydrochloride

Pregnancy category: C

Important contra-indications noted in the prescribing guidelines for: nursing mothers; pediatric patients

Note: Levodopa is always used in conjuntion with carbidopa. Stalevo is levodopa, carbidopa and entacapone. Contra-indicated in patients with narrow-angle glaucoma or those with a history of melanoma.

Skin
Chromhidrosis (<10%)
Edema [2]
Exanthems [2]
Lupus erythematosus [2]
Melanoma [28]
Rash [3]

Hair
Hair pigmentation [2]

Nails
Nail growth [2]

Mucosal
Xerostomia (<10%) [2]

Cardiovascular
Hypotension [2]
Orthostatic hypotension [4]

Central Nervous System
Agitation [2]
Anosmia [2]
Anxiety [2]
Confusion [3]
Delusions [2]
Depression [3]
Dyskinesia [44]
Gait instability [3]
Hallucinations [12]
Insomnia [6]
Narcolepsy [2]
Neuroleptic malignant syndrome [7]
Neurotoxicity [3]
Psychosis [6]
Restless legs syndrome [5]
Somnolence (drowsiness) [5]
Suicidal ideation [2]
Tardive dyskinesia [2]
Vertigo (dizziness) [4]

Neuromuscular/Skeletal
Arthralgia [2]
Asthenia (fatigue) [2]

Back pain [2]

Gastrointestinal/Hepatic
Abdominal pain [2]
Constipation [4]
Diarrhea [2]
Hepatotoxicity [2]
Nausea [9]
Vomiting [4]

Endocrine/Metabolic
Weight loss [2]

Ocular
Hallucinations, visual [2]
Ocular adverse effects [2]

Other
Adverse effects [2]
Hiccups [2]

LEVOFLOXACIN

Trade names: Iquix (Santen), Levaquin (Ortho-McNeil), Quixin (Johnson & Johnson), Tavanic (Sanofi-Aventis)
Indications: Various infections caused by susceptible organisms, inhalational anthrax (post exposure)
Class: Antibiotic, fluoroquinolone
Half-life: 6–8 hours
Clinically important, potentially hazardous interactions with: alfuzosin, aminophylline, amiodarone, antacids, antidiabetics, arsenic, artemether/lumefantrine, BCG vaccine, chloroquine, ciprofloxacin, corticosteroids, cyclosporine, didanosine, dronedarone, gadobutrol, insulin, lanthanum, mycophenolate, nilotinib, NSAIDs, oral iron, oral typhoid vaccine, phenindione, pimozide, probenecid, QT prolonging agents, quinine, strontium ranelate, sucralfate, sulfonylureas, tetrabenazine, thioridazine, vitamin K antagonists, warfarin, zinc, ziprasidone, zolmitriptan
Pregnancy category: C
Important contra-indications noted in the prescribing guidelines for: the elderly; nursing mothers
Note: Fluoroquinolones are associated with an increased risk of tendinitis and tendon rupture in all ages. This risk is further increased in older patients usually over 60 years of age, in patients taking corticosteroid drugs, and in patients with kidney, heart or lung transplants.
Fluoroquinolones may exacerbate muscle weakness in persons with myasthenia gravis.
Warning: SERIOUS ADVERSE REACTIONS INCLUDING TENDINITIS, TENDON RUPTURE, PERIPHERAL NEUROPATHY, CENTRIAL NERVOUS SYSTEM EFFECTS and EXACERBATION OF MYASTHENIA GRAVIS

Skin
Anaphylactoid reactions/Anaphylaxis [6]
Erythema [2]
Erythema nodosum (<3%)
Exanthems [2]
Hypersensitivity [5]
Photosensitivity [3]
Phototoxicity [5]
Pruritus (2%) [3]
Purpura [2]

Radiation recall dermatitis [2]
Rash (2%) [2]
Stevens-Johnson syndrome [2]
Toxic epidermal necrolysis [5]
Vasculitis [3]

Cardiovascular
Myocardial infarction [2]
Palpitation [2]
QT prolongation [5]
Torsades de pointes [6]

Central Nervous System
Anorexia [2]
Delirium [5]
Depression [2]
Dysgeusia (taste perversion) [2]
Headache (6%) [6]
Insomnia (4%) [3]
Peripheral neuropathy [3]
Psychosis [2]
Seizures [9]
Vertigo (dizziness) [6]

Neuromuscular/Skeletal
Arthralgia [4]
Myalgia/Myopathy [4]
Myasthenia gravis (exacerbation) [3]
Rhabdomyolysis [4]
Tendinitis [2]
Tendinopathy/Tendon rupture [35]

Gastrointestinal/Hepatic
Abdominal pain [3]
Constipation (3%)
Diarrhea (5%) [4]
Hepatotoxicity [4]
Nausea (7%) [6]
Vomiting [3]

Endocrine/Metabolic
ALT increased [3]
AST increased [3]
Hypoglycemia [3]

Genitourinary
Vaginitis (2%)

Renal
Nephrotoxicity [5]

Hematologic
Thrombocytopenia [5]

Other
Adverse effects [13]
Death [5]
Side effects [2]

LEVOLEUCOVORIN

See: www.drugeruptiondata.com/drug/id/1297

LEVOMEPROMAZINE

See: www.drugeruptiondata.com/drug/id/2175

LEVOMILNACIPRAN

Trade name: Fetzima (Forest)
Indications: Major depressive disorder
Class: Antidepressant, Serotonin-norepinephrine reuptake inhibitor
Half-life: 12 hours
Clinically important, potentially hazardous interactions with: ketoconazole, MAO inhibitors, NSAIDs
Pregnancy category: C
Important contra-indications noted in the prescribing guidelines for: nursing mothers; pediatric patients
Warning: SUICIDAL THOUGHTS AND BEHAVIORS

Skin
Hyperhidrosis (9%) [8]
Pruritus (<2%)
Rash (2%)
Urticaria (<2%)
Xerosis (<2%)

Mucosal
Xerostomia [4]

Cardiovascular
Angina (<2%)
Extrasystoles (<2%)
Hypertension (3%) [2]
Hypotension (3%)
Palpitation (5%) [4]
Tachycardia (6%) [8]

Central Nervous System
Aggression (<2%)
Agitation (<2%)
Extrapyramidal symptoms (<2%)
Headache [5]
Insomnia [3]
Migraine (<2%)
Panic attack (<2%)
Paresthesias (<2%)
Syncope (<2%)
Vertigo (dizziness) [4]
Yawning (<2%)

Gastrointestinal/Hepatic
Abdominal pain (<2%)
Constipation (9%) [8]
Flatulence (<2%)
Nausea (17%) [9]
Vomiting (5%) [4]

Respiratory
Upper respiratory tract infection [2]

Endocrine/Metabolic
Appetite decreased (3%)

Genitourinary
Ejaculatory dysfunction (5%) [3]
Erectile dysfunction (6%) [6]
Hematuria (<2%)
Pollakiuria (<2%)
Testicular pain (4%)
Urinary hesitancy (4%) [3]

Renal
Proteinuria (<2%)

Ocular
Conjunctival hemorrhage (<2%)
Vision blurred (<2%)
Xerophthalmia (<2%)

Other
Adverse effects [2]
Bruxism (<2%)

LEVONORGESTREL

Trade names: Kyleena (Bayer), Mirena (Bayer), Plan B (Duramed)
Indications: Intrauterine contraception, treatment of heavy menstrual bleeding, emergency contraception
Class: Hormone, Progestogen
Half-life: 17 hours
Clinically important, potentially hazardous interactions with: barbiturates, bosentan, carbamazepine, CYP3A4 inducers and inhibitors, efavirenz, felbamate, griseofulvin, nevirapine, oxcarbazepine, phenytoin, rifabutin, rifampin, St John's wort, topiramate, ulipristal
Pregnancy category: X
Important contra-indications noted in the prescribing guidelines for: the elderly; nursing mothers; pediatric patients

Central Nervous System
Headache (17%) [5]
Vertigo (dizziness) (11%)

Neuromuscular/Skeletal
Asthenia (fatigue) (17%)

Gastrointestinal/Hepatic
Abdominal pain (18%)
Diarrhea (5%)
Nausea (23%) [6]
Vomiting (6%) [3]

Endocrine/Metabolic
Amenorrhea [3]
Mastodynia (11%) [2]
Menstrual irregularities (26%) [7]

Genitourinary
Vaginal bleeding [3]

Other
Adverse effects [2]

LEVOTHYROXINE

Synonyms: L-thyroxine sodium; T_4
Trade names: Levothyroid (Forest), Levoxyl (Monarch), Synthroid (AbbVie), Unithroid (Watson)
Indications: Hypothyroidism
Class: Thyroid hormone, synthetic
Half-life: 6–7 days
Clinically important, potentially hazardous interactions with: colesevelam, dicumarol, lanthanum, oral anticoagulants, orlistat, propranolol, raloxifene, red rice yeast, ritonavir, warfarin
Pregnancy category: A

Skin
Angioedema [2]
Urticaria [3]

Cardiovascular
Circulatory collapse [2]

Central Nervous System
Restless legs syndrome [2]

Neuromuscular/Skeletal
Bone loss [2]
Fractures [2]

Endocrine/Metabolic
Thyrotoxicosis [3]

Other
Adverse effects [2]
Side effects [2]

LIDOCAINE

Synonyms: lignocaine; xylocaine
Trade names: Anamantle HC (Doak), ELA-Max (Ferndale), EMLA (AstraZeneca), Lidoderm (Endo), Xylocaine (AstraZeneca)
Indications: Ventricular arrhythmias, topical anesthesia
Class: Anesthetic, local, Antiarrhythmic, Antiarrhythmic class Ib
Half-life: terminal: 1.5–2 hours
Clinically important, potentially hazardous interactions with: amiodarone, amprenavir, antiarrhythmics, atazanavir, cimetidine, cobicistat/elvitegravir/emtricitabine/tenofovir alafenamide, cobicistat/elvitegravir/emtricitabine/tenofovir disoproxil, darunavir, delavirdine, fosamprenavir, indinavir, lopinavir, mivacurium, nevirapine, nilutamide, oxprenolol, propranolol, telaprevir
Pregnancy category: B
Important contra-indications noted in the prescribing guidelines for: nursing mothers; pediatric patients

Skin
Anaphylactoid reactions/Anaphylaxis [7]
Angioedema [3]
Dermatitis [27]
Eczema [3]
Edema [2]
Erythema [3]
Erythema multiforme [2]
Exanthems [2]
Exfoliative dermatitis [2]
Fixed eruption [2]
Hypersensitivity [9]
Pruritus [3]
Toxicity [3]
Urticaria [5]

Cardiovascular
Bradycardia [2]

Central Nervous System
Hoigne's syndrome [2]
Seizures [14]
Shivering (<10%)

Hematologic
Methemoglobinemia [4]

Otic
Tinnitus [3]

Local
Application-site erythema [2]
Application-site reactions [3]
Injection-site pain [2]

Other
Adverse effects [3]
Death [3]

LIFITEGRAST

Trade name: Xiidra (Shire)
Indications: Ophthalmic solution for dry eye disease
Class: Lymphocyte function-associated antigen-1 (LFA-1) antagonist
Half-life: N/A
Clinically important, potentially hazardous interactions with: none known
Pregnancy category: N/A (No data available)
Important contra-indications noted in the prescribing guidelines for: nursing mothers; pediatric patients

Central Nervous System
Dysgeusia (taste perversion) (5–25%) [3]
Headache (<5%)

Respiratory
Sinusitis (<5%)

Ocular
Conjunctival hyperemia (<5%)
Lacrimation (<5%)
Ocular adverse effects [2]
Ocular burning [2]
Ocular discharge (<5%)
Ocular pruritus (5–25%) [2]
Reduced visual acuity (5–25%) [2]
Vision blurred (<5%)
Xerophthalmia [2]

Local
Application-site reactions [3]

LINACLOTIDE

Trade name: Linzess (Forest)
Indications: Irritable bowel syndrome with constipation and chronic idiopathic constipation
Class: Amino acid, Guanylate cyclase-C agonist
Half-life: N/A
Clinically important, potentially hazardous interactions with: none known
Pregnancy category: C
Important contra-indications noted in the prescribing guidelines for: nursing mothers; pediatric patients
Note: Contra-indicated in patients with known or suspected mechanical gastrointestinal obstruction.
Warning: PEDIATRIC RISK

Central Nervous System
Headache (4%)

Neuromuscular/Skeletal
Asthenia (fatigue) (<2%)

Gastrointestinal/Hepatic
Abdominal distension (2–3%)
Abdominal pain (7%) [3]
Diarrhea (16–20%) [19]
Dyspepsia (<2%)
Flatulence (4–6%) [3]
Gastroenteritis (3%)

Gastroesophageal reflux (<2%)
Vomiting (<2%)

Respiratory
Sinusitis (3%)
Upper respiratory tract infection (5%)

LINAGLIPTIN

Trade names: Glyxambi (Boehringer Ingelheim), Tradjenta (Boehringer Ingelheim)
Indications: Type II diabetes mellitus
Class: Antidiabetic, Dipeptidyl peptidase-4 (DPP-4) inhibitor
Half-life: 12 hours
Clinically important, potentially hazardous interactions with: efavirenz, rifampin
Pregnancy category: B
Important contra-indications noted in the prescribing guidelines for: nursing mothers; pediatric patients
Note: Linagliptin should not be used in patients with Type I diabetes or for the treatment of diabetic ketoacidosis, and has not been studied in combination with insulin. Glyxambi is linagliptin and empagliflozin.

Cardiovascular
Cardiotoxicity [3]
Hypertension [2]

Central Nervous System
Headache [5]

Neuromuscular/Skeletal
Arthralgia [2]
Back pain [3]
Pain in extremities [2]

Gastrointestinal/Hepatic
Diarrhea [2]
Nausea [3]

Respiratory
Cough [4]
Nasopharyngitis [7]
Upper respiratory tract infection [5]

Endocrine/Metabolic
Hyperglycemia [2]
Hyperlipidemia [2]
Hypertriglyceridemia [2]
Hypoglycemia [15]

Genitourinary
Urinary tract infection [3]

Other
Adverse effects [17]
Infection [3]

LINCOMYCIN

Trade name: Lincocin (Pfizer)
Indications: Various infections caused by susceptible organisms
Class: Antibiotic, lincosamide
Half-life: 2–11.5 hours
Clinically important, potentially hazardous interactions with: mivacurium

Pregnancy category: C
Important contra-indications noted in the prescribing guidelines for: nursing mothers; pediatric patients

Skin
AGEP [3]
Dermatitis [2]

Other
Allergic reactions (<5%)

LINDANE

Synonyms: hexachlorocyclohexane; gamma benzene hexachloride
Indications: Scabies, pediculosis capitis, pediculosis pubis
Class: Chemical, Scabicide
Half-life: 17–22 hours
Clinically important, potentially hazardous interactions with: oil-based hair dressings
Pregnancy category: C
Important contra-indications noted in the prescribing guidelines for: nursing mothers; pediatric patients

Skin
Dermatitis [5]
Erythema (2%) [2]
Pruritus (2%) [5]
Toxicity [2]
Urticaria [2]

Central Nervous System
Neurotoxicity [3]
Pseudotumor cerebri [2]
Seizures [11]

Neuromuscular/Skeletal
Rhabdomyolysis [3]

Other
Adverse effects [4]
Death [19]

LINEZOLID

Trade name: Zyvox (Pfizer)
Indications: Various infections caused by susceptible organisms
Class: Antibiotic, oxazolidinone
Half-life: 4–5 hours
Clinically important, potentially hazardous interactions with: alcohol, alpha blockers, altretamine, amitriptyline, amoxapine, amphetamines, anilidopiperidine opioids, antihypertensives, atomoxetine, beta blockers, buprenorphine, bupropion, buspirone, caffeine, carbamazepine, clomipramine, cyclobenzaprine, desipramine, desvenlafaxine, dexmethylphenidate, dextromethorphan, diethylpropion, doxapram, doxepin, fluoxetine, fluvoxamine, hydromorphone, imipramine, levodopa, lithium, MAO inhibitors, maprotiline, meperidine, methadone, methyldopa, methylphenidate, mirtazapine, nortriptyline, oral typhoid vaccine, paroxetine hydrochloride, propoxyphene, protriptyline, reserpine, rifampin, safinamide, serotonin 5-HT1D receptor agonists,

serotonin/norepinephrine reuptake inhibitors, sertraline, sibutramine, SSRIs, tapentadol, tetrabenazine, tetrahydrozoline, tramadol, trazodone, tricyclic antidepressants, trimipramine, tryptophan, venlafaxine
Pregnancy category: C
Important contra-indications noted in the prescribing guidelines for: nursing mothers

Skin
Cellulitis [2]
Edema (2%)
Fungal dermatitis (2%)
Pruritus [2]
Rash (<7%) [3]

Mucosal
Black tongue [2]

Central Nervous System
Dysgeusia (taste perversion) (<2%)
Fever (2–14%)
Headache (<11%) [4]
Insomnia (3%)
Neurotoxicity [5]
Peripheral neuropathy [12]
Seizures (3%)
Serotonin syndrome [27]
Vertigo (dizziness) (2%)

Gastrointestinal/Hepatic
Abdominal pain (<2%)
Constipation (2%) [2]
Diarrhea (3–11%) [9]
Gastrointestinal bleeding (2%)
Gastrointestinal disorder [2]
Loose stools (<2%)
Nausea (3–10%) [9]
Vomiting (<10%) [4]

Respiratory
Apnea (2%)
Cough (<2%)
Dyspnea (3%)
Pneumonia (3%)
Upper respiratory tract infection (4%)

Endocrine/Metabolic
Acidosis [5]
ALP increased (<4%)
ALT increased (2–10%)
AST increased (2–5%)
Hypoglycemia [2]
Hypokalemia (3%)
Hyponatremia [2]

Genitourinary
Candidal vaginitis (<2%)

Renal
Nephrotoxicity [2]

Hematologic
Anemia (<6%) [6]
Leukopenia [2]
Myelosuppression [7]
Pancytopenia [4]
Sepsis (8%)
Thrombocytopenia (<5%) [19]

Ocular
Optic neuropathy [14]

Local
Injection-site reactions (3%)

Other
Adverse effects (4%) [15]

Allergic reactions (4%)
Death [2]

LIOTHYRONINE

Synonym: T$_3$ sodium
Trade names: Cytomel (Pfizer), Triostat (Par)
Indications: Hypothyroidism
Class: Thyroid hormone, synthetic
Half-life: 16–49 hours
Clinically important, potentially hazardous interactions with: anticoagulants, dicumarol, warfarin
Pregnancy category: A

Skin
Urticaria [3]

LIRAGLUTIDE

Trade names: Saxenda (Novo Nordisk), Victoza (Novo Nordisk), Xultophy (Novo Nordisk)
Indications: To improve glycemic control in adults with Type II diabetes mellitus (Victoza), adjunct to diet and exercise for chronic weight management (Saxenda)
Class: Glucagon-like peptide-1 (GLP-1) receptor agonist
Half-life: 13 hours
Clinically important, potentially hazardous interactions with: acetaminophen, atorvastatin, digoxin, griseofulvin, lisinopril, warfarin
Pregnancy category: C
Important contra-indications noted in the prescribing guidelines for: nursing mothers; pediatric patients
Note: Contra-indicated in patients with a personal or family history of medullary thyroid carcinoma or in patients with multiple endocrine neoplasia syndrome Type 2. Xultophy is liraglutide and insulin degludec.
Warning: RISK OF THYROID C-CELL TUMORS

Cardiovascular
Cardiotoxicity [2]
Hypertension (3%)

Central Nervous System
Headache (~5%) [7]
Vertigo (dizziness) (6%) [2]

Neuromuscular/Skeletal
Asthenia (fatigue) [3]
Back pain (5%) [3]

Gastrointestinal/Hepatic
Abdominal pain [3]
Cholelithiasis (gallstones) [3]
Constipation (10%) [12]
Diarrhea (17%) [31]
Dyspepsia [3]
Gastrointestinal disorder [3]
Nausea (28%) [61]
Pancreatitis [10]
Vomiting (11%) [30]

Respiratory
Influenza (7%)
Nasopharyngitis (5%) [6]
Sinusitis (6%)

Upper respiratory tract infection (10%) [3]

Endocrine/Metabolic
Appetite decreased [6]
Hypoglycemia [10]
Weight loss [6]

Genitourinary
Urinary tract infection (6%)

Local
Injection-site reactions (2%) [3]

Other
Adverse effects [13]
Malignant neoplasms (11%)

LISDEXAMFETAMINE

Trade name: Vyvanse (Shire)
Indications: Attention-deficit hyperactivity disorder (ADHD)
Class: CNS stimulant, Dextroamphetamine prodrug
Half-life: 1 hour
Clinically important, potentially hazardous interactions with: acetazolamide, ammonium chloride, analgesics, antacids, antihistamines, antihypertensives, antipsychotics, atomoxetine, cannabinoids, carbonic anhydrase inhibitors, chlorpromazine, epinephrine, ethosuximide, haloperidol, iobenguane, lithium, MAO inhibitors, meperidine, methenamine, phenobarbital, phenytoin, propoxyphene, sympathomimetics, tricyclic antidepressants, urinary alkalinizing agents
Pregnancy category: C
Important contra-indications noted in the prescribing guidelines for: nursing mothers; pediatric patients
Warning: ABUSE AND DEPENDENCE

Skin
Hyperhidrosis (3%)
Rash (3%)

Mucosal
Xerostomia (4–26%) [20]

Cardiovascular
Hypertension (3%)
Tachycardia [3]

Central Nervous System
Agitation (3%)
Anorexia (5%) [3]
Anxiety [8]
Fever (2%)
Headache [29]
Insomnia (13–23%) [28]
Irritability (10%) [19]
Restlessness (3%)
Somnolence (drowsiness) (2%) [2]
Tic disorder (2%) [2]
Vertigo (dizziness) (5%) [6]

Neuromuscular/Skeletal
Asthenia (fatigue) [3]
Back pain [2]
Muscle spasm [2]

Gastrointestinal/Hepatic
Abdominal pain (12%) [12]
Constipation [2]
Diarrhea (7%)

Litt's Drug Eruption & Reaction Manual © 2018 by Taylor & Francis Group, LLC

Nausea (6–7%) [10]
Vomiting (9%) [3]

Respiratory
Dyspnea (2%)
Influenza [2]
Nasopharyngitis [5]
Sinusitis [2]
Upper respiratory tract infection [11]

Endocrine/Metabolic
Appetite decreased (27–39%) [27]
Libido decreased (<2%)
Weight loss (9%) [9]

Genitourinary
Erectile dysfunction (<2%)

Other
Adverse effects [6]

LISINOPRIL

Trade names: Prinivil (Merck), Prinzide (Merck), Zestoretic (AstraZeneca), Zestril (AstraZeneca)
Indications: Hypertension, as adjunctive therapy in the management of heart failure, short-term treatment following myocardial infarction in hemodynamically stable patients
Class: Angiotensin-converting enzyme (ACE) inhibitor
Half-life: 12 hours
Clinically important, potentially hazardous interactions with: alcohol, aldesleukin, allopurinol, alpha blockers, alprostadil, amifostine, amiloride, angiotensin II receptor antagonists, antacids, antidiabetics, antihypertensives, antipsychotics, anxiolytics and hypnotics, aprotinin, azathioprine, baclofen, beta blockers, calcium channel blockers, clonidine, corticosteroids, cyclosporine, diazoxide, diuretics, eplerenone, estrogens, everolimus, general anesthetics, gold & gold compounds, heparins, hydralazine, hypotensives, insulin, levodopa, liraglutide, lithium, MAO inhibitors, metformin, methyldopa, methylphenidate, minoxidil, moxisylyte, moxonidine, nitrates, nitroprusside, NSAIDs, pentoxifylline, phosphodiesterase 5 inhibitors, potassium salts, prostacyclin analogues, rituximab, salicylates, sirolimus, spironolactone, sulfonylureas, temsirolimus, tizanidine, tolvaptan, triamterene, trimethoprim, yohimbine
Pregnancy category: D (category C in first trimester; category D in second and third trimesters)
Important contra-indications noted in the prescribing guidelines for: nursing mothers; pediatric patients
Note: Prinzide and Zestoretic are lisinopril and hydrochlorothiazide. Hydrochlorothiazide is a sulfonamide and can be absorbed systemically. Sulfonamides can produce severe, possibly fatal, reactions such as toxic epidermal necrolysis and Stevens-Johnson syndrome.
Contra-indicated in patients with a history of angioedema related to previous treatment with an ACE inhibitor and in patients with hereditary or idiopathic angioedema.
Warning: FETAL TOXICITY

Skin
Angioedema [43]
Edema of lip [2]
Exanthems (3%) [4]
Exfoliative dermatitis [2]
Kaposi's sarcoma [2]
Lichenoid eruption [2]
Pemphigus foliaceus [2]
Pityriasis rosea [2]
Purpura [2]
Rash (2%) [5]
Urticaria [2]

Mucosal
Tongue edema [2]

Cardiovascular
Flushing [2]
Hypotension (<4%) [3]

Central Nervous System
Headache (4–6%)
Vertigo (dizziness) (5–12%)

Neuromuscular/Skeletal
Asthenia (fatigue) (3%)

Gastrointestinal/Hepatic
Hepatotoxicity [2]
Intestinal angioedema [3]
Pancreatitis [10]

Respiratory
Cough (4–9%) [15]
Upper respiratory tract infection (<2%)

Endocrine/Metabolic
Hyperkalemia [3]

Other
Death [3]

LITHIUM

Trade names: Eskalith (GSK), Lithobid (Solvay)
Indications: Manic-depressive states
Class: Antipsychotic, Mood stabilizer
Half-life: 18–24 hours
Clinically important, potentially hazardous interactions with: aceclofenac, acemetacin, acetazolamide, acitretin, amitriptyline, arsenic, benazepril, bendroflumethiazide, benzthiazide, captopril, celecoxib, chlorothiazide, chlorthalidone, cilazapril, citalopram, clozapine, cyclopenthiazide, desvenlafaxine, dichlorphenamide, diclofenac, enalapril, ethoxzolamide, etoricoxib, fluoxetine, flurbiprofen, fosinopril, haloperidol, hydrochlorothiazide, hydroflumethiazide, indapamide, insulin degludec, insulin detemir, insulin glargine, insulin glulisine, irbesartan, levomepromazine, linezolid, lisdexamfetamine, lisinopril, lorcaserin, lurasidone, meloxicam, meperidine, mesoridazine, methyclothiazide, metolazone, metronidazole, milnacipran, neostigmine, olanzapine, olmesartan, paliperidone, paroxetine hydrochloride, pericyazine, phenylbutazone, piroxicam, polythiazide, quinapril, quinethazone, ramipril, rocuronium, rofecoxib, sibutramine, sulpiride, tenoxicam, tetrabenazine, thalidomide, thiazides, tinidazole, tolmetin, trandolapril, trichlormethiazide, trifluoperazine, valdecoxib, venlafaxine, xipamide, ziprasidone, zofenopril, zuclopenthixol

Pregnancy category: D

Skin
Acneform eruption [20]
Angioedema [2]
Atopic dermatitis (3%)
Darier's disease [3]
Dermatitis [4]
Dermatitis herpetiformis [3]
Edema [3]
Erythema [2]
Exanthems [11]
Exfoliative dermatitis [3]
Follicular keratosis [3]
Folliculitis [5]
Hidradenitis [3]
Ichthyosis [2]
Keratosis pilaris [2]
Linear IgA bullous dermatosis [4]
Lupus erythematosus [5]
Myxedema [10]
Papulo-nodular lesions (elbows) [2]
Pruritus [9]
Psoriasis (2%) [58]
Purpura [2]
Pustules [2]
Rash (<10%)
Seborrheic dermatitis [3]
Toxicity [2]
Ulcerations (lower extremities) [5]
Urticaria [3]
Vasculitis [4]

Hair
Alopecia (10–19%) [17]
Alopecia areata (2%) [3]

Nails
Nail dystrophy [2]

Mucosal
Lichenoid stomatitis [3]
Oral ulceration [4]
Sialorrhea [4]
Stomatitis [2]
Xerostomia [5]

Cardiovascular
Brugada syndrome [5]
QT prolongation [4]

Central Nervous System
Amnesia [2]
Coma [2]
Dysgeusia (taste perversion) (>10%)
Hallucinations [2]
Neuroleptic malignant syndrome [7]
Neurotoxicity [3]
Parkinsonism [8]
Pseudohallucinations [2]
Restless legs syndrome [4]
Serotonin syndrome [5]
Somnambulism [3]
Tardive dyskinesia [2]
Tremor [3]

Neuromuscular/Skeletal
Myasthenia gravis [2]
Rhabdomyolysis [3]

Endocrine/Metabolic
Diabetes insipidus [4]
Hypercalcemia [3]
Hyperparathyroidism [5]
Hyperthyroidism [2]

Hypothyroidism [3]
Thyrotoxicosis [2]
Weight gain [3]

Genitourinary
Polyuria [2]
Priapism [5]

Renal
Nephrogenic diabetes insipidus [2]
Nephrotoxicity [13]

Other
Adverse effects [5]
Side effects (23–33%) [4]
Teratogenicity [3]

LIXISENATIDE

Trade names: Adlyxin (Sanofi-Aventis), Lyxumia (Sanofi-Aventis), Soliqua (Sanofi-Aventis)
Indications: To improve glycemic control in adults with Type II diabetes mellitus
Class: Glucagon-like peptide-1 (GLP-1) receptor agonist
Half-life: 3 hours
Clinically important, potentially hazardous interactions with: none known
Pregnancy category: N/A (Use during pregnancy only if the potential benefit justifies the potential risk to the fetus)
Important contra-indications noted in the prescribing guidelines for: nursing mothers; pediatric patients
Note: Soliqua is lixisenatide and insulin glargine.

Central Nervous System
Headache (9%) [2]
Vertigo (dizziness) (7%) [2]

Gastrointestinal/Hepatic
Abdominal distension (2%)
Abdominal pain (2%)
Constipation (3%)
Diarrhea (8%) [9]
Dyspepsia (3%)
Nausea (25%) [21]
Vomiting (10%) [20]

Endocrine/Metabolic
Hypoglycemia (3%) [7]

Local
Injection-site reactions (4%) [2]

Other
Adverse effects [3]
Allergic reactions [2]

LODOXAMIDE

See: www.drugeruptiondata.com/drug/id/1207

LOMEFLOXACIN

See: www.drugeruptiondata.com/drug/id/407

LOMITAPIDE

Trade name: Juxtapid (Aegerion)
Indications: Homozygous familial hypercholesterolemia
Class: Lipid regulator
Half-life: 39.7 hours
Clinically important, potentially hazardous interactions with: bile acid sequestrants, boceprevir, clarithromycin, conivaptan, grapefruit juice, indinavir, itraconazole, ketoconazole, lopinavir, lovastatin, mibefradil, nefazodone, nelfinavir, oral contraceptives, P-glycoprotein substrates, posaconazole, ritonavir, saquinavir, simvastatin, strong or moderate CYP3A4 inhibitors, telaprevir, telithromycin, voriconazole, warfarin
Pregnancy category: X
Important contra-indications noted in the prescribing guidelines for: nursing mothers; pediatric patients
Warning: RISK OF HEPATOTOXICITY

Mucosal
Nasal congestion (10%)

Cardiovascular
Angina (10%)
Chest pain (24%)
Palpitation (10%)

Central Nervous System
Fever (10%)
Headache (10%)
Vertigo (dizziness) (10%)

Neuromuscular/Skeletal
Asthenia (fatigue) (17%)
Back pain (14%)

Gastrointestinal/Hepatic
Abdominal pain (21–34%)
Constipation (21%)
Defecation (urgency) (10%)
Diarrhea (79%) [3]
Dyspepsia (38%) [3]
Flatulence (21%)
Gastroenteritis (14%)
Gastroesophageal reflux (10%)
Hepatotoxicity [5]
Nausea (65%) [2]
Tenesmus (10%)
Vomiting (34%) [3]

Respiratory
Influenza (21%)
Nasopharyngitis (17%)
Pharyngolaryngeal pain (14%)

Endocrine/Metabolic
ALT increased (17%) [3]
Weight loss (24%)

Other
Adverse effects [5]

LOMUSTINE

See: www.drugeruptiondata.com/drug/id/408

LOPERAMIDE

Trade names: Imodium (McNeil), Maalox (Novartis)
Indications: Diarrhea
Class: Opiate agonist
Half-life: 9–14 hours
Clinically important, potentially hazardous interactions with: St John's wort
Pregnancy category: B
Important contra-indications noted in the prescribing guidelines for: nursing mothers; pediatric patients

Cardiovascular
Torsades de pointes [2]

Gastrointestinal/Hepatic
Abdominal pain [2]
Constipation [3]
Nausea [2]

LOPINAVIR

Trade name: Kaletra (AbbVie)
Indications: HIV-1 infected children above the age of 2 years and adults, in combination with other antiretroviral agents
Class: Antiretroviral, HIV-1 protease inhibitor
Half-life: 5–6 hours
Clinically important, potentially hazardous interactions with: abacavir, alfuzosin, amiodarone, amprenavir, aripiprazole, artemether/lumefantrine, atazanavir, atorvastatin, atovaquone, bepridil, bosentan, brigatinib, bupropion, cabozantinib, carbamazepine, chlorpheniramine, cisapride, clarithromycin, colchicine, copanlisib, cyclosporine, darifenacin, darunavir, dasatinib, delavirdine, dexamethasone, didanosine, digoxin, disulfiram, efavirenz, elbasvir & grazoprevir, eltrombopag, eluxadoline, ergotamine, estradiol, felodipine, fentanyl, flecainide, fluticasone propionate, fosamprenavir, glecaprevir & pibrentasvir, indinavir, itraconazole, ketoconazole, lidocaine, lidocaine, lomitapide, lovastatin, maraviroc, methadone, methylergonovine, metronidazole, midazolam, midostaurin, mifepristone, nelfinavir, neratinib, nevirapine, nicardipine, nifedipine, nilotinib, olaparib, ombitasvir/paritaprevir/ritonavir, palbociclib, phenobarbital, phenytoin, pimozide, pitavastatin, ponatinib, primidone, quinidine, ranolazine, ribociclib, rifabutin, rifampin, rilpivirine, rivaroxaban, rosuvastatin, ruxolitinib, salmeterol, saquinavir, sildenafil, simeprevir, simvastatin, sirolimus, sofosbuvir/velpatasvir/voxilaprevir, St John's wort, tacrolimus, tadalafil, telithromycin, tenofovir disoproxil, tipranavir, tolterodine, trazodone, triazolam, vardenafil, venetoclax, vinblastine, vincristine, voriconazole, warfarin, zidovudine
Pregnancy category: C
Important contra-indications noted in the prescribing guidelines for: nursing mothers
Note: Kaletra is lopinavir and ritonavir.

Skin
Acneform eruption (<10%)
Lipodystrophy (<10%)

Rash (<10%) [5]
Hair
Alopecia [3]
Central Nervous System
Vertigo (dizziness) [2]
Neuromuscular/Skeletal
Asthenia (fatigue) (<10%) [2]
Gastrointestinal/Hepatic
Diarrhea (>10%) [5]
Flatulence (<10%)
Nausea (<10%) [4]
Pancreatitis [2]
Vomiting (<10%) [3]
Renal
Nephrolithiasis [2]

LORACARBEF

See: www.drugeruptiondata.com/drug/id/410

LORATADINE

Trade names: Alavert (Wyeth), Claritin (Schering), Claritin-D (Schering)
Indications: Allergic rhinitis, urticaria
Class: Histamine H1 receptor antagonist
Half-life: 3–20 hours
Clinically important, potentially hazardous interactions with: amiodarone
Pregnancy category: B

Skin
Anaphylactoid reactions/Anaphylaxis (>2%)
Angioedema (>2%)
Dermatitis (>2%)
Diaphoresis (>2%)
Erythema multiforme (>2%)
Fixed eruption [3]
Peripheral edema (>2%)
Photosensitivity (>2%)
Pruritus (>2%)
Purpura (>2%)
Rash (>2%)
Urticaria (>2%) [4]
Xerosis (>2%)
Hair
Alopecia (>2%)
Dry hair (>2%)
Mucosal
Sialorrhea (>2%)
Stomatitis (>2%)
Xerostomia (>10%) [9]
Cardiovascular
Flushing (>2%)
QT prolongation [2]
Torsades de pointes [4]
Central Nervous System
Dysgeusia (taste perversion) (>2%)
Headache (12%) [3]
Hyperesthesia (>2%)
Paresthesias (>2%)
Somnolence (drowsiness) [2]
Neuromuscular/Skeletal
Asthenia (fatigue) (4%) [2]

Myalgia/Myopathy (>2%)
Respiratory
Pharyngitis [2]
Endocrine/Metabolic
Gynecomastia (>2%)
Mastodynia (<10%)
Genitourinary
Vaginitis (>2%)

LORAZEPAM

Trade name: Ativan (Valeant)
Indications: Anxiety, depression
Class: Benzodiazepine
Half-life: 10–20 hours
Clinically important, potentially hazardous interactions with: alcohol, amprenavir, barbiturates, chlorpheniramine, clarithromycin, clozapine, CNS depressants, cobicistat/ elvitegravir/emtricitabine/tenofovir alafenamide, efavirenz, erythromycin, esomeprazole, eszopiclone, imatinib, MAO inhibitors, narcotics, nelfinavir, phenothiazines, valproate
Pregnancy category: D

Skin
Dermatitis (<10%)
Diaphoresis (>10%)
Pseudolymphoma [2]
Rash (>10%)
Mucosal
Nasal congestion (<10%)
Sialopenia (>10%)
Xerostomia (>10%)
Cardiovascular
Hypotension [2]
Central Nervous System
Agitation [2]
Akathisia (<10%)
Amnesia (<10%) [18]
Catatonia [2]
Confusion (<10%)
Delirium [2]
Depression (<10%)
Hallucinations [2]
Headache (<10%)
Somnolence (drowsiness) (<10%) [3]
Tremor (<10%)
Vertigo (dizziness) (<10%) [2]
Respiratory
Apnea (<10%)
Hyperventilation (<10%)
Ocular
Visual disturbances (<10%)
Local
Injection-site pain (>10%)
Injection-site phlebitis (>10%)
Other
Adverse effects [2]

LORCAINIDE

See: www.drugeruptiondata.com/drug/id/1304

LORCASERIN

Trade name: Belviq (Arena)
Indications: Obesity in adults who have at least one weight-related health condition, such as high blood pressure, Type II diabetes, or high cholesterol
Class: Serotonin receptor agonist
Half-life: ~11 hours
Clinically important, potentially hazardous interactions with: antipsychotics, bupropion, dextromethorphan, lithium, MAO inhibitors, SNRIs, SSRIs, St John's wort, tramadol, tricyclic antidepressants, triptans
Pregnancy category: X
Important contra-indications noted in the prescribing guidelines for: nursing mothers; pediatric patients

Skin
Peripheral edema (5%)
Rash (2%)
Mucosal
Nasal congestion (3%)
Oropharyngeal pain (4%)
Xerostomia (5%) [2]
Cardiovascular
Hypertension (5%)
Valvulopathy (2–3%) [5]
Central Nervous System
Anxiety (4%)
Cognitive impairment (2%) [2]
Depression (2%) [2]
Euphoria [2]
Headache (15–17%) [11]
Insomnia (4%)
Vertigo (dizziness) (7–9%) [9]
Neuromuscular/Skeletal
Asthenia (fatigue) (7%) [3]
Back pain (6–12%) [2]
Bone or joint pain (2%)
Muscle spasm (5%)
Gastrointestinal/Hepatic
Constipation (6%)
Diarrhea (7%)
Gastroenteritis (3%)
Nausea (8–9%) [9]
Vomiting (4%)
Respiratory
Cough (4%)
Nasopharyngitis (11–13%) [2]
Upper respiratory tract infection (14%)
Endocrine/Metabolic
Appetite decreased (2%)
Diabetes mellitus (exacerbation) (3%)
Hypoglycemia (29%) [3]
Genitourinary
Urinary tract infection (7–9%)
Other
Toothache (3%)

LOSARTAN

Trade names: Cozaar (Merck), Hyzaar (Merck)
Indications: Hypertension
Class: Angiotensin II receptor antagonist (blocker), Antihypertensive
Half-life: 2 hours
Clinically important, potentially hazardous interactions with: aliskiren, rifampin, voriconazole
Pregnancy category: D (category C in first trimester; category D in second and third trimesters)
Important contra-indications noted in the prescribing guidelines for: nursing mothers
Note: Hyzaar is losartan and hydrochlorothiazide. Hydrochlorothiazide is a sulfonamide and can be absorbed systemically. Sulfonamides can produce severe, possibly fatal, reactions such as toxic epidermal necrolysis and Stevens-Johnson syndrome.
Warning: USE IN PREGNANCY

Skin
Anaphylactoid reactions/Anaphylaxis [2]
Angioedema [11]
Purpura [2]

Mucosal
Nasal congestion (2%)

Central Nervous System
Ageusia (taste loss) [2]
Vertigo (dizziness) (3%)

Neuromuscular/Skeletal
Back pain (2%)

Respiratory
Upper respiratory tract infection (8%)

Endocrine/Metabolic
Hyperkalemia [7]

Other
Adverse effects [7]

LOTEPREDNOL

See: www.drugeruptiondata.com/drug/id/1074

LOVASTATIN

Trade names: Advicor (Kos), Altoprev (Shionogi), Mevacor (Merck)
Indications: Hypercholesterolemia
Class: HMG-CoA reductase inhibitor, Statin
Half-life: 1–2 hours
Clinically important, potentially hazardous interactions with: amprenavir, atazanavir, azithromycin, boceprevir, bosentan, cholestyramine, clarithromycin, cyclosporine, darunavir, dasabuvir/ombitasvir/paritaprevir/ritonavir, delavirdine, efavirenz, elbasvir & grazoprevir, erythromycin, exenatide, fenofibrate, fosamprenavir, gemfibrozil, glecaprevir & pibrentasvir, grapefruit juice, imatinib, indinavir, itraconazole, lomitapide, lopinavir, mifepristone, nelfinavir, ombitasvir/paritaprevir/ritonavir, paclitaxel, posaconazole, red rice yeast,

tacrolimus, telaprevir, telithromycin, ticagrelor, tipranavir, tolvaptan, verapamil
Pregnancy category: X
Important contra-indications noted in the prescribing guidelines for: nursing mothers

Skin
Exanthems (<5%) [3]
Lupus erythematosus [4]
Pruritus (5%) [2]
Rash (5%) [3]

Central Nervous System
Parkinsonism [2]

Neuromuscular/Skeletal
Asthenia (fatigue) [2]
Myalgia/Myopathy (<10%) [6]
Rhabdomyolysis [41]

Gastrointestinal/Hepatic
Hepatotoxicity [2]
Pancreatitis [2]

Endocrine/Metabolic
Gynecomastia (<10%)

LOXAPINE

Trade names: Adasuve (Teva), Loxitane (Watson)
Indications: Psychoses
Class: Antipsychotic, tricyclic
Half-life: 12–19 hours (terminal)
Clinically important, potentially hazardous interactions with: none known
Pregnancy category: C
Important contra-indications noted in the prescribing guidelines for: the elderly; nursing mothers; pediatric patients
Warning: BRONCHOSPASM and INCREASED MORTALITY IN ELDERLY PATIENTS WITH DEMENTIA-RELATED PSYCHOSIS

Skin
Rash (<10%)

Mucosal
Xerostomia (>10%)

Central Nervous System
Dysgeusia (taste perversion) (14%) [8]
Neuroleptic malignant syndrome [3]
Sedation (12%) [4]
Somnolence (drowsiness) [3]
Vertigo (dizziness) [2]

Neuromuscular/Skeletal
Rhabdomyolysis [3]

Gastrointestinal/Hepatic
Dysphagia [2]

Respiratory
Bronchospasm [3]
Pulmonary toxicity [3]

Endocrine/Metabolic
Gynecomastia (<10%)

LUBIPROSTONE

Trade name: Amitiza (Takeda)
Indications: Constipation, irritable bowel syndrome
Class: Chloride channel activator
Half-life: 0–1.4 hours
Clinically important, potentially hazardous interactions with: none known
Pregnancy category: C
Important contra-indications noted in the prescribing guidelines for: nursing mothers; pediatric patients
Note: Contra-indicated in patients with known or suspected mechanical gastrointestinal obstruction.

Skin
Peripheral edema (4%)

Central Nervous System
Headache (13%) [7]

Neuromuscular/Skeletal
Arthralgia (3%)
Asthenia (fatigue) (2%)
Back pain (2%)

Gastrointestinal/Hepatic
Abdominal distension [5]
Abdominal pain (7%) [8]
Diarrhea [18]
Flatulence [3]
Nausea [19]
Vomiting [7]

Respiratory
Dyspnea [3]
Flu-like syndrome (2%)
Sinusitis (5%)
Upper respiratory tract infection (4%)

Other
Adverse effects [3]

LUCINACTANT

See: www.drugeruptiondata.com/drug/id/2847

LULICONAZOLE

Trade name: Luzu (Medicis)
Indications: Interdigital tinea pedis, tinea cruris, and tinea corporis caused by the organisms *Trichophyton rubrum* and *Epidermophyton floccosum*
Class: Antifungal, azole
Half-life: N/A
Clinically important, potentially hazardous interactions with: none known
Pregnancy category: C
Important contra-indications noted in the prescribing guidelines for: nursing mothers; pediatric patients

Skin
Contact dermatitis [2]

Litt's Drug Eruption & Reaction Manual © 2018 by Taylor & Francis Group, LLC

LUMACAFTOR/ IVACAFTOR

Trade name: Orkambi (Vertex)
Indications: Cystic fibrosis in patients aged 12 years and older who are homozygous for the *F508del* mutation in the *CFTR* gene
Class: CFTR potentiator, CYP3A4 inducer
Half-life: 26 hours
Clinically important, potentially hazardous interactions with: rifampin, St John's wort
Pregnancy category: B
Important contra-indications noted in the prescribing guidelines for: nursing mothers; pediatric patients
Note: See also separate profile for ivacaftor.

Skin
  Rash (7%) [2]
Mucosal
  Rhinorrhea (6%)
Neuromuscular/Skeletal
  Asthenia (fatigue) (9%)
Gastrointestinal/Hepatic
  Diarrhea (12%)
  Flatulence (7%)
  Nausea (13%)
Respiratory
  Dyspnea (13%) [3]
  Influenza (5%)
  Nasopharyngitis (13%)
  Upper respiratory tract infection (10%)
Endocrine/Metabolic
  Creatine phosphokinase increased (7%)
  Menstrual irregularities (10%)

Other
  Adverse effects [2]

LUMIRACOXIB

See: www.drugeruptiondata.com/drug/id/1245

LURASIDONE

Trade name: Latuda (Sunovion)
Indications: Schizophrenia, depressive epidodes associated with bipolar I disorder
Class: Antipsychotic
Half-life: 18 hours
Clinically important, potentially hazardous interactions with: alcohol, amphetamines, CNS depressants, dasabuvir/ombitasvir/paritaprevir/ritonavir, dasatinib, deferasirox, diltiazem, disopyramide, dopamine, dopamine agonists, droperidol, efavirenz, epinephrine, hydroxyzine, ketoconazole, levomepromazine, lithium, MAO inhibitors, methylphenidate, metoclopramide, ombitasvir/paritaprevir/ritonavir, pimozide, procainamide, quinagolide, quinidine, rifampin, strong CYP3A4 inducers or inhibitors, tetrabenazine, tocilizumab
Pregnancy category: B
Important contra-indications noted in the prescribing guidelines for: the elderly; nursing mothers; pediatric patients
Warning: INCREASED MORTALITY IN ELDERLY PATIENTS WITH DEMENTIA-RELATED PSYCHOSIS

Mucosal
  Sialorrhea (2%)
Central Nervous System
  Agitation (5%)
  Akathisia (13%) [19]
  Anxiety (5%)
  Extrapyramidal symptoms [2]
  Insomnia (10%) [2]
  Parkinsonism (10%) [5]
  Restlessness (2%) [2]
  Sedation [8]
  Somnolence (drowsiness) (17%) [13]
  Vertigo (dizziness) (4%) [3]
Neuromuscular/Skeletal
  Dystonia (5%)
Gastrointestinal/Hepatic
  Dyspepsia (6%)
  Nausea (10%) [11]
  Vomiting (8%) [3]
Endocrine/Metabolic
  Hyperprolactinemia [2]
  Weight gain (5%) [3]
Other
  Adverse effects [3]

LUTROPIN ALFA

See: www.drugeruptiondata.com/drug/id/1148

LYMECYCLINE

See: www.drugeruptiondata.com/drug/id/1359

MACITENTAN

Trade name: Opsumit (Actelion)
Indications: Pulmonary arterial hypertension
Class: Endothelin receptor (ETR) antagonist
Half-life: 16 hours
Clinically important, potentially hazardous interactions with: ketoconazole, rifampin, ritonavir, strong CYP3A4 inducers or inhibitors
Pregnancy category: X
Important contra-indications noted in the prescribing guidelines for: nursing mothers; pediatric patients
Note: Contra-indicated in pregnancy.
Warning: EMBRYO-FETAL TOXICITY

Skin
 Peripheral edema [3]
Central Nervous System
 Headache (14%) [6]
Gastrointestinal/Hepatic
 Hepatotoxicity [5]
Respiratory
 Bronchitis (12%) [2]
 Influenza (6%)
 Nasopharyngitis (20%) [6]
 Pharyngitis (20%)
 Upper respiratory tract infection [2]
Genitourinary
 Urinary tract infection (9%)
Hematologic
 Anemia (13%) [8]

MAFENIDE

See: www.drugeruptiondata.com/drug/id/931

MAPROTILINE

See: www.drugeruptiondata.com/drug/id/416

MARAVIROC

Trade names: Celsentri (ViiV), Selzentry (ViiV)
Indications: HIV infection
Class: Antiretroviral, CCR5 co-receptor antagonist
Half-life: 14–18 hours
Clinically important, potentially hazardous interactions with: atazanavir, clarithromycin, conivaptan, CYP3A4 inhibitors or inducers, darunavir, dasatinib, deferasirox, delavirdine, efavirenz, etravirine, indinavir, ketoconazole, lopinavir, nelfinavir, oxcarbazepine, rifampin, rifapentine, ritonavir, saquinavir, St John's wort, telithromycin, voriconazole
Pregnancy category: B
Important contra-indications noted in the prescribing guidelines for: the elderly; nursing mothers; pediatric patients
Warning: HEPATOTOXICITY

Skin
 Dermatitis (5%)

 Folliculitis (5%)
 Lipodystrophy (5%)
 Pruritus (6%) [2]
 Rash (17%) [2]
Mucosal
 Stomatitis (4%)
Cardiovascular
 Postural hypotension [2]
Central Nervous System
 Depression (6%)
 Fever (21%) [2]
 Headache [3]
 Pain (8%)
 Paresthesias (8%)
 Peripheral neuropathy (5%)
 Sleep disturbances (12%)
 Vertigo (dizziness) (14%)
Neuromuscular/Skeletal
 Asthenia (fatigue) [2]
 Myalgia/Myopathy (5%)
Gastrointestinal/Hepatic
 Abdominal pain (14%)
 Diarrhea [2]
 Hepatotoxicity [2]
Respiratory
 Cough (22%) [2]
 Flu-like syndrome (3%)
 Nasopharyngitis [2]
 Pneumonia (4%)
 Upper respiratory tract infection (37%) [2]
Genitourinary
 Urinary tract infection (4%)
Other
 Adverse effects [6]

MARIHUANA

Synonyms: marijuana; grass; hashish; pot; cannabis
Indications: Nausea and vomiting, substance abuse drug
Class: Antiemetic, Cannabinoid, Hallucinogen
Half-life: N/A
Clinically important, potentially hazardous interactions with: atazanavir
Pregnancy category: N/A
Note: Marihuana is the popular name for the dried flowering leaves of the hemp plant, *cannabis sativa*. It contains tetrahydrocannabinols.

Cardiovascular
 Cardiotoxicity [4]
 Myocardial infarction [2]
Central Nervous System
 Amnesia [2]
 Hallucinations [2]
 Neurotoxicity [2]
 Schizophrenia [3]
 Seizures [2]
 Stroke [2]
Gastrointestinal/Hepatic
 Pancreatitis [2]
Genitourinary
 Priapism [2]

 Ocular
 Hallucinations, visual [2]
Other
 Adverse effects [2]

MAZINDOL

See: www.drugeruptiondata.com/drug/id/418

MDMA

Synonyms: 3,4-methylenedioxymethamphetamine; ecstasy; E; X; molly; club drug
Indications: N/A
Class: Amphetamine
Half-life: N/A
Clinically important, potentially hazardous interactions with: none known

Skin
 Diaphoresis [4]
Mucosal
 Xerostomia [5]
Cardiovascular
 Cardiotoxicity [2]
 Myocardial infarction [2]
Central Nervous System
 Amnesia [2]
 Confusion [2]
 Depression (37%) [14]
 Hallucinations [4]
 Headache [2]
 Hyperthermia [3]
 Memory loss [3]
 Neuroleptic malignant syndrome [4]
 Neurotoxicity [5]
 Parkinsonism [4]
 Psychosis [4]
 Seizures [3]
 Serotonin syndrome [6]
Neuromuscular/Skeletal
 Myalgia/Myopathy [2]
 Rhabdomyolysis [34]
Gastrointestinal/Hepatic
 Hepatitis [2]
 Hepatotoxicity [4]
 Nausea [2]
Endocrine/Metabolic
 Hyponatremia [5]
 SIADH [8]
Genitourinary
 Priapism [2]
Hematologic
 Coagulopathy [2]
Ocular
 Hallucinations, visual [2]
Other
 Bruxism [8]
 Death [47]
 Dipsia (thirst) [2]
 Multiorgan failure [2]

MEASLES, MUMPS & RUBELLA (MMR) VIRUS VACCINE

Trade name: M-M-R II (Merck)
Indications: Protection against measles (rubeola), mumps and rubella (German measles)
Class: Vaccine
Half-life: N/A
Clinically important, potentially hazardous interactions with: none known
Pregnancy category: C
Important contra-indications noted in the prescribing guidelines for: nursing mothers; pediatric patients
Note: Contra-indicated for pregnant females; patients who have had anaphylactic or anaphylactoid reactions to neomycin; febrile respiratory illness or other active febrile infection; patients receiving immunosuppressive therapy or with blood dyscrasias, leukemia, lymphomas of any type, or other malignant neoplasms affecting the bone marrow or lymphatic systems; primary and acquired immunodeficiency states, or individuals with a family history of congenital or hereditary immunodeficiency, until the immune competence of the potential vaccine recipient is demonstrated.

Skin
Henoch–Schönlein purpura [2]
Rash [4]
Central Nervous System
Fever [7]
Seizures [3]
Neuromuscular/Skeletal
Asthenia (fatigue) [2]
Gastrointestinal/Hepatic
Vomiting [2]
Local
Injection-site erythema [2]
Injection-site pain [2]
Injection-site reactions [3]
Other
Adverse effects [5]
Infection [2]

MEBENDAZOLE

Trade name: Vermox (Janssen)
Indications: Parasitic worm infestations
Class: Anthelmintic, Antibiotic, imidazole
Half-life: 1–12 hours
Clinically important, potentially hazardous interactions with: aminophylline
Pregnancy category: C

Skin
Stevens-Johnson syndrome [2]
Hair
Alopecia [3]
Central Nervous System
Headache [2]
Vertigo (dizziness) [2]

Gastrointestinal/Hepatic
Abdominal pain [4]

MEBEVERINE

See: www.drugeruptiondata.com/drug/id/1418

MECAMYLAMINE

See: www.drugeruptiondata.com/drug/id/965

MECASERMIN

See: www.drugeruptiondata.com/drug/id/1089

MECHLORETHAMINE

Synonyms: mustine; nitrogen mustard
Indications: Hodgkin's disease, mycosis fungoides
Class: Alkylating agent
Half-life: <1 minute
Clinically important, potentially hazardous interactions with: aldesleukin, vaccines
Pregnancy category: D

Skin
Anaphylactoid reactions/Anaphylaxis (<10%) [4]
Bullous dermatitis [3]
Dermatitis [26]
Herpes zoster (>10%)
Hypersensitivity (<10%)
Pigmentation [8]
Pruritus [2]
Squamous cell carcinoma [3]
Urticaria [3]
Hair
Alopecia (<10%)
Central Nervous System
Dysgeusia (taste perversion) (<10%)
Local
Injection-site extravasation (<10%)
Injection-site thrombophlebitis (<10%) [2]

MECLIZINE

See: www.drugeruptiondata.com/drug/id/421

MECLOFENAMATE

See: www.drugeruptiondata.com/drug/id/422

MEDROXY-PROGESTERONE

Trade names: Depo-Provera (Pfizer), Lunelle (Pfizer), Premphase (Wyeth), Prempro (Wyeth), Provera (Pfizer)
Indications: Secondary amenorrhea, renal or endometrial carcinoma
Class: Progestogen
Half-life: 30 days
Clinically important, potentially hazardous interactions with: acitretin, dofetilide
Pregnancy category: X

Skin
Acneform eruption (<5%)
Chloasma (<10%)
Diaphoresis (<31%)
Edema (>10%)
Melasma (<10%)
Pruritus (<10%)
Rash (<5%)
Hair
Alopecia (<5%)
Cardiovascular
Flushing (12%)
Thrombophlebitis (<10%)
Neuromuscular/Skeletal
Osteoporosis [2]
Endocrine/Metabolic
Amenorrhea [3]
Galactorrhea [2]
Mastodynia (<5%)
Weight gain [3]
Genitourinary
Vaginitis (<5%)
Local
Injection-site pain (>10%)

MEFENAMIC ACID

Trade name: Ponstel (First Horizon)
Indications: Pain, dysmenorrhea
Class: Non-steroidal anti-inflammatory (NSAID)
Half-life: 3.5 hours
Clinically important, potentially hazardous interactions with: methotrexate
Pregnancy category: C
Important contra-indications noted in the prescribing guidelines for: nursing mothers; pediatric patients
Note: NSAIDs may cause an increased risk of serious cardiovascular and gastrointestinal adverse events, which can be fatal. This risk may increase with duration of use.
Warning: CARDIOVASCULAR AND GASTROINTESTINAL RISK

Skin
Anaphylactoid reactions/Anaphylaxis [2]
Erythema multiforme [2]
Fixed eruption [12]
Pruritus (<10%)
Rash (>10%)
Toxic epidermal necrolysis [2]

Cardiovascular
Myocardial infarction [2]

Central Nervous System
Seizures [2]

Gastrointestinal/Hepatic
Hepatotoxicity [2]

Renal
Renal failure [2]

Ocular
Glaucoma [2]

MEFLOQUINE

Trade name: Lariam (Roche)
Indications: Malaria
Class: Antimalarial, Antiprotozoal
Half-life: 21–22 days
Clinically important, potentially hazardous interactions with: acebutolol, artemether/ lumefantrine, ethosuximide, halofantrine, ketoconazole, lacosamide, moxifloxacin, oxcarbazepine, quinine, tiagabine, typhoid vaccine, vigabatrin
Pregnancy category: C
Important contra-indications noted in the prescribing guidelines for: nursing mothers
Warning: NEUROPSYCHIATRIC ADVERSE REACTIONS

Skin
Anaphylactoid reactions/Anaphylaxis [2]
Erythema [2]
Exanthems (30%)
Pruritus (4–10%) [2]
Psoriasis [2]
Rash (<10%)
Stevens-Johnson syndrome [2]
Toxic epidermal necrolysis [2]
Vasculitis [3]

Cardiovascular
Palpitation [3]
Tachycardia [2]

Central Nervous System
Abnormal dreams [3]
Aggression [2]
Amnesia [2]
Anorexia [2]
Anxiety [5]
Chills (<10%)
Confusion [2]
Delusions [2]
Depression [7]
Fever (<10%) [2]
Hallucinations [3]
Headache (<10%) [5]
Insomnia [3]
Mania [4]
Neurotoxicity [8]
Psychosis [8]
Seizures [6]
Sleep disturbances [2]
Suicidal ideation [2]
Vertigo (dizziness) (<10%) [20]

Neuromuscular/Skeletal
Arthralgia [2]
Asthenia (fatigue) (<10%) [2]
Myalgia/Myopathy (<10%) [2]

Gastrointestinal/Hepatic
Abdominal pain [4]
Diarrhea [4]
Nausea [8]
Vomiting [14]

Otic
Tinnitus (<10%)

Ocular
Maculopathy [2]

Other
Adverse effects [2]
Death [3]

MELOXICAM

Trade name: Mobic (Boehringer Ingelheim)
Indications: Osteoarthritis
Class: COX-2 inhibitor, Non-steroidal anti-inflammatory (NSAID)
Half-life: 15–20 hours
Clinically important, potentially hazardous interactions with: ACE inhibitors, adrenergic neurone blockers, alcohol, aliskiren, alpha blockers, angiotensin II receptor antagonists, anticoagulants, antidepressants, antiplatelet agents, aspirin, baclofen, beta blockers, bile acid sequestrants, calcium channel blockers, cardiac glycosides, cholestyramine, clonidine, clopidogrel, collagenase, conivaptan, corticosteroids, coumarins, cyclosporine, dabigatran, dasatinib, desmopressin, diazoxide, digoxin, diuretics, drotrecogin alfa, eplerenone, erlotinib, glucosamine, haloperidol, heparins, hydralazine, ibritumomab, iloprost, ketorolac, lithium, methotrexate, methyldopa, mifamurtide, minoxidil, moxonidine, nitrates, nitroprusside, NSAIDs, pemetrexed, penicillamine, pentosan, pentoxifylline, phenindione, pralatrexate, prasugrel, probenecid, prostacyclin analogues, quinolones, ritonavir, serotonin/norepinephrine reuptake inhibitors, SSRIs, sulfonylureas, tacrolimus, thrombolytic agents, tositumomab & iodine[131], treprostinil, vancomycin, venlafaxine, vitamin K antagonists, voriconazole, zidovudine
Pregnancy category: C (category D from 30 weeks gestation)
Important contra-indications noted in the prescribing guidelines for: the elderly; nursing mothers
Note: NSAIDs may cause an increased risk of serious cardiovascular and gastrointestinal adverse events, which can be fatal. This risk may increase with duration of use.
Warning: CARDIOVASCULAR AND GASTROINTESTINAL RISKS

Skin
Anaphylactoid reactions/Anaphylaxis (<2%)
Angioedema (<2%) [3]
Bullous dermatitis (<2%)
Edema (2–5%)
Erythema [2]
Erythema multiforme (<2%)
Exanthems (<2%)
Facial edema (<2%)
Hematoma [3]
Hot flashes (<2%)
Hyperhidrosis (<2%)

Hypersensitivity [2]
Photosensitivity (<2%)
Pruritus (<2%) [3]
Purpura (<2%)
Rash (<3%) [3]
Stevens-Johnson syndrome (<2%)
Toxic epidermal necrolysis (<2%)
Urticaria (<2%) [4]
Vasculitis (<2%)

Hair
Alopecia (<2%)

Mucosal
Ulcerative stomatitis (<2%)
Xerostomia (<2%)

Cardiovascular
Angina (<2%)
Arrhythmias (<2%)
Cardiac failure (<2%)
Hypertension (<2%)
Hypotension (<2%)
Myocardial infarction (<2%)
Palpitation (<2%)
Tachycardia (<2%)

Central Nervous System
Abnormal dreams (<2%)
Anxiety (<2%)
Confusion (<2%)
Depression (<2%)
Dysgeusia (taste perversion) (<2%)
Fever (<2%)
Headache (2–6%) [2]
Insomnia (<4%)
Nervousness (<2%)
Pain (4%)
Paresthesias (<2%)
Seizures (<2%)
Somnolence (drowsiness) (<2%)
Syncope (<2%)
Tremor (<2%)
Vertigo (dizziness) (<3%)

Neuromuscular/Skeletal
Arthralgia (<5%)
Asthenia (fatigue) [2]
Back pain (<3%)
Bone or joint pain (2%)

Gastrointestinal/Hepatic
Abdominal pain (2–5%) [2]
Black stools (<2%)
Colitis (<2%)
Constipation (<3%) [2]
Diarrhea (2–6%) [2]
Dyspepsia (4–10%) [2]
Eructation (belching) (<2%)
Esophagitis (<2%)
Flatulence (<3%)
Gastritis (<2%)
Gastroesophageal reflux (<2%)
Gastrointestinal bleeding [2]
Gastrointestinal perforation (<2%) [2]
Gastrointestinal ulceration (<2%) [3]
Hematemesis (<2%)
Hepatitis (<2%)
Hepatotoxicity [6]
Nausea (3–7%) [4]
Pancreatitis (<2%)
Vomiting (<3%)

Respiratory
Asthma (<2%)

Bronchospasm (<2%)
Cough (<2%)
Dyspnea (<2%)
Flu-like syndrome (2–3%)
Upper respiratory tract infection (<8%)

Endocrine/Metabolic
ALT increased (<2%)
Appetite increased (<2%)
AST increased (<2%)
Dehydration (<2%)
GGT increased (<2%)
Weight gain (<2%)
Weight loss (<2%)

Genitourinary
Albuminuria (<2%)
Hematuria (<2%)
Urinary frequency (<2%)
Urinary tract infection (<7%)

Renal
Nephrotoxicity [2]
Renal failure (<2%)

Hematologic
Anemia (<4%)
Leukopenia (<2%)

Otic
Tinnitus (<2%)

Ocular
Abnormal vision (<2%)
Conjunctivitis (<2%)

Other
Adverse effects (18%) [6]
Allergic reactions (<2%)

MELPHALAN

Trade names: Alkeran (GSK), Evomela (Spectrum)
Indications: Multiple myeloma, carcinomas
Class: Alkylating agent
Half-life: 90 minutes
Clinically important, potentially hazardous interactions with: aldesleukin, PEG-interferon, tasonermin
Pregnancy category: D
Important contra-indications noted in the prescribing guidelines for: the elderly; nursing mothers; pediatric patients
Warning: SEVERE BONE MARROW SUPPRESSION, HYPERSENSITIVITY, and LEUKEMOGENICITY

Skin
Anaphylactoid reactions/Anaphylaxis [2]
Angioedema [2]
Dermatitis [2]
Exanthems (4%) [4]
Hypersensitivity (<10%)
Pruritus (<10%)
Rash (<10%)
Toxicity [3]
Urticaria [3]
Vasculitis (<10%)
Vesiculation (<10%)

Hair
Alopecia (<10%) [2]

Nails
Beau's lines (transverse nail bands) [4]

Mucosal
Mucositis [8]
Oral mucositis [4]
Stomatitis (<10%) [2]

Cardiovascular
Atrial fibrillation [2]

Central Nervous System
Peripheral neuropathy [3]

Neuromuscular/Skeletal
Rhabdomyolysis [2]

Gastrointestinal/Hepatic
Diarrhea [3]
Hepatotoxicity [2]
Nausea [2]

Hematologic
Febrile neutropenia [2]
Neutropenia [5]
Thrombocytopenia [5]

Other
Death [2]

MEMANTINE

Trade names: Ebixa (Lundbeck), Namenda (Forest)
Indications: Alzheimer's disease, vascular dementia
Class: Adamantane, NMDA receptor antagonist
Half-life: 60–80 hours
Clinically important, potentially hazardous interactions with: amantadine, bromocriptine, darifenacin, dextromethorphan, ketamine, levodopa, levomepromazine, oxybutynin, risperidone, rotigotine, tiotropium, trimethoprim, trospium, zuclopenthixol
Pregnancy category: B
Important contra-indications noted in the prescribing guidelines for: nursing mothers; pediatric patients

Skin
Peripheral edema (>2%)

Central Nervous System
Agitation [2]
Confusion [3]
Depression (>2%)
Gait instability [3]
Headache (6%) [3]
Vertigo (dizziness) (7%) [6]

Neuromuscular/Skeletal
Arthralgia (>2%)
Asthenia (fatigue) (2%)
Back pain (3%)
Myoclonus [2]

Gastrointestinal/Hepatic
Constipation [2]
Diarrhea [2]
Vomiting [2]

Respiratory
Cough (4%)
Flu-like syndrome (>2%)
Nasopharyngitis [2]

Genitourinary
Urinary tract infection [2]

Ocular
Hallucinations, visual [2]

Other
Adverse effects [3]

MENADIONE

See: www.drugeruptiondata.com/drug/id/1961

MENINGOCOCCAL GROUP B VACCINE

Trade names: Bexsero (Novartis), Trumenba (Wyeth)
Indications: Immunization to prevent invasive disease caused by *Neisseria meningitidis* serogroup B
Class: Vaccine
Half-life: N/A
Clinically important, potentially hazardous interactions with: none known
Pregnancy category: B
Important contra-indications noted in the prescribing guidelines for: the elderly; nursing mothers; pediatric patients

Central Nervous System
Chills (18–30%)
Fever (2–8%) [3]
Headache (41–57%)

Neuromuscular/Skeletal
Arthralgia (16–22%)
Asthenia (fatigue) (44–65%)
Myalgia/Myopathy (35–41%)

Gastrointestinal/Hepatic
Diarrhea (9–15%)
Vomiting (2–8%)

Respiratory
Upper respiratory tract infection [2]

Local
Injection-site edema (18–22%)
Injection-site erythema (15–20%)
Injection-site pain (85–93%) [2]

MENINGOCOCCAL GROUPS C & Y & HAEMOPHILUS B TETANUS TOXOID CONJUGATE VACCINE

Synonym: HibMenCY
Trade name: Menhibrix (GSK)
Indications: Immunization to prevent invasive disease caused by *Neisseria meningitidis* serogroups C and Y and *Haemophilus influenzae* Type B
Class: Vaccine
Half-life: N/A
Clinically important, potentially hazardous interactions with: immunosuppressants
Pregnancy category: C
Important contra-indications noted in the prescribing guidelines for: pediatric patients

Central Nervous System
    Fever (11–26%)
    Irritability (62–71%)
    Sedation (49–63%)
Endocrine/Metabolic
    Appetite decreased (30–34%)
Local
    Injection-site edema (15–25%) [2]
    Injection-site erythema (21–36%)
    Injection-site pain (42–46%) [2]

MEPENZOLATE

See: www.drugeruptiondata.com/drug/id/1029

MEPERIDINE

Synonym: pethidine
Trade name: Demerol (Sanofi-Aventis)
Indications: Pain
Class: Opiate agonist
Half-life: 3–4 hours
Clinically important, potentially hazardous interactions with: acyclovir, alcohol, amphetamines, barbiturates, CNS depressants, darunavir, duloxetine, fluoxetine, furazolidone, general anesthetics, glycopyrrolate, glycopyrronium, indinavir, isocarboxazid, linezolid, lisdexamfetamine, lithium, MAO inhibitors, moclobemide, phenelzine, phenobarbital, phenothiazines, phenytoin, rasagiline, ritonavir, safinamide, selegiline, sibutramine, SSRIs, tipranavir, tranquilizers, tranylcypromine, tricyclic antidepressants, valacyclovir
Pregnancy category: C
Important contra-indications noted in the prescribing guidelines for: the elderly; nursing mothers; pediatric patients

Skin
    Pruritus [3]

Mucosal
    Xerostomia (<10%)
Central Nervous System
    Catatonia [2]
    Delirium [2]
    Seizures [2]
    Serotonin syndrome [7]
Local
    Injection-site erythema [2]
    Injection-site pain (<10%)

MEPHENYTOIN

See: www.drugeruptiondata.com/drug/id/430

MEPHOBARBITAL

See: www.drugeruptiondata.com/drug/id/431

MEPIVACAINE

See: www.drugeruptiondata.com/drug/id/1781

MEPOLIZUMAB

Trade name: Nucala (GSK)
Indications: Adjunctive treatment for severe eosinophilic asthma
Class: Interleukin-5 antagonist, Monoclonal antibody
Half-life: 16–22 days
Clinically important, potentially hazardous interactions with: none known
Pregnancy category: N/A (Insufficent evidence to inform drug-associated risk)
Important contra-indications noted in the prescribing guidelines for: nursing mothers; pediatric patients

Skin
    Eczema (3%)
    Pruritus (3%)
    Rash (>3%)
Mucosal
    Nasal congestion (>3%)
Central Nervous System
    Fever (>3%)
    Headache (19%) [4]
    Vertigo (dizziness) (>3%)
Neuromuscular/Skeletal
    Asthenia (fatigue) (5%) [2]
    Back pain (5%)
    Bone or joint pain (>3%)
    Muscle spasm (3%)
Gastrointestinal/Hepatic
    Abdominal pain (3%)
    Gastroenteritis (>3%)
    Nausea (>3%) [2]
    Vomiting (>3%)
Respiratory
    Asthma [2]
    Bronchitis (>3%) [2]
    Dyspnea (>3%)
    Influenza (3%)
    Nasopharyngitis (>3%) [3]
    Pharyngitis (>3%)
    Rhinitis (>3%)
    Sinusitis [2]
    Upper respiratory tract infection [2]
Genitourinary
    Cystitis (>3%)
    Urinary tract infection (3%)
Otic
    Ear infection (>3%)
Local
    Injection-site reactions (8%) [2]
Other
    Infection (>3%)
    Toothache (>3%)

MEPROBAMATE

See: www.drugeruptiondata.com/drug/id/432

MEPTAZINOL

See: www.drugeruptiondata.com/drug/id/1340

MERCAPTOPURINE

Synonyms: 6-mercaptopurine; 6-MP
Trade name: Purinethol (Gate)
Indications: Leukemias
Class: Antimetabolite, Antineoplastic
Half-life: triphasic: 45 minutes; 2.5 hours; 10 hours
Clinically important, potentially hazardous interactions with: aldesleukin, allopurinol, balsalazide, febuxostat, influenza vaccine, mycophenolate, natalizumab, olsalazine, trimethoprim, typhoid vaccine, vaccines, yellow fever vaccine
Pregnancy category: D

Skin
    Dermatitis (2%)
    Hand–foot syndrome [3]
    Hypersensitivity [2]
    Neoplasms [2]
    Peripheral edema [2]
    Photosensitivity [2]
    Pigmentation (<10%)
    Rash (<10%) [2]
Hair
    Alopecia [2]
Mucosal
    Mucositis (<10%)
    Oral lesions (<5%) [2]
    Stomatitis (<10%)
Central Nervous System
    Fever [3]
Gastrointestinal/Hepatic
    Hepatotoxicity [5]
    Nausea [2]
    Pancreatitis [9]

Hematologic
Leukopenia [2]
Myelosuppression [2]
Myelotoxicity [3]

Other
Death [2]

MEROPENEM

Trade name: Meronem (AstraZeneca)
Indications: Aerobic and anaerobic infections, febrile neutropenia
Class: Antibiotic, carbapenem, Thienamycin
Half-life: 4–6 hours
Clinically important, potentially hazardous interactions with: oral contraceptives, probenecid, valproic acid
Pregnancy category: B

Skin
AGEP [2]
Hypersensitivity [3]
Rash (2%) [6]

Central Nervous System
Headache (2%)
Seizures [7]

Gastrointestinal/Hepatic
Diarrhea [4]
Hepatotoxicity [3]
Nausea [2]
Vomiting [2]

Endocrine/Metabolic
ALT increased [3]
AST increased [3]

Local
Injection-site pain [3]

Other
Adverse effects [14]
Death [2]

MEROPENEM & VABORBACTAM *

Trade name: Vabomere (Rempex)
Indications: Complicated urinary tract infections caused by susceptible bacteria
Class: Antibiotic, carbapenem (meropenem), Beta-lactamase inhibitor (vaborbactam)
Half-life: 1–2 hours
Clinically important, potentially hazardous interactions with: probenecid, valproic acid
Pregnancy category: N/A (Potential risk to fetus based on animal studies)
Important contra-indications noted in the prescribing guidelines for: pediatric patients
Note: See also separate entry for meropenem.

Skin
Hypersensitivity (2%)

Central Nervous System
Fever (2%)
Headache (9%)

Gastrointestinal/Hepatic
Diarrhea (3%)

Nausea (2%)

Endocrine/Metabolic
ALT increased (2%)
AST increased (2%)

Local
Infusion-site reactions (4%)
Injection-site phlebitis (4%)

MESALAMINE

Synonyms: 5-aminosalicylic acid; 5-ASA; fisalamine; mesalazine
Trade names: Asacol (Procter & Gamble), Canasa (Aptalis), Lialda (Shire), Pentasa (Shire), Rowasa (Solvay)
Indications: Ulcerative colitis
Class: Aminosalicylate
Half-life: 0.5–1.5 hours
Clinically important, potentially hazardous interactions with: azathioprine, NSAIDs, pantoprazole
Pregnancy category: B
Important contra-indications noted in the prescribing guidelines for: the elderly; nursing mothers

Skin
Diaphoresis (3%)
Exanthems [3]
Hypersensitivity [8]
Lupus erythematosus [2]
Photosensitivity [3]
Psoriasis [2]
Rash (3%) [6]

Hair
Alopecia [6]

Cardiovascular
Cardiotoxicity [2]
Myocarditis [6]
Pericarditis [5]

Central Nervous System
Fever (<6%) [6]
Headache (2–25%) [5]
Pain (14%)
Vertigo (dizziness) (2–8%)

Neuromuscular/Skeletal
Myalgia/Myopathy (3%)

Gastrointestinal/Hepatic
Abdominal pain (<18%) [6]
Colitis (ulcerative / exacerbation) [3]
Diarrhea (2–8%) [4]
Eructation (belching) (16%)
Flatulence (<6%) [2]
Nausea (3–13%) [3]
Pancreatitis [20]
Vomiting (<5%) [2]

Respiratory
Eosinophilic pneumonia [4]
Pharyngitis (11%)
Pneumonia [5]
Pneumonitis [2]
Pulmonary toxicity [9]

Renal
Nephrotoxicity [6]

Hematologic
Anemia [2]

Eosinophilia [3]

Otic
Tinnitus (<3%)

Other
Adverse effects [11]
Allergic reactions [2]
Kounis syndrome [2]

MESNA

See: www.drugeruptiondata.com/drug/id/435

MESORIDAZINE

See: www.drugeruptiondata.com/drug/id/436

METAMIZOLE

See: www.drugeruptiondata.com/drug/id/1131

METAXALONE

Trade name: Skelaxin (Elan)
Indications: Muscle spasm
Class: Central muscle relaxant
Half-life: 4–14 hours
Clinically important, potentially hazardous interactions with: alcohol, barbiturates, conivaptan, droperidol, interferon alfa, levomepromazine, St John's wort, tricyclic antidepressants
Pregnancy category: B
Important contra-indications noted in the prescribing guidelines for: nursing mothers; pediatric patients
Note: Contra-indicated in patients with known tendency to drug-induced, hemolytic, or other anemias, or significantly impaired renal or hepatic function.

Cardiovascular
Tachycardia [2]

Central Nervous System
Agitation [2]
Serotonin syndrome [2]
Somnolence (drowsiness) [3]
Vertigo (dizziness) [3]

Gastrointestinal/Hepatic
Nausea [2]
Vomiting [2]

METFORMIN

Trade names: Avandamet (GSK), Fortamet (Andrx), Glucophage (Merck Serono), Glucovance (Merck Serono), Invokamet (Janssen), Janumet (Merck Sharpe & Dohme), Synjardy (Boehringer Ingelheim), Xigduo XR (AstraZeneca)
Indications: Diabetes
Class: Antidiabetic, Biguanide
Half-life: 6 hours
Clinically important, potentially hazardous interactions with: ACE inhibitors, acetazolamide, alcohol, amiloride, anabolic steroids, beta blockers, calcium channel blockers, captopril, cephalexin, cilazapril, cimetidine, corticosteroids, diazoxide, dichlorphenamide, digoxin, disopyramide, diuretics, enalapril, estrogens, fosinopril, iodinated contrast agents, isoniazid, ketotifen, lanreotide, lisinopril, luteinizing hormone releasing hormone analogs, MAO inhibitors, morphine, nicotinic acid, octreotide, oral contraceptives, pegvisomant, phenothiazines, phenytoin, procainamide, progestogens, quinapril, quinidine, quinine, ramipril, ranitidine, somatropin, sympathomimetics, testosterone, thiazides, thyroid products, topiramate, trandolapril, triamterene, trimethoprim, trospium, vancomycin, zonisamide
Pregnancy category: B
Important contra-indications noted in the prescribing guidelines for: the elderly; nursing mothers; pediatric patients
Note: Lactic acidosis is a rare, but serious, metabolic complication that can occur due to metformin accumulation.
Avandamet is metformin and rosiglitazone; Glucovance is metformin and glyburide; Invokamet is metformin and canagliflozin; Janumet is metformin and sitagliptin; Synjardy is metformin and empagliflozin; Xigduo XR is metformin and dapagliflozin.
Warning: LACTIC ACIDOSIS

Skin
Angioedema [2]
Bullous pemphigoid [2]
Erythema (transient) [3]
Fixed eruption [2]
Lichenoid eruption [2]
Peripheral edema [5]
Photosensitivity (<10%)
Rash (<10%) [4]
Urticaria (<10%) [4]
Vasculitis [2]

Cardiovascular
Flushing (<10%)
Hypertension [3]
Palpitation (<10%)

Central Nervous System
Chills (<10%)
Dysgeusia (taste perversion) (3%)
Headache (6%) [10]
Vertigo (dizziness) (<10%) [6]

Neuromuscular/Skeletal
Arthralgia [5]
Asthenia (fatigue) (9%) [2]
Back pain [5]

Myalgia/Myopathy (<10%)
Gastrointestinal/Hepatic
Abdominal pain (6%) [5]
Constipation [3]
Diarrhea (10–35%) [31]
Dyspepsia [5]
Flatulence [2]
Gastroenteritis [2]
Hepatotoxicity [6]
Nausea (7–26%) [25]
Pancreatitis [5]
Vomiting (7–26%) [12]

Respiratory
Bronchitis [3]
Dyspnea (<10%)
Influenza [2]
Nasopharyngitis [6]
Respiratory tract infection (<10%)
Sinusitis [2]
Upper respiratory tract infection [6]

Endocrine/Metabolic
Acidosis [22]
Appetite decreased [5]
Hypoglycemia [15]
Weight gain [2]
Weight loss [5]

Genitourinary
Genital mycotic infections [8]
Pollakiuria [3]
Urinary tract infection [11]

Renal
Nephrotoxicity [5]

Hematologic
Anemia [2]

Other
Adverse effects [24]
Death [2]
Vitamin B-12 deficiency [5]

METHADONE

Trade names: Dolophine (Roxane), Methadose (Mallinckrodt)
Indications: Pain, narcotic addiction
Class: Opiate agonist
Half-life: 15–25 hours
Clinically important, potentially hazardous interactions with: abacavir, amprenavir, boceprevir, citalopram, darunavir, delavirdine, diazepam, efavirenz, erythromycin, fluconazole, fluvoxamine, interferon alfa, ketoconazole, linezolid, lopinavir, nelfinavir, nilotinib, paroxetine hydrochloride, PEG-interferon, quetiapine, ribociclib, rifapentine, rilpivirine, safinamide, St John's wort, tipranavir, vandetanib, voriconazole, zidovudine, zuclopenthixol
Pregnancy category: C
Important contra-indications noted in the prescribing guidelines for: pediatric patients
Note: Methadone is not licensed for use in children though it can be employed for the management of neonatal opiate withdrawal syndrome.

Skin
Diaphoresis (<48%) [4]
Pruritus [2]

Mucosal
Xerostomia (<10%)

Cardiovascular
QT prolongation [36]
Torsades de pointes [27]
Ventricular arrhythmia [2]

Central Nervous System
Hallucinations [2]
Hyperalgesia [2]
Neurotoxicity [2]
Serotonin syndrome [2]
Somnolence (drowsiness) [2]
Syncope [2]

Neuromuscular/Skeletal
Rhabdomyolysis [4]

Respiratory
Respiratory depression [3]

Genitourinary
Sexual dysfunction [2]

Local
Injection-site pain (<10%)

Other
Adverse effects [2]
Death [14]

METHAMPHETAMINE

Trade name: Desoxyn (Recordati)
Indications: Attention deficit disorder, obesity
Class: Amphetamine
Half-life: 4–5 hours
Clinically important, potentially hazardous interactions with: fluoxetine, fluvoxamine, MAO inhibitors, paroxetine hydrochloride, phenelzine, sertraline, tranylcypromine
Pregnancy category: C
Important contra-indications noted in the prescribing guidelines for: nursing mothers; pediatric patients
Warning: POTENTIAL FOR ABUSE

Skin
Diaphoresis (<10%)

Mucosal
Xerostomia (<10%) [5]

Cardiovascular
Polyarteritis nodosa [2]

Central Nervous System
Depression [2]
Hallucinations [4]
Insomnia [2]
Neurotoxicity [6]
Paranoia [2]
Parkinsonism [2]
Psychosis [11]

Neuromuscular/Skeletal
Rhabdomyolysis (43%) [5]

Other
Bruxism [4]
Death [3]
Dental disease [2]

METHANTHELINE

See: www.drugeruptiondata.com/drug/id/441

METHAZOLAMIDE

See: www.drugeruptiondata.com/drug/id/442

METHENAMINE

See: www.drugeruptiondata.com/drug/id/443

METHICILLIN

See: www.drugeruptiondata.com/drug/id/444

METHIMAZOLE

Synonym: thiamazole
Trade name: Tapazole (Paladin)
Indications: Hyperthyroidism
Class: Antithyroid, hormone modifier
Half-life: 4–13 hours
Clinically important, potentially hazardous interactions with: anticoagulants, dicumarol, warfarin
Pregnancy category: D

Skin
Aplasia cutis congenita [4]
Exanthems (<15%) [5]
Hypersensitivity [2]
Lupus erythematosus (<10%) [10]
Pruritus (<5%) [4]
Rash (>10%)
Urticaria (>5%) [2]
Vasculitis [6]

Central Nervous System
Ageusia (taste loss) (<10%)

Neuromuscular/Skeletal
Arthralgia [4]

Gastrointestinal/Hepatic
Hepatotoxicity [11]
Pancreatitis [3]

Respiratory
Pulmonary toxicity [2]

Hematologic
Agranulocytosis [10]
Neutropenia [2]

Other
Side effects (in high dosages) (28%) [2]
Teratogenicity [2]

METHOCARBAMOL

See: www.drugeruptiondata.com/drug/id/446

METHOHEXITAL

See: www.drugeruptiondata.com/drug/id/447

METHOTREXATE

Synonyms: amethopterin; MTX
Trade names: Rasuvo (Medac), Rheumatrex (Stada)
Indications: Carcinomas, leukemias, lymphomas, psoriasis, rheumatoid arthritis
Class: Antimetabolite, Disease-modifying antirheumatic drug (DMARD), Folic acid antagonist
Half-life: 3–10 hours
Clinically important, potentially hazardous interactions with: acemetacin, acitretin, aldesleukin, aminoglycosides, amiodarone, amoxicillin, ampicillin, aspirin, bacampicillin, bismuth, carbenicillin, chloroquine, ciprofloxacin, cisplatin, cloxacillin, co-trimoxazole, cyclopenthiazide, dapsone, demeclocycline, dexamethasone, diclofenac, dicloxacillin, doxycycline, echinacea, etodolac, etoricoxib, etretinate, fenoprofen, flurbiprofen, folic acid antagonists, gadobenate, haloperidol, hydrocortisone, ibuprofen, indomethacin, infliximab, ketoprofen, ketorolac, leflunomide, magnesium trisalicylate, meclofenamate, mefenamic acid, meloxicam, methicillin, mezlocillin, minocycline, nabumetone, nafcillin, naproxen, natalizumab, NSAIDs, omeprazole, oxacillin, oxaprozin, oxtriphylline, oxytetracycline, pantoprazole, paromomycin, penicillin G, penicillin V, penicillins, phenylbutazone, piperacillin, piperacillin/tazobactam, piroxicam, polypeptide antibiotics, prednisolone, prednisone, pristinamycin, probenecid, procarbazine, rofecoxib, salicylates, salsalate, sapropterin, sulfadiazine, sulfamethoxazole, sulfapyridine, sulfasalazine, sulfisoxazole, sulindac, taxobactam, tenoxicam, tetracycline, ticarcillin, tolmetin, trimethoprim, vaccines
Pregnancy category: X
Important contra-indications noted in the prescribing guidelines for: the elderly; nursing mothers; pediatric patients
Warning: SEVERE TOXIC REACTIONS, INCLUDING EMBRYOFETAL TOXICITY AND DEATH

Skin
Abscess (peritoneal) [2]
Acral erythema [13]
Anaphylactoid reactions/Anaphylaxis (<10%) [9]
Bullous acral erythema [2]
Bullous dermatitis [4]
Capillaritis [2]
Carcinoma [2]
Dermatitis [2]
Edema [2]
Erosion of psoriatic plaques [8]
Erythema (>10%)
Erythema multiforme [4]
Erythroderma [2]
Exanthems (15%) [5]
Folliculitis [2]
Hand–foot syndrome [3]
Herpes simplex [2]
Herpes zoster [7]
Hypersensitivity [4]
Lymphoma [5]
Malignant lymphoma [4]
Molluscum contagiosum [2]
Necrosis [6]
Neoplasms [2]
Nodular eruption [15]
Non-Hodgkin's lymphoma [2]
Photosensitivity (5%) [9]
Pigmentation (<10%)
Pruritus (<5%)
Pseudolymphoma [10]
Radiation recall dermatitis [7]
Rash (<3%) [11]
Squamous cell carcinoma [2]
Stevens-Johnson syndrome [4]
Sunburn (reactivation) [6]
Toxic epidermal necrolysis [8]
Toxicity [9]
Ulceration of psoriatic plaques [4]
Ulcerations [12]
Urticaria [4]
Vasculitis (>10%) [9]

Hair
Alopecia (<6%) [25]

Nails
Nail pigmentation [2]
Paronychia [2]

Mucosal
Aphthous stomatitis [2]
Gingivitis (>10%)
Glossitis (>10%)
Mucocutaneous reactions [2]
Mucositis [10]
Nasal septal perforation [2]
Oral mucositis [6]
Oral ulceration [11]
Stomatitis (3–10%) [18]

Cardiovascular
Hypertension [2]
Pericardial effusion [2]
Pericarditis [3]

Central Nervous System
Encephalopathy [5]
Fever [5]
Headache [16]
Leukoencephalopathy [61]
Migraine [2]
Neurotoxicity [11]
Vertigo (dizziness) [2]

Neuromuscular/Skeletal
Arthralgia [5]
Asthenia (fatigue) [13]
Back pain [2]
Bone or joint pain [2]

Gastrointestinal/Hepatic
Abdominal pain [9]
Colitis [2]
Diarrhea [12]
Dyspepsia [3]
Gastroenteritis [2]
Hepatic steatosis [2]
Hepatitis [3]
Hepatotoxicity [54]
Nausea [28]
Vomiting [12]

Respiratory
Cough [3]
Nasopharyngitis [6]
Pharyngitis [2]
Pneumonia [6]

Pneumonitis [8]
Pulmonary toxicity [9]
Upper respiratory tract infection [8]
Endocrine/Metabolic
ALT increased [7]
AST increased [3]
Diabetes mellitus [2]
Gynecomastia [8]
Hypoalbuminemia [2]
Weight gain [2]
Genitourinary
Urinary tract infection [4]
Renal
Nephrotoxicity [25]
Renal failure [2]
Hematologic
Anemia [8]
Febrile neutropenia [3]
Hemotoxicity [2]
Leukopenia [10]
Myelosuppression [6]
Myelotoxicity [4]
Neutropenia [9]
Pancytopenia [9]
Thrombocytopenia [9]
Ocular
Cotton wool spots [2]
Optic neuropathy [2]
Local
Injection-site reactions [2]
Other
Adverse effects [38]
Death [14]
Hodgkin's disease (nodular sclerosing) [2]
Infection [23]
Side effects [3]
Teratogenicity [3]

METHOXSALEN

Trade name: Oxsoralen (Valeant)
Indications: Psoriasis, vitiligo
Class: CYP1A2 inhibitor, Psoralen, Repigmenting agent
Half-life: 1.1 hours
Clinically important, potentially hazardous interactions with: caffeine, chloroquine, cyclosporine, fluoroquinolones, phenothiazines, sulfonamides
Pregnancy category: C
Important contra-indications noted in the prescribing guidelines for: pediatric patients
Note: Potential hazards of long-term therapy include the possibilities of carcinogenicity and cataractogenicity.

Skin
Anaphylactoid reactions/Anaphylaxis [2]
Basal cell carcinoma [3]
Bullous dermatitis (with UVA) [4]
Burning (<10%) [3]
Carcinoma [5]
Dermatitis [4]
Edema (<10%)
Ephelides (<10%) [5]
Erythema (<10%)
Exanthems [2]

Herpes zoster [2]
Hypomelanosis (<10%)
Lupus erythematosus [3]
Photosensitivity [9]
Phototoxicity [7]
Pigmentation [3]
Porokeratosis (actinic) [3]
Pruritus (>10%)
Rash (<10%)
Squamous cell carcinoma [4]
Tumors [2]
Vitiligo [2]
Hair
Hypertrichosis [3]
Nails
Nail pigmentation [5]
Photo-onycholysis [5]
Mucosal
Cheilitis (<10%)
Central Nervous System
Pain [2]

METHOXYFLURANE

See: www.drugeruptiondata.com/drug/id/881

METHSUXIMIDE

See: www.drugeruptiondata.com/drug/id/450

METHYCLOTHIAZIDE

See: www.drugeruptiondata.com/drug/id/451

METHYL SALICYLATE

See: www.drugeruptiondata.com/drug/id/2055

METHYLDOPA

Trade name: Aldoclor (Merck)
Indications: Hypertension
Class: Adrenergic alpha-receptor agonist
Half-life: 1.7 hours
Clinically important, potentially hazardous interactions with: acebutolol, alfuzosin, bromocriptine, captopril, cilazapril, cyclopenthiazide, diclofenac, enalapril, ephedrine, fosinopril, irbesartan, levodopa, levomepromazine, linezolid, lisinopril, meloxicam, olmesartan, quinapril, ramipril, risperidone, rotigotine, trandolapril, triamcinolone, zuclopenthixol
Pregnancy category: B
Important contra-indications noted in the prescribing guidelines for: nursing mothers
Note: Aldoril is methyldopa and hydrochlorothiazide. Hydrochlorothiazide is a sulfonamide and can be absorbed systemically. Sulfonamides can produce severe, possibly fatal, reactions such as toxic epidermal necrolysis and Stevens-Johnson syndrome.

Skin
Eczema [3]
Erythema multiforme [2]
Exanthems (3%) [3]
Lichen planus [3]
Lichenoid eruption [9]
Lupus erythematosus [14]
Peripheral edema (>10%)
Photosensitivity [2]
Pigmentation [3]
Seborrheic dermatitis [3]
Urticaria [2]
Mucosal
Oral lichenoid eruption [3]
Oral ulceration [6]
Xerostomia (<10%)
Central Nervous System
Anxiety (<10%)
Depression (<10%)
Dyskinesia [2]
Fever (<10%)
Headache (<10%)
Nightmares (<10%)
Parkinsonism [2]
Gastrointestinal/Hepatic
Hepatitis [2]
Hepatotoxicity [8]
Endocrine/Metabolic
Amenorrhea [2]
Galactorrhea [4]
Hematologic
Hemolytic anemia [2]

METHYLERGONOVINE

See: www.drugeruptiondata.com/drug/id/1871

METHYLNALTREXONE

See: www.drugeruptiondata.com/drug/id/2907

METHYLPHENIDATE

Trade names: Concerta (Janssen), Metadate CD (Celltech), Methylin (Mallinckrodt), Ritalin (Novartis)
Indications: Attention deficit disorder, narcolepsy
Class: Amphetamine
Half-life: 2–4 hours
Clinically important, potentially hazardous interactions with: amitriptyline, benazepril, bupropion, captopril, citalopram, clevidipine, cyclosporine, enalapril, escitalopram, irbesartan, linezolid, lisinopril, lurasidone, MAO inhibitors, olmesartan, paliperidone, pantoprazole, paroxetine hydrochloride, phenylbutazone, pimozide, quinapril, safinamide, ziprasidone
Pregnancy category: C
Important contra-indications noted in the prescribing guidelines for: the elderly; nursing mothers
Warning: ABUSE AND DEPENDENCE

Skin
Angioedema [2]
Exanthems [2]
Exfoliative dermatitis [2]
Hypersensitivity (<10%)
Leukoderma [2]

Mucosal
Xerostomia [7]

Cardiovascular
Cardiotoxicity [3]
Palpitation [4]
QT prolongation [2]
Tachycardia [5]

Central Nervous System
Agitation [2]
Anorexia [7]
Anxiety [7]
Compulsions [2]
Depression [2]
Fever [2]
Hallucinations [6]
Headache [12]
Insomnia [14]
Irritability [6]
Mood changes [2]
Nervousness [2]
Neurotoxicity [3]
Seizures [3]
Somnolence (drowsiness) [3]
Suicidal ideation [2]
Tic disorder [6]
Tremor [2]
Vertigo (dizziness) [5]

Neuromuscular/Skeletal
Asthenia (fatigue) [2]
Dystonia [2]

Gastrointestinal/Hepatic
Abdominal pain [12]
Nausea [7]
Vomiting [5]

Respiratory
Cough [3]
Nasopharyngitis [4]
Upper respiratory tract infection [3]

Endocrine/Metabolic
Appetite decreased [15]
Weight loss [9]

Genitourinary
Priapism [5]

Ocular
Hallucinations, visual [6]

Other
Adverse effects [7]
Bruxism [2]

METHYL-PREDNISOLONE

Trade names: Advantan (Intendis), Medrol (Pharmacia), Solu-Medrol (Pharmacia)
Indications: Arthralgias, asthma, dermatoses, inflammatory ocular conditions, rhinitis
Class: Corticosteroid, systemic
Half-life: 12–36 hours; 2–4 hours (plasma)
Clinically important, potentially hazardous interactions with: aminophylline, aprepitant, aspirin, carbamazepine, clarithromycin, conivaptan, cyclosporine, daclizumab, darunavir, delavirdine, erythromycin, indinavir, itraconazole, ketoconazole, live vaccines, oral contraceptives, phenobarbital, phenytoin, rifampin, telaprevir, telithromycin, troleandomycin, voriconazole, warfarin
Pregnancy category: C
Important contra-indications noted in the prescribing guidelines for: nursing mothers; pediatric patients

Skin
Anaphylactoid reactions/Anaphylaxis [15]
Dermatitis [5]
Hypersensitivity [3]
Pruritus [2]
Rash [2]
Urticaria [5]

Cardiovascular
Arrhythmias [2]
Bradycardia [6]
Flushing [2]
Hypertension [6]
Myocardial infarction [2]
Myocardial toxicity [2]

Central Nervous System
Depression [5]
Dysgeusia (taste perversion) [4]
Neurotoxicity [2]
Psychosis [3]
Seizures [3]
Vertigo (dizziness) [2]

Neuromuscular/Skeletal
Arthralgia [2]
Myalgia/Myopathy [4]
Osteonecrosis [9]
Osteoporosis [2]
Tendinopathy/Tendon rupture [2]

Gastrointestinal/Hepatic
Abdominal pain [3]
Gastrointestinal bleeding [2]
Hepatotoxicity [8]

Respiratory
Dysphonia [2]

Endocrine/Metabolic
Hyperglycemia [4]

Ocular
Cataract [3]
Glaucoma [2]

Other
Adverse effects [7]
Allergic reactions [3]
Death [2]

Hiccups [2]
Infection [7]

METHYL-TESTOSTERONE

Trade names: Android (Valeant), Estratest (Solvay), Testred (Valeant)
Indications: Hypogonadism, impotence, metastatic breast cancer
Class: Androgen
Half-life: 2.5–3.5 hours
Clinically important, potentially hazardous interactions with: anticoagulants, cyclosporine, warfarin
Pregnancy category: X
Important contra-indications noted in the prescribing guidelines for: nursing mothers; pediatric patients

Skin
Acneform eruption (>10%) [12]
Edema (>10%)

Hair
Alopecia [2]
Hirsutism (in females) (<10%) [9]

Cardiovascular
Flushing (<5%)

Endocrine/Metabolic
Mastodynia (>10%)

Genitourinary
Priapism (>10%)

METHYSERGIDE

Trade name: Sansert (Novartis)
Indications: Vascular (migraine) headaches
Class: Hallucinogen, Psychotomimetic
Half-life: 10 hours
Clinically important, potentially hazardous interactions with: acebutolol, almotriptan, amprenavir, azithromycin, chlortetracycline, clarithromycin, delavirdine, demeclocycline, doxycycline, efavirenz, eletriptan, erythromycin, frovatriptan, indinavir, itraconazole, lymecycline, minocycline, naratriptan, nelfinavir, oxytetracycline, ritonavir, rizatriptan, saquinavir, sibutramine, sumatriptan, telithromycin, tetracycline, tigecycline, troleandomycin, voriconazole, zolmitriptan
Pregnancy category: X
Important contra-indications noted in the prescribing guidelines for: nursing mothers; pediatric patients

Skin
Lupus erythematosus [2]
Peripheral edema (<10%)
Rash (<10%)
Scleroderma [4]

Hair
Alopecia [4]

Cardiovascular
Valvulopathy [3]

METIPRANOLOL

See: www.drugeruptiondata.com/drug/id/998

METOCLOPRAMIDE

See: www.drugeruptiondata.com/drug/id/456

METOLAZONE

See: www.drugeruptiondata.com/drug/id/457

METOPROLOL

Trade names: Lopressor (Novartis), Toprol XL (AstraZeneca)
Indications: Hypertension, angina pectoris
Class: Adrenergic beta-receptor agonist, Antiarrhythmic class II
Half-life: 3–4 hours
Clinically important, potentially hazardous interactions with: cinacalcet, clonidine, cobicistat/elvitegravir/emtricitabine/tenofovir alafenamide, cobicistat/elvitegravir/emtricitabine/tenofovir disoproxil, dronedarone, epinephrine, mirabegron, paroxetine hydrochloride, propoxyphene, tadalafil, telithromycin, tipranavir, venlafaxine, verapamil
Pregnancy category: C
Important contra-indications noted in the prescribing guidelines for: the elderly; pediatric patients
Note: Cutaneous side effects of beta-receptor blockers are clinically polymorphous. They apparently appear after several months of continuous therapy.

Skin
Eczema [2]
Erythroderma [2]
Lichenoid eruption [4]
Pruritus (<5%)
Psoriasis (induction and aggravation of) [8]
Rash (<5%) [3]
Raynaud's phenomenon [3]

Cardiovascular
Arrhythmias [2]
Bradycardia [8]
Hypotension [4]

Central Nervous System
Delirium [3]
Hallucinations [2]
Sleep disturbances [2]

Neuromuscular/Skeletal
Asthenia (fatigue) [2]

Gastrointestinal/Hepatic
Gastrointestinal disorder [2]

Genitourinary
Peyronie's disease [5]

Ocular
Hallucinations, visual [3]

METRONIDAZOLE

Trade names: Flagyl (Pfizer), Metrocream (Galderma), MetroGel (Galderma), Metrolotion (Galderma), Noritate (Dermik), Vandazole (Upsher-Smith)
Indications: Various infections caused by susceptible organisms, rosacea
Class: Antibacterial, Antibiotic, nitroimidazole
Half-life: 6–12 hours
Clinically important, potentially hazardous interactions with: alcohol, anisindione, anticoagulants, astemizole, barbiturates, busulfan, cimetidine, dicumarol, disulfiram, dronabinol, fluorouracil, lithium, lopinavir, mycophenolate, phenytoin, primidone, thalidomide, tipranavir, uracil/tegafur, warfarin
Pregnancy category: B (in patients with trichomoniasis, metronidazole is contra-indicated during the first trimester of pregnancy)
Important contra-indications noted in the prescribing guidelines for: nursing mothers

Skin
AGEP [2]
Dermatitis [2]
Exanthems (<5%) [2]
Fixed eruption [14]
Pruritus (<10%) [6]
Stevens-Johnson syndrome [4]
Toxic epidermal necrolysis [2]
Urticaria [4]

Mucosal
Glossitis [2]
Tongue furry [2]
Xerostomia [2]

Cardiovascular
Flushing [2]
Hypertension [2]
Torsades de pointes [2]

Central Nervous System
Cerebellar syndrome [6]
Dysgeusia (taste perversion) [8]
Encephalopathy [22]
Fever [7]
Headache (7%) [7]
Neurotoxicity [13]
Peripheral neuropathy [2]
Psychosis [3]

Neuromuscular/Skeletal
Ataxia [2]

Gastrointestinal/Hepatic
Abdominal pain (5%) [8]
Diarrhea [15]
Hepatotoxicity [5]
Nausea [19]
Pancreatitis [6]
Vomiting [14]

Endocrine/Metabolic
ALT increased [2]
AST increased [2]

Genitourinary
Vulvovaginal candidiasis [2]

Hematologic
Anemia [2]
Bleeding [2]

Otic
Hearing loss [2]

Ocular
Vision loss [2]

Other
Adverse effects [12]
Death [3]
Infection (fungal) (12%)

MEXILETINE

See: www.drugeruptiondata.com/drug/id/460

MEZLOCILLIN

See: www.drugeruptiondata.com/drug/id/461

MIANSERIN

See: www.drugeruptiondata.com/drug/id/1270

MICAFUNGIN

Trade name: Mycamine (Astellas)
Indications: Invasive candidiasis, esophageal candidiasis
Class: Antifungal
Half-life: 11–21 hours
Clinically important, potentially hazardous interactions with: amphotericin B, conivaptan, cyclosporine, itraconazole, nifedipine, sirolimus
Pregnancy category: C
Important contra-indications noted in the prescribing guidelines for: nursing mothers; pediatric patients

Skin
Anaphylactoid reactions/Anaphylaxis [2]
Peripheral edema (7%)
Pruritus (6%)
Rash (9%) [6]
Ulcerations (5%)

Mucosal
Epistaxis (nosebleed) (6%) [2]
Mucosal inflammation (14%)

Cardiovascular
Bradycardia (3%)
Hypertension (7%) [2]
Hypotension (9%)
Phlebitis (6%)
Tachycardia (8%)

Central Nervous System
Anorexia (6%)
Anxiety (6%)
Fever (20%) [6]
Headache (16%) [3]
Insomnia (10%)
Rigors (9%)
Shock (8%)

Neuromuscular/Skeletal
Asthenia (fatigue) (6%)
Back pain (5%)

Gastrointestinal/Hepatic
Abdominal pain (10%) [3]
Constipation (11%)
Diarrhea (23%) [8]
Dyspepsia (6%)
Hepatotoxicity [8]
Nausea (22%) [6]
Vomiting (22%) [5]

Respiratory
Cough (8%)
Dyspnea (6%)
Pneumonia (2%)

Endocrine/Metabolic
ALP increased (5%) [2]
ALT increased (5%) [6]
AST increased (6%) [4]
Hyperbilirubinemia [3]
Hyperglycemia (6%)
Hyperkalemia (5%)
Hypernatremia (5%)
Hypocalcemia (7%)
Hypoglycemia (6%)
Hypokalemia (18%) [3]
Hypomagnesemia (13%)

Hematologic
Anemia (10%) [3]
Febrile neutropenia (6%)
Hemolysis [3]
Neutropenia (14%)
Sepsis (5%)
Thrombocytopenia (15%) [2]

Local
Infusion-related reactions [2]

Other
Adverse effects [5]
Infection (40%)

MICONAZOLE

Trade names: Monistat (Janssen), Oravig (Dara)
Indications: Fungal infections, oropharyngeal candidiasis
Class: Antibiotic, imidazole, Antifungal, azole
Half-life: initial: 40 minutes; terminal: 24 hours
Clinically important, potentially hazardous interactions with: anisindione, anticoagulants, astemizole, clopidogrel, dicumarol, gliclazide, simvastatin, thioridazine, tolvaptan, vinblastine, vincristine, warfarin
Pregnancy category: C
Important contra-indications noted in the prescribing guidelines for: nursing mothers; pediatric patients

Skin
Angioedema (2%)
Contact dermatitis [2]
Dermatitis [11]
Exanthems (2–87%) [5]
Pruritus (2–36%) [3]
Purpura (3–8%)
Rash (9%)
Toxicity [2]
Urticaria (2%)

Cardiovascular
Flushing (<2%) [2]
Phlebitis (5–79%) [3]

Central Nervous System
Chills (>5%)

Gastrointestinal/Hepatic
Nausea [2]

Local
Injection-site pain (10%)

Other
Adverse effects [2]

MIDAZOLAM

Trade name: Versed (Roche)
Indications: Preoperative sedation
Class: Benzodiazepine
Half-life: 1–4 hours
Clinically important, potentially hazardous interactions with: amprenavir, aprepitant, atazanavir, atorvastatin, boceprevir, carbamazepine, chlorpheniramine, cimetidine, clarithromycin, clorazepate, CNS depressants, cobicistat/elvitegravir/emtricitabine/tenofovir alafenamide, cobicistat/elvitegravir/emtricitabine/tenofovir disoproxil, conivaptan, darunavir, dasabuvir/ombitasvir/paritaprevir/ritonavir, delavirdine, dexamethasone, efavirenz, enzalutamide, erythromycin, esomeprazole, fluconazole, fluoxetine, fosamprenavir, grapefruit juice, griseofulvin, imatinib, indinavir, itraconazole, ivermectin, ketoconazole, lopinavir, nelfinavir, nevirapine, nilotinib, ombitasvir/paritaprevir/ritonavir, phenobarbital, phenytoin, posaconazole, primidone, ribociclib, rifabutin, rifampin, ritonavir, roxithromycin, saquinavir, St John's wort, telaprevir, telithromycin, tibolone, tipranavir, voriconazole
Pregnancy category: D

Skin
Edema [2]
Pruritus [3]
Urticaria [2]

Cardiovascular
Bradycardia [2]
Hypotension [10]

Central Nervous System
Agitation [3]
Amnesia [38]
Dysphoria [2]
Hallucinations [2]
Sedation [2]
Vertigo (dizziness) [2]

Gastrointestinal/Hepatic
Vomiting [3]

Respiratory
Apnea [2]
Hypoxia [2]

Local
Injection-site pain (>10%)
Injection-site reactions (>10%)

Other
Adverse effects [7]
Hiccups [3]

MIDODRINE

See: www.drugeruptiondata.com/drug/id/882

MIDOSTAURIN *

Trade name: Rydapt (Novartis)
Indications: Aggressive systemic mastocytosis, systemic mastocytosis with associated hematological neoplasm, or mast cell leukemia, acute myeloid leukemia (FLT3 mutation-positive) in combination with cytarabine and daunorubicin induction and cytarabine consolidation
Class: Multikinase inhibitor
Half-life: 21 hours
Clinically important, potentially hazardous interactions with: boceprevir, carbamazepine, clarithromycin, cobicistat, conivaptan, danoprevir, dasabuvir/ombitasvir/paritaprevir/ritonavir, diltiazem, elvitegravir, enzalutamide, grapefruit juice, idelalisib, indinavir, itraconazole, ketoconazole, lopinavir, mitotane, nefazodone, nelfinavir, ombitasvir/paritaprevir/ritonavir, phenytoin, posaconazole, rifampin, ritonavir, saquinavir, St John's wort, stong CYP3A inducers and inhibitors, tipranavir, troleandomycin, voriconazole
Pregnancy category: N/A (May cause fetal toxicity based on findings in animal studies)
Important contra-indications noted in the prescribing guidelines for: the elderly; nursing mothers; pediatric patients

Skin
Cellulitis (5%)
Edema (40%)
Erysipelas (5%)
Hematoma (6%)
Herpes zoster (10%)
Hypersensitivity (4%)
Rash (14%)

Mucosal
Epistaxis (nosebleed) (12%)
Oropharyngeal pain (4%)

Cardiovascular
Cardiac failure (6%)
Cardiotoxicity [2]
Hypotension (9%)
Myocardial infarction (4%)
Myocardial ischemia (4%)
Pulmonary edema (3%)
QT prolongation (11%) [3]

Central Nervous System
Altered mental status (4%)
Chills (5%)
Fever (27%)
Headache (26%)
Impaired concentration (7%)
Insomnia (11%)
Tremor (6%)
Vertigo (dizziness) (13%)

Neuromuscular/Skeletal
Arthralgia (19%)
Asthenia (fatigue) (34%) [4]
Bone or joint pain (35%)

Gastrointestinal/Hepatic
Abdominal pain (34%)

Constipation (29%) [2]
Diarrhea (54%) [5]
Dyspepsia (6%)
Gastritis (3%)
Gastrointestinal bleeding (14%)
Nausea (82%) [10]
Vomiting (68%) [10]

Respiratory
Bronchitis (6%)
Cough (18%)
Dyspnea (23%)
Pleural effusion (13%)
Pneumonia (10%)
Pneumonitis (2%)
Upper respiratory tract infection (30%)

Endocrine/Metabolic
ALP increased (39%)
ALT increased (31%)
AST increased (32%)
GGT increased (35%)
Hyperamylasemia (20%)
Hyperbilirubinemia (29%)
Hyperglycemia (80%) [2]
Hyperkalemia (23%)
Hyperuricemia (37%)
Hypoalbuminemia (27%)
Hypocalcemia (39%)
Hypokalemia (25%) [2]
Hypomagnesemia (20%)
Hyponatremia (34%)
Hypophosphatemia (22%)
Serum creatinine increased (25%)
Weight gain (6%)

Genitourinary
Urinary tract infection (16%)

Renal
Nephrotoxicity (11%)

Hematologic
Anemia (60%)
Febrile neutropenia (8%)
Hyperlipasemia (37%)
Leukopenia (61%)
Lymphopenia (66%)
Neutropenia (49%)
Sepsis (9%)
Thrombocytopenia (50%)

MIFEPRISTONE

Trade names: Korlym (Corcept), Mifeprex (Danco)
Indications: Medical termination of intrauterine pregnancy (Mifeprex), Cushing's syndrome in patients with Type II diabetes (Korlym)
Class: Corticosteroid antagonist, CYP3A4 inhibitor, Progestogen antagonist
Half-life: 85 hours
Clinically important, potentially hazardous interactions with: amprenavir, aprepitant, atazanavir, boceprevir, bupropion, carbamazepine, ciclesonide, ciprofloxacin, clarithromycin, conivaptan, cyclosporine, darunavir, dihydroergotamine, diltiazem, efavirenz, ergotamine, erythromycin, fentanyl, fluconazole, fluvastatin, fosamprenavir, grapefruit juice, imatinib, indinavir, itraconazole, lopinavir, lovastatin, mibefradil, nefazodone, nelfinavir, NSAIDs, oral contraceptives, phenobarbital,

phenytoin, pimozide, posaconazole, quinidine, repaglinide, rifabutin, rifampin, rifapentine, ritonavir, ritonavir, saquinavir, simvastatin, sirolimus, St John's wort, tacrolimus, telaprevir, telithromycin, tenoxicam, triamcinolone, verapamil, voriconazole, warfarin
Pregnancy category: X
Important contra-indications noted in the prescribing guidelines for: nursing mothers; pediatric patients
Note: Contra-indicated in pregnancy, with concurrent use of simvastatin or lovastatin and CYP3A substrates with narrow therapeutic range or long-term corticosteroid use, and in women with a history of unexplained vaginal bleeding or with endometrial hyperplasia with atypia or endometrial carcinoma.
Warning: TERMINATION OF PREGNANCY

Skin
Edema (5–10%)
Peripheral edema (26%)
Pruritus (4%)
Rash (4%)

Mucosal
Xerostomia (18%)

Cardiovascular
Chest pain (5–10%)
Hypertension (24%)

Central Nervous System
Anorexia (10%)
Anxiety (10%)
Chills (3–38%)
Fever (4%)
Headache (2–44%)
Insomnia (5–10%)
Pain (14%)
Somnolence (drowsiness) (10%)
Vertigo (dizziness) (<22%)

Neuromuscular/Skeletal
Arthralgia (30%)
Asthenia (fatigue) (<48%)
Back pain (9–16%)
Myalgia/Myopathy (14%)
Pain in extremities (12%)

Gastrointestinal/Hepatic
Abdominal pain (5–89%) [2]
Constipation (10%)
Diarrhea (12–20%)
Gastroesophageal reflux (5–10%)
Nausea (43–61%)
Vomiting (16–26%)

Respiratory
Dyspnea (16%)
Nasopharyngitis (12%)
Sinusitis (14%)

Endocrine/Metabolic
Adrenal insufficiency (4%)
Appetite decreased (20%)
Hypoglycemia (5–10%)
Hypokalemia (44%) [2]
Menstrual irregularities [2]

Genitourinary
Metrorrhagia (5–10%)
Uterine pain (83%)
Vaginal bleeding (5–10%)
Vaginitis (3%)

Other
Dipsia (thirst) (5–10%)
Infection [2]

MIGLITOL

See: www.drugeruptiondata.com/drug/id/466

MIGLUSTAT

See: www.drugeruptiondata.com/drug/id/1006

MILNACIPRAN

Trade name: Savella (Forest)
Indications: Fibromyalgia
Class: Antidepressant, Selective norepinepherine reuptake inhibitor
Half-life: 6–8 hours
Clinically important, potentially hazardous interactions with: alcohol, alpha / beta argonists, antipsychotics, aspirin, clomipramine, clonidine, CNS-active drugs, digoxin, droperidol, epinephrine, levomepromazine, lithium, MAO inhibitors, norepinephrine, NSAIDs, serotonergic drugs, sibutramine, St John's wort, tryptophan, vitamin K antagonists
Pregnancy category: C
Important contra-indications noted in the prescribing guidelines for: the elderly; nursing mothers; pediatric patients
Note: Contra-indicated in patients with uncontrolled narrow-angle glaucoma.
Warning: SUICIDALITY AND ANTIDEPRESSANT DRUGS

Skin
Hot flashes (12%)
Hyperhidrosis (9%) [6]
Pruritus (2%)
Rash (4%)

Mucosal
Xerostomia (5%)

Cardiovascular
Chest pain (2%)
Flushing (4%)
Hypertension (4%) [4]
Palpitation (7%)
Tachycardia (2%) [2]

Central Nervous System
Anxiety (3%)
Chills (2%)
Headache (17%) [7]
Hypoesthesia (2%)
Insomnia (12%) [2]
Migraine (4%)
Paresthesias (3%)
Serotonin syndrome [2]
Tremor (2%)
Vertigo (dizziness) (10%) [3]

Gastrointestinal/Hepatic
Abdominal pain (3%)
Constipation (15%) [6]
Nausea (39%) [17]
Vomiting (7%)

Respiratory
Dyspnea (2%)
Upper respiratory tract infection (6%)

Endocrine/Metabolic
Appetite decreased (2%)

Genitourinary
Dysuria (>2%) [2]
Ejaculatory dysfunction (>2%) [2]

Ocular
Vision blurred (2%)

Other
Adverse effects [3]

MILRINONE

Trade name: Primacor (Sanofi-Aventis)
Indications: Severe congestive heart failure unresponsive to conventional maintenance therapy, acute heart failure, including low output states following cardiac surgery
Class: Phosphodiesterase inhibitor
Half-life: 2.3 hours
Clinically important, potentially hazardous interactions with: anagrelide
Pregnancy category: C
Important contra-indications noted in the prescribing guidelines for: nursing mothers; pediatric patients

Cardiovascular
Hypotension (<10%) [5]
Supraventricular arrhythmias (<10%)
Vasodilation [2]
Ventricular tachycardia (<10%)

Central Nervous System
Headache (<10%)

MILTEFOSINE

See: www.drugeruptiondata.com/drug/id/1336

MINOCYCLINE

Trade names: Dynacin (Medicis), Minocin (Wyeth), Solodyn (Medicis)
Indications: Various infections caused by susceptible organisms
Class: Antibiotic, tetracycline, Disease-modifying antirheumatic drug (DMARD)
Half-life: 11–23 hours
Clinically important, potentially hazardous interactions with: acitretin, aluminum, amoxicillin, ampicillin, antacids, bacampicillin, BCG vaccine, bismuth, carbenicillin, cloxacillin, coumarins, digoxin, ergotamine, estradiol, estrogens, isotretinoin, kaolin, magnesium salts, methotrexate, methoxyflurane, methysergide, mezlocillin, nafcillin, oral iron, oral typhoid vaccine, oxacillin, penicillin G, penicillin V, penicillins, phenindione, piperacillin, quinapril, retinoids, St John's wort, strontium ranelate, sucralfate, sulfonylureas, ticarcillin, tripotassium dicitratobismuthate, vitamin A, zinc

Pregnancy category: D
Important contra-indications noted in the prescribing guidelines for: nursing mothers; pediatric patients

Skin
Anaphylactoid reactions/Anaphylaxis [3]
Angioedema [2]
Candidiasis [2]
Cellulitis [2]
DRESS syndrome [14]
Erythema multiforme [2]
Erythema nodosum [2]
Exanthems [5]
Exfoliative dermatitis [3]
Fixed eruption [8]
Folliculitis [2]
Hypersensitivity [25]
Livedo reticularis [3]
Lupus erythematosus [50]
Photosensitivity (<10%) [9]
Pigmentation [123]
Pruritus [7]
Purpura [4]
Rash [9]
Raynaud's phenomenon [2]
Serum sickness [4]
Serum sickness-like reaction (3–5%) [6]
Stevens-Johnson syndrome [2]
Sweet's syndrome [4]
Urticaria [9]
Vasculitis [13]

Hair
Alopecia [2]

Nails
Nail pigmentation (<5%) [19]
Photo-onycholysis [2]

Mucosal
Black tongue [2]
Gingival pigmentation (8%) [2]
Oral pigmentation (7%) [22]

Cardiovascular
Polyarteritis nodosa [12]

Central Nervous System
Fever [2]
Headache [6]
Intracranial pressure increased [4]
Pseudotumor cerebri [14]
Vertigo (dizziness) [8]

Neuromuscular/Skeletal
Arthralgia [6]
Asthenia (fatigue) [4]
Black bone disease [6]
Myalgia/Myopathy [7]

Gastrointestinal/Hepatic
Abdominal pain [2]
Diarrhea [2]
Hepatitis [10]
Hepatotoxicity [20]
Nausea [5]
Pancreatitis [2]
Vomiting [3]

Respiratory
Eosinophilic pneumonia [5]
Pneumonitis [2]

Endocrine/Metabolic
Black thyroid syndrome [4]

Galactorrhea (black) [2]
Thyroid dysfunction [2]

Otic
Tinnitus [2]

Ocular
Conjunctival pigmentation [2]
Diplopia [2]
Papilledema [2]
Scleral pigmentation [5]

Other
Adverse effects [4]
Tooth pigmentation (primarily in children) (>10%) [22]

MINOXIDIL

Trade names: Loniten (Par), Rogaine (Pfizer) (topical)
Indications: Hypertension, androgenetic alopecia
Class: Vasodilator
Half-life: 4.2 hours
Clinically important, potentially hazardous interactions with: acebutolol, alcohol, alfuzosin, captopril, cilazapril, diclofenac, enalapril, fosinopril, guanethidine, levodopa, levomepromazine, lisinopril, meloxicam, olmesartan, quinapril, ramipril, trandolapril, triamcinolone, trifluoperazine
Pregnancy category: C
Note: Topical [T].

Skin
Bullous dermatitis [2]
Dermatitis [T] (7%) [17]
Eczema [2]
Edema [T] (>10%) [2]
Exanthems [4]
Lupus erythematosus [3]
Peripheral edema (7%)
Pruritus [T] [10]
Stevens-Johnson syndrome [2]

Hair
Alopecia [T] [2]
Hair pigmentation [2]
Hirsutism (in women) (100%) [4]
Hypertrichosis (80–100%) [22]

Cardiovascular
Palpitation [3]
Pericardial effusion [2]

Central Nervous System
Headache [2]
Vertigo (dizziness) [2]

Respiratory
Pleural effusion [2]

MIRABEGRON

Trade name: Myrbetriq (Astellas)
Indications: Overactive bladder
Class: Beta-3 adrenergic agonist
Half-life: 50 hours
Clinically important, potentially hazardous interactions with: antimuscarinics, desipramine, digoxin, flecainide, metoprolol, propafenone, thioridazine
Pregnancy category: C
Important contra-indications noted in the prescribing guidelines for: nursing mothers; pediatric patients

Mucosal
Xerostomia (3%) [3]

Cardiovascular
Hypertension (8–11%) [7]
Tachycardia (<2%) [3]

Central Nervous System
Headache (2–4%) [4]
Vertigo (dizziness) (3%)

Neuromuscular/Skeletal
Arthralgia (<2%)
Back pain (3%)

Gastrointestinal/Hepatic
Constipation (2–3%) [4]
Diarrhea (<2%)
Gastrointestinal disorder [2]

Respiratory
Influenza (3%)
Nasopharyngitis (4%) [2]
Sinusitis (<3%)
Upper respiratory tract infection (2%)

Genitourinary
Cystitis (2%)
Urinary tract infection (3–6%) [4]

Other
Adverse effects [3]

MIRTAZAPINE

Trade name: Remeron (Organon)
Indications: Depression
Class: Adrenergic alpha-receptor agonist, Antidepressant, tetracyclic
Half-life: 20–40 hours
Clinically important, potentially hazardous interactions with: linezolid, tapentadol, venlafaxine
Pregnancy category: C
Warning: SUICIDALITY AND ANTIDEPRESSANT DRUGS

Skin
Diaphoresis [2]
Edema (<10%) [2]
Peripheral edema (<10%)
Pigmentation [2]
Rash (<10%)

Mucosal
Glossitis (<10%)
Xerostomia (25%) [3]

Central Nervous System
Abnormal dreams (4%)
Anorexia (<10%)
Cognitive impairment [2]
Headache [2]
Mania [2]
Neurotoxicity [3]
Nightmares [2]
Restless legs syndrome [9]
Sedation [3]
Seizures [3]
Serotonin syndrome [7]
Somnolence (drowsiness) (54%) [10]
Tremor (<10%) [2]
Vertigo (dizziness) (7%) [2]

Neuromuscular/Skeletal
Arthralgia [4]
Asthenia (fatigue) [7]
Myalgia/Myopathy (<10%)
Rhabdomyolysis [4]

Gastrointestinal/Hepatic
Abdominal pain (<10%)
Constipation (<10%) [2]
Hepatotoxicity [3]
Pancreatitis [2]
Vomiting (<10%)

Respiratory
Flu-like syndrome (<10%)

Endocrine/Metabolic
ALT increased (2%)
Appetite increased (12%) [2]
Galactorrhea [2]
Gynecomastia [2]
Weight gain (12%) [9]

Other
Adverse effects [2]

MISOPROSTOL

Trade names: Arthrotec (Pfizer), Cytotec (Pfizer)
Indications: Prevention of NSAID-induced ulcer
Class: Corticosteroid antagonist, Progestogen antagonist
Half-life: 20–40 minutes
Clinically important, potentially hazardous interactions with: none known
Pregnancy category: X
Important contra-indications noted in the prescribing guidelines for: nursing mothers; pediatric patients
Note: Arthrotec is diclofenac and misoprostol.

Skin
Anaphylactoid reactions/Anaphylaxis [2]

Central Nervous System
Chills [7]
Dysgeusia (taste perversion) [2]
Fever [13]
Headache (2%)
Shivering (17%) [8]

Gastrointestinal/Hepatic
Abdominal pain (7%) [7]
Diarrhea (13%)
Dyspepsia (2%)
Flatulence (3%)
Nausea (3%) [4]

Vomiting [4]

Other
Adverse effects [6]

MITOMYCIN

Synonyms: mitomycin-C; MTC
Trade name: Mutamycin (Bristol-Myers Squibb)
Indications: Carcinomas
Class: Alkylating agent, Antibiotic, anthracycline
Half-life: 23–78 minutes
Clinically important, potentially hazardous interactions with: aldesleukin
Pregnancy category: D
Important contra-indications noted in the prescribing guidelines for: nursing mothers; pediatric patients

Skin
Dermatitis [9]
Erythema multiforme [2]
Exanthems [2]
Exfoliative dermatitis [2]
Hand–foot syndrome [2]
Thrombocytopenic purpura [2]

Hair
Alopecia (<10%)

Nails
Nail pigmentation (purple) (<10%)

Mucosal
Oral lesions (2–8%) [4]
Oral ulceration (<10%)
Stomatitis (>10%)

Cardiovascular
Congestive heart failure (3–15%)

Central Nervous System
Anorexia (14%)
Fever (14%)
Paresthesias (<10%)

Neuromuscular/Skeletal
Asthenia (fatigue) [2]

Gastrointestinal/Hepatic
Nausea (14%)
Vomiting (14%)

Respiratory
Cough (7%)

Renal
Nephrotoxicity [2]

Hematologic
Anemia (19–24%)
Hemolytic uremic syndrome [41]
Neutropenia [2]

Ocular
Epiphora [2]
Keratitis [2]
Ocular toxicity [3]

Local
Injection-site cellulitis (>10%)
Injection-site necrosis (>10%) [3]

MITOTANE

See: www.drugeruptiondata.com/drug/id/473

MITOXANTRONE

Trade name: Novantrone (OSI)
Indications: Acute myelogenous leukemia, multiple sclerosis, prostate cancer
Class: Antibiotic, anthracycline, Antineoplastic
Half-life: median terminal: 75 hours
Clinically important, potentially hazardous interactions with: aldesleukin, safinamide
Pregnancy category: D
Important contra-indications noted in the prescribing guidelines for: nursing mothers; pediatric patients

Skin
  Diaphoresis (<10%)
  Ecchymoses (7%)
  Edema (>10%)
  Fungal dermatitis (>15%)
  Peripheral edema [2]
  Petechiae (>10%)
  Purpura (>10%)
Hair
  Alopecia (20–60%) [6]
Cardiovascular
  Cardiac failure [2]
  Cardiotoxicity [4]
  Congestive heart failure [3]
Central Nervous System
  Chills (<10%)
Gastrointestinal/Hepatic
  Diarrhea [2]
  Nausea [6]
  Vomiting [3]
Endocrine/Metabolic
  Amenorrhea [4]
  Menstrual irregularities [2]
Genitourinary
  Urinary tract infection [2]
Hematologic
  Anemia [2]
  Febrile neutropenia [2]
  Leukemia [4]
  Leukopenia [4]
  Neutropenia [6]
  Thrombocytopenia [2]
Other
  Death [2]
  Infection (>66%) [3]

MIVACURIUM

See: www.drugeruptiondata.com/drug/id/1335

MIZOLASTINE

See: www.drugeruptiondata.com/drug/id/1393

MIZORIBINE

See: www.drugeruptiondata.com/drug/id/1264

MOCLOBEMIDE

See: www.drugeruptiondata.com/drug/id/1275

MODAFINIL

Trade name: Provigil (Cephalon)
Indications: Narcolepsy
Class: Analeptic, CNS stimulant, CYP1A2 inducer, CYP3A4 inducer
Half-life: ~15 hours
Clinically important, potentially hazardous interactions with: elbasvir & grazoprevir, enzalutamide, neratinib, olaparib, oral contraceptives, palbociclib, sonidegib, thalidomide, venetoclax
Pregnancy category: C
Important contra-indications noted in the prescribing guidelines for: the elderly; nursing mothers; pediatric patients

Skin
  Fixed eruption [2]
Mucosal
  Xerostomia (5%)
Cardiovascular
  Hypertension [2]
  Palpitation [2]
Central Nervous System
  Agitation [2]
  Chills (2%)
  Hallucinations [2]
  Headache (28%) [13]
  Insomnia (5%) [6]
  Nervousness [2]
  Paresthesias (3%)
  Psychosis [2]
  Vertigo (dizziness) (5%) [3]
Neuromuscular/Skeletal
  Back pain (6%)
Gastrointestinal/Hepatic
  Abdominal pain [2]
  Diarrhea (6%) [3]
  Nausea (11%) [6]
Respiratory
  Rhinitis (7%)
Ocular
  Hallucinations, visual [2]
Other
  Adverse effects [3]

MOEXIPRIL

See: www.drugeruptiondata.com/drug/id/475

MOLINDONE

See: www.drugeruptiondata.com/drug/id/476

MOMETASONE

See: www.drugeruptiondata.com/drug/id/1094

MONTELUKAST

Trade name: Singulair (Merck)
Indications: Asthma
Class: Leukotriene receptor antagonist
Half-life: 2.7–5.5 hours
Clinically important, potentially hazardous interactions with: prednisone
Pregnancy category: B
Important contra-indications noted in the prescribing guidelines for: nursing mothers

Skin
  Angioedema [3]
  Churg-Strauss syndrome [27]
  Rash (2%) [2]
  Urticaria (2%)
Central Nervous System
  Aggression [3]
  Anxiety [2]
  Depression [2]
  Hallucinations [2]
  Headache [4]
  Irritability [2]
  Neurotoxicity [5]
  Nightmares [2]
  Sleep disturbances [3]
  Suicidal ideation [2]
Gastrointestinal/Hepatic
  Abdominal pain [2]
  Hepatotoxicity [3]
Respiratory
  Cough [2]
  Flu-like syndrome (<10%)
Other
  Adverse effects [3]

MORICIZINE

See: www.drugeruptiondata.com/drug/id/478

MORPHINE

Trade names: Avinza (Ligand), Duramorph (Baxter) (Elkins-Sinn), Infumorph (Baxter), Kadian (aaiPharma), Morphabond (Inspirion), MS Contin (Purdue), MSIR Oral (Purdue), Roxanol (aaiPharma)
Indications: Severe pain, acute myocardial infarction
Class: Opiate agonist
Half-life: 2–4 hours
Clinically important, potentially hazardous interactions with: buprenorphine, cimetidine, furazolidone, MAO inhibitors, metformin, mianserin, pentazocine, rifapentine, trospium

Pregnancy category: C
Important contra-indications noted in the prescribing guidelines for: nursing mothers; pediatric patients
Warning: ADDICTION, ABUSE, AND MISUSE; LIFETHREATENING RESPIRATORY DEPRESSION; ACCIDENTAL INGESTION; NEONATAL OPIOID WITHDRAWAL SYNDROME; and INTERACTION WITH ALCOHOL

Skin
AGEP [3]
Edema [2]
Pruritus (5–65%) [36]

Mucosal
Xerostomia (>10%) [8]

Cardiovascular
Cardiotoxicity [3]
Hypotension [5]

Central Nervous System
Allodynia [4]
Confusion [2]
Hallucinations [4]
Hyperalgesia [10]
Sedation [2]
Somnolence (drowsiness) [4]
Trembling (<10%)
Vertigo (dizziness) [5]

Neuromuscular/Skeletal
Myoclonus [5]
Rhabdomyolysis [2]

Gastrointestinal/Hepatic
Constipation [7]
Nausea [14]
Vomiting [11]

Respiratory
Respiratory depression [5]

Endocrine/Metabolic
Amenorrhea [2]

Genitourinary
Urinary retention [2]

Local
Injection-site pain (>10%)

Other
Adverse effects [2]
Death [3]
Hiccups [3]

MOXIFLOXACIN

Trade names: Avelox (Bayer), Moxeza (Alcon)
Indications: Various infections caused by susceptible organisms
Class: Antibiotic, fluoroquinolone
Half-life: 12 hours
Clinically important, potentially hazardous interactions with: alfuzosin, aminophylline, amiodarone, amitriptyline, antacids, arsenic, artemether/lumefantrine, asenapine, atomoxetine, BCG vaccine, benperidol, bepridil, bretylium, chloroquine, ciprofloxacin, corticosteroids, cyclosporine, degarelix, didanosine, disopyramide, dronedarone, droperidol, erythromycin, gadobutrol, haloperidol, hydroxychloroquine, insulin,

lanthanum, levomepromazine, magnesium salts, mefloquine, mizolastine, mycophenolate, nilotinib, NSAIDs, oral iron, oral typhoid vaccine, pentamidine, phenothiazines, pimavanserin, pimozide, probenecid, procainamide, QT prolonging agents, quinapril, quinidine, quinine, ribociclib, sevelamer, sotalol, strontium ranelate, sucralfate, sulfonylureas, tetrabenazine, thioridazine, tricyclic antidepressants, vandetanib, vitamin K antagonists, warfarin, zinc, ziprasidone, zolmitriptan, zuclopenthixol
Pregnancy category: C
Important contra-indications noted in the prescribing guidelines for: the elderly; nursing mothers; pediatric patients
Note: Fluoroquinolones are associated with an increased risk of tendinitis and tendon rupture in all ages. This risk is further increased in older patients usually over 60 years of age, in patients taking corticosteroid drugs, and in patients with kidney, heart or lung transplants.
Fluoroquinolones may exacerbate muscle weakness in persons with myasthenia gravis. Moxeza is for topical ophthalmic use only.
Warning: SERIOUS ADVERSE REACTIONS INCLUDING TENDINITIS, TENDON RUPTURE, PERIPHERAL NEUROPATHY, CENTRAL NERVOUS SYSTEM EFFECTS and EXACERBATION OF MYASTHENIA GRAVIS

Skin
AGEP [2]
Anaphylactoid reactions/Anaphylaxis [5]
Bullous dermatitis [2]
Hypersensitivity [6]
Photosensitivity [5]
Pruritus [3]
Rash [4]
Thrombocytopenic purpura [2]
Toxic epidermal necrolysis [2]
Urticaria [3]

Cardiovascular
Phlebitis [2]
QT prolongation [13]
Torsades de pointes [7]

Central Nervous System
Dysgeusia (taste perversion) [3]
Hallucinations [2]
Headache (4%) [5]
Somnolence (drowsiness) [2]
Vertigo (dizziness) (3%) [6]

Neuromuscular/Skeletal
Myasthenia gravis (exacerbation) [2]
Tendinopathy/Tendon rupture [3]

Gastrointestinal/Hepatic
Abdominal pain [5]
Diarrhea (6%) [6]
Gastrointestinal disorder [2]
Hepatotoxicity [3]
Nausea (7%) [9]
Vomiting [5]

Local
Injection-site reactions [2]

Other
Adverse effects [8]

MOXISYLYTE

See: www.drugeruptiondata.com/drug/id/1350

MOXONIDINE

See: www.drugeruptiondata.com/drug/id/1392

MUPIROCIN

See: www.drugeruptiondata.com/drug/id/935

MUROMONAB-CD3

See: www.drugeruptiondata.com/drug/id/1251

MYCOPHENOLATE

Synonyms: mycophenolate mofetil, mycophenolate sodium
Trade names: CellCept (Roche), Myfortic (Novartis)
Indications: Prophylaxis of organ rejection
Class: Immunosuppressant
Half-life: 18 hours
Clinically important, potentially hazardous interactions with: antacids, azathioprine, basiliximab, belatacept, cholestyramine, ciprofloxacin, corticosteroids, cyclophosphamide, cyclosporine, daclizumab, gemifloxacin, Hemophilus B vaccine, levofloxacin, mercaptopurine, metronidazole, moxifloxacin, norfloxacin, ofloxacin, pantoprazole, rifapentine, sevelamer, tacrolimus, vaccines
Pregnancy category: D
Important contra-indications noted in the prescribing guidelines for: the elderly; nursing mothers; pediatric patients
Warning: EMBRYOFETAL TOXICITY, MALIGNANCIES AND SERIOUS INFECTIONS

Skin
Acneform eruption (>10%) [3]
Carcinoma (non-melanoma) (4%)
Edema (12%)
Herpes simplex [3]
Herpes zoster [6]
Peripheral edema (29%)
Rash (8%) [2]
Warts [2]

Hair
Alopecia [3]

Mucosal
Gingival hyperplasia/hypertrophy [2]
Oral candidiasis (10%)
Oral ulceration [5]

Cardiovascular
Hypertension [4]
Thrombophlebitis (<10%)

Central Nervous System
Fever [3]
Headache (>20%) [5]
Insomnia [3]

Leukoencephalopathy [4]
Neurotoxicity [2]
Pain (>20%)
Tremor (11%)

Neuromuscular/Skeletal
Arthralgia [4]
Asthenia (fatigue) [6]
Back pain (6%)
Myalgia/Myopathy [4]

Gastrointestinal/Hepatic
Abdominal distension [2]
Abdominal pain [6]
Colitis [3]
Diarrhea [13]
Hepatotoxicity [5]

Nausea [5]
Vomiting [5]

Respiratory
Bronchitis [2]
Cough [2]
Upper respiratory tract infection [3]

Endocrine/Metabolic
Hyperglycemia [4]
Hyperlipidemia [3]

Genitourinary
Urinary tract infection [2]

Renal
Nephrotoxicity [3]

Hematologic
Anemia (>20%)
Bone marrow suppression [2]
Dyslipidemia [2]
Leukopenia [4]
Lymphopenia [3]
Myelotoxicity [2]
Neutropenia [4]
Thrombocytopenia [4]

Other
Adverse effects [19]
Death [2]
Infection (12–20%) [18]
Teratogenicity [4]

NABILONE

Trade name: Cesamet (Valeant)
Indications: Nausea and vomiting
Class: Antiemetic, Cannabinoid
Half-life: 2 hours
Clinically important, potentially hazardous interactions with: CNS depressants
Pregnancy category: C

Mucosal
 Xerostomia [6]

Cardiovascular
 Hypotension [8]

Central Nervous System
 Dyskinesia [3]
 Somnolence (drowsiness) [2]
 Vertigo (dizziness) [15]

Neuromuscular/Skeletal
 Asthenia (fatigue) [5]

NABUMETONE

Trade name: Relafen (GSK)
Indications: Arthritis
Class: Non-steroidal anti-inflammatory (NSAID)
Half-life: 22.5–30 hours
Clinically important, potentially hazardous interactions with: methotrexate
Pregnancy category: C
Important contra-indications noted in the prescribing guidelines for: nursing mothers; pediatric patients
Note: NSAIDs may cause an increased risk of serious cardiovascular and gastrointestinal adverse events, which can be fatal. This risk may increase with duration of use.
Warning: CARDIOVASCULAR AND GASTROINTESTINAL RISKS

Skin
 Diaphoresis (<3%)
 Edema (3–9%)
 Erythema [2]
 Hypersensitivity [3]
 Photosensitivity [2]
 Pruritus (3–9%) [2]
 Rash (3–9%) [4]

Mucosal
 Stomatitis (<3%)
 Xerostomia (<3%)

Central Nervous System
 Headache (3–9%) [2]
 Insomnia (3–9%)
 Nervousness (3–9%)
 Somnolence (drowsiness) (3–9%)
 Vertigo (dizziness) (3–9%)

Gastrointestinal/Hepatic
 Abdominal pain (12%) [5]
 Constipation (3–9%)
 Diarrhea (14%) [5]
 Dyspepsia (13%) [4]
 Flatulence (3–9%)
 Gastrointestinal ulceration [3]
 Hepatotoxicity [2]
 Nausea (3–9%) [2]

 Vomiting (3–9%)

Endocrine/Metabolic
 Pseudoporphyria [8]

Renal
 Nephrotoxicity [2]

Otic
 Tinnitus (<10%)

Other
 Adverse effects [6]

NADOLOL

Trade name: Corzide (Monarch)
Indications: Hypertension, angina pectoris
Class: Adrenergic beta-receptor antagonist, Antiarrhythmic class II
Half-life: 10–24 hours
Clinically important, potentially hazardous interactions with: clonidine, epinephrine, verapamil
Pregnancy category: C
Important contra-indications noted in the prescribing guidelines for: nursing mothers; pediatric patients
Note: Corzide is nadolol and bendroflumethiazide. Cutaneous side effects of beta-receptor blockers are clinically polymorphous. They apparently appear after several months of continuous therapy. Contra-indicated in patients with bronchial asthma, sinus bradycardia and greater than first degree conduction block, cardiogenic shock, and overt cardiac failure.

Skin
 Edema (<5%)
 Psoriasis [4]
 Raynaud's phenomenon (2%) [2]

Cardiovascular
 Bradycardia (2%)

Central Nervous System
 Hypoesthesia (fingers and toes) (>5%)
 Paresthesias (>5%)
 Vertigo (dizziness) (2%)

Neuromuscular/Skeletal
 Asthenia (fatigue) (2%)

Other
 Adverse effects [4]

NAFARELIN

See: www.drugeruptiondata.com/drug/id/484

NAFCILLIN

See: www.drugeruptiondata.com/drug/id/485

NALBUPHINE

Trade name: Nubain (Endo)
Indications: Moderate to severe pain
Class: Opiate agonist
Half-life: 5 hours
Clinically important, potentially hazardous interactions with: CNS depressants, diazepam, hydrocodone, hydromorphone, oxymorphone, pentobarbital, promethazine, tapentadol
Pregnancy category: B
Note: Nalbuphine contains sulfites.

Skin
 Clammy skin (9%)
 Diaphoresis (9%)

Mucosal
 Xerostomia (4%)

Central Nervous System
 Vertigo (dizziness) (5%)

Local
 Injection-site pain [4]

NALDEMEDINE *

Trade name: Symproic (Shionogi)
Indications: Opioid-induced constipation in adult patients with chronic non-cancer pain
Class: Opioid antagonist
Half-life: 11 hours
Clinically important, potentially hazardous interactions with: amiodarone, aprepitant, atazanavir, captopril, carbamazepine, clarithromycin, cyclosporine, diltiazem, erythromycin, fluconazole, itraconazole, ketoconazole, moderate or strong CYP3A inhibitors, other opioid antagonists, P-gp inhibitors, phenytoin, quercetin, quinidine, rifampin, ritonavir, saquinavir, St John's wort, strong CYP3A inducers, verapamil
Pregnancy category: N/A (Potential for opioid withdrawal in fetus)
Important contra-indications noted in the prescribing guidelines for: nursing mothers; pediatric patients
Note: Contra-indicated in patients with known or suspected gastrointestinal obstruction. Opioid withdrawal symptoms have occurred in patients treated with naldemedine.

Skin
 Hypersensitivity (<2%)
 Rash (<2%)

Gastrointestinal/Hepatic
 Abdominal pain (8–11%)
 Diarrhea (7%) [2]
 Gastroenteritis (2–3%)
 Nausea (4–6%)
 Vomiting (3%)

Respiratory
 Bronchospasm (<2%)

Other
 Adverse effects [3]

Litt's Drug Eruption & Reaction Manual © 2018 by Taylor & Francis Group, LLC

NALIDIXIC ACID

See: www.drugeruptiondata.com/drug/id/486

NALMEFENE

See: www.drugeruptiondata.com/drug/id/1303

NALOXEGOL

Trade name: Movantik (AstraZeneca)
Indications: Opioid-induced constipation
Class: Opioid receptor antagonist
Half-life: 6–11 hours
Clinically important, potentially hazardous interactions with: diltiazem, erythromycin, grapefruit juice, verapamil
Pregnancy category: C
Important contra-indications noted in the prescribing guidelines for: nursing mothers; pediatric patients
Note: Contra-indicated in patients with known or suspected gastrointestinal obstruction, patients at increased risk of recurrent gastrointestinal obstruction, and patients concomitantly using strong CYP3A4 inhibitors.

Skin
Hyperhidrosis (<3%)

Central Nervous System
Headache (4%) [3]

Gastrointestinal/Hepatic
Abdominal pain (12–21%) [5]
Diarrhea (6–9%) [5]
Flatulence (3–6%) [2]
Nausea (7–8%) [5]
Vomiting (3–5%)

Other
Adverse effects [2]

NALOXONE

Trade names: Suboxone (Reckitt Benckiser), Talwin-NX (Sanofi-Aventis), Targiniq (Purdue)
Indications: Narcotic overdose
Class: Opioid antagonist
Half-life: <1.5 hours
Clinically important, potentially hazardous interactions with: cobicistat/elvitegravir/emtricitabine/tenofovir alafenamide, cobicistat/elvitegravir/emtricitabine/tenofovir disoproxil, thioridazine
Pregnancy category: C
Important contra-indications noted in the prescribing guidelines for: nursing mothers
Note: Suboxone contains buprenorphine; Targiniq is naloxone and oxycodone.

Skin
Diaphoresis (<10%)
Pruritus [2]
Rash (<10%)

Mucosal
Xerostomia [2]

Cardiovascular
Arrhythmias [2]
Bradycardia [2]
Hypertension [8]
Hypotension [2]
Pulmonary edema [2]

Central Nervous System
Headache [4]
Seizures [5]
Somnolence (drowsiness) [3]

Neuromuscular/Skeletal
Asthenia (fatigue) [3]
Myoclonus [2]

Gastrointestinal/Hepatic
Constipation [6]
Nausea [3]
Vomiting [2]

Other
Adverse effects [4]
Death [2]

NALTREXONE

Trade names: Contrave (Takeda), Depade (Mallinckrodt), Nalorex (Bristol-Myers Squibb), Opizone (Genus), ReVia (Meda), Troxyca (Pfizer), Vivitrex (Alkermes), Vivitrol (Alkermes)
Indications: Substance abuse, opioid dependence, alcohol dependence
Class: Opioid antagonist
Half-life: 4 hours
Clinically important, potentially hazardous interactions with: opioid analgesics, opioid containing medications
Pregnancy category: C
Important contra-indications noted in the prescribing guidelines for: nursing mothers; pediatric patients
Note: Naltrexone has the capacity to cause hepatocellular injury when given in excessive doses.
Troxyca is naltrexone and oxycodone. Contra-indicated in acute hepatitis or liver failure; patients receiving opioid analgesics, with current physiologic opioid dependence, or in acute opioid withdrawal.

Skin
Pruritus [2]
Rash (<10%)

Cardiovascular
Hypertension [3]

Central Nervous System
Chills (<10%)
Compulsions [2]
Depression [2]
Headache [3]
Insomnia [3]
Seizures [2]
Vertigo (dizziness) [4]

Neuromuscular/Skeletal
Arthralgia (>10%)
Asthenia (fatigue) [3]

Gastrointestinal/Hepatic
Constipation [5]
Hepatotoxicity [5]

Nausea [7]
Vomiting [5]

Respiratory
Influenza [2]
Nasopharyngitis [2]

Local
Injection-site pain [2]
Injection-site reactions [4]

Other
Adverse effects [3]

NANDROLONE

Trade name: Deca-Durabolin (Organon)
Indications: Anemia of renal insufficiency, control of metastatic breast cancer, osteoporosis in post-menopausal women
Class: Anabolic steroid
Half-life: 6–14 days
Clinically important, potentially hazardous interactions with: acenocoumarol, anisindione, anticoagulants, dabigatran, danaparoid, fondaparinux, heparin, warfarin
Pregnancy category: X
Important contra-indications noted in the prescribing guidelines for: nursing mothers; pediatric patients
Note: Deca Durabolin contains Arachis oil (peanut oil) and should not be taken / applied by patients known to be allergic to peanut.

Hair
Hirsutism [3]

Other
Adverse effects [2]

NAPHAZOLINE

See: www.drugeruptiondata.com/drug/id/2195

NAPROXEN

Trade names: Aleve (Bayer), Naprosyn (Roche), Synflex (Roche)
Indications: Pain, arthritis
Class: Non-steroidal anti-inflammatory (NSAID)
Half-life: 15 hours
Clinically important, potentially hazardous interactions with: methotrexate, methyl salicylate, prednisolone
Pregnancy category: C
Important contra-indications noted in the prescribing guidelines for: the elderly; nursing mothers; pediatric patients
Note: NSAIDs may cause an increased risk of serious cardiovascular and gastrointestinal adverse events, which can be fatal. This risk may increase with duration of use.

Skin
Anaphylactoid reactions/Anaphylaxis [2]
Angioedema [5]
Bullous dermatitis [5]
Diaphoresis (<3%) [3]
DRESS syndrome [4]

Ecchymoses (3–9%)
Edema (<9%)
Erythema multiforme [2]
Exanthems (<14%) [9]
Fixed eruption [25]
Hypersensitivity [2]
Lichen planus [3]
Lichenoid eruption [3]
Lupus erythematosus [2]
Photosensitivity [16]
Pruritus (3–17%) [5]
Purpura (<3%) [4]
Pustules [2]
Rash (3–9%) [2]
Toxic epidermal necrolysis [5]
Urticaria (<5%) [6]
Vasculitis [9]

Hair
Alopecia [3]

Mucosal
Stomatitis (<3%)
Xerostomia [2]

Cardiovascular
Chest pain [2]
Myocardial infarction [2]

Central Nervous System
Somnolence (drowsiness) [2]
Vertigo (dizziness) [6]

Neuromuscular/Skeletal
Leg cramps [2]

Gastrointestinal/Hepatic
Abdominal pain [4]
Constipation [2]
Diarrhea [3]
Dyspepsia [9]
Hepatotoxicity [4]
Nausea [10]

Respiratory
Nasopharyngitis [2]

Endocrine/Metabolic
Pseudoporphyria [29]

Renal
Nephrotoxicity [3]

Hematologic
Thrombocytopenia [2]

Otic
Tinnitus [2]

Other
Adverse effects [10]
Death [2]
Side effects (5–9%) [3]

NARATRIPTAN

See: www.drugeruptiondata.com/drug/id/489

NATALIZUMAB

Synonym: antegren
Trade name: Tysabri (Biogen)
Indications: Multiple sclerosis, Crohn's disease
Class: Immunomodulator, Monoclonal antibody
Half-life: 11 days
Clinically important, potentially hazardous interactions with: abatacept, alefacept, azacitidine, azathioprine, betamethasone, cabazitaxel, certolizumab, cortocosteroids, cyclosporine, denileukin, docetaxel, fingolimod, gefitinib, leflunomide, lenalidomide, mercaptopurine, methotrexate, oxaliplatin, pazopanib, pemetrexed, rilonacept, temsirolimus, triamcinolone, vedolizumab
Pregnancy category: C
Important contra-indications noted in the prescribing guidelines for: nursing mothers; pediatric patients
Note: Contra-indicated in patients who have or have had progressive multifocal leukoencephalopathy.
Warning: PROGRESSIVE MULTIFOCAL LEUKOENCEPHALOPATHY

Skin
Dermatitis (6%)
Herpes simplex [2]
Hypersensitivity [6]
Pruritus (4%)
Rash (9%)

Central Nervous System
Depression (17%)
Headache (35%) [3]
Leukoencephalopathy [77]
Tremor (3%)

Neuromuscular/Skeletal
Asthenia (fatigue) (24%) [4]

Gastrointestinal/Hepatic
Hepatotoxicity [4]

Genitourinary
Vaginitis (8%)

Local
Application-site reactions (22%)
Infusion-related reactions [3]
Infusion-site reactions [2]

Other
Adverse effects [4]
Allergic reactions (7%) [4]
Death [6]
Infection (2%) [3]

NATEGLINIDE

Trade name: Starlix (Novartis)
Indications: Diabetes Type II
Class: Meglitinide
Half-life: 1.5 hours
Clinically important, potentially hazardous interactions with: none known
Pregnancy category: C
Important contra-indications noted in the prescribing guidelines for: nursing mothers; pediatric patients

Respiratory
Flu-like syndrome (4%)

NEBIVOLOL

Trade names: Bystolic (Forest), Byvalson (Forest), Nebilet (Menarini)
Indications: Hypertension
Class: Adrenergic beta-receptor antagonist, Beta blocker
Half-life: 8 hours
Clinically important, potentially hazardous interactions with: beta blockers, cinacalcet, clonidine, CYP2D6 inhibitors, delavirdine, digitalis glycosides, duloxetine, terbinafine, tipranavir
Pregnancy category: C
Important contra-indications noted in the prescribing guidelines for: nursing mothers; pediatric patients
Note: Byvalson is nebivolol and valsartan.
Warning: Byvalson: FETAL TOXICITY

Cardiovascular
Bradycardia [3]

Central Nervous System
Headache (6–9%) [9]
Vertigo (dizziness) (2–4%) [5]

Neuromuscular/Skeletal
Asthenia (fatigue) (2–5%) [4]

Gastrointestinal/Hepatic
Diarrhea (<2%)
Nausea (<3%)

Respiratory
Nasopharyngitis [3]
Upper respiratory tract infection [3]

Other
Adverse effects [3]

NECITUMUMAB

Trade name: Portrazza (Lilly)
Indications: Metastatic squamous non-small cell lung cancer (in combination with cisplatin and gemcitabine)
Class: Epidermal growth factor receptor (EGFR) inhibitor, Monoclonal antibody
Half-life: 14 days
Clinically important, potentially hazardous interactions with: none known
Pregnancy category: N/A (Can cause fetal harm)
Important contra-indications noted in the prescribing guidelines for: nursing mothers; pediatric patients
Note: See separate entries for cisplatin and gemcitabine.
Warning: CARDIOPULMONARY ARREST and HYPOMAGNESEMIA

Skin
Acneform eruption (9–15%)
Fissures (5%)
Hypersensitivity (2%)
Pruritus (7%) [2]
Rash (44%) [9]
Toxicity (8%) [2]

Xerosis (7%) [2]

Mucosal
Stomatitis (11%)

Cardiovascular
Cardiac arrest (3%)
Phlebitis (2%)
Venous thromboembolism (9%) [4]

Central Nervous System
Headache (11%) [2]

Neuromuscular/Skeletal
Asthenia (fatigue) [3]
Muscle spasm (2%)

Gastrointestinal/Hepatic
Diarrhea (16%) [2]
Dysphagia (3%)
Vomiting (29%)

Respiratory
Hemoptysis (10%)
Pulmonary embolism (5%)
Pulmonary toxicity [2]

Endocrine/Metabolic
Hypocalcemia (45%)
Hypokalemia (28%)
Hypomagnesemia (83%) [8]
Hypophosphatemia (31%)
Weight loss (13%)

Hematologic
Anemia [2]
Febrile neutropenia [2]
Neutropenia [4]
Thrombocytopenia [3]

Ocular
Conjunctivitis (7%)

Local
Infusion-related reactions (2%) [2]

Other
Adverse effects [2]
Death [2]

NEDOCROMIL

See: www.drugeruptiondata.com/drug/id/966

NEFAZODONE

See: www.drugeruptiondata.com/drug/id/491

NELARABINE

See: www.drugeruptiondata.com/drug/id/1121

NELFINAVIR

Trade name: Viracept (ViiV)
Indications: HIV infection
Class: Antiretroviral, CYP3A4 inhibitor, HIV-1 protease inhibitor
Half-life: 3.5–5 hours
Clinically important, potentially hazardous interactions with: abiraterone, afatinib, alfuzosin, amiodarone, amprenavir, aripiprazole, artemether/lumefantrine, atorvastatin, avanafil,

barbiturates, benzodiazepines, brigatinib, cabazitaxel, cabozantinib, calcifediol, carbamazepine, chlordiazepoxide, ciclesonide, cisapride, clonazepam, clorazepate, copanlisib, crizotinib, cyclosporine, darifenacin, dasatinib, delavirdine, diazepam, dihydroergotamine, eletriptan, eplerenone, ergot alkaloids, ergotamine, erlotinib, estrogens, eszopiclone, etravirine, eucalyptus, everolimus, fentanyl, fesoterodine, flibanserin, flurazepam, fluticasone propionate, indinavir, ivabradine, ixabepilone, lapatinib, lomitapide, lopinavir, lorazepam, lovastatin, maraviroc, methadone, methylergonovine, methysergide, midazolam, midostaurin, mifepristone, neratinib, olaparib, omeprazole, oral contraceptives, oxazepam, paclitaxel, palbociclib, pantoprazole, pazopanib, phenytoin, pimozide, ponatinib, primidone, progestogens, quazepam, quinidine, quinine, ranolazine, rifabutin, rifampin, rilpivirine, ritonavir, rivaroxaban, romidepsin, rosuvastatin, ruxolitinib, saquinavir, sildenafil, simeprevir, simvastatin, solifenacin, St John's wort, sunitinib, tacrolimus, tadalafil, telithromycin, temazepam, temsirolimus, ticagrelor, tolterodine, tolvaptan, triazolam, vardenafil, vemurafenib, vorapaxar
Pregnancy category: B
Important contra-indications noted in the prescribing guidelines for: nursing mothers
Note: Protease inhibitors cause dyslipidemia which includes elevated triglycerides and cholesterol and redistribution of body fat centrally to produce the so-called 'protease paunch', breast enlargement, facial atrophy, and 'buffalo hump'.

Skin
Rash (<10%) [4]

Gastrointestinal/Hepatic
Diarrhea [3]
Hepatotoxicity [3]

Genitourinary
Urolithiasis [2]

Hematologic
Lymphopenia [2]

NEOMYCIN

Trade names: Maxitrol (Falcon), Neosporin (Monarch)
Indications: Various infections caused by susceptible organisms
Class: Antibiotic, aminoglycoside
Half-life: 3 hours
Clinically important, potentially hazardous interactions with: acarbose, aldesleukin, aminoglycosides, atracurium, bacitracin, bumetanide, doxacurium, ethacrynic acid, furosemide, methoxyflurane, neostigmine, pancuronium, penicillin V, polypeptide antibiotics, rocuronium, sorafenib, succinylcholine, teicoplanin, torsemide, vecuronium
Pregnancy category: D
Important contra-indications noted in the prescribing guidelines for: nursing mothers; pediatric patients
Note: Aminoglycosides may cause neurotoxicity and/or nephrotoxicity.

Skin
Anaphylactoid reactions/Anaphylaxis [2]
Contact dermatitis (<10%) [72]
Eczema [2]
Exanthems [2]
Rash (<10%)
Toxic epidermal necrolysis [2]
Urticaria (<10%)

Otic
Hearing loss [3]

NEOSTIGMINE

Trade name: Prostigmin (Valeant)
Indications: Myasthenia gravis
Class: Acetylcholinesterase inhibitor, Cholinesterase inhibitor, Parasympathomimetic
Half-life: 52 minutes
Clinically important, potentially hazardous interactions with: aminoglycosides, antiarrhythmics, anticholinergics, chloroquine, clindamycin, hydroxychloroquine, kanamycin, lithium, local and general anesthetics, neomycin, non-depolarising muscle relaxants, polymixins, propafenone, propranolol, streptomycin, succinylcholine
Pregnancy category: C (Anticholinesterase drugs may cause uterine irritability and induce premature labor when given intravenously to pregnant women near term)
Important contra-indications noted in the prescribing guidelines for: nursing mothers; pediatric patients
Note: Neostigmine bromide is given orally; neostigmine methylsulfate is given parenterally. Contra-indicated in patients with a previous history of reaction to bromides, or those with peritonitis or mechanical obstruction of the intestinal or urinary tract.

Skin
Anaphylactoid reactions/Anaphylaxis [3]

Cardiovascular
Atrioventricular block [3]
Bradycardia [3]
Cardiac arrest [3]
Tachycardia [2]

Central Nervous System
Anxiety [2]
Sedation [2]

Gastrointestinal/Hepatic
Abdominal pain [3]
Diarrhea [2]
Nausea [14]
Vomiting [12]

Respiratory
Bronchospasm [3]

NEPAFENAC

See: www.drugeruptiondata.com/drug/id/1090

NERATINIB *

Trade name: Nerlynx (Puma)
Indications: Early stage HER2-overexpressed/amplified breast cancer, to follow adjuvant trastuzumab-based therapy
Class: Kinase inhibitor
Half-life: 7–17 hours
Clinically important, potentially hazardous interactions with: aprepitant, boceprevir, bosentan, carbamazepine, cimetidine, ciprofloxacin, clarithromycin, clotrimazole, cobicistat, conivaptan, crizotinib, cyclosporine, dabigatran, dasabuvir/ombitasvir/paritaprevir/ritonavir, digoxin, diltiazem, dronedarone, efavirenz, enzalutamide, erythromycin, etravirine, fexofenadine, fluconazole, fluvoxamine, grapefruit juice, H2-receptor antagonists, idelalisib, imatinib, indinavir, itraconazole, ketoconazole, lansoprazole, lopinavir, mitotane, modafinil, nefazodone, nelfinavir, ombitasvir/paritaprevir/ritonavir, phenytoin, posaconazole, rifampin, ritonavir, saquinavir, St John's wort, strong or moderate CYP3A4 inhibitors or inducers, tipranavir, tofisopam, troleandomycin, verapamil, voriconazole
Pregnancy category: N/A (Can cause fetal harm)
Important contra-indications noted in the prescribing guidelines for: nursing mothers; pediatric patients

Skin
Fissures (2%)
Rash (18%)
Xerosis (6%)

Nails
Nail disorder (8%)

Mucosal
Epistaxis (nosebleed) (5%)
Stomatitis (14%)
Xerostomia (3%)

Cardiovascular
Cardiotoxicity [2]

Central Nervous System
Anorexia [4]
Peripheral neuropathy [2]

Neuromuscular/Skeletal
Asthenia (fatigue) (27%) [4]
Muscle spasm (11%)

Gastrointestinal/Hepatic
Abdominal distension (5%)
Abdominal pain (36%)
Diarrhea (95%) [13]
Dyspepsia (10%)
Hepatotoxicity (<2%)
Nausea (43%) [8]
Vomiting (26%) [5]

Endocrine/Metabolic
ALT increased (9%)
Appetite decreased (12%)
AST increased (7%)
Dehydration (4%)
Weight loss (5%)

Genitourinary
Urinary tract infection (5%)

Hematologic
Anemia [2]
Leukopenia [2]
Neutropenia [3]

NESIRITIDE

See: www.drugeruptiondata.com/drug/id/852

NETUPITANT & PALONOSETRON

Synonym: NEPA
Trade name: Akynzeo (Helsinn)
Indications: Acute and delayed nausea and vomiting associated with cancer chemotherapy
Class: Neurokinin 1 receptor antagonist (netupitant), Serotonin type 3 receptor antagonist (palonosetron)
Half-life: 40 hours
Clinically important, potentially hazardous interactions with: rifampin
Pregnancy category: C
Important contra-indications noted in the prescribing guidelines for: nursing mothers; pediatric patients

Skin
Erythema (3%)

Central Nervous System
Headache (9%) [7]

Neuromuscular/Skeletal
Asthenia (fatigue) (4–8%)

Gastrointestinal/Hepatic
Constipation (3%) [6]
Dyspepsia (4%) [2]

Other
Adverse effects [2]
Hiccups [2]

NEVIRAPINE

Trade name: Viramune (Boehringer Ingelheim)
Indications: HIV infection
Class: Antiretroviral, CYP3A4 inducer, Non-nucleoside reverse transcriptase inhibitor
Half-life: 45 hours
Clinically important, potentially hazardous interactions with: amiodarone, amprenavir, atazanavir, carbamazepine, caspofungin, clarithromycin, clonazepam, cyclosporine, diltiazem, disopyramide, efavirenz, ethosuximide, etravirine, fentanyl, fluconazole, fosamprenavir, indinavir, itraconazole, ketoconazole, levonorgestrel, lidocaine, lopinavir, midazolam, nifedipine, rifampin, rilpivirine, simeprevir, St John's wort, verapamil
Pregnancy category: B
Important contra-indications noted in the prescribing guidelines for: nursing mothers
Warning: LIFE-THREATENING (INCLUDING FATAL) HEPATOTOXICITY and SKIN REACTIONS

Skin
Angioedema [2]
DRESS syndrome [12]
Exanthems [6]
Hypersensitivity [15]
Lipodystrophy [2]
Rash (<48%) [31]
Stevens-Johnson syndrome [34]
Toxic epidermal necrolysis [16]
Toxicity [3]

Mucosal
Gingivitis (<3%)
Ulcerative stomatitis (4%)

Central Nervous System
Fever [2]
Paresthesias (2%)
Peripheral neuropathy [2]

Neuromuscular/Skeletal
Myalgia/Myopathy (<10%)

Gastrointestinal/Hepatic
Hepatic failure [2]
Hepatotoxicity [30]

Endocrine/Metabolic
Acidosis [2]

Other
Adverse effects [7]
Death [3]

NIACIN

Synonyms: nicotinic acid; vitamin B₃
Trade names: Advicor (Kos), Niacor (Upsher-Smith), Niaspan (Merck), Simcor (AbbVie), Slo-Niacin (Upsher-Smith)
Indications: Hyperlipidemia
Class: Vitamin
Half-life: 45 minutes
Clinically important, potentially hazardous interactions with: antihypertensives, atorvastatin, bile acid sequestrants, insulin aspart, insulin degludec, insulin detemir, insulin glargine, insulin glulisine, pitavastatin, rosuvastatin, selenium
Pregnancy category: C (Where niacin is co-administered with a statin, refer to the pregnancy category for the statin)
Important contra-indications noted in the prescribing guidelines for: nursing mothers; pediatric patients
Note: Contra-indicated in patients with active liver or peptic ulcer disease, or arterial bleeding. Simcor is niacin and simvastatin.

Skin
Acanthosis nigricans (8%) [14]
Exanthems (<3%)
Pruritus (<5%) [9]
Rash [5]

Cardiovascular
Flushing (<30%) [31]

Central Nervous System
Paresthesias (<10%) [2]

Neuromuscular/Skeletal
Myalgia/Myopathy [5]

Gastrointestinal/Hepatic
Hepatotoxicity [3]

Endocrine/Metabolic
Hyperglycemia [2]

Ocular
Maculopathy [3]

NIACINAMIDE

Synonyms: nicotinamide; vitamin B_3
Indications: Prophylaxis and treatment of pellagra
Class: Vitamin
Half-life: 45 minutes
Clinically important, potentially hazardous interactions with: atorvastatin, primidone, rosuvastatin
Pregnancy category: A (the pregnancy category will be C if used in doses above the RDA)

Skin
Pruritus (<5%) [2]

Central Nervous System
Paresthesias (<10%)

Hematologic
Thrombocytopenia [2]

NICARDIPINE

Trade name: Cardene (Roche)
Indications: Angina, hypertension
Class: Calcium channel blocker
Half-life: 2–4 hours
Clinically important, potentially hazardous interactions with: amprenavir, atazanavir, boceprevir, cobicistat/elvitegravir/emtricitabine/tenofovir alafenamide, cobicistat/elvitegravir/emtricitabine/tenofovir disoproxil, delavirdine, epirubicin, imatinib, indinavir, lopinavir, posaconazole, propranolol, telaprevir
Pregnancy category: C
Important contra-indications noted in the prescribing guidelines for: the elderly; pediatric patients

Skin
Peripheral edema (7%) [2]
Rash [3]
Urticaria [3]

Mucosal
Gingival hyperplasia/hypertrophy [2]

Cardiovascular
Erythromelalgia [2]
Flushing (6%) [2]
Pulmonary edema [5]

Endocrine/Metabolic
Gynecomastia [2]

Other
Adverse effects [2]
Side effects [2]

NICORANDIL

See: www.drugeruptiondata.com/drug/id/1081

NICOTINE

Trade names: Habitrol Patch (Novartis), Nicoderm (GSK), Nicorette (GSK), Nicotrol (Pfizer)
Indications: Aid to smoking cessation
Class: Alkaloid
Half-life: varies with the delivery system
Clinically important, potentially hazardous interactions with: adenosine, bendamustine, heparin, horsetail
Pregnancy category: D
Important contra-indications noted in the prescribing guidelines for: nursing mothers; pediatric patients
Note: Smoking cessation therapy has various delivery systems. These include: transdermal patches, chewing gum, nasal spray, inhaler, and oral forms.

Skin
Acneform eruption (3%)
Diaphoresis (<3%)
Erythema (>10%)
Pigmentation [3]
Pruritus (>10%)

Mucosal
Sialorrhea (>10%)
Stomatitis (>10%)
Xerostomia (<3%)

Central Nervous System
Headache (18–26%)

Neuromuscular/Skeletal
Arthralgia (5%)
Back pain (6%)
Myalgia/Myopathy (<10%)

Gastrointestinal/Hepatic
Dyspepsia (18%)
Flatulence (4%)
Pancreatitis [2]
Throat irritation/pain (66%)

Respiratory
Cough (32%) [2]
Rhinitis (23%)

Other
Death [2]
Hiccups [2]

NIFEDIPINE

Trade names: Adalat (Bayer), Coracten (UCB), Procardia (Pfizer), Tenif (AstraZeneca), Tensipine MR (Genus), Valni XL (Winthrop)
Indications: Angina, hypertension
Class: Calcium channel blocker
Half-life: 2–5 hours (immediate release products)
Clinically important, potentially hazardous interactions with: acebutolol, amprenavir, atazanavir, beta blockers, boceprevir, carbamazepine, cobicistat/elvitegravir/emtricitabine/tenofovir alafenamide, cobicistat/elvitegravir/emtricitabine/tenofovir disoproxil, cyclosporine, delavirdine, digoxin, diltiazem, dronedarone, efavirenz, epirubicin, fentanyl, fluoxetine, grapefruit juice, imatinib, indinavir, insulin, lopinavir, micafungin, mizolastine, nevirapine, oxcarbazepine, parenteral magnesium, phenytoin, posaconazole, propranolol, rifampin, ritonavir, St John's wort, tacrolimus, vardenafil, vincristine
Pregnancy category: C
Important contra-indications noted in the prescribing guidelines for: the elderly; nursing mothers; pediatric patients
Note: Tenif is atenolol and nifedipine.

Skin
AGEP [3]
Angioedema [2]
Bullous dermatitis [2]
Dermatitis (<2%)
Diaphoresis (<2%) [2]
Edema [3]
Erysipelas [2]
Erythema [2]
Erythema multiforme [5]
Erythema nodosum [2]
Exanthems [9]
Exfoliative dermatitis [5]
Fixed eruption [2]
Lichenoid eruption [3]
Lupus erythematosus [3]
Peripheral edema [12]
Photosensitivity [5]
Pruritus (<2%) [3]
Purpura (<2%) [3]
Rash (<3%) [2]
Stevens-Johnson syndrome [3]
Telangiectasia [2]
Toxic epidermal necrolysis [2]
Urticaria [7]
Vasculitis [4]

Hair
Alopecia [4]

Mucosal
Gingival hyperplasia/hypertrophy (6–10%) [75]
Xerostomia (<3%)

Cardiovascular
Erythromelalgia [4]
Flushing (3–25%) [9]
Hypotension [9]
Pulmonary edema [3]
Tachycardia [4]

Central Nervous System
Chills (2%)
Headache (19%) [7]
Paresthesias (<3%)
Tremor (2–8%)
Vertigo (dizziness) [5]

Neuromuscular/Skeletal
Asthenia (fatigue) (4%)

Gastrointestinal/Hepatic
Hepatotoxicity [3]
Nausea (2%) [2]

Endocrine/Metabolic
Gynecomastia [6]

Other
Adverse effects [4]
Side effects [3]

NILOTINIB

Trade name: Tasigna (Novartis)
Indications: Chronic myelogenous leukemia
Class: Antineoplastic, Epidermal growth factor receptor (EGFR) inhibitor, Tyrosine kinase inhibitor
Half-life: 17 hours
Clinically important, potentially hazardous interactions with: amiodarone, amitriptyline, amoxapine, arsenic, astemizole, bepridil, carbamazepine, chloroquine, cisapride, citalopram, clarithromycin, clozapine, conivaptan, darunavir, dasatinib, degarelix, delavirdine, digoxin, dihydroergotamine, disopyramide, dolasetron, efavirenz, ergotamine, grapefruit juice, halofantrine, haloperidol, indinavir, itraconazole, ketoconazole, lapatinib, levofloxacin, lopinavir, methadone, midazolam, moxifloxacin, oxcarbazepine, pazopanib, phenobarbital, phenytoin, pimozide, procainamide, quinidine, rifampin, rifapentine, ritonavir, sotalol, St John's wort, telavancin, telithromycin, terfenadine, voriconazole, vorinostat, ziprasidone
Pregnancy category: D
Important contra-indications noted in the prescribing guidelines for: nursing mothers; pediatric patients
Note: Contra-indicated in patients with hypokalemia, hypomagnesemia, or long QT syndrome.
Warning: QT PROLONGATION AND SUDDEN DEATHS

Skin
Acneform eruption (<10%)
Dermatitis (<10%)
Eczema (<10%)
Edema [3]
Erythema (<10%) [2]
Exanthems [2]
Folliculitis (<10%)
Hematoma (<10%)
Hyperhidrosis (<10%)
Peripheral edema (<10%)
Pruritus (<10%) [13]
Rash (<10%) [16]
Sweet's syndrome [3]
Toxicity [7]
Urticaria (<10%)
Xerosis [2]

Hair
Alopecia (<10%) [4]

Cardiovascular
Angina (<10%)
Arrhythmias (<10%) [2]
Arterial occlusion [5]
Atrial fibrillation (<10%)
Atrioventricular block (<10%)
Bradycardia (<10%)
Cardiotoxicity [4]
Chest pain (<10%)
Extrasystoles (<10%)
Flushing (<10%)
Hypertension (<10%)
Myocardial infarction [2]
Palpitation (<10%)
QT prolongation (<10%) [8]

Central Nervous System
Anorexia (<10%)
Depression (<10%) [2]
Fever (<10%) [2]
Headache (~10%) [13]
Hypoesthesia (<10%)
Insomnia (<10%)
Pain [2]
Paresthesias (<10%)
Stroke [2]
Vertigo (dizziness) (<10%)

Neuromuscular/Skeletal
Arthralgia (<10%) [3]
Asthenia (fatigue) (<10%) [9]
Bone or joint pain (<10%)
Muscle spasm [3]
Myalgia/Myopathy (<10%) [5]
Neck pain (<10%)

Gastrointestinal/Hepatic
Abdominal distension (<10%)
Abdominal pain (<10%) [2]
Constipation (~10%) [2]
Diarrhea (~10%) [4]
Dyspepsia (<10%)
Flatulence (<10%)
Hepatotoxicity [5]
Nausea (~10%) [8]
Pancreatitis (<10%) [4]
Vomiting (~10%)

Respiratory
Cough (<10%)
Dysphonia (<10%)
Dyspnea (<10%)
Nasopharyngitis [2]
Pleural effusion [2]
Pulmonary hypertension [2]

Endocrine/Metabolic
ALT increased (4%) [3]
AST increased (<3%) [2]
Diabetes mellitus (<10%)
Hyperamylasemia [2]
Hyperbilirubinemia [6]
Hypercalcemia (<10%)
Hypercholesterolemia (<10%)
Hyperglycemia (6–12%) [5]
Hyperkalemia (2–6%)
Hyperlipidemia (<10%)
Hypocalcemia (<10%)
Hypokalemia (<10%) [2]
Hypomagnesemia (<10%)
Hyponatremia (<10%)
Hypophosphatemia (5–17%) [3]
Hypothyroidism [2]
Weight gain (<10%)
Weight loss (<10%)

Genitourinary
Pollakiuria (<10%)

Hematologic
Anemia (4–27%) [8]
Febrile neutropenia (<10%)
Hyperlipasemia [3]
Lymphopenia (<10%)
Neutropenia (12–42%) [8]
Pancytopenia (<10%)
Thrombocytopenia (10–42%) [9]

Ocular
Conjunctivitis (<10%)
Ocular hemorrhage (<10%)
Periorbital edema (<10%)
Xerophthalmia (<10%)

Other
Adverse effects [3]
Death [3]
Side effects [3]

NILUTAMIDE

See: www.drugeruptiondata.com/drug/id/1212

NIMESULIDE

See: www.drugeruptiondata.com/drug/id/1228

NIMODIPINE

See: www.drugeruptiondata.com/drug/id/500

NINTEDANIB

Trade name: Ofev (Boehringer Ingelheim)
Indications: Idiopathic pulmonary fibrosis
Class: Tyrosine kinase inhibitor
Half-life: 9.5 hours
Clinically important, potentially hazardous interactions with: anticoagulants, carbamazepine, erythromycin, phenytoin, St John's wort
Pregnancy category: D
Important contra-indications noted in the prescribing guidelines for: nursing mothers; pediatric patients

Skin
Hand–foot syndrome [2]
Rash [4]

Hair
Alopecia [2]

Mucosal
Epistaxis (nosebleed) [2]

Cardiovascular
Cardiotoxicity [2]
Hypertension (5%) [7]
Myocardial infarction (2%)

Central Nervous System
Anorexia [6]
Headache (8%)
Peripheral neuropathy [2]

Neuromuscular/Skeletal
Asthenia (fatigue) [15]

Gastrointestinal/Hepatic
Abdominal pain (15%) [6]
Diarrhea (62%) [28]
Gastrointestinal disorder [4]
Hepatotoxicity (14%) [10]
Nausea (24%) [21]
Vomiting (12%) [18]

Respiratory
Bronchitis [3]
Cough [3]
Dyspnea [4]

Nasopharyngitis [3]
Pneumonia [3]
Upper respiratory tract infection [2]
Endocrine/Metabolic
ALT increased [11]
Appetite decreased (11%) [6]
AST increased [9]
Weight loss (10%) [2]
Hematologic
Anemia [3]
Bleeding (10%) [3]
Leukopenia [2]
Neutropenia [4]
Thrombocytopenia [2]
Other
Adverse effects [5]
Death [3]

NIRAPARIB *

Trade name: Zejula (Tesaro)
Indications: Maintenance treatment of adult
patients with recurrent epithelial ovarian, fallopian
tube, or primary peritoneal cancer who are in a
complete or partial response to platinum-based
chemotherapy
Class: Poly (ADP-ribose) polymerase (PARP)
inhibitor
Half-life: 36 hours
**Clinically important, potentially hazardous
interactions with:** none known
Pregnancy category: N/A (Can cause fetal
harm)
**Important contra-indications noted in the
prescribing guidelines for:** nursing mothers;
pediatric patients

Skin
Peripheral edema (<10%)
Rash (21%)
Mucosal
Epistaxis (nosebleed) (<10%)
Mucositis (20%)
Stomatitis (20%)
Xerostomia (10%)
Cardiovascular
Hypertension (20%)
Palpitation (10%)
Tachycardia (<10%)
Central Nervous System
Anxiety (11%)
Depression (<10%)
Dysgeusia (taste perversion) (10%)
Headache (26%)
Insomnia (27%)
Vertigo (dizziness) (18%)
Neuromuscular/Skeletal
Arthralgia (13%)
Asthenia (fatigue) (57%)
Back pain (18%)
Myalgia/Myopathy (19%)
Gastrointestinal/Hepatic
Abdominal distension (33%)
Abdominal pain (33%)
Constipation (40%)
Diarrhea (20%)

Dyspepsia (18%)
Nausea (74%)
Vomiting (34%)
Respiratory
Bronchitis (<10%)
Dyspnea (20%)
Nasopharyngitis (23%)
Endocrine/Metabolic
ALT increased (10%)
Appetite decreased (25%)
AST increased (10%)
Creatine phosphokinase increased (<10%)
GGT increased (<10%)
Hypokalemia (<10%)
Serum creatinine increased (<10%)
Weight loss (<10%)
Genitourinary
Urinary tract infection (13%)
Hematologic
Anemia (50%) [2]
Leukopenia (17%)
Neutropenia (30%) [2]
Thrombocytopenia (61%) [2]
Ocular
Conjunctivitis (<10%)

NISOLDIPINE

Trade name: Sular (First Horizon)
Indications: Hypertension
Class: Calcium channel blocker
Half-life: 7–12 hours
**Clinically important, potentially hazardous
interactions with:** amprenavir, conivaptan,
cyclosporine, darunavir, delavirdine, efavirenz,
epirubicin, grapefruit juice, imatinib, indinavir,
itraconazole, ketoconazole, oxcarbazepine,
propranolol, telaprevir, telithromycin,
voriconazole
Pregnancy category: C

Skin
Peripheral edema (22%) [6]
Rash (2%)
Central Nervous System
Headache [4]
Endocrine/Metabolic
Gynecomastia [2]

NITAZOXANIDE

Trade name: Alinia (Romark)
Indications: Diarrhea caused by *Cryptosporidium
parvum* or *Giardia lamblia* (in children)
Class: Antiprotozoal
Half-life: N/A
**Clinically important, potentially hazardous
interactions with:** none known
Pregnancy category: B

Central Nervous System
Headache [2]
Gastrointestinal/Hepatic
Abdominal pain [3]
Diarrhea [2]

NITISINONE

See: www.drugeruptiondata.com/drug/id/926

NITRAZEPAM

See: www.drugeruptiondata.com/drug/id/1262

NITROFURANTOIN

Trade names: Furadantin (First Horizon),
Macrobid (Procter & Gamble), Macrodantin
(Procter & Gamble)
Indications: Various urinary tract infections
caused by susceptible organisms
Class: Antibiotic
Half-life: 1–2 minutes
**Clinically important, potentially hazardous
interactions with:** norfloxacin
Pregnancy category: B
**Important contra-indications noted in the
prescribing guidelines for:** nursing mothers;
pediatric patients

Skin
Anaphylactoid reactions/Anaphylaxis [2]
Angioedema [4]
Dermatitis [3]
DRESS syndrome [4]
Eczema [2]
Erythema multiforme [3]
Exanthems (<5%) [9]
Exfoliative dermatitis [3]
Lupus erythematosus [8]
Purpura [2]
Rash [2]
Stevens-Johnson syndrome [2]
Toxic epidermal necrolysis [5]
Urticaria [8]
Hair
Alopecia [5]
Central Nervous System
Neurotoxicity [2]
Paresthesias (<10%)
Gastrointestinal/Hepatic
Hepatitis [2]
Hepatotoxicity [14]
Respiratory
Pneumonitis [3]
Pulmonary toxicity [8]
Other
Adverse effects [3]
Death [3]

NITROFURAZONE

See: www.drugeruptiondata.com/drug/id/1022

NITROGLYCERIN

Synonyms: glyceryl trinitrate; nitroglycerol; NTG
Trade names: Minitran (3M), Nitrodur (Schering) (Key), Nitrolingual (First Horizon), Nitrostat (Pfizer)
Indications: Acute angina
Class: Nitrate, Vasodilator
Half-life: 1–4 minutes
Clinically important, potentially hazardous interactions with: acetylcysteine, alteplase, heparin, sildenafil, tadalafil, vardenafil
Pregnancy category: C
Important contra-indications noted in the prescribing guidelines for: nursing mothers; pediatric patients

Skin

Dermatitis (to topical systems) [25]
Eczema [2]
Erythema (to transdermal delivery system) [2]
Exfoliative dermatitis (<10%)
Purpura [2]
Rash (<10%)
Urticaria [2]

Cardiovascular

Bradycardia [2]
Flushing (>10%)
Hypotension [4]

Central Nervous System

Headache [14]
Migraine [2]

NITROPRUSSIDE

See: www.drugeruptiondata.com/drug/id/1214

NIVOLUMAB

Trade name: Opdivo (Bristol-Myers Squibb)
Indications: Metastatic squamous non-small cell lung cancer with progression on or after platinum-based chemotherapy, unresectable or metastatic melanoma and disease progression following ipilimumab and, if BRAF V600 mutation positive, a BRAF inhibitor, advanced renal cell carcinoma with prior anti-angiogenic therapy, Hodgkin lymphoma that has relapsed or progressed after autologous hematopoietic stem cell transplantation and post-transplantation brentuximab vedotin
Class: Monoclonal antibody, Programmed death receptor-1 (PD-1) inhibitor
Half-life: 27 days
Clinically important, potentially hazardous interactions with: none known
Pregnancy category: N/A (Can cause fetal harm)
Important contra-indications noted in the prescribing guidelines for: nursing mothers; pediatric patients

Skin

Bullous pemphigoid [5]
Dermatitis [3]

Edema (17%) [2]
Erythema [3]
Erythema multiforme (<10%)
Exanthems [2]
Exfoliative dermatitis (<10%)
Hypersensitivity [2]
Lichenoid eruption [2]
Pruritus (11–19%) [25]
Psoriasis (<10%) [3]
Rash (16–21%) [33]
Sarcoidosis [6]
Thrombocytopenic purpura [2]
Toxicity [4]
Vitiligo (<10%) [13]

Mucosal

Stomatitis (<10%)
Xerostomia [2]

Cardiovascular

Chest pain (13%)
Myocarditis [5]
Ventricular arrhythmia (<10%)

Central Nervous System

Encephalopathy [6]
Fever (17%) [8]
Neurotoxicity [4]
Pain (10%)
Peripheral neuropathy (<10%)
Vertigo (dizziness) (<10%)

Neuromuscular/Skeletal

Arthralgia (13%) [7]
Asthenia (fatigue) (19–50%) [26]
Bone or joint pain (36%)
Myalgia/Myopathy [9]
Myasthenia gravis [11]
Polymyositis [2]
Synovial effusions [2]

Gastrointestinal/Hepatic

Abdominal pain (16%)
Colitis [20]
Constipation (24%)
Diarrhea (18%) [26]
Hepatitis [9]
Hepatotoxicity [12]
Nausea (29%) [13]
Pancreatitis [4]
Vomiting (19%) [2]

Respiratory

Bronchitis (<10%)
Cough (17–32%) [2]
Dyspnea (38%) [3]
Pneumonia (10%) [4]
Pneumonitis [27]
Pulmonary toxicity [2]
Upper respiratory tract infection (11%)

Endocrine/Metabolic

Adrenal insufficiency [3]
ALP increased (14–22%)
ALT increased (12–16%) [5]
Appetite decreased (35%) [9]
AST increased (16–28%) [4]
Diabetes mellitus [10]
Hyperamylasemia [2]
Hypercalcemia (20%)
Hyperkalemia (15–18%)
Hyperthyroidism [9]
Hypocalcemia (18%)
Hypokalemia (20%)
Hypomagnesemia (20%)

Hyponatremia (25–38%)
Hypophosphatemia [2]
Hypophysitis [10]
Hypothyroidism [16]
Serum creatinine increased (22%) [2]
Thyroid dysfunction [7]
Thyroiditis [7]
Weight loss (13%)

Renal

Nephrotoxicity [10]
Renal failure [4]

Hematologic

Anemia (28%) [4]
Hemolytic anemia [4]
Hyperlipasemia [4]
Lymphopenia (47%) [3]
Neutropenia [6]
Thrombocytopenia (14%) [5]

Ocular

Iridocyclitis (<10%)
Uveitis [3]

Local

Infusion-related reactions (<10%) [5]

Other

Adverse effects [25]
Death [11]
Side effects [2]

NIZATIDINE

See: www.drugeruptiondata.com/drug/id/504

NORFLOXACIN

Trade names: Chibroxin (Merck), Noroxin (Merck)
Indications: Various urinary tract infections caused by susceptible organisms, conjunctivitis
Class: Antibiotic, fluoroquinolone, CYP3A4 inhibitor
Half-life: 3–4 hours
Clinically important, potentially hazardous interactions with: aminophylline, amiodarone, antacids, arsenic, artemether/lumefantrine, bepridil, bretylium, caffeine, ciprofibrate, clozapine, cyclosporine, dairy products, didanosine, disopyramide, erythromycin, glyburide, lanthanum, mycophenolate, nitrofurantoin, NSAIDs, oral iron, oral typhoid vaccine, oxtriphylline, phenothiazines, probenecid, procainamide, quinidine, ropinirole, sotalol, strontium ranelate, sucralfate, tacrine, tamoxifen, tizanidine, tricyclic antidepressants, warfarin, zinc, zolmitriptan
Pregnancy category: C
Important contra-indications noted in the prescribing guidelines for: the elderly; nursing mothers; pediatric patients
Note: Fluoroquinolones are associated with an increased risk of tendinitis and tendon rupture in all ages. This risk is further increased in older patients usually over 60 years of age, in patients taking corticosteroid drugs, and in patients with kidney, heart or lung transplants.
Fluoroquinolones may exacerbate muscle weakness in persons with myasthenia gravis.

Skin
Exanthems [2]
Fixed eruption [3]
Phototoxicity [4]
Toxic epidermal necrolysis [2]

Nails
Photo-onycholysis [2]

Neuromuscular/Skeletal
Rhabdomyolysis [2]
Tendinopathy/Tendon rupture [4]

Other
Adverse effects [2]

NORTRIPTYLINE

Trade names: Aventyl (Ranbaxy), Pamelor (Mallinckrodt)
Indications: Depression
Class: Antidepressant, tricyclic
Half-life: 28–31 hours
Clinically important, potentially hazardous interactions with: amprenavir, arbutamine, clonidine, cobicistat/elvitegravir/emtricitabine/tenofovir alafenamide, cobicistat/elvitegravir/emtricitabine/tenofovir disoproxil, epinephrine, fluoxetine, formoterol, guanethidine, isocarboxazid, linezolid, MAO inhibitors, phenelzine, quinolones, sparfloxacin, tranylcypromine

Pregnancy category: D
Important contra-indications noted in the prescribing guidelines for: pediatric patients
Warning: SUICIDALITY AND ANTIDEPRESSANT DRUGS

Skin
Diaphoresis (<10%)
Photosensitivity [2]

Mucosal
Xerostomia (>10%) [9]

Central Nervous System
Dysgeusia (taste perversion) (>10%)
Parkinsonism (<10%)
Vertigo (dizziness) [2]

Other
Adverse effects [2]

NUSINERSEN *

Trade name: Spinraza (Biogen)
Indications: Spinal muscular atrophy
Class: Survival motor neuron-2 (SMN2)-directed antisense oligonucleotide
Half-life: 63–87 days (in plasma)
Clinically important, potentially hazardous interactions with: none known
Pregnancy category: N/A (No data available)
Important contra-indications noted in the prescribing guidelines for: nursing mothers

Central Nervous System
Headache (50%)

Neuromuscular/Skeletal
Back pain (41%)
Scoliosis (5%)

Gastrointestinal/Hepatic
Constipation (30%)

Respiratory
Bronchitis (>5%)
Upper respiratory tract infection (39%)

Otic
Ear infection (5%)

NYSTATIN

Trade names: Mycology-II (Bristol-Myers Squibb), Mycostatin (Bristol-Myers Squibb)
Indications: Candidiasis
Class: Antifungal
Half-life: ~2–3 hours
Clinically important, potentially hazardous interactions with: none known
Pregnancy category: C
Important contra-indications noted in the prescribing guidelines for: nursing mothers

Skin
AGEP [5]
Dermatitis [12]
Eczema [2]
Fixed eruption [2]

OBETICHOLIC ACID

Trade name: Ocaliva (Intercept)
Indications: Primary biliary cholangitis
Class: Farnesoid X receptor (FXR) agonist
Half-life: N/A
Clinically important, potentially hazardous interactions with: aminophylline, tizanidine, warfarin
Pregnancy category: N/A (Insufficient evidence to inform drug-associated risk)
Important contra-indications noted in the prescribing guidelines for: nursing mothers; pediatric patients
Note: Contra-indicated in patients with complete biliary obstruction.

Skin
Eczema (3–6%)
Peripheral edema (3–7%)
Pruritus (56–70%) [4]
Rash (7–10%)
Urticaria (<10%)
Mucosal
Oropharyngeal pain (7–8%)
Cardiovascular
Palpitation (3–7%)
Central Nervous System
Fever (<7%)
Syncope (<7%)
Vertigo (dizziness) (7%)
Neuromuscular/Skeletal
Arthralgia (6–10%)
Asthenia (fatigue) (19–25%)
Gastrointestinal/Hepatic
Abdominal pain (10–19%)
Constipation (7%)
Endocrine/Metabolic
Thyroid dysfunction (4–6%)

OBINUTUZUMAB

Trade name: Gazyva (Genentech)
Indications: Chronic lymphocytic leukemia (in combination with chlorambucil), follicular lymphoma (firstly with bendamustine then as monotherapy)
Class: CD20-directed cytolytic monoclonal antibody, Monoclonal antibody
Half-life: 28 days
Clinically important, potentially hazardous interactions with: live vaccines
Pregnancy category: N/A (Insufficient evidence to inform drug-associated risk)
Important contra-indications noted in the prescribing guidelines for: nursing mothers; pediatric patients
Warning: HEPATITIS B VIRUS REACTIVATION AND PROGRESSIVE MULTIFOCAL LEUKOENCEPHALOPATHY

Skin
Tumor lysis syndrome [5]
Central Nervous System
Fever (10%) [4]
Headache [2]

Leukoencephalopathy [2]
Gastrointestinal/Hepatic
Nausea [3]
Respiratory
Cough (10%) [2]
Endocrine/Metabolic
ALP increased (16%)
AST increased (25%)
Hyperkalemia (31%)
Hypoalbuminemia (22%)
Hypocalcemia (32%)
Hypokalemia (13%)
Hematologic
Anemia (12%) [4]
Leukopenia (7%)
Neutropenia (40%) [12]
Thrombocytopenia (15%) [7]
Local
Infusion-related reactions (69%) [15]
Other
Infection (38%) [8]

OCRELIZUMAB *

Trade name: Ocrevus (Genentech)
Indications: Relapsing or primary progressive forms of multiple sclerosis
Class: CD20-directed cytolytic monoclonal antibody, Monoclonal antibody
Half-life: 26 days
Clinically important, potentially hazardous interactions with: none known
Pregnancy category: N/A (May cause fetal toxicity based on findings in animal studies)
Important contra-indications noted in the prescribing guidelines for: nursing mothers; pediatric patients
Note: Contra-indicated in active hepatitis B virus infection.

Central Nervous System
Depression (8%)
Neuromuscular/Skeletal
Back pain (6%)
Pain in extremities (5%)
Respiratory
Upper respiratory tract infection (40–49%) [2]
Hematologic
Neutropenia (13%)
Local
Infusion-related reactions (34–40%) [6]
Other
Infection (58%) [3]

OCRIPLASMIN

Trade name: Jetrea (ThromboGenics)
Indications: Symptomatic vitreomacular adhesion
Class: Enzyme
Half-life: N/A
Clinically important, potentially hazardous interactions with: none known

Pregnancy category: C
Important contra-indications noted in the prescribing guidelines for: nursing mothers; pediatric patients

Ocular
Cataract (2–4%)
Conjunctival hemorrhage (5–20%)
Conjunctival hyperemia (2–4%)
Dyschromatopsia (2%)
Intraocular inflammation (7%)
Intraocular pressure increased (4%)
Iritis (2–4%)
Macular edema (2–4%)
Macular hole (5–20%)
Ocular adverse effects [2]
Ocular hemorrhage (2%)
Ocular pain (5–20%) [2]
Photophobia (2–4%)
Photopsia (5–20%) [4]
Reduced visual acuity (5–20%) [2]
Retinal edema (5–20%)
Vision blurred (5–20%)
Vision impaired (5–20%)
Vision loss [3]
Vitreous detachment (2–4%)
Vitreous floaters (5–20%) [4]
Xerophthalmia (2–4%)

OCTREOTIDE

Trade name: Sandostatin (Novartis)
Indications: Diarrhea, sulfonylurea poisoning
Class: Somatostatin analog
Half-life: 1.5 hours
Clinically important, potentially hazardous interactions with: bromocriptine, insulin aspart, insulin degludec, metformin
Pregnancy category: B
Important contra-indications noted in the prescribing guidelines for: the elderly; nursing mothers; pediatric patients

Skin
Cellulitis (<4%)
Diaphoresis (5–15%)
Edema (<10%)
Petechiae (<4%)
Pruritus (18%)
Purpura (<4%)
Rash (5–15%)
Raynaud's phenomenon (<4%)
Urticaria (<4%)
Hair
Alopecia (~13%) [4]
Cardiovascular
Arrhythmias (3–9%)
Bradycardia (19–25%) [4]
Chest pain (20%)
Flushing (<4%)
Hypertension (13%) [3]
QT prolongation [2]
Thrombophlebitis (<4%)
Central Nervous System
Anorexia (4–6%)
Headache [3]
Pain (4–6%)
Rigors (5–15%)

Vertigo (dizziness) [2]

Neuromuscular/Skeletal
Arthralgia (5–15%)
Asthenia (fatigue) [4]
Myalgia/Myopathy (5–15%) [2]

Gastrointestinal/Hepatic
Abdominal pain (5–61%) [4]
Diarrhea (34–58%) [4]
Flatulence (38%)
Hepatotoxicity [3]
Loose stools [2]
Nausea (5–61%) [6]
Pancreatitis [2]
Vomiting (4–21%)

Respiratory
Cough (5–15%)
Pharyngitis (5–15%)
Rhinitis (5–15%)
Sinusitis (5–15%)

Endocrine/Metabolic
Galactorrhea (<4%)
Gynecomastia (<4%)
Hyperglycemia [6]
Hypothyroidism (12%)

Genitourinary
Vaginitis (<4%)

Hematologic
Anemia (15%)
Neutropenia [2]
Thrombocytopenia [3]

Otic
Ear pain (5–15%)

Local
Injection-site granuloma [2]
Injection-site pain (8%) [2]

OFATUMUMAB

Trade name: Arzerra (Novartis)
Indications: Chronic lymphocytic leukemia
Class: CD20-directed cytolytic monoclonal antibody, Monoclonal antibody
Half-life: 14 days
Clinically important, potentially hazardous interactions with: live vaccines
Pregnancy category: N/A (May cause fetal B-cell depletion)
Important contra-indications noted in the prescribing guidelines for: nursing mothers; pediatric patients
Warning: HEPATITIS B VIRUS REACTIVATION AND PROGRESSIVE MULTIFOCAL LEUKOENCEPHALOPATHY

Skin
Herpes (6%)
Hyperhidrosis (5%)
Peripheral edema (9%)
Rash (14%) [2]
Toxicity [3]
Urticaria (8%)

Cardiovascular
Angina [2]
Hypertension (5%)
Hypotension (5%)
Tachycardia (5%)

Central Nervous System
Chills (8%)
Fever (20%) [2]
Headache (6%)
Insomnia (7%)
Peripheral neuropathy [2]

Neuromuscular/Skeletal
Asthenia (fatigue) (15%) [4]
Back pain (8%)

Gastrointestinal/Hepatic
Diarrhea (18%) [2]
Nausea (11%) [3]

Respiratory
Bronchitis (11%)
Cough (19%)
Dyspnea (14%)
Nasopharyngitis (8%)
Pneumonia (23%)
Pulmonary toxicity [3]
Upper respiratory tract infection (11%)

Hematologic
Anemia (16%) [4]
Hemolysis [2]
Hemolytic anemia [2]
Leukopenia [2]
Lymphopenia [2]
Neutropenia (>10%) [11]
Sepsis (8%)
Thrombocytopenia [5]

Local
Infusion-related reactions [10]
Infusion-site reactions [2]

Other
Adverse effects [2]
Infection (70%) [10]

OFLOXACIN

Trade names: Floxin (Ortho-McNeil), Ocuflox (Allergan), Taravid (Sanofi-Aventis)
Indications: Various infections caused by susceptible organisms
Class: Antibiotic, fluoroquinolone
Half-life: 4–8 hours
Clinically important, potentially hazardous interactions with: aminophylline, amiodarone, antacids, arsenic, artemether/lumefantrine, BCG vaccine, bendamustine, bepridil, bretylium, calcium salts, clozapine, corticosteroids, cyclosporine, CYP1A2 substrates, didanosine, disopyramide, erythromycin, insulin, lanthanum, magnesiuim salts, mycophenolate, NSAIDs, oral iron, oral typhoid vaccine, oxtriphylline, phenothiazines, probenecid, procainamide, quinapril, quinidine, sevelamer, sotalol, St John's wort, strontium ranelate, sucralfate, sulfonylureas, tricyclic antidepressants, vitamin K antagonists, warfarin, zinc, zolmitriptan
Pregnancy category: C
Important contra-indications noted in the prescribing guidelines for: the elderly; nursing mothers; pediatric patients
Note: Fluoroquinolones are associated with an increased risk of tendinitis and tendon rupture in all ages. This risk is further increased in older patients usually over 60 years of age, in patients taking corticosteroid drugs, and in patients with kidney, heart or lung transplants. Fluoroquinolones may exacerbate muscle weakness in persons with myasthenia gravis.
Warning: SERIOUS ADVERSE REACTIONS INCLUDING TENDINITIS, TENDON RUPTURE, PERIPHERAL NEUROPATHY, CENTRAL NERVOUS SYSTEM EFFECTS and EXACERBATION OF MYASTHENIA GRAVIS

Skin
Anaphylactoid reactions/Anaphylaxis [4]
Angioedema [3]
Exanthems [3]
Fixed eruption [4]
Hypersensitivity [2]
Photosensitivity [8]
Phototoxicity [3]
Pruritus (<3%) [5]
Pruritus ani et vulvae (<3%)
Rash (<10%) [5]
Stevens-Johnson syndrome [4]
Toxic epidermal necrolysis [3]
Urticaria [3]
Vasculitis [4]

Nails
Photo-onycholysis [2]

Mucosal
Oral mucosal eruption [3]
Xerostomia (<3%)

Cardiovascular
QT prolongation [3]

Central Nervous System
Dysgeusia (taste perversion) (<3%) [2]
Hallucinations [2]
Headache [3]
Insomnia [2]
Peripheral neuropathy [2]
Psychosis [2]
Seizures [2]
Vertigo (dizziness) [3]

Neuromuscular/Skeletal
Arthralgia [2]
Arthropathy [2]
Asthenia (fatigue) [2]
Myalgia/Myopathy [2]
Rhabdomyolysis [2]
Tendinopathy/Tendon rupture [7]

Gastrointestinal/Hepatic
Abdominal pain [3]
Diarrhea [2]
Nausea [4]
Vomiting [2]

Genitourinary
Vaginitis (<10%)

Local
Injection-site pain (<10%)

Other
Adverse effects [10]
Death [2]
Side effects [2]

OLANZAPINE

Trade names: Symbyax (Lilly), Zyprexa (Lilly), Zyprexa Relprevv (Lilly)
Indications: Schizophrenia, bipolar I disorder
Class: Antipsychotic, Muscarinic antagonist
Half-life: 21–54 hours
Clinically important, potentially hazardous interactions with: alcohol, antihypertensive agents, carbamazepine, ciprofloxacin, CNS acting drugs, diazepam, dopamine agonists, eszopiclone, fluoxetine, fluvoxamine, insulin degludec, insulin detemir, insulin glargine, levodopa, lithium, tetrabenazine, valproic acid
Pregnancy category: C
Important contra-indications noted in the prescribing guidelines for: the elderly; nursing mothers; pediatric patients
Note: Can cause DRESS and other serious skin reactions.
Symbyax is olanzapine and fluoxetine; Zyprexa Relprevv is olanzapine pamoate.
Warning: INCREASED MORTALITY IN ELDERLY PATIENTS WITH DEMENTIA-RELATED PSYCHOSIS
POST-INJECTION DELIRIUM/SEDATION SYNDROME (Zyprexa Relprevv)

Skin
Angioedema [2]
Edema [3]
Hypersensitivity [2]
Peripheral edema (<10%) [5]
Psoriasis [2]
Purpura (<10%)
Rash (>2%) [2]
Vesiculobullous eruption (2%)
Xanthomas [2]

Hair
Alopecia [3]

Mucosal
Epistaxis (nosebleed) (<10%)
Sialorrhea [4]
Xerostomia (13%) [11]

Cardiovascular
Hypertension (<10%)
Hypotension (<10%) [4]
Orthostatic hypotension [2]
QT prolongation [6]
Tachycardia (<10%)
Torsades de pointes [3]
Venous thromboembolism [4]

Central Nervous System
Akathisia (<10%) [7]
Amnesia [2]
Compulsions [2]
Confusion [2]
Delirium [6]
Extrapyramidal symptoms [3]
Fever [2]
Hallucinations [2]
Headache (17%) [3]
Insomnia (12%) [3]
Neuroleptic malignant syndrome [35]
Parkinsonism (<10%) [6]
Psychosis [2]
Restless legs syndrome [7]
Restlessness [2]

Sedation [17]
Seizures [8]
Serotonin syndrome [2]
Somnolence (drowsiness) (20–39%) [11]
Suicidal ideation [2]
Tardive dyskinesia [5]
Tremor (<10%) [5]
Twitching (2%)
Vertigo (dizziness) [5]

Neuromuscular/Skeletal
Asthenia (fatigue) (8–20%) [4]
Back pain (<10%)
Dystonia [6]
Myalgia/Myopathy [2]
Rhabdomyolysis [9]

Gastrointestinal/Hepatic
Abdominal pain (<10%)
Constipation (9–11%) [2]
Diarrhea (<10%) [2]
Dyspepsia (7–11%)
Flatulence (<10%)
Hepatotoxicity [4]
Nausea (<10%)
Pancreatitis [7]
Vomiting (<10%)

Respiratory
Cough (<10%)
Nasopharyngitis [2]
Pharyngitis (<10%)
Pneumonia [2]
Pulmonary embolism [3]
Rhinitis (<10%)
Sinusitis (<10%)

Endocrine/Metabolic
Appetite increased [2]
Diabetes mellitus [7]
Diabetic ketoacidosis [2]
Galactorrhea [2]
Glucose dysregulation [3]
Gynecomastia [2]
Hypercholesterolemia [2]
Hyperglycemia [6]
Hyperprolactinemia [2]
Metabolic syndrome [11]
Weight gain (5–40%) [60]

Genitourinary
Priapism [19]
Sexual dysfunction [2]
Urinary incontinence (<10%)
Urinary tract infection (<10%)

Hematologic
Agranulocytosis [2]
Dyslipidemia [4]
Eosinophilia [2]
Neutropenia [4]
Pancytopenia [2]

Ocular
Amblyopia (<10%)
Oculogyric crisis [2]
Vision blurred [2]

Other
Adverse effects [9]
Death [7]

OLAPARIB

Trade name: Lynparza (AstraZeneca)
Indications: BRCA-mutated ovarian cancer
Class: Poly (ADP-ribose) polymerase (PARP) inhibitor
Half-life: 7–17 hours
Clinically important, potentially hazardous interactions with: amprenavir, aprepitant, atazanavir, boceprevir, bosentan, carbamazepine, ciprofloxacin, clarithromycin, crizotinib, darunavir, diltiazem, efavirenz, erythromycin, etravirine, fluconazole, fosamprenavir, grapefruit juice, imatinib, indinavir, itraconazole, ketoconazole, lopinavir, modafinil, nafcillin, nefazodone, nelfinavir, phenytoin, posaconazole, rifampin, ritonavir, saquinavir, St John's wort, strong and moderate CYP3A inhibitors, telaprevir, telithromycin, verapamil, voriconazole
Pregnancy category: D
Important contra-indications noted in the prescribing guidelines for: nursing mothers; pediatric patients

Skin
Eczema (<10%)
Hot flashes (<10%)
Peripheral edema (10–20%)
Pruritus (<10%)
Rash (25%) [2]
Xerosis (<10%)

Hair
Alopecia [2]

Mucosal
Stomatitis (<10%)

Cardiovascular
Hypertension (<10%) [2]
Venous thromboembolism (<10%)

Central Nervous System
Anxiety (<10%)
Depression (<10%)
Dysgeusia (taste perversion) (21%) [2]
Fever (<10%)
Headache (25%) [4]
Insomnia (<10%)
Peripheral neuropathy (<10%) [2]

Neuromuscular/Skeletal
Arthralgia (21–32%)
Asthenia (fatigue) (66–68%) [18]
Back pain (25%)
Myalgia/Myopathy (22–25%)

Gastrointestinal/Hepatic
Abdominal pain (43–47%) [3]
Constipation (10–20%) [2]
Diarrhea (28–31%) [8]
Dyspepsia (25%) [3]
Gastric obstruction [2]
Nausea (64–75%) [14]
Vomiting (32–43%) [10]

Respiratory
Cough (21%) [2]
Dyspnea (10–20%)
Nasopharyngitis (26–43%)
Pharyngitis (43%)
Pulmonary embolism (<10%)
Upper respiratory tract infection (26–43%)

Endocrine/Metabolic
ALT increased [2]
Appetite decreased (22–25%) [4]
Creatine phosphokinase increased (26–30%)
Hyperglycemia (<10%)
Hypomagnesemia (<10%)

Genitourinary
Dysuria (<10%)
Urinary incontinence (<10%)
Urinary tract infection (10–20%)

Hematologic
Anemia (25–34%) [17]
Febrile neutropenia [2]
Leukopenia (<10%) [3]
Lymphopenia (56%)
Myelodysplastic syndrome [2]
Myeloid leukemia [2]
Neutropenia (25–32%) [12]
Thrombocytopenia (26–30%) [8]

Other
Adverse effects [5]
Death [3]

OLARATUMAB

Trade name: Lartruvo (Lilly)
Indications: Treatment of adult patients with soft tissue sarcoma (with doxorubicin) with a histologic subtype for which an anthracycline-containing regimen is appropriate and which is not amenable to curative treatment with radiotherapy or surgery
Class: Monoclonal antibody, Platelet-derived growth factor receptor alpha blocking antibody
Half-life: ~11 days
Clinically important, potentially hazardous interactions with: none known
Pregnancy category: N/A (Can cause fetal harm)
Important contra-indications noted in the prescribing guidelines for: the elderly; nursing mothers; pediatric patients
Note: See separate entry for doxorubicin.

Hair
Alopecia (52%)

Mucosal
Mucositis (53%) [2]

Central Nervous System
Anxiety (11%)
Headache (20%)
Neurotoxicity (22%)

Neuromuscular/Skeletal
Asthenia (fatigue) (64%)
Bone or joint pain (64%)

Gastrointestinal/Hepatic
Abdominal pain (23%)
Diarrhea (34%) [3]
Nausea (73%) [2]
Vomiting (45%) [2]

Endocrine/Metabolic
ALP increased (16%)
Appetite decreased (31%)
Hyperglycemia (52%)
Hypokalemia (21%)
Hypomagnesemia (16%)

Hematologic
Lymphopenia (77%)
Neutropenia (65%) [2]
Prothrombin time increased (33%)
Thrombocytopenia (63%)

Ocular
Xerophthalmia (11%)

Local
Infusion-related reactions (13%)

OLMESARTAN

Trade names: Benicar (Sankyo), Olmetec (Daiichi Sankyo)
Indications: Hypertension
Class: Angiotensin II receptor antagonist (blocker), Antihypertensive
Half-life: ~13 hours
Clinically important, potentially hazardous interactions with: ACE inhibitors, adrenergic neurone blockers, aldesleukin, aliskiren, alprostadil, amifostine, antihypertensives, antipsychotics, anxiolytics and hypnotics, baclofen, beta blockers, calcium channel blockers, clonidine, colesevelam, corticosteroids, cyclosporine, diazoxide, diuretics, eltrombopag, eplerenone, estrogens, general anesthetics, heparins, hydralazine, levodopa, lithium, MAO inhibitors, methyldopa, methylphenidate, minoxidil, moxisylyte, moxonidine, nitrates, nitroprusside, NSAIDs, pentoxifylline, phosphodiesterase 5 inhibitors, potassium salts, quinine, rituximab, tacrolimus, tizanidine, tolvaptan, trimethoprim
Pregnancy category: D (category C in first trimester; category D in second and third trimesters)
Important contra-indications noted in the prescribing guidelines for: nursing mothers; pediatric patients
Note: Contra-indicated in patients with diabetes.
Warning: FETAL TOXICITY

Skin
Angioedema [3]
Edema [2]
Peripheral edema [2]

Cardiovascular
Hypotension [2]

Central Nervous System
Vertigo (dizziness) (3%) [8]

Neuromuscular/Skeletal
Asthenia (fatigue) [2]

Gastrointestinal/Hepatic
Diarrhea [4]
Enteropathy [20]
Gastrointestinal disorder [6]

Respiratory
Upper respiratory tract infection [2]

Endocrine/Metabolic
Hyperkalemia [3]

Other
Adverse effects [6]

OLODATEROL

Trade names: Stiolto Respimat (Boehringer Ingelheim), Striverdi Respimat (Boehringer Ingelheim)
Indications: Chronic obstructive pulmonary disease including chronic bronchitis and emphysema
Class: Beta-2 adrenergic agonist
Half-life: 8 hours
Clinically important, potentially hazardous interactions with: adrenergics, beta blockers, diuretics, MAO inhibitors, QT interval prolonging agents, steroids, tricyclic antidepressants, xanthine derivatives
Pregnancy category: C
Important contra-indications noted in the prescribing guidelines for: nursing mothers; pediatric patients
Note: Stiolto Respimat is olodaterol and tiotropium.
Warning: ASTHMA-RELATED DEATH

Skin
Rash (2%)

Cardiovascular
Hypertension [2]

Central Nervous System
Fever (>2%)
Headache [3]
Vertigo (dizziness) (2%) [2]

Neuromuscular/Skeletal
Arthralgia (2%) [2]
Back pain (4%) [4]

Gastrointestinal/Hepatic
Constipation (>2%)
Diarrhea (3%) [3]

Respiratory
Bronchitis (5%) [4]
COPD [2]
Cough (4%) [3]
Dyspnea [3]
Nasopharyngitis (11%) [4]
Pneumonia (>2%) [3]
Upper respiratory tract infection (8%) [4]

Genitourinary
Urinary tract infection (3%) [3]

OLOPATADINE

Trade names: Pataday (Alcon), Patanol (Alcon)
Indications: Pruritus due to allergic conjunctivitis, rhinitis
Class: Histamine H1 receptor antagonist
Half-life: 3 hours
Clinically important, potentially hazardous interactions with: none known
Pregnancy category: C
Important contra-indications noted in the prescribing guidelines for: nursing mothers; pediatric patients

Central Nervous System
Headache (7%) [2]

Ocular
Eyelid burning (<5%)

Eyelid edema (<5%)
Eyelid stinging (<5%)

OLSALAZINE

See: www.drugeruptiondata.com/drug/id/512

OMACETAXINE

Trade name: Synribo (Ivax)
Indications: Chronic myeloid leukemia (CML) in patients with resistance and/or intolerance to two or more tyrosine kinase inhibitors
Class: Protein synthesis inhibitor
Half-life: ~6 hours
Clinically important, potentially hazardous interactions with: none known
Pregnancy category: D
Important contra-indications noted in the prescribing guidelines for: the elderly; nursing mothers; pediatric patients

Skin
Burning (<10%)
Ecchymoses (<10%)
Edema (<10%)
Erythema (<10%)
Exfoliative dermatitis (<10%)
Hematoma (<10%)
Hot flashes (<10%)
Hyperhidrosis (<10%)
Hypersensitivity (<10%)
Lesions (<10%)
Peripheral edema (13%)
Petechiae (<10%)
Pigmentation (<10%)
Pruritus (<10%)
Purpura (<10%)
Rash (10%)
Ulcerations (<10%)
Xerosis (<10%)

Hair
Alopecia (15%)

Mucosal
Aphthous stomatitis (<10%)
Epistaxis (nosebleed) (11–15%)
Gingival bleeding (<10%)
Nasal congestion (<10%)
Oral bleeding (<10%)
Oral ulceration (<10%)
Rhinorrhea (<10%)
Stomatitis (<10%)
Xerostomia (<10%)

Cardiovascular
Acute coronary syndrome (<10%)
Angina (<10%)
Arrhythmias (<10%)
Bradycardia (<10%)
Extrasystoles (<10%)
Hypertension (<10%)
Hypotension (<10%)
Palpitation (<10%)
Tachycardia (<10%)

Central Nervous System
Agitation (<10%)
Anorexia (13%)

Anxiety (<10%)
Cerebral hemorrhage (<10%)
Chills (13%)
Confusion (<10%)
Depression (<10%)
Dysgeusia (taste perversion) (<10%)
Fever (24–29%) [4]
Headache (13%) [4]
Hypoesthesia (<10%)
Insomnia (10%)
Mood changes (<10%)
Paresthesias (<10%)
Seizures (<10%)
Tremor (<10%)
Vertigo (dizziness) (<10%)

Neuromuscular/Skeletal
Arthralgia (19%)
Asthenia (fatigue) (23–31%) [5]
Back pain (11%)
Bone or joint pain (<10%)
Gouty tophi (<10%)
Muscle spasm (<10%)
Myalgia/Myopathy (<10%)
Pain in extremities (11–13%)

Gastrointestinal/Hepatic
Abdominal distension (<10%)
Abdominal pain (13–14%)
Black stools (<10%)
Constipation (15%)
Diarrhea (35–42%) [6]
Dyspepsia (<10%)
Gastritis (<10%)
Gastroesophageal reflux (<10%)
Gastrointestinal bleeding (<10%)
Hemorrhoids (<10%)
Nausea (32%) [6]
Vomiting (12–15%)

Respiratory
Cough (15–16%)
Dysphonia (<10%)
Dyspnea (11%)
Hemoptysis (<10%)
Pharyngolaryngeal pain (<10%)

Endocrine/Metabolic
ALT increased (2–6%)
Appetite decreased (<10%)
Creatine phosphokinase increased (9–16%)
Dehydration (<10%)
Diabetes mellitus (<10%)

Genitourinary
Dysuria (<10%)

Hematologic
Anemia (51–61%) [6]
Bone marrow suppression (10%)
Febrile neutropenia (10–20%)
Hemoglobin decreased (62–80%)
Leukocytosis (6%)
Myelosuppression [2]
Neutropenia (50%) [7]
Platelets decreased (85–88%)
Thrombocytopenia (56–74%) [8]

Otic
Ear pain (<10%)
Ototoxicity (<10%)
Tinnitus (<10%)

Ocular
Cataract (<10%)
Conjunctival hemorrhage (<10%)

Conjunctivitis (<10%)
Diplopia (<10%)
Eyelid edema (<10%)
Lacrimation (<10%)
Ocular pain (<10%)
Vision blurred (<10%)
Xerophthalmia (<10%)

Local
Infusion-site reactions (22–34%)
Injection-site reactions (22–34%)

Other
Infection (46–56%) [3]

OMALIZUMAB

Trade name: Xolair (Genentech)
Indications: Asthma
Class: IgE-targeting monoclonal antibody, Monoclonal antibody
Half-life: 26 days
Clinically important, potentially hazardous interactions with: none known
Pregnancy category: B
Important contra-indications noted in the prescribing guidelines for: nursing mothers
Warning: ANAPHYLAXIS

Skin
Anaphylactoid reactions/Anaphylaxis [10]
Angioedema [2]
Churg-Strauss syndrome [13]
Dermatitis (2%)
Pruritus (2%)
Rash [2]
Serum sickness [2]
Serum sickness-like reaction [2]
Urticaria (7%) [3]

Central Nervous System
Headache (15%) [8]
Pain (7%)
Vertigo (dizziness) (3%)

Neuromuscular/Skeletal
Arthralgia (8%) [2]
Asthenia (fatigue) (3%) [2]
Myalgia/Myopathy [2]

Gastrointestinal/Hepatic
Abdominal pain [3]
Diarrhea [2]
Nausea [3]

Respiratory
Cough [2]
Nasopharyngitis [4]
Sinusitis (16%) [4]
Upper respiratory tract infection (20%) [5]

Local
Injection-site pain [2]
Injection-site reactions (45%) [7]

Other
Adverse effects [5]
Infection [2]

OMBITASVIR/ PARITAPREVIR/ RITONAVIR

Trade names: Technivie (AbbVie), Viekira Pak (AbbVie), Viekirax (AbbVie)
Indications: Genotype 4 chronic hepatitis C virus infection in patients without cirrhosis (in combination with ribavirin)
Class: CYP3A4 inhibitor (ritonavir), Direct-acting antiviral, Hepatitis C virus NS3/4A protease inhibitor (paritaprevir), Hepatitis C virus NS5A inhibitor (ombitasvir)
Half-life: 21–25 hours (ombitasvir); 6 hours (paritaprevir); 4 hours (ritonavir)
Clinically important, potentially hazardous interactions with: atazanavir, carbamazepine, cisapride, colchicine, dihydroergotamine, dronedarone, efavirenz, ergotamine, ethinyl estradiol-containing medications, lopinavir, lovastatin, lurasidone, methylergonovine, midazolam, midostaurin, neratinib, phenobarbital, phenytoin, pimozide, ranolazine, rifampin, rilpivirine, salmeterol, sildenafil, simvastatin, St John's wort, triazolam, voriconazole
Pregnancy category: B (pregnancy category will be X when administered with ribavirin)
Important contra-indications noted in the prescribing guidelines for: nursing mothers; pediatric patients
Note: Contra-indicated in patients with moderate or severe hepatic impairment or with known hypersensitivity to ritonavir (see separate entry). See also separate entry for ribavirin. Viekira Pak is ombitasvir/paritaprevir/ritonavir co-packaged with dasabuvir.

Skin
Dermatitis (<5%)
Eczema (<5%)
Erythema (<5%)
Exfoliative dermatitis (<5%)
Photosensitivity (<5%)
Pruritus (5%) [8]
Psoriasis (<5%)
Rash (<5%) [4]
Ulcerations (<5%)
Urticaria (<5%)

Central Nervous System
Headache [17]
Insomnia (5%) [11]
Irritability [2]
Vertigo (dizziness) [2]

Neuromuscular/Skeletal
Arthralgia [2]
Asthenia (fatigue) (7–25%) [17]

Gastrointestinal/Hepatic
Diarrhea [10]
Nausea (9%) [13]
Vomiting [2]

Respiratory
Cough [3]
Dyspnea [2]
Nasopharyngitis [2]

Endocrine/Metabolic
Acidosis [2]

ALT increased [3]
AST increased [3]
Hematologic
Anemia [6]
Hemoglobin decreased [2]
Other
Adverse effects [2]
Death [2]

OMEPRAZOLE

Trade names: Prilosec (AstraZeneca), Yosprala (Aralez)
Indications: Duodenal ulcer, gastric ulcer, gastroesophageal reflux disease (GERD), erosive esophagitis
Class: CYP1A2 inducer, Proton pump inhibitor (PPI)
Half-life: 0.5–1 hour
Clinically important, potentially hazardous interactions with: amoxicillin, atazanavir, bendamustine, benzodiazepines, cilostazol, clarithromycin, clobazam, clopidogrel, clozapine, coumarins, cyclosporine, dasatinib, delavirdine, diazepam, digoxin, disulfiram, enzalutamide, erlotinib, escitalopram, itraconazole, ketoconazole, lapatinib, methotrexate, nelfinavir, phenytoin, posaconazole, prednisone, raltegravir, rilpivirine, saquinavir, sofosbuvir & velpatasvir, St John's wort, tacrolimus, tipranavir, ulipristal, voriconazole, warfarin
Pregnancy category: C
Important contra-indications noted in the prescribing guidelines for: nursing mothers; pediatric patients
Note: Yosprala is omeprazole and aspirin.

Skin
AGEP [2]
Anaphylactoid reactions/Anaphylaxis [7]
Angioedema [5]
Baboon syndrome (SDRIFE) [2]
Bullous pemphigoid [2]
Contact dermatitis [2]
Eczema [2]
Edema (<10%) [2]
Erythroderma [2]
Exfoliative dermatitis [3]
Hypersensitivity [2]
Lichen planus [2]
Lichen spinulosus [2]
Lichenoid eruption [2]
Lupus erythematosus [5]
Pemphigus (exacerbation) [2]
Peripheral edema [2]
Pruritus (<10%) [8]
Rash (2%) [6]
Toxic epidermal necrolysis [5]
Urticaria (<10%) [9]
Vasculitis [2]
Xerosis [2]

Hair
Alopecia [2]

Mucosal
Oral candidiasis [3]
Xerostomia (<10%) [2]

Central Nervous System
Anorexia [3]
Dysgeusia (taste perversion) (<10%) [4]
Headache (7%) [2]
Paresthesias [2]
Somnolence (drowsiness) [2]
Vertigo (dizziness) (2%)

Neuromuscular/Skeletal
Asthenia (fatigue) [2]
Myalgia/Myopathy (<10%)
Rhabdomyolysis [2]

Gastrointestinal/Hepatic
Abdominal distension [2]
Abdominal pain (5%) [4]
Constipation [3]
Diarrhea (4%) [9]
Flatulence (3%)
Hepatitis [4]
Hepatotoxicity [3]
Nausea (4%) [7]
Pancreatitis [2]
Vomiting (3%) [6]

Respiratory
Cough [2]
Upper respiratory tract infection (2%)

Endocrine/Metabolic
Gynecomastia [11]
Hypomagnesemia [7]

Renal
Nephrotoxicity [9]

Hematologic
Agranulocytosis [3]
Hemolytic anemia [2]
Leukopenia [3]
Neutropenia [3]

Ocular
Visual disturbances [2]

Other
Adverse effects [9]

ONDANSETRON

Trade names: Zofran (GSK), Zuplenz (Par)
Indications: Nausea and vomiting
Class: 5-HT3 antagonist, Antiemetic, Serotonin type 3 receptor antagonist
Half-life: 3–6 hours
Clinically important, potentially hazardous interactions with: apomorphine, carbamazepine, phenytoin, ribociclib, rifampin, tramadol
Pregnancy category: B
Important contra-indications noted in the prescribing guidelines for: nursing mothers; pediatric patients

Skin
Anaphylactoid reactions/Anaphylaxis [5]
Fixed eruption [2]
Pruritus (5%)

Mucosal
Sialopenia (<5%)
Xerostomia (<10%) [3]

Cardiovascular
Bradycardia [2]
Flushing [2]

Hypotension [3]
Myocardial ischemia [2]
QT prolongation [11]
Torsades de pointes [3]
Ventricular tachycardia [2]

Central Nervous System
Anxiety (6%)
Chills (5–10%)
Fever (2–8%)
Headache (17–25%) [14]
Paresthesias (2%)
Seizures [3]
Somnolence (drowsiness) (8%) [4]
Vertigo (dizziness) (4–7%) [8]

Neuromuscular/Skeletal
Asthenia (fatigue) (9–13%)

Gastrointestinal/Hepatic
Abdominal pain [2]
Constipation (6–11%) [7]
Diarrhea (8–16%) [3]

Respiratory
Hypoxia (9%)

Endocrine/Metabolic
ALT increased [2]

Local
Injection-site reactions (4%)

Other
Adverse effects [3]
Death [2]
Hiccups [2]

ORAL CONTRACEPTIVES

Trade names: Alesse (Wyeth), Aviane (Barr), Brevicon (Watson), Demulen (Pfizer), Desogen (Organon), Estrostep (Pfizer), Evra (Johnson & Johnson), Levlen (Bayer), Levlite (Bayer), Levora (Watson), Lo/Ovral (Wyeth), Loestrin (Barr), Lunelle (Pfizer), Mircette (Organon), Modicon (Ortho), Necon (Watson), Nordette (Monarch), Norinyl (Watson), Ortho Tri-Cyclen (Ortho-McNeil), Ortho-Cept (Ortho-McNeil), Ortho-Cyclen (Ortho-McNeil), Ortho-Novum (Ortho-McNeil), Ovcon (Warner Chilcott), Ovral (Wyeth), Tri-Levlen (Bayer), Tri-Norinyl (Watson), Triphasil (Wyeth), Trivora (Watson), Yasmin (Bayer), Yaz (Bayer), Zovia (Watson)
Indications: Prevention of pregnancy
Class: Hormone
Half-life: N/A
Clinically important, potentially hazardous interactions with: aminophylline, amprenavir, anticonvulsants, aprepitant, atazanavir, atorvastatin, beclomethasone, bexarotene, bosentan, budesonide, cigarette smoking, danazol, doxycycline, efavirenz, eslicarbazepine, exenatide, flucloxacillin, flunisolide, fluticasone propionate, glecaprevir & pibrentasvir, hydrocortisone, insulin aspart, insulin degludec, insulin detemir, insulin glargine, insulin glulisine, isotretinoin, lamotrigine, lomitapide, lymecycline, metformin, methylprednisolone, mifepristone, modafinil, naratriptan, nelfinavir, oxcarbazepine, perampanel, prednisolone, prednisone, rifabutin, rifampin, ritonavir, roflumilast, selegiline, St John's

wort, teriflunomide, tigecycline, triamcinolone, troleandomycin, tuberculostatics, ursodiol, zolmitriptan
Warning: CIGARETTE SMOKING AND SERIOUS CARDIOVASCULAR EVENTS

Skin
Acneform eruption [17]
Angioedema [4]
Candidiasis [9]
Chloasma [13]
Erythema multiforme [2]
Erythema nodosum [18]
Exanthems [2]
Herpes gestationis [3]
Lupus erythematosus [29]
Melanoma [5]
Melasma [8]
Perioral dermatitis [8]
Photosensitivity [12]
Pigmentation [18]
Pruritus [5]
Purpura [3]
Seborrhea [3]
Spider angioma [2]
Sweet's syndrome [2]
Telangiectasia [6]
Urticaria [2]

Hair
Alopecia [19]
Alopecia areata [4]
Hirsutism [12]

Mucosal
Gingival hyperplasia/hypertrophy [2]

Cardiovascular
Thrombophlebitis [2]
Venous thromboembolism [6]

Central Nervous System
Chorea [2]
Depression [2]
Headache [3]

Gastrointestinal/Hepatic
Colitis [3]
Nausea [4]

Endocrine/Metabolic
Acute intermittent porphyria [5]
Galactorrhea [2]
Mastodynia [3]
Porphyria cutanea tarda [28]
Porphyria variegata [2]

Genitourinary
Vaginal bleeding [4]

Local
Application-site reactions (92%) [2]

Other
Adverse effects [3]

ORITAVANCIN

Trade name: Orbactiv (Medicines Co)
Indications: Acute bacterial skin and skin structure infections caused or suspected to be caused by susceptible isolates of designated Gram-positive microorganisms
Class: Antibiotic, lipoglycopeptide
Half-life: 245 hours
Clinically important, potentially hazardous interactions with: warfarin
Pregnancy category: C
Important contra-indications noted in the prescribing guidelines for: nursing mothers; pediatric patients

Skin
Abscess (4%) [3]
Angioedema (<2%)
Cellulitis [4]
Erythema multiforme (<2%)
Hypersensitivity (<2%)
Leukocytoclastic vasculitis (<2%)
Pruritus (<2%) [3]
Rash (<2%)
Urticaria (<2%)

Cardiovascular
Phlebitis [2]
Tachycardia (3%)

Central Nervous System
Fever [4]
Headache (7%) [6]
Vertigo (dizziness) (3%) [4]

Neuromuscular/Skeletal
Myalgia/Myopathy (<2%)
Osteomyelitis (<2%)

Gastrointestinal/Hepatic
Constipation [5]
Diarrhea (4%) [6]
Nausea (10%) [7]
Vomiting (5%) [5]

Respiratory
Bronchospasm (<2%)
Wheezing (<2%)

Endocrine/Metabolic
ALT increased (3%) [4]
AST increased (2%) [2]
Hyperuricemia (<2%)
Hypoglycemia (<2%)

Hematologic
Anemia (<2%)
Eosinophilia (<2%)

Local
Infusion-site reactions (2%) [3]
Injection-site extravasation [3]
Injection-site phlebitis [3]
Injection-site reactions [2]

ORLISTAT

Trade names: Alli (GSK), Xenical (Roche)
Indications: Obesity, weight reduction
Class: Lipase inhibitor
Half-life: 1–2 hours
Clinically important, potentially hazardous interactions with: acarbose, amiodarone, antiepileptics, coumarins, cyclosporine, ergocalciferol, ethosuximide, lacosamide, levothyroxine, oxcarbazepine, paricalcitol, phytonadione, tiagabine, vigabatrin, vitamin A, vitamin E, warfarin
Pregnancy category: B
Important contra-indications noted in the prescribing guidelines for: nursing mothers; pediatric patients
Note: Contra-indicated in organ transplant recipients. Orlistat interferes with the medicines used to prevent transplant rejection.

Skin
 Lichenoid eruption [2]
 Peripheral edema (3%)
 Rash (4%)
 Xerosis (2%)
Mucosal
 Gingivitis (2–4%)
Central Nervous System
 Anxiety (3–5%)
 Depression (3%)
 Headache (31%) [2]
 Sleep related disorder (4%)
 Vertigo (dizziness) (5%)
Neuromuscular/Skeletal
 Arthralgia (5%)
 Asthenia (fatigue) (3–7%)
 Back pain (14%)
 Bone or joint pain (2%)
 Myalgia/Myopathy (4%)
 Tendinitis (2%)
Gastrointestinal/Hepatic
 Abdominal pain (26%) [4]
 Cholelithiasis (gallstones) (3%)
 Defecation (increased) (3–11%) [2]
 Fecal incontinence (2–8%)
 Fecal urgency (3–23%) [2]
 Flatulence (with discharge) (2–24%) [2]
 Hepatic failure [2]
 Hepatitis [3]
 Hepatotoxicity [4]
 Nausea (4–8%)
 Pancreatitis [5]
 Vomiting (4%)
Respiratory
 Influenza (40%)
 Upper respiratory tract infection (26–38%) [2]
Endocrine/Metabolic
 Hypoglycemia (in diabetic patients) [2]
 Menstrual irregularities (10%)
Genitourinary
 Urinary tract infection (6–8%)
 Vaginitis (3–4%)
Renal
 Nephrotoxicity [9]
 Renal failure [2]

Otic
 Otitis media (3–4%)
Other
 Adverse effects [7]
 Tooth disorder (3–4%)

ORPHENADRINE

See: www.drugeruptiondata.com/drug/id/517

OSELTAMIVIR

Trade name: Tamiflu (Roche)
Indications: Influenza infection
Class: Antiviral, Neuraminidase inhibitor
Half-life: 6–10 hours
Clinically important, potentially hazardous interactions with: none known
Pregnancy category: C

Skin
 Rash [5]
 Toxic epidermal necrolysis [2]
Central Nervous System
 Delirium [5]
 Hallucinations [3]
 Headache [2]
 Insomnia [2]
 Neuropsychiatric disturbances [3]
 Neurotoxicity [5]
 Seizures [2]
 Suicidal ideation [2]
Gastrointestinal/Hepatic
 Abdominal pain (2–5%) [2]
 Diarrhea (<3%) [8]
 Hemorrhagic colitis [5]
 Nausea (4–10%) [16]
 Vomiting (2–15%) [16]
Respiratory
 Respiratory failure [2]
 Upper respiratory tract infection [2]
Hematologic
 Thrombocytopenia [2]
Other
 Adverse effects [7]

OSIMERTINIB

Trade name: Tagrisso (AstraZeneca)
Indications: Metastatic epidermal growth factor receptor T790M mutation-positive non-small cell lung cancer
Class: Kinase inhibitor
Half-life: 48 hours
Clinically important, potentially hazardous interactions with: carbamazepine, cyclosporine, ergot alkaloids, fentanyl, itraconazole, nefazodone, phenytoin, quinidine, rifampin, ritonavir, St John's wort, strong CYP3A inhibitors or inducers, telithromycin

Pregnancy category: N/A (Can cause fetal harm)
Important contra-indications noted in the prescribing guidelines for: nursing mothers; pediatric patients

Skin
 Rash (41%) [7]
 Xerosis (31%) [2]
Nails
 Nail toxicity (25%)
 Paronychia [2]
Mucosal
 Stomatitis (12%)
Cardiovascular
 QT prolongation (3%)
 Venous thromboembolism (7%)
Central Nervous System
 Cerebrovascular accident (3%)
 Headache (10%)
Neuromuscular/Skeletal
 Asthenia (fatigue) (14%) [2]
 Back pain (13%)
Gastrointestinal/Hepatic
 Constipation (15%)
 Diarrhea (42%) [7]
 Nausea (17%) [2]
Respiratory
 Cough (14%)
 Dyspnea [2]
 Pneumonia (4%)
 Pneumonitis (3%)
 Pulmonary toxicity [5]
Endocrine/Metabolic
 Appetite decreased (16%) [2]
 Hypermagnesemia (20%)
 Hyponatremia (26%)
Hematologic
 Anemia (44%)
 Lymphopenia (63%)
 Neutropenia (33%)
 Thrombocytopenia (54%)
Ocular
 Ocular adverse effects (18%)

OSPEMIFENE

Trade name: Osphena (Shionogi)
Indications: Dyspareunia due to menopausal vulvar and vaginal atrophy
Class: Estrogen agonist, Estrogen antagonist, Selective estrogen receptor modulator (SERM)
Half-life: 26 hours
Clinically important, potentially hazardous interactions with: fluconazole, ketoconazole, other estrogen agonists or antagonists, rifampin
Pregnancy category: X
Important contra-indications noted in the prescribing guidelines for: nursing mothers; pediatric patients
Note: Contra-indicated in patients with undiagnosed abnormal genital bleeding, known or suspected estrogen-dependent neoplasia, active DVT or pulmonary embolism, or active arterial thromboembolic disease.

Warning: ENDOMETRIAL CANCER AND CARDIOVASCULAR DISORDERS

Skin
Hot flashes (8%) [7]
Hyperhidrosis (2%)

Neuromuscular/Skeletal
Muscle spasm (3%)

Genitourinary
Urinary tract infection [2]
Vaginal discharge (4%)

OXACILLIN

Indications: Various infections caused by susceptible organisms
Class: Antibiotic, penicillin
Half-life: 23–60 minutes
Clinically important, potentially hazardous interactions with: anticoagulants, cyclosporine, demeclocycline, doxycycline, imipenem/cilastatin, methotrexate, minocycline, oxytetracycline, tetracycline
Pregnancy category: B
Important contra-indications noted in the prescribing guidelines for: the elderly; nursing mothers; pediatric patients

Skin
Exanthems [2]
Rash (<22%)

Other
Adverse effects [2]

OXALIPLATIN

Trade name: Eloxatin (Sanofi-Aventis)
Indications: Metastatic carcinoma of the colon or rectum (in combination with fluorouracil/leucovorin (FOLFOX))
Class: Alkylating agent, Antineoplastic
Half-life: 391 hours
Clinically important, potentially hazardous interactions with: aminoglycosides, BCG vaccine, capreomycin, cardiac glycosides, clozapine, denosumab, diuretics, leflunomide, natalizumab, pimecrolimus, polymyxins, sipuleucel-T, tacrolimus, taxanes, topotecan, trastuzumab, vaccines, vitamin K antagonists
Pregnancy category: D
Important contra-indications noted in the prescribing guidelines for: nursing mothers; pediatric patients
Warning: ANAPHYLACTIC REACTIONS

Skin
Anaphylactoid reactions/Anaphylaxis [11]
Diaphoresis (5%) [2]
Edema (13–15%) [2]
Erythema [4]
Exanthems (2–5%)
Hand–foot syndrome (7–13%) [12]
Hot flashes (2–5%)
Hypersensitivity (12%) [29]
Peripheral edema (11%)
Pruritus (6%) [5]

Purpura (2–5%)
Radiation recall dermatitis [3]
Rash (5–11%) [11]
Thrombocytopenic purpura [2]
Toxicity [2]
Urticaria [2]
Xerosis (6%)

Hair
Alopecia (3–38%) [3]

Mucosal
Epistaxis (nosebleed) (<16%)
Gingivitis (2–5%)
Mucositis (10%) [4]
Oral mucositis [2]
Stomatitis (32–42%) [3]
Xerostomia (5%)

Cardiovascular
Chest pain (4%) [2]
Flushing (2–7%) [2]
Hypertension [5]
Hypotension (5%) [2]
Tachycardia [3]
Thromboembolism (4%)

Central Nervous System
Anorexia (13–35%) [4]
Anxiety (5%)
Chills [3]
Depression (9%)
Dysesthesia (often cold-induced or cold-exacerbated) (38%) [7]
Dysgeusia (taste perversion) (<14%)
Dysphasia (5%)
Fever (16–27%) [9]
Headache (7–13%)
Hyperalgesia [2]
Hypoesthesia [2]
Insomnia (4–13%)
Leukoencephalopathy [4]
Neurotoxicity (48%) [37]
Pain (5–9%)
Paresthesias (77%) [7]
Peripheral neuropathy (92%) [38]
Rigors (8%)
Sensory disturbances (8%)
Vertigo (dizziness) (7–8%)

Neuromuscular/Skeletal
Arthralgia (5–10%)
Asthenia (fatigue) (44–70%) [21]
Ataxia [2]
Back pain (11–16%)
Myalgia/Myopathy (14%)

Gastrointestinal/Hepatic
Abdominal pain (18–31%) [4]
Constipation (22–32%) [2]
Diarrhea (44–56%) [41]
Dyspepsia (8–12%)
Flatulence (6–9%)
Gastroesophageal reflux (3%)
Hepatotoxicity [8]
Nausea (59–74%) [23]
Sinusoidal obstruction syndrome [2]
Vomiting (27–47%) [19]

Respiratory
Cough (9–35%)
Dyspnea (5–18%) [2]
Pharyngitis (10%)
Pneumonia [2]
Pulmonary embolism [2]

Pulmonary fibrosis [2]
Pulmonary toxicity [2]
Rhinitis (4–10%)
Upper respiratory tract infection (4%)

Endocrine/Metabolic
ALP increased (42%)
ALT increased (57%)
AST increased [2]
Dehydration (9%)
Hyperglycemia (14%)
Hypoalbuminemia (8%)
Hypocalcemia (7%)
Hypokalemia (11%)
Hyponatremia (8%) [2]
Serum creatinine increased (4%) [2]
Weight gain (10%)
Weight loss (11%)

Genitourinary
Urinary frequency (5%)

Renal
Nephrotoxicity [3]

Hematologic
Anemia (27–76%) [24]
Febrile neutropenia (<4%) [7]
Hemolytic anemia [4]
Leukocytopenia [2]
Leukopenia (34–85%) [14]
Lymphopenia (6%)
Myelosuppression [4]
Neutropenia (25–81%) [52]
Thrombocytopenia (20–77%) [38]
Thrombosis (6%)

Ocular
Abnormal vision (5%)
Conjunctivitis (9%)
Epiphora [3]
Lacrimation (4–9%)
Vision blurred [2]

Local
Injection-site reactions (5–11%) [2]

Other
Adverse effects [2]
Allergic reactions (3%) [4]
Death [3]
Hiccups (5%)
Infection (8–25%) [2]

OXAPROZIN

Trade name: Daypro (Pfizer)
Indications: Arthritis
Class: Non-steroidal anti-inflammatory (NSAID)
Half-life: 42–50 hours
Clinically important, potentially hazardous interactions with: methotrexate
Pregnancy category: C
Important contra-indications noted in the prescribing guidelines for: nursing mothers; pediatric patients
Note: NSAIDs may cause an increased risk of serious cardiovascular and gastrointestinal adverse events, which can be fatal. This risk may increase with duration of use.

Skin
Pruritus (<10%)
Rash (>10%) [2]

Stevens-Johnson syndrome [2]
Toxic epidermal necrolysis [4]

Gastrointestinal/Hepatic
Hepatotoxicity [3]

Endocrine/Metabolic
Pseudoporphyria [3]

Renal
Nephrotoxicity [2]

Other
Adverse effects [3]

OXAZEPAM

Trade name: Serax (Mayne)
Indications: Anxiety, depression
Class: Benzodiazepine
Half-life: 3–6 hours
Clinically important, potentially hazardous interactions with: amprenavir, chlorpheniramine, clarithromycin, efavirenz, esomeprazole, imatinib, nelfinavir
Pregnancy category: D
Important contra-indications noted in the prescribing guidelines for: pediatric patients

Skin
Dermatitis (<10%)
Diaphoresis (>10%)
Rash (>10%)

Mucosal
Sialopenia (>10%)
Sialorrhea (<10%)
Xerostomia (>10%)

OXCARBAZEPINE

Trade names: Oxtellar XR (Supernus), Trileptal (Novartis)
Indications: Partial epileptic seizures
Class: Anticonvulsant, CYP3A4 inducer, Mood stabilizer
Half-life: 1–2.5 hours
Clinically important, potentially hazardous interactions with: alcohol, antipsychotics, carbamazepine, chloroquine, clopidogrel, cobicistat/elvitegravir/emtricitabine/tenofovir alafenamide, cobicistat/elvitegravir/emtricitabine/ tenofovir disoproxil, cyclosporine, CYP3A4 substrates, dronedarone, emtricitabine/rilpivirine/ tenofovir alafenamide, eslicarbazepine, everolimus, exemestane, guanfacine, hydroxychloroquine, imatinib, ixabepilone, ledipasvir & sofosbuvir, levomepromazine, levonorgestrel, MAO inhibitors, maraviroc, mefloquine, nifedipine, nilotinib, nisoldipine, oral contraceptives, orlistat, pazopanib, perampanel, phenobarbital, phenytoin, praziquantel, ranolazine, rilpivirine, risperidone, romidepsin, saxagliptin, selegiline, simeprevir, sofosbuvir, sofosbuvir & velpatasvir, sofosbuvir/velpatasvir/ voxilaprevir, sorafenib, SSRIs, St John's wort, tadalafil, tenofovir alafenamide, thiazide diuretics, tolvaptan, tricyclic antidepressants, ulipristal, valproic acid, zuclopenthixol

Pregnancy category: C
Important contra-indications noted in the prescribing guidelines for: nursing mothers; pediatric patients

Skin
Acneform eruption (<2%)
Diaphoresis (3%)
DRESS syndrome [6]
Ecchymoses (4%)
Edema (<2%)
Exanthems [4]
Hot flashes (<2%)
Hyperhidrosis (3%)
Hypersensitivity [6]
Lymphadenopathy (2%)
Purpura (2%)
Rash (<6%) [11]
Stevens-Johnson syndrome [10]
Toxic epidermal necrolysis [4]

Mucosal
Epistaxis (nosebleed) (4%)
Rectal hemorrhage (2%)
Xerostomia (3%)

Cardiovascular
Chest pain (2%)
Hypotension (<3%)

Central Nervous System
Agitation (<2%)
Amnesia (4%)
Anorexia (3–5%)
Anxiety (5–7%)
Coma [2]
Confusion (<7%)
Dysgeusia (taste perversion) (5%)
Emotional lability (2–3%)
Fever (3%)
Gait instability (5–17%)
Headache (13–32%) [8]
Hyperesthesia (3%)
Hypoesthesia (<3%)
Incoordination (<4%)
Insomnia (2–6%)
Nervousness (2–4%)
Seizures (2–5%) [5]
Somnolence (drowsiness) (5–36%) [5]
Speech disorder (<3%)
Tremor (3–16%) [2]
Vertigo (dizziness) (3–49%) [12]

Neuromuscular/Skeletal
Asthenia (fatigue) (3–15%) [5]
Ataxia (<31%) [2]
Back pain (4%)
Myoclonus [3]
Osteoporosis [2]

Gastrointestinal/Hepatic
Abdominal pain (3–13%)
Constipation (2–6%)
Diarrhea (5–7%)
Dyspepsia (5–6%)
Gastritis (<2%)
Nausea (15–29%) [8]
Vomiting (13–36%) [4]

Respiratory
Cough (5%)
Pharyngitis (3%)
Pneumonia (2%)
Rhinitis (2–5%)

Sinusitis (4%)
Upper respiratory tract infection (5–10%)

Endocrine/Metabolic
Hyponatremia (<5%) [16]
SIADH [3]
Weight gain (<2%)

Genitourinary
Ejaculatory dysfunction [3]
Urinary frequency (<2%)
Urinary tract infection (<5%)
Vaginitis (2%)

Hematologic
Leukopenia [3]
Thrombocytopenia [2]

Otic
Ear pain (<2%)

Ocular
Abnormal vision (2–14%)
Accommodation disorder (<3%)
Diplopia (<40%) [10]
Nystagmus (2–26%)

Other
Adverse effects [7]
Allergic reactions (2%) [3]
Dipsia (thirst) (2%)
Infection (2–7%)
Teratogenicity [3]
Toothache (2%)

OXERUTINS

See: www.drugeruptiondata.com/drug/id/1358

OXILAN

See: www.drugeruptiondata.com/drug/id/1149

OXPRENOLOL

See: www.drugeruptiondata.com/drug/id/1391

OXTRIPHYLLINE

See: www.drugeruptiondata.com/drug/id/1971

OXYBUTYNIN

Trade names: Cystrin (Sanofi-Aventis), Ditropan (Ortho-McNeil), Lyrinel (Janssen-Cilag)
Indications: Neurogenic bladder, urinary incontinence, palmar and axillary hyperhidrosis
Class: Anticholinergic, Antimuscarinic, Muscarinic antagonist
Half-life: 2–3 hours
Clinically important, potentially hazardous interactions with: alcohol, anticholinergics, antihistamines, arbutamine, cannabinoids, clozapine, conivaptan, diphenoxylate, disopyramide, domperidone, haloperidol, ketoconazole, levodopa, MAO inhibitors, memantine, metoclopramide, nefopam, nitrates,

parasympathomimetics, pramlintide, secretin, tricyclic antidepressants
Pregnancy category: B
Important contra-indications noted in the prescribing guidelines for: nursing mothers
Note: Contra-indicated in patients with urinary retention, gastric retention and other severe decreased gastrointestinal motility conditions, uncontrolled narrow-angle glaucoma and in patients who are at risk for these conditions.

Skin
Hot flashes (<10%)
Pruritus [2]
Rash (<10%)

Mucosal
Sialopenia [2]
Xerostomia (71%) [31]

Central Nervous System
Cognitive impairment [4]
Headache (8%) [2]
Insomnia (6%)
Nervousness (7%)
Somnolence (drowsiness) (14%)
Vertigo (dizziness) (17%) [2]

Gastrointestinal/Hepatic
Constipation (15%) [4]
Dyspepsia (6%)
Nausea [3]

Genitourinary
Urinary retention (6%)
Urinary tract infection (7%)

Ocular
Vision blurred (10%)

Other
Adverse effects [4]
Allergic reactions [2]

OXYCODONE

Trade names: OxyContin (Purdue), OxyIR (Purdue), Percocet (Endo), Roxicodone (aaiPharma), Targiniq (Purdue), Troxyca (Pfizer), Tylox (Ortho-McNeil), Xtampza ER (Collegium)
Indications: Pain
Class: Opiate agonist
Half-life: 4.6 hours
Clinically important, potentially hazardous interactions with: cimetidine, clonazepam, telithromycin, voriconazole
Pregnancy category: B
Important contra-indications noted in the prescribing guidelines for: the elderly; nursing mothers; pediatric patients
Note: Oxycodone is often combined with acetaminophen (Percocet, Roxicet, Tylox) or aspirin (Percodan, Roxiprin); Targiniq is oxycodone and naloxone; Troxyca is oxycodone and naltrexone. Contra-indicated in patients with significant respiratory depression, acute or severe bronchial asthma, or with known or suspected gastrointestinal obstruction, including paralytic ileus.

Warning: ADDICTION, ABUSE and MISUSE; LIFETHREATENING RESPIRATORY DEPRESSION; ACCIDENTAL INGESTION; NEONATAL OPIOID WITHDRAWAL SYNDROME; and CYTOCHROME P450 3A4 INTERACTION

Skin
Pruritus [7]

Mucosal
Xerostomia [2]

Central Nervous System
Fever [2]
Headache [6]
Insomnia [3]
Sedation [2]
Serotonin syndrome [2]
Somnolence (drowsiness) [13]
Vertigo (dizziness) [8]

Neuromuscular/Skeletal
Asthenia (fatigue) [9]

Gastrointestinal/Hepatic
Abdominal pain [3]
Constipation [12]
Diarrhea [2]
Ileus [2]
Nausea [21]
Vomiting [18]

Ocular
Hallucinations, visual [2]

Local
Injection-site pain (<10%)

Other
Adverse effects [9]
Death [3]
Tooth disorder [2]

OXYMETAZOLINE *

Trade name: Rhofade (Allergan)
Indications: Persistant facial erythema associated with rosacea
Class: Alpha adrenoceptor agonist
Half-life: N/A
Clinically important, potentially hazardous interactions with: none known
Pregnancy category: N/A (No available data to inform drug-associated risk)
Important contra-indications noted in the prescribing guidelines for: nursing mothers; pediatric patients
Note: For topical use only. See separate entry for tetracaine & oxymetazoline as intranasal formulation.
Oxymetazoline is also available as an ophthalmic solution and a nasal decongestant in over-the-counter products.

Skin
Rosacea (exacerbation) (<3%)

Local
Application-site dermatitis (<3%)
Application-site pain (<2%)
Application-site pruritus (<2%)

OXYMORPHONE

Trade name: Opana (Endo)
Indications: Pain (moderate to severe)
Class: Analgesic, Opiate agonist
Half-life: 7–9 hours
Clinically important, potentially hazardous interactions with: anticholinergics, buprenorphine, butorphanol, cimetidine, CNS depressants, MAO inhibitors, nalbuphine, pentazocine
Pregnancy category: C
Important contra-indications noted in the prescribing guidelines for: the elderly; nursing mothers; pediatric patients
Note: Contra-indicated in patients with a known hypersensitivity to morphine analogs such as codeine; in patients with respiratory depression, except in monitored settings and in the presence of resuscitative equipment; in patients with acute or severe bronchial asthma or hypercarbia; in any patient who has or is suspected of having paralytic ileus; and in patients with moderate or severe hepatic impairment.

Skin
Hyperhidrosis (<10%)
Pruritus (8%) [2]

Mucosal
Xerostomia (<10%)

Cardiovascular
Hypotension (<10%)
Tachycardia (<10%)

Central Nervous System
Anxiety (<10%)
Confusion (3%)
Fever (14%)
Headache (7%)
Sedation (<10%)
Somnolence (drowsiness) (9%) [2]
Vertigo (dizziness) (7%)

Gastrointestinal/Hepatic
Abdominal distension (<10%)
Constipation (4%) [3]
Flatulence (<10%)
Nausea (19%) [4]
Vomiting (9%) [2]

Respiratory
Hypoxia (<10%)

Local
Injection-site reactions (<10%)

OXYTETRACYCLINE

See: www.drugeruptiondata.com/drug/id/525

OXYTOCIN

Trade name: Pitocin (Par)
Indications: Induction of labor
Class: Oxytocic
Half-life: N/A
Clinically important, potentially hazardous interactions with: cyclopropane, gemeprost, halothane, prostaglandins

Pregnancy category: X

_____

Skin
 Anaphylactoid reactions/Anaphylaxis [7]

Mucosal
 Xerostomia [3]

Cardiovascular
 Bradycardia [2]

Respiratory
 Hypoxia [2]

Genitourinary
 Urinary frequency [3]
 Uterine hyperstimulation [2]

PACLITAXEL

Trade name: Taxol (Bristol-Myers Squibb)
Indications: Breast cancer and metastatic carcinoma of the ovary
Class: Antineoplastic, Taxane
Half-life: 5–17 hours
Clinically important, potentially hazardous interactions with: atazanavir, bexarotene, buspirone, carbamazepine, cisplatin, clarithromycin, delavirdine, doxorubicin, efavirenz, eletriptan, felodipine, gadobenate, gemfibrozil, indinavir, itraconazole, ketoconazole, lapatinib, lovastatin, nefazodone, nelfinavir, repaglinide, rifampin, ritonavir, rosiglitazone, saquinavir, sildenafil, simvastatin, telithromycin, teriflunomide, thalidomide, trastuzumab, triazolam
Pregnancy category: D
Important contra-indications noted in the prescribing guidelines for: the elderly; nursing mothers; pediatric patients
Note: Studies have shown that elderly patients have an increased risk of severe myelosuppression, severe neuropathy and a higher incidence of cardiovascular events.

Skin
Acneform eruption [6]
Acral erythema [4]
Anaphylactoid reactions/Anaphylaxis [3]
Dermatitis [2]
Desquamation (7%)
Edema (21%) [2]
Erythema [6]
Exanthems [2]
Fixed eruption [2]
Folliculitis [2]
Hand–foot syndrome [17]
Hypersensitivity (31–45%) [25]
Lupus erythematosus [5]
Photosensitivity [4]
Pigmentation [3]
Pruritus [6]
Pustules [2]
Radiation recall dermatitis [10]
Rash (12%) [18]
Recall reaction [2]
Scleroderma [6]
Toxicity [9]
Tumor lysis syndrome [2]
Urticaria (2–4%) [4]

Hair
Alopecia (87–100%) [47]

Nails
Leukonychia (Mees' lines) [2]
Nail changes (2%) [6]
Nail pigmentation (2%) [2]
Onycholysis [9]
Pyogenic granuloma [2]

Mucosal
Epistaxis (nosebleed) [2]
Mucosal inflammation [3]
Mucositis (17–35%) [12]
Oral lesions (3–8%)
Stomatitis (2–39%) [9]

Cardiovascular
Atrial fibrillation [2]
Bradycardia (3%)
Cardiotoxicity [3]
Congestive heart failure [3]
Flushing (28%) [3]
Hypertension [12]
Hypotension (4–12%)
Myocardial infarction [2]
Tachycardia (2%)

Central Nervous System
Anorexia [6]
Dysgeusia (taste perversion) [3]
Fever [4]
Headache [2]
Insomnia [2]
Neurotoxicity [39]
Pain [9]
Paresthesias (>10%) [5]
Peripheral neuropathy (42–70%) [35]
Seizures [2]
Vertigo (dizziness) [7]

Neuromuscular/Skeletal
Arthralgia (60%) [15]
Asthenia (fatigue) (17%) [54]
Bone or joint pain [3]
Myalgia/Myopathy (19–60%) [23]

Gastrointestinal/Hepatic
Abdominal pain (>10%) [2]
Constipation [6]
Diarrhea (38%) [39]
Dyspepsia [2]
Gastrointestinal bleeding [2]
Gastrointestinal disorder [2]
Gastrointestinal perforation [3]
Hepatotoxicity [5]
Nausea (52%) [33]
Pancreatitis [4]
Vomiting [26]

Respiratory
Cough [3]
Dyspnea (2%) [4]
Pneumonia [5]
Pneumonitis [4]
Pulmonary toxicity [5]

Endocrine/Metabolic
ALP increased [2]
ALT increased [10]
Appetite decreased [4]
AST increased [7]
Hyperglycemia [4]
SIADH [3]

Renal
Proteinuria [3]

Hematologic
Anemia (47%) [34]
Bleeding [2]
Febrile neutropenia [19]
Hemotoxicity [10]
Leukopenia (90%) [27]
Lymphopenia [2]
Myelosuppression [4]
Myelotoxicity [3]
Neutropenia (78–98%) [83]
Thrombocytopenia (4–20%) [29]

Ocular
Macular edema [10]
Maculopathy [2]

Local
Injection-site cellulitis (>10%)
Injection-site extravasation (>10%) [4]
Injection-site pain (>10%)
Injection-site reactions (13%) [2]

Other
Adverse effects [8]
Allergic reactions (15%) [8]
Death [12]
Infection (3–22%) [12]
Kounis syndrome [2]

PALBOCICLIB

Trade name: Ibrance (Pfizer)
Indications: Treatment of postmenopausal women with estrogen receptor (ER)-positive, human epidermal growth factor receptor 2 (HER2)-negative advanced breast cancer (in combination with letrozole)
Class: Kinase inhibitor
Half-life: 29 hours
Clinically important, potentially hazardous interactions with: bosentan, carbamazepine, clarithromycin, efavirenz, etravirine, grapefruit juice, indinavir, itraconazole, ketoconazole, lopinavir, modafinil, nafcillin, nefazodone, nelfinavir, phenytoin, posaconazole, rifampin, ritonavir, saquinavir, St John's wort, telaprevir, telithromycin, verapamil, voriconazole
Pregnancy category: N/A (Can cause fetal harm)
Important contra-indications noted in the prescribing guidelines for: nursing mothers; pediatric patients

Skin
Peripheral edema [2]
Rash [4]

Hair
Alopecia (22%)

Mucosal
Epistaxis (nosebleed) (11%) [2]
Stomatitis (25%)

Central Nervous System
Fever [2]
Headache [2]
Peripheral neuropathy (13%)

Neuromuscular/Skeletal
Asthenia (fatigue) (13–41%) [10]

Gastrointestinal/Hepatic
Constipation [2]
Diarrhea (21%) [6]
Nausea (25%) [7]
Vomiting (15%) [3]

Respiratory
Dyspnea [2]
Upper respiratory tract infection (31%)

Endocrine/Metabolic
Appetite decreased (16%)

Hematologic
Anemia (35%) [9]
Febrile neutropenia [7]
Leukopenia (43%) [11]
Lymphopenia [2]
Neutropenia (75%) [21]
Thrombocytopenia (17%) [6]

Other

Adverse effects [3]
Infection [2]

PALIFERMIN

Trade name: Kepivance (Amgen)
Indications: Severe oral mucositis in cancer patients
Class: Keratinocyte growth factor
Half-life: 4.5 hours
Clinically important, potentially hazardous interactions with: heparin
Pregnancy category: C
Important contra-indications noted in the prescribing guidelines for: nursing mothers

Skin

Acanthosis nigricans [2]
Edema (28%) [2]
Erythema (32%) [2]
Hand–foot syndrome [3]
Pruritus (35%) [3]
Rash (62%) [7]

Mucosal

Tongue edema (17%) [3]
Tongue pigmentation (17%)

Cardiovascular

Hypertension (~12%)

Central Nervous System

Dysesthesia (12%)
Dysgeusia (taste perversion) (16%) [4]
Fever (39%)
Pain (16%)
Paresthesias (12%)

Neuromuscular/Skeletal

Arthralgia (10%)

PALIPERIDONE

Trade name: Invega (Janssen)
Indications: Schizophrenia
Class: Antipsychotic
Half-life: ~23 hours
Clinically important, potentially hazardous interactions with: ACE inhibitors, alcohol, alpha blockers, amphetamines, angiotensin II receptor antagonists, carbamazepine, CNS depressants, dopamine agonists, droperidol, general anesthetics, itraconazole, levodopa, levomepromazine, lithium, methylphenidate, metoclopramide, myleosuppressives, P-glycoprotein inhibitors or inducers, quinagolide, risperidone, tetrabenazine, valproic acid
Pregnancy category: C
Important contra-indications noted in the prescribing guidelines for: the elderly; nursing mothers; pediatric patients
Note: Invega is not recommended for patients with creatinine clearance below 10 mL/min. Paliperidone is the active metabolite of risperidone (see separate entry).
Warning: INCREASED MORTALITY IN ELDERLY PATIENTS WITH DEMENTIA-RELATED PSYCHOSIS

Skin

Anaphylactoid reactions/Anaphylaxis (<2%)
Edema (<2%)
Peripheral edema [4]
Pruritus (<2%)
Rash (<2%)

Mucosal

Nasal congestion (<2%)
Sialorrhea (<6%) [2]
Tongue edema (3%)
Xerostomia (<4%)

Cardiovascular

Arrhythmias (<2%)
Atrioventricular block (<2%)
Bradycardia (<2%)
Bundle branch block (<3%)
Hypertension (<2%)
Palpitation (<2%) [2]
Tachycardia (<14%) [6]

Central Nervous System

Agitation (<2%) [6]
Akathisia (3–17%) [22]
Anxiety (2–9%) [9]
Depression [2]
Dysarthria (<4%) [2]
Extrapyramidal symptoms (4–23%) [15]
Headache (4–14%) [16]
Insomnia (<2%) [22]
Neuroleptic malignant syndrome [6]
Nightmares (<2%)
Parkinsonism [4]
Psychosis [3]
Schizophrenia [6]
Sleep related disorder (2–3%)
Somnolence (drowsiness) (6–26%) [13]
Tardive dyskinesia [3]
Tremor [7]
Vertigo (dizziness) (2–6%) [3]

Neuromuscular/Skeletal

Asthenia (fatigue) (<4%) [3]
Dystonia [6]
Hyperkinesia [2]
Rhabdomyolysis [3]

Gastrointestinal/Hepatic

Abdominal pain (<3%)
Constipation (4–5%) [3]
Dyspepsia (5–6%)
Flatulence (<2%)
Nausea [3]
Vomiting (3–11%)

Respiratory

Cough (<3%)
Nasopharyngitis (2–5%) [6]
Pharyngolaryngeal pain (<2%)
Pulmonary embolism [2]
Rhinitis (<3%)

Endocrine/Metabolic

ALT increased (<2%)
Amenorrhea (6%) [3]
Appetite decreased (<2%)
Appetite increased (2–3%)
AST increased (<2%)
Galactorrhea (4%) [5]
Gynecomastia (3%)
Hyperprolactinemia [10]
Hyponatremia [2]
Menstrual irregularities (<2%)
Weight gain (2–7%) [19]

Genitourinary

Ejaculatory dysfunction (<2%)
Erectile dysfunction [2]
Sexual dysfunction [3]
Urinary tract infection (<2%)

Ocular

Vision blurred (3%)

Local

Injection-site pain [9]

Other

Adverse effects [7]
Death [3]

PALIVIZUMAB

Trade name: Synagis (Medimmune)
Indications: Prophylaxis of serious lower respiratory tract disease caused by respiratory syncytial virus in pediatric patients
Class: Immunomodulator, Monoclonal antibody
Half-life: 18 days
Clinically important, potentially hazardous interactions with: none known
Pregnancy category: C

Skin

Anaphylactoid reactions/Anaphylaxis [3]
Rash (26%)

Central Nervous System

Fever [2]

Local

Injection-site bruising (<3%)
Injection-site edema (<3%)
Injection-site erythema [3]
Injection-site induration (<3%)
Injection-site pain (<9%) [2]
Injection-site reactions [2]

PALONOSETRON

Trade name: Aloxi (MGI)
Indications: Antiemetic (for cancer chemotherapy)
Class: 5-HT3 antagonist, Antiemetic, Serotonin type 3 receptor antagonist
Half-life: 40 hours
Clinically important, potentially hazardous interactions with: none known
Pregnancy category: B
Note: See also the fixed drug combination Netupitant & Palonosetron (separate entry).

Skin

Hot flashes (<15)
Pruritus (8–22%)
Rash (6%)

Central Nervous System

Anorexia [2]
Fever [2]
Headache (9%) [13]
Vertigo (dizziness) [4]

Neuromuscular/Skeletal

Asthenia (fatigue) [3]
Osteonecrosis (jaw) [13]

Gastrointestinal/Hepatic
Abdominal pain [2]
Constipation [10]
Diarrhea [2]

Endocrine/Metabolic
AST increased [2]

Renal
Nephrotoxicity [3]

Other
Hiccups [3]

PAMIDRONATE

Trade name: Aredia (Novartis)
Indications: Hypercalcemia, Paget's disease, osteogenesis imperfecta
Class: Bisphosphonate
Half-life: 1.6 hours
Clinically important, potentially hazardous interactions with: none known
Pregnancy category: D
Important contra-indications noted in the prescribing guidelines for: nursing mothers; pediatric patients

Skin
Candidiasis (6%)

Cardiovascular
Atrial fibrillation (6%)
Hypertension (6%)
Tachycardia (6%)

Central Nervous System
Anorexia (26%)
Fever (18–39%) [8]
Headache (26%)
Insomnia (22%)
Somnolence (drowsiness) (6%)

Neuromuscular/Skeletal
Arthralgia (14%) [2]
Asthenia (fatigue) (37%) [2]
Bone or joint pain [3]
Fractures [3]
Myalgia/Myopathy [3]
Osteonecrosis [19]

Gastrointestinal/Hepatic
Abdominal pain (23%)
Constipation (6%)
Dyspepsia (23%)
Nausea (54%)
Vomiting (36%) [2]

Respiratory
Cough (26%)
Flu-like syndrome [3]
Rhinitis (6%)
Sinusitis (16%)

Endocrine/Metabolic
Hypocalcemia [10]
Hypophosphatemia [2]
Hypothyroidism (6%)

Genitourinary
Azotemia (prerenal) (4%)
Urinary tract infection (19%)

Renal
Nephrotoxicity [11]

Hematologic
Anemia (43%)
Granulocytopenia (20%)

Ocular
Conjunctivitis [5]
Episcleritis [2]
Orbital inflammation [2]
Scleritis [4]
Uveitis [12]
Vision blurred [2]

Local
Injection-site reactions (18%)

PANCREATIN

See: www.drugeruptiondata.com/drug/id/1389

PANCRELIPASE

See: www.drugeruptiondata.com/drug/id/1180

PANCURONIUM

See: www.drugeruptiondata.com/drug/id/886

PANDEMIC INFLUENZA VACCINE (H1N1)

Trade names: Celvapan (Baxter), Focetria (Novartis), Pandemrix (GSK), Tamiflu (Roche)
Indications: Pandemic influenza vaccine (H1N1)
Class: Vaccine
Half-life: N/A
Clinically important, potentially hazardous interactions with: none known
Pregnancy category: C
Note: This is the vaccine for swine flu.

Skin
Lymphadenopathy (<10%)

Central Nervous System
Fever [3]
Guillain–Barré syndrome [2]
Headache (>10%)
Seizures [2]

Neuromuscular/Skeletal
Asthenia (fatigue) [2]

Other
Adverse effects [4]

PANITUMUMAB

Trade name: Vectibix (Amgen)
Indications: Metastatic colorectal carcinoma progression
Class: Antineoplastic, Biologic, Epidermal growth factor receptor (EGFR) inhibitor, Monoclonal antibody
Half-life: ~7.5 days
Clinically important, potentially hazardous interactions with: none known

Pregnancy category: C
Important contra-indications noted in the prescribing guidelines for: nursing mothers; pediatric patients
Warning: DERMATOLOGIC TOXICITY and INFUSION REACTIONS

Skin
Acneform eruption (57%) [18]
Desquamation [3]
Eczema [2]
Erythema (65%) [5]
Exfoliative dermatitis (25%) [2]
Fissures (20%) [4]
Folliculitis [3]
Hand–foot syndrome [3]
Papulopustular eruption [4]
Peripheral edema (12%)
Pruritus (57%) [9]
Rash (22%) [30]
Toxicity (90%) [26]
Xerosis (10%) [12]

Hair
Alopecia [3]
Hair changes (9%) [2]

Nails
Nail changes (9–29%) [2]
Paronychia (25%) [13]

Mucosal
Mucosal inflammation (6%)
Mucositis [4]
Stomatitis (7%) [4]

Central Nervous System
Anorexia [3]
Fever [2]
Neurotoxicity [2]

Neuromuscular/Skeletal
Asthenia (fatigue) (26%) [15]

Gastrointestinal/Hepatic
Abdominal pain (25%) [3]
Constipation (21%) [4]
Diarrhea (21%) [19]
Nausea (23%) [8]
Vomiting (19%) [8]

Respiratory
Cough (14%)
Dyspnea [2]
Pulmonary embolism [3]
Pulmonary fibrosis [3]
Pulmonary toxicity [7]

Endocrine/Metabolic
Dehydration [3]
Hypocalcemia [3]
Hypokalemia [6]
Hypomagnesemia [20]

Hematologic
Anemia [2]
Neutropenia [5]
Thrombocytopenia [3]

Ocular
Conjunctivitis (4%) [2]
Corneal perforation [2]
Eyelashes – hypertrichosis (6%)
Lacrimation (2%)
Ocular toxicity (15%) [2]
Trichomegaly [3]

Local
Infusion-related reactions (3%) [5]
Injection-site reactions (4%)

Other
Adverse effects [5]
Death [2]
Infection [3]

PANOBINOSTAT

Trade name: Farydak (Novartis)
Indications: Multiple myeloma (in combination with bortezomib and dexamethasone)
Class: Histone deacetylase (HDAC) inhibitor
Half-life: 37 hours
Clinically important, potentially hazardous interactions with: antiarrhythmics, QT prolonging agents, sensitive CYP2D6 substrates, strong CYP3A4 inducers
Pregnancy category: N/A (can cause fetal harm)
Important contra-indications noted in the prescribing guidelines for: the elderly; pediatric patients
Warning: FATAL AND SERIOUS TOXICITIES: SEVERE DIARRHEA AND CARDIAC TOXICITIES

Skin
Edema (<10%)
Erythema (<10%)
Lesions (<10%)
Peripheral edema (29%) [3]
Rash (<10%) [5]

Mucosal
Cheilitis (<10%)
Xerostomia (<10%)

Cardiovascular
Arrhythmias (12%)
Hypertension (<10%)
Hypotension (<10%) [2]
Orthostatic hypotension (<10%)
Palpitation (<10%)
QT prolongation [7]

Central Nervous System
Anorexia [5]
Chills (<10%)
Dysgeusia (taste perversion) (<10%) [3]
Fever (26%) [3]
Headache (<10%) [3]
Insomnia (<10%)
Peripheral neuropathy [8]
Syncope (<10%) [2]
Tremor (<10%)
Vertigo (dizziness) (<10%) [2]

Neuromuscular/Skeletal
Asthenia (fatigue) (60%) [29]
Back pain [2]
Joint disorder (<10%)

Gastrointestinal/Hepatic
Abdominal distension (<10%)
Abdominal pain (<10%) [4]
Colitis (<10%)
Constipation [5]
Diarrhea (68%) [27]
Dyspepsia (<10%) [2]
Flatulence (<10%)
Gastritis (<10%)

Nausea (36%) [17]
Vomiting (26%) [11]

Respiratory
Cough (<10%)
Dyspnea (<10%) [5]
Pneumonia [5]
Respiratory failure (<10%)
Wheezing (<10%)

Endocrine/Metabolic
ALP increased (<10%)
Appetite decreased (28%) [4]
Creatine phosphokinase increased (41%) [4]
Dehydration (<10%) [2]
Hyperbilirubinemia (21%) [3]
Hyperglycemia (<10%)
Hypermagnesemia (27%)
Hyperphosphatemia (29%)
Hyperuricemia (<10%)
Hypoalbuminemia (63%)
Hypocalcemia (67%) [2]
Hypokalemia (52%) [7]
Hypomagnesemia (<10%)
Hyponatremia (49%) [2]
Hypophosphatemia (63%) [4]
Hypothyroidism (<10%)
Weight loss (12%) [3]

Genitourinary
Urinary incontinence (<10%)

Renal
Renal failure (<10%)

Hematologic
Anemia (62%) [13]
Febrile neutropenia [2]
Leukopenia (81%) [5]
Lymphopenia (82%) [6]
Myelosuppression [5]
Neutropenia (75%) [20]
Sepsis [2]
Thrombocytopenia (97%) [34]

Other
Adverse effects [2]
Death (8%)

PANTOPRAZOLE

Trade names: Protium (Nycomed), Protonix (Wyeth)
Indications: Esophagitis associated with gastroesophageal reflux disease (GERD), Zollinger-Ellison syndrome, erosive esophagitis
Class: Proton pump inhibitor (PPI)
Half-life: 1 hour
Clinically important, potentially hazardous interactions with: alcohol, allopurinol, atazanavir, cefditoren, clopidogrel, conivaptan, CYP2C19 inducers and substrates, dabigatran, dasatinib, delavirdine, dexmethylphenidate, digoxin, erlotinib, eucalyptus, fluconazole, indinavir, iron salts, itraconazole, ketoconazole, lapatinib, mesalamine, methotrexate, methylphenidate, mycophenolate, nelfinavir, PEG-interferon, posaconazole, raltegravir, rilpivirine, saquinavir, tipranavir, topotecan, ulipristal, voriconazole, warfarin

Pregnancy category: B
Important contra-indications noted in the prescribing guidelines for: nursing mothers

Skin
Anaphylactoid reactions/Anaphylaxis [7]
Edema (<2%)
Facial edema (<4%)
Lupus erythematosus (discoid) [3]
Peripheral edema [2]
Photosensitivity (<2%)
Pruritus (<2%)
Rash (<2%) [3]
Urticaria (<4%) [2]

Mucosal
Xerostomia (<2%)

Central Nervous System
Depression (<2%)
Fever (>4%) [3]
Headache (12%) [2]
Vertigo (dizziness) (3%)

Neuromuscular/Skeletal
Arthralgia (<4%)
Myalgia/Myopathy (<4%)

Gastrointestinal/Hepatic
Abdominal pain (6%)
Constipation (<4%)
Diarrhea (9%)
Flatulence (<4%)
Hepatitis (<2%)
Nausea (7%)
Pancreatitis [2]
Vomiting (4%)

Respiratory
Flu-like syndrome (<10%)
Upper respiratory tract infection (>4%)

Endocrine/Metabolic
Creatine phosphokinase increased (<2%)
Hypomagnesemia [3]

Renal
Nephrotoxicity [4]

Hematologic
Leukopenia (<2%)
Thrombocytopenia (<2%) [5]

Ocular
Vision blurred (<2%)

Other
Adverse effects [2]
Allergic reactions (<4%)
Infection (<10%)
Kounis syndrome [2]

PANTOTHENIC ACID

See: www.drugeruptiondata.com/drug/id/529

PAPAVERINE

Indications: Peripheral and cerebral ischemia
Class: Opium alkaloid, Vasodilator, peripheral
Half-life: 0.5–2 hours
Clinically important, potentially hazardous interactions with: levodopa, reboxetine

Pregnancy category: C
Important contra-indications noted in the prescribing guidelines for: nursing mothers; pediatric patients

Cardiovascular
Hypotension [2]
Genitourinary
Priapism (11%) [16]

PARAMETHADIONE

See: www.drugeruptiondata.com/drug/id/532

PARICALCITOL

See: www.drugeruptiondata.com/drug/id/943

PAROMOMYCIN

Trade name: Humatin (Pfizer)
Indications: Intestinal amebiasis
Class: Antibiotic, aminoglycoside
Half-life: N/A
Clinically important, potentially hazardous interactions with: methotrexate, succinylcholine
Pregnancy category: C

Skin
Pruritus [2]

Central Nervous System
Pain [2]

Gastrointestinal/Hepatic
Abdominal pain [2]

Local
Injection-site pain [2]

PAROXETINE HYDRO-CHLORIDE

Trade names: Paxil (GSK), Paxil CR (GSK), Seroxat (GSK)
Indications: Depression, obsessive-compulsive disorder, panic disorder, social and generalized anxiety disorders, post-traumatic stress disorder
Class: Antidepressant, Selective serotonin reuptake inhibitor (SSRI)
Half-life: 21 hours
Clinically important, potentially hazardous interactions with: alcohol, amitriptyline, amphetamines, antiepileptics, aprepitant, aripiprazole, artemether/lumefantrine, asenapine, aspirin, astemizole, atomoxetine, barbiturates, clarithromycin, clozapine, cobicistat/elvitegravir/emtricitabine/tenofovir alafenamide, cobicistat/elvitegravir/emtricitabine/tenofovir disoproxil, coumarins, cyproheptadine, darifenacin, darunavir, deutetrabenazine, dexibuprofen, dextroamphetamine, diethylpropion, digitalis, digoxin, duloxetine, eluxadoline, entacapone, erythromycin, galantamine, iloperidone, isocarboxazid, linezolid, lithium, MAO inhibitors,

mazindol, methadone, methamphetamine, methylene blue, methylphenidate, metoprolol, moclobemide, molindone, NSAIDs, perphenazine, phendimetrazine, phenelzine, phenobarbital, phentermine, phenylpropanolamine, phenytoin, pimozide, primidone, procyclidine, propafenone, propranolol, pseudoephedrine, ranolazine, rasagiline, risperidone, ritonavir, selegiline, sibutramine, St John's wort, sumatriptan, sympathomimetics, tamoxifen, tamsulosin, tetrabenazine, thioridazine, tramadol, tranylcypromine, trazodone, tricyclic antidepressants, troleandomycin, tryptophan, valbenazine, vortioxetine
Pregnancy category: D
Important contra-indications noted in the prescribing guidelines for: nursing mothers; pediatric patients
Note: For menopausal indications see separate entry for paroxetine mesylate.
Warning: SUICIDALITY AND ANTIDEPRESSANT DRUGS

Skin
Diaphoresis (11%) [10]
Ecchymoses [2]
Exanthems [2]
Hyperhidrosis [2]
Photosensitivity [3]
Pruritus [3]
Rash (2%)
Vasculitis [2]

Mucosal
Xerostomia (18%) [16]

Cardiovascular
Venous thromboembolism [2]

Central Nervous System
Abnormal dreams (3–4%)
Agitation (3–6%)
Akathisia [3]
Anxiety (5%) [2]
Chills (2%) [2]
Delirium [3]
Depression [3]
Dysarthria [2]
Dysgeusia (taste perversion) (2%)
Extrapyramidal symptoms [2]
Headache (17–28%) [12]
Insomnia (11–24%) [5]
Irritability [2]
Mania [2]
Nervousness (4–9%)
Neuroleptic malignant syndrome [4]
Paresthesias (4%)
Parkinsonism [3]
Restless legs syndrome [7]
Serotonin syndrome [19]
Somnolence (drowsiness) (15–24%) [4]
Suicidal ideation [4]
Tic disorder [3]
Tremor (4–11%) [5]
Vertigo (dizziness) (6–14%) [7]
Yawning (2–4%)

Neuromuscular/Skeletal
Asthenia (fatigue) [4]
Myalgia/Myopathy (<10%)

Gastrointestinal/Hepatic
Abdominal pain (4%) [2]

Constipation (5–18%) [2]
Diarrhea (9–12%) [3]
Nausea (26%) [6]
Vomiting [2]
Respiratory
Pharyngitis (4%)
Rhinitis (3%)
Sinusitis (4%)
Endocrine/Metabolic
Galactorrhea [4]
Gynecomastia [2]
Libido decreased (3–15%)
SIADH [18]
Weight gain [8]
Genitourinary
Ejaculatory dysfunction (13–28%)
Erectile dysfunction [2]
Priapism [4]
Sexual dysfunction [7]
Otic
Hallucinations, auditory [3]
Ocular
Glaucoma [2]
Hallucinations, visual [2]
Vision impaired [2]
Other
Adverse effects [2]
Bruxism [4]
Congenital malformations [2]
Death [2]
Infection (5–6%)

PAROXETINE MESYLATE

Trade name: Brisdelle (Noven)
Indications: Vasomotor symptoms associated with the menopause
Class: Selective serotonin reuptake inhibitor (SSRI)
Half-life: N/A
Clinically important, potentially hazardous interactions with: eluxadoline, linezolid, MAO inhibitors, methylene blue, pimozide, tamoxifen, thioridazine
Pregnancy category: X
Important contra-indications noted in the prescribing guidelines for: the elderly; nursing mothers; pediatric patients
Note: Brisdelle contains a low dose of paroxetine and is not indicated for psychiatric conditions. Paroxetine mesylate is also available as Pexeva. For psychiatric indications see separate entry for paroxetine hydrochloride.
Warning: SUICIDAL THOUGHTS AND BEHAVIORS

Central Nervous System
Headache (6%)

Neuromuscular/Skeletal
Asthenia (fatigue) (5%)

Gastrointestinal/Hepatic
Nausea (4%) [2]
Vomiting (4%)

Other

Adverse effects [2]

PASIREOTIDE

See: www.drugeruptiondata.com/drug/id/3135

PATIROMER

Trade name: Veltassa (Relypsa)
Indications: Hyperkalemia
Class: Potassium binder
Half-life: N/A
Clinically important, potentially hazardous interactions with: none known
Pregnancy category: N/A (Not expected to cause fetal risk)
Important contra-indications noted in the prescribing guidelines for: pediatric patients
Warning: BINDING TO OTHER ORAL MEDICATIONS

Gastrointestinal/Hepatic

Abdominal pain (2%)
Constipation (7%) [11]
Diarrhea (5%) [5]
Flatulence (2%) [3]
Nausea (2%) [2]
Vomiting (<2%) [3]

Endocrine/Metabolic

Hypokalemia (5%) [5]
Hypomagnesemia (5–9%) [6]

PAZOPANIB

See: www.drugeruptiondata.com/drug/id/1430

PEG-INTERFERON

Trade names: PegIntron (Schering), Sylatron (Schering)
Indications: Chronic hepatitis C, melanoma
Class: Immunomodulator, Interferon
Half-life: ~40 hours
Clinically important, potentially hazardous interactions with: ACE inhibitors, acetaminophen, aldesleukin, bupivacaine, cilostazol, cinacalcet, CYP2C9 substrates, CYP2D6 substrates, delavirdine, duloxetine, estradiol, fesoterodine, fingolimod, fluoxetine, indinavir, melphalan, methadone, methylnaltrexone, pantoprazole, pegloticase, ribavirin, sildenafil, tapentadol, telbivudine, theophylline, theophylline derivatives, tiotropium, trimethoprim, voriconazole, warfarin, zidovudine
Pregnancy category: C (pregnancy category will be X when used in combination with ribavirin)
Important contra-indications noted in the prescribing guidelines for: nursing mothers; pediatric patients
Note: PEG-interferon is commonly administered with ribavirin and many of the reactions listed below are in combination therapy with this drug. Contra-indicated in patients with known hypersensitivity reactions, such as urticaria, angioedema, bronchoconstriction, anaphylaxis, Stevens-Johnson syndrome, and toxic epidermal necrolysis to interferon alpha or any other product component; or with autoimmune hepatitis.
Warning: RISK OF SERIOUS DISORDERS AND RIBAVIRIN-ASSOCIATED EFFECTS DEPRESSION AND OTHER NEUROPSYCHIA-TRIC DISORDERS

Skin

Dermatitis (7%)
Diaphoresis (6%)
DRESS syndrome [2]
Eczema [2]
Exanthems [5]
Fixed eruption [2]
Lupus erythematosus [3]
Nummular eczema [2]
Photosensitivity [4]
Pruritus (12%) [11]
Psoriasis [4]
Rash (6%) [24]
Rosacea fulminans [2]
Sarcoidosis [9]
Stevens-Johnson syndrome [2]
Toxic epidermal necrolysis [2]
Toxicity [3]
Vasculitis [2]
Vitiligo [3]
Xerosis (11%) [2]

Hair

Alopecia (22%) [5]
Alopecia areata [2]

Cardiovascular

Flushing (6%)

Central Nervous System

Anorexia (17%) [2]
Chills [2]
Cognitive impairment [2]
Depression (16–29%) [10]
Dysgeusia (taste perversion) (<10%) [5]
Fever (37%) [8]
Headache (54%) [16]
Insomnia (19%) [4]
Irritability [2]
Neurotoxicity [2]
Pain (12%)
Parkinsonism [2]
Psychosis [2]
Vertigo (dizziness) (16%) [3]

Neuromuscular/Skeletal

Arthralgia (28%) [2]
Asthenia (fatigue) (56%) [24]
Back pain (9%)
Myalgia/Myopathy (38–42%) [4]

Gastrointestinal/Hepatic

Abdominal pain (15%)
Diarrhea (16%) [4]
Hepatotoxicity [5]
Nausea (24%) [12]
Pancreatitis [4]
Vomiting (24%) [2]

Respiratory

Cough (6%)
Dyspnea (13%) [2]
Flu-like syndrome (46%) [11]

Pneumonitis [2]

Endocrine/Metabolic

ALT increased [3]
Appetite decreased [2]
AST increased [3]
Diabetes mellitus [2]
Thyroid dysfunction [2]
Weight loss (16%) [3]

Genitourinary

Urinary tract infection [2]

Renal

Nephrotoxicity [4]

Hematologic

Anemia (14%) [44]
Hemotoxicity [2]
Leukopenia [6]
Lymphopenia (14%) [2]
Neutropenia (21%) [20]
Sepsis [2]
Thrombocytopenia (5%) [15]

Otic

Hearing loss [2]
Tinnitus [2]

Ocular

Retinopathy [7]
Vision blurred (4%)

Local

Injection-site pain (2%)
Injection-site reactions (22%) [4]

Other

Adverse effects [26]
Death [2]
Infection (3%) [4]

PEGAPTANIB

Trade name: Macugen (Valeant)
Indications: Neovascular (wet) age-related macular degeneration
Class: Vascular endothelial growth factor antagonist
Half-life: 10±4 days
Clinically important, potentially hazardous interactions with: none known
Pregnancy category: B
Important contra-indications noted in the prescribing guidelines for: nursing mothers; pediatric patients
Note: Contra-indicated in patients with ocular or periocular infections.

Skin

Dermatitis (<5%)

Cardiovascular

Arterial occlusion (carotid) (<5%)
Chest pain (<5%)
Hypertension (10–40%)
Myocardial ischemia (transient) (<5%)

Central Nervous System

Cerebrovascular accident (<5%)
Headache (6–10%)
Ischemic injury (transient) (<5%)
Vertigo (dizziness) (<10%)

Neuromuscular/Skeletal

Arthralgia (<5%)

Gastrointestinal/Hepatic
Diarrhea (6–10%)
Nausea (6–10%)
Vomiting (<5%)

Respiratory
Bronchitis (6–10%)
Pleural effusion (<5%)

Endocrine/Metabolic
Diabetes mellitus (<5%)

Genitourinary
Urinary retention (<5%)
Urinary tract infection (6–10%)

Otic
Hearing loss (<5%)
Otitis media (<5%)

Ocular
Blepharitis (6–10%)
Cataract (10–40%) [2]
Conjunctival edema (<5%)
Conjunctival hemorrhage (10–40%)
Conjunctivitis (<10%)
Corneal abnormalities (<5%)
Corneal deposits (<5%)
Corneal edema (10–40%)
Endophthalmitis (<5%) [4]
Eyelid irritation (<5%)
Intraocular pressure increased (10–40%)
Meibomianitis (<5%)
Mydriasis (<5%)
Ocular edema (<5%)
Ocular hypertension (10–40%)
Ocular inflammation (<5%) [2]
Ocular pain (10–40%)
Ocular stinging (10–40%)
Ophthalmitis (<5%)
Periorbital hematoma (<5%)
Photopsia (6–10%)
Punctate keratitis (10–40%)
Reduced visual acuity (10–40%)
Retinal detachment (<10%) [5]
Retinal edema (<5%)
Vision blurred (10–40%)
Visual disturbances (10–40%)
Vitreous floaters (10–40%)

PEGASPARGASE

Trade name: Oncaspar (Enzon)
Indications: Acute lymphoblastic leukemia
Class: Antineoplastic
Half-life: 5.7 days
Clinically important, potentially hazardous interactions with: none known
Pregnancy category: C

Skin
Anaphylactoid reactions/Anaphylaxis (<5%) [2]
Angioedema (<5%)
Edema (>5%)
Rash (<5%)
Urticaria (<5%)

Cardiovascular
Hypotension (>5%)
Tachycardia (>5%)

Central Nervous System
Chills (<5%)

Fever (>5%)
Headache (<5%)
Paresthesias (<5%)
Seizures (<5%) [2]

Neuromuscular/Skeletal
Arthralgia (<5%)
Myalgia/Myopathy (<5%)

Gastrointestinal/Hepatic
Abdominal pain (<5%)
Hepatotoxicity [3]
Pancreatitis [3]

Hematologic
Leukopenia [2]
Neutropenia [2]
Thrombocytopenia [2]

Other
Allergic reactions (>5%) [6]

PEGINESATIDE

See: www.drugeruptiondata.com/drug/id/2887

PEGLOTICASE

Trade name: Krystexxa (Savient)
Indications: Chronic gout
Class: Enzyme
Half-life: N/A
Clinically important, potentially hazardous interactions with: PEG-interferon
Pregnancy category: C
Important contra-indications noted in the prescribing guidelines for: nursing mothers; pediatric patients
Note: Contra-indicated for patients at higher risk for G6PD deficiency (e.g. those of African and Mediterranean ancestry) who should be screened due to the risk of hemolysis and methemoglobinemia.
Warning: ANAPHYLAXIS and INFUSION REACTIONS

Skin
Anaphylactoid reactions/Anaphylaxis (5%) [3]
Ecchymoses (11%)

Cardiovascular
Chest pain (6%)

Central Nervous System
Vertigo (dizziness) [3]

Neuromuscular/Skeletal
Arthralgia [3]
Back pain [2]
Gouty tophi (flare) (77%) [7]

Gastrointestinal/Hepatic
Constipation (6%)
Nausea (12%) [3]
Vomiting (5%)

Respiratory
Dyspnea [2]
Nasopharyngitis (7%)

Local
Infusion-related reactions [4]
Infusion-site reactions (26%) [4]

Other
Adverse effects [2]

PEGVISOMANT

Trade name: Somavert (Pfizer)
Indications: Acromegaly
Class: Growth hormone analog
Half-life: 6 days
Clinically important, potentially hazardous interactions with: acarbose, exenatide, hydromorphone, insulin, latex, metformin, opioids, oral hypoglycemics, pioglitazone, saxagliptin, tapentadol
Pregnancy category: B
Important contra-indications noted in the prescribing guidelines for: the elderly; nursing mothers; pediatric patients

Skin
Lipohypertrophy (<5%) [2]
Peripheral edema (4–8%)

Cardiovascular
Chest pain (4–8%)
Hypertension (8%)

Central Nervous System
Pain (4–14%)
Paresthesias (7%)
Vertigo (dizziness) (4–8%)

Neuromuscular/Skeletal
Back pain (4–8%)

Gastrointestinal/Hepatic
Diarrhea (4–14%)
Hepatitis [2]
Hepatotoxicity [6]
Nausea (8–14%)

Respiratory
Flu-like syndrome (4–12%)
Sinusitis (4–8%)

Local
Injection-site reactions (8–11%) [4]

Other
Adverse effects [3]
Infection (23%)

PEMBROLIZUMAB

Synonym: lambrolizumab
Trade name: Keytruda (Merck Sharpe & Dohme)
Indications: Unresectable or metastatic melanoma and disease progression following ipilimumab and, if BRAF V600 mutation positive, a BRAF inhibitor
Class: Monoclonal antibody, Programmed death receptor-1 (PD-1) inhibitor
Half-life: 26 days
Clinically important, potentially hazardous interactions with: none known
Pregnancy category: D
Important contra-indications noted in the prescribing guidelines for: nursing mothers; pediatric patients

Skin
Bullous pemphigoid [4]
Dermatitis [2]
Exanthems [3]
Lichen planus [2]
Lichenoid eruption [3]
Peripheral edema (17%)
Pruritus (30%) [15]
Psoriasis [3]
Rash (29%) [14]
Sarcoidosis [4]
Scleroderma [2]
Toxicity [5]
Vasculitis [2]
Vitiligo (11%) [9]

Hair
Alopecia [2]

Central Nervous System
Chills (14%)
Encephalopathy [3]
Fever (11%) [5]
Headache (16%) [3]
Insomnia (14%)
Neurotoxicity [3]
Peripheral neuropathy [2]
Vertigo (dizziness) (11%)

Neuromuscular/Skeletal
Arthralgia (20%) [8]
Asthenia (fatigue) (47%) [20]
Back pain (12%)
Myalgia/Myopathy (14%) [6]
Myasthenia gravis [5]
Pain in extremities (18%)

Gastrointestinal/Hepatic
Abdominal pain (12%) [2]
Colitis [11]
Constipation (21%)
Diarrhea (20%) [11]
Hepatitis [5]
Hepatotoxicity [6]
Nausea (30%) [9]
Pancreatitis [6]
Vomiting (16%) [3]

Respiratory
Cough (30%) [5]
Dyspnea (18%) [4]
Pneumonia [4]
Pneumonitis (3%) [15]
Upper respiratory tract infection (11%)

Endocrine/Metabolic
ALT increased [4]
Appetite decreased (26%) [7]
AST increased (24%) [4]
Diabetes mellitus [5]
Hyperglycemia (40%)
Hyperthyroidism [5]
Hypertriglyceridemia (25%)
Hypoalbuminemia (34%)
Hypocalcemia (24%)
Hyponatremia (35%) [2]
Hypophysitis [7]
Hypothyroidism (8%) [13]
Thyroid dysfunction [5]
Thyroiditis [4]

Renal
Nephrotoxicity [5]
Renal failure [3]

Hematologic
Anemia (14–55%) [6]
Neutropenia [3]
Sepsis (<10%) [2]
Thrombocytopenia [4]

Ocular
Iridocyclitis [2]
Uveitis [5]

Local
Infusion-related reactions [2]

Other
Adverse effects [17]
Death [6]
Side effects [3]

PEMETREXED

Trade name: Alimta (Lilly)
Indications: Non-squamous non-small cell lung cancer, mesothelioma (in combination with cisplatin)
Class: Antimetabolite, Folic acid antagonist
Half-life: 3.5 hours
Clinically important, potentially hazardous interactions with: clozapine, digoxin, leflunomide, meloxicam, natalizumab, nephrotoxic drugs, NSAIDs, phenytoin, pimecrolimus, probenecid, pyrimethamine, sipuleucel-T, tacrolimus, trastuzumab, vaccines
Pregnancy category: D
Important contra-indications noted in the prescribing guidelines for: nursing mothers; pediatric patients

Skin
AGEP [4]
Cellulitis [3]
Desquamation (10–14%)
Edema (<5%)
Erythema multiforme (<5%)
Hypersensitivity (<5%)
Peripheral edema [4]
Pruritus (<7%)
Radiation recall dermatitis [7]
Rash (10–14%) [20]
Toxic epidermal necrolysis [5]
Toxicity [2]
Urticaria [3]
Vasculitis [2]

Hair
Alopecia (<6%) [5]

Mucosal
Epistaxis (nosebleed) [2]
Mucositis (7%) [6]
Stomatitis (7–15%) [6]

Cardiovascular
Hypertension [6]
Venous thromboembolism [2]

Central Nervous System
Anorexia (19–22%) [8]
Depression (14%)
Dysgeusia (taste perversion) [2]
Fever (<8%) [2]
Headache [4]
Insomnia [2]
Neurotoxicity (<9%)
Peripheral neuropathy [2]

Neuromuscular/Skeletal
Asthenia (fatigue) (25–34%) [34]

Gastrointestinal/Hepatic
Abdominal pain (<5%)
Constipation (<6%) [4]
Diarrhea (5–13%) [13]
Hepatotoxicity [7]
Nausea (19–31%) [17]
Vomiting (9–16%) [10]

Respiratory
Cough [2]
Dysphonia [2]
Dyspnea [4]
Hemoptysis [2]
Pharyngitis (15%)
Pulmonary toxicity [2]

Endocrine/Metabolic
ALT increased (8–10%) [3]
Appetite decreased [5]
AST increased (7–8%) [3]
Creatine phosphokinase increased (<5%) [3]
Hyperglycemia [2]
Hyperkalemia [2]
Hypokalemia [2]
Hypomagnesemia [3]
Hyponatremia [3]

Renal
Nephrotoxicity [3]

Hematologic
Anemia (15–19%) [22]
Febrile neutropenia (<5%) [10]
Hemotoxicity [3]
Leukocytopenia [2]
Leukopenia (6–12%) [11]
Lymphocytopenia [2]
Myelosuppression [3]
Neutropenia (6–11%) [22]
Sepsis [2]
Thrombocytopenia (<8%) [14]
Thrombotic complications [2]

Ocular
Conjunctivitis (<5%)
Eyelid edema [3]
Lacrimation (<5%)

Other
Adverse effects (53%) [14]
Allergic reactions (<5%)
Death [5]
Hiccups [2]
Infection (<5%) [7]

PEMIROLAST

See: www.drugeruptiondata.com/drug/id/887

PEMOLINE

See: www.drugeruptiondata.com/drug/id/534

PENBUTOLOL

See: www.drugeruptiondata.com/drug/id/535

PENCICLOVIR

See: www.drugeruptiondata.com/drug/id/1178

PENICILLAMINE

Trade name: Depen (MedPointe)
Indications: Wilson's disease, rheumatoid arthritis
Class: Antidote, Chelator, Disease-modifying antirheumatic drug (DMARD)
Half-life: 1.7–3.2 hours
Clinically important, potentially hazardous interactions with: aluminum, antacids, ascorbic acid, bone marrow suppressants, chloroquine, clozapine, cytotoxic agents, diclofenac, ferrous sulfate, food, gold & gold compounds, hydroxychloroquine, iron, magnesium, meloxicam, primaquine, probenecid, sodium picosulfate
Pregnancy category: D
Important contra-indications noted in the prescribing guidelines for: nursing mothers; pediatric patients
Note: As an antidote, it is difficult to differentiate side effects due to the drug from those due to the effects of the poison.

Skin
Bullous dermatitis [3]
Bullous pemphigoid [6]
Cicatricial pemphigoid [2]
Cutis laxa [13]
Dermatitis [4]
Dermatomyositis [14]
Edema of lip (<10%)
Ehlers–Danlos syndrome [2]
Elastosis perforans serpiginosa [43]
Epidermolysis bullosa [4]
Epidermolysis bullosa acquisita [2]
Erythema multiforme (<5%)
Exanthems [8]
Fragility [2]
Hypersensitivity [3]
Lichen planus [4]
Lichenoid eruption [7]
Lupus erythematosus [43]
Morphea [2]
Pemphigus [75]
Pemphigus erythematodes (Senear–Usher) [10]
Pemphigus foliaceus [16]
Pemphigus herpetiformis [3]
Pemphigus vulgaris [2]
Peripheral edema (<10%)
Pruritus (44–50%) [2]
Pseudoxanthoma elasticum [16]
Psoriasis [4]
Purpura [5]
Rash (44–50%) [6]
Scleroderma [7]
Toxic epidermal necrolysis [2]
Urticaria (44–50%) [2]
Vasculitis [7]

Hair
Alopecia [3]
Hirsutism [2]

Nails
Nail pigmentation [4]

Mucosal
Aphthous stomatitis [2]
Mucosal lesions (pemphigus-like) [2]
Oral ulceration [5]
Stomatitis [6]

Central Nervous System
Ageusia (taste loss) (12%) [2]
Dysgeusia (taste perversion) (metallic taste) [8]
Hypogeusia (25–33%) [2]

Neuromuscular/Skeletal
Dystonia [4]
Myasthenia gravis [73]
Polymyositis [8]

Respiratory
Pulmonary toxicity [2]

Endocrine/Metabolic
Gynecomastia [5]

Renal
Glomerulonephritis [3]
Nephrotoxicity [5]
Proteinuria [2]

Hematologic
Hemotoxicity [2]

Other
Adverse effects [2]

PENICILLIN G

Trade name: Crystapen (Britannia)
Indications: Anthrax, cellulitis, endocarditis, infections, otitis media, rheumatic fever, respiratory infections, septicemia
Class: Antibiotic, penicillin
Half-life: 4 hours
Clinically important, potentially hazardous interactions with: estrogens, methotrexate, minocycline, phenindione, probenecid, sulfinpyrazone, warfarin
Pregnancy category: B
Important contra-indications noted in the prescribing guidelines for: nursing mothers

Skin
Anaphylactoid reactions/Anaphylaxis [5]
Dermatitis [2]
Hypersensitivity [4]
Jarisch–Herxheimer reaction [21]
Nicolau syndrome [2]
Rash [4]
Serum sickness-like reaction [2]

Central Nervous System
Hoigne's syndrome [16]
Seizures [2]

Gastrointestinal/Hepatic
Hepatotoxicity [2]

Genitourinary
Cystitis [3]

Renal
Nephrotoxicity [2]

Hematologic
Thrombosis [2]

PENICILLIN V

Trade name: V-cillin K (Lilly)
Indications: Cellulitis, endocarditis, erysipelas, oral infections, otitis media, rheumatic fever, scarlet fever, tonsillitis
Class: Antibiotic, penicillin
Half-life: 4 hours
Clinically important, potentially hazardous interactions with: estrogens, methotrexate, minocycline, neomycin, phenindione, probenecid, sulfinpyrazone, warfarin
Pregnancy category: B

Skin
Anaphylactoid reactions/Anaphylaxis [2]
DRESS syndrome [2]
Hypersensitivity [3]
Serum sickness [2]
Serum sickness-like reaction [2]
Urticaria [3]

Central Nervous System
Fever [3]

Neuromuscular/Skeletal
Arthralgia [2]

Gastrointestinal/Hepatic
Diarrhea [2]

PENTAGASTRIN

See: www.drugeruptiondata.com/drug/id/538

PENTAMIDINE

Trade names: NebuPent (Astellas), Pentacarinat (Sanofi-Aventis), Pentam 300 (Astellas)
Indications: *Pneumocystis jiroveci* infection, trypanosomiasis, leishmaniasis
Class: Antiprotozoal
Half-life: 9.1–13.2 hours (intramuscular); 6.5 hours (intravenous)
Clinically important, potentially hazardous interactions with: adefovir, aminoglycosides, amiodarone, amisulpride, amitriptyline, amphotericin B, cisplatin, droperidol, erythromycin, foscarnet, insulin aspart, insulin degludec, insulin detemir, insulin glargine, insulin glulisine, ivabradine, levomepromazine, moxifloxacin, phenothiazines, saquinavir, sparfloxacin, sulpiride, tricyclic antidepressants, trifluoperazine, vancomycin
Pregnancy category: C
Important contra-indications noted in the prescribing guidelines for: nursing mothers; pediatric patients
Note: The rate of adverse side effects is increased in patients with AIDS.

Skin
Exanthems (<15%) [10]
Pruritus [2]
Rash (<47%) [4]
Toxic epidermal necrolysis [3]
Urticaria [3]

Cardiovascular
  QT prolongation [8]
  Torsades de pointes [4]

Central Nervous System
  Dysgeusia (taste perversion) (metallic taste) (2%)
  Paresthesias [2]
  Vertigo (dizziness) [2]

Neuromuscular/Skeletal
  Myalgia/Myopathy (<5%)
  Rhabdomyolysis [4]

Gastrointestinal/Hepatic
  Pancreatitis [6]

Local
  Injection-site irritation [2]
  Injection-site pain [2]
  Injection-site reactions (>10%)

Other
  Adverse effects [4]

PENTAZOCINE

See: www.drugeruptiondata.com/drug/id/540

PENTOBARBITAL

See: www.drugeruptiondata.com/drug/id/541

PENTOSAN

See: www.drugeruptiondata.com/drug/id/542

PENTOSTATIN

See: www.drugeruptiondata.com/drug/id/543

PENTOXIFYLLINE

Trade names: Pentoxil (Upsher-Smith), Trental (Sanofi-Aventis)
Indications: Peripheral vascular disease, intermittent claudication
Class: Vasodilator, peripheral, Xanthine alkaloid
Half-life: 0.4–0.8 hours
Clinically important, potentially hazardous interactions with: abciximab, benazepril, captopril, ceftobiprole, cilostazol, ciprofloxacin, citalopram, clevidipine, clopidogrel, diclofenac, enalapril, eptifibatide, fosinopril, insulin degludec, insulin glargine, insulin glulisine, irbesartan, lisinopril, meloxicam, olmesartan, quinapril, ramipril, tinzaparin
Pregnancy category: C

Mucosal
  Xerostomia [2]

Cardiovascular
  Flushing (2%) [2]

PEPLOMYCIN

See: www.drugeruptiondata.com/drug/id/1129

PERAMIVIR

Trade name: Rapivab (BioCryst)
Indications: Influenza
Class: Antiviral, Neuraminidase inhibitor
Half-life: ~20 hours
Clinically important, potentially hazardous interactions with: live attenuated influenza vaccine
Pregnancy category: C
Important contra-indications noted in the prescribing guidelines for: nursing mothers; pediatric patients

Cardiovascular
  Hypertension (2%)

Central Nervous System
  Behavioral disturbances [2]
  Insomnia (3%)

Gastrointestinal/Hepatic
  Constipation (4%)
  Diarrhea (8%) [6]
  Nausea [4]
  Vomiting [4]

Endocrine/Metabolic
  ALT increased (3%)
  AST increased (3%)
  Creatine phosphokinase increased (4%)
  Hyperglycemia (5%)

Hematologic
  Neutropenia (8%) [4]
  Thrombocytopenia [2]

PERAMPANEL

Trade name: Fycompa (Eisai)
Indications: Partial-onset seizures, primary generalized tonic-clonic seizures
Class: AMPA glutamate receptor antagonist, Anticonvulsant, Antiepileptic
Half-life: ~105 hours
Clinically important, potentially hazardous interactions with: alcohol, carbamazepine, oral contraceptives, oxcarbazepine, phenobarbital, phenytoin, primidone, rifampin, St John's wort
Pregnancy category: C
Important contra-indications noted in the prescribing guidelines for: the elderly; nursing mothers; pediatric patients
Warning: SERIOUS PSYCHIATRIC AND BEHAVIORAL REACTIONS

Skin
  Peripheral edema (<2%)

Mucosal
  Oropharyngeal pain (2%)

Central Nervous System
  Aggression (<3%) [11]
  Anxiety (2–4%)
  Balance disorder (<5%)
  Behavioral disturbances [4]
  Confusion (<2%)
  Depression [2]
  Dysarthria (<4%)
  Euphoria (<2%)
  Gait instability (<4%) [11]
  Headache (11–13%) [15]
  Hypersomnia (<3%)
  Hypoesthesia (<3%)
  Incoordination (<2%)
  Irritability (4–12%) [16]
  Memory loss (<2%)
  Mood changes (<2%)
  Neurotoxicity [2]
  Paresthesias (<2%)
  Sedation [2]
  Seizures [3]
  Somnolence (drowsiness) (9–18%) [27]
  Suicidal ideation [3]
  Vertigo (dizziness) (16–43%) [32]

Neuromuscular/Skeletal
  Arthralgia (<3%)
  Asthenia (fatigue) (<12%) [18]
  Ataxia (<8%) [6]
  Back pain (2–5%)
  Bone or joint pain (<2%)
  Myalgia/Myopathy (<3%)
  Pain in extremities (<3%)

Gastrointestinal/Hepatic
  Constipation (2–3%)
  Nausea (3–8%) [6]
  Vomiting (2–4%) [2]

Respiratory
  Cough (<4%)
  Nasopharyngitis [2]
  Upper respiratory tract infection (3–4%)

Endocrine/Metabolic
  Hyponatremia (<2%)
  Weight gain (4%) [8]

Ocular
  Diplopia (<3%)
  Vision blurred (<4%)

Other
  Adverse effects [6]

PERFLUTREN

See: www.drugeruptiondata.com/drug/id/1057

PERGOLIDE

See: www.drugeruptiondata.com/drug/id/545

PERICYAZINE

See: www.drugeruptiondata.com/drug/id/1411

PERINDOPRIL

Trade names: Aceon (Solvay), Prestalia (Symplmed)
Indications: Hypertension, coronary disease
Class: Angiotensin-converting enzyme (ACE) inhibitor, Antihypertensive
Half-life: 1.5–3 hours
Clinically important, potentially hazardous interactions with: none known
Pregnancy category: D (category C in first trimester; category D in second and third trimesters)
Important contra-indications noted in the prescribing guidelines for: nursing mothers; pediatric patients
Note: Prestalia is perindopril and amlodipine.
Warning: FETAL TOXICITY

Skin
Angioedema [6]
Edema (4%)
Peripheral edema [3]
Pruritus (<10%)
Rash (<10%)
Mucosal
Tongue edema [2]
Central Nervous System
Paresthesias (2%)
Vertigo (dizziness) [2]
Neuromuscular/Skeletal
Back pain (6%)
Respiratory
Cough (12%) [16]
Other
Adverse effects [2]

PERMETHRIN

See: www.drugeruptiondata.com/drug/id/1363

PERPHENAZINE

Trade names: Decentan (Merck), Fentazin (Goldshield), Trilafon (Schering)
Indications: Psychotic disorders, nausea and vomiting
Class: Antiemetic, Antipsychotic, Phenothiazine
Half-life: 9 hours
Clinically important, potentially hazardous interactions with: cobicistat/elvitegravir/emtricitabine/tenofovir alafenamide, cobicistat/elvitegravir/emtricitabine/tenofovir disoproxil, paroxetine hydrochloride, sparfloxacin
Pregnancy category: C
Note: Perphenazine is also used in combination with amitriptyline.

Skin
Exanthems [2]
Lupus erythematosus [4]
Rash (<10%)
Central Nervous System
Tardive dyskinesia [2]

Neuromuscular/Skeletal
Rhabdomyolysis [2]
Endocrine/Metabolic
Mastodynia (<10%)
Genitourinary
Priapism [2]

PERTUZUMAB

See: www.drugeruptiondata.com/drug/id/2937

PHENACEMIDE

See: www.drugeruptiondata.com/drug/id/1981

PHENAZOPYRIDINE

See: www.drugeruptiondata.com/drug/id/548

PHENDIMETRAZINE

See: www.drugeruptiondata.com/drug/id/549

PHENELZINE

See: www.drugeruptiondata.com/drug/id/550

PHENINDAMINE

See: www.drugeruptiondata.com/drug/id/551

PHENOBARBITAL

Synonyms: phenobarbitone; phenylethylmalonylurea
Trade name: Luminal (Sanofi-Aventis)
Indications: Insomnia, seizures
Class: Anticonvulsant, Barbiturate, CYP3A4 inducer
Half-life: 2–6 days
Clinically important, potentially hazardous interactions with: abacavir, abiraterone, afatinib, alcohol, amprenavir, anticoagulants, antihistamines, apremilast, aprepitant, betamethasone, boceprevir, brompheniramine, buclizine, buprenorphine, cabazitaxel, cabozantinib, caffeine, calcifediol, chlorpheniramine, cobicistat/elvitegravir/emtricitabine/tenofovir disoproxil, crizotinib, darunavir, dasabuvir/ombitasvir/paritaprevir/ritonavir, dasatinib, deferasirox, delavirdine, dexamethasone, dicumarol, doxercalciferol, dronedarone, eliglustat, emtricitabine/rilpivirine/tenofovir alafenamide, enzalutamide, estradiol, ethanolamine, ethosuximide, etravirine, fesoterodine, flibanserin, fluconazole, flunisolide, fosamprenavir, gefitinib, hydrocortisone, imatinib, indinavir, influenza vaccine, itraconazole, ixabepilone, lacosamide, lapatinib, ledipasvir & sofosbuvir, lisdexamfetamine, lopinavir, meperidine, methsuximide, methylprednisolone,

midazolam, mifepristone, nilotinib, ombitasvir/paritaprevir/ritonavir, oxcarbazepine, oxtriphylline, paroxetine hydrochloride, perampanel, piracetam, pizotifen, prednisolone, prednisone, propranolol, ranolazine, regorafenib, rilpivirine, riociguat, rivaroxaban, roflumilast, romidepsin, rufinamide, simeprevir, sodium oxybate, sofosbuvir, sofosbuvir & velpatasvir, sofosbuvir/velpatasvir/voxilaprevir, solifenacin, sonidegib, sorafenib, sunitinib, telaprevir, telithromycin, temsirolimus, teniposide, tenofovir alafenamide, tiagabine, ticagrelor, tipranavir, trabectedin, triamcinolone, ulipristal, vandetanib, vemurafenib, voriconazole, warfarin
Pregnancy category: D
Important contra-indications noted in the prescribing guidelines for: the elderly; nursing mothers
Note: Aromatic antiepileptic drugs, phenytoin, phenobarbital, carbamazepine and primidone, are a frequent cause of severe cutaneous adverse reactions. A strong genetic association between HLA-B*1502 and phenobarbital-induced Stevens-Johnson syndrome and toxic epidermal necrolysis has been shown in Han Chinese patients.

Skin
Anticonvulsant hypersensitivity syndrome [10]
Bullous dermatitis [5]
DRESS syndrome [13]
Erythema multiforme [7]
Erythroderma [2]
Exanthems [13]
Exfoliative dermatitis [6]
Fixed eruption [9]
Hypersensitivity [12]
Lupus erythematosus [2]
Purpura [2]
Rash [4]
Stevens-Johnson syndrome [21]
Toxic epidermal necrolysis [26]
Nails
Nail hypoplasia [2]
Mucosal
Gingival hyperplasia/hypertrophy [4]
Central Nervous System
Behavioral disturbances [3]
Somnolence (drowsiness) [2]
Vertigo (dizziness) [2]
Neuromuscular/Skeletal
Asthenia (fatigue) [2]
Hypoplasia of phalanges [2]
Gastrointestinal/Hepatic
Hepatotoxicity [2]
Local
Injection-site pain (>10%)
Injection-site thrombophlebitis (>10%)
Other
Allergic reactions [2]
Death [2]
Side effects [2]
Teratogenicity [5]

PHENOLPHTHALEIN

See: www.drugeruptiondata.com/drug/id/553

PHENOXY-BENZAMINE

See: www.drugeruptiondata.com/drug/id/554

PHENSUXIMIDE

See: www.drugeruptiondata.com/drug/id/555

PHENTERMINE

Trade names: Adipex-P (Teva), Ionamin (Celltech), Lomaira (Avanthi), Qsymia (Vivus)
Indications: Obesity
Class: Amphetamine
Half-life: 19–24 hours
Clinically important, potentially hazardous interactions with: fluoxetine, fluvoxamine, MAO inhibitors, paroxetine hydrochloride, phenelzine, sertraline, tranylcypromine
Pregnancy category: X
Important contra-indications noted in the prescribing guidelines for: the elderly; nursing mothers; pediatric patients
Note: Qsymia is phentermine and topiramate.

Mucosal
Xerostomia [6]

Cardiovascular
Cardiotoxicity [3]
Hypertension [11]
Palpitation [3]
Tachycardia [4]
Valvulopathy [17]

Central Nervous System
Anxiety [2]
Cognitive impairment [4]
Depression [3]
Dysgeusia (taste perversion) [4]
Headache [2]
Insomnia [7]
Paresthesias [6]
Vertigo (dizziness) [4]

Gastrointestinal/Hepatic
Constipation [5]

Endocrine/Metabolic
Acidosis [3]

Renal
Nephrotoxicity [2]

Other
Death [4]
Teratogenicity [2]

PHENTOLAMINE

Trade name: Regitine (Novartis)
Indications: Hypertensive episodes in pheochromocytoma
Class: Adrenergic alpha-receptor antagonist
Half-life: 19 minutes
Clinically important, potentially hazardous interactions with: none known

Pregnancy category: C
Important contra-indications noted in the prescribing guidelines for: nursing mothers

Cardiovascular
Flushing (<10%) [2]

Central Nervous System
Headache [2]

Genitourinary
Priapism [4]

PHENYLBUTAZONE

See: www.drugeruptiondata.com/drug/id/1257

PHENYLEPHRINE

Trade names: Rynatan (MedPointe), Tussi-12D (MedPointe)
Indications: Nasal congestion, glaucoma, hypotension
Class: Adrenergic alpha-receptor agonist, Sympathomimetic
Half-life: 2.5 hours
Clinically important, potentially hazardous interactions with: epinephrine, furazolidone, iobenguane, MAO inhibitors, oxprenolol, phenelzine, tranylcypromine
Pregnancy category: C
Important contra-indications noted in the prescribing guidelines for: nursing mothers; pediatric patients

Skin
Dermatitis [16]
Hypersensitivity [2]
Stinging (from nasal or ophthalmic preparations) (<10%)

Cardiovascular
Bradycardia [3]
Hypertension [2]

Ocular
Blepharoconjunctivitis [4]
Periorbital dermatitis [4]

Other
Adverse effects [2]

PHENYL-PROPANOLAMINE

See: www.drugeruptiondata.com/drug/id/872

PHENYTOIN

Synonyms: diphenylhydantoin; DPH; phenytoin sodium
Trade name: Dilantin (Pfizer)
Indications: Grand mal seizures
Class: Antiarrhythmic class Ib, Anticonvulsant, Antiepileptic, hydantoin, CYP3A4 inducer
Half-life: 7–42 hours (dose dependent)
Clinically important, potentially hazardous interactions with: abacavir, abiraterone, acitretin, afatinib, amiodarone, amitriptyline, amlodipine, amprenavir, apixaban, apremilast, aprepitant, artemether/lumefantrine, beclomethasone, boceprevir, brigatinib, brivaracetam, buprenorphine, cabazitaxel, cabozantinib, caffeine, calcium, capecitabine, caspofungin, cefazolin, ceritinib, chloramphenicol, cimetidine, ciprofloxacin, citalopram, clobazam, clorazepate, cobicistat/elvitegravir/emtricitabine/tenofovir disoproxil, cobimetinib, colesevelam, copanlisib, crizotinib, cyclosporine, cyproterone, dabigatran, daclatasvir, darunavir, dasabuvir/ombitasvir/paritaprevir/ritonavir, dasatinib, deferasirox, deflazacort, delavirdine, dexamethasone, diazoxide, disulfiram, dopamine, doxycycline, dronedarone, efavirenz, elbasvir & grazoprevir, eliglustat, emtricitabine/rilpivirine/tenofovir alafenamide, enzalutamide, erlotinib, eslicarbazepine, ethosuximide, etravirine, everolimus, ezogabine, fesoterodine, flibanserin, floxuridine, fluconazole, flunisolide, fluoxetine, fosamprenavir, gefitinib, gold & gold compounds, hydrocortisone, ibrutinib, idelalisib, imatinib, indinavir, influenza vaccine, isoniazid, isotretinoin, isradipine, itraconazole, ixabepilone, ixazomib, lacosamide, lapatinib, ledipasvir & sofosbuvir, leflunomide, levodopa, levomepromazine, levonorgestrel, lisdexamfetamine, lomustine, lopinavir, meperidine, metformin, methsuximide, methylprednisolone, metronidazole, midazolam, midostaurin, mifepristone, mivacurium, naldemedine, nelfinavir, neratinib, nifedipine, nilotinib, nilutamide, nintedanib, olaparib, ombitasvir/paritaprevir/ritonavir, omeprazole, ondansetron, osimertinib, oxcarbazepine, oxtriphylline, palbociclib, paroxetine hydrochloride, pemetrexed, perampanel, phenylbutazone, pimavanserin, piracetam, ponatinib, posaconazole, prednisolone, prednisone, propranolol, regorafenib, rifapentine, rilpivirine, riociguat, risperidone, ritonavir, rivaroxaban, roflumilast, romidepsin, saquinavir, simeprevir, sofosbuvir, sofosbuvir & velpatasvir, sofosbuvir/velpatasvir/voxilaprevir, solifenacin, sonidegib, sorafenib, St John's wort, sucralfate, sunitinib, tegafur/gimeracil/oteracil, telaprevir, telithromycin, temsirolimus, teniposide, tenofovir alafenamide, thalidomide, tiagabine, ticagrelor, ticlopidine, tinidazole, tipranavir, tizanidine, tolvaptan, triamcinolone, trimethoprim, ulipristal, uracil/tegafur, valbenazine, vandetanib, vemurafenib, venetoclax, vigabatrin, vorapaxar, voriconazole, vortioxetine, zidovudine, zuclopenthixol
Pregnancy category: D
Note: Aromatic antiepileptic drugs, phenytoin, phenobarbital, carbamazepine and primidone, are a frequent cause of severe cutaneous adverse reactions. A strong genetic association between

HLA-B*1502 and phenytoin-induced Stevens-Johnson syndrome and toxic epidermal necrolysis has been shown in Han Chinese patients. Children whose mothers receive phenytoin during pregnancy are born with fetal hydantoin syndrome. The main features of this syndrome are mental and growth retardation, unusual facies, digital and nail hypoplasia, and coarse scalp hair. Occasionally neonatal acne will be present.

Skin
Acne keloid [2]
Acneform eruption [8]
AGEP [5]
Angioedema [2]
Anticonvulsant hypersensitivity syndrome [10]
Coarse facies [4]
Dermatomyositis [2]
DRESS syndrome [32]
Erythema multiforme [11]
Erythroderma [9]
Exanthems (6–71%) [22]
Exfoliative dermatitis [15]
Fixed eruption [5]
Hypersensitivity [47]
Kaposi's varicelliform eruption [2]
Linear IgA bullous dermatosis [8]
Lupus erythematosus [19]
Lymphoma [6]
Mycosis fungoides [7]
Pemphigus [2]
Pigmentation [4]
Pruritus [5]
Pseudolymphoma [31]
Purple glove syndrome [10]
Purpura [4]
Pustules [3]
Rash (<10%) [13]
Reticular hyperplasia [2]
Serum sickness-like reaction [2]
Stevens-Johnson syndrome (14%) [58]
Toxic epidermal necrolysis (2%) [65]
Urticaria [5]
Vasculitis (2%) [11]

Hair
Alopecia [3]
Hirsutism [8]

Nails
Nail changes [2]
Nail hypoplasia [3]

Mucosal
Gingival hyperplasia/hypertrophy (>10%) [57]
Mucocutaneous eruption [2]

Cardiovascular
Bradycardia [2]
Polyarteritis nodosa [2]

Central Nervous System
Ageusia (taste loss) [2]
Fetal hydantoin syndrome [8]
Hallucinations [2]
Neurotoxicity [2]
Paresthesias [2]
Restless legs syndrome [2]

Neuromuscular/Skeletal
Digital malformations [4]
Myalgia/Myopathy [2]
Myasthenia gravis [2]
Osteoporosis [2]
Rhabdomyolysis [6]

Gastrointestinal/Hepatic
Hepatotoxicity [10]

Respiratory
Cough [2]

Ocular
Hallucinations, visual [2]

Local
Injection-site extravasation [2]
Injection-site necrosis [2]

Other
Adverse effects [3]
Death [4]
Hiccups [2]
Teratogenicity [3]

PHYSOSTIGMINE

Synonym: eserine
Indications: Miotic in glaucoma treatment, reverses toxic CNS effects caused by anticholinergic drugs
Class: Cholinesterase inhibitor
Half-life: 15–40 minutes
Clinically important, potentially hazardous interactions with: bethanechol, corticosteroids, galantamine, methacholine, succinylcholine
Pregnancy category: C
Important contra-indications noted in the prescribing guidelines for: nursing mothers
Note: Antilirium is a derivative of the Calabar bean, and its active moiety, physostigmine, is also known as eserine. Physostigmine is used to reverse the effect upon the nervous system caused by clinical or toxic dosages of drugs and herbs capable of producing the anticholinergic syndrome. Some of the drugs responsible are: amitriptyline, amoxapine, atropine, benztropine, biperiden, clidinium, cyclobenzaprine, desipramine, doxepin, hyoscyamine, imipramine, lorazepam, maprotiline, nortriptyline, protriptyline, propantheline, scopolamine, trimipramine. Some herbals that can elicit the anticholinergic syndrome are black henbane, deadly nightshade, Devil's apple, Jimson weed, Loco seeds or weeds, Matrimony vine, night blooming jessamine, stinkweed.

Skin
Diaphoresis (>10%)
Erythema (<10%)

Mucosal
Sialorrhea (>10%)

Cardiovascular
Atrial fibrillation [2]
Bradycardia [3]

Central Nervous System
Seizures (<10%) [4]
Twitching (<10%)

Gastrointestinal/Hepatic
Nausea [4]
Vomiting [3]

Ocular
Epiphora (>10%)
Ocular burning (<10%)
Ocular stinging (>10%)

PHYTONADIONE

Synonym: vitamin K₁
Trade names: Mephyton (Valeant), Vitamin K (AbbVie)
Indications: Coagulation disorders
Class: Vitamin
Half-life: 2–4 hours
Clinically important, potentially hazardous interactions with: cholestyramine, orlistat, warfarin
Pregnancy category: C
Important contra-indications noted in the prescribing guidelines for: nursing mothers; pediatric patients

Skin
Anaphylactoid reactions/Anaphylaxis [4]
Dermatitis [9]
Eczema [2]
Nicolau syndrome [2]
Scleroderma [12]
Urticaria [4]

Local
Injection-site eczematous eruption [10]
Injection-site erythema [2]
Injection-site induration [15]

Other
Allergic reactions [2]

PILOCARPINE

Trade names: Ocusert Pilo (Akorn), Pilopine (Alcon), Salagen (MGI)
Indications: Glaucoma, miosis induction, xerostomia
Class: Miotic, Muscarinic cholinergic agonist
Half-life: N/A
Clinically important, potentially hazardous interactions with: acebutolol, galantamine
Pregnancy category: C
Important contra-indications noted in the prescribing guidelines for: nursing mothers; pediatric patients

Skin
Burning (<10%)
Dermatitis [4]
Diaphoresis [5]
Edema (4%)
Hyperhidrosis [2]
Hypersensitivity (<10%)
Stinging (<10%)

Central Nervous System
Dysgeusia (taste perversion) (2%)
Headache [2]

Ocular
Cataract [2]

PIMAVANSERIN

Trade name: Nuplazid (Acadia)
Indications: Hallucinations and delusions associated with Parkinson's disease psychosis
Class: Antipsychotic
Half-life: 57 hours
Clinically important, potentially hazardous interactions with: amiodarone, carbamazepine, chlorpromazine, clarithromycin, disopyramide, drugs known to prolong the QT interval, gatifloxacin, indinavir, itraconazole, ketoconazole, moxifloxacin, phenytoin, procainamide, quinidine, rifampin, sotalol, St John's wort, strong CYP3A4 inhibitors and inducers, thioridazine, ziprasidone
Pregnancy category: N/A (No data available)
Important contra-indications noted in the prescribing guidelines for: the elderly; nursing mothers; pediatric patients
Warning: INCREASED MORTALITY IN ELDERLY PATIENTS WITH DEMENTIA-RELATED PSYCHOSIS

Skin
Peripheral edema (7%) [2]

Central Nervous System
Confusion (6%)
Gait instability (2%) [3]
Hallucinations (5%) [2]

Gastrointestinal/Hepatic
Constipation (4%)
Nausea (7%)

Genitourinary
Urinary tract infection [2]

PIMECROLIMUS

Trade name: Elidel (Valeant)
Indications: Second-line therapy for the short-term and non-continuous chronic treatment of mild to moderate atopic dermatitis
Class: Immunomodulator, Macrolactam
Half-life: N/A
Clinically important, potentially hazardous interactions with: abatacept, alcohol, alefacept, aprepitant, azacitidine, betamethasone, cabazitaxel, calcium channel blockers, cimetidine, conivaptan, CYP3A4 inhibitors, darunavir, delavirdine, denileukin, docetaxel, efavirenz, erythromycin, fingolimod, fluconazole, gefitinib, immunosuppressants, indinavir, itraconazole, ketoconazole, lapatinib, leflunomide, lenalidomide, oxaliplatin, pazopanib, pemetrexed, telithromycin, temsirolimus, triamcinolone, voriconazole
Pregnancy category: C
Important contra-indications noted in the prescribing guidelines for: nursing mothers; pediatric patients
Warning: LONG-TERM SAFETY OF TOPICAL CALCINEURIN INHIBITORS HAS NOT BEEN ESTABLISHED.

Skin
Burning [4]
Dermatitis [2]
Peripheral edema [3]

Rosacea [5]
Tinea [3]

Cardiovascular
Cardiac arrest [2]

Respiratory
Upper respiratory tract infection (19%)

Local
Application-site burning (8–26%)
Application-site reactions (2%)

Other
Infection (5%) [2]

PIMOZIDE

Trade name: Orap (Teva)
Indications: Tourette's syndrome, schizophrenia
Class: Antipsychotic
Half-life: 50 hours
Clinically important, potentially hazardous interactions with: amitriptyline, amoxapine, amphetamines, amprenavir, aprepitant, arsenic, artemether/lumefantrine, astemizole, atazanavir, azithromycin, azole antifungals, boceprevir, ceritinib, citalopram, clarithromycin, crizotinib, darunavir, dasabuvir/ombitasvir/paritaprevir/ritonavir, dasatinib, degarelix, delavirdine, dirithromycin, dolasetron, droperidol, efavirenz, eluxadoline, enzalutamide, erythromycin, fluoxetine, fosamprenavir, grapefruit juice, imatinib, indinavir, itraconazole, ketoconazole, lapatinib, levofloxacin, levomepromazine, lopinavir, lurasidone, methylphenidate, mifepristone, moxifloxacin, nefazodone, nelfinavir, nilotinib, ombitasvir/paritaprevir/ritonavir, paroxetine hydrochloride, pazopanib, pemoline, phenothiazines, posaconazole, protease inhibitors, quinidine, quinine, ribociclib, ritonavir, saquinavir, sertraline, sotalol, sparfloxacin, sulpiride, telaprevir, telavancin, telithromycin, thioridazine, tipranavir, tricyclic antidepressants, trifluoperazine, troleandomycin, vandetanib, voriconazole, vorinostat, zileuton, ziprasidone
Pregnancy category: C
Important contra-indications noted in the prescribing guidelines for: nursing mothers; pediatric patients

Skin
Facial edema (<10%)
Rash (8%)

Mucosal
Sialorrhea (14%)
Xerostomia (>10%) [3]

Cardiovascular
QT prolongation [4]

Neuromuscular/Skeletal
Myalgia/Myopathy (3%)

Endocrine/Metabolic
Gynecomastia (>10%)

PINDOLOL

See: www.drugeruptiondata.com/drug/id/563

PIOGLITAZONE

Trade name: Actos (Takeda)
Indications: Type II diabetes
Class: Antidiabetic, CYP3A4 inducer, Thiazolidinedione
Half-life: 3–7 hours
Clinically important, potentially hazardous interactions with: alcohol, conivaptan, corticosteroids, CYP2C8 inhibitors and inducers, dapagliflozin, deferasirox, gemfibrozil, insulin, pegvisomant, pregabalin, rifampin, saxagliptin, somatropin, teriflunomide, trimethoprim
Pregnancy category: C
Important contra-indications noted in the prescribing guidelines for: nursing mothers; pediatric patients
Note: Contra-indicated in patients with established NYHA Class III or IV heart failure.
Warning: CONGESTIVE HEART FAILURE

Skin
Edema (4–11%) [29]
Peripheral edema [12]

Cardiovascular
Cardiac failure (<10%) [14]
Cardiomyopathy [3]
Cardiotoxicity [2]
Myocardial infarction [3]

Central Nervous System
Headache (9%) [4]
Stroke [2]

Neuromuscular/Skeletal
Asthenia (fatigue) (4%)
Bone loss [4]
Fractures [10]
Myalgia/Myopathy (5%)

Gastrointestinal/Hepatic
Diarrhea [4]
Hepatotoxicity [8]
Nausea [3]
Vomiting [2]

Respiratory
Nasopharyngitis [3]
Pharyngitis (5%)
Sinusitis (6%)
Upper respiratory tract infection (13%)

Endocrine/Metabolic
Hypoglycemia [10]
Weight gain [19]

Genitourinary
Bladder cancer [7]

Hematologic
Anemia (<2%) [2]
Pancytopenia [2]

Ocular
Macular edema [2]

Other
Adverse effects [4]
Death [3]
Tooth disorder (5%)

PIPECURONIUM

See: www.drugeruptiondata.com/drug/id/949

PIPERACILLIN

See: www.drugeruptiondata.com/drug/id/565

PIPERACILLIN/ TAZOBACTAM

Trade name: Zosyn (Wyeth)
Indications: Moderate to severe infections
Class: Antibacterial
Half-life: 0.7-1.2 hours
Clinically important, potentially hazardous interactions with: heparin, methotrexate
Pregnancy category: B
Important contra-indications noted in the prescribing guidelines for: nursing mothers

Skin
AGEP [2]
DRESS syndrome [3]
Hypersensitivity [2]
Rash [5]

Central Nervous System
Fever [3]
Neurotoxicity [2]

Gastrointestinal/Hepatic
Diarrhea [4]
Hepatotoxicity [3]
Nausea [2]
Vomiting [2]

Endocrine/Metabolic
Hypokalemia [3]

Renal
Nephrotoxicity [4]

Hematologic
Hemolytic anemia [3]
Hemotoxicity [2]
Thrombocytopenia [4]

Other
Adverse effects [3]

PIRACETAM

See: www.drugeruptiondata.com/drug/id/1328

PIRBUTEROL

See: www.drugeruptiondata.com/drug/id/566

PIRFENIDONE

Trade name: Esbriet (Intermune)
Indications: Idiopathic pulmonary fibrosis
Class: Immunosuppressant, Pyridone
Half-life: 3 hours
Clinically important, potentially hazardous interactions with: ciprofloxacin, fluvoxamine
Pregnancy category: C
Important contra-indications noted in the prescribing guidelines for: nursing mothers; pediatric patients

Skin
Photosensitivity (9%) [21]
Phototoxicity [2]
Pruritus (8%) [3]
Rash (30%) [13]

Cardiovascular
Chest pain (5%) [3]

Central Nervous System
Anorexia (13%) [10]
Dysgeusia (taste perversion) (6%)
Headache (22%) [3]
Insomnia (10%)
Sedation [2]
Vertigo (dizziness) (18%) [6]

Neuromuscular/Skeletal
Arthralgia (10%)
Asthenia (fatigue) (6–26%) [8]

Gastrointestinal/Hepatic
Abdominal pain (24%) [7]
Diarrhea (26%) [10]
Dyspepsia (19%) [9]
Gastroesophageal reflux (11%) [5]
Gastrointestinal disorder [2]
Hepatotoxicity [4]
Nausea (36%) [17]
Vomiting (13%) [6]

Respiratory
Cough [2]
Dyspnea [2]
Nasopharyngitis [2]
Sinusitis (11%)
Upper respiratory tract infection (27%) [2]

Endocrine/Metabolic
ALT increased [5]
Appetite decreased (8%) [3]
AST increased [5]
Weight loss (10%) [3]

Other
Adverse effects [9]

PIROXICAM

Trade name: Feldene (Pfizer)
Indications: Arthritis
Class: Non-steroidal anti-inflammatory (NSAID)
Half-life: 50 hours
Clinically important, potentially hazardous interactions with: ACE inhibitors, aspirin, furosemide, lithium, methotrexate, ritonavir, warfarin
Pregnancy category: D (pregnancy category C prior to 30 weeks gestation; category D starting at 30 weeks gestation)
Important contra-indications noted in the prescribing guidelines for: the elderly; nursing mothers
Note: NSAIDs may cause an increased risk of serious cardiovascular and gastrointestinal adverse events, which can be fatal. This risk may increase with duration of use.
Elderly patients are at greater risk for serious gastrointestinal events.
Warning: CARDIOVASCULAR AND GASTROINTESTINAL RISKS

Skin
AGEP [2]

Angioedema [3]
Dermatitis [5]
Erythema multiforme [12]
Erythroderma [2]
Exanthems (>5%) [8]
Fixed eruption [15]
Lichenoid eruption [5]
Linear IgA bullous dermatosis [3]
Pemphigus [3]
Photosensitivity [40]
Pruritus (<10%) [6]
Purpura [3]
Rash (>10%)
Stevens-Johnson syndrome [2]
Toxic epidermal necrolysis [12]
Urticaria [7]
Vasculitis [3]
Vesiculation [2]

Hair
Alopecia [3]

Mucosal
Aphthous stomatitis [4]

Central Nervous System
Anorexia (<10%)
Vertigo (dizziness) (<10%)

Gastrointestinal/Hepatic
Abdominal pain (<10%)
Constipation (<10%)
Diarrhea (<10%)
Dyspepsia (<10%)
Flatulence (<10%)
Gastrointestinal ulceration (<10%)
Nausea (<10%)
Vomiting (<10%)

Renal
Renal function abnormal (<10%)

Otic
Hearing loss [2]
Tinnitus [2]

Other
Adverse effects [2]
Side effects (47%)

PITAVASTATIN

Trade name: Livalo (Kowa)
Indications: Primary hyperlipidemia, mixed dyslipidemia
Class: Statin
Half-life: 12 hours
Clinically important, potentially hazardous interactions with: alcohol, cyclosporine, erythromycin, gemfibrozil, lopinavir, niacin, rifampin, ritonavir, sofosbuvir/velpatasvir/voxilaprevir
Pregnancy category: X
Important contra-indications noted in the prescribing guidelines for: nursing mothers; pediatric patients
Note: Contra-indicated in patients with active liver disease.

Skin
Hypersensitivity (<2%)
Rash (<2%)
Urticaria (<2%)

Central Nervous System
Headache (<2%)

Neuromuscular/Skeletal
Arthralgia (<2%)
Back pain (2–4%)
Myalgia/Myopathy (2–3%) [5]
Pain in extremities (<2%)

Gastrointestinal/Hepatic
Constipation (2–4%)
Diarrhea (2–3%)

Respiratory
Influenza (<2%)
Nasopharyngitis (<2%) [2]

Endocrine/Metabolic
ALT increased [2]
AST increased [2]
Creatine phosphokinase increased [2]

Other
Adverse effects [4]

PIZOTIFEN

See: www.drugeruptiondata.com/drug/id/1369

PLASMA (HUMAN) BLOOD PRODUCT

See: www.drugeruptiondata.com/drug/id/3195

PLECANATIDE *

Trade name: Trulance (Synergy)
Indications: Chronic idiopathic constipation
Class: Guanylate cyclase-C agonist
Half-life: N/A
Clinically important, potentially hazardous interactions with: none known
Pregnancy category: N/A (Insufficient data to inform drug-associated risks)
Important contra-indications noted in the prescribing guidelines for: the elderly; nursing mothers; pediatric patients
Warning: RISK OF SERIOUS DEHYDRATION IN PEDIATRIC PATIENTS

Gastrointestinal/Hepatic
Abdominal distension (<2%)
Abdominal pain [2]
Diarrhea (5%) [5]
Flatulence (<2%)
Nausea [2]
Vomiting [2]

Respiratory
Sinusitis (<2%)
Upper respiratory tract infection (<2%)

Endocrine/Metabolic
ALT increased (<2%)
AST increased (<2%)

PLICAMYCIN

See: www.drugeruptiondata.com/drug/id/568

PNEUMOCOCCAL VACCINE

Trade names: PCV (Lederle), PncOMP (Merck), Pneumovax II (Sanofi-Aventis), Pnu-Immune (Lederle), PPV (Lederle), Prevnar (Wyeth)
Indications: Prevention of bacteremia, meningitis, pneumonia, respiratory tract infections, otitis media, sinusitis
Class: Vaccine
Half-life: N/A
Clinically important, potentially hazardous interactions with: none known
Pregnancy category: C

Skin
Anaphylactoid reactions/Anaphylaxis [2]
Rash [2]
Serum sickness [2]
Sweet's syndrome [2]
Urticaria [5]

Central Nervous System
Fever [21]
Headache [4]
Irritability [3]
Seizures [4]
Sleep disturbances [2]

Neuromuscular/Skeletal
Arthralgia [3]
Asthenia (fatigue) [7]
Myalgia/Myopathy [4]

Respiratory
Respiratory tract infection [2]

Endocrine/Metabolic
Appetite decreased [3]

Local
Injection-site edema [8]
Injection-site erythema [10]
Injection-site induration [3]
Injection-site pain [10]
Injection-site reactions [10]

Other
Adverse effects [3]

PODOPHYLLOTOXIN

See: www.drugeruptiondata.com/drug/id/1364

POLIDOCANOL

Trade names: Asclera (Chemische Fabrik Kreussler), Varithena (BTG)
Indications: Uncomplicated spider veins and uncomplicated reticular veins in the lower extremity
Class: Sclerosant, local
Half-life: 1.5 hours
Clinically important, potentially hazardous interactions with: none known

Pregnancy category: C
Important contra-indications noted in the prescribing guidelines for: nursing mothers; pediatric patients
Note: Severe allergic reactions have been reported following polidocanol use, including anaphylactic reactions, some of them fatal. Severe reactions are more frequent with use of larger volumes (>3 mL).
Contra-indicated in patients with acute thromboembolic diseases.

Skin
Anaphylactoid reactions/Anaphylaxis [4]
Pigmentation [2]
Urticaria [2]

Cardiovascular
Cardiac arrest [2]
Phlebitis [2]

Central Nervous System
Migraine [2]

Neuromuscular/Skeletal
Leg pain [2]

Hematologic
Thrombosis [2]

Local
Injection-site hematoma (42%)
Injection-site irritation (41%)
Injection-site pain (24%)
Injection-site pigmentation (38%)
Injection-site pruritus (19%)
Injection-site reactions [3]
Injection-site thrombosis (6%)

POLYTHIAZIDE

See: www.drugeruptiondata.com/drug/id/569

POMALIDOMIDE

Trade name: Pomalyst (Celgene)
Indications: Multiple myeloma in patients who have received at least two prior therapies including lenalidomide and bortezomib
Class: Immunomodulator, Thalidomide analog
Half-life: 7.5–9.5 hours
Clinically important, potentially hazardous interactions with: ketoconazole, P-glycoprotein, rifampin
Pregnancy category: X
Important contra-indications noted in the prescribing guidelines for: nursing mothers; pediatric patients
Warning: EMBRYO-FETAL TOXICITY and VENOUS AND ARTERIAL THROMBOEMBOLISM

Skin
Edema [4]
Hyperhidrosis (6%)
Peripheral edema (23%)
Pruritus (15%)
Rash (22%) [2]
Xerosis (9%)

Mucosal
  Epistaxis (nosebleed) (15%)
Cardiovascular
  Chest pain (22%)
  Venous thromboembolism [8]
Central Nervous System
  Anxiety (11%)
  Chills (9%)
  Confusion (10%)
  Fever (19%) [3]
  Headache (13%)
  Insomnia (7%)
  Neurotoxicity (18%) [3]
  Pain (6%)
  Peripheral neuropathy (10%) [2]
  Tremor (9%) [2]
  Vertigo (dizziness) (20%)
Neuromuscular/Skeletal
  Arthralgia (16%)
  Asthenia (fatigue) (12–55%) [10]
  Back pain (32%) [3]
  Bone or joint pain (11–12%) [2]
  Muscle spasm (19%)
  Myalgia/Myopathy [2]
  Pain in extremities (5%)
Gastrointestinal/Hepatic
  Constipation (36%) [2]
  Diarrhea (34%) [2]
  Nausea (36%)
  Vomiting (14%)
Respiratory
  Cough (14%)
  Dyspnea (34%) [5]
  Pneumonia (23%) [7]
  Upper respiratory tract infection (32%)
Endocrine/Metabolic
  Appetite decreased (22%)
  Dehydration [2]
  Hypercalcemia (21%)
  Hyperglycemia (12%) [2]
  Hypocalcemia (6%)
  Hypokalemia (10%)
  Hyponatremia (10%)
  Serum creatinine increased (15%)
  Weight loss (14%)
Genitourinary
  Urinary tract infection (8%)
Renal
  Renal failure (15%)
Hematologic
  Anemia (38%) [13]
  Febrile neutropenia [2]
  Leukopenia (11%) [3]
  Lymphopenia (4%) [2]
  Myelosuppression [4]
  Neutropenia (52%) [22]
  Sepsis [2]
  Thrombocytopenia (25%) [14]
Other
  Death [3]
  Infection [9]

PONATINIB

See: www.drugeruptiondata.com/drug/id/3145

PORFIMER

See: www.drugeruptiondata.com/drug/id/1177

POSACONAZOLE

Trade name: Noxafil (Schering)
Indications: *Aspergillus* and *Candida* infection prophylaxis in immunocompromised patients
Class: Antibiotic, triazole, Antifungal, azole
Half-life: 35 hours
Clinically important, potentially hazardous interactions with: alprazolam, atazanavir, atorvastatin, boceprevir, brigatinib, cabozantinib, calcium channel blockers, cimetidine, copanlisib, cyclosporine, digoxin, dihydroergotamine, diltiazem, dronedarone, efavirenz, ergotamine, esomeprazole, everolimus, felodipine, flibanserin, fosamprenavir, HMG-CoA reductase inhibitors, ibrutinib, lapatinib, lomitapide, lovastatin, metoclopramide, midazolam, midostaurin, mifepristone, neratinib, nicardipine, nifedipine, olaparib, omeprazole, palbociclib, pantoprazole, phenytoin, pimozide, ponatinib, quinidine, regorafenib, rifabutin, rilpivirine, ritonavir, rivaroxaban, ruxolitinib, simeprevir, simvastatin, sirolimus, sonidegib, tacrolimus, telaprevir, temsirolimus, triazolam, venetoclax, verapamil, vinblastine, vincristine, vorapaxar
Pregnancy category: C
Important contra-indications noted in the prescribing guidelines for: nursing mothers; pediatric patients

Skin
  Edema (9%)
  Herpes (14%)
  Herpes simplex (3–15%)
  Hyperhidrosis (2–10%)
  Jaundice (<5%)
  Peripheral edema (15%)
  Petechiae (11%)
  Pruritus (11%)
  Rash (3–19%) [3]
  Thrombocytopenic purpura (<5%)
Mucosal
  Epistaxis (nosebleed) (14%)
  Mucositis (17%)
  Oral candidiasis (<12%)
Cardiovascular
  Hypertension (18%)
  Hypotension (14%)
  QT prolongation [3]
  Tachycardia (12%)
  Torsades de pointes (<5%)
Central Nervous System
  Anorexia (2–19%)
  Anxiety (9%)
  Dysgeusia (taste perversion) (~2%)
  Fever (6–45%)
  Headache (8–28%) [6]
  Insomnia (<17%)
  Neurotoxicity [2]
  Paresthesias (<5%)
  Rigors (<20%)
  Tremor (~2%)
  Vertigo (dizziness) (11%) [3]

Neuromuscular/Skeletal
  Arthralgia (11%)
  Asthenia (fatigue) (3–17%) [2]
  Back pain (10%)
  Bone or joint pain (16%)
  Myalgia/Myopathy (16%)
Gastrointestinal/Hepatic
  Abdominal pain (5–27%) [3]
  Constipation (21%)
  Diarrhea (10–42%) [6]
  Dyspepsia (10%)
  Flatulence [2]
  Hepatitis (<5%)
  Hepatomegaly (<5%)
  Hepatotoxicity (<5%) [6]
  Nausea (9–38%) [11]
  Vomiting (7–29%) [5]
Respiratory
  Cough (3–25%)
  Dyspnea (<20%)
  Pharyngitis (12%)
  Pneumonia (3–10%)
  Pulmonary embolism (<5%)
  Upper respiratory tract infection (7%)
Endocrine/Metabolic
  Adrenal insufficiency (<5%)
  ALP increased (3–13%)
  ALT increased (3–11%) [2]
  AST increased (6–17%) [2]
  Dehydration (<11%)
  Hyperbilirubinemia [2]
  Hyperglycemia (11%)
  Hypocalcemia (9%)
  Hypokalemia (30%)
  Hypomagnesemia (18%)
  Weight loss (<14%)
Genitourinary
  Vaginal bleeding (10%)
Renal
  Renal failure (<5%)
Hematologic
  Anemia (2–25%)
  Febrile neutropenia (20%)
  Hemolytic uremic syndrome (<5%)
  Neutropenia (4–23%)
  Thrombocytopenia (29%)
Ocular
  Vision blurred (~2%)
Other
  Adverse effects [11]
  Allergic reactions (<5%)
  Infection (18%)

POTASSIUM IODIDE

Synonyms: KI; Lugol's solution
Trade name: SSKI (Upsher-Smith)
Indications: Hyperthyroidism, erythema nodosum, sporotrichosis
Class: Antihyperthyroid, Antimycobacterial
Half-life: N/A
Clinically important, potentially hazardous interactions with: ACE inhibitors, potassium-sparing diuretics, spironolactone, triamterene

Pregnancy category: D
Important contra-indications noted in the prescribing guidelines for: nursing mothers

Skin
Acneform eruption (<10%) [3]
Angioedema (<10%)
Bullous pemphigoid [2]
Dermatitis herpetiformis [2]
Iododerma [17]
Psoriasis [2]
Urticaria (<10%)
Vasculitis [3]

Central Nervous System
Dysgeusia (taste perversion) (<10%) [2]

Gastrointestinal/Hepatic
Gastrointestinal disorder [2]

Endocrine/Metabolic
Hypothyroidism [2]

PRALATREXATE

See: www.drugeruptiondata.com/drug/id/1431

PRALIDOXIME

Trade name: Protopam (Baxter)
Indications: Muscle weakness and respiratory depression caused by organophosphate drugs which have anticholinesterase activity, antidote to overdose of anticholinesterase drugs
Class: Antidote
Half-life: 2.4–5.3 hours
Clinically important, potentially hazardous interactions with: succinylcholine
Pregnancy category: C
Important contra-indications noted in the prescribing guidelines for: the elderly; nursing mothers
Note: Pralidoxime is not effective in the treatment of poisoning due to phosphorus, inorganic phosphates, or organophosphates not having anticholinesterase activity. Pralidoxime is not indicated as an antidote for intoxication by pesticides of the carbamate class since it may increase the toxicity of carbaryl. In therapy it has been difficult to differentiate side effects due to the drug from those due to the effects of the poison.

PRAMIPEXOLE

Trade name: Mirapex (Boehringer Ingelheim)
Indications: Parkinsonism, restless legs syndrome
Class: Dopamine receptor agonist
Half-life: ~8 hours
Clinically important, potentially hazardous interactions with: levomepromazine, risperidone, zuclopenthixol
Pregnancy category: C
Important contra-indications noted in the prescribing guidelines for: nursing mothers; pediatric patients

Skin
Edema (5%)
Peripheral edema (5%) [3]

Mucosal
Xerostomia (7%) [3]

Cardiovascular
Chest pain (3%)
Hypotension (~53%) [2]
Orthostatic hypotension [2]

Central Nervous System
Abnormal dreams (11%)
Akathisia (2–3%)
Amnesia (4–6%)
Anorexia (<5%)
Compulsions [6]
Confusion [2]
Depression (2%)
Dyskinesia (17–47%) [3]
Hallucinations (5–17%) [6]
Headache (4–7%) [3]
Hyperesthesia (3%)
Impulse control disorder [10]
Insomnia (4–27%) [2]
Restless legs syndrome [2]
Somnolence (drowsiness) (9–36%) [9]
Tremor (4%)
Twitching (2%)
Vertigo (dizziness) (2–26%) [6]

Neuromuscular/Skeletal
Antecollis [2]
Arthralgia (4%)
Asthenia (fatigue) (<14%) [2]

Gastrointestinal/Hepatic
Constipation [5]
Nausea [9]
Vomiting (4%) [3]

Respiratory
Cough (3%)
Dyspnea (4%)
Rhinitis (3%)

Genitourinary
Urinary frequency (6%)
Urinary tract infection (4%)

Other
Adverse effects (2%) [5]

PRAMLINTIDE

See: www.drugeruptiondata.com/drug/id/1069

PRANLUKAST

See: www.drugeruptiondata.com/drug/id/1269

PRANOPROFEN

See: www.drugeruptiondata.com/drug/id/1278

PRASTERONE *

Trade name: Intrarosa (Endoceutics)
Indications: Moderate to severe dyspareunia, a symptom of vulvar and vaginal atrophy, due to menopause
Class: Steroid
Half-life: N/A
Clinically important, potentially hazardous interactions with: none known
Pregnancy category: N/A (Indicated for post-menopausal women only)
Note: Contra-indicated in patients with undiagnosed abnormal genital bleeding or with a known or suspected history of breast cancer.

Genitourinary
Vaginal discharge (5–14%) [2]

PRASUGREL

Trade name: Effient (Lilly)
Indications: Acute coronary syndrome in patients who are to be managed with percutaneous coronary intervention
Class: Antiplatelet, thienopyridine
Half-life: 2–15 hours
Clinically important, potentially hazardous interactions with: cangrelor, clopidogrel, conivaptan, coumarins, darunavir, delavirdine, diclofenac, indinavir, meloxicam, NSAIDs, phenindione, telithromycin, voriconazole, warfarin
Pregnancy category: B
Important contra-indications noted in the prescribing guidelines for: the elderly; nursing mothers; pediatric patients
Note: Contra-indicated in patients with active pathological bleeding, prior transient ischemic attack or stroke.
Warning: BLEEDING RISK

Skin
Hypersensitivity [2]
Peripheral edema (3%)
Rash (3%) [4]

Mucosal
Epistaxis (nosebleed) (6%)

Cardiovascular
Atrial fibrillation (3%)
Bradycardia (3%)
Chest pain (3%)
Hypertension (8%)
Hypotension (4%)

Central Nervous System
Fever (3%)
Headache (6%)
Vertigo (dizziness) (4%)

Neuromuscular/Skeletal
Asthenia (fatigue) (4%)
Back pain (5%)
Pain in extremities (3%)

Gastrointestinal/Hepatic
Diarrhea (3%)
Gastrointestinal bleeding (2%)
Nausea (5%)

Respiratory
Cough (4%)
Dyspnea (5%)
Respiratory distress [2]

Endocrine/Metabolic
Hypercholesterolemia (7%)
Hyperlipidemia (7%)

Hematologic
Anemia (2%)
Bleeding (<14%) [24]
Hemorrhage [2]
Leukopenia (3%)

Other
Adverse effects [2]
Malignant neoplasms (2%)

PRAVASTATIN

Trade names: Lipostat (Bristol-Myers Squibb), Pravachol (Bristol-Myers Squibb)
Indications: Hypercholesterolemia
Class: HMG-CoA reductase inhibitor, Statin
Half-life: ~2–3 hours
Clinically important, potentially hazardous interactions with: azithromycin, ciprofibrate, clarithromycin, colchicine, cyclosporine, darunavir, efavirenz, erythromycin, gemfibrozil, imatinib, red rice yeast, telithromycin
Pregnancy category: X
Important contra-indications noted in the prescribing guidelines for: nursing mothers

Skin
Dermatomyositis [2]
Eczema (generalized) [2]
Edema (3%)
Lichenoid eruption [2]
Pruritus [2]
Rash (5–7%) [7]

Cardiovascular
Angina (5%)
Chest pain (3–10%)

Central Nervous System
Anxiety (5%)
Fever (2%)
Headache (6%)
Nervousness (5%)
Paresthesias (3%)
Sleep disturbances (3%)
Vertigo (dizziness) (4–7%)

Neuromuscular/Skeletal
Asthenia (fatigue) (3–8%)
Bone or joint pain (25%)
Cramps (5%)
Myalgia/Myopathy (2–3%) [9]
Rhabdomyolysis [24]

Gastrointestinal/Hepatic
Abdominal distension (2%)
Diarrhea (7%)
Dyspepsia (3%)
Flatulence (3%)
Nausea (7%)
Pancreatitis [4]
Vomiting (7%)

Respiratory
Bronchitis (3%)

Cough (3–8%)
Influenza (9%)
Pharyngitis (2%)
Pulmonary toxicity (4%)
Rhinitis (4%)
Upper respiratory tract infection (6–21%)

Endocrine/Metabolic
ALT increased (3%)
Creatine phosphokinase increased (4%) [3]
GGT increased (2%)
Weight gain (4%)
Weight loss (3%)

Genitourinary
Urinary tract infection (3%)

Renal
Renal failure [2]

Ocular
Diplopia (3%)
Vision blurred (3%)

Other
Adverse effects [2]
Infection (3%)

PRAZEPAM

See: www.drugeruptiondata.com/drug/id/573

PRAZIQUANTEL

Trade name: Biltricide (Bayer)
Indications: Helmintic infections
Class: Anthelmintic
Half-life: 0.8–1.5 hours
Clinically important, potentially hazardous interactions with: dexamethasone, efavirenz, oxcarbazepine, rifampin, rifapentine
Pregnancy category: B
Important contra-indications noted in the prescribing guidelines for: nursing mothers

Skin
Diaphoresis (<10%)
Edema [2]
Pruritus [3]
Rash [2]
Urticaria [5]

Central Nervous System
Fever [2]
Headache [7]
Seizures [2]
Somnolence (drowsiness) [2]
Vertigo (dizziness) [7]

Neuromuscular/Skeletal
Asthenia (fatigue) [3]

Gastrointestinal/Hepatic
Abdominal pain [9]
Diarrhea [5]
Nausea [5]
Vomiting [6]

Other
Adverse effects [2]
Allergic reactions [2]

PRAZOSIN

See: www.drugeruptiondata.com/drug/id/575

PREDNICARBATE

See: www.drugeruptiondata.com/drug/id/1095

PREDNISOLONE

Trade names: Blephamide (Allergan), Delta-Cortef (Pharmacia), Hydeltrasol (Merck), Inflamase (Novartis), Pediapred (UCB), Prelone (Teva)
Indications: Arthralgias, asthma, dermatoses, inflammatory ocular conditions
Class: Corticosteroid, systemic
Half-life: 2–4 hours
Clinically important, potentially hazardous interactions with: aluminum, aminophylline, carbamazepine, carbimazole, cyclosporine, daclizumab, diuretics, etoposide, etretinate, grapefruit juice, indomethacin, isoniazid, itraconazole, ketoconazole, live vaccines, methotrexate, naproxen, oral contraceptives, pancuronium, phenobarbital, phenytoin, rifampin, troleandomycin
Pregnancy category: C

Skin
Acneform eruption [4]
AGEP [2]
Candidiasis [2]
Dermatitis [3]
Edema [7]
Erythema [2]
Erythema multiforme [2]
Exanthems [3]
Kaposi's sarcoma [3]
Pruritus [2]
Stevens-Johnson syndrome [2]
Toxicity [2]

Hair
Alopecia [2]

Cardiovascular
Atrial fibrillation [2]
Cardiotoxicity [4]
Flushing [2]
Hypertension [13]
Tachycardia [2]

Central Nervous System
Behavioral disturbances [2]
Depression [4]

Neuromuscular/Skeletal
Arthralgia [4]
Asthenia (fatigue) [5]
Back pain [4]
Bone or joint pain [5]
Myalgia/Myopathy [2]
Osteonecrosis [4]
Osteoporosis [32]

Gastrointestinal/Hepatic
Constipation [3]
Diarrhea [2]
Hepatotoxicity [6]

Nausea [2]
Pancreatitis [2]

Respiratory
Upper respiratory tract infection [2]

Endocrine/Metabolic
Cushing's syndrome [2]
Diabetes mellitus [4]
Hyperglycemia [3]
Hypokalemia [7]

Hematologic
Anemia [3]
Febrile neutropenia [3]
Neutropenia [4]
Thrombocytopenia [2]

Ocular
Cataract [5]
Chorioretinopathy [2]
Glaucoma [2]
Intraocular pressure increased [4]

Other
Adverse effects [11]
Allergic reactions [2]
Death [2]
Infection [17]
Side effects [4]

PREDNISONE

Trade names: Deltasone (Pharmacia),
Meticorten (Schering)
Indications: Arthralgias, asthma, dermatoses,
inflammatory ocular conditions
Class: Corticosteroid, systemic
Half-life: N/A
**Clinically important, potentially hazardous
interactions with:** aluminum, aminophylline,
aspirin, chlorambucil, cimetidine, clarithromycin,
cyclophosphamide, cyclosporine, dicumarol,
diuretics, docetaxel, estrogens, grapefruit juice,
indomethacin, influenza vaccine, itraconazole,
ketoconazole, lansoprazole, live vaccines,
methotrexate, montelukast, omeprazole, oral
contraceptives, pancuronium, phenobarbital,
phenytoin, ranitidine, rifampin, timolol,
tolbutamide, vitamin A, yellow fever vaccine
Pregnancy category: B
**Important contra-indications noted in the
prescribing guidelines for:** the elderly; nursing
mothers

Skin
Dermatitis [4]
Ecchymoses [2]
Erythema [3]
Kaposi's sarcoma [7]
Squamous cell carcinoma [2]
Thinning [2]
Toxicity [2]

Hair
Alopecia [2]

Mucosal
Stomatitis [2]

Cardiovascular
Cardiotoxicity [2]
Hypertension [7]

Central Nervous System
Headache [3]
Leukoencephalopathy [3]
Peripheral neuropathy [4]

Neuromuscular/Skeletal
Arthralgia [2]
Asthenia (fatigue) [7]
Bone or joint pain [2]
Fractures [3]
Myalgia/Myopathy [3]
Osteonecrosis [3]
Osteoporosis [23]

Gastrointestinal/Hepatic
Constipation [3]
Diarrhea [4]
Nausea [4]
Vomiting [2]

Respiratory
Cough [2]

Endocrine/Metabolic
Diabetes mellitus [2]
Hyperglycemia [3]
Weight gain [2]

Hematologic
Anemia [5]
Febrile neutropenia [3]
Leukopenia [3]
Lymphopenia [3]
Neutropenia [15]
Thrombocytopenia [10]

Ocular
Cataract [3]

Other
Adverse effects [10]
Death [3]
Infection [12]
Side effects [3]

PREGABALIN

Trade name: Lyrica (Pfizer)
Indications: Neuropathy, post-herpetic
neuralgia, partial epilepsy, fibromyalgia
Class: Anticonvulsant, GABA analog
Half-life: 6 hours
**Clinically important, potentially hazardous
interactions with:** lacosamide, pioglitazone
Pregnancy category: C
**Important contra-indications noted in the
prescribing guidelines for:** nursing mothers;
pediatric patients

Skin
Edema (2%) [9]
Peripheral edema (9%) [14]

Mucosal
Xerostomia (5%) [11]

Cardiovascular
Cardiac failure [3]
Chest pain (2%)

Central Nervous System
Anorgasmia [2]
Confusion [2]
Depression [2]
Gait instability [4]
Headache (7%) [8]

Impaired concentration [2]
Insomnia [3]
Memory loss [2]
Neurotoxicity [3]
Pain (5%)
Sedation [6]
Somnolence (drowsiness) [45]
Suicidal ideation [4]
Tremor [2]
Vertigo (dizziness) (4%) [58]

Neuromuscular/Skeletal
Asthenia (fatigue) (5%) [8]
Ataxia [8]
Back pain (2%)
Muscle spasm [2]
Myoclonus [4]
Rhabdomyolysis [3]

Gastrointestinal/Hepatic
Constipation [5]
Diarrhea [2]
Nausea [9]
Vomiting [3]

Endocrine/Metabolic
Appetite increased [2]
Weight gain [21]

Genitourinary
Erectile dysfunction [3]

Ocular
Diplopia (9%) [2]
Ocular edema [2]
Vision blurred (6%) [7]

Other
Adverse effects [6]
Infection (7%)
Side effects [2]

PRENYLAMINE

See: www.drugeruptiondata.com/drug/id/1985

PRILOCAINE

Trade name: Citanest (AstraZeneca)
Indications: Local anesthetic
Class: Membrane integrity antagonist, Potassium
channel antagonist, Sodium channel antagonist
Half-life: 2 hours
**Clinically important, potentially hazardous
interactions with:** adenosine, amide-type
anesthetics, antimalarials, co-trimoxazole,
dronedarone, nitric compounds, sulfonamides
Pregnancy category: B
**Important contra-indications noted in the
prescribing guidelines for:** nursing mothers;
pediatric patients

Skin
Angioedema [3]
Contact dermatitis [3]
Hypersensitivity [2]
Petechiae [3]
Purpura [3]

Central Nervous System
Coma [4]
Paresthesias [3]

Seizures [2]
Hematologic
Methemoglobinemia [11]
Other
Adverse effects [2]

PRIMAQUINE

See: www.drugeruptiondata.com/drug/id/576

PRIMIDONE

See: www.drugeruptiondata.com/drug/id/577

PRISTINAMYCIN

See: www.drugeruptiondata.com/drug/id/1311

PROBENECID

Indications: Gouty arthritis
Class: Uricosuric
Half-life: 6–12 hours (dose-dependent)
Clinically important, potentially hazardous interactions with: acemetacin, acetaminophen, amphotericin B, ampicillin/sulbactam, benzodiazepines, captopril, cefazolin, cefditoren, cefixime, ceftaroline fosamil, ceftazidime & avibactam, ceftriaxone, ciprofloxacin, deferiprone, doripenem, ertapenem, flucloxacillin, furosemide, gemifloxacin, glibenclamide, ketoprofen, ketorolac, levodopa, levofloxacin, meloxicam, meropenem & vaborbactam, methotrexate, moxifloxacin, norfloxacin, NSAIDs, ofloxacin, pemetrexed, penicillamine, penicillin G, penicillin V, salicylates, sulfamethoxazole, sulfonamides, torsemide, zidovudine
Pregnancy category: C
Important contra-indications noted in the prescribing guidelines for: nursing mothers; pediatric patients

Skin
Pruritus (<10%)
Rash (<10%)
Urticaria (<5%)
Mucosal
Gingivitis (<10%)
Cardiovascular
Flushing (<10%)
Renal
Nephrotoxicity [3]
Hematologic
Thrombocytopenia [2]

PROCAINAMIDE

Trade names: Procan (Pfizer), Procanbid (Pfizer)
Indications: Ventricular arrhythmias
Class: Antiarrhythmic, Antiarrhythmic class Ia
Half-life: 2.5–4.5 hours
Clinically important, potentially hazardous interactions with: abarelix, amiodarone, amisulpride, arsenic, artemether/lumefantrine, asenapine, astemizole, ciprofloxacin, enoxacin, ethoxzolamide, gatifloxacin, glycopyrrolate, glycopyrronium, imidapril, lomefloxacin, lurasidone, metformin, mivacurium, moxifloxacin, nilotinib, norfloxacin, ofloxacin, pimavanserin, quinine, quinolones, ribociclib, rocuronium, sotalol, sparfloxacin, tetrabenazine, trimethoprim, trospium, vandetanib, zofenopril
Pregnancy category: C
Important contra-indications noted in the prescribing guidelines for: nursing mothers; pediatric patients

Skin
Dermatitis (6%)
Exanthems (<8%) [5]
Hypersensitivity [2]
Lupus erythematosus (>10%) [175]
Purpura [3]
Urticaria (<5%)
Vasculitis [5]
Mucosal
Oral mucosal eruption (2%)
Cardiovascular
Hypotension [2]
QT prolongation [4]
Torsades de pointes [3]
Central Nervous System
Dysgeusia (taste perversion) (3–4%)
Psychosis [2]
Neuromuscular/Skeletal
Myalgia/Myopathy [2]
Myasthenia gravis [3]
Gastrointestinal/Hepatic
Hepatotoxicity [3]
Nausea [3]
Respiratory
Pulmonary toxicity [2]
Hematologic
Agranulocytosis [4]
Neutropenia [3]
Pancytopenia [2]
Pure red cell aplasia [3]

PROCARBAZINE

See: www.drugeruptiondata.com/drug/id/580

PROCHLORPERAZINE

Trade name: Compazine (GSK)
Indications: Psychotic disorders, control of severe nausea and vomiting
Class: Antiemetic, Antipsychotic, Muscarinic antagonist, Phenothiazine
Half-life: 23 hours
Clinically important, potentially hazardous interactions with: antihistamines, arsenic, chlorpheniramine, dofetilide, pericyazine, piperazine, quinine, quinolones, sparfloxacin
Pregnancy category: C
Important contra-indications noted in the prescribing guidelines for: the elderly; nursing mothers; pediatric patients

Skin
Anaphylactoid reactions/Anaphylaxis (<10%)
Fixed eruption [3]
Photosensitivity (<10%) [3]
Pruritus (<10%)
Rash (<10%)
Toxic epidermal necrolysis [2]
Mucosal
Xerostomia (>10%)
Central Nervous System
Akathisia [14]
Extrapyramidal symptoms [3]
Neuroleptic malignant syndrome [3]
Parkinsonism [4]
Neuromuscular/Skeletal
Dystonia [6]
Endocrine/Metabolic
Gynecomastia (<10%)

PROCYCLIDINE

See: www.drugeruptiondata.com/drug/id/582

PROGESTINS

Trade names: Aygestin (Barr), Megace (Bristol-Myers Squibb), Micronor (Ortho), Ovrette (Wyeth), Provera (Pfizer)
Indications: Prevention of pregnancy
Class: Progestogen
Half-life: N/A
Clinically important, potentially hazardous interactions with: acitretin, aprepitant, dofetilide, rosuvastatin, voriconazole

Skin
Acneform eruption [3]
Dermatitis [4]
Diaphoresis (31%)
Erythema multiforme [2]
Urticaria [2]
Cardiovascular
Flushing (12%)
Endocrine/Metabolic
Amenorrhea [2]

PROMAZINE

See: www.drugeruptiondata.com/drug/id/584

PROMETHAZINE

Trade name: Phenergan (Wyeth)
Indications: Allergic rhinitis, urticaria
Class: Histamine H1 receptor antagonist
Half-life: 10–14 hours
Clinically important, potentially hazardous interactions with: antihistamines, arsenic, chlorpheniramine, dofetilide, nalbuphine, piperazine, quinolones, sparfloxacin, zaleplon
Pregnancy category: C
Important contra-indications noted in the prescribing guidelines for: the elderly; nursing mothers; pediatric patients
Note: Not for intra-arterial or subcutaneous injection and contra-indicated in comatose states.
Warning: RESPIRATORY DEPRESSION and SEVERE TISSUE INJURY, INCLUDING GANGRENE

Skin
Dermatitis [3]
Erythema multiforme [2]
Lupus erythematosus [2]
Photosensitivity [12]
Purpura [2]
Toxic epidermal necrolysis [2]
Urticaria [3]

Mucosal
Xerostomia (<10%) [2]

Cardiovascular
QT prolongation [2]

Central Nervous System
Neuroleptic malignant syndrome [2]
Seizures [2]
Somnolence (drowsiness) [3]

PROPAFENONE

Trade name: Rythmol (Reliant)
Indications: Ventricular arrhythmias
Class: Antiarrhythmic, Antiarrhythmic class Ic
Half-life: 10–32 hours
Clinically important, potentially hazardous interactions with: amitriptyline, boceprevir, carvedilol, clozapine, cobicistat/elvitegravir/emtricitabine/tenofovir alafenamide, cobicistat/elvitegravir/emtricitabine/tenofovir disoproxil, delavirdine, digoxin, efavirenz, fosamprenavir, grapefruit juice, mirabegron, neostigmine, paroxetine hydrochloride, propranolol, pyridostigmine, rifapentine, ritonavir, telaprevir, tipranavir
Pregnancy category: C
Important contra-indications noted in the prescribing guidelines for: nursing mothers; pediatric patients

Skin
Lupus erythematosus [3]
Psoriasis [2]
Rash (<3%)

Mucosal
Oral lesions (>5%)
Xerostomia (2%)

Cardiovascular
Bradycardia [3]
Brugada syndrome [7]
Cardiotoxicity [3]
Congestive heart failure [2]
Hypotension [3]

Central Nervous System
Dysgeusia (taste perversion) (3–23%)
Seizures [3]
Syncope [2]

Gastrointestinal/Hepatic
Hepatotoxicity [8]

Local
Injection-site pain (28–90%) [4]

PROPANTHELINE

See: www.drugeruptiondata.com/drug/id/587

PROPOFOL

Trade name: Diprivan (AstraZeneca)
Indications: Induction and maintenance of anesthesia
Class: Anesthetic, general
Half-life: initial: 40 minutes; terminal: 3 days
Clinically important, potentially hazardous interactions with: zinc
Pregnancy category: B
Important contra-indications noted in the prescribing guidelines for: nursing mothers; pediatric patients

Skin
Anaphylactoid reactions/Anaphylaxis (<10%) [8]
Angioedema [2]
Exanthems (6%) [2]
Rash (5%)
Urticaria [2]

Hair
Hair pigmentation [3]

Cardiovascular
Bradycardia [14]
Brugada syndrome [2]
Cardiac failure [2]
Hypotension [17]
Tachycardia [2]

Central Nervous System
Amnesia [10]
Hallucinations [3]
Seizures [8]
Twitching (<10%)

Neuromuscular/Skeletal
Ataxia [2]
Rhabdomyolysis [9]

Gastrointestinal/Hepatic
Nausea [3]
Pancreatitis [7]
Vomiting [4]

Respiratory
Apnea [4]
Cough [2]
Hypoxia [7]
Respiratory depression [2]

Endocrine/Metabolic
Acidosis [2]

Renal
Green urine [8]

Local
Infusion-related reactions [3]
Injection-site pain (>10%) [35]

Other
Adverse effects [4]
Death [8]
Hiccups [3]

PROPOXYPHENE

See: www.drugeruptiondata.com/drug/id/589

PROPRANOLOL

Trade names: Hemangeol (Pierre Fabre), Inderal (Wyeth)
Indications: Hypertension, angina pectoris, atrial fibrillation, myocardial infarction, migraine, tremor, infantile hemangioma
Class: Antiarrhythmic, Antiarrhythmic class II, Beta adrenergic blocker, Beta blocker
Half-life: 2–6 hours
Clinically important, potentially hazardous interactions with: alcohol, aluminum hydroxide, aminophylline, amiodarone, barbiturates, bupivacaine, chlorpromazine, cholestyramine, cimetidine, ciprofloxacin, clonidine, colestipol, delavirdine, diazepam, dronedarone, epinephrine, ethanol, fluconazole, fluoxetine, fluvoxamine, haloperidol, imipramine, insulin, insulin detemir, insulin glargine, insulin glulisine, isoniazid, levothyroxine, lidocaine, neostigmine, nicardipine, nifedipine, nilutamide, nisoldipine, oxtriphylline, paroxetine hydrochloride, phenobarbital, phenytoin, propafenone, pyridostigmine, quinidine, rifampin, ritonavir, rizatriptan, sodium iodide I-131, teniposide, terbutaline, tolbutamide, verapamil, warfarin, zileuton, zolmitriptan
Pregnancy category: C
Important contra-indications noted in the prescribing guidelines for: nursing mothers; pediatric patients
Note: Cutaneous side effects of beta-receptor blockers are clinically polymorphous. They apparently appear after several months of continuous therapy.

Skin
Acneform eruption [2]
Angioedema [2]
Cold extremities [6]
Dermatitis [2]
Eczema [2]
Exanthems [4]
Lichenoid eruption [3]
Lupus erythematosus [2]
Necrosis [3]

Pemphigus [2]
Psoriasis [21]
Rash (<10%) [2]
Raynaud's phenomenon [3]
Stevens-Johnson syndrome [2]
Urticaria [3]

Hair
Alopecia [6]

Nails
Nail thickening [2]

Cardiovascular
Bradycardia [19]
Cardiac arrest [2]
Flushing [2]
Hypertension [2]
Hypotension [19]

Central Nervous System
Agitation [2]
Amnesia [2]
Confusion [2]
Delirium [3]
Hallucinations [5]
Headache [2]
Insomnia [2]
Nightmares [2]
Psychosis [3]
Sleep disturbances [9]
Somnolence (drowsiness) [4]
Vertigo (dizziness) [3]

Neuromuscular/Skeletal
Asthenia (fatigue) [4]
Myalgia/Myopathy [3]

Gastrointestinal/Hepatic
Constipation [2]
Diarrhea [6]
Gastroesophageal reflux [2]
Nausea [2]

Respiratory
Bronchospasm [3]
Wheezing [3]

Endocrine/Metabolic
Hyperkalemia [4]
Hypoglycemia [15]
Weight gain [2]

Genitourinary
Peyronie's disease [6]

Ocular
Hallucinations, visual [4]

Other
Adverse effects [10]
Death [3]
Tooth decay [2]

PROPYLTHIOURACIL

See: www.drugeruptiondata.com/drug/id/591

PROPYPHENAZONE

See: www.drugeruptiondata.com/drug/id/1405

PROTAMINE SULFATE

Indications: Heparin overdose
Class: Heparin antagonist
Half-life: 2 hours
Clinically important, potentially hazardous interactions with: none known
Pregnancy category: C

Skin
Anaphylactoid reactions/Anaphylaxis [42]
Angioedema [3]
Hypersensitivity [10]
Rash [2]
Urticaria [5]

Cardiovascular
Hypertension [2]
Hypotension [6]

Other
Adverse effects [2]
Allergic reactions [13]
Death [13]

PROTEIN C CONCENTRATE (HUMAN)

See: www.drugeruptiondata.com/drug/id/1247

PROTHROMBIN COMPLEX CONCENTRATE (HUMAN)

Synonym: PCC
Trade name: Kcentra (CSL Behring)
Indications: Urgent reversal of acquired coagulation factor deficiency induced by vitamin K antagonist therapy in adult patients with acute major bleeding
Class: Coagulant
Half-life: 4–60 hours
Clinically important, potentially hazardous interactions with: none known
Pregnancy category: C
Important contra-indications noted in the prescribing guidelines for: nursing mothers; pediatric patients
Warning: ARTERIAL AND VENOUS THROMBOEMBOLIC COMPLICATIONS

Skin
Hematoma (3%)

Cardiovascular
Hypertension (3%)
Hypotension (5%)
Orthostatic hypotension (4%)
Tachycardia (3%)

Central Nervous System
Headache (8%)
Intracranial hemorrhage (3%)
Neurotoxicity (3%)

Neuromuscular/Skeletal
Arthralgia (4%)

Gastrointestinal/Hepatic
Constipation (2%)
Nausea (4%)
Vomiting (4%)

Respiratory
Dyspnea (2%)
Hypoxia (2%)
Respiratory distress (2%)

Endocrine/Metabolic
Hypokalemia (2%)

Hematologic
Prothrombin time increased (3%)

PROTRIPTYLINE

See: www.drugeruptiondata.com/drug/id/594

PSEUDOEPHEDRINE

Trade names: Allegra-D (Sanofi-Aventis), Benadryl (Pfizer), Bromfed (Muro), Entex (Andrx), Robitussin-CF (Wyeth), Sudafed (Pfizer), Trinalin (Schering)
Indications: Nasal congestion
Class: Adrenergic alpha-receptor agonist
Half-life: 9–16 hours
Clinically important, potentially hazardous interactions with: bromocriptine, fluoxetine, fluvoxamine, furazolidone, iobenguane, MAO inhibitors, paroxetine hydrochloride, phenelzine, rasagiline, sertraline, tranylcypromine
Pregnancy category: C

Skin
AGEP [3]
Baboon syndrome (SDRIFE) [2]
Dermatitis [3]
Diaphoresis (<10%)
Erythroderma [2]
Exanthems [4]
Fixed eruption [14]

Cardiovascular
Myocardial infarction [2]
Palpitation [2]

Central Nervous System
Somnolence (drowsiness) [2]

Ocular
Hallucinations, visual [2]

PSORALENS

Trade names: Oxsoralen (Valeant), Trisoralen (Valeant)
Indications: Psoriasis, eczema, vitiligo, cutaneous T-cell lymphoma
Class: Psoralen
Half-life: 2 hours
Clinically important, potentially hazardous interactions with: none known
Pregnancy category: C

Skin
Anaphylactoid reactions/Anaphylaxis [2]
Basal cell carcinoma [3]
Bullous pemphigoid (with UVA) [13]
Burning (<10%) [3]
Dermatitis [11]
Eczema [2]
Edema (<10%)
Ephelides (<10%) [5]
Erythema [2]
Herpes simplex [2]
Herpes zoster [2]
Hypomelanosis (<10%)
Lupus erythematosus [5]
Melanoma [3]
Photosensitivity [14]
Phototoxicity [14]
Pigmentation [9]
Porokeratosis (actinic) [3]
Pruritus (>10%) [4]
Rash (<10%)
Squamous cell carcinoma [4]
Tumors (for the most part malignant) [18]
Vesiculation [2]
Vitiligo [2]

Hair
Hypertrichosis [4]

Nails
Nail pigmentation [4]
Photo-onycholysis [3]

Mucosal
Cheilitis (<10%)

Central Nervous System
Pain [3]

PYRAZINAMIDE

See: www.drugeruptiondata.com/drug/id/597

PYRIDOSTIGMINE

Trade names: Mestinon (Valeant), Regonol (Novartis)
Indications: Myasthenia gravis
Class: Acetylcholinesterase inhibitor
Half-life: ~2 hours
Clinically important, potentially hazardous interactions with: aminoglycosides, bacitracin, clindamycin, colistin, edrophonium, polymyxin B, propafenone, propranolol, quinidine, tetracyclines
Pregnancy category: B
Important contra-indications noted in the prescribing guidelines for: nursing mothers; pediatric patients

Central Nervous System
Neurotoxicity [3]
Parkinsonism [2]

Gastrointestinal/Hepatic
Abdominal pain [5]
Diarrhea [2]
Nausea [3]

Other
Adverse effects [2]
Side effects [2]

PYRIDOXINE

See: www.drugeruptiondata.com/drug/id/598

PYRILAMINE

See: www.drugeruptiondata.com/drug/id/599

PYRIMETHAMINE

Trade names: Daraprim (GSK), Fansidar (Roche)
Indications: Malaria
Class: Antimalarial, Antiprotozoal
Half-life: 80–95 hours
Clinically important, potentially hazardous interactions with: dapsone, pemetrexed, trimethoprim, zidovudine
Pregnancy category: C
Important contra-indications noted in the prescribing guidelines for: the elderly; nursing mothers
Note: Fansidar is pyrimethamine and sulfadoxine. Sulfadoxine is a sulfonamide and can be absorbed systemically. Sulfonamides can produce severe, possibly fatal, reactions such as toxic epidermal necrolysis and Stevens-Johnson syndrome.

Skin
Angioedema [2]
Bullous dermatitis [2]
DRESS syndrome [2]
Erythema multiforme [4]
Exanthems [3]
Exfoliative dermatitis [2]
Fixed eruption [3]
Hypersensitivity (>10%)
Lichenoid eruption [2]
Photosensitivity (>10%) [3]
Pigmentation [5]
Pruritus [2]
Stevens-Johnson syndrome (<10%) [25]
Toxic epidermal necrolysis [15]

Central Nervous System
Vertigo (dizziness) [2]

Neuromuscular/Skeletal
Asthenia (fatigue) [2]

Gastrointestinal/Hepatic
Diarrhea [2]
Nausea [2]
Vomiting [2]

Other
Adverse effects [2]
Death [4]

QUAZEPAM

See: www.drugeruptiondata.com/drug/id/601

QUETIAPINE

Trade name: Seroquel (AstraZeneca)
Indications: Schizophrenia, bipolar I disorder
Class: Antipsychotic, Mood stabilizer
Half-life: ~6 hours
Clinically important, potentially hazardous interactions with: alcohol, amoxapine, antihypertensive agents, arsenic, atazanavir, azithromycin, CNS acting drugs, darunavir, dolasetron, dopamine, drugs known to cause electrolyte imbalance or increase QT interval, erythromycin, fluconazole, hepatic enzyme inducers, itraconazole, ketoconazole, levodopa, methadone, P4503A inhibitors, pazopanib, telavancin, tipranavir, tricyclic antidepressants, voriconazole
Pregnancy category: C
Important contra-indications noted in the prescribing guidelines for: the elderly; nursing mothers; pediatric patients
Warning: INCREASED MORTALITY IN ELDERLY PATIENTS WITH DEMENTIA-RELATED PSYCHOSIS
SUICIDALITY AND ANTIDEPRESSANT DRUGS

Skin
  Diaphoresis (<10%)
  Hyperhidrosis (2%)
  Peripheral edema [5]
  Rash (4%)
Mucosal
  Sialorrhea [3]
  Xerostomia (9%) [22]
Cardiovascular
  Bradycardia [2]
  Hypertension (41%)
  Hypotension [6]
  Postural hypotension [2]
  QT prolongation [7]
  Tachycardia (6%) [3]
Central Nervous System
  Abnormal dreams (2–3%)
  Agitation (20%) [2]
  Akathisia (8%) [6]
  Anxiety (2–4%)
  Compulsions [3]
  Confusion [2]
  Delirium [2]
  Depression (3%) [3]
  Extrapyramidal symptoms [3]
  Headache (21%) [6]
  Hypoesthesia (2%)
  Hypomania [3]
  Impulse control disorder [2]
  Insomnia (9%)
  Mania [2]
  Neuroleptic malignant syndrome [15]
  Pain (7%)
  Paresthesias (3%)
  Parkinsonism (4%) [4]
  Psychosis [2]
  Restless legs syndrome [7]

  Sedation [15]
  Seizures [7]
  Serotonin syndrome [2]
  Sleep related disorder [2]
  Somnambulism [2]
  Somnolence (drowsiness) (18%) [23]
  Suicidal ideation [3]
  Tardive dyskinesia (5%) [3]
  Tic disorder [3]
  Tremor [3]
  Vertigo (dizziness) (11%) [13]
Neuromuscular/Skeletal
  Asthenia (fatigue) (5%) [5]
  Ataxia (2%)
  Dystonia [2]
  Pisa syndrome [2]
  Rhabdomyolysis [4]
Gastrointestinal/Hepatic
  Abdominal pain (4–7%)
  Colitis [3]
  Constipation (8%) [4]
  Dyspepsia (5%)
  Hepatotoxicity [2]
  Nausea (7%)
  Pancreatitis [4]
  Vomiting (6%)
Respiratory
  Pneumonia [2]
Endocrine/Metabolic
  ALT increased (5%)
  Appetite increased [3]
  Diabetes mellitus [2]
  Hyperglycemia [3]
  Hypertriglyceridemia [3]
  Libido decreased (2%)
  Metabolic syndrome [2]
  SIADH [2]
  Weight gain (5%) [23]
Genitourinary
  Priapism [14]
  Sexual dysfunction [2]
  Urinary retention [2]
Hematologic
  Leukopenia [2]
  Neutropenia [2]
  Thrombocytopenia [3]
Ocular
  Amblyopia (2–3%)
  Vision blurred (<4%)
Other
  Adverse effects [11]
  Death [8]
  Toothache (2–3%)

QUINACRINE

Synonym: mepacrine
Trade name: Atabrine (Winthrop)
Indications: Various infections caused by susceptible helminths
Class: Antibiotic, Antimalarial
Half-life: 4–10 hours
Clinically important, potentially hazardous interactions with: none known
Pregnancy category: N/A

Skin
  Exanthems [3]
  Exfoliative dermatitis (8%) [3]
  Fixed eruption [3]
  Lichenoid eruption (12%) [6]
  Ochronosis [2]
  Pigmentation [9]
  Squamous cell carcinoma [2]
Hair
  Alopecia (80%) [2]
Nails
  Nail pigmentation (ala nasi) (blue-gray) [2]
Mucosal
  Oral pigmentation [4]
Gastrointestinal/Hepatic
  Nausea [2]
  Vomiting [2]

QUINAGOLIDE

See: www.drugeruptiondata.com/drug/id/1377

QUINAPRIL

Trade names: Accupril (Pfizer), Accupro (Pfizer), Accuretic (Pfizer)
Indications: Hypertension, heart failure
Class: Angiotensin-converting enzyme (ACE) inhibitor, Antihypertensive, Vasodilator
Half-life: 2 hours
Clinically important, potentially hazardous interactions with: alcohol, aldesleukin, allopurinol, alpha blockers, alprostadil, amifostine, amiloride, angiotensin II receptor antagonists, antacids, antidiabetics, antihypertensives, antipsychotics, anxiolytics and hypnotics, aprotinin, azathioprine, baclofen, beta blockers, calcium channel blockers, chlortetracycline, ciprofloxacin, clonidine, corticosteroids, cyclosporine, demeclocycline, diazoxide, diuretics, doxycycline, eplerenone, estrogens, everolimus, gemifloxacin, general anesthetics, gold & gold compounds, heparins, hydralazine, insulin, levodopa, lithium, lymecycline, MAO inhibitors, metformin, methyldopa, methylphenidate, minocycline, minoxidil, moxifloxacin, moxisylyte, moxonidine, nitrates, nitroprusside, NSAIDs, ofloxacin, oxytetracycline, pentoxifylline, phosphodiesterase 5 inhibitors, potassium salts, prostacyclin analogues, quinine, quinolones, rituximab, salicylates, sirolimus, spironolactone, sulfonylureas, temsirolimus, tetracycline, tetracyclines, tigecycline, tizanidine, tolvaptan, triamterene, trimethoprim
Pregnancy category: D (category C in first trimester; category D in second and third trimesters)
Important contra-indications noted in the prescribing guidelines for: nursing mothers; pediatric patients
Note: Contra-indicated in patients with a history of angioedema related to previous treatment with an ACE inhibitor.
Warning: FETAL TOXICITY

Skin

Angioedema [9]
Diaphoresis [3]
Edema [4]
Peripheral edema [3]
Photosensitivity [2]
Pruritus [7]
Rash [5]

Central Nervous System

Dysgeusia (taste perversion) [3]

Neuromuscular/Skeletal

Myalgia/Myopathy (2%)

Respiratory

Cough [9]

Other

Adverse effects [2]

QUINESTROL

See: www.drugeruptiondata.com/drug/id/605

QUINETHAZONE

See: www.drugeruptiondata.com/drug/id/606

QUINIDINE

Indications: Tachycardia, atrial fibrillation
Class: Antiarrhythmic, Antiarrhythmic class Ia, Antimalarial, Antiprotozoal
Half-life: 6–8 hours
Clinically important, potentially hazardous interactions with: abarelix, afatinib, amiloride, amiodarone, amisulpride, amitriptyline, amprenavir, anisindione, anticoagulants, aripiprazole, arsenic, artemether/lumefantrine, asenapine, astemizole, atazanavir, boceprevir, celiprolol, ceritinib, ciprofloxacin, clevidipine, clozapine, cobicistat/elvitegravir/emtricitabine/tenofovir alafenamide, cobicistat/elvitegravir/emtricitabine/tenofovir disoproxil, crizotinib, dabigatran, darunavir, dasatinib, degarelix, delavirdine, deutetrabenazine, dicumarol, digoxin, duloxetine, eluxadoline, enoxacin, enzalutamide, ethoxzolamide, fosamprenavir, gatifloxacin, glycopyrrolate, glycopyrronium, indinavir, itraconazole, ketoconazole, lomefloxacin, lopinavir, lurasidone, metformin, mifepristone, mivacurium, moxifloxacin, naldemedine, nelfinavir, nilotinib, norfloxacin, ofloxacin, osimertinib, oxprenolol, pimavanserin, pimozide, pipecuronium, posaconazole, pristinamycin, propranolol, pyridostigmine, quinine, quinolones, ranolazine, ribociclib, rifapentine, ritonavir, rocuronium, sertindole, sotalol, sparfloxacin, sulpiride, telaprevir, telithromycin, tetrabenazine, tipranavir, tramadol, valbenazine, vecuronium, venetoclax, verapamil, voriconazole, vortioxetine, warfarin, zuclopenthixol
Pregnancy category: C
Important contra-indications noted in the prescribing guidelines for: nursing mothers; pediatric patients

Skin

Acneform eruption [2]
AGEP [2]
Dermatitis [4]
Exanthems [6]
Exfoliative dermatitis [5]
Fixed eruption [2]
Lichen planus [7]
Lichenoid eruption [6]
Livedo reticularis [6]
Lupus erythematosus [35]
Photosensitivity [21]
Pigmentation [3]
Pruritus [3]
Psoriasis [5]
Purpura [13]
Rash (<10%)
Toxic epidermal necrolysis [2]
Vasculitis [5]

Mucosal

Oral mucosal eruption [2]

Cardiovascular

Congestive heart failure [2]
Flushing [2]
QT prolongation [8]
Torsades de pointes [13]

Central Nervous System

Dysgeusia (taste perversion) (>10%)
Headache (<10%)
Syncope [2]
Tremor (2%)

Gastrointestinal/Hepatic

Diarrhea (>10%) [5]

Genitourinary

Urinary tract infection [2]

Hematologic

Thrombocytopenia [2]

QUININE

Trade name: Qualaquin (URL Pharma)
Indications: Malaria
Class: Antimalarial, Antiprotozoal
Half-life: 8–14 hours
Clinically important, potentially hazardous interactions with: amantadine, amiodarone, amitriptyline, amoxapine, anisindione, anticoagulants, arsenic, artemether/lumefantrine, astemizole, atazanavir, atorvastatin, cimetidine, cisapride, citalopram, class Ia or III antiarrhythmics, clevidipine, CYP3A4 and CYP2D6 substrates, CYP3A4 inducers or inhibitors, darunavir, dasatinib, degarelix, dicumarol, digoxin, disopyramide, dofetilide, dolasetron, droperidol, enalapril, flecainide, fosamprenavir, halofantrine, haloperidol, histamine, indinavir, lapatinib, levofloxacin, mefloquine, metformin, moxifloxacin, nelfinavir, neuromuscular blocking agents, olmesartan, oral typhoid vaccine, pazopanib, pimozide, procainamide, prochlorperazine, quinapril, quinidine, ramipril, rifampin, ritonavir, saquinavir, sotalol, succinylcholine, telavancin, telithromycin, terfenadine, tipranavir, voriconazole, vorinostat, warfarin, ziprasidone

Pregnancy category: C
Important contra-indications noted in the prescribing guidelines for: nursing mothers; pediatric patients
Note: Qualaquin (quinine sulfate) is not idicated for the prevention or treatment of nocturnal leg cramps.
Contra-indicated in patients with prolongation of QT interval, G6PD deficiency, myasthenia gravis, or optic neuritis.

Skin

Acneform eruption [2]
Acral necrosis [2]
Dermatitis [6]
Erythema multiforme [2]
Exanthems (<5%) [3]
Exfoliative dermatitis [2]
Fixed eruption [12]
Lichen planus [3]
Lichenoid eruption [3]
Livedo reticularis (photosensitive) [3]
Photosensitivity [19]
Pigmentation [6]
Purpura [13]
Raynaud's phenomenon [2]
Stevens-Johnson syndrome [2]
Thrombocytopenic purpura [8]
Toxic epidermal necrolysis [3]
Urticaria [2]
Vasculitis [5]

Cardiovascular

Cardiotoxicity [2]

Neuromuscular/Skeletal

Leg cramps [2]
Rhabdomyolysis [2]

Endocrine/Metabolic

Hypoglycemia [3]

Renal

Nephrotoxicity [2]

Hematologic

Hemolytic anemia [2]
Hemolytic uremic syndrome [16]
Thrombocytopenia [11]
Thrombotic microangiopathy [2]

Otic

Hearing loss [4]
Ototoxicity [2]
Tinnitus [9]

Ocular

Amblyopia [8]

Other

Adverse effects [3]
Death [2]

QUINUPRISTIN/ DALFOPRISTIN

See: www.drugeruptiondata.com/drug/id/609

RABEPRAZOLE

Trade name: Aciphex (Eisai) (Janssen)
Indications: Gastroesophageal reflux disease (GERD), duodenal ulcers, Zollinger-Ellison syndrome
Class: Proton pump inhibitor (PPI)
Half-life: 1–2 hours
Clinically important, potentially hazardous interactions with: atazanavir, clopidogrel, cyclosporine, digoxin, ketoconazole, rilpivirine, simvastatin, warfarin
Pregnancy category: B
Important contra-indications noted in the prescribing guidelines for: nursing mothers

Skin
Pruritus [2]
Rash [2]

Central Nervous System
Dysgeusia (taste perversion) [2]
Headache (2–5%) [4]
Pain (3%)
Vertigo (dizziness) [4]

Neuromuscular/Skeletal
Asthenia (fatigue) [3]

Gastrointestinal/Hepatic
Abdominal pain [6]
Constipation (2%)
Diarrhea (3%) [8]
Dyspepsia [3]
Flatulence [2]
Gastrointestinal bleeding [2]
Nausea [5]
Vomiting [5]

Respiratory
Cough [3]
Upper respiratory tract infection [2]

Endocrine/Metabolic
Hypomagnesemia [2]

Renal
Nephrotoxicity [2]

Other
Adverse effects [4]

RADIUM-223 DICHLORIDE

Synonym: Ra-223 dichloride
Trade name: Xofigo (Bayer)
Indications: Castration-resistant prostate cancer
Class: Radiopharmaceutical, alpha-emitting
Half-life: 11.4 days
Clinically important, potentially hazardous interactions with: none known
Pregnancy category: X
Important contra-indications noted in the prescribing guidelines for: nursing mothers; pediatric patients

Skin
Peripheral edema (13%) [3]

Central Nervous System
Anorexia [2]

Neuromuscular/Skeletal
Bone or joint pain [3]

Gastrointestinal/Hepatic
Diarrhea (25%) [6]
Nausea (36%) [5]
Vomiting (19%) [4]

Endocrine/Metabolic
Dehydration (3%)

Renal
Renal failure (3%)
Renal function abnormal (<3%)

Hematologic
Anemia (93%) [7]
Leukopenia (35%) [3]
Lymphocytopenia (72%) [3]
Myelosuppression [2]
Neutropenia (18%) [6]
Pancytopenia (2%)
Thrombocytopenia (31%) [6]

Other
Adverse effects [2]

RALOXIFENE

Trade name: Evista (Lilly)
Indications: Osteoporosis, reduction in risk of invasive breast cancer in postmenopausal women with osteoporosis or at high risk for invasive breast cancer
Class: Selective estrogen receptor modulator (SERM)
Half-life: 27.7 hours
Clinically important, potentially hazardous interactions with: cholestyramine, levothyroxine
Pregnancy category: X
Important contra-indications noted in the prescribing guidelines for: nursing mothers; pediatric patients
Warning: INCREASED RISK OF VENOUS THROMBOEMBOLISM AND DEATH FROM STROKE

Skin
Diaphoresis (3%)
Hot flashes (8–29%) [14]
Peripheral edema (3–5%) [4]
Rash (6%)

Cardiovascular
Chest pain (3%)
Venous thromboembolism [5]

Central Nervous System
Insomnia (6%)
Stroke [4]

Neuromuscular/Skeletal
Arthralgia (11–16%)
Leg cramps (6–12%) [5]
Myalgia/Myopathy (8%)

Gastrointestinal/Hepatic
Abdominal pain (7%)
Vomiting (5%)

Respiratory
Bronchitis (10%)
Flu-like syndrome (~2%)
Pharyngitis (8%)
Pneumonia (3%)

Sinusitis (10%)

Endocrine/Metabolic
Mastodynia (4%) [2]
Weight gain (9%)

Genitourinary
Vaginal bleeding (6%)
Vaginitis (4%)

Hematologic
Thrombosis [2]

Other
Adverse effects [2]
Infection (11%)

RALTEGRAVIR

Trade name: Isentress (Merck)
Indications: HIV-1 infection
Class: Antiretroviral, Integrase strand transfer inhibitor
Half-life: 9 hours
Clinically important, potentially hazardous interactions with: atazanavir, efavirenz, histamine H_2 antagonists, omeprazole, pantoprazole, proton pump inhibitors, rifampin, St John's wort, strong UGT inducers, tipranavir
Pregnancy category: C
Important contra-indications noted in the prescribing guidelines for: nursing mothers; pediatric patients

Skin
DRESS syndrome [4]
Herpes zoster (<2%)
Hypersensitivity (<2%) [7]
Pruritus (4%)
Rash [8]

Central Nervous System
Depression (<2%) [2]
Headache (2%) [9]
Insomnia (4%) [4]
Neurotoxicity [2]
Vertigo (dizziness) (<2%)

Neuromuscular/Skeletal
Asthenia (fatigue) (<2%) [4]
Myalgia/Myopathy [3]
Rhabdomyolysis [8]

Gastrointestinal/Hepatic
Abdominal pain (<2%) [2]
Diarrhea [7]
Dyspepsia (<2%)
Gastritis (<2%)
Hepatitis [2]
Hepatotoxicity (<2%) [3]
Nausea (<2%) [8]
Vomiting (<2%)

Endocrine/Metabolic
ALT increased [3]
Creatine phosphokinase increased [3]

Renal
Nephrolithiasis (<2%)
Renal failure (<2%)

Other
Adverse effects [6]

RALTITREXED

See: www.drugeruptiondata.com/drug/id/1298

RAMELTEON

Trade name: Rozerem (Takeda)
Indications: Insomnia
Class: Hypnotic, Melatonin receptor agonist
Half-life: 1–2.6 hours
Clinically important, potentially hazardous interactions with: alcohol, antifungals, CNS depressants, conivaptan, CYP1A2 inhibitors, donepezil, doxepin, droperidol, fluconazole, fluvoxamine, food, ketoconazole, levomepromazine, rifampin, rifapentine, St John's wort, voriconazole, zolpidem
Pregnancy category: C
Important contra-indications noted in the prescribing guidelines for: nursing mothers; pediatric patients

Central Nervous System
Depression (2%)
Dysgeusia (taste perversion) (2%)
Headache (7%) [8]
Insomnia (exacerbation) (3%)
Somnolence (drowsiness) (3%) [9]
Vertigo (dizziness) (4%) [6]

Neuromuscular/Skeletal
Arthralgia (2%)
Asthenia (fatigue) (3%) [4]
Myalgia/Myopathy (2%)

Gastrointestinal/Hepatic
Nausea (3%) [3]

Respiratory
Upper respiratory tract infection (3%)

Genitourinary
Urinary tract infection [2]

Other
Adverse effects [7]

RAMIPRIL

Trade names: Altace (Monarch), Tritace (Sanofi-Aventis)
Indications: Hypertension
Class: Angiotensin-converting enzyme (ACE) inhibitor, Antihypertensive, Vasodilator
Half-life: 2–17 hours
Clinically important, potentially hazardous interactions with: alcohol, aldesleukin, allopurinol, alpha blockers, alprostadil, amifostine, amiloride, angiotensin II receptor antagonists, antacids, antihypertensives, antipsychotics, azathioprine, baclofen, beta blockers, calcium channel blockers, clonidine, corticosteroids, cyclosporine, diazoxide, diuretics, eplerenone, estrogens, everolimus, general anesthetics, gold & gold compounds, heparins, hydralazine, hypotensives, insulin, levodopa, lithium, MAO inhibitors, metformin, methyldopa, minoxidil, moxisylyte, moxonidine, nitrates, nitroprusside, NSAIDs, pentoxifylline, phosphodiasterase 5 inhibitors, potassium salts, prostacyclin analogues, quinine, rituximab, sirolimus, spironolactone, sulfonylureas, telmisartan, temsirolimus, tizanidine, tolvaptan, triamterene, trimethoprim
Pregnancy category: D (category C in first trimester; category D in second and third trimesters)
Important contra-indications noted in the prescribing guidelines for: nursing mothers; pediatric patients
Note: Contra-indicated in patients with a history of angioedema related to previous treatment with an ACE inhibitor, or a history of hereditary or idiopathic angioedema.
Warning: FETAL TOXICITY

Skin
Angioedema [11]
Diaphoresis [2]
Lichen planus pemphigoides [3]
Photosensitivity [2]
Pruritus [3]
Rash [4]

Hair
Alopecia (<10%)

Cardiovascular
Angina (3%)
Flushing [2]
Hypotension (11%) [3]
Postural hypotension (2%)

Central Nervous System
Headache (5%) [2]
Syncope (2%)
Vertigo (dizziness) (2–4%) [4]

Neuromuscular/Skeletal
Asthenia (fatigue) (2%)

Gastrointestinal/Hepatic
Hepatotoxicity [2]
Nausea (2%)
Pancreatitis [2]
Vomiting (2%)

Respiratory
Cough (8–12%) [22]

Endocrine/Metabolic
Hyperkalemia [2]

Other
Adverse effects [4]

RAMUCIRUMAB

Trade name: Cyramza (Lilly)
Indications: Gastric cancer
Class: Monoclonal antibody, Vascular endothelial growth factor antagonist
Half-life: N/A
Clinically important, potentially hazardous interactions with: none known
Pregnancy category: C
Important contra-indications noted in the prescribing guidelines for: nursing mothers; pediatric patients
Warning: HEMORRHAGE, GASTROINSTINAL PERFORATION, AND IMPAIRED WOUND HEALING

Skin
Peripheral edema [2]

Rash (4%)

Mucosal
Epistaxis (nosebleed) (5%) [2]
Stomatitis [3]

Cardiovascular
Hypertension (16%) [21]
Thromboembolism (2%) [2]
Venous thromboembolism [2]

Central Nervous System
Anorexia [2]
Headache (9%) [3]

Neuromuscular/Skeletal
Asthenia (fatigue) [13]

Gastrointestinal/Hepatic
Abdominal pain [2]
Ascites [2]
Constipation [3]
Diarrhea (14%) [7]
Gastric obstruction (2%)
Gastrointestinal perforation [4]
Hepatotoxicity [2]
Nausea [4]
Vomiting [4]

Respiratory
Dyspnea [3]

Endocrine/Metabolic
Appetite decreased [2]
Hyponatremia (6%)

Renal
Proteinuria [10]

Hematologic
Anemia [5]
Bleeding [5]
Febrile neutropenia [9]
Hemorrhage [3]
Leukopenia [6]
Neutropenia (5%) [12]
Thrombocytopenia [5]

Local
Infusion-related reactions [4]

Other
Adverse effects [2]
Death [3]

RANIBIZUMAB

Trade name: Lucentis (Genentech)
Indications: Neovascular (wet) age-related macular degeneration, macular edema (following retinal vein occlusion)
Class: Monoclonal antibody, Vascular endothelial growth factor antagonist
Half-life: 9 days
Clinically important, potentially hazardous interactions with: none known
Pregnancy category: C
Important contra-indications noted in the prescribing guidelines for: nursing mothers; pediatric patients
Note: Contra-indicated in patients with ocular or periocular infections.

Cardiovascular
Atrial fibrillation (<5%)
Hypertension [4]

Myocardial infarction [2]
Thromboembolism [3]

Central Nervous System
Anxiety (<4%)
Headache (3–12%)
Insomnia (<5%)
Stroke [3]

Neuromuscular/Skeletal
Arthralgia (2–11%)
Pain in extremities (<5%)

Gastrointestinal/Hepatic
Gastroenteritis (<4%)
Nausea (<9%)

Respiratory
Bronchitis (<12%)
COPD (<7%)
Cough (2–9%)
Dyspnea (<5%)
Influenza (3–7%)
Nasopharyngitis (5–16%) [2]
Sinusitis (3–8%)
Upper respiratory tract infection (2–9%)

Endocrine/Metabolic
Hypercholesterolemia (<5%)

Genitourinary
Urinary tract infection (<9%)

Hematologic
Anemia (<8%)

Ocular
Blepharitis (<13%)
Cataract (2–17%) [4]
Conjunctival hemorrhage (48–74%) [4]
Conjunctival hyperemia (<8%)
Endophthalmitis [9]
Hallucinations, visual [2]
Intraocular inflammation (<18%) [5]
Intraocular pressure increased (7–24%) [7]
Iridocyclitis [2]
Lacrimation (increased) (2–14%)
Maculopathy (6–11%)
Ocular adverse effects [3]
Ocular hemorrhage [5]
Ocular hyperemia (5–11%)
Ocular pain (17–35%) [3]
Ocular pruritus (<12%)
Ocular stinging (7–15%)
Posterior capsule opacification (<8%)
Retinal atrophy [2]
Retinal detachment [2]
Retinal vein occlusion [2]
Vision blurred (5–18%)
Visual disturbances (5–18%)
Vitreous detachment (4–21%)
Vitreous floaters (7–27%) [2]
Xerophthalmia (3–12%)

Local
Injection-site bleeding (<6%)

Other
Adverse effects [5]
Systemic reactions [2]

RANITIDINE

Trade name: Zantac (Concordia)
Indications: Duodenal ulcer
Class: Histamine H2 receptor antagonist
Half-life: 2.5 hours
Clinically important, potentially hazardous interactions with: alfentanil, delavirdine, fentanyl, gefitinib, metformin, prednisone, rilpivirine, risperidone
Pregnancy category: B
Important contra-indications noted in the prescribing guidelines for: nursing mothers

Skin
AGEP [2]
Anaphylactoid reactions/Anaphylaxis [18]
Dermatitis [6]
Eczema [2]
Exanthems [5]
Hypersensitivity [2]
Photosensitivity [2]
Pseudolymphoma [2]
Purpura [2]
Rash (<10%)
Toxic epidermal necrolysis [2]
Urticaria [4]

Central Nervous System
Confusion [2]
Somnolence (drowsiness) [2]

Respiratory
Pneumonia [2]

Endocrine/Metabolic
Gynecomastia [3]
Porphyria [3]

Other
Adverse effects [3]

RANOLAZINE

Trade name: Ranexa (CV Therapeutics)
Indications: Angina
Class: Anti-ischemic, Fatty acid oxidation inhibitor
Half-life: 7 hours
Clinically important, potentially hazardous interactions with: aprepitant, atazanavir, clarithromycin, conivaptan, cyclosporine, CYP3A inducers, CYP3A inhibitors, darunavir, dasabuvir/ombitasvir/paritaprevir/ritonavir, delavirdine, diltiazem, dofetilide, efavirenz, erythromycin, grapefruit juice, indinavir, itraconazole, ketoconazole, lopinavir, nelfinavir, ombitasvir/paritaprevir/ritonavir, oxcarbazepine, paroxetine hydrochloride, phenobarbital, quinidine, rifampin, rifapentine, ritonavir, simvastatin, sotalol, telithromycin, thioridazine, tipranavir, venetoclax, verapamil, voriconazole, ziprasidone
Pregnancy category: C
Important contra-indications noted in the prescribing guidelines for: nursing mothers
Note: Contra-indicated in patients with existing QT prolongation, and in patients with liver disease.

Mucosal
Xerostomia (<2%)

Cardiovascular
Palpitation (<2%)
QT prolongation [7]
Torsades de pointes [2]

Central Nervous System
Headache (3%) [4]
Vertigo (dizziness) [10]

Neuromuscular/Skeletal
Asthenia (fatigue) [3]

Gastrointestinal/Hepatic
Abdominal pain (<2%)
Constipation [8]
Nausea [9]
Vomiting [2]

Otic
Tinnitus (<2%)

RAPACURONIUM

See: www.drugeruptiondata.com/drug/id/806

RASAGILINE

Trade name: Azilect (Teva)
Indications: Parkinsonism
Class: Monoamine oxidase B inhibitor
Half-life: 0.6–2.0 hours
Clinically important, potentially hazardous interactions with: aminophylline, amitriptyline, ciprofloxacin, citalopram, dextromethorphan, entacapone, fluoxetine, fluvoxamine, MAO inhibitors, meperidine, paroxetine hydrochloride, pethidine, pseudoephedrine, SSRIs
Pregnancy category: C
Important contra-indications noted in the prescribing guidelines for: nursing mothers; pediatric patients

Skin
Ecchymoses (2%)

Mucosal
Xerostomia (3%)

Cardiovascular
Hypotension (5%)

Central Nervous System
Depression (5%) [2]
Dyskinesia (>10%)
Fever (3%)
Gait instability (5%)
Headache (14%) [2]
Paresthesias (2%)
Somnolence (drowsiness) [3]
Vertigo (dizziness) (2%) [3]

Neuromuscular/Skeletal
Arthralgia (7%) [2]
Asthenia (fatigue) (2%)
Dystonia (2%)
Neck pain (2%)

Gastrointestinal/Hepatic
Dyspepsia (7%)
Gastroenteritis (3%)
Nausea [2]

Respiratory
Flu-like syndrome (5%)

Rhinitis (3%)
Ocular
Conjunctivitis (3%)

RASBURICASE

See: www.drugeruptiondata.com/drug/id/942

REBOXETINE

Trade name: Edronax (Pfizer)
Indications: Clinical depression, panic disorder
Class: Antidepressant, Noradrenaline reuptake inhibitor
Half-life: 13 hours
Clinically important, potentially hazardous interactions with: azithromycin, bosentan, itraconazole, ketoconazole, MAO inhibitors, papaverine, voriconazole
Pregnancy category: N/A (not recommended in pregnancy)
Important contra-indications noted in the prescribing guidelines for: the elderly; nursing mothers; pediatric patients

Skin
Diaphoresis [8]
Mucosal
Xerostomia [12]
Central Nervous System
Headache [5]
Insomnia [9]
Somnolence (drowsiness) [2]
Genitourinary
Ejaculatory dysfunction [2]

REGADENOSON

See: www.drugeruptiondata.com/drug/id/1293

REGORAFENIB

See: www.drugeruptiondata.com/drug/id/3067

REMIFENTANIL

See: www.drugeruptiondata.com/drug/id/1414

REPAGLINIDE

See: www.drugeruptiondata.com/drug/id/614

RESERPINE

See: www.drugeruptiondata.com/drug/id/615

RESLIZUMAB

Trade name: Cinqair (Teva)
Indications: Adjunctive treatment for severe eosinophilic asthma
Class: Interleukin-5 antagonist, Monoclonal antibody
Half-life: 24 days
Clinically important, potentially hazardous interactions with: none known
Pregnancy category: N/A (Insufficient evidence to inform drug-associated risk)
Important contra-indications noted in the prescribing guidelines for: nursing mothers; pediatric patients
Warning: ANAPHYLAXIS

Mucosal
Oropharyngeal pain (3%)
Central Nervous System
Headache [3]
Respiratory
Asthma (exacerbation) [3]
Nasopharyngitis [4]
Upper respiratory tract infection [3]
Endocrine/Metabolic
Creatine phosphokinase increased (14%)

RETAPAMULIN

See: www.drugeruptiondata.com/drug/id/1248

RETEPLASE

See: www.drugeruptiondata.com/drug/id/616

RIBAVIRIN

Trade names: Copegus (Roche), Rebetol (Schering-Plough), Rebetron (Schering), Virazole (Valeant)
Indications: Respiratory syncytial viral infections
Class: Antiviral, nucleoside analog
Half-life: 24 hours
Clinically important, potentially hazardous interactions with: abacavir, azathioprine, didanosine, emtricitabine, interferon alfa, PEG-interferon, stavudine, zidovudine
Pregnancy category: X
Important contra-indications noted in the prescribing guidelines for: nursing mothers
Note: [INH] = Inhalation; [O] = Oral. Rebetron is ribavirin and interferon.
Warning: RISK OF SERIOUS DISORDERS AND RIBAVIRIN-ASSOCIATED EFFECTS

Skin
Dermatitis [O] (16%)
DRESS syndrome [2]
Eczema [O] (4–5%) [3]
Exanthems [5]
Lichenoid eruption [2]
Nummular eczema [2]
Peripheral edema [2]
Photosensitivity [6]
Pruritus [O] (13–29%) [26]
Psoriasis [2]
Rash [O] (5–28%) [38]
Sarcoidosis [16]
Stevens-Johnson syndrome [2]
Toxic epidermal necrolysis [2]
Toxicity [2]
Vasculitis [2]
Vitiligo [2]
Xerosis [O] (10–24%) [2]
Hair
Alopecia [O] (27–36%) [5]
Alopecia areata [2]
Cardiovascular
Flushing [O] (4%)
Central Nervous System
Depression [O] (20–36%) [10]
Dysgeusia (taste perversion) [O] (4–9%) [4]
Fever [O] (32–55%) [7]
Headache [INH] (Insomnia [O] (25–41%) [26]
Irritability [9]
Neurotoxicity [2]
Pain [O] (10%)
Rigors [O] (25–48%)
Suicidal ideation [O] (2%) [2]
Vertigo (dizziness) [O] (14–26%) [6]
Neuromuscular/Skeletal
Arthralgia [INH] (22–34%) [7]
Asthenia (fatigue) [59]
Muscle spasm [3]
Myalgia/Myopathy [INH] (40–64%) [4]
Gastrointestinal/Hepatic
Diarrhea [16]
Hepatotoxicity [6]
Nausea [INH] (<10%) [37]
Pancreatitis [4]
Vomiting [O] (9–25%) [3]
Respiratory
Cough [O] (7–23%) [9]
Dyspnea [O] (13–26%) [5]
Flu-like syndrome [O] (13–18%) [8]
Nasopharyngitis [3]
Pneumonitis [2]
Rhinitis [O] (8%)
Upper respiratory tract infection [3]
Endocrine/Metabolic
ALT increased [6]
Appetite decreased [2]
AST increased [5]
Diabetes mellitus [2]
Hyperbilirubinemia [3]
Hyperuricemia [O] (33–38%)
Thyroid dysfunction [2]
Weight loss [O] (10–29%) [2]
Genitourinary
Erectile dysfunction [2]
Renal
Nephrotoxicity [5]
Hematologic
Anemia [INH] (<10%) [74]
Hemoglobin decreased [3]
Hemotoxicity [2]
Leukopenia [O] (6–45%) [3]
Lymphopenia [O] (12–14%) [2]
Neutropenia [O] (8–42%) [18]

Thrombocytopenia [INH] (<15%) [10]

Otic
Hearing loss [2]
Tinnitus [2]

Ocular
Retinopathy [6]

Local
Injection-site reactions [2]

Other
Adverse effects [24]
Death [4]
Infection [INH] [4]
Vogt-Koyanagi-Harada syndrome [6]

RIBOCICLIB *

Trade name: Kisqali (Novartis)
Indications: Treatment of postmenopausal
women with hormone receptor (HR)-positive,
human epidermal growth factor receptor 2
(HER2)-negative advanced or metastatic breast
cancer (in combination with an aromatase
inhibitor)
Class: Kinase inhibitor
Half-life: 30–55 hours
**Clinically important, potentially hazardous
interactions with:** alfentanil, amiodarone,
bepridil, boceprevir, chloroquine, clarithromycin,
conivaptan, cyclosporine, CYP3A4 substrates,
dihydroergotamine, disopyramide, ergotamine,
everolimus, fentanyl, grapefruit juice, halofantrine,
haloperidol, indinavir, itraconazole, ketoconazole,
lopinavir, methadone, midazolam, moxifloxacin,
ondansetron, pimozide, procainamide, QT
prolonging drugs, quinidine, rifampin, ritonavir,
saquinavir, sirolimus, sotalol, strong CYP3A4
inducers and inhibitors, tacrolimus, voriconazole
Pregnancy category: N/A (Can cause fetal
harm)
**Important contra-indications noted in the
prescribing guidelines for:** nursing mothers;
pediatric patients

Skin
Peripheral edema (12%)
Pruritus (14%)
Rash (17%)

Hair
Alopecia (33%)

Mucosal
Stomatitis (12%)

Central Nervous System
Fever (13%)
Headache (22%)
Insomnia (12%)

Neuromuscular/Skeletal
Asthenia (fatigue) (37%) [3]
Back pain (20%)

Gastrointestinal/Hepatic
Abdominal pain (11%)
Constipation (25%)
Diarrhea (35%)
Nausea (52%) [5]
Vomiting (29%) [2]

Respiratory
Dyspnea (12%)

Endocrine/Metabolic
ALT increased (46%)
Appetite decreased (19%)
AST increased (44%)
Hyperbilirubinemia (18%)
Serum creatinine increased (20%)

Genitourinary
Urinary tract infection (11%)

Hematologic
Anemia (18%)
Leukopenia (33%) [5]
Lymphopenia (11%) [2]
Neutropenia (75%) [8]

RIBOFLAVIN

See: www.drugeruptiondata.com/drug/id/618

RIFABUTIN

Trade name: Mycobutin (Pfizer)
Indications: Disseminated *Mycobacterium avium*
infection
Class: Antibiotic, rifamycin, CYP3A4 inducer
Half-life: 45 hours
**Clinically important, potentially hazardous
interactions with:** abiraterone, amiodarone,
amprenavir, anisindione, anticoagulants,
atazanavir, atovaquone, atovaquone/proguanil,
azithromycin, bedaquiline, boceprevir,
cabazitaxel, cabozantinib, cobicistat/elvitegravir/
emtricitabine/tenofovir alafenamide, cobicistat/
elvitegravir/emtricitabine/tenofovir disoproxil,
corticosteroids, crizotinib, cyclosporine, dapsone,
darunavir, delavirdine, dicumarol, efavirenz,
enzalutamide, etravirine, flibanserin,
fosamprenavir, indinavir, itraconazole,
ixabepilone, lapatinib, ledipasvir & sofosbuvir,
levonorgestrel, lopinavir, midazolam,
mifepristone, nelfinavir, oral contraceptives,
posaconazole, rilpivirine, ritonavir, romidepsin,
simeprevir, sofosbuvir, sofosbuvir & velpatasvir,
sofosbuvir/velpatasvir/voxilaprevir, solifenacin,
sonidegib, sorafenib, sunitinib, tacrolimus,
temsirolimus, tenofovir alafenamide, thalidomide,
tipranavir, tolvaptan, vandetanib, vemurafenib,
voriconazole
Pregnancy category: B
**Important contra-indications noted in the
prescribing guidelines for:** the elderly; nursing
mothers; pediatric patients

Skin
Lupus erythematosus [2]
Pigmentation [2]
Rash (11%) [2]

Central Nervous System
Anorexia (2%)
Dysgeusia (taste perversion) (3%)
Fever (2%)
Headache (3%)

Neuromuscular/Skeletal
Arthralgia [6]
Myalgia/Myopathy (2%)

Gastrointestinal/Hepatic
Abdominal pain (4%)

Diarrhea (3%)
Dyspepsia (3%)
Eructation (belching) (3%)
Flatulence (2%)
Hepatotoxicity [2]
Nausea (6%)

Ocular
Intraocular inflammation [2]
Ocular toxicity [2]
Uveitis [31]
Visual disturbances [2]

RIFAMPIN

Synonym: rifampicin
Trade names: Rifadin (Sanofi-Aventis),
Rimactane (Novartis)
Indications: Tuberculosis
Class: Antibiotic, rifamycin, CYP1A2 inducer,
CYP3A4 inducer
Half-life: 3–5 hours
**Clinically important, potentially hazardous
interactions with:** abacavir, abiraterone, afatinib,
amiodarone, amprenavir, anisindione, antacids,
anticoagulants, apixaban, apremilast, aprepitant,
artemether/lumefantrine, atazanavir, atorvastatin,
atovaquone, atovaquone/proguanil,
beclomethasone, bedaquiline, betamethasone,
bisoprolol, boceprevir, bosentan, brentuximab
vedotin, brigatinib, brivaracetam, buprenorphine,
cabazitaxel, cabozantinib, canagliflozin,
caspofungin, ceritinib, clobazam, clozapine,
cobimetinib, copanlisib, corticosteroids,
cortisone, crizotinib, cyclosporine, cyproterone,
dabigatran, daclatasvir, dapsone, darunavir,
dasabuvir/ombitasvir/paritaprevir/ritonavir,
dasatinib, deferasirox, deflazacort, delavirdine,
dexamethasone, diclofenac, dicumarol, digoxin,
doxycycline, dronedarone, edoxaban, efavirenz,
elbasvir & grazoprevir, eliglustat, eluxadoline,
emtricitabine/rilpivirine/tenofovir alafenamide,
enzalutamide, estradiol, eszopiclone, etoricoxib,
etravirine, everolimus, fesoterodine, flibanserin,
fludrocortisone, flunisolide, fosamprenavir,
gadoxetate, gefitinib, gestrinone, glecaprevir &
pibrentasvir, halothane, hydrocortisone, ibrutinib,
idelalisib, imatinib, indinavir, isavuconazonium
sulfate, isoniazid, itraconazole, ixabepilone,
ixazomib, ketoconazole, lapatinib, ledipasvir &
sofosbuvir, leflunomide, lesinurad, levodopa,
levonorgestrel, linagliptin, linezolid, lopinavir,
lorcainide, losartan, lumacaftor/ivacaftor,
lurasidone, macitentan, maraviroc,
methylprednisolone, midazolam, midostaurin,
mifepristone, naldemedine, nelfinavir, neratinib,
netupitant & palonosetron, nevirapine, nifedipine,
nilotinib, olaparib, ombitasvir/paritaprevir/
ritonavir, ondansetron, oral contraceptives,
osimertinib, ospemifene, oxtriphylline, paclitaxel,
palbociclib, pazopanib, perampanel,
phenylbutazone, pimavanserin, pioglitazone,
pitavastatin, pomalidomide, ponatinib,
praziquantel, prednisolone, prednisone,
propranolol, propyphenazone, protease
inhibitors, pyrazinamide, quinine, raltegravir,
ramelteon, ranolazine, regorafenib, ribociclib,
rilpivirine, riociguat, ritonavir, rivaroxaban,
roflumilast, romidepsin, rosiglitazone, saquinavir,
simeprevir, simvastatin, sofosbuvir, sofosbuvir &

velpatasvir, sofosbuvir/velpatasvir/voxilaprevir, solifenacin, sonidegib, sorafenib, sunitinib, tacrolimus, tadalafil, tasimelteon, telaprevir, telithromycin, temsirolimus, tenofovir alafenamide, terbinafine, thalidomide, ticagrelor, tipranavir, tofacitinib, tolvaptan, trabectedin, treprostinil, triamcinolone, triazolam, trimethoprim, troleandomycin, ulipristal, valbenazine, vandetanib, vemurafenib, venetoclax, vorapaxar, voriconazole, vortioxetine, warfarin, zaleplon, zidovudine, zolpidem

Pregnancy category: C

Skin
Acneform eruption [3]
AGEP [2]
Anaphylactoid reactions/Anaphylaxis [8]
Dermatitis [3]
Diaphoresis (<10%)
DRESS syndrome [5]
Erythema multiforme [4]
Exanthems (<5%) [6]
Fixed eruption [6]
Hypersensitivity [5]
Linear IgA bullous dermatosis [3]
Pemphigus [9]
Pruritus (<62%) [9]
Purpura [6]
Rash (<5%) [5]
Red man syndrome [7]
Serum sickness-like reaction [2]
Stevens-Johnson syndrome [5]
Thrombocytopenic purpura [2]
Toxic epidermal necrolysis [6]
Urticaria [8]
Vasculitis [5]

Cardiovascular
Flushing (7%) [8]

Central Nervous System
Fever [2]
Seizures [3]
Vertigo (dizziness) [2]

Neuromuscular/Skeletal
Asthenia (fatigue) [3]

Gastrointestinal/Hepatic
Abdominal pain [3]
Diarrhea [2]
Hepatitis [3]
Hepatotoxicity [18]
Nausea [4]
Vomiting [2]

Respiratory
Pneumonitis [2]

Endocrine/Metabolic
Amenorrhea [2]
Porphyria [2]

Renal
Nephrotoxicity [10]

Hematologic
Agranulocytosis [2]
Anemia [3]
Thrombocytopenia [11]

Other
Adverse effects [12]
Death [7]
Side effects (5%)

RIFAPENTINE

See: www.drugeruptiondata.com/drug/id/621

RIFAXIMIN

Trade names: Xifaxan (Salix), Xifaxanta (Norgine)
Indications: Diarrhea in travelers (caused by non-invasive strains of *E. coli*), reduction in risk of overt hepatic encephalopathy recurrence (in adults)
Class: Antibiotic, rifamycin
Half-life: 2–5 hours
Clinically important, potentially hazardous interactions with: BCG vaccine
Pregnancy category: C
Important contra-indications noted in the prescribing guidelines for: nursing mothers; pediatric patients

Skin
Cellulitis (2–5%)
Clammy skin (<2%)
Diaphoresis (<2%)
Edema (2–5%)
Hot flashes (<2%)
Hyperhidrosis (<2%)
Peripheral edema (15%) [2]
Pruritus (9%)
Rash (<5%)
Sunburn (<2%)

Mucosal
Epistaxis (nosebleed) (2–5%)
Gingival lesions (<2%)
Rhinorrhea (<2%)
Xerostomia (2–5%)

Cardiovascular
Chest pain (<5%) [2]
Hypotension (2–5%)

Central Nervous System
Abnormal dreams (<2%)
Ageusia (taste loss) (<2%)
Amnesia (2–5%)
Anorexia (<5%)
Confusion (2–5%)
Depression (7%)
Dysgeusia (taste perversion) (<2%) [2]
Fever (3–6%)
Headache (10%) [8]
Hypoesthesia (2–5%)
Impaired concentration (2–5%)
Insomnia (<7%)
Migraine (<2%)
Pain (<5%)
Syncope (<2%)
Tremor (2–5%)
Vertigo (dizziness) (<13%) [3]

Neuromuscular/Skeletal
Arthralgia (<6%)
Asthenia (fatigue) (<12%) [3]
Back pain (6%)
Muscle spasm (<9%)
Myalgia/Myopathy (<5%)
Neck pain (<2%)
Pain in extremities (2–5%)

Gastrointestinal/Hepatic
Abdominal distension (<8%)
Abdominal pain (2–9%) [10]
Ascites (11%)
Black stools (<2%)
Constipation (4–6%)
Diarrhea (<2%) [6]
Fecal urgency (6%)
Flatulence (11%) [2]
Hernia (<2%)
Nausea (5–14%) [8]
Tenesmus (7%)
Vomiting (2%) [3]

Respiratory
Cough (7%)
Dyspnea (<6%)
Flu-like syndrome (2–5%)
Nasopharyngitis (<7%) [4]
Pharyngitis (<2%)
Pharyngolaryngeal pain (<2%)
Pneumonia (2–5%)
Rhinitis (<5%)
Sinusitis [2]
Upper respiratory tract infection (2–5%) [6]

Endocrine/Metabolic
AST increased (<2%)
Dehydration (<5%)
Hyperglycemia (2–5%)
Hyperkalemia (2–5%)
Hypoglycemia (2–5%)
Hyponatremia (2–5%)
Weight gain (2–5%)

Genitourinary
Dysuria (<2%)
Hematuria (<2%)
Polyuria (<2%)
Urinary frequency (<2%)

Renal
Proteinuria (<2%)

Hematologic
Anemia (8%)
Lymphocytosis (<2%)
Monocytosis (<2%)
Neutropenia (<2%)

Otic
Ear pain (<2%)
Tinnitus (<2%)

Other
Breast cancer [2]

RILONACEPT

See: www.drugeruptiondata.com/drug/id/1307

RILPIVIRINE

See: www.drugeruptiondata.com/drug/id/2507

RILUZOLE

See: www.drugeruptiondata.com/drug/id/622

RIMANTADINE

See: www.drugeruptiondata.com/drug/id/623

RIMONABANT

See: www.drugeruptiondata.com/drug/id/1236

RIOCIGUAT

Trade name: Adempas (Bayer)
Indications: Pulmonary hypertension
Class: Soluble guanylate cyclase (sGC) stimulator
Half-life: 7–12 hours
Clinically important, potentially hazardous interactions with: antacids, carbamazepine, dipyridamole, nitrates or nitric oxide donors, nitroprusside, phenobarbital, phenytoin, rifampin, sildenafil, St John's wort, tadalafil, theophylline, vardenafil
Pregnancy category: X
Important contra-indications noted in the prescribing guidelines for: nursing mothers; pediatric patients
Warning: EMBRYO-FETAL TOXICITY

Skin
Peripheral edema [2]

Cardiovascular
Hypotension (10%) [6]

Central Nervous System
Headache (27%) [3]
Syncope [2]
Vertigo (dizziness) (20%)

Gastrointestinal/Hepatic
Constipation (5%)
Diarrhea (12%)
Dyspepsia (21%) [2]
Gastroesophageal reflux (5%)
Nausea (14%)
Vomiting (10%)

Hematologic
Anemia (7%)
Bleeding (2%) [2]

Other
Adverse effects [5]

RISEDRONATE

Trade names: Actonel (Procter & Gamble), Atelvia (Warner Chilcott)
Indications: Paget's disease of bone, osteoporosis
Class: Bisphosphonate
Half-life: terminal: 220 hours
Clinically important, potentially hazardous interactions with: antacids, calcium supplements, iron preparations, laxatives, magnesium-based supplements
Pregnancy category: C
Important contra-indications noted in the prescribing guidelines for: nursing mothers; pediatric patients

Skin
Ecchymoses (4%)
Peripheral edema (8%)
Pruritus (3%)
Rash (8%)

Cardiovascular
Chest pain (5%)
Hypertension (11%)

Central Nervous System
Depression (7%)
Fever [2]
Headache (10%) [3]
Insomnia (5%)
Pain (14%)
Paresthesias (2%)
Vertigo (dizziness) (7%)

Neuromuscular/Skeletal
Arthralgia (10–24%) [6]
Asthenia (fatigue) (5%)
Back pain (28%) [4]
Bone or joint pain (7%) [5]
Fractures (9%) [9]
Myalgia/Myopathy (7%) [3]
Neck pain (5%) [3]
Osteonecrosis [5]
Tendinopathy/Tendon rupture (3%)

Gastrointestinal/Hepatic
Abdominal pain (12%) [3]
Constipation (13%) [3]
Diarrhea (11%) [4]
Dyspepsia (11%) [2]
Esophagitis [2]
Gastrointestinal disorder [3]
Hepatotoxicity [6]
Nausea (11%) [2]

Respiratory
Bronchitis (10%)
Cough (6%)
Flu-like syndrome (11%) [2]
Influenza [3]
Nasopharyngitis [3]
Pharyngitis (6%)
Rhinitis (6%)
Sinusitis (9%)

Genitourinary
Urinary tract infection (11%)

Ocular
Cataract (7%)
Ocular adverse effects [3]
Scleritis [2]

Other
Adverse effects [5]
Allergic reactions (4%)
Infection (31%) [2]
Tooth disorder (2%)

RISPERIDONE

Trade names: Risperdal (Ortho-McNeil) (Janssen), Risperdal Consta (Ortho-McNeil) (Janssen)
Indications: Schizophrenia, bipolar mania, irritability associated with autistic disorder
Class: Antipsychotic, Mood stabilizer
Half-life: 3–30 hours
Clinically important, potentially hazardous interactions with: ACE inhibitors, alcohol, alpha blockers, amantadine, angiotensin II receptor antagonists, anxiolytics and hypnotics, apomorphine, artemether/lumefantrine, barbiturates, bromocriptine, cabergoline, calcium channel blockers, carbamazepine, cimetidine, citalopram, clozapine, cobicistat/elvitegravir/emtricitabine/tenofovir alafenamide, cobicistat/elvitegravir/emtricitabine/tenofovir disoproxil, ethosuximide, fluoxetine, general anesthetics, histamine, levodopa, memantine, methyldopa, metoclopramide, opioid analgesics, oxcarbazepine, paliperidone, paroxetine hydrochloride, pergolide, phenytoin, pramipexole, primidone, ranitidine, ritonavir, ropinirole, rotigotine, sodium oxybate, sympathomimetics, tetrabenazine, tramadol, tricyclics, valproic acid
Pregnancy category: C
Important contra-indications noted in the prescribing guidelines for: nursing mothers; pediatric patients
Note: Safety and effectiveness have not been established for pediatric patients with schizophrenia <13 years of age, for bipolar mania <10 years of age, and for autistic disorder <5 years of age. [C] = in children.
Warning: INCREASED MORTALITY IN ELDERLY PATIENTS WITH DEMENTIA-RELATED PSYCHOSIS

Skin
Angioedema [6]
Edema [3]
Peripheral edema (16%) [4]
Photosensitivity (<10%) [2]
Rash [C] (11%) (2–4%)
Seborrhea (2%)
Urticaria [2]
Xerosis (2%)

Hair
Alopecia [2]

Mucosal
Sialopenia (5%)
Sialorrhea [C] (22%) (<3%) [11]
Xerostomia [C] (13%) (4%) [7]

Cardiovascular
Bradycardia [2]
Cardiotoxicity [2]
Hypotension [2]
QT prolongation [4]
Tachycardia [C] (7%) (<5%)
Venous thromboembolism [6]
Ventricular arrhythmia [2]

Central Nervous System
Agitation [2]
Akathisia [C] (16%) (5–9%) [18]
Anorexia [C] (8%) (2%)

Anxiety [C] (16%) (2–16%) [5]
Catatonia [2]
Compulsions [3]
Depression (14%) [7]
Extrapyramidal symptoms [16]
Fever [C] (20%) (<2%)
Headache [9]
Insomnia [9]
Neuroleptic malignant syndrome [25]
Neurotoxicity [2]
Parkinsonism [C] (2–16%) (12–20%) [7]
Psychosis [3]
Rabbit syndrome [3]
Restless legs syndrome [2]
Schizophrenia [2]
Sedation [4]
Seizures [3]
Serotonin syndrome [3]
Somnolence (drowsiness) [C] (12–67%) (5–14%) [16]
Stuttering [2]
Suicidal ideation [3]
Tardive dyskinesia [5]
Tremor [C] (10–12%) (6%) [6]
Vertigo (dizziness) [C] (7–16%) (4–10%) [5]

Neuromuscular/Skeletal
Arthralgia (2–3%)
Asthenia (fatigue) [C] (18–42%) (<3%) [4]
Back pain (2–3%)
Dystonia [C] (9–18%) (5–11%) [4]
Pisa syndrome [3]
Rhabdomyolysis [7]

Gastrointestinal/Hepatic
Abdominal pain [C] (15–18%) (3–4%)
Constipation [C] (21%) (8–9%) [4]
Diarrhea [C] (7%) (73%)
Dyspepsia [C] (5–16%) (4–10%)
Dysphagia [2]
Nausea [C] (8–16%) (4–9%) [4]
Pancreatitis [2]
Vomiting [C] (10–25%)

Respiratory
Cough [C] (34%) (3%)
Dyspnea [C] (2–5%) (2%)
Pneumonia [2]
Pulmonary embolism [3]
Rhinitis [C] (13–36%) (7–11%)
Upper respiratory tract infection [C] (34%) (2–3%)

Endocrine/Metabolic
Amenorrhea [6]
Appetite decreased [2]
Appetite increased [C] (49%) [3]
Diabetes mellitus [2]
Galactorrhea (<10%) [14]
Gynecomastia (<10%) [6]
Hyperprolactinemia [22]
Metabolic syndrome [5]
Weight gain [C] (5%) [33]

Genitourinary
Priapism (<10%) [27]
Sexual dysfunction [3]
Urinary incontinence [C] (5–22%) (2%)
Urinary tract infection (3%)

Renal
Enuresis [4]

Hematologic
Neutropenia [2]

Ocular
Abnormal vision [C] (4–7%) (<3%)
Vision blurred [3]

Local
Injection-site pain [2]

Other
Adverse effects [11]
Death [3]
Tooth disorder (<3%)

RITODRINE

Indications: Preterm labor
Class: Beta-2 adrenergic agonist, Tocolytic
Half-life: 1.3–12 hours
Clinically important, potentially hazardous interactions with: glycopyrrolate
Pregnancy category: B

Skin
Anaphylactoid reactions/Anaphylaxis (<3%)
Diaphoresis (<14%)
Erythema (10–15%) [2]
Pustules [2]
Rash (<3%)
Toxic epidermal necrolysis [2]
Vasculitis [2]

Cardiovascular
Chest pain [2]
Myocardial ischemia [2]
Pulmonary edema [3]

Central Nervous System
Chills (3–10%)
Tremor (>10%)

Neuromuscular/Skeletal
Rhabdomyolysis [4]

Gastrointestinal/Hepatic
Hepatotoxicity [3]

Endocrine/Metabolic
Hypokalemia [2]

Ocular
Glaucoma [2]

Other
Adverse effects [2]

RITONAVIR

Trade names: Kaletra (AbbVie), Norvir (AbbVie)
Indications: HIV infection
Class: Antiretroviral, CYP3A4 inhibitor, HIV-1 protease inhibitor
Half-life: 3–5 hours
Clinically important, potentially hazardous interactions with: abiraterone, afatinib, alfentanil, alfuzosin, alprazolam, amiodarone, amitriptyline, amprenavir, aprepitant, astemizole, atazanavir, atorvastatin, atovaquone, atovaquone/proguanil, avanafil, azithromycin, bepridil, boceprevir, bosentan, brigatinib, buprenorphine, bupropion, buspirone, cabazitaxel, cabozantinib, calcifediol, carbamazepine, ceritinib, chlordiazepoxide, ciclesonide, citalopram, clozapine, cobicistat/elvitegravir/emtricitabine/tenofovir disoproxil, colchicine, conivaptan, copanlisib, crizotinib, cyclosporine, cyproterone, darifenacin, dasatinib, deferasirox, delavirdine, diazepam, diclofenac, dihydroergotamine, docetaxel, dronedarone, dutasteride, efavirenz, eletriptan, eluxadoline, ergot alkaloids, ergotamine, erlotinib, estazolam, estradiol, eszopiclone, etravirine, everolimus, ezetimibe, fentanyl, fesoterodine, flecainide, flibanserin, flurazepam, fluticasone propionate, glecaprevir & pibrentasvir, halazepam, indacaterol, isavuconazonium sulfate, itraconazole, ivabradine, ixabepilone, ketoconazole, lapatinib, ledipasvir & sofosbuvir, levomepromazine, levothyroxine, lomitapide, macitentan, maraviroc, meloxicam, meperidine, meptazinol, methylergonovine, methysergide, midazolam, midostaurin, mifepristone, naldemedine, nelfinavir, neratinib, nifedipine, nilotinib, olaparib, oral contraceptives, osimertinib, paclitaxel, palbociclib, paroxetine hydrochloride, pazopanib, phenytoin, pimozide, piroxicam, pitavastatin, ponatinib, posaconazole, propafenone, propoxyphene, propranolol, quazepam, quinidine, quinine, ranolazine, ribociclib, rifabutin, rifampin, rifapentine, rilpivirine, rimonabant, risperidone, rivaroxaban, romidepsin, rosuvastatin, ruxolitinib, saquinavir, sildenafil, silodosin, simeprevir, simvastatin, sofosbuvir, sofosbuvir/velpatasvir/voxilaprevir, solifenacin, St John's wort, sunitinib, tadalafil, telaprevir, telithromycin, temsirolimus, tenofovir disoproxil, ticagrelor, tolvaptan, trabectedin, triazolam, ulipristal, vardenafil, vemurafenib, venetoclax, vorapaxar, voriconazole, zolpidem, zuclopenthixol
Pregnancy category: B
Important contra-indications noted in the prescribing guidelines for: nursing mothers
Note: Protease inhibitors cause dyslipidemia which includes elevated triglycerides and cholesterol and redistribution of body fat centrally to produce the so-called 'protease paunch', breast enlargement, facial atrophy, and 'buffalo hump'. Kaletra is ritonavir and lopinavir. See also separate entry for ombitasvir/paritaprevir/ritonavir.
Warning: DRUG-DRUG INTERACTIONS LEADING TO POTENTIALLY SERIOUS AND/OR LIFE THREATENING REACTIONS

Skin
Acneform eruption (4%)
Bullous dermatitis (<2%)
Dermatitis (<2%)
Diaphoresis (<10%)
Ecchymoses (<2%)
Eczema (<2%)
Edema (6%)
Exanthems (<2%) [2]
Facial edema (8%)
Folliculitis (<2%)
Hypersensitivity (8%)
Jaundice [3]
Lipodystrophy [4]
Peripheral edema (6%)
Photosensitivity (<2%)
Pruritus (12%)
Psoriasis (<2%)
Rash (27%) [12]
Seborrhea (<2%)
Toxicity [2]
Urticaria (8%)

Xanthomas [2]
Xerosis (<2%)

Hair
Alopecia [2]

Mucosal
Cheilitis (<2%)
Gingivitis (<2%)
Oral candidiasis (<2%)
Oral ulceration (<2%)
Oropharyngeal pain (16%)
Xerostomia (<2%)

Cardiovascular
Cardiotoxicity [2]
Flushing (13%)
Hypertension (3%)
Hypotension (2%)
Orthostatic hypotension (2%)

Central Nervous System
Ageusia (taste loss) (<2%)
Confusion (3%)
Dysgeusia (taste perversion) (16%)
Headache [8]
Hyperesthesia (<2%)
Impaired concentration (3%)
Insomnia [2]
Neurotoxicity [2]
Paresthesias (51%)
Parosmia (<2%)
Peripheral neuropathy (10%)
Syncope (3%)
Vertigo (dizziness) (16%) [2]

Neuromuscular/Skeletal
Arthralgia (19%)
Asthenia (fatigue) (46%) [3]
Back pain (19%)
Myalgia/Myopathy (4–9%)
Rhabdomyolysis [2]

Gastrointestinal/Hepatic
Abdominal pain (26%) [2]
Diarrhea (68%) [14]
Dyspepsia (12%)
Flatulence (8%)
Gastrointestinal bleeding (2%)
Gastrointestinal disorder [4]
Hepatotoxicity (9%) [5]
Nausea (57%) [12]
Vomiting (32%) [7]

Respiratory
Cough (22%)
Nasopharyngitis [2]
Upper respiratory tract infection [2]

Endocrine/Metabolic
ALT increased [3]
Cushing's syndrome [7]
Gynecomastia [2]
Hyperbilirubinemia [5]
Hypercholesterolemia (3%) [2]
Hyperlipidemia [2]
Hypertriglyceridemia (9%) [2]

Genitourinary
Urinary frequency (4%)

Renal
Fanconi syndrome [4]
Nephrolithiasis [3]
Nephrotoxicity [2]
Renal failure [2]

Ocular
Vision blurred (6%)

Other
Adverse effects [9]
Allergic reactions (<2%)

RITUXIMAB

Trade names: MabThera (Roche), Rituxan (Genentech)
Indications: Non-Hodgkin's lymphoma, chronic lymphocytic leukemia, rheumatoid arthritis (in combination with methotrexate), granulomatosis with polyangiitis and mycroscopic polyangiitis (in combination with glucocorticoids)
Class: Biologic, CD20-directed cytolytic monoclonal antibody, Disease-modifying antirheumatic drug (DMARD), Immunosuppressant, Monoclonal antibody
Half-life: 60 hours (after first infusion)
Clinically important, potentially hazardous interactions with: benazepril, captopril, certolizumab, cisplatin, clevidipine, enalapril, fosinopril, irbesartan, lisinopril, olmesartan, quinapril, ramipril
Pregnancy category: C
Important contra-indications noted in the prescribing guidelines for: nursing mothers; pediatric patients
Warning: FATAL INFUSION REACTIONS, SEVERE MUCOCUTANEOUS REACTIONS, HEPATITIS B VIRUS REACTIVATION and PROGRESSIVE MULTIFOCAL LEUKOENCEPHALOPATHY

Skin
Anaphylactoid reactions/Anaphylaxis [7]
Angioedema (11%) [4]
Dermatitis [2]
Diaphoresis (15%) [2]
Erythema [2]
Herpes simplex [2]
Herpes zoster [7]
Hypersensitivity [5]
Kaposi's sarcoma [3]
Paraneoplastic pemphigus [2]
Peripheral edema (8%)
Pruritus (14%) [8]
Psoriasis [4]
Pyoderma gangrenosum [3]
Rash (15%) [12]
Sarcoidosis [2]
Serum sickness [21]
Serum sickness-like reaction [5]
Stevens-Johnson syndrome [5]
Toxic epidermal necrolysis [3]
Toxicity [3]
Tumor lysis syndrome [3]
Urticaria (8%) [5]
Vasculitis [4]

Mucosal
Mucocutaneous reactions [2]
Stomatitis [2]

Cardiovascular
Cardiotoxicity [5]
Flushing (5%)
Hypertension (6%) [2]
Hypotension (10%) [10]

Myocardial infarction [2]

Central Nervous System
Anxiety (5%)
Chills (33%) [15]
Encephalitis [3]
Fever (53%) [23]
Headache (19%) [4]
Leukoencephalopathy [27]
Neurotoxicity [3]
Pain (12%)
Peripheral neuropathy [5]
Rigors [4]
Vertigo (dizziness) (10%)

Neuromuscular/Skeletal
Arthralgia (10%) [2]
Asthenia (fatigue) (26%) [16]
Back pain (10%)
Myalgia/Myopathy (10%) [2]

Gastrointestinal/Hepatic
Abdominal pain (14%)
Colitis [4]
Constipation [2]
Diarrhea (10%) [9]
Hepatitis [3]
Hepatotoxicity [7]
Nausea (23%) [12]
Pancreatitis [2]
Vomiting (10%) [8]

Respiratory
Acute respiratory distress syndrome [3]
Bronchospasm (8%) [6]
Cough (increased) (13%) [6]
Dyspnea (7%) [7]
Flu-like syndrome [3]
Nasopharyngitis [3]
Pneumonia [20]
Pneumonitis [2]
Pulmonary toxicity [14]
Rhinitis (12%) [2]
Sinusitis (6%) [5]
Upper respiratory tract infection [9]

Endocrine/Metabolic
ALT increased [2]
AST increased [2]
Hyperglycemia (9%)
Hyponatremia [2]

Genitourinary
Urinary tract infection [8]

Renal
Nephrotoxicity [3]

Hematologic
Anemia (8%) [12]
Cytopenia [3]
Febrile neutropenia [15]
Hemotoxicity [3]
Hypogammaglobulinemia [6]
Leukopenia (14%) [14]
Lymphocytopenia [2]
Lymphopenia (48%) [10]
Myelosuppression [5]
Myelotoxicity [2]
Neutropenia (14%) [49]
Sepsis [3]
Thrombocytopenia (12%) [37]
Thrombosis [2]

Local
Application-site reactions [4]
Infusion-related reactions [22]

Infusion-site reactions [11]
Injection-site pain [2]
Injection-site reactions [4]

Other
Adverse effects [28]
Allergic reactions [4]
Death [26]
Infection (31%) [51]

RIVAROXABAN

Trade name: Xarelto (Janssen)
Indications: Prevention of venous thromboembolism in patients undergoing knee or hip replacement surgery, treatment of deep vein thrombosis and pulmonary embolism
Class: Anticoagulant, Direct factor Xa inhibitor
Half-life: 5–9 hours
Clinically important, potentially hazardous interactions with: anticoagulants, aspirin, atazanavir, atorvastatin, carbamazepine, clarithromycin, clopidogrel, combined P-glycoprotein and strong CYP3A4 inhibitors and inducers, conivaptan, dabigatran, darunavir, delavirdine, diclofenac, efavirenz, enoxaparin, erythromycin, fosamprenavir, HIV protease inhibitors, indinavir, itraconazole, ketoconazole, ketorolac, lapatinib, lopinavir, nelfinavir, phenobarbital, phenytoin, posaconazole, rifampin, ritonavir, saquinavir, St John's wort, telithromycin, tipranavir, voriconazole
Pregnancy category: C
Important contra-indications noted in the prescribing guidelines for: nursing mothers; pediatric patients
Note: Contra-indicated in patients with active pathological bleeding.
Warning: PREMATURE DISCONTINUATION OF XARELTO INCREASES THE RISK OF THROMBOTIC EVENTS
SPINAL/EPIDURAL HEMATOMA

Skin
Hematoma [3]
Pruritus (2%)
Rash [3]

Mucosal
Epistaxis (nosebleed) [6]
Gingival bleeding [2]

Gastrointestinal/Hepatic
Abdominal pain [2]
Black stools [2]
Gastrointestinal bleeding [3]
Hepatotoxicity [4]

Genitourinary
Hematuria [5]

Hematologic
Anemia (3%)
Bleeding [13]
Hemorrhage [5]

Other
Adverse effects [4]

RIVASTIGMINE

Trade name: Exelon (Novartis)
Indications: Alzheimer's disease and dementia
Class: Acetylcholinesterase inhibitor, Cholinesterase inhibitor
Half-life: 1–2 hours
Clinically important, potentially hazardous interactions with: galantamine
Pregnancy category: B
Important contra-indications noted in the prescribing guidelines for: nursing mothers; pediatric patients

Skin
Dermatitis [2]
Diaphoresis (10%)
Exanthems [2]
Hyperhidrosis (4%)
Peripheral edema (>2%)
Rash (>2%) [2]

Cardiovascular
Bradycardia [5]
Chest pain (>2%)
Hypertension (3%)
QT prolongation [2]
Thrombophlebitis (<2%)

Central Nervous System
Aggression (3%)
Agitation (>2%)
Anorexia (6–17%) [2]
Anxiety (4–5%)
Confusion (8%)
Delusions of parasitosis (>2%)
Depression (6%)
Hallucinations (4%)
Headache (4–17%)
Insomnia (3–9%)
Nervousness (>2%)
Pain (>2%)
Parkinsonism (2%)
Restlessness [2]
Somnolence (drowsiness) (3–5%)
Syncope (3%) [3]
Tremor (4–10%) [3]
Vertigo (dizziness) (6–21%) [4]

Neuromuscular/Skeletal
Arthralgia (>2%)
Asthenia (fatigue) (2–9%)
Back pain (>2%)
Dystonia [2]
Fractures (>2%)
Myalgia/Myopathy (20%)
Pisa syndrome [2]

Gastrointestinal/Hepatic
Abdominal pain (4–13%)
Constipation (5%) [2]
Diarrhea (7–19%) [4]
Dyspepsia (9%)
Eructation (belching) (2%)
Flatulence (4%)
Nausea (29–47%) [12]
Vomiting (17–31%) [12]

Respiratory
Bronchitis (>2%)
Cough (>2%)
Flu-like syndrome (3%)
Pharyngitis (>2%)

Rhinitis (4%)

Endocrine/Metabolic
Dehydration (2%)
Weight loss (3%) [2]

Genitourinary
Urinary incontinence (>2%)
Urinary tract infection (7%)

Local
Application-site pruritus [2]
Application-site reactions [3]

Other
Adverse effects [5]
Death [2]
Infection (>2%)

RIZATRIPTAN

Trade name: Maxalt (Merck)
Indications: Migraine
Class: 5-HT1 agonist, Serotonin receptor agonist, Triptan
Half-life: 2–3 hours
Clinically important, potentially hazardous interactions with: dihydroergotamine, ergot-containing drugs, isocarboxazid, MAO inhibitors, methysergide, naratriptan, phenelzine, propranolol, sibutramine, SSRIs, St John's wort, sumatriptan, tranylcypromine, zolmitriptan
Pregnancy category: C
Important contra-indications noted in the prescribing guidelines for: nursing mothers
Note: Safety and effectiveness in pediatric patients <6 years of age have not been established.

Mucosal
Xerostomia (3%)

Cardiovascular
Chest pain (<3%) [2]

Central Nervous System
Headache (<2%)
Neurotoxicity [2]
Pain (3%)
Paresthesias (3–4%)
Somnolence (drowsiness) (4–6%)
Vertigo (dizziness) (4–9%) [10]

Neuromuscular/Skeletal
Asthenia (fatigue) (4–7%) [9]
Jaw pain (<2%)
Neck pain (<2%)

Gastrointestinal/Hepatic
Nausea (4–6%)

Other
Adverse effects [4]

ROCURONIUM

See: www.drugeruptiondata.com/drug/id/1187

ROFECOXIB

See: www.drugeruptiondata.com/drug/id/631

ROFLUMILAST

Trade names: Daliresp (Takeda), Daxas (Takeda)
Indications: To reduce the risk of COPD exacerbations in patients with severe COPD associated with chronic bronchitis and a history of exacerbations
Class: Anti-inflammatory, Phosphodiesterase inhibitor, Phosphodiesterase type 4 (PDE4) inhibitor
Half-life: 17 hours
Clinically important, potentially hazardous interactions with: aminophylline, carbamazepine, cimetidine, denileukin, efavirenz, enoxacin, erythromycin, fingolimod, fluvoxamine, ketoconazole, oral contraceptives, pazopanib, phenobarbital, phenytoin, rifampin
Pregnancy category: C
Important contra-indications noted in the prescribing guidelines for: nursing mothers; pediatric patients
Note: Contra-indicated in patients with moderate to severe liver impairment (Child-Pugh B or C class).

Cardiovascular
  Cardiotoxicity [2]
  Hypertension [3]
Central Nervous System
  Anorexia [2]
  Anxiety (<2%) [2]
  Depression (<2%)
  Headache (4%) [21]
  Insomnia (2%) [6]
  Neurotoxicity [3]
  Suicidal ideation [2]
  Tremor (<2%)
  Vertigo (dizziness) [3]
Neuromuscular/Skeletal
  Back pain (3%) [4]
  Muscle spasm (<2%)
Gastrointestinal/Hepatic
  Abdominal pain (<2%) [2]
  Diarrhea (10%) [25]
  Dyspepsia (<2%)
  Gastritis (<2%)
  Nausea (5%) [24]
  Vomiting (<2%) [2]
Respiratory
  Bronchitis [3]
  COPD [3]
  Dyspnea [3]
  Influenza (3%) [3]
  Nasopharyngitis [4]
  Pneumonia [3]
  Rhinitis (<2%)
  Sinusitis (<2%)
  Upper respiratory tract infection [4]
Endocrine/Metabolic
  Appetite decreased (2%) [4]
  Weight loss (8%) [24]
Genitourinary
  Urinary tract infection (<2%)
Other
  Adverse effects [6]

ROLAPITANT

Trade name: Varubi (Tesaro)
Indications: Delayed nausea and vomiting from chemotherapy, in combination with dexamethasone and a 5HT3-receptor antagonist
Class: Antiemetic, Neurokinin 1 receptor antagonist
Half-life: ~7 days
Clinically important, potentially hazardous interactions with: thioridazine
Pregnancy category: N/A (No data available)
Important contra-indications noted in the prescribing guidelines for: nursing mothers; pediatric patients

Mucosal
  Stomatitis (4%)
Central Nervous System
  Headache [5]
  Vertigo (dizziness) (6%)
Neuromuscular/Skeletal
  Asthenia (fatigue) [5]
Gastrointestinal/Hepatic
  Abdominal pain (3%)
  Constipation [6]
  Dyspepsia (4%) [3]
Endocrine/Metabolic
  Appetite decreased (9%)
Genitourinary
  Urinary tract infection (4%)
Hematologic
  Anemia (3%)
  Neutropenia (7–9%) [2]
Other
  Hiccups (5%) [3]

ROMIDEPSIN

Trade name: Istodax (Celgene)
Indications: Cutaneous T-cell lymphoma (CTCL)
Class: Histone deacetylase (HDAC) inhibitor
Half-life: 3 hours
Clinically important, potentially hazardous interactions with: atazanavir, carbamazepine, clarithromycin, conivaptan, coumadin derivatives, CYP3A4 inhibitors and inducers, darunavir, delavirdine, dexamethasone, efavirenz, indinavir, itraconazole, ketoconazole, nefazodone, nelfinavir, oxcarbazepine, phenobarbital, phenytoin, rifabutin, rifampin, rifapentine, ritonavir, saquinavir, St John's wort, telithromycin, voriconazole, warfarin
Pregnancy category: D
Important contra-indications noted in the prescribing guidelines for: nursing mothers; pediatric patients

Skin
  Dermatitis (4–27%)
  Edema (>2%)
  Exfoliative dermatitis (4–27%)
  Peripheral edema (6–10%)
  Pruritus (7–31%)

Mucosal
  Stomatitis (6–10%)
Cardiovascular
  Hypotension (7–23%)
  Supraventricular arrhythmias (>2%)
  Tachycardia (10%)
  Ventricular arrhythmia (>2%)
Central Nervous System
  Anorexia (23–54%) [5]
  Chills (11–17%)
  Dysgeusia (taste perversion) (15–40%)
  Fever (20–47%)
  Headache (15–34%)
Neuromuscular/Skeletal
  Asthenia (fatigue) (53–77%) [10]
Gastrointestinal/Hepatic
  Abdominal pain (13–14%)
  Constipation (12–40%)
  Diarrhea (20–36%)
  Nausea (56–86%) [9]
  Vomiting (34–52%) [5]
Respiratory
  Cough (18–21%)
  Dyspnea (13–21%)
Endocrine/Metabolic
  ALT increased (3–22%)
  AST increased (3–28%)
  Hyperglycemia (2–51%)
  Hypermagnesemia (27%)
  Hyperuricemia (33%)
  Hypoalbuminemia (3–48%)
  Hypocalcemia (4–52%)
  Hypokalemia (6–20%)
  Hypomagnesemia (22–28%)
  Hyponatremia (<20%)
  Hypophosphatemia (27%)
  Weight loss (10–15%)
Hematologic
  Anemia (19–72%) [3]
  Leukopenia (4–55%) [2]
  Lymphopenia (4–57%) [2]
  Neutropenia (11–66%) [5]
  Sepsis (>2%)
  Thrombocytopenia (17–72%) [8]
Other
  Adverse effects [2]
  Infection (46–54%) [2]

ROMIPLOSTIM

See: www.drugeruptiondata.com/drug/id/1305

ROPINIROLE

Trade name: Requip (GSK)
Indications: Parkinsonism
Class: Dopamine receptor agonist
Half-life: ~6 hours
Clinically important, potentially hazardous interactions with: ciprofloxacin, estradiol, levomepromazine, norfloxacin, risperidone, warfarin, zuclopenthixol

Pregnancy category: C
Important contra-indications noted in the prescribing guidelines for: nursing mothers; pediatric patients

Skin
Diaphoresis (3–6%)
Herpes simplex (5%)
Hyperhidrosis (3%)
Peripheral edema (2–7%) [2]
Rash [2]

Mucosal
Xerostomia (5%)

Cardiovascular
Cardiotoxicity [2]
Chest pain (4%)
Flushing (3%)
Hypotension [2]
Orthostatic hypotension [4]

Central Nervous System
Amnesia (3%)
Dyskinesia [9]
Hallucinations (<5%) [7]
Headache (6%) [5]
Hyperesthesia (4%)
Impulse control disorder [3]
Insomnia [2]
Pain (3–8%)
Paresthesias (5%)
Psychosis [5]
Sleep related disorder [2]
Somnolence (drowsiness) (11–40%) [13]
Syncope (<12%) [3]
Tremor (6%)
Vertigo (dizziness) (6–40%) [16]
Yawning (3%)

Neuromuscular/Skeletal
Arthralgia (4%)
Asthenia (fatigue) (8–11%) [4]
Back pain [2]
Myalgia/Myopathy (3%)

Gastrointestinal/Hepatic
Abdominal pain (3–7%) [2]
Constipation [2]
Diarrhea (5%)
Dyspepsia (4–10%) [3]
Nausea (40–60%) [18]
Vomiting (11%) [3]

Respiratory
Cough (3%)
Dyspnea (3%)
Flu-like syndrome (3%)
Pharyngitis (6–9%)
Rhinitis (4%)
Sinusitis (4%)

Genitourinary
Impotence (3%)
Urinary tract infection (5%)

Ocular
Abnormal vision (6%)
Xerophthalmia (2%)

Other
Adverse effects [5]
Infection (viral) (11%)

ROPIVACAINE

See: www.drugeruptiondata.com/drug/id/1771

ROSIGLITAZONE

Trade names: Avandamet (GSK), Avandaryl (GSK), Avandia (GSK)
Indications: Type II diabetes
Class: Antidiabetic, Thiazolidinedione
Half-life: 3–4 hours
Clinically important, potentially hazardous interactions with: CYP2C8 inhibitors and inducers, gemfibrozil, grapefruit juice, paclitaxel, rifampin, teriflunomide
Pregnancy category: C
Important contra-indications noted in the prescribing guidelines for: nursing mothers
Note: Thiazolidinediones, including rosiglitazone, cause or exacerbate congestive heart failure in some patients.
Contra-indicated in patients with established NYHA Class III or IV heart failure. Avandaryl is rosiglitazone and glimepiride; Avandamet is rosiglitazone and metformin.
Warning: CONGESTIVE HEART FAILURE

Skin
Edema (5%) [12]
Peripheral edema [11]

Cardiovascular
Cardiac failure [13]
Congestive heart failure [2]
Myocardial infarction [9]
Myocardial ischemia [3]

Central Nervous System
Headache (6%)
Stroke [2]

Neuromuscular/Skeletal
Arthralgia (5%)
Back pain (4%)
Fractures [5]

Gastrointestinal/Hepatic
Hepatotoxicity [9]
Nausea [2]

Respiratory
Dyspnea [2]
Nasopharyngitis (6%)
Respiratory tract infection (10%)

Endocrine/Metabolic
Weight gain [4]

Genitourinary
Bladder disorder [2]

Hematologic
Anemia [2]

Ocular
Macular edema [8]
Proptosis [2]

Other
Adverse effects [3]
Death [6]

ROSUVASTATIN

Trade name: Crestor (AstraZeneca)
Indications: Hypercholesterolemia, mixed dyslipidemia
Class: HMG-CoA reductase inhibitor, Statin
Half-life: ~19 hours
Clinically important, potentially hazardous interactions with: alcohol, amiodarone, antacids, atazanavir, ciprofibrate, colchicine, conivaptan, coumarins, cyclosporine, daptomycin, darunavir, dronedarone, elbasvir & grazoprevir, eltrombopag, eluxadoline, erythromycin, ethinylestradiol, fenofibrate, fibrates, fosamprenavir, fusidic acid, gemfibrozil, indinavir, ledipasvir & sofosbuvir, lopinavir, nelfinavir, niacin, niacinamide, phenindione, progestins, protease inhibitors, ritonavir, safinamide, saquinavir, sofosbuvir/velpatasvir/voxilaprevir, tipranavir, trabectedin, vitamin K antagonists, warfarin
Pregnancy category: X
Important contra-indications noted in the prescribing guidelines for: nursing mothers

Skin
Peripheral edema (>2%)
Rash (>2%)

Central Nervous System
Depression (>2%)
Headache (6%)
Pain (>2%)
Paresthesias (>2%)
Vertigo (dizziness) (4%) [3]

Neuromuscular/Skeletal
Arthralgia (>2%)
Asthenia (fatigue) (3%) [2]
Back pain (>2%)
Myalgia/Myopathy (3%) [18]
Rhabdomyolysis [16]

Gastrointestinal/Hepatic
Abdominal pain (>2%)
Constipation (2%)
Hepatitis [2]
Hepatotoxicity [5]
Nausea (3%)

Respiratory
Cough (>2%)
Flu-like syndrome (2%)
Rhinitis (2%)
Sinusitis (2%)

Endocrine/Metabolic
Creatine phosphokinase increased [2]
Diabetes mellitus [3]

Renal
Nephrotoxicity [4]
Renal failure [3]

Other
Adverse effects [8]

ROTAVIRUS VACCINE

Trade names: Rotarix (GSK), RotaTeq (Merck)
Indications: Prevention of rotavirus gastroenteritis
Half-life: N/A
Clinically important, potentially hazardous interactions with: none known
Pregnancy category: C

Central Nervous System
Fever [3]

Gastrointestinal/Hepatic
Intussusception [2]

ROTIGOTINE

Trade name: Neupro (Schwarz)
Indications: Parkinsonism, restless legs syndrome
Class: Dopamine receptor agonist
Half-life: 5–7 hours
Clinically important, potentially hazardous interactions with: antipsychotics, levomepromazine, memantine, methyldopa, metoclopramide, risperidone, zuclopenthixol
Pregnancy category: C
Important contra-indications noted in the prescribing guidelines for: nursing mothers; pediatric patients
Note: Neupro contains sodium metabisulfite which is capable of causing anaphylactoid reactions in patients with sulfite allergy.

Skin
Diaphoresis (4%)
Erythema (2%)
Peripheral edema (7%) [3]
Rash (2%) [3]

Mucosal
Xerostomia (3%) [3]

Cardiovascular
Chest pain (>2%)
Hypertension (3%)
Hypotension [2]

Central Nervous System
Abnormal dreams (3%)
Anorexia (3%)
Anxiety (>2%)
Depression (>2%)
Dyskinesia [4]
Gait instability [2]
Hallucinations (2%) [3]
Headache (14%) [8]
Impulse control disorder [4]
Insomnia (10%) [3]
Somnolence (drowsiness) (25%) [16]

Tremor (>2%) [2]
Vertigo (dizziness) (3–18%) [7]

Neuromuscular/Skeletal
Arthralgia (4%)
Asthenia (fatigue) (8%) [10]
Back pain (6%)
Myalgia/Myopathy (2%)

Gastrointestinal/Hepatic
Abdominal pain (>2%)
Constipation (5%)
Diarrhea (>2%)
Dyspepsia (4%)
Gastrointestinal disorder [2]
Nausea (38%) [24]
Vomiting (13%) [6]

Respiratory
Cough (>2%)
Flu-like syndrome (>2%)
Rhinitis (>2%)
Sinusitis (3%)
Upper respiratory tract infection (>2%)

Genitourinary
Urinary frequency (>2%)
Urinary tract infection (3%)

Ocular
Abnormal vision (3%)
Hallucinations, visual (2%) [2]
Visual disturbances (3%)

Local
Application-site erythema [4]
Application-site pruritus [4]
Application-site reactions (37%) [31]

Other
Adverse effects [6]

ROXATIDINE

See: www.drugeruptiondata.com/drug/id/1080

ROXITHROMYCIN

See: www.drugeruptiondata.com/drug/id/1117

RUCAPARIB *

Trade name: Rubraca (Clovis)
Indications: Advanced BRCA-mutated ovarian cancer
Class: Poly (ADP-ribose) polymerase (PARP) inhibitor
Half-life: 17 hours
Clinically important, potentially hazardous interactions with: none known

Pregnancy category: N/A (Can cause fetal harm)
Important contra-indications noted in the prescribing guidelines for: nursing mothers; pediatric patients

Skin
Dermatitis (13%)
Erythema (13%)
Exanthems (13%)
Hand–foot syndrome (2%)
Photosensitivity (10%)
Pruritus (9%)
Rash (13%)

Central Nervous System
Dysgeusia (taste perversion) (39%) [2]
Fever (11%)
Vertigo (dizziness) (17%)

Neuromuscular/Skeletal
Asthenia (fatigue) (77%) [4]

Gastrointestinal/Hepatic
Abdominal pain (32%) [2]
Constipation (40%) [2]
Diarrhea (34%) [2]
Nausea (77%) [4]
Vomiting (46%) [4]

Respiratory
Dyspnea (21%)

Endocrine/Metabolic
ALT increased (74%) [3]
Appetite decreased (39%)
AST increased (73%) [4]
Hypercholesterolemia (40%)
Serum creatinine increased (92%)

Hematologic
Anemia (44%) [6]
Lymphocytopenia (45%)
Neutropenia (15%) [2]
Thrombocytopenia (21%) [2]

RUFINAMIDE

See: www.drugeruptiondata.com/drug/id/1320

RUPATADINE

See: www.drugeruptiondata.com/drug/id/1387

RUXOLITINIB

See: www.drugeruptiondata.com/drug/id/2717

SACCHARIN

Indications: Sugar substitute
Class: Sweetening agent
Half-life: N/A
Clinically important, potentially hazardous interactions with: none known
Pregnancy category: N/A
Note: Saccharin is a sulfonamide and can be absorbed systemically. Sulfonamides can produce severe, possibly fatal, reactions such as toxic epidermal necrolysis and Stevens-Johnson syndrome.

Skin
Dermatitis [3]
Exanthems [2]
Photosensitivity [3]
Pruritus [3]
Urticaria [5]

SACUBITRIL/ VALSARTAN

Trade name: Entresto (Novartis)
Indications: To reduce risk of cardiovascular death and hospitalization for heart failure in chronic heart failure
Class: Angiotensin receptor neprilysin inhibitor (ARNI)
Half-life: <12 hours
Clinically important, potentially hazardous interactions with: ACE inhibitors, aliskiren, lithium, NSAIDs, potassium-sparing diuretics
Pregnancy category: N/A (Can cause fetal harm)
Important contra-indications noted in the prescribing guidelines for: nursing mothers; pediatric patients
Note: Contra-indicated in patients with a history of angioedema related to previous therapy with angiotensin-converting enzyme inhibitor or angiotensin II receptor blocker. See also separate profile for valsartan.
Warning: FETAL TOXICITY

Skin
Angioedema (<2%) [2]
Peripheral edema [2]

Cardiovascular
Hypotension (18%) [4]
Orthostatic hypotension (2%)

Central Nervous System
Gait instability (2%)
Vertigo (dizziness) (6%) [2]

Neuromuscular/Skeletal
Arthralgia [2]

Gastrointestinal/Hepatic
Constipation [2]

Respiratory
Cough (9%) [4]
Nasopharyngitis [2]

Endocrine/Metabolic
Hyperkalemia (12%) [4]
Serum creatinine increased [2]

Renal
Nephrotoxicity [3]
Renal failure (5%)

Other
Adverse effects [2]

SAFINAMIDE *

Trade name: Xadago (Newron)
Indications: Adjunctive treatment to levodopa/ carbidopa in patients with Parkinson's disease experiencing 'off' episodes
Class: Monoamine oxidase B inhibitor
Half-life: 20–26 hours
Clinically important, potentially hazardous interactions with: cyclobenzaprine, dextromethorphan, dopaminergic antagonists, imatinib, irinotecan, isoniazid, lapatinib, linezolid, meperidine, methadone, methylphenidate, metoclopramide, mitoxantrone, other MAO inhibitors, propoxyphene, rosuvastatin, serotonergic drugs, St John's wort, sulfasalazine, sympathomimetics, topotecan, tramadol, tricyclic or tetracyclic antidepressants
Pregnancy category: C
Important contra-indications noted in the prescribing guidelines for: nursing mothers; pediatric patients

Skin
Peripheral edema [2]

Cardiovascular
Hypertension [3]
Orthostatic hypotension (2%)

Central Nervous System
Anxiety (2%)
Dyskinesia (17–21%) [5]
Fever [3]
Gait instability (4–6%) [2]
Headache [3]
Insomnia (<4%) [2]
Parkinsonism (exacerbation) [2]
Tremor [2]
Vertigo (dizziness) [2]

Neuromuscular/Skeletal
Asthenia (fatigue) [2]
Back pain [3]

Gastrointestinal/Hepatic
Abdominal pain [2]
Constipation [2]
Dyspepsia (<2%)
Nausea (3–6%) [2]
Vomiting [2]

Respiratory
Cough (2%) [2]
Nasopharyngitis [2]

Endocrine/Metabolic
ALT increased (3–7%)
AST increased (6–7%)
Weight loss [2]

Ocular
Cataract [3]
Vision blurred [2]

SALMETEROL

See: www.drugeruptiondata.com/drug/id/635

SALSALATE

Trade name: Mono-Gesic (Schwarz)
Indications: Arthritis
Class: Non-steroidal anti-inflammatory (NSAID), Salicylate
Half-life: 7–8 hours
Clinically important, potentially hazardous interactions with: dichlorphenamide, methotrexate
Pregnancy category: C
Important contra-indications noted in the prescribing guidelines for: nursing mothers; pediatric patients
Note: NSAIDs may cause an increased risk of serious cardiovascular and gastrointestinal adverse events, which can be fatal. This risk may increase with duration of use.

Skin
Anaphylactoid reactions/Anaphylaxis (<10%)
Rash (<10%)

SAPROPTERIN

See: www.drugeruptiondata.com/drug/id/1271

SAQUINAVIR

Trade name: Invirase (Roche)
Indications: Advanced HIV infection
Class: Antiretroviral, CYP3A4 inhibitor, HIV-1 protease inhibitor
Half-life: 12 hours
Clinically important, potentially hazardous interactions with: abiraterone, afatinib, alprazolam, amitriptyline, amprenavir, astemizole, atazanavir, atorvastatin, avanafil, brigatinib, cabazitaxel, cabozantinib, calcifediol, clindamycin, clozapine, copanlisib, crizotinib, darifenacin, darunavir, dasatinib, delavirdine, dihydroergotamine, dronedarone, efavirenz, elbasvir & grazoprevir, eluxadoline, eplerenone, ergot derivatives, everolimus, fentanyl, fesoterodine, flibanserin, fluticasone propionate, itraconazole, ixabepilone, ketoconazole, lapatinib, levomepromazine, lomitapide, lopinavir, maraviroc, methysergide, midazolam, midostaurin, mifepristone, naldemedine, nelfinavir, neratinib, olaparib, omeprazole, paclitaxel, palbociclib, pantoprazole, pazopanib, pentamidine, phenytoin, pimozide, ponatinib, quinine, ribociclib, rifampin, rilpivirine, ritonavir, rivaroxaban, romidepsin, rosuvastatin, ruxolitinib, sildenafil, simeprevir, simvastatin, solifenacin, sonidegib, St John's wort, sunitinib, tadalafil, telithromycin, temsirolimus, ticagrelor, tipranavir, tolvaptan, vardenafil, vemurafenib, vorapaxar, voriconazole

Pregnancy category: B
Important contra-indications noted in the prescribing guidelines for: nursing mothers
Note: Protease inhibitors cause dyslipidemia which includes elevated triglycerides and cholesterol and redistribution of body fat centrally to produce the so-called 'protease paunch', breast enlargement, facial atrophy, and 'buffalo hump'.

Skin
Acneform eruption (<2%)
Candidiasis (<2%)
Dermatitis (<2%)
Diaphoresis (<2%)
Eczema (<2%)
Erythema (<2%)
Exanthems (<2%)
Folliculitis (<2%)
Herpes simplex (<2%)
Herpes zoster (<2%)
Photosensitivity (<2%)
Pigmentation (<2%)
Seborrheic dermatitis (<2%)
Ulcerations (<2%)
Urticaria (<2%)
Verrucae (<2%)
Xerosis (<2%)

Hair
Hair changes (<2%)

Mucosal
Cheilitis (<2%)
Gingivitis (<2%)
Glossitis (<2%)
Oral ulceration (2%)
Stomatitis (<2%)
Xerostomia (<2%)

Cardiovascular
QT prolongation [3]

Central Nervous System
Dysesthesia (<2%)
Dysgeusia (taste perversion) (<2%)
Hyperesthesia (<2%)
Paresthesias (3%)

Gastrointestinal/Hepatic
Hepatotoxicity [2]

Endocrine/Metabolic
Gynecomastia [2]

SARILUMAB *

Trade name: Kevzara (Sanofi)
Indications: Rheumatoid arthritis
Class: Anti-interleukin-6 receptor monoclonal antibody, Monoclonal antibody
Half-life: 8–10 days (concentration-dependent)
Clinically important, potentially hazardous interactions with: live vaccines
Pregnancy category: N/A (Based on animal data, may cause fetal harm)
Important contra-indications noted in the prescribing guidelines for: the elderly; nursing mothers; pediatric patients
Warning: RISK OF SERIOUS INFECTIONS

Respiratory
Nasopharyngitis (>3%)

Upper respiratory tract infection (3–4%)
Endocrine/Metabolic
ALT increased (5%) [3]
AST increased (38–43%)
Hypertriglyceridemia (<3%)

Genitourinary
Urinary tract infection (3%)

Hematologic
Leukopenia (<2%)
Neutropenia (7–10%) [5]

Local
Injection-site erythema (4–5%)
Injection-site pruritus (2%)
Injection-site reactions (6–7%)

Other
Infection [5]

SAXAGLIPTIN

Trade names: Onglyza (Bristol-Myers Squibb), Qtern (AstraZeneca)
Indications: Type II diabetes mellitus
Class: Antidiabetic, Dipeptidyl peptidase-4 (DPP-4) inhibitor
Half-life: 2.5–3.1 hours
Clinically important, potentially hazardous interactions with: ACE inhibitors, alcohol, aprepitant, beta blockers, bexarotene, colchicine, conivaptan, corticosteroids, CYP3A4 inducers, darunavir, dasatinib, delavirdine, diazoxide, diuretics, efavirenz, estradiol, estrogens, hypoglycemic agents, indinavir, ketoconazole, lapatinib, MAO inhibitors, oxcarbazepine, P-glycoprotein inhibitors and inducers, pegvisomant, pioglitazone, rifapentine, somatropin, strong CYP3A4/5 inhibitors, telithromycin, terbinafine, testosterone, voriconazole
Pregnancy category: B
Important contra-indications noted in the prescribing guidelines for: nursing mothers; pediatric patients
Note: Qtern is saxagliptin and dapagliflozin.

Skin
Hypersensitivity (<2%)
Peripheral edema (2–3%)

Cardiovascular
Cardiac disorder [2]
Cardiac failure [2]

Central Nervous System
Headache (7%) [7]

Gastrointestinal/Hepatic
Abdominal pain (2%)
Diarrhea [5]
Gastroenteritis (2%)
Vomiting (2%)

Respiratory
Nasopharyngitis [4]
Sinusitis (3%) [2]
Upper respiratory tract infection (8%) [8]

Endocrine/Metabolic
Hypoglycemia [9]

Genitourinary
Urinary tract infection (7%) [7]

Other
Adverse effects [7]
Infection [2]

SCOPOLAMINE

See: www.drugeruptiondata.com/drug/id/639

SEBELIPASE ALFA

Trade name: Kanuma (Alexion)
Indications: Lysosomal acid lipase deficiency
Class: Enzyme replacement
Half-life: 5–7 minutes
Clinically important, potentially hazardous interactions with: none known
Pregnancy category: N/A (No available data)
Important contra-indications noted in the prescribing guidelines for: nursing mothers

Skin
Hypersensitivity (20%)
Urticaria (33%)

Mucosal
Oropharyngeal pain (17%)

Cardiovascular
Chest pain (<8%)
Tachycardia (<30%)

Central Nervous System
Anxiety (<8%)
Fever (25–56%)
Headache (28%)

Neuromuscular/Skeletal
Asthenia (fatigue) (8%)
Hypotonia (<30%)

Gastrointestinal/Hepatic
Constipation (8%)
Diarrhea (67%)
Nausea (8%)
Vomiting (67%)

Respiratory
Cough (33%)
Nasopharyngitis (11–33%)
Rhinitis (56%)

Hematologic
Anemia (44%)

Other
Sneezing (<30%)

SECNIDAZOLE *

Trade name: Solosec (Symbiomix)
Indications: Bacterial vaginosis
Class: Antibiotic, nitroimidazole
Half-life: ~17 hours
Clinically important, potentially hazardous interactions with: none known
Pregnancy category: N/A (Insufficient evidence to inform drug-associated risk)
Important contra-indications noted in the prescribing guidelines for: nursing mothers; pediatric patients
Note: Potential risk for carcinogenicity from animal studies – avoid chronic use.

Central Nervous System
Dysgeusia (taste perversion) (3%)
Headache (4%) [3]

Gastrointestinal/Hepatic
Abdominal pain (2%)
Diarrhea (3%)
Nausea [3]

Genitourinary
Vulvovaginal candidiasis (10%)
Vulvovaginal pruritus (2%)

SECOBARBITAL

See: www.drugeruptiondata.com/drug/id/640

SECRETIN

See: www.drugeruptiondata.com/drug/id/641

SECUKINUMAB

Trade name: Cosentyx (Novartis)
Indications: Plaque psoriasis, psoriatic arthritis, ankylosing spondylitis
Class: Interleukin-17A (IL-17A) antagonist, Monoclonal antibody
Half-life: 22–31 days
Clinically important, potentially hazardous interactions with: live vaccines
Pregnancy category: B
Important contra-indications noted in the prescribing guidelines for: nursing mothers; pediatric patients
Note: Use with caution in patients with inflammatory bowel disease.

Skin
Candidiasis [4]
Neoplasms [2]
Pruritus [3]
Psoriasis (exacerbation) [2]

Cardiovascular
Hypertension [2]

Central Nervous System
Headache [13]

Neuromuscular/Skeletal
Arthralgia [3]

Gastrointestinal/Hepatic
Diarrhea (3–4%) [4]

Respiratory
Nasopharyngitis (11–12%) [19]
Upper respiratory tract infection (3%) [12]

Hematologic
Neutropenia [4]

Local
Injection-site reactions [3]

Other
Adverse effects [5]
Infection (29%) [12]

SELEGILINE

Synonyms: deprenyl; L-deprenyl
Trade names: Eldepryl (Somerset), Emsam (Mylan Specialty), Zelapar (Valeant)
Indications: Parkinsonism
Class: Antidepressant, Monoamine oxidase B inhibitor
Half-life: 9 minutes
Clinically important, potentially hazardous interactions with: amitriptyline, carbidopa, citalopram, doxepin, ephedra, ephedrine, escitalopram, fluoxetine, fluvoxamine, levodopa, meperidine, methadone, moclobemide, naratriptan, nefazodone, oral contraceptives, oxcarbazepine, paroxetine hydrochloride, propoxyphene, sertraline, tramadol, valbenazine, venlafaxine
Pregnancy category: C
Important contra-indications noted in the prescribing guidelines for: nursing mothers; pediatric patients
Warning: SUICIDALITY IN CHILDREN AND ADOLESCENTS

Mucosal
Xerostomia (>10%) [2]

Cardiovascular
Hypertension [2]

Central Nervous System
Hallucinations [2]
Headache [2]
Serotonin syndrome [2]

Gastrointestinal/Hepatic
Nausea [2]

Local
Application-site reactions [5]

Other
Bruxism (<10%)

SELENIUM

See: www.drugeruptiondata.com/drug/id/915

SELEXIPAG

Trade name: Uptravi (Actelion)
Indications: Pulmonary arterial hypertension
Class: Prostacyclin receptor agonist
Half-life: <3 hours
Clinically important, potentially hazardous interactions with: gemfibrozil, strong CYP2C8 inhibitors
Pregnancy category: N/A (No data available)
Important contra-indications noted in the prescribing guidelines for: nursing mothers

Skin
Rash (11%)

Cardiovascular
Flushing (12%)

Central Nervous System
Headache (65%) [7]

Neuromuscular/Skeletal
Arthralgia (11%)
Jaw pain (26%) [5]
Myalgia/Myopathy (16%)
Pain in extremities (17%)

Gastrointestinal/Hepatic
Diarrhea (42%) [3]
Nausea (33%) [5]
Vomiting (18%)

Endocrine/Metabolic
Appetite decreased (6%)

Hematologic
Anemia (8%)

SERMORELIN

See: www.drugeruptiondata.com/drug/id/961

SERTACONAZOLE

See: www.drugeruptiondata.com/drug/id/1023

SERTINDOLE

See: www.drugeruptiondata.com/drug/id/2455

SERTRALINE

Trade name: Zoloft (Pfizer)
Indications: Depression, panic disorders, obsessive compulsive disorders
Class: Antidepressant, Selective serotonin reuptake inhibitor (SSRI)
Half-life: 24–26 hours
Clinically important, potentially hazardous interactions with: amphetamines, astemizole, clarithromycin, clozapine, darunavir, dextroamphetamine, diethylpropion, droperidol, efavirenz, erythromycin, isocarboxazid, linezolid, MAO inhibitors, mazindol, methamphetamine, metoclopramide, phendimetrazine, phenelzine, phentermine, phenylpropanolamine, pimozide, pseudoephedrine, selegiline, sibutramine, St John's wort, sumatriptan, sympathomimetics, tranylcypromine, trazodone, troleandomycin, zolmitriptan
Pregnancy category: C

Skin
Angioedema [3]
Diaphoresis (8%) [6]
Rash (<10%)
Stevens-Johnson syndrome [2]

Hair
Alopecia [3]

Mucosal
Xerostomia (16%) [7]

Cardiovascular
Chest pain (<10%)
Flushing (2%)
Palpitation (<10%)
QT prolongation [3]
Torsades de pointes [2]

Central Nervous System
Akathisia [6]
Anxiety (<10%)
Coma [2]
Headache (>10%)
Hypoesthesia (5%)
Insomnia (>10%)
Mania [4]
Pain (<10%)
Paresthesias (<10%)
Restless legs syndrome [3]
Seizures [2]
Serotonin syndrome [10]
Somnolence (drowsiness) (>10%)
Tremor (<10%) [3]
Vertigo (dizziness) (>10%) [3]
Yawning (<10%)

Neuromuscular/Skeletal
Asthenia (fatigue) (>10%)
Back pain (<10%)

Gastrointestinal/Hepatic
Constipation (<10%)
Diarrhea (>10%) [3]
Hepatotoxicity [4]
Nausea (10%) [2]
Vomiting (>10%)

Respiratory
Rhinitis (<10%)

Endocrine/Metabolic
Galactorrhea [4]
Gynecomastia [2]
Hyponatremia [4]
Libido decreased (>10%)
SIADH [14]
Weight gain (<10%)

Genitourinary
Impotence (<10%)
Priapism [5]
Sexual dysfunction (10%) [4]

Otic
Tinnitus (<10%)

Ocular
Abnormal vision (<10%)
Hallucinations, visual [3]

Other
Adverse effects [4]
Allergic reactions [2]
Bruxism [3]
Death [5]

SEVELAMER

See: www.drugeruptiondata.com/drug/id/1402

SEVOFLURANE

See: www.drugeruptiondata.com/drug/id/1197

SIBUTRAMINE

See: www.drugeruptiondata.com/drug/id/644

SILDENAFIL

Trade names: Revatio (Pfizer), Viagra (Pfizer)
Indications: Erectile dysfunction, hypertension
Class: Phosphodiesterase type 5 (PDE5) inhibitor
Half-life: 4 hours
Clinically important, potentially hazardous interactions with: alfuzosin, alpha blockers, amlodipine, amprenavir, amyl nitrite, antifungals, antihypertensives, atazanavir, boceprevir, bosentan, cimetidine, clarithromycin, cobicistat/elvitegravir/emtricitabine/tenofovir alafenamide, cobicistat/elvitegravir/emtricitabine/tenofovir disoproxil, conivaptan, CYP3A4 inhibitors and inducers, darunavir, dasabuvir/ombitasvir/paritaprevir/ritonavir, dasatinib, deferasirox, delavirdine, disopyramide, erythromycin, etravirine, fosamprenavir, grapefruit juice, high-fat foods, HMG-CoA reductase inhibitors, indinavir, isosorbide, isosorbide dinitrate, isosorbide mononitrate, itraconazole, ketoconazole, lopinavir, macrolide antibiotics, nelfinavir, nicorandil, nitrates, nitroglycerin, ombitasvir/paritaprevir/ritonavir, other phosphodiesterase 5 inhibitors, paclitaxel, PEG-interferon, riociguat, ritonavir, saproterin, saquinavir, St John's wort, telaprevir, telithromycin, tipranavir
Pregnancy category: B
Important contra-indications noted in the prescribing guidelines for: nursing mothers; pediatric patients

Skin
Dermatitis (<2%)
Diaphoresis (<2%)
Edema (<2%)
Erythema (6%)
Exfoliative dermatitis (<2%)
Facial edema (<2%)
Genital edema (<2%)
Herpes simplex (<2%)
Lichenoid eruption [2]
Peripheral edema (<2%)
Photosensitivity (<2%)
Pruritus (<2%)
Rash (2%)
Ulcerations (<2%)
Urticaria (<2%)

Mucosal
Epistaxis (nosebleed) (9–13%) [2]
Gingivitis (<2%)
Glossitis (<2%)
Nasal congestion [7]
Rectal hemorrhage (<2%)
Stomatitis (<2%)
Xerostomia (<2%)

Cardiovascular
Angina (<2%)
Atrial fibrillation [2]
Atrioventricular block (<2%)
Cardiac arrest (<2%) [2]
Cardiac failure (<2%)
Cardiomyopathy (<2%)
Chest pain (<2%) [2]
Congestive heart failure [2]
Flushing (10–25%) [34]
Hypotension (<2%) [5]
Myocardial infarction [4]
Myocardial ischemia (<2%)

Palpitation (<2%)
Postural hypotension (<2%)
Tachycardia (<2%)
Vasodilation [3]
Ventricular arrhythmia [2]

Central Nervous System
Abnormal dreams (<2%)
Amnesia [3]
Anorgasmia (<2%)
Chills (<2%)
Depression (<2%)
Fever (6%)
Headache (16–46%) [40]
Hyperesthesia (<2%)
Insomnia (7%)
Migraine (<2%)
Neurotoxicity (<2%)
Pain (<2%)
Paresthesias (3%)
Seizures [3]
Somnolence (drowsiness) (<2%)
Stroke [2]
Subarachnoid hemorrhage [2]
Syncope (<2%)
Tremor (<2%)
Vertigo (dizziness) (2%) [7]

Neuromuscular/Skeletal
Arthralgia (<2%)
Asthenia (fatigue) (<2%) [2]
Ataxia (<2%)
Back pain [3]
Bone or joint pain (<2%)
Gouty tophi (<2%)
Hypertonia (<2%)
Myalgia/Myopathy (7%) [4]
Tendinopathy/Tendon rupture (<2%)

Gastrointestinal/Hepatic
Abdominal pain (<2%) [3]
Colitis (<2%)
Diarrhea (3–9%) [4]
Dyspepsia (7–17%) [15]
Dysphagia (<2%)
Esophagitis (<2%)
Gastritis (<2%)
Gastroenteritis (<2%)
Hepatotoxicity [2]
Nausea [4]
Vomiting (<2%)

Respiratory
Asthma (<2%)
Bronchitis (<2%)
Cough (<2%)
Dyspnea (7%) [4]
Hemoptysis [2]
Hypoxia [3]
Laryngitis (<2%)
Pharyngitis (<2%)
Pneumonia [2]
Respiratory failure [3]
Rhinitis (4%) [6]
Sinusitis (<2%)
Stridor [2]
Upper respiratory tract infection [2]

Endocrine/Metabolic
Gynecomastia (<2%)
Hyperglycemia (<2%)
Hypernatremia (<2%)
Hyperuricemia (<2%)

Genitourinary
Cystitis (<2%)
Ejaculatory dysfunction (<2%)
Nocturia (<2%)
Priapism [6]
Urinary frequency (<2%)
Urinary incontinence (<2%)
Urinary tract infection (3%)

Hematologic
Anemia (<2%)
Leukopenia (<2%)

Otic
Ear pain (<2%)
Hearing loss (<2%) [4]
Tinnitus (<2%) [2]

Ocular
Abnormal vision [3]
Cataract (<2%)
Conjunctivitis (<2%)
Dyschromatopsia (blue-green vision) (3–11%) [5]
Mydriasis (<2%)
Ocular hemorrhage (<2%)
Ocular pain (<2%)
Ocular pigmentation (<2%)
Optic neuropathy [18]
Photophobia (<2%)
Retinal vein occlusion [2]
Vision blurred [4]
Visual disturbances [5]
Xerophthalmia (<2%)

Other
Adverse effects [5]
Allergic reactions (<2%)
Death [3]
Dipsia (thirst) (<2%)

SILODOSIN

Trade names: Rapaflo (Watson), Urief (Kissei)
Indications: Benign prostatic hyperplasia
Class: Adrenergic alpha-receptor antagonist
Half-life: 4.7–6 hours
Clinically important, potentially hazardous interactions with: alpha blockers, antihypertensives, atorvastatin, clarithromycin, conivaptan, cyclosporine, darunavir, delavirdine, diltiazem, erythromycin, indinavir, itraconazole, ketoconazole, lapatinib, ritonavir, stong CYP3A4 inhibitors, telithromycin, vasodilators, verapamil, voriconazole
Pregnancy category: B (Not indicated for use in women)
Important contra-indications noted in the prescribing guidelines for: pediatric patients
Note: Contra-indicated in patients with severe hepatic or renal impairment.

Mucosal
Nasal congestion (2%) [3]
Rhinorrhea (<2%)

Cardiovascular
Orthostatic hypotension (3%) [9]
Postural hypotension [2]

Central Nervous System
Headache (2%) [3]
Insomnia (<2%)

Vertigo (dizziness) (3%) [8]

Neuromuscular/Skeletal
Asthenia (fatigue) (<2%)

Gastrointestinal/Hepatic
Abdominal pain (<2%)
Diarrhea (3%) [2]

Respiratory
Nasopharyngitis (2%)
Sinusitis (<2%)

Genitourinary
Ejaculatory dysfunction (25%) [28]
Retrograde ejaculation (28%) [4]

Other
Adverse effects [2]
Dipsia (thirst) (7%) [2]

SILTUXIMAB

See: www.drugeruptiondata.com/drug/id/3515

SIMEPREVIR

Trade name: Olysio (Janssen)
Indications: Hepatitis C
Class: Direct-acting antiviral, Hepatitis C virus NS3/4A protease inhibitor
Half-life: 10–13 hours
Clinically important, potentially hazardous interactions with: atazanavir, carbamazepine, cisapride, clarithromycin, cobicistat/elvitegravir/emtricitabine/tenofovir disoproxil, darunavir, delavirdine, dexamethasone, efavirenz, erythromycin, etravirine, fluconazole, fosamprenavir, indinavir, itraconazole, ketoconazole, ledipasvir & sofosbuvir, lopinavir, milk thistle, nelfinavir, nevirapine, oxcarbazepine, phenobarbital, phenytoin, posaconazole, rifabutin, rifampin, rifapentine, ritonavir, saquinavir, St John's wort, telithromycin, tipranavir, voriconazole
Pregnancy category: X (simeprevir is pregnancy category C but must not be used in monotherapy)
Important contra-indications noted in the prescribing guidelines for: nursing mothers; pediatric patients
Note: Must be used in combination with PEG-interferon and ribavirin (see separate entries).
Warning: RISK OF HEPATITIS B VIRUS REACTIVATION IN PATIENTS COINFECTED WITH HCV AND HBV

Skin
Photosensitivity (28%) [5]
Pruritus (22%) [8]
Rash (28%) [10]

Central Nervous System
Fever [2]
Headache [13]
Insomnia [3]

Neuromuscular/Skeletal
Asthenia (fatigue) [10]
Myalgia/Myopathy (16%)

Gastrointestinal/Hepatic
Nausea (22%) [9]

Vomiting [2]

Respiratory
Dyspnea (12%)
Flu-like syndrome [3]

Endocrine/Metabolic
Hyperbilirubinemia [9]

Hematologic
Anemia [11]
Neutropenia [3]

Other
Adverse effects [7]

SIMVASTATIN

Trade names: Inegy (MSD), Simcor (AbbVie), Vytorin (MSD), Zocor (Merck)
Indications: Hypercholesterolemia
Class: HMG-CoA reductase inhibitor, Statin
Half-life: 1.9 hours
Clinically important, potentially hazardous interactions with: alitretinoin, amiodarone, amlodipine, amprenavir, atazanavir, azithromycin, boceprevir, bosentan, carbamazepine, ciprofibrate, clarithromycin, clopidogrel, colchicine, conivaptan, coumarins, cyclosporine, danazol, darunavir, dasabuvir/ombitasvir/paritaprevir/ritonavir, dasatinib, delavirdine, diltiazem, dronedarone, efavirenz, elbasvir & grazoprevir, erythromycin, fosamprenavir, fusidic acid, gemfibrozil, glecaprevir & pibrentasvir, grapefruit juice, HIV protease inhibitors, imatinib, imidazoles, indinavir, itraconazole, ketoconazole, lomitapide, lopinavir, miconazole, mifepristone, nefazodone, nelfinavir, ombitasvir/paritaprevir/ritonavir, paclitaxel, pazopanib, posaconazole, rabeprazole, ranolazine, red rice yeast, rifampin, ritonavir, roxithromycin, saquinavir, selenium, St John's wort, tacrolimus, telaprevir, telithromycin, ticagrelor, tipranavir, triazoles, verapamil, voriconazole, warfarin
Pregnancy category: X
Important contra-indications noted in the prescribing guidelines for: nursing mothers; pediatric patients
Note: Simcor is simvastatin and niacin; Vytorin is simvastatin and ezetimibe.

Skin
Dermatomyositis [5]
Eczema (5%) [4]
Edema (3%)
Eosinophilic fasciitis [2]
Erythema multiforme [2]
Lichen planus pemphigoides [2]
Lupus erythematosus [5]
Peripheral edema [2]
Photosensitivity [7]
Pruritus [3]
Purpura [3]
Rash (<10%) [4]
Vasculitis [2]

Mucosal
Stomatitis [2]

Cardiovascular
Atrial fibrillation (6%)

Central Nervous System
Cognitive impairment [3]

Headache (3–7%)
Memory loss [2]
Vertigo (dizziness) (5%)

Neuromuscular/Skeletal
Asthenia (fatigue) (9%) [3]
Compartment syndrome [2]
Myalgia/Myopathy (<10%) [37]
Rhabdomyolysis [87]
Tendinopathy/Tendon rupture [3]

Gastrointestinal/Hepatic
Abdominal pain (7%)
Constipation (2–7%)
Diarrhea [5]
Gastritis (5%)
Hepatitis [4]
Hepatotoxicity [7]
Nausea (5%)
Pancreatitis [7]

Respiratory
Bronchitis (7%)
Upper respiratory tract infection (9%)

Endocrine/Metabolic
Creatine phosphokinase increased [2]
Diabetes mellitus [4]

Renal
Nephrotoxicity [2]
Renal failure [9]

Hematologic
Leukopenia [2]

Other
Adverse effects [9]
Death [5]

SINCALIDE

See: www.drugeruptiondata.com/drug/id/1165

SINECATECHINS

See: www.drugeruptiondata.com/drug/id/1300

SIPULEUCEL-T

See: www.drugeruptiondata.com/drug/id/2647

SIROLIMUS

Synonym: rapamycin
Trade name: Rapamune (Wyeth)
Indications: Prophylaxis of organ rejection in renal transplants, lymphangioleiomyomatosis
Class: Immunosuppressant, Macrolactam, Non-calcineurin inhibitor
Half-life: 62 hours
Clinically important, potentially hazardous interactions with: atazanavir, benazepril, boceprevir, captopril, ceritinib, cobicistat/elvitegravir/emtricitabine/tenofovir disoproxil, crizotinib, cyclosporine, darunavir, dasatinib, delavirdine, dronedarone, efavirenz, eluxadoline, enalapril, enzalutamide, fosinopril, Hemophilus B vaccine, indinavir, itraconazole, lisinopril, lopinavir, micafungin, mifepristone, posaconazole, quinapril,

ramipril, ribociclib, St John's wort, tacrolimus, telaprevir, telithromycin, tipranavir, venetoclax, voriconazole, zotarolimus
Pregnancy category: C
Important contra-indications noted in the prescribing guidelines for: the elderly; nursing mothers; pediatric patients
Warning: IMMUNOSUPPRESSION, USE IS NOT RECOMMENDED IN LIVER OR LUNG TRANSPLANT PATIENTS

Skin
Abscess (3–20%)
Acneform eruption (20–31%) [9]
Angioedema [5]
Cellulitis (3–20%)
Dermatitis [3]
Diaphoresis (3–20%)
Ecchymoses (3–20%)
Edema (16–24%) [6]
Facial edema (3–20%) [2]
Folliculitis [3]
Fungal dermatitis (3–20%)
Hypertrophy (3–20%)
Lymphedema [2]
Peripheral edema (54–64%) [3]
Pruritus (3–20%)
Purpura (3–20%)
Rash (10–20%) [5]
Toxicity [2]
Ulcerations (3–20%)
Vasculitis [2]

Hair
Hirsutism (3–20%)

Nails
Onychopathy [2]

Mucosal
Aphthous stomatitis (9%) [8]
Gingival hyperplasia/hypertrophy (3–20%) [2]
Gingivitis (3–20%)
Mucositis [2]
Oral candidiasis (3–20%)
Oral ulceration (3–20%) [8]
Stomatitis (3–20%) [6]

Cardiovascular
Thrombophlebitis (3–20%)

Central Nervous System
Chills (3–20%)
Depression (3–20%)
Fever [2]
Hyperesthesia (3–20%)
Paresthesias (3–20%)
Tremor (21–31%)

Neuromuscular/Skeletal
Arthralgia (25–31%) [3]
Asthenia (fatigue) [3]
Myalgia/Myopathy [2]

Gastrointestinal/Hepatic
Diarrhea [3]
Hepatitis [2]
Hepatotoxicity [3]

Respiratory
Cough [2]
Flu-like syndrome (3–20%)
Pneumonitis [7]
Pulmonary toxicity [3]

Upper respiratory tract infection (20–26%) [2]

Endocrine/Metabolic
Hypercholesterolemia [2]
Hyperlipidemia [2]
Hypertriglyceridemia [2]

Renal
Nephrotoxicity [2]
Proteinuria [5]

Hematologic
Anemia [3]
Dyslipidemia [4]
Hemolytic uremic syndrome [2]
Leukopenia [2]
Neutropenia [2]
Thrombosis [2]

Otic
Tinnitus (3–20%)

Ocular
Eyelid edema (40%) [2]

Local
Application-site pruritus [2]

Other
Adverse effects [5]
Death [3]
Infection [5]

SITAGLIPTIN

Trade names: Janumet (Merck Sharpe & Dohme), Januvia (Merck Sharpe & Dohme)
Indications: Type II diabetes mellitus
Class: Antidiabetic, Dipeptidyl peptidase-4 (DPP-4) inhibitor
Half-life: 12 hours
Clinically important, potentially hazardous interactions with: alcohol, anabolic steroids, beta blockers, corticosteroids, diazoxide, digoxin, estrogens, loop diuretics, MAO inhibitors, progestogens, testosterone, thiazides
Pregnancy category: B
Important contra-indications noted in the prescribing guidelines for: the elderly; nursing mothers; pediatric patients
Note: Janumet is sitagliptin and metformin.

Skin
Angioedema [3]
Bullous pemphigoid [2]
Edema [3]
Rash [2]

Central Nervous System
Headache [5]

Neuromuscular/Skeletal
Arthralgia [2]
Bone or joint pain [2]
Rhabdomyolysis [4]

Gastrointestinal/Hepatic
Abdominal pain (2%)
Constipation [3]
Diarrhea [9]
Hepatotoxicity [2]
Nausea [10]
Pancreatitis [9]
Vomiting [6]

Respiratory
Nasopharyngitis [5]
Upper respiratory tract infection [2]

Endocrine/Metabolic
Creatine phosphokinase increased [2]
Hypoglycemia [10]
Weight gain [3]
Weight loss [2]

Renal
Renal failure [2]

Other
Adverse effects [7]
Cancer [3]

SITAXENTAN

See: www.drugeruptiondata.com/drug/id/1222

SMALLPOX VACCINE

Trade name: Dryvax (Wyeth)
Indications: Prevention of smallpox (variola)
Class: Vaccine
Half-life: ~5 years
Clinically important, potentially hazardous interactions with: corticosteroids
Pregnancy category: C

Skin
Basal cell carcinoma [4]
Bullous dermatitis [2]
Carcinoma [2]
Dermatitis [2]
Eczema vaccinatum [13]
Erythema multiforme [8]
Exanthems [7]
Folliculitis [2]
Herpes simplex [2]
Herpes zoster [2]
Melanoma [2]
Photosensitivity [2]
Purpura [11]
Rash [3]
Scar [2]
Stevens-Johnson syndrome [3]
Toxic epidermal necrolysis [5]
Tumors [3]
Urticaria [5]
Vaccinia [25]
Vaccinia gangrenosum [3]
Vaccinia necrosum [6]

Central Nervous System
Headache [2]

Other
Allergic reactions [2]
Death [8]

SODIUM IODIDE I-131

See: www.drugeruptiondata.com/drug/id/2657

SODIUM NITRITE

See: www.drugeruptiondata.com/drug/id/2797

SODIUM OXYBATE

See: www.drugeruptiondata.com/drug/id/919

SODIUM PICOSULFATE

See: www.drugeruptiondata.com/drug/id/2988

SODIUM THIOSULFATE

See: www.drugeruptiondata.com/drug/id/2807

SOFOSBUVIR

Trade name: Sovaldi (Gilead)
Indications: Hepatitis C
Class: Direct-acting antiviral, Hepatitis C virus nucleotide analog NS5B polymerase inhibitor
Half-life: <27 hours
Clinically important, potentially hazardous interactions with: carbamazepine, oxcarbazepine, phenobarbital, phenytoin, rifabutin, rifampin, rifapentine, ritonavir, St John's wort, tipranavir
Pregnancy category: N/A (May cause fetal harm)
Important contra-indications noted in the prescribing guidelines for: nursing mothers; pediatric patients
Note: Used in combination with daclatasvir, ledipasvir, ribavirin, velpatasvir or with PEG-interferon and ribavirin (see separate entries).

Skin
Pruritus (11–27%) [11]
Rash (8–18%) [9]

Cardiovascular
Bradyarrhythmia [2]
Bradycardia [2]

Central Nervous System
Chills (2–18%) [2]
Fever (4–18%) [3]
Headache (24–44%) [48]
Insomnia (15–29%) [19]
Irritability (10–16%) [5]
Vertigo (dizziness) [3]

Neuromuscular/Skeletal
Arthralgia [2]
Asthenia (fatigue) (30–59%) [47]
Back pain [2]
Myalgia/Myopathy (6–16%) [4]

Gastrointestinal/Hepatic
Diarrhea (9–17%) [6]
Nausea (13–34%) [35]
Vomiting [2]

Respiratory
Cough [4]
Flu-like syndrome (3–18%) [3]
Nasopharyngitis [2]

Upper respiratory tract infection [4]

Endocrine/Metabolic
Appetite decreased (6–18%)

Hematologic
Anemia (6–21%) [32]
Lymphopenia [2]
Neutropenia (<17%) [5]

Other
Adverse effects [8]
Infection [2]

SOFOSBUVIR & VELPATASVIR

Trade name: Epclusa (Gilead)
Indications: Hepatitis C
Class: Direct-acting antiviral, Hepatitis C virus NS5A inhibitor (velpatasvir), Hepatitis C virus nucleotide analog NS5B polymerase inhibitor (sofosbuvir)
Half-life: <27 hours (sofosbuvir); 15 hours (velpatasvir)
Clinically important, potentially hazardous interactions with: amiodarone, carbamazepine, efavirenz, omeprazole, oxcarbazepine, phenobarbital, phenytoin, rifabutin, rifampin, rifapentine, St John's wort, topotecan
Pregnancy category: N/A (Insufficient evidence to inform drug-associated risk; contra-indicated in pregnancy when given with ribavirin)
Important contra-indications noted in the prescribing guidelines for: nursing mothers; pediatric patients
Note: See also separate entry for sofosbuvir.

Skin
Rash (2%)

Central Nervous System
Headache (22%) [13]
Insomnia (5%) [6]

Neuromuscular/Skeletal
Arthralgia [2]
Asthenia (fatigue) (5–15%) [13]

Gastrointestinal/Hepatic
Hepatotoxicity (2–6%)
Nausea (9%) [11]

Respiratory
Nasopharyngitis [4]

Endocrine/Metabolic
Creatine phosphokinase increased (<2%)

Hematologic
Anemia [3]
Thrombocytopenia [2]

SOFOSBUVIR/ VELPATASVIR/ VOXILAPREVIR *

Trade name: Vosevi (Gilead)
Indications: Chronic HCV infection
Class: Direct-acting antiviral, Hepatitis C virus NS3/4A protease inhibitor (voxilaprevir), Hepatitis C virus NS5A inhibitor (velpatasvir), Hepatitis C virus nucleotide analog NS5B polymerase inhibitor (sofosbuvir)
Half-life: <29 hours (sofosbuvir); 17 hours (velpatasvir); 33 hours (voxilaprevir)
Clinically important, potentially hazardous interactions with: amiodarone, atazanavir, carbamazepine, cyclosporine, efavirenz, lopinavir, oxcarbazepine, phenobarbital, phenytoin, pitavastatin, rifabutin, rifampin, rifapentine, ritonavir, rosuvastatin, St John's wort, tipranavir
Pregnancy category: N/A (Insufficient evidence to inform drug-associated risk)
Important contra-indications noted in the prescribing guidelines for: nursing mothers; pediatric patients
Note: See also separate entries for sofosbuvir and sofosbuvir & velpatasvir.
Warning: RISK OF HEPATITIS B VIRUS REACTIVATION IN PATIENTS COINFECTED WITH HCV AND HBV

Skin
Rash (<2%)

Central Nervous System
Headache (21–23%) [6]
Insomnia (3–6%)

Neuromuscular/Skeletal
Asthenia (fatigue) (6–19%) [7]

Gastrointestinal/Hepatic
Diarrhea (13–14%) [6]
Nausea (10–13%) [6]

Endocrine/Metabolic
Hyperbilirubinemia (4–13%)

Hematologic
Hyperlipasemia (2–3%)

SOLIFENACIN

Trade name: Vesicare (Astellas)
Indications: Overactive bladder
Class: Antimuscarinic, Muscarinic antagonist
Half-life: 45–68 hours
Clinically important, potentially hazardous interactions with: atazanavir, carbamazepine, clarithromycin, indinavir, itraconazole, ketoconazole, nefazodone, nelfinavir, phenobarbital, phenytoin, rifabutin, rifampin, rifapentine, ritonavir, saquinavir, St John's wort, troleandomycin, voriconazole
Pregnancy category: C
Important contra-indications noted in the prescribing guidelines for: nursing mothers; pediatric patients

Mucosal
Xerostomia (11–27%) [21]

Cardiovascular
QT prolongation [3]

Central Nervous System
Vertigo (dizziness) (2%) [3]

Neuromuscular/Skeletal
Asthenia (fatigue) (<2%)

Gastrointestinal/Hepatic
Abdominal pain (2%)
Constipation [11]

Ocular
Vision blurred (4–5%) [5]
Xerophthalmia (2%)

Other
Adverse effects [5]

SOMATROPIN

See: www.drugeruptiondata.com/drug/id/1035

SONIDEGIB

Trade name: Odomzo (Novartis)
Indications: Basal cell carcinoma
Class: Hedgehog (Hh) signaling pathway inhibitor
Half-life: 28 days
Clinically important, potentially hazardous interactions with: atazanavir, carbamazepine, diltiazem, efavirenz, fluconazole, itraconazole, ketoconazole, modafinil, nefazodone, phenobarbital, phenytoin, posaconazole, rifabutin, rifampin, saquinavir, St John's wort, telithromycin, voriconazole
Pregnancy category: N/A (Can cause fetal harm)
Important contra-indications noted in the prescribing guidelines for: nursing mothers; pediatric patients
Note: Patients should not donate blood or blood products while receiving sonidegib and for at least 20 months after the last dose.
Warning: EMBRYO-FETAL TOXICITY

Skin
Pruritus (10%)

Hair
Alopecia (53%) [6]

Central Nervous System
Anorexia [2]
Dysgeusia (taste perversion) (46%) [6]
Headache (15%)
Pain (14%)
Vertigo (dizziness) [2]

Neuromuscular/Skeletal
Asthenia (fatigue) (41%) [5]
Bone or joint pain (32%)
Muscle spasm (54%) [6]
Myalgia/Myopathy (19%) [5]

Gastrointestinal/Hepatic
Abdominal pain (18%)
Diarrhea (32%)
Hepatotoxicity [2]
Nausea (39%) [4]
Vomiting (11%) [3]

Endocrine/Metabolic
ALT increased (19%)
Appetite decreased (30%)
AST increased (19%)
Creatine phosphokinase increased (61%) [7]
Hyperbilirubinemia [2]
Hyperglycemia (51%)
Weight loss (30%) [3]

Hematologic
Anemia (32%)
Lymphopenia (28%)

SORAFENIB

Trade name: Nexavar (Bayer)
Indications: Advanced renal cell carcinoma
Class: Antineoplastic, Epidermal growth factor receptor (EGFR) inhibitor, Tyrosine kinase inhibitor
Half-life: 25–48 hours
Clinically important, potentially hazardous interactions with: bevacizumab, carbamazepine, clozapine, conivaptan, coumarins, CYP3A4 inducers, darunavir, delavirdine, dexamethasone, digoxin, docetaxel, doxorubicin, efavirenz, indinavir, irinotecan, neomycin, oxcarbazepine, phenobarbital, phenytoin, rifabutin, rifampin, rifapentine, St John's wort, telithromycin, voriconazole, warfarin
Pregnancy category: D
Important contra-indications noted in the prescribing guidelines for: nursing mothers; pediatric patients
Note: In combination with carboplatin and paclitaxel, Nexavar is contra-indicated in patients with squamous cell lung cancer.

Skin
Acneform eruption (<10%) [6]
Actinic keratoses [4]
AGEP [2]
Desquamation (19–40%) [9]
Eczema [2]
Edema [3]
Erythema (>10%) [4]
Erythema multiforme [11]
Exanthems [3]
Exfoliative dermatitis (<10%)
Facial erythema [3]
Folliculitis [3]
Hand–foot syndrome (21–30%) [113]
Hyperkeratosis [4]
Hypersensitivity [2]
Keratoacanthoma [4]
Keratosis pilaris [2]
Milia [2]
Nevi [3]
Palmar–plantar toxicity [2]
Pigmentation [2]
Pruritus (14–19%) [10]
Psoriasis [2]
Radiation recall dermatitis [3]
Rash (19–40%) [51]
Recall reaction [2]
Seborrheic dermatitis [2]
Squamous cell carcinoma [8]
Stevens-Johnson syndrome [2]
Toxicity [16]
Xerosis (10–11%) [6]

Hair
Alopecia (14–27%) [26]
Hair pigmentation [2]

Nails
Splinter hemorrhage [4]
Subungual hemorrhage [2]

Mucosal
Epistaxis (nosebleed) [2]
Glossodynia (<10%)
Mucositis (<10%) [12]
Stomatitis (<10%) [13]
Xerostomia (<10%)

Cardiovascular
Cardiac failure [2]
Cardiotoxicity (3%) [3]
Congestive heart failure (<10%)
Flushing (<10%)
Hypertension (9–17%) [52]
Myocardial infarction (<10%)

Central Nervous System
Anorexia (16–29%) [15]
Depression (<10%)
Encephalopathy [2]
Fever (<10%) [6]
Headache (10%) [5]
Neurotoxicity (2–40%) [4]
Pain (>10%) [4]

Neuromuscular/Skeletal
Arthralgia (<10%)
Asthenia (fatigue) (37–46%) [53]
Back pain [3]
Bone or joint pain (>10%) [3]
Myalgia/Myopathy (<10%)

Gastrointestinal/Hepatic
Abdominal pain (11–31%) [9]
Ascites [2]
Constipation (14–15%) [4]
Diarrhea (43–55%) [64]
Dyspepsia (<10%)
Dysphagia (<10%)
Gastrointestinal bleeding [5]
Hepatotoxicity (11%) [24]
Nausea (23–24%) [14]
Pancreatitis [7]
Pneumatosis intestinalis [2]
Vomiting (15–16%) [8]

Respiratory
Cough (13%) [2]
Dysphonia [5]
Dyspnea (14%) [4]
Flu-like syndrome (<10%)
Hoarseness (<10%)
Pulmonary toxicity [2]

Endocrine/Metabolic
ALT increased [9]
Appetite decreased (<10%) [5]
AST increased [8]
Creatine phosphokinase increased [2]
Hyperbilirubinemia [4]
Hypoalbuminemia (56%)
Hypocalcemia [2]
Hypokalemia [2]
Hyponatremia [2]
Hypophosphatemia (35–45%) [7]
Hypothyroidism [8]
Thyroid dysfunction [4]
Weight loss (10–30%) [12]

Genitourinary
Erectile dysfunction (<10%)

Renal
Proteinuria [3]
Renal failure (<10%) [2]

Hematologic
Anemia (44%) [10]
Hemorrhage (15–18%) [4]
Hemotoxicity [2]
Leukopenia (>10%) [3]
Lymphopenia (23–47%) [5]
Myelosuppression [2]
Neutropenia (<10%) [7]
Thrombocytopenia (12–46%) [17]
Thrombosis [2]

Other
Adverse effects [15]
Death [9]
Infection [2]
Side effects (71%) [4]

SOTALOL

Trade name: Betapace (Bayer)
Indications: Ventricular arrhythmias
Class: Antiarrhythmic, Antiarrhythmic class II, Antiarrhythmic class III, Beta adrenergic blocker, Beta blocker
Half-life: 7–18 hours
Clinically important, potentially hazardous interactions with: abarelix, amiodarone, amisulpride, amitriptyline, arsenic, artemether/lumefantrine, asenapine, astemizole, atomoxetine, bepridil, ciprofloxacin, class I and class III antiarrhythmics, clonidine, degarelix, disopyramide, dronedarone, droperidol, enoxacin, gatifloxacin, guanethidine, haloperidol, insulin, isoprenaline, ivabradine, levomepromazine, lomefloxacin, loop diuretics, mizolastine, moxifloxacin, nilotinib, norfloxacin, ofloxacin, oral macrolides, phenothiazines, pimavanserin, pimozide, procainamide, quinidine, quinine, quinolones, ranolazine, reserpine, ribociclib, salbutamol, sertindole, sparfloxacin, sulpiride, terbutaline, tetrabenazine, thiazides and related diruetics, tolterodine, tricyclic antidepressants, trifluoperazine, vandetanib, zuclopenthixol
Pregnancy category: B
Important contra-indications noted in the prescribing guidelines for: nursing mothers; pediatric patients
Note: Contra-indicated in patients with bronchial asthma, sinus bradycardia, second and third degree AV block, unless a functioning pacemaker is present, congenital or acquired long QT syndromes, cardiogenic shock, or uncontrolled congestive heart failure.

Skin
Edema (5%)
Pruritus (<10%)
Psoriasis [3]
Rash (3%)
Scleroderma [3]

Cardiovascular
Arrhythmias [2]
Atrioventricular block [2]

Bradycardia [9]
Cardiac failure [2]
Cardiogenic shock [2]
Cardiotoxicity [2]
Hypotension [3]
QT prolongation [18]
Torsades de pointes [24]

Central Nervous System
Depression [2]
Paresthesias (3%)

Neuromuscular/Skeletal
Asthenia (fatigue) (6%) [2]

Other
Adverse effects [2]

SPARFLOXACIN

See: www.drugeruptiondata.com/drug/id/650

SPECTINOMYCIN

See: www.drugeruptiondata.com/drug/id/651

SPINOSAD

See: www.drugeruptiondata.com/drug/id/2185

SPIRONOLACTONE

Trade names: Aldactazide (Pfizer), Aldactone (Pfizer)
Indications: Hyperaldosteronism, hirsutism, hypertension, edema for patients with congestive heart failure, cirrhosis of the liver or nephrotic syndrome
Class: Aldosterone antagonist, Diuretic
Half-life: 78–84 minutes
Clinically important, potentially hazardous interactions with: ACE inhibitors, alcohol, amiloride, barbiturates, benazepril, captopril, cyclosporine, enalapril, fosinopril, lisinopril, mitotane, moexipril, narcotics, NSAIDs, potassium chloride, potassium iodide, quinapril, ramipril, trandolapril, triamterene, zofenopril
Pregnancy category: C
Important contra-indications noted in the prescribing guidelines for: nursing mothers; pediatric patients
Note: Aldactazide is spironolactone and hydrochlorothiazide. Hydrochlorothiazide is a sulfonamide and can be absorbed systemically. Sulfonamides can produce severe, possibly fatal, reactions such as toxic epidermal necrolysis and Stevens-Johnson syndrome.
Warning: Spironolactone has been shown to be a tumorigen in chronic toxicity studies in rats

Skin
Bullous pemphigoid [2]
Dermatitis [6]
Eczema [2]
Exanthems (<5%) [6]
Lichenoid eruption [2]
Melasma [2]

Pigmentation [3]
Pruritus [3]
Rash (<10%) [2]
Urticaria [2]
Xerosis (40%) [2]

Hair
Alopecia [2]

Endocrine/Metabolic
Amenorrhea [2]
Gynecomastia [29]
Hyperkalemia [9]

Renal
Renal function abnormal [2]

STANOZOLOL

Trade name: Winstrol (Ovation)
Indications: Hereditary angioedema
Class: Anabolic steroid
Half-life: N/A
Clinically important, potentially hazardous interactions with: anticoagulants, warfarin
Pregnancy category: X
Important contra-indications noted in the prescribing guidelines for: nursing mothers

Skin
Acneform eruption (>10%) [2]
Pigmentation (<10%)

Hair
Hirsutism (in women) [3]

Cardiovascular
Cardiomyopathy [2]
Hypertension [2]
Myocardial infarction [2]
Myocardial ischemia [2]

Central Nervous System
Chills (<10%)

Gastrointestinal/Hepatic
Hepatotoxicity [3]

Endocrine/Metabolic
Gynecomastia (>10%)

Genitourinary
Priapism (>10%)

Renal
Nephrotoxicity [3]

Other
Death [3]

STAVUDINE

Synonym: D4T
Trade name: Zerit (Bristol-Myers Squibb)
Indications: HIV infection
Class: Antiretroviral, Nucleoside analog reverse transcriptase inhibitor
Half-life: 1.44 hours
Clinically important, potentially hazardous interactions with: doxorubicin, ribavirin, zidovudine

Pregnancy category: C
Important contra-indications noted in the prescribing guidelines for: nursing mothers
Warning: LACTIC ACIDOSIS and HEPATOMEGALY with STEATOSIS; PANCREATITIS

Skin
Diaphoresis (19%)
Lipoatrophy [7]
Lipodystrophy [8]
Rash (40%)
Toxic epidermal necrolysis [2]
Toxicity [2]

Central Nervous System
Chills (50%)
Neurotoxicity [4]
Peripheral neuropathy (52%) [11]

Neuromuscular/Skeletal
Myalgia/Myopathy (32%) [2]

Gastrointestinal/Hepatic
Diarrhea (50%)
Hepatotoxicity [2]
Nausea (39%)
Pancreatitis [6]
Vomiting (39%)

Endocrine/Metabolic
Acidosis [11]
Diabetes mellitus [2]
Fat distribution abnormality [4]
Gynecomastia [4]

Renal
Fanconi syndrome [2]

Other
Adverse effects [3]
Allergic reactions (9%)

STREPTOKINASE

Trade names: Kabikinase (Pfizer), Streptase (AstraZeneca)
Indications: Pulmonary embolism, acute myocardial infarction
Class: Fibrinolytic
Half-life: 83 minutes
Clinically important, potentially hazardous interactions with: bivalirudin, lepirudin
Pregnancy category: C

Skin
Anaphylactoid reactions/Anaphylaxis [2]
Angioedema (>10%) [2]
Diaphoresis (<10%)
Exanthems (<5%) [2]
Pruritus (<10%)
Purpura [2]
Rash (<10%)
Serum sickness [4]
Serum sickness-like reaction [3]
Urticaria (<5%)
Vasculitis [7]

Neuromuscular/Skeletal
Rhabdomyolysis [2]

Ocular
Periorbital edema (>10%)

Other
Allergic reactions (4%) [4]

STREPTOMYCIN

Trade name: Streptomycin (Pfizer)
Indications: Tuberculosis
Class: Antibiotic, aminoglycoside
Half-life: 2–5 hours
Clinically important, potentially hazardous interactions with: aldesleukin, aminoglycosides, atracurium, bacitracin, bumetanide, doxacurium, ethacrynic acid, furosemide, methoxyflurane, neostigmine, non-depolarizing muscle relaxants, pancuronium, polypeptide antibiotics, rocuronium, succinylcholine, teicoplanin, torsemide, vecuronium
Pregnancy category: D
Important contra-indications noted in the prescribing guidelines for: nursing mothers
Note: Aminoglycosides may cause neurotoxicity and/or nephrotoxicity.

Skin
Anaphylactoid reactions/Anaphylaxis [3]
Dermatitis [2]
DRESS syndrome [3]
Erythema multiforme [4]
Exanthems (>5%) [8]
Exfoliative dermatitis [11]
Lupus erythematosus [5]
Nicolau syndrome [2]
Photosensitivity [2]
Pruritus [2]
Purpura [3]
Stevens-Johnson syndrome [3]
Toxic epidermal necrolysis [9]
Urticaria [3]

Mucosal
Cheilitis (2%)
Glossitis (2%)
Oral mucosal eruption [2]
Stomatitis [2]

Renal
Nephrotoxicity [2]

Otic
Ototoxicity [6]

Ocular
Optic neuropathy [2]

Other
Adverse effects [2]
Allergic reactions [2]

STREPTOZOCIN

Trade name: Zanosar (Gensia)
Indications: Carcinoma of the pancreas, carcinoid tumor, Hodgkin's disease
Class: Alkylating agent, Antineoplastic
Half-life: 35 minutes
Clinically important, potentially hazardous interactions with: aldesleukin
Pregnancy category: D
Important contra-indications noted in the prescribing guidelines for: nursing mothers

Neuromuscular/Skeletal
Asthenia (fatigue) [2]

Gastrointestinal/Hepatic
Abdominal pain [2]
Nausea [2]
Vomiting [2]

Renal
Nephrotoxicity [2]

Hematologic
Neutropenia [2]

Local
Injection-site pain (<10%)

STRONTIUM RANELATE

See: www.drugeruptiondata.com/drug/id/1386

SUCCIMER

Synonym: DMSA
Trade name: Chemet (Sanofi-Aventis)
Indications: Heavy metal poisoning
Class: Chelator
Half-life: 2 days
Clinically important, potentially hazardous interactions with: other chelating agents
Pregnancy category: C
Important contra-indications noted in the prescribing guidelines for: nursing mothers; pediatric patients

Skin
Candidiasis (16%)
Exanthems (11%)
Pruritus (11%)
Rash (<11%) [2]

Mucosal
Mucocutaneous eruption (11%)

Central Nervous System
Chills (16%)
Dysgeusia (taste perversion) (metallic) (21%)
Fever (16%)
Headache (16%)
Pain (3%)
Paresthesias (13%)

Neuromuscular/Skeletal
Back pain (16%)

Gastrointestinal/Hepatic
Abdominal pain (16%)

Respiratory
Flu-like syndrome (16%)

SUCCINYLCHOLINE

Synonym: suxamethonium
Trade name: Anectine (Sabex)
Indications: Skeletal muscle relaxation during general anesthesia
Class: Cholinesterase inhibitor, Depolarizing muscle relaxant
Half-life: N/A
Clinically important, potentially hazardous interactions with: amikacin, aminoglycosides, donepezil, galantamine, gentamicin, hydromorphone, kanamycin, levomepromazine, neomycin, neostigmine, paromomycin, physostigmine, pipecuronium, pralidoxime, quinine, streptomycin, tapentadol, thalidomide, tobramycin, vancomycin, vecuronium
Pregnancy category: C
Important contra-indications noted in the prescribing guidelines for: the elderly; nursing mothers
Warning: RISK OF CARDIAC ARREST FROM HYPERKALEMIC RHABDOMYOLYSIS

Skin
Anaphylactoid reactions/Anaphylaxis [13]

Mucosal
Sialorrhea (<10%)

Cardiovascular
Bradycardia [2]

Central Nervous System
Malignant hyperthermia [7]
Paralysis [3]
Twitching [4]

Neuromuscular/Skeletal
Myalgia/Myopathy [11]
Rhabdomyolysis [26]

Endocrine/Metabolic
Hyperkalemia [8]

Other
Death [3]

SUCRALFATE

Trade name: Carafate (Aptalis)
Indications: Duodenal ulcer
Class: Chelator
Half-life: N/A
Clinically important, potentially hazardous interactions with: anagrelide, chlortetracycline, ciprofloxacin, clorazepate, demeclocycline, doxycycline, gemifloxacin, ketoconazole, lansoprazole, levofloxacin, lomefloxacin, lymecycline, minocycline, moxifloxacin, norfloxacin, ofloxacin, oxtriphylline, oxytetracycline, paricalcitol, phenytoin, sparfloxacin, tetracycline, tigecycline, voriconazole
Pregnancy category: B
Important contra-indications noted in the prescribing guidelines for: the elderly; nursing mothers; pediatric patients
Note: Sucralfate use can lead to symptoms of aluminum toxicity.

Mucosal
Xerostomia [2]

Gastrointestinal/Hepatic
Constipation (2%)

SUCRALOSE

Trade name: Splenda (McNeil)
Indications: Weight reduction
Class: Sweetening agent
Half-life: 2–5 hours
Clinically important, potentially hazardous interactions with: none known
Pregnancy category: N/A

Central Nervous System
Migraine [3]

SUFENTANIL

See: www.drugeruptiondata.com/drug/id/660

SUGAMMADEX

Trade name: Bridion (Organon)
Indications: Reversal of neuromuscular blockade induced by rocuronium bromide and vecuronium bromide in adults undergoing surgery
Class: Cyclodextrin, Selective relaxant binding agent
Half-life: ~2 hours
Clinically important, potentially hazardous interactions with: toremifene
Pregnancy category: N/A (No data available)
Important contra-indications noted in the prescribing guidelines for: the elderly; nursing mothers; pediatric patients

Skin
Anaphylactoid reactions/Anaphylaxis [8]
Erythema (<2%)
Hypersensitivity [7]
Pruritus (2–3%)

Mucosal
Oropharyngeal pain (3–5%)
Xerostomia (<2%) [2]

Cardiovascular
Bradycardia (<5%)
QT prolongation (<6%) [2]
Tachycardia (2–5%)

Central Nervous System
Anxiety (<3%)
Chills (3–7%)
Depression (<2%)
Dysgeusia (taste perversion) [3]
Fever (5–9%)
Headache (5–10%) [2]
Hypoesthesia (<3%)
Insomnia (2–5%)
Pain (36–52%)
Restlessness (<2%)
Somnolence (drowsiness) [2]
Vertigo (dizziness) (3–6%)

Neuromuscular/Skeletal
Bone or joint pain (<2%)
Myalgia/Myopathy (<2%)
Pain in extremities (<6%)

Gastrointestinal/Hepatic
Abdominal pain (4–6%)
Diarrhea [2]
Flatulence (<3%)
Nausea (23–26%) [3]
Vomiting (11–15%) [2]

Respiratory
Bronchospasm [2]
Cough (<8%)

Endocrine/Metabolic
Creatine phosphokinase increased (<2%)
Hypocalcemia (<2%)

Hematologic
Anemia (<2%)

Local
Injection-site pain (4–6%)

Other
Allergic reactions [2]

SULFACETAMIDE

See: www.drugeruptiondata.com/drug/id/894

SULFADIAZINE

See: www.drugeruptiondata.com/drug/id/661

SULFADOXINE

Trade name: Fansidar (Roche)
Indications: Malaria
Class: Antibiotic, sulfonamide, Antimalarial
Half-life: 5–8 days
Clinically important, potentially hazardous interactions with: none known
Pregnancy category: C
Important contra-indications noted in the prescribing guidelines for: the elderly; nursing mothers; pediatric patients
Note: Sulfadoxine is a sulfonamide and can be absorbed systemically. Sulfonamides can produce severe, possibly fatal, reactions such as toxic epidermal necrolysis and Stevens-Johnson syndrome.
Fansidar is sulfadoxine and pyrimethamine (this combination is almost always prescribed).

Skin
Erythema multiforme [3]
Exfoliative dermatitis [3]
Fixed eruption [2]
Hypersensitivity (>10%)
Photosensitivity (>10%) [2]
Pruritus [2]
Stevens-Johnson syndrome (<10%) [24]
Toxic epidermal necrolysis [17]

Mucosal
Glossitis (>10%)

Central Nervous System
Tremor (>10%)

Vertigo (dizziness) [2]
Neuromuscular/Skeletal
Asthenia (fatigue) [2]
Gastrointestinal/Hepatic
Diarrhea [2]
Other
Death [7]

SULFA-METHOXAZOLE

Trade names: Bactrim (Women First), Septra (Monarch)
Indications: Various infections caused by susceptible organisms
Class: Antibiotic, sulfonamide, Folic acid antagonist
Half-life: 7–12 hours
Clinically important, potentially hazardous interactions with: anticoagulants, azathioprine, cyclosporine, methotrexate, pralatrexate, probenecid, warfarin
Pregnancy category: C
Note: Sulfamethoxazole is a sulfonamide and can be absorbed systemically. Sulfonamides can produce severe, possibly fatal, reactions such as toxic epidermal necrolysis and Stevens-Johnson syndrome.
Sulfamethoxazole is commonly used in conjunction with trimethoprim (see separate entry for co-trimoxazole).

Skin
AGEP [3]
Anaphylactoid reactions/Anaphylaxis [4]
Angioedema (<5%)
Dermatitis [4]
DRESS syndrome [4]
Erythema multiforme [15]
Erythema nodosum [2]
Exanthems (<5%) [30]
Exfoliative dermatitis [3]
Fixed eruption [29]
Hypersensitivity [6]
Linear IgA bullous dermatosis [3]
Lupus erythematosus [3]
Photosensitivity (>10%) [3]
Pruritus (10%) [7]
Purpura [3]
Pustules [6]
Radiation recall dermatitis [3]
Rash (>10%) [3]
Stevens-Johnson syndrome (<10%) [22]
Sweet's syndrome [3]
Toxic epidermal necrolysis (<10%) [32]
Urticaria [9]
Vasculitis [6]

Mucosal
Oral mucosal eruption [2]
Oral ulceration [2]

Neuromuscular/Skeletal
Rhabdomyolysis [4]

Renal
Nephrotoxicity [2]

Hematologic
Thrombocytopenia [2]

Other
Allergic reactions [2]
Side effects (2%) [2]

SULFASALAZINE

Synonyms: salicylazosulfapyridine; salazopyrin
Trade name: Azulfidine (Pfizer)
Indications: Inflammatory bowel disease, ulcerative colitis, rheumatoid arthritis
Class: Aminosalicylate, Disease-modifying antirheumatic drug (DMARD), Sulfonamide
Half-life: 5–10 hours
Clinically important, potentially hazardous interactions with: cholestyramine, methotrexate, safinamide
Pregnancy category: B
Important contra-indications noted in the prescribing guidelines for: nursing mothers; pediatric patients
Note: Sulfasalazine is a sulfonamide and can be absorbed systemically. Sulfonamides can produce severe, possibly fatal, reactions such as toxic epidermal necrolysis and Stevens-Johnson syndrome.
Contra-indicated in patients with intestinal or urinary obstruction, or with porphyria.

Skin
AGEP [3]
Anaphylactoid reactions/Anaphylaxis [4]
Angioedema [3]
Bullous pemphigoid [3]
Cyanosis (<10%)
Dermatitis [2]
DRESS syndrome [31]
Erythema multiforme [8]
Erythema nodosum [2]
Exanthems (2–23%) [23]
Exfoliative dermatitis [5]
Fixed eruption [7]
Hypersensitivity (<5%) [21]
Lichen planus [3]
Lupus erythematosus [34]
Photosensitivity (10%) [4]
Pigmentation [3]
Pruritus (10%) [8]
Pseudolymphoma [2]
Pustules [3]
Rash (>10%) [19]
Raynaud's phenomenon [3]
Stevens-Johnson syndrome [9]
Toxic epidermal necrolysis (<10%) [13]
Urticaria (<5%) [11]
Vasculitis [4]

Hair
Alopecia [6]

Mucosal
Mucocutaneous reactions (6%) [2]
Oral mucosal eruption [4]
Oral ulceration [3]
Stomatitis (<10%)

Cardiovascular
Flushing [2]

Central Nervous System
Anorexia (10%)
Aseptic meningitis [3]
Fever [4]

Headache (10%) [7]
Vertigo (dizziness) (<10%)

Neuromuscular/Skeletal
Arthralgia [2]
Asthenia (fatigue) [5]

Gastrointestinal/Hepatic
Abdominal pain (<10%)
Dyspepsia (10%) [3]
Hepatotoxicity [14]
Nausea (10%) [7]
Pancreatitis [6]
Vomiting (10%) [2]

Respiratory
Pulmonary toxicity [3]
Upper respiratory tract infection [3]

Renal
Nephrotoxicity [4]
Renal failure [2]

Hematologic
Agranulocytosis [5]
Anemia (<10%)
Leukopenia (<10%) [4]
Neutropenia [2]
Thrombocytopenia (<10%)

Ocular
Conjunctival pigmentation [2]

Other
Adverse effects [9]
Death [4]
Side effects (5%)

SULFINPYRAZONE

See: www.drugeruptiondata.com/drug/id/665

SULFISOXAZOLE

See: www.drugeruptiondata.com/drug/id/666

SULINDAC

Trade name: Clinoril (Merck)
Indications: Arthritis
Class: Non-steroidal anti-inflammatory (NSAID)
Half-life: 7.8–16.4 hours
Clinically important, potentially hazardous interactions with: methotrexate, warfarin
Pregnancy category: C (category C in first and second trimesters; category D in third trimester)
Important contra-indications noted in the prescribing guidelines for: nursing mothers; pediatric patients
Note: NSAIDs may cause an increased risk of serious cardiovascular and gastrointestinal adverse events, which can be fatal. This risk may increase with duration of use.

Skin
Anaphylactoid reactions/Anaphylaxis [4]
Erythema multiforme [8]
Exanthems (<5%) [9]
Fixed eruption [5]
Photosensitivity [2]
Pruritus (<10%) [5]

Purpura [2]
Rash (>10%)
Stevens-Johnson syndrome [5]
Toxic epidermal necrolysis [13]
Urticaria [4]

Mucosal
Oral mucosal eruption (3%) [2]
Stomatitis [2]
Xerostomia [2]

Gastrointestinal/Hepatic
Hepatotoxicity [4]
Pancreatitis [3]

SULPIRIDE

See: www.drugeruptiondata.com/drug/id/1351

SUMATRIPTAN

Trade names: Alsuma (King), Imigran (GSK), Imitrex (GSK), Onzetra Xsail (Avanir), Sumavel DosePro (Endo), Zecuity (Teva)
Indications: Migraine attacks, cluster headaches
Class: 5-HT1 agonist, Serotonin receptor agonist, Triptan
Half-life: 2.5 hours
Clinically important, potentially hazardous interactions with: citalopram, dihydroergotamine, ergot-containing drugs, escitalopram, fluoxetine, fluvoxamine, isocarboxazid, MAO inhibitors, methysergide, naratriptan, nefazodone, paroxetine hydrochloride, phenelzine, rizatriptan, sertraline, sibutramine, SNRIs, SSRIs, St John's wort, tranylcypromine, venlafaxine, zolmitriptan
Pregnancy category: C
Important contra-indications noted in the prescribing guidelines for: the elderly; nursing mothers; pediatric patients
Note: Contra-indicated in patients with Wolff-Parkinson-White syndrome, peripheral vascular disease, ischemic bowel disease, uncontrolled hypertension, severe hepatic impairment or a history of coronary artery disease, coronary vasospasm, stroke, transient ischemic attack, or hemiplegic or basilar migraine; or with recent (within 24 hours) use of another 5-HT1 agonist (e.g. another triptan) or an ergotamine-containing medication, or current or recent (past 2 weeks) use of a monoamine oxidase-A inhibitor.

Skin
Burning (<10%)
Diaphoresis (2%)
Hot flashes (>10%)

Mucosal
Nasal discomfort [2]
Xerostomia [2]

Cardiovascular
Chest pain (<2%) [7]
Flushing (7%) [4]
Hypertension [2]
Myocardial infarction [5]

Central Nervous System
Dysgeusia (taste perversion) [10]
Headache [2]

Neurotoxicity [3]
Pain (<2%) [2]
Paresthesias (3–5%) [11]
Somnolence (drowsiness) [3]
Stroke [2]
Vertigo (dizziness) (<2%) [10]
Warm feeling (2–3%)

Neuromuscular/Skeletal
Asthenia (fatigue) (2–3%) [5]
Jaw pain (<3%)
Muscle spasm [2]
Myalgia/Myopathy (2%) [2]
Neck pain (<3%)

Gastrointestinal/Hepatic
Colitis [2]
Nausea [12]

Respiratory
Nasopharyngitis [2]
Upper respiratory tract infection [2]

Local
Application-site erythema [2]
Injection-site reactions (10–58%) [2]

Other
Adverse effects [10]

SUNITINIB

Trade name: Sutent (Pfizer)
Indications: Gastrointestinal stromal tumor, advanced renal cell carcinoma, advanced pancreatic neuroendocrine tumor
Class: Antineoplastic, Epidermal growth factor receptor (EGFR) inhibitor, Tyrosine kinase inhibitor
Half-life: 40–60 hours
Clinically important, potentially hazardous interactions with: atazanavir, bevacizumab, carbamazepine, clarithromycin, clozapine, dexamethasone, digoxin, efavirenz, grapefruit juice, indinavir, itraconazole, ketoconazole, nefazodone, nelfinavir, phenobarbital, phenytoin, rifabutin, rifampin, rifapentine, ritonavir, saquinavir, St John's wort, telithromycin, temsirolimus, voriconazole
Pregnancy category: D
Important contra-indications noted in the prescribing guidelines for: nursing mothers; pediatric patients
Note: [G] = treated for gastrointestinal tumor; [R] = treated for renal cell carcinoma; [P] treated for pancreatic neuroendocrine tumor.
Warning: HEPATOTOXICITY

Skin
Acral erythema [2]
Edema [6]
Erythema [6]
Facial edema [3]
Hand–foot syndrome (12–14%) [68]
Lesions [2]
Nevi [2]
Peripheral edema [R] (17%)
Pigmentation [14]
Pruritus [R] [3]
Pyoderma gangrenosum [8]
Rash (14–38%) [17]
Thrombocytopenic purpura [4]

Toxicity [24]
Xerosis (17%) [3]

Hair
Alopecia (5–12%) [5]
Hair pigmentation [G] [8]

Nails
Splinter hemorrhage [2]
Subungual hemorrhage [4]

Mucosal
Epistaxis (nosebleed) [2]
Glossodynia [R] [P] (15%)
Mucosal inflammation [4]
Mucositis (29–53%) [18]
Stomatitis [17]
Xerostomia [R] [P] [2]

Cardiovascular
Aortic dissection [3]
Cardiac failure [2]
Cardiomyopathy [2]
Cardiotoxicity [7]
Congestive heart failure [2]
Hypertension [56]
QT prolongation [2]
Ventricular arrhythmia [2]

Central Nervous System
Anorexia [8]
Dysgeusia (taste perversion) (21–43%) [6]
Fever [R] (15–18%) [2]
Headache (13–25%) [4]
Leukoencephalopathy [3]
Neurotoxicity [R] (10%)
Pain [R] (18%)
Vertigo (dizziness) [R] (16%)

Neuromuscular/Skeletal
Arthralgia [R] (12–28%)
Asthenia (fatigue) (22%) [69]
Back pain [R] (11–17%)
Myalgia/Myopathy [G] (14–17%)
Osteonecrosis [3]

Gastrointestinal/Hepatic
Abdominal pain (20–33%) [2]
Constipation [3]
Diarrhea [36]
Dyspepsia [R] [P] [3]
Esophagitis [2]
Gastrointestinal bleeding [4]
Gastrointestinal disorder [2]
Hepatotoxicity [7]
Nausea [17]
Pneumatosis intestinalis [2]
Vomiting [14]

Respiratory
Cough [R] (8–17%) [2]
Dyspnea [5]
Pulmonary toxicity [3]
Radiation recall pneumonitis [2]

Endocrine/Metabolic
ALT increased [4]
Appetite decreased [2]
AST increased [2]
Hypothyroidism [R] [29]
Serum creatinine increased [2]
Thyroid dysfunction [8]

Renal
Nephrotoxicity [4]
Proteinuria [3]

Hematologic
Anemia [20]
Bleeding [5]
Bone marrow suppression [2]
Cytopenia [2]
Hemorrhage [2]
Hemotoxicity [3]
Hyperlipasemia [2]
Leukopenia [16]
Lymphocytopenia [2]
Lymphopenia [8]
Myelosuppression [3]
Neutropenia [44]

Thrombocytopenia [39]

Ocular
Epiphora [R] (6%)
Periorbital edema [R] (7%)

Other
Adverse effects [17]
Death [7]
Side effects [3]

SUVOREXANT

Trade name: Belsomra (Merck Sharpe & Dohme)
Indications: Insomnia
Class: Orexin receptor antagonist
Half-life: 10–22 hours
Clinically important, potentially hazardous interactions with: none known
Pregnancy category: C
Important contra-indications noted in the prescribing guidelines for: nursing mothers; pediatric patients
Note: Contra-indicated in patients with narcolepsy.

Mucosal
Xerostomia (2%)

Central Nervous System
Abnormal dreams (2%) [2]
Headache (7%) [2]
Sedation [2]
Somnolence (drowsiness) (7%) [6]
Vertigo (dizziness) (3%)

Gastrointestinal/Hepatic
Diarrhea (2%)

Respiratory
Cough (2%)
Upper respiratory tract infection (2%)

TACRINE

See: www.drugeruptiondata.com/drug/id/669

TACROLIMUS

Trade names: Envarsus XR (Veloxis), Prograf (Astellas), Protopic (Astellas)
Indications: Prophylaxis of organ rejection, atopic dermatitis (topical)
Class: Calcineurin inhibitor, Immunosuppressant, Macrolactam
Half-life: ~8.7 hours
Clinically important, potentially hazardous interactions with: abatacept, afatinib, alefacept, amiodarone, amprenavir, atazanavir, azacitidine, beta blockers, betamethasone, boceprevir, bosentan, cabazitaxel, caspofungin, ceritinib, cinacalcet, cobicistat/elvitegravir/emtricitabine/ tenofovir disoproxil, crizotinib, cyclosporine, CYP3A4 inhibitors and inducers, dabigatran, dairy products, danazol, darunavir, dasatinib, delavirdine, denileukin, dexlansoprazole, diclofenac, docetaxel, dronedarone, efavirenz, elbasvir & grazoprevir, eluxadoline, enzalutamide, erythromycin, etoricoxib, fingolimod, gefitinib, grapefruit juice, Hemophilus B vaccine, HMG-CoA reductase inhibitors, ibuprofen, immunosuppressants, indinavir, irbesartan, itraconazole, ketoconazole, leflunomide, lenalidomide, lopinavir, lovastatin, meloxicam, mifepristone, mycophenolate, nelfinavir, nifedipine, olmesartan, omeprazole, oxaliplatin, pazopanib, pemetrexed, posaconazole, potassium, potassium-sparing diuretics, pralatrexate, ribociclib, rifabutin, rifampin, rifapentine, sevelamer, simvastatin, sirolimus, St John's wort, telaprevir, telithromycin, temsirolimus, tinidazole, tipranavir, tofacitinib, triamcinolone, vaccines, voriconazole
Pregnancy category: C
Important contra-indications noted in the prescribing guidelines for: the elderly; nursing mothers; pediatric patients
Warning: MALIGNANCIES AND SERIOUS INFECTIONS

Skin
Anaphylactoid reactions/Anaphylaxis [3]
Burning (46%) [13]
Dermatitis [2]
Diaphoresis (>3%)
Ecchymoses (>3%)
Edema (>10%)
Erythema (12%) [3]
Exanthems (4%) [2]
Folliculitis (10%) [2]
Graft-versus-host reaction [2]
Herpes simplex (13%) [4]
Kaposi's sarcoma [2]
Kaposi's varicelliform eruption [2]
Lymphoma [2]
Peripheral edema (26%)
Photosensitivity (>3%)
Pigmentation [2]
Pruritus (25–36%) [11]
Pustules (6%)
Rash (24%) [2]

Rosacea [5]
Thrombocytopenic purpura [2]
Toxicity [3]

Hair
Alopecia (>3%) [6]
Hypertrichosis [2]

Mucosal
Gingival hyperplasia/hypertrophy [6]
Oral candidiasis (>3%)
Oral pigmentation [2]
Oral ulceration [2]

Cardiovascular
Cardiomyopathy [3]
Flushing [4]
Hypertension (49%) [8]
QT prolongation [2]

Central Nervous System
Encephalopathy [10]
Fever (>10%) [2]
Headache [9]
Leukoencephalopathy [14]
Neurotoxicity [10]
Pain [2]
Paresthesias (40%) [4]
Parkinsonism [2]
Seizures (<10%) [4]
Tremor (>10%) [9]
Vertigo (dizziness) [3]

Neuromuscular/Skeletal
Arthralgia (>10%) [2]
Asthenia (fatigue) (>10%) [3]
Back pain (>10%)
Bone or joint pain [2]
Myalgia/Myopathy (>3%)

Gastrointestinal/Hepatic
Abdominal pain [3]
Constipation (>10%)
Diarrhea (>10%) [5]
Dyspepsia (>10%)
Dysphagia (>3%)
Hepatotoxicity [11]
Nausea (>10%) [3]
Pancreatitis [3]
Vomiting (>10%)

Respiratory
Cough (>10%)
Dyspnea (>10%)
Pulmonary toxicity [2]

Endocrine/Metabolic
Creatine phosphokinase increased (>10%) [3]
Diabetes mellitus [6]
Diabetic ketoacidosis [5]
Gynecomastia [3]
Hyperglycemia [10]
Hyperkalemia [3]
Hyperlipidemia [2]
Hypomagnesemia (>10%) [2]
Hypophosphatemia (>10%)
SIADH [2]

Genitourinary
Urinary tract infection [2]

Renal
Nephrotoxicity [42]
Renal failure [2]
Renal function abnormal [3]

Hematologic
Anemia (>10%) [2]
Angiopathy [4]
Dyslipidemia [3]
Hemolytic anemia [2]
Hemolytic uremic syndrome [18]
Leukopenia (>10%) [5]
Neutropenia [3]
Thrombotic microangiopathy [5]

Otic
Tinnitus [2]

Ocular
Diplopia [2]
Ocular burning [3]
Optic neuropathy [2]
Vision blurred [2]
Vision loss [3]

Local
Application-site burning [6]
Application-site erythema [3]
Application-site infection [2]
Application-site irritation [2]
Application-site pruritus [7]

Other
Adverse effects [13]
Cancer [2]
Infection (>10%) [15]

TADALAFIL

Trade names: Adcirca (Lilly), Cialis (Lilly)
Indications: Erectile dysfunction, pulmonary arterial hypertension
Class: Phosphodiesterase type 5 (PDE5) inhibitor
Half-life: 15–18 hours
Clinically important, potentially hazardous interactions with: alcohol, alfuzosin, alpha blockers, amlodipine, amyl nitrite, angiotensin II receptor blockers, antifungals, antihypertensives, atazanavir, bendroflumethiazide, boceprevir, bosentan, clarithromycin, cobicistat/elvitegravir/ emtricitabine/tenofovir alafenamide, cobicistat/ elvitegravir/emtricitabine/tenofovir disoproxil, conivaptan, CYP3A4 inhibitors or inducers, darunavir, dasatinib, delavirdine, disopyramide, doxazosin, efavirenz, enalapril, erythromycin, etravirine, fosamprenavir, grapefruit juice, indinavir, itraconazole, ketoconazole, lopinavir, macrolide antibiotics, metoprolol, nelfinavir, nicorandil, nitrates, nitroglycerin, nitroprusside, oxcarbazepine, phosphodiesterase 5 inhibitors, rifampin, rifapentine, riociguat, ritonavir, saproterin, saquinavir, St John's wort, tamsulosin, telaprevir, telithromycin, voriconazole
Pregnancy category: B (Cialis is not indicated for use in women)
Important contra-indications noted in the prescribing guidelines for: pediatric patients

Skin
Diaphoresis (<2%)
Facial edema (<2%)
Peripheral edema [2]
Pruritus (<2%)
Rash (<2%)

Mucosal
Epistaxis (nosebleed) (<2%) [2]

Nasal congestion [4]
Rectal hemorrhage (<2%)
Xerostomia (<2%)

Cardiovascular
Angina (<2%)
Chest pain (<2%)
Flushing (2–3%) [16]
Hypotension (<2%)
Myocardial infarction (<2%)
Palpitation (<2%)
Postural hypotension (<2%)
Tachycardia (<2%)

Central Nervous System
Amnesia [3]
Headache (4–15%) [36]
Hyperesthesia (<2%)
Hypoesthesia (<2%)
Insomnia (<2%)
Pain (<3%)
Paresthesias (<2%)
Somnolence (drowsiness) (<2%)
Syncope (<2%)
Vertigo (dizziness) (<2%) [6]

Neuromuscular/Skeletal
Arthralgia (<2%)
Asthenia (fatigue) (<2%)
Back pain (2–6%) [21]
Myalgia/Myopathy (<4%) [15]
Neck pain (<2%)

Gastrointestinal/Hepatic
Diarrhea [2]
Dyspepsia [8]
Dysphagia (<2%)
Esophagitis (<2%)
Gastritis (<2%)
Gastroesophageal reflux (<2%)
Hepatotoxicity [2]
Loose stools (<2%)
Nausea (<2%) [3]
Vomiting (<2%)

Respiratory
Dyspnea (<2%)
Pharyngitis (<2%)

Endocrine/Metabolic
GGT increased (<2%)

Genitourinary
Erection (<2%)
Priapism (spontaneous) (<2%) [2]

Hematologic
Anemia [2]
Platelets decreased [2]

Otic
Hearing loss (<2%) [4]
Tinnitus (<2%)

Ocular
Chorioretinopathy [2]
Conjunctival hyperemia (<2%)
Conjunctivitis (<2%)
Dyschromatopsia (<2%)
Eyelid edema (<2%)
Eyelid pain (<2%)
Lacrimation (<2%)
Optic neuropathy [7]
Vision blurred (<2%)

Other
Adverse effects [4]

TAFLUPROST

Trade names: Saflutan (Merck Sharpe & Dohme), Zioptan (Merck Sharpe & Dohme)
Indications: Reduction of elevated intraocular pressure in open angle glaucoma or ocular hypertension
Class: Antiglaucoma, Prostaglandin analog
Half-life: 0.5 hours
Clinically important, potentially hazardous interactions with: none known
Pregnancy category: C
Important contra-indications noted in the prescribing guidelines for: nursing mothers; pediatric patients

Central Nervous System
Headache (6%)

Respiratory
Cough (3%)

Genitourinary
Urinary tract infection (2%)

Ocular
Cataract (3%)
Conjunctival hyperemia (4–20%) [7]
Conjunctivitis (5%)
Deepening of upper lid sulcus [4]
Eyelashes – hypertrichosis (2%)
Eyelashes – pigmentation (2%) [2]
Eyelid erythema (<10%)
Eyelid pigmentation [3]
Keratoconjunctivitis (<10%)
Lacrimation (<10%)
Ocular burning [3]
Ocular hyperemia [2]
Ocular itching [5]
Ocular pain (3%)
Ocular pigmentation (<10%)
Ocular pruritus (5%) [2]
Ocular stinging (7%) [4]
Photophobia (<10%)
Vision blurred (2%)
Visual disturbances (<10%)
Xerophthalmia (3%)

Other
Adverse effects [5]

TALIGLUCERASE

See: www.drugeruptiondata.com/drug/id/2927

TALIMOGENE LAHERPAREPVEC

Synonym: T-VEC
Trade name: Imlygic (Amgen)
Indications: Unresectable cutaneous, subcutaneous, and nodal lesions in patients with melanoma recurrent after initial surgery
Class: Oncolytic virus immunotherapy
Half-life: N/A
Clinically important, potentially hazardous interactions with: none known

Pregnancy category: N/A (Contraception advised to prevent pregnancy during treatment)
Important contra-indications noted in the prescribing guidelines for: nursing mothers; pediatric patients

Skin
Cellulitis (<5%) [3]
Herpes (oral) (<5%)
Vitiligo (<5%)

Mucosal
Oropharyngeal pain (6%)

Central Nervous System
Chills (49%) [4]
Fever (43%) [3]
Headache (19%)
Vertigo (dizziness) (10%)

Neuromuscular/Skeletal
Arthralgia (17%)
Asthenia (fatigue) (50%) [4]
Myalgia/Myopathy (18%)
Pain in extremities (16%)

Gastrointestinal/Hepatic
Abdominal pain (9%)
Constipation (12%)
Diarrhea (19%)
Nausea (36%)
Vomiting (21%)

Respiratory
Flu-like syndrome (31%) [2]

Endocrine/Metabolic
Weight loss (6%)

Renal
Glomerulonephritis (<5%)

Local
Injection-site pain (28%)

TAMOXIFEN

Trade name: Nolvadex (AstraZeneca)
Indications: Advanced breast cancer
Class: Selective estrogen receptor modulator (SERM)
Half-life: 5–7 days
Clinically important, potentially hazardous interactions with: anastrozole, bexarotene, cinacalcet, delavirdine, droperidol, duloxetine, gadobenate, paroxetine hydrochloride, rifapentine, terbinafine, tipranavir
Pregnancy category: D
Important contra-indications noted in the prescribing guidelines for: nursing mothers; pediatric patients

Skin
Carcinosarcoma [2]
Diaphoresis [4]
Edema (2–6%) [3]
Exanthems (3%) [3]
Hot flashes [18]
Lupus erythematosus [2]
Pruritus ani et vulvae [2]
Radiation recall dermatitis [6]
Rash (<10%) [2]
Sarcoma [9]
Toxicity [3]

Tumors [3]
Vasculitis [5]
Xerosis (7%)

Hair
Alopecia [7]
Hirsutism [2]

Mucosal
Stomatitis [2]
Xerostomia (7%) [2]

Cardiovascular
Flushing (>10%) [9]
Myocardial ischemia [2]
QT prolongation [3]
Thromboembolism [6]
Thrombophlebitis [3]
Venous thromboembolism [6]

Central Nervous System
Depression [5]
Headache [3]
Insomnia [4]
Mood changes [3]
Parkinsonism [2]
Stroke [4]
Vertigo (dizziness) [3]

Neuromuscular/Skeletal
Asthenia (fatigue) [5]
Bone or joint pain [3]
Fractures [2]
Leg cramps [2]
Myalgia/Myopathy [4]

Gastrointestinal/Hepatic
Hepatic steatosis [2]
Hepatotoxicity [10]
Nausea [4]
Pancreatitis [4]
Vomiting [3]

Respiratory
Pulmonary embolism [7]

Endocrine/Metabolic
ALP increased [2]
Amenorrhea [8]
Galactorrhea (<10%)
Hypercholesterolemia [2]
Hypertriglyceridemia [7]
Libido decreased [4]
Weight gain [4]

Genitourinary
Dyspareunia [4]
Endometrial cancer [5]
Ovarian hyperstimulation syndrome [2]
Sexual dysfunction [2]
Vaginal bleeding [4]
Vaginal discharge [5]
Vaginal dryness [5]

Hematologic
Hemolytic uremic syndrome [2]
Thrombosis [9]

Ocular
Cataract [9]
Keratopathy [4]
Macular edema [2]
Maculopathy [5]
Ocular adverse effects [5]
Ocular toxicity [5]
Retinopathy [5]
Vision impaired [3]

TAMSULOSIN

Trade names: Flomax (Boehringer Ingelheim), Jalyn (GSK)
Indications: Benign prostatic hypertrophy
Class: Adrenergic alpha-receptor antagonist
Half-life: 9–13 hours
Clinically important, potentially hazardous interactions with: alpha adrenergic blockers, cimetidine, conivaptan, darunavir, delavirdine, erythromycin, indinavir, ketoconazole, paroxetine hydrochloride, phosphodiesterase 5 inhibitors, tadalafil, telithromycin, terbinafine, vardenafil, voriconazole, warfarin
Pregnancy category: B (not indicated for use in women; Jalyn is pregnancy category X)
Important contra-indications noted in the prescribing guidelines for: nursing mothers; pediatric patients
Note: Jalyn is tamsulosin and dutasteride.

Mucosal
Xerostomia [4]

Cardiovascular
Chest pain (4%)
Hypotension (6–19%) [3]
Postural hypotension [3]

Central Nervous System
Headache (19–21%) [6]
Insomnia (<2%)
Somnolence (drowsiness) (3–4%)
Vertigo (dizziness) (15–17%) [16]

Neuromuscular/Skeletal
Asthenia (fatigue) (8–9%) [2]
Back pain (7–8%)

Gastrointestinal/Hepatic
Constipation [2]
Diarrhea (4–6%)
Nausea (3–4%)

Respiratory
Cough (3–5%)
Pharyngitis (5–6%)
Rhinitis (13–18%) [2]
Sinusitis (2–4%)

Endocrine/Metabolic
Libido decreased (<2%)

Genitourinary
Ejaculatory dysfunction (8–18%) [9]
Erectile dysfunction [2]
Priapism [4]
Urinary retention [3]

Ocular
Floppy iris syndrome [34]
Vision blurred (<2%)

Other
Adverse effects [3]
Infection (9–11%)
Tooth disorder (<2%)

TAPENTADOL

Trade names: Nucynta (Janssen), Nucynta ER (Janssen), Palexia (Grunenthal)
Indications: Immediate release formulation: moderate to severe acute pain, extended release formulation: moderate to severe chronic pain and neuropathic pain associated with diabetic peripheral neuropathy when a continuous analgesic is needed for an extended period of time
Class: Analgesic, opioid
Half-life: 5 hours
Clinically important, potentially hazardous interactions with: alcohol, alvimopan, amphetamines, anesthetics, anitemetics, anticholinergics, buprenorphine, butorphanol, CNS depressants, desmopressin, droperidol, hypnotics, linezolid, MAO inhibitors, mirtazapine, nalbuphine, PEG-interferon, pegvisomant, pentazocine, phenothiazines, sedatives, sibutramine, SNRIs, SSRIs, St John's wort, succinylcholine, thiazide diuretics, tramadol, tranquilizers, trazodone, tricyclic antidepressants, triptans
Pregnancy category: C
Important contra-indications noted in the prescribing guidelines for: the elderly; nursing mothers; pediatric patients
Note: Contra-indicated in patients with impaired pulmonary function or paralytic ileus. Should not be used in patients currently using or within 14 days of using a monoamine oxidase inhibitor.
Warning: For extended release oral tablets: ABUSE POTENTIAL, LIFE-THREATENING RESPIRATORY DEPRESSION, ACCIDENTAL EXPOSURE, and INTERACTION WITH ALCOHOL

Mucosal
Xerostomia [4]

Central Nervous System
Headache [4]
Neurotoxicity [2]
Somnolence (drowsiness) [8]
Vertigo (dizziness) (4%) [9]

Neuromuscular/Skeletal
Asthenia (fatigue) [3]

Gastrointestinal/Hepatic
Constipation [15]
Diarrhea [2]
Gastrointestinal disorder [2]
Nausea (4%) [21]
Vomiting (3%) [14]

Other
Adverse effects [4]

TARTRAZINE

Class: Food additive
Half-life: N/A
Clinically important, potentially hazardous interactions with: none known
Note: Tartrazine intolerance has been estimated to affect between 0.01% and 0.1% of the population. Adverse reactions are most common in people who are sensitive to aspirin.

Banned in Austria and Norway.

Skin
Anaphylactoid reactions/Anaphylaxis [8]
Angioedema [11]
Atopic dermatitis [2]
Hypersensitivity [9]
Pruritus [2]
Purpura [5]
Urticaria (often related to aspirin
  intolerance) [33]
Vasculitis [3]

Other
Adverse effects [3]
Allergic reactions [9]

TASIMELTEON

Trade name: Hetlioz (Vanda)
Indications: Non-24-hour sleep-wake disorder
Class: Melatonin receptor agonist
Half-life: 2–3 hours
Clinically important, potentially hazardous interactions with: fluvoxamine, ketoconazole, rifampin
Pregnancy category: C
Important contra-indications noted in the prescribing guidelines for: the elderly; nursing mothers; pediatric patients

Central Nervous System
Abnormal dreams (10%) [3]
Headache (17%) [3]
Nightmares (10%) [3]

Respiratory
Upper respiratory tract infection (7%) [2]

Endocrine/Metabolic
ALT increased (10%) [2]

Genitourinary
Urinary tract infection (7%) [3]

TASONERMIN

See: www.drugeruptiondata.com/drug/id/1400

TAVABOROLE

Indications: Onychomycosis
Class: Antifungal, oxaborole
Half-life: N/A
Clinically important, potentially hazardous interactions with: none known
Pregnancy category: C
Important contra-indications noted in the prescribing guidelines for: nursing mothers; pediatric patients

Nails
Onychocryptosis (3%)

Local
Application-site erythema (2%) [2]
Application-site exfoliation (3%)

TAZAROTENE

Trade names: Avage (Allergan), Fabior (GSK), Tazorac (Allergan), Zorac (Allergan)
Indications: Acne vulgaris, mild to moderate plaque psoriasis involving up to 10% body surface area
Half-life: 18 hours
Clinically important, potentially hazardous interactions with: none known
Pregnancy category: X
Important contra-indications noted in the prescribing guidelines for: the elderly; nursing mothers; pediatric patients

Skin
Burning (10–20%) [5]
Contact dermatitis (5–10%)
Desquamation (5–10%)
Erythema (10–20%) [5]
Pruritus (10–25%) [11]
Psoriasis (5–10%)
Rash (5–10%)
Scaling [2]
Stinging (<3%) [2]
Xerosis (<3%) [5]

Local
Application-site reactions [2]

Other
Adverse effects [2]
Side effects [2]

TEDIZOLID

Trade name: Sivextro (Cubist)
Indications: Acute bacterial skin and skin structure infections caused by susceptible bacteria
Class: Antibiotic, oxazolidinone
Half-life: 12 hours
Clinically important, potentially hazardous interactions with: none known
Pregnancy category: C
Important contra-indications noted in the prescribing guidelines for: nursing mothers; pediatric patients

Skin
Dermatitis (<2%)
Hypersensitivity (<2%)
Pruritus (<2%)
Urticaria (<2%)

Cardiovascular
Flushing (<2%)
Hypertension (<2%)
Palpitation (<2%)
Tachycardia (<2%)

Central Nervous System
Headache (6%) [3]
Hypoesthesia (<2%)
Insomnia (<2%)
Vertigo (dizziness) (2%) [3]

Gastrointestinal/Hepatic
Diarrhea (4%) [4]
Nausea (8%) [5]
Vomiting (3%) [4]

Hematologic
Anemia (<2%)

Ocular
Asthenopia (<2%)
Vision blurred (<2%)
Vision impaired (<2%)
Vitreous floaters (<2%)

Local
Infusion-related reactions (<2%)

Other
Adverse effects [2]
Infection (<2%)

TEDUGLUTIDE

Trade name: Gattex (Hospira)
Indications: Treatment of short bowel syndrome in adult patients dependent on parenteral support
Class: Glucagon-like peptide-2 (GLP-2) analog
Half-life: 1–2 hours
Clinically important, potentially hazardous interactions with: none known
Pregnancy category: B
Important contra-indications noted in the prescribing guidelines for: nursing mothers; pediatric patients

Skin
Edema [4]
Hypersensitivity (<10%)

Central Nervous System
Headache (16%) [6]
Sleep disturbances (<10%)

Gastrointestinal/Hepatic
Abdominal distension (14%) [4]
Abdominal pain (30%) [8]
Constipation [3]
Flatulence (<10%)
Gastrointestinal disorder [2]
Hepatotoxicity [3]
Nausea (18%) [7]
Vomiting (<10%) [2]

Respiratory
Cough (<10%)
Nasopharyngitis [2]
Upper respiratory tract infection (12%)

Local
Injection-site erythema [2]
Injection-site reactions (22%)

Other
Adverse effects [9]

TEGAFUR/GIMERACIL/ OTERACIL

Synonyms: TS-1; S-1
Trade name: Teysuno (Taiho Pharma)
Indications: Gastric, colorectal, head and neck cancers, non-small cell lung cancer, inoperable or recurrent breast cancer, pancreatic cancer
Class: Antineoplastic
Half-life: N/A
Clinically important, potentially hazardous interactions with: capecitabine, flucytosine, fluorouracil, other fluoropyrimidine-group antineoplastics, phenytoin, uracil/tegafur, warfarin
Pregnancy category: N/A (Contra-indicated in pregnancy)
Important contra-indications noted in the prescribing guidelines for: the elderly; nursing mothers; pediatric patients
Note: Contra-indicated in patients with severe bone marrow depression, hepatic or renal impairment.
Not available in the USA.

Skin
Dermatitis (<5%)
Desquamation (<5%)
Edema (<5%) [3]
Erythema (<5%)
Hand–foot syndrome (<5%) [12]
Herpes simplex (<5%)
Jaundice (<5%)
Pigmentation (21%) [9]
Pruritus (<5%)
Rash (12%) [6]
Raynaud's phenomenon (<5%)
Ulcerations (<5%)
Xerosis (<5%) [2]

Hair
Alopecia (<5%) [4]

Nails
Nail disorder (<5%)
Paronychia (<5%) [2]

Mucosal
Mucositis [7]
Stomatitis (17%) [9]

Cardiovascular
Flushing (<5%)
Hypertension (<5%)
Hypotension (<5%)

Central Nervous System
Anorexia (34%) [25]
Fever (<5%) [2]
Headache (<5%)
Neurotoxicity [4]
Paresthesias (<5%)
Peripheral neuropathy [3]
Vertigo (dizziness) (<5%)
Warm feeling (<5%)

Neuromuscular/Skeletal
Arthralgia (<5%)
Asthenia (fatigue) (22%) [14]
Myalgia/Myopathy (<5%)

Gastrointestinal/Hepatic
Diarrhea (19%) [37]
Hepatotoxicity [6]
Nausea (23%) [18]
Vomiting (8%) [13]

Respiratory
Pharyngitis (<5%)
Pneumonitis [4]
Rhinitis (<5%)

Endocrine/Metabolic
ALT increased (12%) [5]
Appetite decreased [5]
AST increased (12%) [3]
Hyperbilirubinemia [3]
Hyponatremia [4]
Weight loss (<5%)

Genitourinary
Glycosuria (<5%)
Hematuria (<5%)

Renal
Nephrotoxicity [2]
Proteinuria (<5%)

Hematologic
Anemia [26]
Bleeding (<5%)
Bone marrow suppression [2]
Febrile neutropenia [12]
Hemotoxicity [5]
Leukocytopenia [2]
Leukopenia (87%) [25]
Myelosuppression [6]
Neutropenia (44%) [48]
Thrombocytopenia (11%) [18]

Ocular
Conjunctivitis (<5%)
Keratitis (<5%)
Lacrimation (<5%)
Ocular adverse effects [2]
Ocular pain (<5%)
Reduced visual acuity (<5%)

Other
Adverse effects [21]
Death [3]

TEGASEROD

See: www.drugeruptiondata.com/drug/id/936

TEICOPLANIN

Trade name: Targocid (Sanofi-Aventis)
Indications: Staphylococcal infections
Class: Antibiotic, glycopeptide
Half-life: 150 hours
Clinically important, potentially hazardous interactions with: amikacin, cephaloridine, colistin, gentamicin, kanamycin, neomycin, streptomycin, tobramycin, vancomycin
Pregnancy category: N/A (Not recommended in pregnancy)
Important contra-indications noted in the prescribing guidelines for: nursing mothers

Skin
DRESS syndrome [3]
Erythema (<10%)
Exanthems [2]
Hypersensitivity [3]
Pruritus (<10%)
Rash (<10%) [4]
Red man syndrome [3]
Urticaria [2]

Central Nervous System
Fever (<10%)

Gastrointestinal/Hepatic
Hepatotoxicity (2%) [2]

Renal
Nephrotoxicity [2]

Hematologic
Neutropenia [2]

Otic
Ototoxicity [2]

Other
Adverse effects [2]

TELAPREVIR

Trade name: Incivek (Vertex)
Indications: Hepatitis C (must only be used in combination with PEG-interferon alfa and ribavirin)
Class: CYP3A4 inhibitor, Direct-acting antiviral, Hepatitis C virus NS3/4A protease inhibitor
Half-life: 4–11 hours
Clinically important, potentially hazardous interactions with: alfuzosin, alprazolam, amiodarone, amlodipine, atazanavir, atorvastatin, bepridil, bosentan, budesonide, carbamazepine, cisapride, dabigatran, darunavir, desipramine, dexamethasone, digoxin, dihydroergotamine, diltiazem, efavirenz, ergotamine, escitalopram, estradiol, felodipine, flecainide, flibanserin, fluticasone propionate, fosamprenavir, itraconazole, ketoconazole, lidocaine, lomitapide, lovastatin, methylergonovine, methylprednisolone, midazolam, mifepristone, nicardipine, nisoldipine, olaparib, palbociclib, phenobarbital, phenytoin, pimozide, ponatinib, posaconazole, propafenone, quinidine, rifampin, ritonavir, ruxolitinib, salmeterol, sildenafil, simvastatin, sirolimus, St John's wort, tacrolimus, tadalafil, telithromycin, tenofovir disoproxil, trazodone, triazolam, vardenafil, venetoclax, verapamil, vorapaxar, voriconazole, warfarin, zolpidem
Pregnancy category: X
Important contra-indications noted in the prescribing guidelines for: the elderly; nursing mothers; pediatric patients
Note: Must be used in combination with PEG-interferon alfa and ribavirin (see separate entries).
Warning: SERIOUS SKIN REACTIONS

Skin
Dermatitis [2]
DRESS syndrome [6]
Exanthems [6]
Pruritus (including anal pruritus) (53%) [14]
Rash (56%) [38]
Stevens-Johnson syndrome [3]
Toxic epidermal necrolysis [2]
Toxicity [2]

Central Nervous System
Dysgeusia (taste perversion) (10%)

Neuromuscular/Skeletal
Asthenia (fatigue) (56%) [4]

Gastrointestinal/Hepatic
Anorectal discomfort (11%)
Diarrhea (26%) [2]
Hemorrhoids (12%)
Hepatotoxicity [5]
Nausea (39%) [4]
Vomiting (13%)

Renal
Nephrotoxicity [3]

Hematologic
Anemia [36]
Neutropenia [6]
Thrombocytopenia [6]

Other
Adverse effects [19]
Infection [4]

TELAVANCIN

See: www.drugeruptiondata.com/drug/id/1751

TELBIVUDINE

Trade names: Sebvio (Novartis), Tyzeka (Novartis)
Indications: Hepatitis B (chronic)
Class: Nucleoside analog reverse transcriptase inhibitor
Half-life: ~15 hours
Clinically important, potentially hazardous interactions with: interferon alfa, PEG-interferon
Pregnancy category: B
Important contra-indications noted in the prescribing guidelines for: the elderly; nursing mothers; pediatric patients

Skin
Pruritus (2%)
Rash (4%)

Cardiovascular
Arrhythmias [2]

Central Nervous System
Fever (4%)
Headache (11%)
Insomnia (3%)
Neurotoxicity [2]
Vertigo (dizziness) (4%)

Neuromuscular/Skeletal
Arthralgia (4%)
Asthenia (fatigue) (>5%) [2]
Back pain (4%)
Myalgia/Myopathy (3%) [8]

Gastrointestinal/Hepatic
Abdominal distension (3%)
Abdominal pain (12%)
Diarrhea [2]
Dyspepsia (3%)
Hepatitis (exacerbation) (2%)

Respiratory
Cough (7%)
Flu-like syndrome (7%)
Pharyngolaryngeal pain (5%)

Upper respiratory tract infection (>5%)

Endocrine/Metabolic
ALT increased (3%)
Creatine phosphokinase increased [4]

Hematologic
Neutropenia (2%)

TELITHROMYCIN

See: www.drugeruptiondata.com/drug/id/1038

TELMISARTAN

Trade name: Micardis (Boehringer Ingelheim)
Indications: Hypertension
Class: Angiotensin II receptor antagonist (blocker), Antihypertensive
Half-life: 24 hours
Clinically important, potentially hazardous interactions with: ramipril
Pregnancy category: D (category C in first trimester; category D in second and third trimesters)
Important contra-indications noted in the prescribing guidelines for: nursing mothers; pediatric patients
Warning: FETAL TOXICITY

Skin
Angioedema [2]
Peripheral edema [2]

Cardiovascular
Hypotension [2]

Central Nervous System
Headache [4]
Vertigo (dizziness) [5]

Neuromuscular/Skeletal
Asthenia (fatigue) [4]

Respiratory
Cough [9]

Endocrine/Metabolic
Hyperkalemia [2]

TELOTRISTAT ETHYL *

Trade name: Xermelo (Lexicon)
Indications: Carcinoid syndrome diarrhea in combination with somatostatin analog (SSA) therapy for adults inadequately controlled by SSA therapy
Class: Tryptophan hydroxylase inhibitor
Half-life: <1 hour
Clinically important, potentially hazardous interactions with: CYP3A4 substrates
Pregnancy category: N/A (No data available)
Important contra-indications noted in the prescribing guidelines for: nursing mothers; pediatric patients

Central Nervous System
Depression (9%)
Fever (7%)
Headache (11%)

Gastrointestinal/Hepatic
Abdominal distension (>5%)
Abdominal pain (>5%)
Constipation (>5%)
Flatulence (7%)
Nausea (13%) [2]

Endocrine/Metabolic
ALP increased (<5%)
ALT increased (<5%)
Appetite decreased (7%)
AST increased (<5%)
GGT increased (9%)

TEMAZEPAM

Trade name: Restoril (Mallinckrodt)
Indications: Insomnia, anxiety
Class: Benzodiazepine
Half-life: 8–15 hours
Clinically important, potentially hazardous interactions with: amprenavir, chlorpheniramine, clarithromycin, efavirenz, esomeprazole, imatinib, mianserin, nelfinavir
Pregnancy category: X
Important contra-indications noted in the prescribing guidelines for: the elderly; nursing mothers; pediatric patients

Skin
Dermatitis (<10%)
Diaphoresis (>10%)
Rash (>10%)

Mucosal
Sialopenia (>10%)
Sialorrhea (<10%)
Xerostomia (2%)

Other
Adverse effects [2]

TEMOZOLOMIDE

Trade name: Temodar (MSD)
Indications: Anaplastic astrocytoma, newly diagnosed glioblastoma multiforme concomitantly with radiotherapy and then as maintenance treatment
Class: Alkylating agent, Antineoplastic
Half-life: 1.8 hours
Clinically important, potentially hazardous interactions with: clozapine, digoxin, valproic acid
Pregnancy category: D
Important contra-indications noted in the prescribing guidelines for: the elderly; nursing mothers; pediatric patients

Skin
Peripheral edema (11%)
Pruritus (8%)
Rash (8%) [8]
Toxicity [3]

Hair
Alopecia [3]

Cardiovascular
Thromboembolism [2]

Central Nervous System
Anorexia [3]
Fever [2]
Headache [3]
Paresthesias (9%)

Neuromuscular/Skeletal
Asthenia (fatigue) [14]
Myalgia/Myopathy (5%)

Gastrointestinal/Hepatic
Constipation [2]
Diarrhea [8]
Hepatotoxicity [6]
Nausea [9]
Vomiting [4]

Endocrine/Metabolic
Mastodynia (6%)

Hematologic
Anemia [3]
Febrile neutropenia [2]
Hemotoxicity [5]
Leukopenia [6]
Lymphocytopenia [4]
Lymphopenia [4]
Myelosuppression [3]
Neutropenia [10]
Thrombocytopenia [11]

Other
Death [7]
Infection [5]

TEMSIROLIMUS

Trade name: Torisel (Wyeth)
Indications: Renal cell carcinoma, other cancers
Class: Analog of sirolimus, Antineoplastic, mTOR inhibitor
Half-life: 17 hours
Clinically important, potentially hazardous interactions with: ACE inhibitors, atazanavir, BCG vaccine, benazepril, captopril, carbamazepine, clarithromycin, clozapine, conivaptan, cyclosporine, darunavir, dasatinib, denosumab, dexamethasone, digoxin, enalapril, fluconazole, fosinopril, grapefruit juice, hypoglycemic agents, indinavir, itraconazole, ketoconazole, leflunomide, lisinopril, live and inactive vaccines, macolide antibiotics, natalizumab, nefazodone, nelfinavir, P-glycoprotein inhibitors, phenobarbital, phenytoin, pimecrolimus, posaconazole, protease inhibitors, quinapril, ramipril, rifabutin, rifampin, rifapentine, ritonavir, saquinavir, St John's wort, sunitinib, tacrolimus, telithromycin, tipranavir, trastuzumab, voriconazole
Pregnancy category: D
Important contra-indications noted in the prescribing guidelines for: the elderly; nursing mothers; pediatric patients
Note: Contra-indicated in patients with bilirubin >1.5xULN.

Skin
Acneform eruption (10%) [4]
Edema [2]
Exanthems [3]
Hypersensitivity (9%) [3]
Pruritus (19%) [3]

Rash (47%) [14]
Toxicity [3]
Xerosis (11%)

Nails
Nail disorder (14%)
Paronychia [2]

Mucosal
Mucositis (30%) [12]
Oral mucositis [2]
Stomatitis [16]

Cardiovascular
Chest pain (16%)
Hypertension (7%) [3]

Central Nervous System
Anorexia (30%) [3]
Chills (8%)
Depression (4%)
Dysgeusia (taste perversion) (20%) [2]
Fever (24%)
Headache (15%)
Insomnia (12%)
Neurotoxicity [2]
Pain (28%)

Neuromuscular/Skeletal
Arthralgia (18%)
Asthenia (fatigue) (30%) [20]
Back pain (20%)
Myalgia/Myopathy (8%)

Gastrointestinal/Hepatic
Abdominal pain (21%)
Diarrhea [7]
Nausea [7]
Vomiting [2]

Respiratory
Cough (26%) [3]
Dyspnea [7]
Pharyngitis (12%)
Pneumonia [2]
Pneumonitis (36%) [11]
Rhinitis (10%)
Upper respiratory tract infection (7%)

Endocrine/Metabolic
ALT increased [4]
AST increased [2]
Dehydration [2]
Hypercholesterolemia [4]
Hyperglycemia [14]
Hyperlipidemia [2]
Hypertriglyceridemia [5]
Hypokalemia [3]
Hypophosphatemia [4]
Serum creatinine increased [2]

Genitourinary
Urinary tract infection (15%)

Hematologic
Anemia [10]
Febrile neutropenia [3]
Hemorrhage [2]
Hemotoxicity [2]
Immunosupression [2]
Leukopenia [4]
Lymphopenia [4]
Neutropenia [5]
Thrombocytopenia [16]

Ocular
Conjunctivitis (7%)

Other
Adverse effects [9]
Death [2]
Infection (20%) [5]

TENECTEPLASE

See: www.drugeruptiondata.com/drug/id/812

TENIPOSIDE

See: www.drugeruptiondata.com/drug/id/1204

TENOFOVIR ALAFENAMIDE

Trade names: Descovy (Gilead), Vemlidy (Gilead)
Indications: Hepatitis B
Class: Antiviral, Hepatitis B virus necleoside analog reverse transcriptase inhibitor
Half-life: <1 hour
Clinically important, potentially hazardous interactions with: carbamazepine, oxcarbazepine, phenobarbital, phenytoin, rifabutin, rifampin, rifapentine, St John's wort
Pregnancy category: N/A (No data available)
Important contra-indications noted in the prescribing guidelines for: nursing mothers; pediatric patients
Note: Descovy is tenofovir alafenamide and emtricitabine. See also separate profile for tenofovir alafenamide in combination with cobicistat, elvitegravir and emtricitabine.
Warning: LACTIC ACIDOSIS/SEVERE HEPATOMEGALY WITH STEATOSIS and POST TREATMENT SEVERE ACUTE EXACERBATION OF HEPATITIS B

Central Nervous System
Headache (9%) [3]

Neuromuscular/Skeletal
Asthenia (fatigue) (6%)
Back pain (5%)

Gastrointestinal/Hepatic
Abdominal pain (7%)
Nausea (5%)

Respiratory
Cough (6%)
Nasopharyngitis [2]
Upper respiratory tract infection [2]

Endocrine/Metabolic
ALT increased (8%)
AST increased (3%)
Creatine phosphokinase increased (3%)
Hyperamylasemia (3%)
Hypercholesterolemia (4%)

Genitourinary
Glycosuria (5%)

Other
Adverse effects [2]

TENOFOVIR DISOPROXIL

Trade names: Atripla (Gilead), Complera (Gilead), Truvada (Gilead), Viread (Gilead)
Indications: HIV infection in combination with at least two other antiretroviral agents
Class: Antiretroviral, Nucleoside analog reverse transcriptase inhibitor
Half-life: 12–18 hours
Clinically important, potentially hazardous interactions with: acyclovir, adefovir, atazanavir, cidofovir, cobicistat/elvitegravir/emtricitabine/ tenofovir disoproxil, darunavir, didanosine, ganciclovir, high-fat foods, indinavir, ledipasvir & sofosbuvir, lopinavir, protease inhibitors, ritonavir, telaprevir, tipranavir, trospium, valacyclovir, valganciclovir
Pregnancy category: B
Important contra-indications noted in the prescribing guidelines for: nursing mothers; pediatric patients
Note: Atripla is tenofovir disoproxil, efavirenz and emtricitabine; Complera is tenofovir disoproxil, emtricitabine and rilpivirine; Truvada is tenofovir disoproxil and emtricitabine. See also separate profile for tenofovir disoproxil in combination with cobicistat, elvitegravir and emtricitabine.
Warning: LACTIC ACIDOSIS/SEVERE HEPATOMEGALY WITH STEATOSIS and POST TREATMENT EXACERBATION OF HEPATITIS

Skin
Diaphoresis (3%)
Lichenoid eruption [2]
Rash (5–18%) [4]
Stevens-Johnson syndrome [2]

Cardiovascular
Chest pain (3%)

Central Nervous System
Abnormal dreams [3]
Anorexia (3%)
Anxiety (6%) [2]
Depression (4–11%)
Fever (2–8%)
Headache (5–14%) [10]
Insomnia (3–5%) [2]
Neurotoxicity (3%) [6]
Pain (7–13%)
Peripheral neuropathy (<3%)
Somnolence (drowsiness) [2]
Vertigo (dizziness) (<3%) [4]

Neuromuscular/Skeletal
Arthralgia (5%)
Asthenia (fatigue) (6–7%) [6]
Back pain (3–9%)
Bone or joint pain [4]
Fractures [2]
Myalgia/Myopathy (3%) [2]
Osteomalacia [5]

Gastrointestinal/Hepatic
Abdominal pain (4–7%) [2]
Diarrhea (11%) [7]
Dyspepsia (3–4%)
Flatulence (3%)
Hepatic failure [2]
Hepatotoxicity [3]
Nausea (8%) [10]
Pancreatitis [5]
Vomiting (4–5%) [5]

Respiratory
Nasopharyngitis [3]
Pneumonia (2–5%)
Upper respiratory tract infection [2]

Endocrine/Metabolic
Acidosis [3]
ALT increased [3]
Creatine phosphokinase increased [3]
Hypokalemia [2]
Hypophosphatemia [3]
Weight loss (2%)

Renal
Fanconi syndrome [25]
Nephrotoxicity [41]
Proteinuria [4]
Renal failure [10]
Renal tubular necrosis [2]

Other
Adverse effects [11]

TENOXICAM

See: www.drugeruptiondata.com/drug/id/1346

TERAZOSIN

Trade name: Hytrin (AbbVie)
Indications: Hypertension, benign prostatic hypertrophy
Class: Adrenergic alpha-receptor antagonist
Half-life: 12 hours
Clinically important, potentially hazardous interactions with: vardenafil
Pregnancy category: C

Skin
Edema (<10%)
Lichenoid eruption [2]
Peripheral edema (6%)

Mucosal
Xerostomia (<10%)

Cardiovascular
Postural hypotension [2]

Central Nervous System
Paresthesias (3%)
Vertigo (dizziness) [3]

Genitourinary
Priapism [2]

Ocular
Floppy iris syndrome [2]

TERBINAFINE

Trade name: Lamisil (Novartis)
Indications: Fungal infections of the skin and nails
Class: Antifungal
Half-life: ~36 hours
Clinically important, potentially hazardous interactions with: amitriptyline, amphotericin B, atomoxetine, caffeine, carbamazepine, cimetidine, codeine, conivaptan, cyclosporine, CYP2D6 substrates, desipramine, estrogens, fesoterodine, fluconazole, nebivolol, progestogens, rifampin, rifapentine, saxagliptin, tamoxifen, tamsulosin, tetrabenazine, thioridazine, tramadol, tricyclic antidepressants
Pregnancy category: B
Important contra-indications noted in the prescribing guidelines for: nursing mothers; pediatric patients

Skin
AGEP [24]
Baboon syndrome (SDRIFE) [2]
Dermatitis (<10%)
Eczema [2]
Erythema multiforme [9]
Erythroderma [2]
Exanthems [5]
Fixed eruption [3]
Hypersensitivity [3]
Lichenoid eruption [2]
Lupus erythematosus [30]
Pityriasis rosea [2]
Pruritus (3%) [6]
Psoriasis [14]
Pustules [3]
Rash (6%) [3]
Stevens-Johnson syndrome [2]
Toxic epidermal necrolysis [3]
Urticaria [7]

Hair
Alopecia (<10%)

Nails
Onychocryptosis [2]

Central Nervous System
Ageusia (taste loss) [17]
Dysgeusia (taste perversion) (3%) [8]
Headache (13%)

Gastrointestinal/Hepatic
Abdominal pain (2%)
Diarrhea (6%)
Dyspepsia (4%)
Flatulence (2%)
Hepatotoxicity [11]
Nausea (3%)

Other
Adverse effects [3]
Allergic reactions (<10%)
Side effects (3%)

TERBUTALINE

Trade names: Brethine (aaiPharma), Bricanyl (AstraZeneca)
Indications: Bronchospasm
Class: Beta-2 adrenergic agonist, Bronchodilator, Tocolytic
Half-life: 11–16 hours
Clinically important, potentially hazardous interactions with: alpha blockers, atomoxetine, beta blockers, betahistine, cannabinoids, epinephrine, insulin aspart, insulin degludec, insulin detemir, insulin glargine, insulin glulisine, iobenguane, loop diuretics, MAO inhibitors, propranolol, sotalol, sympathomimetics, tricyclic antidepressants, yohimbine
Pregnancy category: C
Important contra-indications noted in the prescribing guidelines for: nursing mothers; pediatric patients
Warning: PROLONGED TOCOLYSIS

Skin
  Diaphoresis (<10%)

Mucosal
  Xerostomia (<10%)

Cardiovascular
  Arrhythmias [2]

Central Nervous System
  Dysgeusia (taste perversion) (<10%)
  Tremor [2]

Gastrointestinal/Hepatic
  Nausea [2]

Other
  Side effects [2]

TERCONAZOLE

See: www.drugeruptiondata.com/drug/id/679

TERFENADINE

See: www.drugeruptiondata.com/drug/id/680

TERIFLUNOMIDE

Trade name: Aubagio (Sanofi-Aventis)
Indications: Relapsing forms of multiple sclerosis
Class: Pyrimidine synthesis inhibitor
Half-life: N/A
Clinically important, potentially hazardous interactions with: alosetron, caffeine, duloxetine, ethinylestradiol, leflunomide, live vaccines, oral contraceptives, paclitaxel, pioglitazone, repaglinide, rosiglitazone, theophylline, tizanidine, warfarin
Pregnancy category: X
Important contra-indications noted in the prescribing guidelines for: the elderly; nursing mothers; pediatric patients
Warning: HEPATOTOXICITY and RISK OF TERATOGENICITY

Skin
  Acneform eruption (<3%)
  Burning (2–3%)
  Herpes (oral) (2–4%)
  Pruritus (3–4%)

Hair
  Alopecia (10–13%) [14]

Cardiovascular
  Hypertension (4%) [3]
  Palpitation (2–3%)

Central Nervous System
  Anxiety (3–4%)
  Carpal tunnel syndrome (<3%)
  Headache (19–22%) [4]
  Paresthesias (9–10%) [3]
  Peripheral neuropathy (<2%) [2]

Neuromuscular/Skeletal
  Asthenia (fatigue) [2]
  Back pain (<3%) [2]
  Bone or joint pain (4–5%)
  Myalgia/Myopathy (3–4%)

Gastrointestinal/Hepatic
  Abdominal distension (<2%)
  Abdominal pain (5–6%)
  Diarrhea (15–18%) [11]
  Gastroenteritis (2–4%)
  Hepatotoxicity [4]
  Nausea (9–14%) [9]

Respiratory
  Bronchitis (5–8%)
  Influenza (9–12%) [2]
  Nasopharyngitis [2]
  Sinusitis (4–6%)
  Upper respiratory tract infection (9%)

Endocrine/Metabolic
  ALT increased (12–14%) [11]
  AST increased (2–3%)
  GGT increased (3–5%)
  Hypophosphatemia (mild) (18%)
  Weight loss (2–3%)

Genitourinary
  Cystitis (2–4%)

Renal
  Renal failure [2]

Hematologic
  Immunosupression (10–15%)
  Leukopenia (<2%) [2]
  Lymphopenia [2]
  Neutropenia (2–4%) [4]

Ocular
  Conjunctivitis (<3%)
  Vision blurred (3%)

Other
  Adverse effects [4]
  Allergic reactions (2–3%)
  Infection [5]
  Side effects [2]
  Toothache (4%)

TERIPARATIDE

Trade name: Forteo (Lilly)
Indications: Osteoporosis in postmenopausal women and men at increased risk of fractures
Class: Parathyroid hormone analog
Half-life: 1 hour
Clinically important, potentially hazardous interactions with: alcohol, digoxin
Pregnancy category: C
Important contra-indications noted in the prescribing guidelines for: nursing mothers; pediatric patients
Warning: POTENTIAL RISK OF OSTEOSARCOMA

Skin
  Diaphoresis (2%)
  Herpes zoster (3%)
  Rash (5%)

Cardiovascular
  Angina (3%)
  Hypertension (7%)

Central Nervous System
  Anxiety (4%)
  Depression (4%)
  Dysgeusia (taste perversion) (<2%)
  Headache (8%) [8]
  Insomnia (4–5%)
  Pain (21%)
  Paresthesias (<2%)
  Syncope (3%)
  Vertigo (dizziness) (4–8%) [7]

Neuromuscular/Skeletal
  Arthralgia (10%) [3]
  Asthenia (fatigue) (9%)
  Bone tumor [2]
  Leg cramps (3%) [4]
  Myalgia/Myopathy [2]
  Neck pain (3%)
  Pain in extremities [3]

Gastrointestinal/Hepatic
  Constipation (5%)
  Diarrhea (5%)
  Dyspepsia (5%)
  Gastritis (2–7%)
  Nausea (9–14%) [8]
  Vomiting (3%)

Respiratory
  Cough (6%)
  Dyspnea (4–6%)
  Pharyngitis (6%)
  Pneumonia (4–6%)
  Rhinitis (10%)

Endocrine/Metabolic
  Hypercalcemia [6]

Local
  Injection-site pain (<2%)

Other
  Adverse effects [4]
  Tooth disorder (2%)

TERLIPRESSIN

Trade names: Glypressin (IS Pharma), Terlipressin (Ferring) (Bissendorf Peptide)
Indications: Esophageal variceal hemorrhage
Class: Vasopressin agonist
Half-life: 50–70 minutes
Clinically important, potentially hazardous interactions with: none known
Pregnancy category: N/A (Contra-indicated in pregnancy)

Skin
  Gangrene [2]
  Necrosis [12]
Cardiovascular
  Myocardial infarction [3]
  QT prolongation [2]
  Torsades de pointes [2]
Central Nervous System
  Seizures [3]
Neuromuscular/Skeletal
  Rhabdomyolysis [3]
Endocrine/Metabolic
  Hyponatremia [8]
Other
  Adverse effects [2]

TESAMORELIN

See: www.drugeruptiondata.com/drug/id/2155

TESTOLACTONE

See: www.drugeruptiondata.com/drug/id/1172

TESTOSTERONE

Trade names: Androderm (Actavis), AndroGel (AbbVie), Delatestryl (Endo), Fortesta (Endo), Natesto (Endo), Testim (Auxilium)
Indications: Androgen replacement, hypogonadism, postpartum breast pain
Class: Androgen
Half-life: 10–100 minutes
Clinically important, potentially hazardous interactions with: acarbose, anisindione, anticoagulants, cyclosporine, dicumarol, metformin, saxagliptin, sitagliptin, warfarin
Pregnancy category: N/A (Contra-indicated in pregnancy)
Important contra-indications noted in the prescribing guidelines for: nursing mothers; pediatric patients
Note: Contra-indicated in men with carcinoma of the breast or known or suspected carcinoma of the prostate.
Warning: SECONDARY EXPOSURE TO TESTOSTERONE

Skin
  Acneform eruption (>10%) [20]
  Carcinoma [2]
  Dermatitis (4%) [2]
  Edema (<10%)
  Rash (2%)
Hair
  Alopecia [3]
  Hirsutism (<10%) [12]
Cardiovascular
  Cardiotoxicity [2]
  Flushing (<10%)
  Myocardial infarction [3]
Endocrine/Metabolic
  Gynecomastia [2]
  Mastodynia (>10%)
Genitourinary
  Priapism (>10%) [10]
Hematologic
  Thrombosis [2]
Local
  Application-site bullae (12%)
  Application-site burning (3%)
  Application-site erythema (7%)
  Application-site induration (3%)
  Application-site pruritus (37%)
  Application-site vesicles (6%)
  Injection-site pain [2]
Other
  Adverse effects [3]

TETRABENAZINE

See: www.drugeruptiondata.com/drug/id/1301

TETRACAINE & OXYMETAZOLINE *

Trade name: Kovanaze (St Renatus)
Indications: Regional anesthesia in restorative dentistry
Class: Alpha adrenoceptor agonist (oxymetazoline), Anesthetic, local (tetracaine)
Half-life: <2 hours
Clinically important, potentially hazardous interactions with: beta blockers, MAO inhibitors, other intranasal products, tricyclic antidepressants
Pregnancy category: N/A (Insufficient evidence to inform drug-associated risk)
Important contra-indications noted in the prescribing guidelines for: the elderly; nursing mothers; pediatric patients
Note: For intranasal use only. See separate entry for oxymetazoline as topical formulation.

Mucosal
  Epistaxis (nosebleed) (2%)
  Mucosal ulceration (2–3%)
  Nasal congestion (32%) [3]
  Nasal discomfort (26%)
  Nasal dryness (2%)
  Oropharyngeal pain (14%)
  Rhinorrhea (52%) [3]
Cardiovascular
  Blood pressure variations (3–5%)
  Bradycardia (3%)
  Hypertension (3%)
Central Nervous System
  Dysgeusia (taste perversion) (8%)
  Headache (10%)
  Hypoesthesia (intranasal and pharyngeal) (10%)
  Sensory disturbances (2%)
  Vertigo (dizziness) (3%)
Ocular
  Lacrimation (13%)
Other
  Sneezing (4%)

TETRACYCLINE

Trade names: Helidac (Prometheus), Sumycin (Par)
Indications: Various infections caused by susceptible organisms
Class: Antibiotic, tetracycline
Half-life: 6–11 hours
Clinically important, potentially hazardous interactions with: ACE inhibitors, acitretin, aluminum, amoxicillin, ampicillin, antacids, atovaquone, atovaquone/proguanil, bacampicillin, betamethasone, bismuth, bromelain, calcium salts, carbenicillin, cholestyramine, cloxacillin, colestipol, corticosteroids, coumarins, dairy products, dicloxacillin, didanosine, digoxin, ergotamine, food, gliclazide, isotretinoin, kaolin, methicillin, methotrexate, methoxyflurane, methysergide, mezlocillin, nafcillin, oral iron, oral typhoid vaccine, oxacillin, penicillins, phenindione, piperacillin, quinapril, retinoids, rocuronium, sodium picosulfate, strontium ranelate, sucralfate, sulfonylureas, ticarcillin, tripotassium dicitratobismuthate, vitamin A, zinc
Pregnancy category: D

Skin
  Acneform eruption [2]
  Angioedema [2]
  Candidiasis [2]
  Erythema multiforme [7]
  Exanthems [3]
  Exfoliative dermatitis [2]
  Fixed eruption (15%) [43]
  Hypersensitivity [2]
  Jarisch–Herxheimer reaction [3]
  Lichenoid eruption [3]
  Lupus erythematosus [6]
  Photosensitivity (<10%) [12]
  Phototoxicity [4]
  Pigmentation [4]
  Psoriasis (exacerbation) [2]
  Stevens-Johnson syndrome [4]
  Toxic epidermal necrolysis [13]
  Urticaria [5]
Nails
  Onycholysis [5]
  Photo-onycholysis [8]
Central Nervous System
  Pseudotumor cerebri [6]
Gastrointestinal/Hepatic
  Diarrhea [2]
  Hepatotoxicity [2]
  Pancreatitis [3]

Genitourinary
Vaginitis [3]

Other
Adverse effects [4]
Tooth pigmentation (commonly in under 8-year-olds) (>10%) [12]

TETRAZEPAM

See: www.drugeruptiondata.com/drug/id/2015

THALIDOMIDE

Trade name: Thalomid (Celgene)
Indications: Graft-versus-host reactions, recalcitrant aphthous stomatitis
Class: Immunosuppressant, TNF modulator
Half-life: 5–7 hours
Clinically important, potentially hazardous interactions with: alcohol, amiodarone, antihistamines, antipsychotics, bortezomib, calcium channel blockers, carbamazepine, cimetidine, cisplatin, CNS depressants, digoxin, disulfiram, docetaxel, famotidine, griseofulvin, lithium, metronidazole, modafinil, opioids, paclitaxel, penicillins, phenytoin, rifabutin, rifampin, St John's wort, succinylcholine, vincristine
Pregnancy category: X
Important contra-indications noted in the prescribing guidelines for: nursing mothers; pediatric patients
Note: Thalidomide is a potent teratogen, an agent that causes congenital malformations and developmental abnormalities if introduced during gestation. Some of these teratogenic side effects of thalidomide include fetal limb growth retardation (arms, legs, hands, feet), ingrown genitalia, absence of lung, partial/total loss of hearing or sight, malformed digestive tract, heart, kidney, and stillborn infant.
Warning: FETAL RISK AND VENOUS THROMBOEMBOLIC EVENTS

Skin
Bullous dermatitis (5%)
Dermatitis [2]
Diaphoresis (13%)
Edema (57%) [11]
Erythema [2]
Erythema nodosum [2]
Erythroderma [2]
Exanthems [2]
Exfoliative dermatitis [4]
Facial erythema (<5%) [2]
Hypersensitivity [3]
Peripheral edema (3–8%) [4]
Pruritus (3–8%) [3]
Psoriasis [2]
Purpura [2]
Rash (11–50%) [24]
Stevens-Johnson syndrome [2]
Toxic epidermal necrolysis [4]
Urticaria (3%) [2]
Vasculitis [2]
Xerosis (21%) [5]

Mucosal
Oral candidiasis (4–11%)
Xerostomia (8%) [9]

Cardiovascular
Bradycardia [5]
Cardiotoxicity [2]
Hypotension (16%)
Thromboembolism [2]
Venous thromboembolism [5]

Central Nervous System
Agitation (9–26%)
Fever (19–23%) [2]
Hyperesthesia [2]
Insomnia (9%)
Neurotoxicity (22%) [24]
Paresthesias (6–16%) [8]
Parkinsonism [2]
Peripheral neuropathy [26]
Somnolence (drowsiness) (36%) [13]
Tremor (4–26%) [6]
Vertigo (dizziness) (4–20%) [16]

Neuromuscular/Skeletal
Arthralgia (13%)
Asthenia (fatigue) (79%) [16]
Myalgia/Myopathy (7%)

Gastrointestinal/Hepatic
Abdominal pain (3%)
Constipation [13]
Diarrhea (4–19%)
Flatulence (8%)
Hepatotoxicity [4]
Pancreatitis [2]

Respiratory
Dyspnea (42%)
Pharyngitis (4–8%)
Pneumonia [2]
Rhinitis (4%)
Sinusitis (3–8%)

Endocrine/Metabolic
Amenorrhea [6]
Gynecomastia [2]
Weight gain (22%)
Weight loss (23%)

Genitourinary
Erectile dysfunction [2]
Impotence (38%)
Leukorrhea (17–35%)

Hematologic
Anemia (6–13%) [4]
Neutropenia (31%) [9]
Thrombocytopenia [6]
Thrombosis [13]

Other
Adverse effects [8]
Death [2]
Infection (6–8%) [6]
Teratogenicity [6]
Toothache (4%)

THALLIUM

Indications: For diagnostic use in myocardial perfusion imaging
Class: Radioactive element
Half-life: 73.1 hours
Clinically important, potentially hazardous interactions with: none known
Pregnancy category: C

Hair
Alopecia [11]

Nails
Leukonychia (Mees' lines) [2]

Cardiovascular
Tachycardia [3]

Central Nervous System
Encephalopathy [5]
Peripheral neuropathy [5]

Gastrointestinal/Hepatic
Abdominal pain [5]

Other
Death [2]

THIABENDAZOLE

Synonym: tiabendazole
Indications: Various infections caused by susceptible helminths
Class: Anthelmintic, Antibiotic, imidazole
Half-life: 1.2 hours
Clinically important, potentially hazardous interactions with: none known
Pregnancy category: C

Skin
Dermatitis [3]
Erythema multiforme [3]
Exanthems (>5%) [4]
Fixed eruption [2]
Rash (<10%)
Sjögren's syndrome [3]
Stevens-Johnson syndrome (<10%)
Toxic epidermal necrolysis [2]
Urticaria (<5%)

Central Nervous System
Vertigo (dizziness) [3]

Gastrointestinal/Hepatic
Abdominal pain [2]
Nausea [2]

THIAMINE

See: www.drugeruptiondata.com/drug/id/686

THIMEROSAL

See: www.drugeruptiondata.com/drug/id/848

THIOGUANINE

See: www.drugeruptiondata.com/drug/id/687

THIOPENTAL

See: www.drugeruptiondata.com/drug/id/688

THIORIDAZINE

See: www.drugeruptiondata.com/drug/id/689

THIOTEPA

See: www.drugeruptiondata.com/drug/id/690

THIOTHIXENE

See: www.drugeruptiondata.com/drug/id/691

THYROTROPIN ALFA

See: www.drugeruptiondata.com/drug/id/1357

TIAGABINE

Trade name: Gabitril (Cephalon)
Indications: Partial seizures
Class: Anticonvulsant, Mood stabilizer
Half-life: 7–9 hours
Clinically important, potentially hazardous interactions with: alcohol, antipsychotics, carbamazepine, chloroquine, conivaptan, CYP3A4 inhibitors and inducers, dasatinib, deferasirox, droperidol, hydroxychloroquine, ketorolac, levomepromazine, MAO inhibitors, mefloquine, orlistat, phenobarbital, phenytoin, SSRIs, St John's wort, tricyclic antidepressants
Pregnancy category: C
Important contra-indications noted in the prescribing guidelines for: the elderly; nursing mothers; pediatric patients

Skin
  Ecchymoses (<6%)
  Pruritus (2%)
  Rash (5%) [2]
Cardiovascular
  Vasodilation (2%)
Central Nervous System
  Confusion (5%)
  Depression (<7%) [4]
  Emotional lability (3%)
  Gait instability (3–5%)
  Headache [8]
  Hostility (2–5%)
  Impaired concentration (6–14%) [2]
  Insomnia (5–6%)
  Nervousness (10–14%) [10]
  Pain (2–7%)
  Paresthesias (4%)
  Seizures [4]
  Somnolence (drowsiness) (18–21%) [9]
  Speech disorder (4%)
  Status epilepticus (non-convulsive) [17]
  Syncope [2]
  Tremor (9–21%) [7]
  Vertigo (dizziness) (27–31%) [22]
Neuromuscular/Skeletal
  Asthenia (fatigue) (18–23%) [16]
  Ataxia (5–9%)
  Dystonia [5]
  Myalgia/Myopathy (2–5%)
Gastrointestinal/Hepatic
  Abdominal pain (5–7%)
  Diarrhea (2–10%)
  Nausea (11%) [7]
  Vomiting (7%)
Respiratory
  Cough (4%)
  Flu-like syndrome (6–9%)
  Pharyngitis (7–8%)
Endocrine/Metabolic
  Appetite increased (2%)
Genitourinary
  Urinary tract infection (<5%)
Ocular
  Amblyopia (4–9%)
  Nystagmus (2%)
Other
  Adverse effects [6]
  Infection (10–19%) [3]

TIANEPTINE

See: www.drugeruptiondata.com/drug/id/2065

TIBOLONE

See: www.drugeruptiondata.com/drug/id/1310

TICAGRELOR

Trade name: Brilinta (AstraZeneca)
Indications: Thrombotic cardiovascular events
Class: Antiplatelet, Antiplatelet, cyclopentyl triazolo-pyrimidine (CPTP)
Half-life: 7 hours
Clinically important, potentially hazardous interactions with: atazanavir, carbamazepine, clarithromycin, dexamethasone, digoxin, efavirenz, indinavir, itraconazole, ketoconazole, lovastatin, nefazodone, nelfinavir, phenobarbital, phenytoin, rifampin, ritonavir, saquinavir, simvastatin, telithromycin, venetoclax, voriconazole
Pregnancy category: C
Important contra-indications noted in the prescribing guidelines for: nursing mothers; pediatric patients
Note: Maintenance doses of aspirin above 100 mg reduce the effectiveness of ticagrelor and should be avoided. Contra-indicated in patients with a history of intracranial hemorrhage, or active pathological bleeding, and in patients with severe hepatic impairment.
Warning: BLEEDING RISK

Cardiovascular
  Atrial fibrillation (4%)
  Bradycardia [2]
  Chest pain (3–4%)
  Hypertension (4%)
  Hypotension (3%)
  Ventricular arrhythmia [7]
Central Nervous System
  Headache (7%)
  Vertigo (dizziness) (5%)
Neuromuscular/Skeletal
  Asthenia (fatigue) (3%)
  Back pain (4%)
  Rhabdomyolysis [2]
Gastrointestinal/Hepatic
  Diarrhea (4%)
  Nausea (4%)
Respiratory
  Cough (5%)
  Dyspnea (14%) [19]
  Pneumonitis [2]
Hematologic
  Bleeding (12%) [11]
Other
  Adverse effects [2]

TICARCILLIN

See: www.drugeruptiondata.com/drug/id/693

TICLOPIDINE

See: www.drugeruptiondata.com/drug/id/694

TIGECYCLINE

See: www.drugeruptiondata.com/drug/id/1078

TILUDRONATE

See: www.drugeruptiondata.com/drug/id/1203

TIMOLOL

See: www.drugeruptiondata.com/drug/id/695

TINIDAZOLE

See: www.drugeruptiondata.com/drug/id/1051

TINZAPARIN

Trade name: Innohep (Leo Pharma)
Indications: Acute symptomatic deep vein thrombosis
Class: Anticoagulant, Heparin, low molecular weight
Half-life: 3–4 hours
Clinically important, potentially hazardous interactions with: aliskiren, angiotensin II recepton antagonists, aspirin, butabarbital,

clopidogrel, collagenase, dasatinib, dextran, diclofenac, dipyridamole, drotrecogin alfa, glyceryl trinitrate, ibritumomab, iloprost, ketorolac, NSAIDs, oral anticoagulants, pentosan, pentoxifylline, platelet inhibitors, prostacyclin analogues, salicylates, sulfinpyrazone, throbolytics, ticlopidine, tositumomab & iodine[131]
Pregnancy category: B
Important contra-indications noted in the prescribing guidelines for: the elderly; nursing mothers; pediatric patients
Warning: SPINAL / EPIDURAL HEMATOMAS

Skin
Bullous dermatitis (<10%)
Pruritus (<10%)
Mucosal
Epistaxis (nosebleed) (2%)
Cardiovascular
Chest pain (2%)
Central Nervous System
Fever (2%)
Headache (2%)
Pain (2%)
Neuromuscular/Skeletal
Back pain (2%)
Respiratory
Pulmonary embolism (2%)
Endocrine/Metabolic
ALT increased (13%)
AST increased (9%)
Genitourinary
Urinary tract infection (4%)
Hematologic
Bleeding [4]
Hemorrhage (2%)
Local
Injection-site hematoma (16%)

TIOPRONIN

See: www.drugeruptiondata.com/drug/id/696

TIOTROPIUM

Trade names: Spiriva (Boehringer Ingelheim), Stiolto Respimat (Boehringer Ingelheim)
Indications: Bronchospasm (associated with COPD)
Class: Anticholinergic, Muscarinic antagonist
Half-life: 5–6 days
Clinically important, potentially hazardous interactions with: acetylcholinesterase inhibitors, anticholinergics, antihistamines, botulinum toxin (A & B), cannabinoids, conivaptan, disopyramide, domperidone, haloperidol, ketoconazole, levodopa, MAO inhibitors, memantine, metoclopramide, nefopam, parasympathomimetics, PEG-interferon, phenothiazines, potassium chloride, pramlintide, secretin, sublingual nitrates, tricyclic antidepressants

Pregnancy category: C
Important contra-indications noted in the prescribing guidelines for: nursing mothers; pediatric patients
Note: Stiolto Respimat is tiotropium and olodaterol.

Skin
Candidiasis (4%)
Edema (5%)
Herpes zoster (<3%)
Rash (4%)
Mucosal
Epistaxis (nosebleed) (4%)
Oral candidiasis [2]
Stomatitis (<3%)
Xerostomia (10–16%) [22]
Cardiovascular
Angina (<3%)
Cardiotoxicity [2]
Chest pain (7%) [2]
Hypertension [2]
Central Nervous System
Depression (<3%)
Headache [6]
Paresthesias (<3%)
Vertigo (dizziness) [2]
Neuromuscular/Skeletal
Arthralgia (>3%)
Back pain [4]
Bone or joint pain (<3%)
Leg pain (<3%)
Myalgia/Myopathy (4%)
Gastrointestinal/Hepatic
Abdominal pain (5%)
Constipation (4%) [2]
Diarrhea [3]
Dyspepsia (6%)
Gastroesophageal reflux (<3%)
Vomiting (4%)
Respiratory
Asthma [4]
Bronchitis [4]
COPD (exacerbation) [5]
Cough (>3%) [8]
Dysphonia (<3%)
Dyspnea [4]
Flu-like syndrome (>3%)
Influenza [3]
Laryngitis (<3%)
Nasopharyngitis [11]
Pharyngitis (9%)
Pneumonia [3]
Rhinitis (6%) [3]
Sinusitis (11%)
Upper respiratory tract infection (41%) [4]
Endocrine/Metabolic
Hypercholesterolemia (<3%)
Hyperglycemia (<3%)
Genitourinary
Urinary tract infection (7%)
Ocular
Cataract (<3%)
Other
Adverse effects [12]
Allergic reactions (<3%)

Death [7]
Infection (4%)

TIPRANAVIR

Trade name: Aptivus (Boehringer Ingelheim)
Indications: Antiretroviral treatment of HIV-1
Class: HIV-1 protease inhibitor, Sulfonamide
Half-life: 4.8–6.0 hours
Clinically important, potentially hazardous interactions with: abacavir, alcohol, alfuzosin, alprazolam, amiodarone, antacids, antifungals, apixaban, artemether/lumefantrine, atazanavir, atomoxetine, atorvastatin, bepridil, bosentan, buprenorphine, calcium channel blockers, carbamazepine, cisapride, clarithromycin, codeine, conivaptan, copanlisib, corticosteroids, cyclosporine, CYP2D6 substrates, CYP3A4 inducers, dabigatran, darifenacin, deferasirox, delavirdine, didanosine, digoxin, dihydroergotamine, disulfiram, efavirenz, elbasvir & grazoprevir, eluxadoline, enfuvirtide, eplerenone, ergotamine, esomeprazole, estradiol, estrogens, etravirine, fesoterodine, flecainide, fluconazole, fosamprenavir, fusidic acid, garlic, HMG-CoA reductase inhibitors, lopinavir, lovastatin, meperidine, methadone, metoprolol, metronidazole, midazolam, midostaurin, nebivolol, nefazodone, neratinib, omeprazole, P-glycoprotein substrates, pantoprazole, phenobarbital, phenytoin, pimozide, propafenone, protease inhibitors, proton pump inhibitors, quetiapine, quinidine, quinine, raltegravir, ranolazine, rifabutin, rifampin, rilpivirine, rivaroxaban, rosuvastatin, salmeterol, saquinavir, sildenafil, simeprevir, simvastatin, sirolimus, sofosbuvir, sofosbuvir/velpatasvir/voxilaprevir, St John's wort, tacrolimus, tamoxifen, telithromycin, temsirolimus, tenofovir disoproxil, tetrabenazine, theophylline, thioridazine, tramadol, trazodone, triazolam, tricyclic antidepressants, valproic acid, vardenafil, vitamin E, zidovudine
Pregnancy category: C
Important contra-indications noted in the prescribing guidelines for: the elderly; nursing mothers; pediatric patients
Note: Tipranavir is a sulfonamide and can be absorbed systemically. Sulfonamides can produce severe, possibly fatal, reactions such as toxic epidermal necrolysis and Stevens-Johnson syndrome.
Tipranavir is co-administered with ritonavir.
Contra-indicated in patients with moderate or severe (Child-Pugh Class B or C) hepatic impairment.
Warning: HEPATOTOXICITY and INTRACRANIAL HEMORRHAGE

Skin
Exanthems (<2%)
Herpes simplex (<2%)
Herpes zoster (<2%)
Hypersensitivity (<2%)
Lipoatrophy (<2%)
Lipodystrophy (<2%)
Lipohypertrophy (<2%)
Pruritus (<2%)
Rash (3%) [2]

Central Nervous System
Anorexia (<2%)
Depression (2%)
Fever (14%)
Headache (5%)
Insomnia (2%)
Intracranial hemorrhage (<2%) [3]
Neurotoxicity (<2%)
Peripheral neuropathy (2%)
Sleep related disorder (<2%)
Somnolence (drowsiness) (<2%)
Vertigo (dizziness) (<2%)

Neuromuscular/Skeletal
Asthenia (fatigue) (2%)
Cramps (<2%)
Myalgia/Myopathy (2%)

Gastrointestinal/Hepatic
Abdominal distension (<2%)
Abdominal pain (6%)
Dyspepsia (<2%)
Flatulence (<2%)
Gastroesophageal reflux (<2%)
Hepatic failure (<2%)
Hepatitis (<2%)
Hepatotoxicity [4]
Nausea (9%)
Pancreatitis (<2%)
Vomiting (6%)

Respiratory
Dyspnea (2%)
Flu-like syndrome (<2%)

Endocrine/Metabolic
ALT increased (2%) [2]
Appetite decreased (<2%)
Dehydration (2%)
Diabetes mellitus (<2%)
GGT increased (2%)
Hyperamylasemia (<2%)
Hypercholesterolemia (<2%)
Hyperglycemia (<2%)
Hyperlipidemia (3%)
Hypertriglyceridemia (4%) [2]
Weight loss (3%)

Hematologic
Anemia (3%)
Neutropenia (2%)
Thrombocytopenia (<2%)

Other
Adverse effects [3]

TIROFIBAN

See: www.drugeruptiondata.com/drug/id/697

TIXOCORTOL

See: www.drugeruptiondata.com/drug/id/1099

TIZANIDINE

Trade name: Zanaflex (Acorda)
Indications: Muscle spasticity, multiple sclerosis
Class: Adrenergic alpha2-receptor agonist
Half-life: 2.5 hours
Clinically important, potentially hazardous interactions with: acebutolol, alfuzosin, benazepril, captopril, cilazapril, ciprofloxacin, enalapril, fluvoxamine, fosinopril, irbesartan, lisinopril, norfloxacin, obeticholic acid, olmesartan, phenytoin, quinapril, ramipril, rofecoxib, teriflunomide, trandolapril
Pregnancy category: C
Important contra-indications noted in the prescribing guidelines for: the elderly; pediatric patients

Skin
Pallor [2]
Pruritus (<10%)
Rash (<10%)

Mucosal
Xerostomia (49–88%) [14]

Cardiovascular
Bradycardia (<10%) [5]
Hypotension (16–33%) [3]

Central Nervous System
Dyskinesia (3%)
Nervousness (3%)
Somnolence (drowsiness) (48–92%) [4]
Speech disorder (3%)
Tremor (<10%)
Vertigo (dizziness) (41–45%) [3]

Neuromuscular/Skeletal
Asthenia (fatigue) (41–78%) [5]

Gastrointestinal/Hepatic
Constipation (4%)
Hepatotoxicity (6%) [4]
Vomiting (3%)

Respiratory
Flu-like syndrome (3%)
Pharyngitis (3%)
Rhinitis (3%)

Genitourinary
Urinary frequency (3%)
Urinary tract infection (10%)

Ocular
Amblyopia (3%)

Other
Infection (6%)

TOBRAMYCIN

Trade names: TOBI (Chiron), TobraDex (Alcon)
Indications: Various serious infections caused by susceptible organisms, superficial ocular infections
Class: Antibiotic, aminoglycoside
Half-life: 2–3 hours
Clinically important, potentially hazardous interactions with: adefovir, aldesleukin, aminoglycosides, atracurium, bumetanide, daptomycin, doxacurium, ethacrynic acid, furosemide, neuromuscular blockers, pancuronium, polypeptide antibiotics, rocuronium, succinylcholine, teicoplanin, torsemide, vecuronium
Pregnancy category: D (category D for injection and inhalation; category B for ophthalmic use)
Important contra-indications noted in the prescribing guidelines for: the elderly; nursing mothers; pediatric patients
Note: Aminoglycosides may cause neurotoxicity and/or nephrotoxicity.
TobraDex is tobramycin and dexamethasone.

Skin
Exanthems [4]
Hypersensitivity [3]
Rash [2]

Central Nervous System
Dysgeusia (taste perversion) [2]
Fever [2]

Respiratory
Cough [3]

Renal
Nephrotoxicity [6]

Ocular
Conjunctivitis [2]
Eyelid dermatitis [2]
Intraocular pressure increased [2]

TOCAINIDE

See: www.drugeruptiondata.com/drug/id/700

TOCILIZUMAB

Trade name: Actemra (Roche)
Indications: Rheumatoid arthritis, juvenile idiopathic arthritis, Castleman's disease
Class: Anti-interleukin-6 receptor monoclonal antibody, Disease-modifying antirheumatic drug (DMARD), Monoclonal antibody
Half-life: 8–14 days
Clinically important, potentially hazardous interactions with: efavirenz, fesoterodine, fingolimod, infliximab, lurasidone, paricalcitol, pazopanib, typhoid vaccine, yellow fever vaccine
Pregnancy category: N/A (Based on animal data, may cause fetal harm)
Important contra-indications noted in the prescribing guidelines for: nursing mothers; pediatric patients
Warning: RISK OF SERIOUS INFECTIONS

Skin
Anaphylactoid reactions/Anaphylaxis [5]
Cellulitis [9]
Herpes zoster [8]
Hypersensitivity [5]
Malignancies [2]
Peripheral edema (<2%)
Psoriasis [2]
Rash (2%) [6]
Urticaria [2]

Mucosal
Mucosal ulceration [2]
Oral ulceration (2%)
Stomatitis (<2%)

Cardiovascular
Cardiotoxicity [3]
Hypertension (6%) [3]

Central Nervous System
Headache (7%) [7]
Neurotoxicity [2]
Vertigo (dizziness) (3%)

Neuromuscular/Skeletal
Arthralgia [4]
Fractures [2]

Gastrointestinal/Hepatic
Abdominal pain (2%)
Diarrhea [2]
Gastroenteritis [6]
Gastrointestinal bleeding [3]
Gastrointestinal perforation [8]
Gastrointestinal ulceration (<2%)
Hepatotoxicity [15]
Nausea [3]
Pancreatitis [2]

Respiratory
Bronchitis (3%) [6]
Cough (<2%)
Dyspnea (<2%)
Influenza [3]
Nasopharyngitis (7%) [7]
Pharyngitis [3]
Pneumonia [12]
Pneumothorax [2]
Pulmonary toxicity [5]
Upper respiratory tract infection (7%) [10]

Endocrine/Metabolic
ALT increased (6%) [10]
AST increased [4]
Hypercholesterolemia [4]
Hyperlipidemia [5]
Hypertriglyceridemia [2]
Hypothyroidism (<2%)
Weight gain (<2%)

Genitourinary
Urinary tract infection [3]

Renal
Nephrolithiasis (<2%)
Pyelonephritis [3]

Hematologic
Hemotoxicity [2]
Leukopenia (<2%) [5]
Lymphopenia [2]
Neutropenia [19]
Sepsis [2]

Ocular
Conjunctivitis (<2%)

Local
Infusion-related reactions [3]
Infusion-site reactions [2]

Other
Adverse effects [11]
Death [5]
Infection [39]

TOFACITINIB

Trade name: Xeljanz (Pfizer)
Indications: Rheumatoid arthritis
Class: Janus kinase (JAK) inhibitor
Half-life: ~3 hours
Clinically important, potentially hazardous interactions with: azathioprine, biologic disease-modifying antirheumatics, cyclosporine, CYP3A4 inhibitors, fluconazole, ketoconazole, live vaccines, potent immunosuppressives, rifampin, strong CYP inducers, strong CYP2C19 inhibitors, tacrolimus
Pregnancy category: C
Important contra-indications noted in the prescribing guidelines for: the elderly; nursing mothers; pediatric patients
Warning: SERIOUS INFECTIONS AND MALIGNANCY

Skin
Erythema (<2%)
Herpes zoster [5]
Peripheral edema (<2%)
Pruritus (<2%)
Rash (<2%) [3]

Mucosal
Nasal congestion (<2%)

Cardiovascular
Hypertension (2%)

Central Nervous System
Fever (<2%)
Headache (3–4%) [10]
Insomnia (<2%)
Paresthesias (<2%)

Neuromuscular/Skeletal
Arthralgia (<2%)
Bone or joint pain (<2%)
Tendinitis (<2%)

Gastrointestinal/Hepatic
Abdominal pain (<2%) [2]
Diarrhea (3–4%) [8]
Dyspepsia (<2%) [2]
Gastritis (<2%)
Nausea (<2%) [3]
Vomiting (<2%)

Respiratory
Bronchitis [3]
Cough (<2%)
Dyspnea (<2%)
Influenza [2]
Nasopharyngitis (3–4%) [8]
Tuberculosis [3]
Upper respiratory tract infection (4–5%) [8]

Endocrine/Metabolic
ALT increased [2]
AST increased [2]
Creatine phosphokinase increased [2]
Dehydration (<2%)

Genitourinary
Urinary tract infection (2%) [5]

Hematologic
Anemia (<2%)
Neutropenia [3]

Other
Adverse effects [8]
Infection (20–22%) [11]

TOLAZAMIDE

See: www.drugeruptiondata.com/drug/id/701

TOLAZOLINE

See: www.drugeruptiondata.com/drug/id/702

TOLBUTAMIDE

See: www.drugeruptiondata.com/drug/id/703

TOLCAPONE

See: www.drugeruptiondata.com/drug/id/704

TOLMETIN

See: www.drugeruptiondata.com/drug/id/705

TOLTERODINE

Trade name: Detrol (Pharmacia & Upjohn)
Indications: Urinary incontinence
Class: Muscarinic antagonist
Half-life: 2–4 hours
Clinically important, potentially hazardous interactions with: itraconazole, ketoconazole, lopinavir, nelfinavir, sotalol, voriconazole, warfarin
Pregnancy category: C
Important contra-indications noted in the prescribing guidelines for: nursing mothers; pediatric patients

---

Skin
Erythema (2%)
Rash (2%)

Mucosal
Xerostomia (35%) [38]

Cardiovascular
Chest pain (2%)

Central Nervous System
Headache (7%) [4]
Somnolence (drowsiness) (3%)
Vertigo (dizziness) (5%) [4]

Neuromuscular/Skeletal
Arthralgia (2%)
Asthenia (fatigue) (4%)

Gastrointestinal/Hepatic
Abdominal pain (5%) [2]
Constipation (7%) [13]
Diarrhea (4%)
Dyspepsia (4%)

Respiratory
Flu-like syndrome (3%)
Upper respiratory tract infection (6%)

Genitourinary
Dysuria (2%)

Ocular
Vision blurred [3]
Xerophthalmia (3%) [2]

Other
Adverse effects [6]

TOLVAPTAN

See: www.drugeruptiondata.com/drug/id/1384

TOPIRAMATE

Trade names: Qsymia (Vivus), Qudexy (Upsher-Smith), Topamax (Janssen), Trokendi XR (Supernus)
Indications: Partial onset seizures, migraine
Class: Anticonvulsant, Mood stabilizer
Half-life: 21 hours
Clinically important, potentially hazardous interactions with: eslicarbazepine, levonorgestrel, metformin, rufinamide, ulipristal, valproic acid
Pregnancy category: D
Important contra-indications noted in the prescribing guidelines for: nursing mothers; pediatric patients
Note: Qsymia is topiramate and phentermine.

Skin
Anhidrosis [2]
Bromhidrosis (2%)
Diaphoresis (2%)
Edema (2%)
Fixed eruption [2]
Hot flashes (<10%)
Hypohidrosis [2]
Palmar erythema [2]
Pruritus (2%) [3]
Rash (4%) [3]

Hair
Alopecia [2]

Mucosal
Gingival hyperplasia/hypertrophy [2]
Gingivitis (2%)
Xerostomia (3%) [5]

Cardiovascular
Flushing (>5%)
Tachycardia [3]

Central Nervous System
Anorexia (>5%) [4]
Anxiety [3]
Cognitive impairment (>5%) [16]
Confusion (>5%)
Depression [11]
Dysgeusia (taste perversion) (>5%) [9]
Encephalopathy [3]
Fever (>5%)
Headache [2]
Hyperthermia [3]
Impaired concentration [3]
Insomnia [7]
Irritability [2]
Nervousness (>5%)
Neurotoxicity [5]
Palinopsia [3]

Paresthesias (>5%) [33]
Psychosis [3]
Seizures [3]
Somnambulism [2]
Somnolence (drowsiness) (>5%) [5]
Suicidal ideation [2]
Tremor (>10%)
Vertigo (dizziness) (>5%) [12]

Neuromuscular/Skeletal
Asthenia (fatigue) (>5%) [9]
Ataxia [2]

Gastrointestinal/Hepatic
Constipation [5]
Diarrhea [3]
Nausea [5]

Respiratory
Flu-like syndrome (<2%)

Endocrine/Metabolic
Acidosis [4]
Appetite decreased [4]
Gynecomastia (8%)
Hyperammonemia [2]
Mastodynia (3–9%)
Weight gain [2]
Weight loss (>5%) [15]

Genitourinary
Erectile dysfunction [2]

Renal
Nephrolithiasis [5]

Ocular
Diplopia [2]
Glaucoma [16]
Myopia [9]
Uveitis [5]
Vision loss [3]

Other
Adverse effects [11]
Death [2]
Infection (>5%)
Side effects [3]
Teratogenicity [8]

TOPOTECAN

Trade name: Hycamtin (GSK)
Indications: Metastatic ovarian carcinoma
Class: Antineoplastic, Topoisomerase 1 inhibitor
Half-life: 3–6 hours
Clinically important, potentially hazardous interactions with: atorvastatin, darunavir, gefitinib, lapatinib, oxaliplatin, pantoprazole, safinamide, sofosbuvir & velpatasvir
Pregnancy category: D
Important contra-indications noted in the prescribing guidelines for: nursing mothers; pediatric patients
Warning: BONE MARROW SUPPRESSION

Hair
Alopecia (59%) [7]

Mucosal
Mucositis [2]
Stomatitis (24%) [4]

Central Nervous System
Fever [2]
Paresthesias (9%)

Neuromuscular/Skeletal
Asthenia (fatigue) [9]

Gastrointestinal/Hepatic
Abdominal pain [2]
Diarrhea [5]
Hepatotoxicity [3]
Nausea [3]
Vomiting [4]

Respiratory
Dyspnea [3]

Renal
Nephrotoxicity [2]

Hematologic
Anemia [11]
Febrile neutropenia [5]
Granulocytopenia [2]
Myelosuppression [2]
Neutropenia [16]
Thrombocytopenia [15]

Other
Adverse effects [2]
Death [5]
Infection [2]

TOREMIFENE

Trade name: Fareston (ProStrakan)
Indications: Metastatic breast cancer
Class: Selective estrogen receptor modulator (SERM)
Half-life: ~5 days
Clinically important, potentially hazardous interactions with: amoxapine, arsenic, dolasetron, efavirenz, pazopanib, sugammadex, telavancin
Pregnancy category: D
Important contra-indications noted in the prescribing guidelines for: nursing mothers; pediatric patients
Warning: QT PROLONGATION

Skin
Diaphoresis (20%) [6]
Edema (5%) [2]
Hot flashes (35%) [4]

Cardiovascular
Flushing [3]
Thromboembolism [3]
Venous thromboembolism [2]

Central Nervous System
Headache [2]
Vertigo (dizziness) [2]

Gastrointestinal/Hepatic
Hepatotoxicity [3]
Nausea [2]
Vomiting [2]

Endocrine/Metabolic
ALP increased [2]
Galactorrhea (<10%)

Genitourinary
Priapism (<10%)
Vaginal bleeding [2]
Vaginal discharge [2]

Ocular
Cataract [3]

TORSEMIDE

Trade names: Demadex (Roche), Torem (Roche)
Indications: Essential hypertension, edema due to congestive heart failure, hepatic, pulmonary or renal edema
Class: Diuretic, loop
Half-life: 2–4 hours
Clinically important, potentially hazardous interactions with: ACE inhibitors, amikacin, aminoglycosides, aminophylline, anti-diabetics, antihypertensives, cephalosporins, cisplatin, gentamicin, indomethacin, kanamycin, neomycin, probenecid, salicylates, streptomycin, tobramycin
Pregnancy category: B
Important contra-indications noted in the prescribing guidelines for: nursing mothers; pediatric patients
Note: Torsemide is a sulfonamide and can be absorbed systemically. Sulfonamides can produce severe, possibly fatal, reactions such as toxic epidermal necrolysis and Stevens-Johnson syndrome.

Skin
Photosensitivity (<10%)
Urticaria (<10%)
Vasculitis [2]

Central Nervous System
Headache (7%)
Vertigo (dizziness) (3%)

Neuromuscular/Skeletal
Arthralgia (2%)
Asthenia (fatigue) (2%)
Myalgia/Myopathy (2%)

Gastrointestinal/Hepatic
Constipation (2%)
Diarrhea (2%)
Dyspepsia (2%)
Nausea (2%)

Respiratory
Cough (2%)
Pharyngolaryngeal pain (2%)
Rhinitis (3%)

Endocrine/Metabolic
Pseudoporphyria [2]

TOSITUMOMAB & IODINE[131]

See: www.drugeruptiondata.com/drug/id/1015

TOSUFLOXACIN

See: www.drugeruptiondata.com/drug/id/1309

TRABECTEDIN

See: www.drugeruptiondata.com/drug/id/1385

TRAMADOL

Trade names: Rybix ODT (Victory Pharma), Ultracet (Ortho-McNeil), Ultram (Ortho-McNeil)
Indications: Pain
Class: Opiate agonist
Half-life: 6–7 hours
Clinically important, potentially hazardous interactions with: alcohol, amitriptyline, carbamazepine, cinacalcet, citalopram, delavirdine, desflurane, desvenlafaxine, duloxetine, erythromycin, fluoxetine, fluvoxamine, ketoconazole, levomepromazine, linezolid, lorcaserin, MAO inhibitors, nefazodone, ondansetron, paroxetine hydrochloride, phenelzine, quinidine, risperidone, safinamide, tapentadol, terbinafine, tianeptine, tipranavir, tranylcypromine, venlafaxine, vilazodone, zuclopenthixol
Pregnancy category: C
Important contra-indications noted in the prescribing guidelines for: the elderly; nursing mothers; pediatric patients

Skin
Anaphylactoid reactions/Anaphylaxis [2]
Angioedema [2]
Contact dermatitis [2]
Diaphoresis (9%) [3]
Hypersensitivity [2]
Peripheral edema [2]
Pruritus (<10%) [4]
Rash (<5%) [2]
Urticaria (<18%)

Mucosal
Xerostomia (10%) [5]

Cardiovascular
Flushing [2]
Vasodilation (<5%)

Central Nervous System
Anorexia (<5%)
Anxiety (<5%)
Catatonia [2]
Confusion (<5%)
Euphoria (<5%)
Fever [2]
Headache [8]
Insomnia [3]
Nervousness (<5%)
Restless legs syndrome [5]
Seizures [16]
Serotonin syndrome [16]
Sleep related disorder (<5%)
Somnolence (drowsiness) [7]
Tremor (5–10%)
Vertigo (dizziness) [18]

Neuromuscular/Skeletal
Asthenia (fatigue) (<5%) [3]
Hypertonia (<5%)

Gastrointestinal/Hepatic
Abdominal pain (<5%) [3]
Constipation [8]
Diarrhea [2]
Flatulence (<5%)
Nausea [25]
Vomiting [23]

Respiratory
Apnea [2]

Respiratory depression [2]

Endocrine/Metabolic
Adrenal insufficiency [2]
Hypoglycemia [7]
Hyponatremia [3]

Genitourinary
Urinary frequency (<5%)
Urinary retention (<5%)

Otic
Hallucinations, auditory [2]

Ocular
Hallucinations, visual [3]
Mydriasis [2]
Visual disturbances (<5%)

Other
Adverse effects [8]
Death [2]

TRAMETINIB

Trade name: Mekinist (Novartis)
Indications: Melanoma (unresectable or metastatic) in patients with BRAF V600E or V600K mutations
Class: MEK inhibitor
Half-life: 4–5 days
Clinically important, potentially hazardous interactions with: none known
Pregnancy category: D
Important contra-indications noted in the prescribing guidelines for: nursing mothers; pediatric patients

Skin
Acneform eruption (19%) [7]
Actinic keratoses [2]
Cellulitis (<10%)
Dermatitis (19%) [2]
Edema (32%)
Erythema [2]
Exanthems [2]
Folliculitis (<10%)
Keratosis pilaris [2]
Lymphedema (32%)
Panniculitis [4]
Papulopustular eruption [2]
Peripheral edema (32%) [7]
Pruritus (10%) [3]
Pustules (<10%)
Rash (57%) [16]
Squamous cell carcinoma [3]
Toxicity (87%) [5]
Xerosis (11%) [2]

Hair
Alopecia [3]

Nails
Paronychia (10%)

Mucosal
Aphthous stomatitis (15%)
Epistaxis (nosebleed) (13%)
Gingival bleeding (13%)
Mucosal inflammation (15%)
Oral ulceration (15%)
Rectal hemorrhage (13%)
Stomatitis (15%) [2]
Xerostomia (<10%)

Cardiovascular
Bradycardia (<10%)
Cardiomyopathy (7%)
Cardiotoxicity [5]
Hypertension (15%) [6]

Central Nervous System
Chills [2]
Dysgeusia (taste perversion) (<10%)
Fever [7]
Headache [3]
Vertigo (dizziness) (<10%)

Neuromuscular/Skeletal
Arthralgia [3]
Asthenia (fatigue) [13]
Rhabdomyolysis (<10%)

Gastrointestinal/Hepatic
Abdominal pain (13%)
Black stools (13%)
Constipation [2]
Diarrhea (43%) [15]
Hepatotoxicity [2]
Nausea [11]
Vomiting [5]

Respiratory
Pneumonitis (2%)

Endocrine/Metabolic
ALP increased (24%)
ALT increased (39%) [3]
Appetite decreased [2]
AST increased (60%) [3]
Hypoalbuminemia (42%)

Genitourinary
Hematuria (13%)
Vaginal bleeding (13%)

Hematologic
Anemia (38%) [3]
Hemorrhage (13%)
Neutropenia [2]
Thrombocytopenia [3]

Ocular
Chorioretinopathy [2]
Conjunctival hemorrhage (13%)
Retinopathy [2]
Vision blurred (<10%) [2]
Xerophthalmia (<10%)

Other
Adverse effects [5]

TRANDOLAPRIL

Trade names: Mavik (AbbVie), Tarka (AbbVie)
Indications: Hypertension
Class: Angiotensin-converting enzyme (ACE) inhibitor, Antihypertensive, Vasodilator
Half-life: 6 hours
Clinically important, potentially hazardous interactions with: alcohol, aldesleukin, aliskiren, allopurinol, alpha blockers, amiloride, angiotensin II receptor antagonists, antacids, antidiabetics, antipsychotics, anxiolytics and hypnotics, baclofen, beta blockers, calcium channel blockers, clonidine, corticosteroids, cyclosporine, diazoxide, diuretics, estrogens, general anesthetics, gold & gold compounds, heparins, hydralazine, insulin, levodopa, lithium, MAO inhibitors, metformin, methyldopa, minoxidil, moxisylyte, moxonidine, nitrates, nitroprusside, NSAIDs, potassium salts, spironolactone,

sulfonylureas, tizanidine, triamterene, trimethoprim
Pregnancy category: D (category C in first trimester; category D in second and third trimesters)
Important contra-indications noted in the prescribing guidelines for: nursing mothers; pediatric patients
Note: Contra-indicated in patients with hereditary/idiopathic angioedema and in patients with a history of angioedema related to previous treatment with an ACE inhibitor. Tarka is trandolapril and verapamil.
Warning: FETAL TOXICITY

Skin
Angioedema [3]
Edema (>3%)

Mucosal
Xerostomia (>3%)

Cardiovascular
Bradycardia (5%)
Cardiogenic shock (4%)
Hypotension (11%)

Central Nervous System
Hyperesthesia (>3%)
Stroke (3%)
Syncope (6%)
Vertigo (dizziness) (23%)

Neuromuscular/Skeletal
Asthenia (fatigue) (3%)
Myalgia/Myopathy (5%)

Gastrointestinal/Hepatic
Dyspepsia (6%)
Gastritis (4%)

Respiratory
Cough (35%) [5]

Endocrine/Metabolic
Creatine phosphokinase increased (5%)
Hyperkalemia (5%)
Hypocalcemia (5%)

TRANEXAMIC ACID

Trade name: Cyklokapron (Pharmacia)
Indications: Fibrinolysis
Class: Antifibrinolytic
Half-life: 2 hours
Clinically important, potentially hazardous interactions with: none known
Pregnancy category: B

Skin
Fixed eruption [2]

Central Nervous System
Headache [3]
Seizures [11]

Gastrointestinal/Hepatic
Abdominal pain [2]

Endocrine/Metabolic
Menstrual irregularities [3]

Renal
Nephrotoxicity [3]

Other
Adverse effects [2]

TRANYLCYPROMINE

See: www.drugeruptiondata.com/drug/id/713

TRASTUZUMAB

Trade name: Herceptin (Genentech)
Indications: Metastatic breast cancer
Class: Antineoplastic, HER2/neu receptor antagonist, Monoclonal antibody
Half-life: 2–16 days (dose dependent)
Clinically important, potentially hazardous interactions with: abatacept, abciximab, alefacept, antineoplastics, azacitidine, betamethasone, cabazitaxel, denileukin, docetaxel, doxorubicin, fingolimod, gefitinib, immunosuppressants, leflunomide, lenalidomide, oxaliplatin, paclitaxel, pazopanib, pemetrexed, temsirolimus
Pregnancy category: D
Important contra-indications noted in the prescribing guidelines for: nursing mothers; pediatric patients
Warning: CARDIOMYOPATHY, INFUSION REACTIONS, EMBRYO-FETAL TOXICITY, and PULMONARY TOXICITY

Skin
Acneform eruption (2%) [4]
Edema (8%)
Erythema [2]
Hand–foot syndrome [10]
Herpes simplex (2%)
Hypersensitivity [2]
Peripheral edema (5–10%)
Photosensitivity [2]
Pruritus (2%)
Radiation recall dermatitis [2]
Rash (4–18%) [11]
Toxicity [3]

Hair
Alopecia [6]

Nails
Nail disorder (2%)

Mucosal
Epistaxis (nosebleed) (2%)
Mucositis [3]
Stomatitis [4]

Cardiovascular
Arrhythmias (3%)
Cardiac disorder [4]
Cardiac failure [4]
Cardiomyopathy [2]
Cardiotoxicity [26]
Congestive heart failure (2–7%) [7]
Hypertension (4%) [3]
Myocardial toxicity [3]
Palpitation (3%)
Tachycardia (5%)

Central Nervous System
Anorexia (14%) [3]
Chills (5–32%) [8]
Depression (6%)
Fever (6–36%) [6]
Headache (10–26%) [2]
Insomnia (14%)
Neurotoxicity [4]

Pain (47%) [2]
Paresthesias (2–9%)
Peripheral neuropathy [5]
Vertigo (dizziness) (4–13%)

Neuromuscular/Skeletal
Arthralgia (6–8%) [4]
Asthenia (fatigue) (5–47%) [17]
Back pain (5–22%)
Bone or joint pain (3–7%)
Muscle spasm (3%)
Myalgia/Myopathy (4%) [3]

Gastrointestinal/Hepatic
Abdominal pain (2–22%)
Constipation (2%)
Diarrhea (7–25%) [29]
Dyspepsia (2%)
Hepatotoxicity [8]
Nausea (6–33%) [8]
Vomiting (4–23%) [4]

Respiratory
Cough (5–26%)
Dyspnea (3–22%)
Flu-like syndrome (10%) [3]
Influenza (4%)
Nasopharyngitis (8%)
Pharyngitis (12%)
Pharyngolaryngeal pain (2%)
Pneumonia [2]
Pneumonitis [2]
Pulmonary toxicity [4]
Rhinitis (2–14%)
Sinusitis (2–9%)
Upper respiratory tract infection (3%)

Endocrine/Metabolic
ALT increased [5]
Appetite decreased [2]
AST increased [3]
Hyperbilirubinemia [2]
Hyperglycemia [3]

Genitourinary
Urinary tract infection (3–5%)

Hematologic
Anemia (4%) [7]
Febrile neutropenia [15]
Leukopenia (3%) [10]
Neutropenia [27]
Thrombocytopenia [6]

Local
Infusion-related reactions [4]
Injection-site reactions (21–40%) [6]

Other
Adverse effects [4]
Allergic reactions (3%) [2]
Death [5]
Infection (20%) [2]

TRAVOPROST

Trade names: Izba (Alcon), Travatan (Alcon), Travatan Z (Alcon)
Indications: Reduction of elevated intraocular pressure in open-angle glaucoma or ocular hypertension
Class: Prostaglandin analog
Half-life: N/A
Clinically important, potentially hazardous interactions with: none known

Pregnancy category: C
Important contra-indications noted in the prescribing guidelines for: nursing mothers; pediatric patients

Cardiovascular
Angina (<5%)
Bradycardia (<5%)
Chest pain (<5%)
Hypertension (<5%) [2]
Hypotension (<5%)

Central Nervous System
Anxiety (<5%)
Depression (<5%)
Dysgeusia (taste perversion) [3]
Headache (<5%)
Pain (<5%)

Neuromuscular/Skeletal
Arthralgia (<5%)
Back pain (<5%)

Gastrointestinal/Hepatic
Dyspepsia (<5%)
Gastrointestinal disorder (<5%)
Nausea [2]

Respiratory
Bronchitis (<5%)
Flu-like syndrome (<5%)
Sinusitis (<5%)

Endocrine/Metabolic
Hypercholesterolemia (<5%)

Genitourinary
Prostatitis (<5%)
Urinary incontinence (<5%)
Urinary tract infection (<5%)

Ocular
Abnormal vision (<4%)
Blepharitis (<4%)
Cataract (<4%)
Conjunctival hyperemia [10]
Conjunctivitis (<4%)
Corneal staining (<4%)
Deepening of upper lid sulcus [7]
Eyelashes – hypertrichosis [3]
Eyelid crusting (<4%)
Foreign body sensation (5–10%)
Iris pigmentation (<4%) [2]
Keratitis (<4%)
Lacrimation (<4%)
Ocular adverse effects [4]
Ocular hemorrhage (35–50%)
Ocular hyperemia [7]
Ocular inflammation (<4%)
Ocular pain (5–10%)
Ocular pigmentation (<5%) [4]
Ocular pruritus (5–10%) [6]
Ocular stinging (5–10%)
Photophobia (<4%)
Reduced visual acuity (5–10%)
Subconjunctival hemorrhage (<4%)
Uveitis [5]
Vision blurred [2]
Xerophthalmia (<4%)

Other
Allergic reactions (<5%)
Infection (<5%)

TRAZODONE

Trade names: Desyrel (Bristol-Myers Squibb), Oleptro (Angelini)
Indications: Depression
Class: Antidepressant, tricyclic, Serotonin reuptake inhibitor
Half-life: 3–6 hours
Clinically important, potentially hazardous interactions with: amiodarone, amprenavir, atazanavir, boceprevir, citalopram, cobicistat/elvitegravir/emtricitabine/tenofovir alafenamide, cobicistat/elvitegravir/emtricitabine/tenofovir disoproxil, darunavir, delavirdine, fluoxetine, fluvoxamine, ginkgo biloba, indinavir, linezolid, lopinavir, MAO inhibitors, nefazodone, paroxetine hydrochloride, sertraline, tapentadol, telaprevir, tipranavir, venlafaxine
Pregnancy category: C
Important contra-indications noted in the prescribing guidelines for: nursing mothers; pediatric patients
Warning: SUICIDALITY IN CHILDREN AND ADOLESCENTS

Skin
Edema (<10%)
Exanthems [6]
Photosensitivity [2]
Psoriasis (exacerbation) [2]
Urticaria [3]

Hair
Alopecia [2]

Mucosal
Xerostomia (>10%) [6]

Cardiovascular
Arrhythmias [2]
QT prolongation [2]

Central Nervous System
Dysgeusia (taste perversion) (>10%)
Headache [3]
Sedation (>5%)
Serotonin syndrome [7]
Somnolence (drowsiness) (>5%) [3]
Tremor (<10%)
Vertigo (dizziness) (>5%) [4]

Neuromuscular/Skeletal
Myalgia/Myopathy (<10%)

Gastrointestinal/Hepatic
Constipation (>5%)
Nausea [2]

Genitourinary
Priapism (12%) [23]
Sexual dysfunction [2]

Ocular
Vision blurred (>5%)

TREPROSTINIL

See: www.drugeruptiondata.com/drug/id/953

TRETINOIN

Synonyms: all-trans-retinoic acid; ATRA
Trade names: Aknemycin Plus (EM Industries), Renova (Ortho), Retin-A Micro (Ortho), Solage (Galderma), Vesanoid (Roche)
Indications: Acne vulgaris, skin aging, facial roughness, fine wrinkles, hyperpigmentation [T], acute promyelocytic leukemia [O]
Class: Antineoplastic, Retinoid
Half-life: 0.5–2 hours
Clinically important, potentially hazardous interactions with: aldesleukin, bexarotene
Pregnancy category: D (category B (topical), category C (oral), category D in third trimester)
Important contra-indications noted in the prescribing guidelines for: nursing mothers; pediatric patients
Note: Oral retinoids can cause birth defects, and women should avoid tretinoin when pregnant or trying to conceive. Avoid prolonged exposure to sunlight.
[T] = Topical; [O] = Oral.

Skin
Bullous dermatitis [2]
Burning [O][T] (10–40%) [20]
Cellulitis [O] (<10%)
Crusting [2]
Dermatitis [7]
Desquamation (14%)
Diaphoresis (20%)
Differentiation syndrome [O] (25%) [19]
Edema (29%) [8]
Erythema [O][T] (<49%) [19]
Erythema nodosum [4]
Exfoliative dermatitis [O] (8%) [3]
Facial edema [O] (<10%)
Flaking [O] (23%)
Hyperkeratosis [O] (78%)
Hypomelanosis (5%) [2]
Pallor [O] (<10%)
Palmar–plantar desquamation [O] (<10%)
Peeling [4]
Photosensitivity [O][T] (10%) [3]
Pigmentation (5%) [3]
Pruritus [O][T] (5–40%) [14]
Rash [O][T] (54%) [3]
Scaling (10–40%) [16]
Stinging (<26%) [8]
Sweet's syndrome [21]
Ulcerations (scrotal) [9]
Vasculitis [2]
Xerosis [O] (49–100%) [19]

Hair
Alopecia areata [O] (14%)

Nails
Pyogenic granuloma [3]

Mucosal
Cheilitis [O] (10%)
Xerostomia [O] (10%)

Cardiovascular
Phlebitis (11%)

Central Nervous System
Depression [O] (14%)
Fever [O] [6]
Headache [2]
Intracranial pressure increased [2]

Pain [O] (37%)
Paresthesias [O] (17%)
Pseudotumor cerebri [O] [11]
Shivering [O] (63%)
Tremor [O] (<10%)

Neuromuscular/Skeletal
Arthralgia [O] (10%) [3]
Bone or joint pain [O] (77%) [3]
Myalgia/Myopathy (14%) [3]

Gastrointestinal/Hepatic
Hepatotoxicity [3]
Pancreatitis [2]

Hematologic
Hemorrhage [2]

Ocular
Diplopia [2]
Ocular pigmentation [O] (<10%)
Ocular pruritus [O] (10%)
Xerophthalmia [O] (<10%) [2]

Local
Injection-site reactions (17%)

Other
Death [O] [2]
Infection [O] (58%)

TRIAMCINOLONE

See: www.drugeruptiondata.com/drug/id/1108

TRIAMTERENE

Trade names: Dyazide (GSK), Dyrenium (Concordia)
Indications: Edema
Class: Diuretic, potassium-sparing
Half-life: 1–2 hours
Clinically important, potentially hazardous interactions with: ACE inhibitors, acemetacin, benazepril, captopril, cyclosporine, enalapril, fosinopril, indomethacin, lisinopril, metformin, moexipril, potassium iodide, potassium salts, quinapril, ramipril, spironolactone, trandolapril, zofenopril
Pregnancy category: C
Important contra-indications noted in the prescribing guidelines for: nursing mothers; pediatric patients
Note: Dyazide and Maxzide are triamterene and hydrochlorothiazide. Hydrochlorothiazide is a sulfonamide and can be absorbed systemically. Sulfonamides can produce severe, possibly fatal, reactions such as toxic epidermal necrolysis and Stevens-Johnson syndrome.

Skin
Edema (<10%)
Lupus erythematosus (with hydrochlorothiazide) [2]
Photosensitivity [2]
Rash (<10%)

TRIAZOLAM

See: www.drugeruptiondata.com/drug/id/716

TRICHLORMETHIAZIDE

See: www.drugeruptiondata.com/drug/id/717

TRIENTINE

See: www.drugeruptiondata.com/drug/id/718

TRIFLUOPERAZINE

See: www.drugeruptiondata.com/drug/id/719

TRIFLURIDINE

See: www.drugeruptiondata.com/drug/id/1205

TRIFLURIDINE & TIPIRACIL

Trade name: Lonsurf (Monarch)
Indications: Metastatic colorectal cancer in patients who have been previously treated with fluoropyrimidine-, oxaliplatin-and irinotecan-based chemotherapy, an anti-VEGF biological therapy, and if RAS wild-type, an anti-EGFR therapy
Class: Antineoplastic, Thymidine phosphorylase inhibitor, Thymidine-based nucleoside analogue
Half-life: 2 hours
Clinically important, potentially hazardous interactions with: none known
Pregnancy category: N/A (Can cause fetal harm)
Important contra-indications noted in the prescribing guidelines for: nursing mothers; pediatric patients
Note: See also separate entry for trifluridine.

Hair
Alopecia (7%)

Mucosal
Stomatitis (8%)

Central Nervous System
Dysgeusia (taste perversion) (7%)
Fever (19%)

Neuromuscular/Skeletal
Asthenia (fatigue) (52%) [3]

Gastrointestinal/Hepatic
Abdominal pain (21%) [2]
Diarrhea (32%) [2]
Nausea (48%) [3]
Vomiting (28%)

Respiratory
Nasopharyngitis (4%)
Pulmonary embolism (2%)

Endocrine/Metabolic
Appetite decreased (39%)
Genitourinary
Urinary tract infection (4%)
Hematologic
Anemia (77%) [7]
Febrile neutropenia [3]
Granulocytopenia [3]
Leukopenia [7]
Neutropenia (67%) [9]
Thrombocytopenia (42%) [3]
Other
Infection (27%)

TRIHEXYPHENIDYL

See: www.drugeruptiondata.com/drug/id/720

TRIMEPRAZINE

See: www.drugeruptiondata.com/drug/id/721

TRIMETHADIONE

See: www.drugeruptiondata.com/drug/id/722

TRIMETHOBENZAMIDE

See: www.drugeruptiondata.com/drug/id/723

TRIMETHOPRIM

Trade names: Bactrim (Women First), Septra (Monarch)
Indications: Various urinary tract infections caused by susceptible organisms, acute otitis media in children, acute and chronic bronchitis
Class: Antibiotic
Half-life: 8–10 hours
Clinically important, potentially hazardous interactions with: ACE inhibitors, amantadine, angiotensin II receptor antagonists, antidiabetics, azathioprine, benazepril, captopril, carvedilol, cilazapril, conivaptan, coumarins, cyclosporine, CYP2C8 substrates, CYP2C9 inhibitors, CYP3A4 inducers, dapsone, deferasirox, digoxin, dofetilide, enalapril, eplerenone, fosinopril, irbesartan, lamivudine, leucovorin, levoleucovorin, lisinopril, memantine, mercaptopurine, metformin, methotrexate, olmesartan, oral typhoid vaccine, PEG-interferon, phenytoin, pioglitazone, pralatrexate, procainamide, pyrimethamine, quinapril, ramipril, repaglinide, rifampin, sulfonylureas, trandolapril
Pregnancy category: C
Important contra-indications noted in the prescribing guidelines for: nursing mothers
Note: Although trimethoprim has been known to elicit occasional adverse reactions by itself, it is most commonly used in conjunction with sulfamethoxazole (co-trimoxazole - see separate entry).

Skin
DRESS syndrome [2]
Fixed eruption [6]
Pruritus (<10%)
Rash (3–7%)
Stevens-Johnson syndrome [5]
Toxic epidermal necrolysis [3]
Central Nervous System
Aseptic meningitis [3]
Neuromuscular/Skeletal
Rhabdomyolysis [3]
Gastrointestinal/Hepatic
Hepatotoxicity [2]
Endocrine/Metabolic
Hyperkalemia [3]
Hyponatremia [2]
Hematologic
Anemia [2]
Thrombocytopenia [2]

TRIMETREXATE

See: www.drugeruptiondata.com/drug/id/725

TRIMIPRAMINE

Trade name: Surmontil (Odyssey)
Indications: Major depression
Class: Antidepressant, tricyclic
Half-life: 20–26 hours
Clinically important, potentially hazardous interactions with: amprenavir, arbutamine, bupropion, clonidine, epinephrine, formoterol, guanethidine, isocarboxazid, linezolid, MAO inhibitors, phenelzine, quinolones, sparfloxacin, tranylcypromine, venlafaxine
Pregnancy category: C
Important contra-indications noted in the prescribing guidelines for: pediatric patients
Warning: SUICIDALITY AND ANTIDEPRESSANT DRUGS

Skin
Diaphoresis (<10%)
Mucosal
Xerostomia (>10%) [2]
Cardiovascular
QT prolongation [2]
Central Nervous System
Dysgeusia (taste perversion) (>10%)
Parkinsonism (<10%)
Seizures [4]

TRIOXSALEN

See: www.drugeruptiondata.com/drug/id/727

TRIPELENNAMINE

See: www.drugeruptiondata.com/drug/id/728

TRIPROLIDINE

See: www.drugeruptiondata.com/drug/id/729

TRIPTORELIN

See: www.drugeruptiondata.com/drug/id/814

TROGLITAZONE

See: www.drugeruptiondata.com/drug/id/1861

TROLEANDOMYCIN

See: www.drugeruptiondata.com/drug/id/731

TROSPIUM

See: www.drugeruptiondata.com/drug/id/1173

TROVAFLOXACIN

See: www.drugeruptiondata.com/drug/id/732

TRYPTOPHAN

See: www.drugeruptiondata.com/drug/id/798

TYPHOID VACCINE

Trade names: Typherix (GSK), Typhim Vi (Sanofi Pasteur), Vivotif (Berna Biotech)
Indications: Immunization against typhoid fever
Class: Vaccine
Half-life: N/A
Clinically important, potentially hazardous interactions with: alcohol, antibiotics, antimalarials, atovaquone/proguanil, azathioprine, belimumab, cefixime, ceftaroline fosamil, ceftobiprole, chloroquine, ciprofloxacin, corticosteroids, daptomycin, fingolimod, gemifloxacin, hydroxychloroquine, immunosuppressants, interferon gamma, leflunomide, mefloquine, mercaptopurine, sulfonamides, telavancin, tigecycline, tinidazole, tocilizumab, ustekinumab
Pregnancy category: C
Important contra-indications noted in the prescribing guidelines for: nursing mothers; pediatric patients
Note: Vivotif is a live oral vaccine.

Skin
Anaphylactoid reactions/Anaphylaxis [2]

Central Nervous System
Fever (<3%) [5]
Headache (5–20%) [3]
Myelitis [2]

Neuromuscular/Skeletal
Asthenia (fatigue) (4–24%) [3]
Myalgia/Myopathy (3–7%) [3]

Gastrointestinal/Hepatic
Abdominal pain (6%) [2]
Diarrhea (<3%)
Nausea (2–8%)
Vomiting (2%)

Local
Injection-site edema [3]

Injection-site erythema (4–5%) [2]
Injection-site induration (5–15%)
Injection-site pain (27–41%) [5]

Other
Adverse effects [4]
Death [2]

Litt's Drug Eruption & Reaction Manual © 2018 by Taylor & Francis Group, LLC

ULIPRISTAL

See: www.drugeruptiondata.com/drug/id/1421

UMECLIDINIUM

Trade name: Incruse (GSK)
Indications: Chronic obstructive pulmonary disease (COPD)
Class: Anticholinergic, Muscarinic antagonist
Half-life: 11 hours
Clinically important, potentially hazardous interactions with: anticholinergics
Pregnancy category: C
Important contra-indications noted in the prescribing guidelines for: nursing mothers; pediatric patients

Mucosal
Oropharyngeal pain [2]

Cardiovascular
Angina [2]
Arrhythmias [2]
Extrasystoles [3]
Hypertension [3]
Supraventricular tachycardia [2]
Tachycardia [2]

Central Nervous System
Dysgeusia (taste perversion) [3]
Headache [12]

Neuromuscular/Skeletal
Arthralgia (2%) [2]
Back pain [5]

Gastrointestinal/Hepatic
Constipation [2]

Respiratory
Bronchitis [2]
COPD (exacerbation) [5]
Cough (3%) [6]
Dysphonia [4]
Influenza [2]
Nasopharyngitis (8%) [12]
Pharyngitis [2]
Pneumonia [4]
Sinusitis [3]
Upper respiratory tract infection [5]

Genitourinary
Urinary tract infection [2]

Other
Adverse effects [4]

UNOPROSTONE

See: www.drugeruptiondata.com/drug/id/819

URACIL/TEGAFUR

See: www.drugeruptiondata.com/drug/id/1118

URAPIDIL

See: www.drugeruptiondata.com/drug/id/1302

URIDINE TRIACETATE

See: www.drugeruptiondata.com/drug/id/3997

UROFOLLITROPIN

See: www.drugeruptiondata.com/drug/id/990

UROKINASE

See: www.drugeruptiondata.com/drug/id/733

URSODIOL

Synonyms: ursodeoxycholic acid; UDCA
Trade names: Actigall (Watson), Destolit (Norgine), Urdox (Wockhardt), Urso 250 (Aptalis), Urso Forte (Aptalis), Ursogal (Galen)
Indications: The dissolution of radiolucent (i.e. non-radio opaque) cholesterol gallstones in patients with a functioning gallbladder, primary biliary cirrhosis, biliary calculus, cholelithiasis
Class: Cholesterol antagonist, Urolithic
Half-life: 100 hours
Clinically important, potentially hazardous interactions with: aluminum based antacids, aluminum hydroxide, charcoal, cholestyramine, clofibrate, colestimide, colestipol, cyclosporine, dapsone, estradiol, estrogens, nitrendipine, oral contraceptives, P4503A substrates
Pregnancy category: B
Important contra-indications noted in the prescribing guidelines for: the elderly; nursing mothers; pediatric patients

Skin
Lichenoid eruption [3]
Pruritus [3]
Rash (3%)

Hair
Alopecia (<5%)

Cardiovascular
Chest pain (3%)

Central Nervous System
Headache (18–25%)
Insomnia (2%)
Vertigo (dizziness) (17%)

Neuromuscular/Skeletal
Arthralgia (7%)
Asthenia (fatigue) (3–7%)
Back pain (7–12%)
Bone or joint pain (6%)
Myalgia/Myopathy (5%)

Gastrointestinal/Hepatic
Abdominal pain (43%)
Cholecystitis (5%)
Constipation (26%)
Diarrhea (27%) [4]
Dyspepsia (16%) [2]
Flatulence (7%)
Nausea (14%) [4]
Vomiting (9–14%) [3]

Respiratory
Bronchitis (6%)
Cough (7%)

Flu-like syndrome (6%)
Pharyngitis (8%)
Rhinitis (5%)
Sinusitis (5–11%)
Upper respiratory tract infection (12–15%)

Endocrine/Metabolic
Weight gain [2]

Genitourinary
Dysmenorrhea (5%)
Urinary tract infection (6%)

Hematologic
Leukopenia (3%)

Other
Adverse effects [3]
Allergic reactions (5%)
Infection (viral) (9–19%)

USTEKINUMAB

Trade name: Stelara (Centocor)
Indications: Plaque psoriasis (moderate to severe), active psoriatic arthritis, active Crohn's disease (moderate to severe)
Class: Interleukin-12/23 antagonist, Monoclonal antibody
Half-life: 15–32 days
Clinically important, potentially hazardous interactions with: live vaccines
Pregnancy category: B
Important contra-indications noted in the prescribing guidelines for: nursing mothers; pediatric patients

Skin
Cellulitis (<10%)
Herpes zoster [2]
Malignancies [2]
Pruritus (<10%)
Psoriasis [3]

Mucosal
Nasal congestion (<10%)

Cardiovascular
Cardiotoxicity [3]

Central Nervous System
Depression (<10%)
Headache (<10%) [8]
Leukoencephalopathy [3]
Vertigo (dizziness) (<10%)

Neuromuscular/Skeletal
Arthralgia [3]
Asthenia (fatigue) (<10%) [2]
Back pain (<10%)
Myalgia/Myopathy (<10%)
Psoriatic arthralgia [2]

Gastrointestinal/Hepatic
Diarrhea (<10%)
Hepatotoxicity [2]

Respiratory
Nasopharyngitis (10%) [9]
Pharyngolaryngeal pain (<10%)
Upper respiratory tract infection (10%) [8]

Local
Injection-site reactions [6]

Other
Adverse effects [11]
Infection [12]

VALACYCLOVIR

Trade name: Valtrex (GSK)
Indications: Genital herpes, herpes simplex, herpes zoster
Class: Antiviral, Guanine nucleoside analog
Half-life: 3 hours
Clinically important, potentially hazardous interactions with: cobicistat/elvitegravir/emtricitabine/tenofovir alafenamide, cobicistat/elvitegravir/emtricitabine/tenofovir disoproxil, immunosuppressants, meperidine, tenofovir disoproxil
Pregnancy category: B
Important contra-indications noted in the prescribing guidelines for: the elderly; pediatric patients

Central Nervous System
Hallucinations [2]
Headache [5]
Neurotoxicity [4]

Gastrointestinal/Hepatic
Abdominal pain [2]
Nausea [4]
Vomiting [3]

Renal
Nephrotoxicity [2]

VALBENAZINE *

Trade name: Ingrezza (Neurocrine Biosciences)
Indications: Tardive dyskinesia
Class: Vesicular monoamine transporter 2 inhibitor
Half-life: 15–22 hours
Clinically important, potentially hazardous interactions with: carbamazepine, clarithromycin, digoxin, fluoxetine, isocarboxazid, itraconazole, ketoconazole, MAO inhibitors, paroxetine hydrochloride, phenelzine, phenytoin, quinidine, rifampin, selegiline, St John's wort, strong CYP2D6 inducers, strong CYP3A4 inducers or inhibitors
Pregnancy category: N/A (May cause fetal harm)
Important contra-indications noted in the prescribing guidelines for: nursing mothers; pediatric patients

Mucosal
Xerostomia (<5%)

Central Nervous System
Akathisia (<3%)
Gait instability (<4%)
Headache (3%) [4]
Impaired concentration (<5%)
Restlessness (<3%)
Sedation (<11%)
Somnolence (drowsiness) (<11%) [4]
Vertigo (dizziness) (<4%)

Neuromuscular/Skeletal
Arthralgia (2%)
Asthenia (fatigue) (<11%) [5]

Gastrointestinal/Hepatic
Constipation (<5%) [2]

Nausea (2%) [2]
Vomiting (3%)

Genitourinary
Urinary retention (<5%)
Urinary tract infection [2]

Ocular
Vision blurred (<5%)

VALDECOXIB

See: www.drugeruptiondata.com/drug/id/902

VALGANCICLOVIR

Trade name: Valcyte (Roche)
Indications: Cytomegalovirus retinitis (CMV) in patients with AIDS, prevention of CMV disease in high-risk transplant patients
Class: Antiviral, Guanine nucleoside analog
Half-life: 4 hours (in severe renal impairment up to 68%)
Clinically important, potentially hazardous interactions with: abacavir, cobicistat/elvitegravir/emtricitabine/tenofovir alafenamide, cobicistat/elvitegravir/emtricitabine/tenofovir disoproxil, emtricitabine, tenofovir disoproxil
Pregnancy category: N/A (May cause fetal toxicity based on findings in animal studies)
Important contra-indications noted in the prescribing guidelines for: nursing mothers
Note: Valganciclovir is rapidly converted to ganciclovir in the body.
Warning: HEMATOLOGIC TOXICITY, IMPAIRMENT OF FERTILITY, FETAL TOXICITY, MUTAGENESIS AND CARCINOGENESIS

Mucosal
Oral candidiasis [2]

Central Nervous System
Fever [3]
Headache [2]
Neurotoxicity [2]
Paresthesias (8%)

Hematologic
Neutropenia [8]

Other
Allergic reactions (<5%)
Infection (<5%)

VALPROIC ACID

Synonyms: valproate sodium; divalproex
Trade names: Depacon (AbbVie), Depakene (AbbVie), Depakote (AbbVie)
Indications: Seizures, migraine
Class: Anticonvulsant, Antipsychotic
Half-life: 6–16 hours
Clinically important, potentially hazardous interactions with: amitriptyline, aspirin, ceftobiprole, cholestyramine, clobazam, clozapine, doripenem, eslicarbazepine, ethosuximide, indinavir, ivermectin, lesinurad, levomepromazine, meropenem & vaborbactam, olanzapine, oxcarbazepine, paliperidone, risperidone, rufinamide, temozolomide,

tipranavir, vorinostat, zidovudine, zinc, zuclopenthixol
Pregnancy category: D
Warning: LIFE THREATENING ADVERSE REACTIONS

Skin
Anticonvulsant hypersensitivity syndrome [6]
DRESS syndrome [9]
Ecchymoses (<5%) [4]
Edema [3]
Erythema multiforme [3]
Erythroderma [3]
Exanthems (5%) [3]
Facial edema (>5%)
Furunculosis (<5%)
Hypersensitivity [5]
Lupus erythematosus [5]
Peripheral edema (<5%)
Petechiae (<5%)
Pruritus (>5%)
Pseudolymphoma [2]
Purpura [2]
Rash (>5%) [7]
Stevens-Johnson syndrome [11]
Toxic epidermal necrolysis [7]
Vasculitis [3]

Hair
Alopecia (7%) [22]
Curly hair [6]
Hirsutism [2]

Nails
Nail pigmentation [2]

Mucosal
Gingival hyperplasia/hypertrophy [8]
Glossitis (<5%)
Stomatitis (<5%)
Xerostomia (<5%) [2]

Central Nervous System
Brain atrophy [2]
Cerebral edema [2]
Cognitive impairment [2]
Coma [3]
Confusion [2]
Delirium [2]
Dysgeusia (taste perversion) (<5%)
Encephalopathy [17]
Gait instability [2]
Headache [2]
Neurotoxicity [4]
Paresthesias (<5%)
Parkinsonism [15]
Sedation [3]
Seizures [10]
Somnolence (drowsiness) [11]
Tremor [14]
Vertigo (dizziness) [7]

Neuromuscular/Skeletal
Asthenia (fatigue) [4]
Osteoporosis [3]
Rhabdomyolysis [3]

Gastrointestinal/Hepatic
Constipation [2]
Dyspepsia [2]
Hepatic steatosis [2]
Hepatotoxicity [19]
Nausea [4]
Pancreatitis [32]

Vomiting [2]

Respiratory
Pleural effusion [3]
Pneumonitis [2]

Endocrine/Metabolic
Acute intermittent porphyria [2]
Appetite increased [2]
Hyperammonemia [13]
Hyponatremia [2]
Metabolic syndrome [3]
Porphyria [2]
SIADH [6]
Weight gain [23]

Genitourinary
Vaginitis (<5%)

Renal
Enuresis [2]
Fanconi syndrome [4]

Hematologic
Bone marrow suppression [4]
Coagulopathy [2]
Eosinophilia [2]
Hemotoxicity [3]
Neutropenia [3]
Thrombocytopenia [4]

Otic
Hearing loss [2]

Ocular
Ocular adverse effects [2]

Other
Adverse effects [8]
Allergic reactions (<5%)
Congenital malformations [4]
Death [8]
Teratogenicity [31]

VALRUBICIN

See: www.drugeruptiondata.com/drug/id/964

VALSARTAN

Trade names: Byvalson (Forest), Diovan (Novartis), Diovan HCT (Novartis), Exforge (Novartis), Valturna (Novartis)
Indications: Hypertension
Class: Angiotensin II receptor antagonist (blocker), Antihypertensive
Half-life: 9 hours
Clinically important, potentially hazardous interactions with: none known
Pregnancy category: D
Important contra-indications noted in the prescribing guidelines for: nursing mothers; pediatric patients
Note: Byvalson is valsartan and nebivolol; Exforge is valsartan and amlodipine; Valturna is valsartan and aliskiren; Diovan HCT is valsartan and hydrochlorothiazide. Hydrochlorothiazide is a sulfonamide and can be absorbed systemically. Sulfonamides can produce severe, possibly fatal, reactions such as toxic epidermal necrolysis and Stevens-Johnson syndrome.
See also separate profile for Sacubitril/Valsartan.

Warning: FETAL TOXICITY

Skin
Angioedema (>2%) [9]
Edema [5]
Peripheral edema [3]
Photosensitivity [2]
Pruritus (>2%)
Pseudolymphoma [2]
Rash (>2%)

Mucosal
Aphthous stomatitis (<10%)
Xerostomia (>10%)

Cardiovascular
Hypotension [2]

Central Nervous System
Dysgeusia (taste perversion) (>10%)
Headache [7]
Paresthesias (>2%)
Vertigo (dizziness) [9]

Neuromuscular/Skeletal
Arthralgia (<10%)
Myalgia/Myopathy (10–29%)

Gastrointestinal/Hepatic
Enteropathy [2]

Respiratory
Cough [2]
Nasopharyngitis [3]
Upper respiratory tract infection [2]

Endocrine/Metabolic
Hyperkalemia [3]

Other
Adverse effects [5]
Allergic reactions (>2%)

VANCOMYCIN

Trade name: Vancocin (Lilly)
Indications: Various infections caused by susceptible organisms
Class: Antibiotic, glycopeptide
Half-life: 5–11 hours
Clinically important, potentially hazardous interactions with: meloxicam, metformin, pentamidine, rocuronium, succinylcholine, teicoplanin, trospium
Pregnancy category: C

Skin
Abscess [2]
AGEP [8]
Anaphylactoid reactions/Anaphylaxis [14]
Angioedema [3]
Bullous dermatitis [5]
Cellulitis [3]
DRESS syndrome [18]
Erythema multiforme [5]
Exanthems [16]
Exfoliative dermatitis [4]
Fixed eruption [2]
Hypersensitivity [8]
Leukocytoclastic vasculitis [4]
Linear IgA bullous dermatosis [50]
Lupus erythematosus [2]
Pruritus [12]
Rash [19]

Red man syndrome (<14%) [50]
Red neck syndrome [2]
Stevens-Johnson syndrome [10]
Toxic epidermal necrolysis [10]
Urticaria [8]
Vasculitis [2]

Cardiovascular
Cardiac arrest [2]
Extravasation [2]
Flushing (<10%)
Hypotension [3]
Phlebitis (14–23%) [6]

Central Nervous System
Chills (>10%) [2]
Dysgeusia (taste perversion) (>10%)
Fever [7]
Headache [4]
Vertigo (dizziness) [2]

Gastrointestinal/Hepatic
Constipation [3]
Diarrhea [7]
Gastrointestinal disorder [2]
Nausea [11]
Vomiting [5]

Endocrine/Metabolic
ALT increased [2]
AST increased [2]

Renal
Nephrotoxicity [32]
Renal failure [3]

Hematologic
Anemia [2]
Eosinophilia [3]
Leukopenia [2]
Neutropenia [7]
Thrombocytopenia [16]

Otic
Ototoxicity [5]
Tinnitus [2]

Local
Infusion-related reactions [2]

Other
Adverse effects [5]
Allergic reactions (<5%) [5]
Death [5]

VANDETANIB

Trade name: Caprelsa (AstraZeneca)
Indications: Medullary thyroid cancer
Class: Tyrosine kinase inhibitor
Half-life: 19 days
Clinically important, potentially hazardous interactions with: amiodarone, amoxapine, antiarrhythmics, arsenic, carbamazepine, chloroquine, clarithromycin, CYP3A4 inducers, dexamethasone, disopyramide, dofetilide, dolasetron, efavirenz, granisetron, haloperidol, methadone, moxifloxacin, pazopanib, phenobarbital, phenytoin, pimozide, procainamide, QT prolonging agents, rifabutin, rifampin, rifapentine, sotalol, St John's wort, telavancin

Pregnancy category: D
Important contra-indications noted in the prescribing guidelines for: nursing mothers; pediatric patients
Note: Contra-indicated in patients with congenital long QT syndrome.
Warning: QT PROLONGATION, TORSADES DE POINTES, AND SUDDEN DEATH

Skin
Acneform eruption (35%) [4]
Folliculitis [5]
Hand–foot syndrome [4]
Photosensitivity (13%) [8]
Phototoxicity [3]
Pigmentation [6]
Pruritus (11%) [2]
Rash (53%) [34]
Stevens-Johnson syndrome [2]
Toxicity [9]
Xerosis (15%) [3]

Hair
Hair changes [2]

Nails
Paronychia [5]
Splinter hemorrhage [2]

Mucosal
Mucositis [2]
Stomatitis [2]

Cardiovascular
Hypertension (33%) [24]
QT prolongation (14%) [25]

Central Nervous System
Anorexia [3]
Depression (10%)
Headache (26%) [4]
Insomnia (13%)
Neurotoxicity [2]

Neuromuscular/Skeletal
Asthenia (fatigue) (15–24%) [17]

Gastrointestinal/Hepatic
Abdominal pain (21%)
Constipation [2]
Diarrhea (57%) [44]
Dyspepsia (11%)
Hepatotoxicity [4]
Nausea (33%) [14]
Vomiting (15%) [6]

Respiratory
Cough (11%)
Dyspnea [3]
Nasopharyngitis (11%)

Endocrine/Metabolic
ALT increased (51%) [2]
Appetite decreased (21%) [3]
Hypocalcemia (11%)
Hypothyroidism [2]
Thyroid dysfunction [2]
Weight loss (10%) [2]

Renal
Proteinuria (10%) [2]

Hematologic
Anemia [3]
Hemorrhage [2]
Hemotoxicity [2]
Myelosuppression [2]
Neutropenia [5]

Platelets decreased (9%)

Other
Adverse effects [6]
Death [3]

VARDENAFIL

Trade name: Levitra (Bayer)
Indications: Erectile dysfunction
Class: Phosphodiesterase type 5 (PDE5) inhibitor
Half-life: 4–5 hours
Clinically important, potentially hazardous interactions with: alfuzosin, alpha blockers, amyl nitrite, antifungals, antihypertensives, atazanavir, boceprevir, bosentan, cobicistat/elvitegravir/emtricitabine/tenofovir alafenamide, cobicistat/elvitegravir/emtricitabine/tenofovir disoproxil, conivaptan, CYP3A4 inhibitors, darunavir, dasatinib, disopyramide, doxazosin, erythromycin, etravirine, fosamprenavir, grapefruit juice, high-fat foods, indinavir, itraconazole, ketoconazole, lopinavir, macrolide antibiotics, nelfinavir, nicorandil, nifedipine, nitrates, nitroglycerin, nitroprusside, phosphodiesterase 5 inhibitors, protease inhibitors, riociguat, ritonavir, sapropterin, saquinavir, tamsulosin, telaprevir, terazosin, tipranavir
Pregnancy category: B (not indicated for use in women)
Important contra-indications noted in the prescribing guidelines for: pediatric patients

Skin
Anaphylactoid reactions/Anaphylaxis (<2%)
Angioedema (<2%)
Diaphoresis (<2%)
Erythema (<2%)
Facial edema (<2%)
Photosensitivity (<2%)
Pruritus (<2%)
Rash (<2%)

Mucosal
Nasal congestion [4]
Xerostomia (<2%)

Cardiovascular
Angina (<2%)
Chest pain (<2%)
Flushing (11%) [14]
Hypotension (<2%)
Myocardial infarction (<2%)
Palpitation (<2%)
QT prolongation [2]
Tachycardia (<2%)
Ventricular arrhythmia (<2%)

Central Nervous System
Amnesia (<2%)
Dysesthesia (<2%)
Headache (7–15%) [16]
Pain (<2%)
Paresthesias (<2%)
Seizures (<2%)
Sleep related disorder (<2%)
Somnolence (drowsiness) (<2%)
Syncope (<2%)
Vertigo (dizziness) (2%) [3]

Neuromuscular/Skeletal
Arthralgia (<2%)
Back pain (<2%)
Cramps (<2%)
Myalgia/Myopathy (<2%)

Gastrointestinal/Hepatic
Abdominal pain (<2%)
Diarrhea (<2%)
Dyspepsia [3]
Gastritis (<2%)
Gastroesophageal reflux (<2%)
Nausea (<2%)
Vomiting (<2%)

Respiratory
Dyspnea (<2%)
Flu-like syndrome (3%)
Rhinitis (9%) [10]
Sinusitis (3%)

Endocrine/Metabolic
ALT increased (<2%)
Creatine phosphokinase increased (<2%)

Genitourinary
Erection (<2%)
Priapism (<2%)

Otic
Hearing loss [2]
Tinnitus (<2%)

Ocular
Conjunctivitis (<2%)
Dyschromatopsia (<2%)
Intraocular pressure increased (<2%)
Ocular hyperemia (<2%)
Ocular pain (<2%)
Photophobia (<2%)
Visual disturbances (<2%)

Other
Allergic reactions (<2%)

VARENICLINE

Trade names: Champix (Pfizer), Chantix (Pfizer)
Indications: Smoking deterrent
Class: Nicotinic antagonist
Half-life: 24 hours
Clinically important, potentially hazardous interactions with: none known
Pregnancy category: C
Important contra-indications noted in the prescribing guidelines for: nursing mothers; pediatric patients
Warning: SERIOUS NEUROPSYCHIATRIC EVENTS

Skin
AGEP [3]
Rash (<3%)

Mucosal
Xerostomia (4–6%)

Cardiovascular
Cardiotoxicity [5]

Central Nervous System
Abnormal dreams (9–13%) [16]
Aggression [3]
Anorexia (<2%)
Anxiety [5]
Depression [9]

Dysgeusia (taste perversion) (5–8%)
Hallucinations [2]
Headache (15–19%) [12]
Insomnia (18–19%) [15]
Mania [5]
Mood changes [4]
Neuropsychiatric disturbances [2]
Nightmares (<2%)
Psychosis [7]
Sleep disturbances [7]
Sleep related disorder (2–5%) [3]
Somnolence (drowsiness) (3%) [2]
Suicidal ideation [7]

Neuromuscular/Skeletal
Asthenia (fatigue) (<7%) [5]

Gastrointestinal/Hepatic
Abdominal pain (5–7%) [3]
Constipation (5–8%) [4]
Dyspepsia (5%) [2]
Flatulence (6–9%)
Hepatotoxicity [2]
Nausea (16–30%) [28]
Vomiting (<5%) [2]

Respiratory
Dyspnea (<2%)
Upper respiratory tract infection (5–7%)

Endocrine/Metabolic
Appetite decreased (<2%)
Appetite increased (3–4%)

Ocular
Hallucinations, visual [2]

Other
Adverse effects [10]
Death [3]

VARICELLA VACCINE

Trade names: Varilrix (GSK), Varivax (Merck)
Indications: Immunization, varicella
Class: Vaccine
Half-life: N/A
Clinically important, potentially hazardous interactions with: none known
Pregnancy category: C

Skin
Herpes zoster [10]
Rash [10]
Stevens-Johnson syndrome [2]

Central Nervous System
Fever (15%) [3]

Ocular
Uveitis [2]

Local
Injection-site edema (19%)
Injection-site erythema (19%)
Injection-site hematoma (19%)
Injection-site induration (19%)
Injection-site pain (19%)
Injection-site pruritus (19%)
Injection-site reactions [4]

VASOPRESSIN

Trade name: Vasostrict (Par)
Indications: Diabetes insipidus, prevention and treatment of postoperative abdominal distension, hypotension in adults with vasodilatory shock (Vasostrict)
Class: Antidiuretic hormone
Half-life: 10–20 minutes
Clinically important, potentially hazardous interactions with: none known
Pregnancy category: C
Important contra-indications noted in the prescribing guidelines for: pediatric patients

Skin
Bullous dermatitis [4]
Diaphoresis (<10%)
Ecchymoses [2]
Pallor (<10%)
Purpura [2]
Urticaria (<10%)

Central Nervous System
Tremor (<10%)

Neuromuscular/Skeletal
Rhabdomyolysis [6]

Endocrine/Metabolic
SIADH [2]

Local
Injection-site inflammation [7]

Other
Death [3]

VECURONIUM

See: www.drugeruptiondata.com/drug/id/991

VEDOLIZUMAB

Trade name: Entyvio (Takeda)
Indications: Ulcerative colitis, Crohn's disease
Class: Integrin receptor antagonist, Monoclonal antibody
Half-life: 25 days
Clinically important, potentially hazardous interactions with: live vaccines, natalizumab, TNF blockers
Pregnancy category: B
Important contra-indications noted in the prescribing guidelines for: nursing mothers; pediatric patients

Skin
Pruritus (3%)
Rash (3%) [2]

Mucosal
Oropharyngeal pain (3%)

Central Nervous System
Fever (9%) [5]
Headache (12%) [11]

Neuromuscular/Skeletal
Arthralgia (12%) [8]
Asthenia (fatigue) (6%) [6]
Back pain (4%) [3]

Pain in extremities (3%)
Gastrointestinal/Hepatic
Abdominal pain [7]
Colitis [5]
Crohn's disease (exacerbation) [2]
Nausea (9%) [9]
Vomiting [4]

Respiratory
Bronchitis (4%)
Cough (5%) [3]
Influenza (4%)
Nasopharyngitis (13%) [11]
Sinusitis (3%)
Upper respiratory tract infection (7%) [7]

Hematologic
Anemia [4]

Local
Infusion-related reactions (4%) [4]

Other
Adverse effects [7]
Cancer [2]
Infection [5]

VELAGLUCERASE ALFA

See: www.drugeruptiondata.com/drug/id/1651

VEMURAFENIB

Trade name: Zelboraf (Roche)
Indications: Melanoma (metastatic or unresectable)
Class: BRAF inhibitor
Half-life: 57 hours
Clinically important, potentially hazardous interactions with: amoxapine, arsenic, atazanavir, carbamazepine, clarithromycin, CYP substrates, dolasetron, efavirenz, indinavir, itraconazole, ketoconazole, nefazodone, nelfinavir, pazopanib, phenobarbital, phenytoin, rifabutin, rifampin, rifapentine, ritonavir, saquinavir, telavancin, telithromycin, voriconazole, warfarin
Pregnancy category: D
Important contra-indications noted in the prescribing guidelines for: nursing mothers; pediatric patients

Skin
Acneform eruption [6]
Actinic keratoses [4]
DRESS syndrome [4]
Eccrine squamous syringometaplasia [2]
Erythema (14%) [2]
Exanthems [8]
Granulomas [2]
Grover's disease [4]
Hand–foot syndrome [8]
Hyperkeratosis (24%) [17]
Keratoacanthoma [27]
Keratoses [4]
Keratosis pilaris [10]
Lymphoma [2]
Melanoma [2]
Milia [2]
Neoplasms [2]

Nevi [6]
Panniculitis [9]
Papillomas (21%)
Papular lesions (5%)
Peripheral edema (17%)
Photosensitivity (33%) [27]
Pruritus (23%) [10]
Radiation recall dermatitis [2]
Rash (37%) [23]
Squamous cell carcinoma (24%) [35]
Stevens-Johnson syndrome [4]
Sunburn (10%)
Toxic epidermal necrolysis [5]
Toxicity [10]
Vasculitis [2]
Verruca vulgaris [2]
Verrucous lesions [3]
Vitiligo [2]
Warts [2]
Xerosis [5]

Hair
Alopecia (45%) [18]
Hair changes [2]

Nails
Paronychia [3]
Pyogenic granuloma [2]

Mucosal
Gingival hyperplasia/hypertrophy [2]

Cardiovascular
QT prolongation [2]

Central Nervous System
Dysgeusia (taste perversion) (14%)
Fever (19%) [5]
Headache (23%) [2]
Paralysis [2]

Neuromuscular/Skeletal
Arthralgia (53%) [19]
Asthenia (fatigue) (38%) [18]
Back pain (8%)
Bone or joint pain (8%)
Myalgia/Myopathy (8–13%) [2]
Pain in extremities (18%)

Gastrointestinal/Hepatic
Constipation (12%)
Diarrhea (28%) [7]
Hepatotoxicity [4]
Nausea (35%) [8]
Vomiting (18%) [3]

Respiratory
Cough (8%)

Endocrine/Metabolic
ALT increased [5]
Appetite decreased (18%) [2]
AST increased [5]
GGT increased [2]

Ocular
Chorioretinopathy [2]
Uveitis [3]
Vision blurred [2]

Other
Adverse effects [11]

VENETOCLAX

Trade name: Venclexta (AbbVie)
Indications: Chronic lymphocytic leukemia in patients with 17p deletion, as detected by an FDA approved test, who have received at least one prior therapy
Class: BCL-2 inhibitor
Half-life: 26 hours
Clinically important, potentially hazardous interactions with: amiodarone, azithromycin, bosentan, captopril, carbamazepine, carvedilol, ciprofloxacin, clarithromycin, conivaptan, cyclosporine, digoxin, diltiazem, dronedarone, efavirenz, erythromycin, etravirine, everolimus, felodipine, fluconazole, grapefruit juice, indinavir, itraconazole, ketoconazole, live vaccines, lopinavir, modafinil, nafcillin, phenytoin, posaconazole, quercetin, quinidine, ranolazine, rifampin, ritonavir, sirolimus, St John's wort, stong or moderate P-gp inhibitors or substrates, strong or moderate CYP3A inducers or inhibitors, telaprevir, ticagrelor, verapamil, voriconazole
Pregnancy category: N/A (May cause fetal harm)
Important contra-indications noted in the prescribing guidelines for: nursing mothers; pediatric patients
Note: Concomitant use of strong CYP3A inhibitors during initiation and ramp-up phase is contra-indicated.

Skin
Peripheral edema (11%)
Tumor lysis syndrome (6%) [7]

Central Nervous System
Fever (16%) [3]
Headache (15%) [2]

Neuromuscular/Skeletal
Asthenia (fatigue) (21%) [3]
Back pain (10%)

Gastrointestinal/Hepatic
Constipation (14%)
Diarrhea (35%) [5]
Nausea (33%) [6]
Vomiting (15%)

Respiratory
Cough (13%)
Pneumonia (8%) [3]
Upper respiratory tract infection (22%) [3]

Endocrine/Metabolic
Hyperkalemia (20%)
Hyperphosphatemia (15%)
Hyperuricemia (6%)
Hypocalcemia (9%)
Hypokalemia (12%)

Hematologic
Anemia (29%) [5]
Febrile neutropenia [3]
Neutropenia (45%) [7]
Thrombocytopenia (22%) [5]

Other
Death [3]

VENLAFAXINE

Trade names: Effexor (Wyeth), Effexor XL (Wyeth)
Indications: Major depressive disorder
Class: Antidepressant, Serotonin-norepinephrine reuptake inhibitor
Half-life: 3–7 hours
Clinically important, potentially hazardous interactions with: 5HT1 agonists, artemether/lumefantrine, aspirin, atomoxetine, clozapine, desvenlafaxine, dexibuprofen, diclofenac, duloxetine, entacapone, haloperidol, indinavir, isocarboxazid, ketoconazole, linezolid, lithium, MAO inhibitors, meloxicam, metoclopramide, metoprolol, mirtazapine, moclobemide, naratriptan, NSAIDs, phenelzine, selegiline, sibutramine, SNRIs, SSRIs, St John's wort, sumatriptan, tramadol, tranylcypromine, trazodone, trimipramine, triptans, voriconazole, warfarin
Pregnancy category: C
Important contra-indications noted in the prescribing guidelines for: the elderly; nursing mothers; pediatric patients
Warning: SUICIDALITY AND ANTIDEPRESSANT DRUGS

Skin
Diaphoresis [7]
Ecchymoses [2]
Hyperhidrosis [2]
Pruritus (<10%)
Rash (3%)

Hair
Alopecia [2]

Mucosal
Xerostomia (22%) [10]

Cardiovascular
Cardiac failure [2]
Cardiomyopathy [3]
Hypertension [7]
Myocardial infarction [2]
Orthostatic hypotension [2]
Preeclampsia [2]
QT prolongation [6]
Tachycardia [2]

Central Nervous System
Akathisia [2]
Delirium [2]
Dysgeusia (taste perversion) (2%)
Headache [8]
Insomnia [5]
Mania [10]
Paresthesias (3%)
Psychosis [3]
Restless legs syndrome [3]
Seizures [7]
Serotonin syndrome [22]
Somnolence (drowsiness) [9]
Tremor (<10%) [3]
Vertigo (dizziness) [10]
Yawning [2]

Neuromuscular/Skeletal
Asthenia (fatigue) [5]
Dystonia [2]
Rhabdomyolysis [3]

Gastrointestinal/Hepatic
Constipation [6]
Hepatotoxicity [8]
Nausea [16]
Vomiting [3]

Respiratory
Pneumonitis [3]

Endocrine/Metabolic
Appetite decreased [2]
Galactorrhea [4]
Hyponatremia [4]
Libido increased [2]
Mastodynia [2]
SIADH [6]
Weight gain [2]

Genitourinary
Ejaculatory dysfunction [2]
Sexual dysfunction [8]
Urinary incontinence [2]

Ocular
Glaucoma [2]
Hallucinations, visual [3]

Other
Adverse effects [3]
Bruxism [7]

VERAPAMIL

Trade names: Calan (Pfizer), Covera-HS (Pfizer), Isoptin (AbbVie), Tarka (AbbVie), Verelan (Schwarz)
Indications: Angina, arrhythmias, hypertension
Class: Antiarrhythmic class IV, Calcium channel blocker, CYP3A4 inhibitor
Half-life: 2–8 hours
Clinically important, potentially hazardous interactions with: acebutolol, afatinib, aliskiren, amiodarone, amitriptyline, amprenavir, aspirin, atazanavir, atenolol, atorvastatin, avanafil, betaxolol, betrixaban, bisoprolol, carbamazepine, carteolol, celiprolol, clonidine, cobicistat/ elvitegravir/emtricitabine/tenofovir alafenamide, cobicistat/elvitegravir/emtricitabine/tenofovir disoproxil, colchicine, dabigatran, dantrolene, darifenacin, deflazacort, delavirdine, digoxin, dofetilide, dronedarone, dutasteride, epirubicin, eplerenone, erythromycin, esmolol, everolimus, fingolimod, flibanserin, indacaterol, lovastatin, metoprolol, mifepristone, nadolol, naldemedine, naloxegol, neratinib, nevirapine, olaparib, oxprenolol, oxtriphylline, palbociclib, penbutolol, pindolol, posaconazole, propranolol, quinidine, ranolazine, sibutramine, silodosin, simvastatin, telaprevir, telithromycin, timolol, trabectedin, venetoclax
Pregnancy category: C
Important contra-indications noted in the prescribing guidelines for: nursing mothers; pediatric patients
Note: Tarka is verapamil and trandolapril.

Skin
Angioedema [3]
Diaphoresis [2]
Edema (2%)
Erythema multiforme [4]
Exanthems [8]

Exfoliative dermatitis [2]
Hyperkeratosis (palms) [2]
Lupus erythematosus [2]
Peripheral edema (<10%)
Photosensitivity [4]
Pruritus [6]
Rash [2]
Stevens-Johnson syndrome [5]
Urticaria [5]
Vasculitis [2]

Hair
Alopecia [5]

Mucosal
Gingival hyperplasia/hypertrophy (19%) [10]

Cardiovascular
Atrial fibrillation [2]
Atrioventricular block [2]
Bradycardia [10]
Congestive heart failure [2]
Flushing (<7%) [4]
Hypotension [2]
Torsades de pointes [2]

Central Nervous System
Parkinsonism [2]
Seizures [3]

Neuromuscular/Skeletal
Rhabdomyolysis [2]

Endocrine/Metabolic
Gynecomastia [8]

Other
Side effects [2]

VERNAKALANT

See: www.drugeruptiondata.com/drug/id/1406

VERTEPORFIN

Trade name: Visudyne (Novartis)
Indications: Neovascular (wet) age-related macular degeneration
Class: Photosensitizer
Half-life: 5–6 hours
Clinically important, potentially hazardous interactions with: none known
Pregnancy category: C
Important contra-indications noted in the prescribing guidelines for: nursing mothers; pediatric patients

Skin
Eczema (<10%)
Photosensitivity (<10%) [2]

Mucosal
Burning mouth syndrome (<10%)

Cardiovascular
Atrial fibrillation (<10%)
Chest pain [2]
Hypertension (<10%)

Central Nervous System
Fever (<10%)
Hypoesthesia (<10%)
Sleep related disorder (<10%)
Vertigo (dizziness) (<10%)

Neuromuscular/Skeletal
Arthralgia (<10%)
Asthenia (fatigue) (<10%)
Back pain (<10%)
Myasthenia gravis (<10%)

Gastrointestinal/Hepatic
Constipation (<10%)
Nausea (<10%)

Respiratory
Flu-like syndrome (<10%)
Pharyngitis (<10%)

Endocrine/Metabolic
Creatine phosphokinase increased (<10%)

Genitourinary
Albuminuria (<10%)

Hematologic
Anemia (<10%)
Leukocytosis (<10%)
Leukopenia (<10%)

Otic
Hearing loss (<10%)

Ocular
Blepharitis (<10%)
Cataract (<10%)
Conjunctivitis (<10%)
Diplopia (<10%)
Endophthalmitis [2]
Intraocular inflammation [2]
Lacrimation (<10%)
Ocular itching (<10%)
Vision loss (severe) (<5%)
Visual disturbances (10–30%)
Xerophthalmia (<10%)

Local
Infusion-site pain (<10%)
Injection-site reactions (10–30%)

Other
Cancer (gastrointestinal) (<10%)

VIDARABINE

See: www.drugeruptiondata.com/drug/id/739

VIGABATRIN

Trade name: Sabril (Lundbeck)
Indications: Epilepsy, infantile spasms (West's syndrome)
Class: Anticonvulsant, Antiepileptic
Half-life: 7.5 hours
Clinically important, potentially hazardous interactions with: antipsychotics, chloroquine, hydroxychloroquine, MAO inhibitors, mefloquine, orlistat, phenytoin, rufinamide, SSRIs, St John's wort, tricyclic antidepressants
Pregnancy category: C
Important contra-indications noted in the prescribing guidelines for: nursing mothers; pediatric patients
Warning: VISION LOSS

Skin
Peripheral edema (5–7%)
Rash (6%) [2]

Cardiovascular
Chest pain (<5%)

Central Nervous System
Abnormal dreams (<5%)
Anxiety (4%)
Confusion (4–14%)
Depression (8%) [4]
Dysarthria (2%)
Encephalopathy [4]
Fever (4–7%)
Gait instability (6–12%)
Headache (18%)
Hypoesthesia (4–5%)
Hyporeflexia (4–5%)
Impaired concentration (9%)
Incoordination (7%)
Insomnia (7%)
Irritability (7%)
Memory loss (7%)
Nervousness (2–5%)
Peripheral neuropathy (4%)
Psychosis [2]
Sedation (4%)
Seizures (11%) [4]
Somnolence (drowsiness) (17%) [3]
Status epilepticus (2–5%)
Tremor (7%)
Vertigo (dizziness) (15%)

Neuromuscular/Skeletal
Arthralgia (5–10%)
Asthenia (fatigue) (16%) [2]
Back pain (4–7%)
Muscle spasm (3%)
Myalgia/Myopathy (3–5%)
Pain in extremities (2–6%)

Gastrointestinal/Hepatic
Abdominal distension (2%)
Abdominal pain (2–3%)
Constipation (5–8%)
Diarrhea (7%)
Dyspepsia (4–5%)
Nausea (7%)
Vomiting (6%)

Respiratory
Bronchitis (5%)
Cough (2–14%)
Influenza (5–7%)
Nasopharyngitis (10%)
Pharyngolaryngeal pain (7–14%)
Upper respiratory tract infection (10%)

Endocrine/Metabolic
Appetite increased (<5%)
Weight gain (10%) [4]

Genitourinary
Dysmenorrhea (5–9%)
Erectile dysfunction (5%)
Urinary tract infection (4–5%)

Hematologic
Anemia (6%)

Otic
Tinnitus (2%)

Ocular
Diplopia (6%)
Nystagmus (7%)
Ocular pain (5%)
Optic atrophy [2]
Retinopathy [12]
Vision blurred (6%)

Vision impaired [20]

Other
Adverse effects [3]
Dipsia (thirst) (2%)
Toothache (2–5%)

VILAZODONE

Trade name: Viibryd (Merck KGaA)
Indications: Major depressive disorder
Class: Antidepressant, Serotonin-norepinephrine reuptake inhibitor
Half-life: 25 hours
Clinically important, potentially hazardous interactions with: anticoagulants, aspirin, buspirone, CNS-active agents, CYP3A4 inhibitors or inducers, efavirenz, erythromycin, ketoconazole, MAO inhibitors, NSAIDs, SNRIs, SSRIs, tramadol, triptans, tryptophan, warfarin
Pregnancy category: C
Important contra-indications noted in the prescribing guidelines for: nursing mothers; pediatric patients
Warning: SUICIDALITY AND ANTIDEPRESSANT DRUGS

Mucosal
Xerostomia (8%)

Cardiovascular
Palpitation (2%)

Central Nervous System
Abnormal dreams (4%)
Headache [3]
Insomnia (6%) [4]
Paresthesias (3%)
Restlessness (3%)
Somnolence (drowsiness) (3%) [2]
Tremor (2%)
Vertigo (dizziness) (9%) [2]

Neuromuscular/Skeletal
Arthralgia (3%)
Asthenia (fatigue) (4%)

Gastrointestinal/Hepatic
Diarrhea (28%) [14]
Dyspepsia (3%)
Flatulence (3%)
Gastroenteritis (3%)
Nausea (23%) [14]
Vomiting (5%) [4]

Endocrine/Metabolic
Appetite increased (2%)
Libido decreased (4–5%)

Genitourinary
Ejaculatory dysfunction (2%)
Erectile dysfunction (2%)
Sexual dysfunction (3%) [2]

Other
Adverse effects [3]

VILDAGLIPTIN

See: www.drugeruptiondata.com/drug/id/1338

VINBLASTINE

Trade names: Velban (Lilly), Velbe (Lilly), Velsar (Lilly)
Indications: Lymphomas, melanoma, carcinomas
Class: Antimitotic, Vinca alkaloid
Half-life: initial: 3.7 minutes; terminal: 24.8 hours
Clinically important, potentially hazardous interactions with: aldesleukin, aprepitant, erythromycin, fluconazole, itraconazole, ketoconazole, lopinavir, miconazole, posaconazole
Pregnancy category: D
Important contra-indications noted in the prescribing guidelines for: nursing mothers

Skin
Acral necrosis [2]
Dermatitis (<10%)
Photosensitivity (<10%) [2]
Pigmentation [3]
Radiation recall dermatitis [2]
Rash (<10%)
Raynaud's phenomenon (<10%) [17]

Hair
Alopecia (>10%)

Mucosal
Mucositis [2]
Oral lesions (<5%)
Stomatitis (>10%)

Central Nervous System
Dysgeusia (taste perversion) (metallic taste) (>10%)
Paresthesias (<10%)

Neuromuscular/Skeletal
Myalgia/Myopathy (<10%)

Endocrine/Metabolic
SIADH [4]

Renal
Nephrotoxicity [2]

Hematologic
Hemolytic uremic syndrome [2]
Neutropenia [2]

Otic
Tinnitus [2]

Local
Injection-site necrosis [2]

Other
Adverse effects [2]

VINCRISTINE

Synonym: oncovin
Trade name: Vincasar (Teva)
Indications: Leukemias, lymphomas, neuroblastoma, Wilm's tumor
Class: Antimitotic, Vinca alkaloid
Half-life: 24 hours
Clinically important, potentially hazardous interactions with: aldesleukin, aprepitant, bromelain, fluconazole, gadobenate, influenza vaccine, itraconazole, ketoconazole, lopinavir, miconazole, nifedipine, posaconazole, thalidomide

Pregnancy category: D
Important contra-indications noted in the prescribing guidelines for: nursing mothers

Skin
Erythroderma [2]
Exanthems [3]
Hand–foot syndrome [2]
Rash (<10%)
Raynaud's phenomenon [2]

Hair
Alopecia (20–70%) [9]

Nails
Beau's lines (transverse nail bands) [2]
Leukonychia (Mees' lines) [5]

Mucosal
Oral lesions (<10%) [2]
Oral ulceration (<10%)

Cardiovascular
Hypertension [2]
Phlebitis (<10%)

Central Nervous System
Anorexia [2]
Dysgeusia (taste perversion) (<10%)
Neurotoxicity [16]
Paresthesias (<10%)
Peripheral neuropathy [10]
Seizures [6]

Neuromuscular/Skeletal
Asthenia (fatigue) [2]
Myalgia/Myopathy (<10%)

Gastrointestinal/Hepatic
Abdominal pain [2]

Respiratory
Pneumonia [2]

Endocrine/Metabolic
Hyponatremia [2]
SIADH [10]

Hematologic
Febrile neutropenia [5]
Hemolytic uremic syndrome [4]
Hemotoxicity [2]
Leukopenia [3]
Neutropenia [9]
Thrombocytopenia [9]

Ocular
Ptosis [4]

Local
Injection-site cellulitis (>10%)
Injection-site necrosis (>10%)

Other
Adverse effects [7]
Death [6]
Infection [3]

VINORELBINE

Trade name: Navelbine (Kyowa)
Indications: Non-small cell lung cancer
Class: Antimitotic, Vinca alkaloid
Half-life: 28–44 hours
Clinically important, potentially hazardous interactions with: aldesleukin, itraconazole

Pregnancy category: D
Important contra-indications noted in the prescribing guidelines for: nursing mothers; pediatric patients
Warning: MYELOSUPPRESSION

Skin
Acneform eruption [3]
Hand–foot syndrome [7]
Rash (<5%) [2]
Recall reaction [2]

Hair
Alopecia (12%) [5]

Mucosal
Mucositis [2]
Stomatitis (>10%) [6]

Cardiovascular
Extravasation [2]
Hypertension [2]
Phlebitis (7%)

Central Nervous System
Anorexia [7]
Dysgeusia (taste perversion) (metallic taste) (>10%)
Hyperesthesia (<10%)
Neurotoxicity [4]
Paresthesias (<10%)

Neuromuscular/Skeletal
Asthenia (fatigue) [14]
Bone or joint pain [3]
Myalgia/Myopathy (<5%)

Gastrointestinal/Hepatic
Constipation [4]
Diarrhea [13]
Hepatotoxicity [2]
Nausea [11]
Vomiting [7]

Endocrine/Metabolic
ALT increased [2]
AST increased [2]
SIADH [3]

Hematologic
Anemia [7]
Febrile neutropenia [5]
Leukopenia [8]
Myelotoxicity [2]
Neutropenia [26]
Thrombocytopenia [4]

Local
Injection-site irritation (<10%)
Injection-site necrosis (<10%)
Injection-site phlebitis (12%) [2]

Other
Adverse effects [2]
Death [2]
Infection [4]

VISMODEGIB

Trade name: Erivedge (Genentech)
Indications: Basal cell carcinoma
Class: Hedgehog (Hh) signaling pathway inhibitor
Half-life: 4–12 days
Clinically important, potentially hazardous interactions with: none known

Pregnancy category: D
Important contra-indications noted in the prescribing guidelines for: nursing mothers; pediatric patients
Note: Patients should not donate blood or blood products while receiving vismodegib and for at least 7 months after the last dose.
Warning: EMBRYO-FETAL TOXICITY

Skin
Squamous cell carcinoma [2]
Toxicity [2]

Hair
Alopecia (64%) [22]

Central Nervous System
Ageusia (taste loss) (11%) [6]
Anorexia [2]
Dysgeusia (taste perversion) (55%) [19]

Neuromuscular/Skeletal
Arthralgia (16%) [2]
Asthenia (fatigue) (40%) [15]
Muscle spasm (72%) [19]
Myalgia/Myopathy [5]

Gastrointestinal/Hepatic
Constipation (21%)
Diarrhea (29%) [7]
Hepatotoxicity [3]
Nausea (30%) [7]
Vomiting (14%) [2]

Endocrine/Metabolic
Amenorrhea [2]
Appetite decreased (25%) [6]
Hyperglycemia [2]
Hyponatremia (4%) [3]
Hypophosphatemia [2]
Weight loss (45%) [15]

Genitourinary
Azotemia (2%)

Other
Adverse effects [9]
Death [3]

VITAMIN A

Trade name: Aquasol A (aaiPharma)
Indications: Vitamin A deficiency
Class: Vitamin
Half-life: N/A
Clinically important, potentially hazardous interactions with: acitretin, alitretinoin, bexarotene, cholestyramine, fish oil supplements, isotretinoin, minocycline, orlistat, prednisone, tetracycline, warfarin
Pregnancy category: A (the pregnancy category will be X if used in doses above the RDA)

Skin
Dermatitis [7]
Pruritus [2]
Xerosis (<10%)

Hair
Alopecia [11]

Mucosal
Oral mucosal eruption [2]

VITAMIN E

Synonym: alpha tocopherol
Trade name: Aquasol E (aaiPharma)
Indications: Vitamin E deficiency
Class: Vitamin
Half-life: N/A
Clinically important, potentially hazardous interactions with: amprenavir, cholestyramine, orlistat, tipranavir, warfarin
Pregnancy category: A (the pregnancy category will be C if used in doses above the RDA)

Skin
Dermatitis [13]
Erythema multiforme [3]
Sclerosing lipogranuloma [2]

Genitourinary
Prostate cancer (increased risk) [4]

VORAPAXAR

Trade name: Zontivity (Merck)
Indications: Reduction of thrombotic cardiovascular events in patients with a history of myocardial infarction or with peripheral arterial disease
Class: Protease-activated receptor-1 (PAR-1) antagonist
Half-life: 3–4 days
Clinically important, potentially hazardous interactions with: boceprevir, carbamazepine, clarithromycin, conivaptan, indinavir, itraconazole, ketoconazole, nefazodone, nelfinavir, phenytoin, posaconazole, rifampin, ritonavir, saquinavir, St John's wort, strong CYP3A inhibitors or inducers, telaprevir, telithromycin
Pregnancy category: B
Important contra-indications noted in the prescribing guidelines for: nursing mothers; pediatric patients
Note: Contra-indicated in patients with a history of stroke, transient ischemic attack, or intracranial hemorrhage, or with active pathological bleeding.
Warning: BLEEDING RISK

Skin
Exanthems (2%)
Rash (2%)

Cardiovascular
Cardiotoxicity [2]

Central Nervous System
Depression (2%)
Intracranial hemorrhage [5]

Hematologic
Anemia (5%)
Bleeding (25%) [10]

Ocular
Diplopia (<2%)
Retinopathy (<2%)

Other
Adverse effects [3]

VORICONAZOLE

Trade name: Vfend (Pfizer)
Indications: Invasive aspergillosis
Class: Antibiotic, triazole, Antifungal, azole, CYP3A4 inhibitor
Half-life: 6–24 hours (dose dependent)
Clinically important, potentially hazardous interactions with: abiraterone, alfentanil, alfuzosin, almotriptan, alosetron, amphotericin B, antineoplastics, apixaban, aprepitant, artemether/lumefantrine, astemizole, atazanavir, atorvastatin, barbiturates, benzodiazepines, boceprevir, bortezomib, bosentan, brigatinib, brinzolamide, buspirone, busulfan, cabazitaxel, cabozantinib, calcifediol, calcium channel blockers, carbamazepine, carvedilol, chloramphenicol, chloroquine, ciclesonide, cilostazol, cinacalcet, ciprofloxacin, cisapride, clopidogrel, cobicistat/elvitegravir/emtricitabine/tenofovir alafenamide, cobicistat/elvitegravir/emtricitabine/tenofovir disoproxil, colchicine, conivaptan, copanlisib, coumarins, crizotinib, cyclosporine, CYP2C19 inhibitors and inducers, CYP2C9 inhibitors and substrates, CYP3A4 substrates, darunavir, diazepam, diclofenac, didanosine, dienogest, docetaxel, dofetilide, dronedarone, dutasteride, efavirenz, eletriptan, eplerenone, ergot alkaloids, ergotamine, erlotinib, esomeprazole, estrogens, eszopiclone, etravirine, everolimus, fentanyl, fesoterodine, food, gadobutrol, gefitinib, grapefruit juice, guanfacine, halofantrine, HMG-CoA reductase inhibitors, ibrutinib, ibuprofen, imatinib, irinotecan, ixabepilone, lapatinib, lomitapide, lopinavir, losartan, macrolide antibiotics, maraviroc, meloxicam, methadone, methylergonovine, methylprednisolone, methysergide, midazolam, midostaurin, mifepristone, mometasone, neratinib, nilotinib, nisoldipine, olaparib, ombitasvir/paritaprevir/ritonavir, omeprazole, oxycodone, palbociclib, pantoprazole, paricalcitol, pazopanib, PEG-interferon, phenobarbital, phenytoin, phosphodiesterase 5 inhibitors, pimecrolimus, pimozide, ponatinib, prasugrel, progestins, progestogens, protease inhibitors, proton pump inhibitors, QT prolonging agents, quetiapine, quinidine, quinine, ramelteon, ranolazine, reboxetine, regorafenib, repaglinide, ribociclib, rifabutin, rifampin, rifapentine, rilpivirine, ritonavir, rivaroxaban, romidepsin, ruxolitinib, salmeterol, saquinavir, saxagliptin, silodosin, simeprevir, simvastatin, sirolimus, solifenacin, sonidegib, sorafenib, St John's wort, sucralfate, sulfonylureas, sunitinib, tacrolimus, tadalafil, tamsulosin, telaprevir, temsirolimus, tetrabenazine, thioridazine, ticagrelor, tolterodine, tolvaptan, vemurafenib, venetoclax, venlafaxine, vitamin K antagonists, ziprasidone, zolpidem
Pregnancy category: D
Important contra-indications noted in the prescribing guidelines for: nursing mothers; pediatric patients
Note: Safety and effectiveness in pediatric patients <12 years of age have not been established.

Skin
Actinic keratoses [2]
Anaphylactoid reactions/Anaphylaxis (<2%)
Angioedema (<2%)
Cellulitis (<2%)
Contact dermatitis (<2%)
Cyanosis (<2%)
Dermatitis (<2%)
Diaphoresis (<2%) [2]
Ecchymoses (<2%)
Eczema (<2%)
Edema (<2%)
Erythema [5]
Erythema multiforme (<2%)
Exfoliative dermatitis (<2%)
Facial edema (<2%)
Fixed eruption (<2%)
Furunculosis (<2%)
Graft-versus-host reaction (<2%)
Granulomas (<2%)
Herpes simplex (<2%)
Lentigo [2]
Lupus erythematosus (<2%) [5]
Lymphadenopathy (<2%)
Malignancies [2]
Melanoma (<2%)
Melanosis (<2%)
Peripheral edema (<2%)
Petechiae (<2%)
Photosensitivity (8%) [18]
Phototoxicity [13]
Pigmentation (<2%)
Pruritus (8%)
Psoriasis (<2%)
Purpura (<2%)
Rash (5%) [7]
Squamous cell carcinoma (<2%) [8]
Stevens-Johnson syndrome (<2%) [4]
Toxic epidermal necrolysis (<2%) [4]
Urticaria (<2%)
Xerosis (<2%) [2]

Hair
Alopecia (<2%) [4]

Nails
Nail changes [3]

Mucosal
Cheilitis (<2%) [4]
Gingival bleeding (<2%)
Gingival hyperplasia/hypertrophy (<2%)
Gingivitis (<2%)
Glossitis (<2%)
Rectal hemorrhage (<2%)
Stomatitis (<2%)
Tongue edema (<2%)
Xerostomia (<2%)

Cardiovascular
Arrhythmias (<2%)
Atrial fibrillation (<2%)
Atrioventricular block (<2%)
Bradycardia (<2%)
Bundle branch block (<2%)
Cardiac arrest (<2%)
Cardiomyopathy (<2%)
Chest pain (<2%)
Congestive heart failure (<2%)
Extrasystoles (<2%)
Hypertension (<2%)
Hypotension (<2%)
Myocardial infarction (<2%)
Palpitation (<2%)
Phlebitis (<2%)

Postural hypotension (<2%)
QT prolongation (<2%) [11]
Supraventricular tachycardia (<2%)
Tachycardia (2%) [2]
Thrombophlebitis (<2%)
Torsades de pointes [7]
Vasodilation (<2%)
Ventricular arrhythmia (<2%)
Ventricular fibrillation (<2%)
Ventricular tachycardia (<2%)

Central Nervous System
Abnormal dreams (<2%)
Ageusia (taste loss) (<2%)
Agitation (<2%)
Akathisia (<2%)
Amnesia (<2%)
Anorexia (<2%)
Anxiety (<2%)
Cerebral edema (<2%)
Cerebral hemorrhage (<2%)
Cerebral ischemia (<2%)
Cerebrovascular accident (<2%)
Chills (4%)
Coma (<2%)
Confusion (<2%) [2]
Delirium (<2%) [2]
Dementia (<2%)
Depersonalization (<2%)
Depression (<2%)
Dysgeusia (taste perversion) (<2%)
Encephalitis (<2%)
Encephalopathy (<2%) [3]
Euphoria (<2%)
Extrapyramidal symptoms (<2%)
Fever (6%)
Guillain–Barré syndrome (<2%)
Hallucinations (2%) [8]
Headache (3%) [3]
Hypoesthesia (<2%)
Insomnia (<2%)
Intracranial pressure increased (<2%)
Neurotoxicity [6]
Paresthesias (<2%)
Peripheral neuropathy [4]
Psychosis (<2%) [2]
Seizures (<2%)
Somnolence (drowsiness) (<2%)
Status epilepticus (<2%)
Suicidal ideation (<2%)
Syncope (<2%)
Tremor (<2%)
Vertigo (dizziness) (<2%)

Neuromuscular/Skeletal
Arthralgia (<2%) [2]
Asthenia (fatigue) (<2%) [2]
Ataxia (<2%)
Back pain (<2%)
Bone or joint pain (<2%)
Hypertonia (<2%)
Leg cramps (<2%)
Myalgia/Myopathy (<2%)
Osteomalacia (<2%)
Osteoporosis (<2%)
Periostitis deformans [22]
Skeletal fluorosis [2]

Gastrointestinal/Hepatic
Abdominal pain (<2%)
Ascites (<2%)
Black stools (<2%)
Cholecystitis (<2%)

Cholelithiasis (gallstones) (<2%)
Constipation (<2%)
Diarrhea (<2%) [2]
Duodentitis (<2%)
Dyspepsia (<2%)
Dysphagia (<2%)
Esophagitis (<2%)
Flatulence (<2%)
Gastroenteritis (<2%)
Gastrointestinal bleeding (<2%)
Gastrointestinal perforation (<2%)
Gastrointestinal ulceration (<2%)
Hematemesis (<2%)
Hepatic failure (<2%)
Hepatotoxicity [18]
Nausea (5%) [3]
Pancreatitis (<2%)
Peritonitis (<2%)
Pseudomembranous colitis (<2%)
Vomiting (4%) [2]

Respiratory
Cough (<2%)
Dysphonia (<2%)
Dyspnea (<2%)
Flu-like syndrome (<2%)
Hemoptysis (<2%)
Hypoxia (<2%)
Pharyngitis (<2%)
Pleural effusion (<2%)
Pneumonia (<2%)
Pneumonitis [2]
Pulmonary embolism (<2%)
Respiratory distress (<2%)
Rhinitis (<2%)
Sinusitis (<2%)
Upper respiratory tract infection (<2%)

Endocrine/Metabolic
ALP increased (4%)
ALT increased [2]
AST increased [2]
Creatine phosphokinase increased (<2%)
Diabetes insipidus (<2%)
GGT increased (<2%)
Hypercalcemia (<2%)
Hypercholesterolemia (<2%)
Hyperglycemia (<2%)
Hyperkalemia (<2%)
Hypermagnesemia (<2%)
Hypernatremia (<2%)
Hyperthyroidism (<2%)
Hyperuricemia (<2%)
Hypervolemia (<2%)
Hypocalcemia (<2%)
Hypoglycemia (<2%)
Hypokalemia (2%) [3]
Hypomagnesemia (<2%)
Hyponatremia (<2%)
Hypophosphatemia (<2%)
Hypothyroidism (<2%)
Libido decreased (<2%)
Pseudoporphyria [6]

Genitourinary
Anuria (<2%)
Cystitis (<2%)
Dysmenorrhea (<2%)
Dysuria (<2%)
Epididymitis (<2%)
Glycosuria (<2%)
Hematuria (<2%)
Impotence (<2%)

Oliguria (<2%)
Urinary incontinence (<2%)
Urinary retention (<2%)
Urinary tract infection (<2%)
Uterine bleeding (<2%)
Vaginal bleeding (<2%)

Renal
Nephrotoxicity (<2%) [3]
Renal tubular necrosis (<2%)

Hematologic
Agranulocytosis (<2%)
Anemia (<2%)
Bone marrow suppression (<2%)
Eosinophilia (<2%)
Hemolytic anemia (<2%)
Leukopenia (<2%)
Pancytopenia (<2%)
Prothrombin time increased (<2%)
Sepsis (<2%)
Thrombocytopenia (<2%)

Otic
Ear pain (<2%)
Hearing loss (<2%)
Hypoacusis (<2%)
Tinnitus (<2%)

Ocular
Abnormal vision (19%)
Accommodation disorder (<2%)
Blepharitis (<2%)
Conjunctivitis (<2%)
Corneal opacity (<2%)
Diplopia (<2%)
Hallucinations, visual [4]
Keratitis (<2%)
Keratoconjunctivitis (<2%)
Mydriasis (<2%)
Night blindness (<2%)
Nystagmus (<2%)
Ocular adverse effects [2]
Ocular hemorrhage (<2%)
Ocular pain (<2%)
Oculogyric crisis (<2%)
Optic atrophy (<2%)
Optic neuritis (<2%)
Papilledema (<2%)
Photophobia (2%)
Retinitis (<2%)
Scleritis (<2%)
Uveitis (<2%)
Visual disturbances (19%) [14]
Xerophthalmia (<2%)

Local
Injection-site infection (<2%)
Injection-site inflammation (<2%)
Injection-site pain (<2%)

Other
Adverse effects (20%) [11]
Infection (<2%)
Multiorgan failure (<2%)
Periodontal infection (<2%)

VORINOSTAT

Trade name: Zolinza (Merck)
Indications: Cutaneous T-cell lymphoma
Class: Antineoplastic, Histone deacetylase (HDAC) inhibitor
Half-life: ~2 hours
Clinically important, potentially hazardous interactions with: alfuzosin, artemether/lumefantrine, chloroquine, ciprofloxacin, coumarins, dronedarone, gadobutrol, nilotinib, pimozide, QT prolonging agents, quinine, tetrabenazine, thioridazine, valproic acid, vitamin K antagonists, ziprasidone
Pregnancy category: D
Important contra-indications noted in the prescribing guidelines for: nursing mothers; pediatric patients

Skin
Exanthems [2]
Peripheral edema (13%)
Pruritus (12%)

Hair
Alopecia (19%) [2]

Mucosal
Mucositis [2]
Xerostomia (16%)

Cardiovascular
QT prolongation [3]

Central Nervous System
Anorexia [5]
Chills (16%)
Dysgeusia (taste perversion) (28%)
Fever (10%)
Headache (12%)
Vertigo (dizziness) (15%)

Neuromuscular/Skeletal
Asthenia (fatigue) (52%) [11]

Gastrointestinal/Hepatic
Abdominal pain [2]
Constipation [2]
Diarrhea [7]
Nausea [10]
Vomiting [4]

Respiratory
Cough (11%)
Upper respiratory tract infection (10%)

Endocrine/Metabolic
Creatine phosphokinase increased [2]
Dehydration [2]
Hyperglycemia [3]
Weight loss [4]

Renal
Renal failure [2]

Hematologic
Anemia (14%) [7]
Febrile neutropenia [2]
Hemotoxicity [2]
Leukopenia [2]
Lymphopenia [5]
Neutropenia [9]
Thrombocytopenia [15]

Other
Adverse effects [2]

VORTIOXETINE

Trade name: Trintellix (formerly Brintellix) (Takeda)
Indications: Major depressive disorder
Class: Antidepressant, Serotonin receptor agonist, Serotonin receptor antagonist, Serotonin reuptake inhibitor
Half-life: ~66 hours
Clinically important, potentially hazardous interactions with: bupropion, carbamazepine, fluoxetine, MAO inhibitors, paroxetine hydrochloride, phenytoin, quinidine, rifampin

Pregnancy category: C
Important contra-indications noted in the prescribing guidelines for: nursing mothers; pediatric patients
Warning: SUICIDAL THOUGHTS AND BEHAVIORS

Skin
Hyperhidrosis [6]
Pruritus (<3%)

Mucosal
Xerostomia (6–8%) [16]

Central Nervous System
Abnormal dreams (<3%) [2]
Agitation [2]
Anxiety [2]
Headache [24]
Insomnia [6]
Somnolence (drowsiness) [3]
Vertigo (dizziness) (6–9%) [15]

Neuromuscular/Skeletal
Asthenia (fatigue) [7]

Gastrointestinal/Hepatic
Constipation (3–6%) [11]
Diarrhea (7–10%) [13]
Flatulence (<3%)
Nausea (21–32%) [32]
Vomiting (3–6%) [15]

Respiratory
Nasopharyngitis [5]
Upper respiratory tract infection [2]

Endocrine/Metabolic
Weight gain [2]

Genitourinary
Sexual dysfunction (<5%) [10]

Other
Adverse effects [2]

WARFARIN

Trade name: Coumadin (Bristol-Myers Squibb)
Indications: Thromboembolic disease, pulmonary embolism
Class: Anticoagulant, Coumarin
Half-life: 1.5–2.5 days (highly variable)
Clinically important, potentially hazardous interactions with: acemetacin, amiodarone, amobarbital, amprenavir, antithyroid agents, aprepitant, aprobarbital, aspirin, atazanavir, atorvastatin, azathioprine, azithromycin, barbiturates, beclomethasone, betamethasone, bezafibrate, bismuth, bivalirudin, boceprevir, bosentan, butabarbital, capecitabine, cefixime, celecoxib, ceritinib, chondroitin, cimetidine, ciprofloxacin, clarithromycin, clofibrate, clopidogrel, clorazepate, co-trimoxazole, cobicistat/elvitegravir/emtricitabine/tenofovir alafenamide, cobicistat/elvitegravir/emtricitabine/tenofovir disoproxil, colesevelam, cyclosporine, danazol, daptomycin, darunavir, delavirdine, desvenlafaxine, dexamethasone, dexibuprofen, dexlansoprazole, diclofenac, dicloxacillin, dirithromycin, disulfiram, dronedarone, duloxetine, econazole, efavirenz, enzalutamide, ergotamine, erlotinib, erythromycin, eslicarbazepine, etoricoxib, exenatide, fenofibrate, fluconazole, flunisolide, fluoxymesterone, fosamprenavir, gefitinib, gemfibrozil, glucagon, grapefruit juice, heparin, imatinib, influenza vaccine, itraconazole, ketoconazole, leflunomide, lepirudin, levofloxacin, levothyroxine, liothyronine, liraglutide, lomitapide, lopinavir, menadione, mephobarbital, methimazole, methyl salicylate, methylprednisolone, methyltestosterone, metronidazole, miconazole, mifepristone, moricizine, moxifloxacin, nafcillin, nalidixic acid, nandrolone, nilutamide, norfloxacin, obeticholic acid, ofloxacin, omeprazole, oritavancin, orlistat, pantoprazole, PEG-interferon, penicillin G, penicillin V, penicillins, pentobarbital, phenobarbital, phenylbutazones, phytonadione, piperacillin, piroxicam, prasugrel, primidone, propoxyphene, propranolol, propylthiouracil, quinidine, quinine, rabeprazole, resveratrol, rifampin, rifapentine, rofecoxib, romidepsin, ropinirole, rosuvastatin, roxithromycin, salicylates, secobarbital, simvastatin, sitaxentan, sorafenib, St John's wort, stanozolol, sulfamethoxazole, sulfinpyrazone, sulfisoxazole, sulfonamides, sulindac, tamsulosin, tegafur/gimeracil/oteracil, telaprevir, telithromycin, teriflunomide, testosterone, tibolone, tigecycline, tinidazole, tolmetin, tolterodine, triamcinolone, troleandomycin, uracil/tegafur, valdecoxib, vemurafenib, venlafaxine, vilazodone, vitamin A, vitamin E, zafirlukast, zileuton
Pregnancy category: X (category D for women with mechanical heart valves)
Note: Alternative remedies, including herbals, may potentially increase the risk of bleeding or potentiate the effects of warfarin therapy. Some of these include the following: angelica root, arnica flower, anise, asafetida, bogbean, borage seed oil, bromelain, dan-shen, devil's claw, fenugreek, feverfew, garlic, ginger, ginkgo biloba, ginseng, horse chestnut, lovage root, meadowsweet, onion, parsley, passionflower herb, poplar, quassia, red clover, rue, turmeric and willow bark.
Warning: BLEEDING RISK

Skin
Bullous dermatitis [2]
Calcification [3]
Dermatitis [2]
Ecchymoses [2]
Exanthems [7]
Gangrene [6]
Hematoma [2]
Hypersensitivity [3]
Necrosis (>10%) [117]
Pruritus [2]
Purplish erythema (feet and toes) [8]
Purpura [3]
Rash [2]
Urticaria [3]
Vasculitis [7]

Hair
Alopecia (>10%) [6]

Central Nervous System
Headache [2]
Intracranial hemorrhage [2]
Vertigo (dizziness) [2]

Neuromuscular/Skeletal
Rhabdomyolysis [2]

Gastrointestinal/Hepatic
Black stools [2]
Gastrointestinal bleeding [5]
Hematemesis [2]

Genitourinary
Priapism [4]

Renal
Nephrotoxicity [3]

Hematologic
Anticoagulation [3]
Bleeding [17]
Hemorrhage [8]
Prothrombin time increased [5]

Other
Adverse effects [8]
Death [2]

XIPAMIDE

See: www.drugeruptiondata.com/drug/id/1354

XYLOMETAZOLINE

Trade name: Otrivine (Novartis)
Indications: Nasal congestion, perennial and allergic rhinitis, sinusitis
Class: Alpha adrenoceptor agonist
Half-life: N/A
Clinically important, potentially hazardous interactions with: none known
Pregnancy category: C
Important contra-indications noted in the prescribing guidelines for: nursing mothers

Mucosal
Epistaxis (nosebleed) [2]
Mucosal bleeding [2]

YELLOW FEVER VACCINE

Trade names: Stamaril (Sanofi Pasteur), YF-VAX (Sanofi Pasteur)
Indications: Immunization against yellow fever
Class: Vaccine
Half-life: N/A
Clinically important, potentially hazardous interactions with: azathioprine, belimumab, corticosteroids, fingolimod, hydroxychloroquine, immunosuppressants, interferon-gamma, leflunomide, mercaptopurine, prednisone, tocilizumab, ustekinumab
Pregnancy category: C
Important contra-indications noted in the prescribing guidelines for: the elderly; nursing mothers; pediatric patients
Note: Contra-indicated in patients with hypersensitivity to egg or chick embryo protein.

Skin
Anaphylactoid reactions/Anaphylaxis [8]
Hypersensitivity [2]
Rash (3%)
Urticaria [2]

Central Nervous System
Encephalopathy [4]
Fever (low-grade) (<5%) [3]
Headache (<30%) [2]
Myelitis [2]
Neurotoxicity [11]

Neuromuscular/Skeletal
Asthenia (fatigue) (10–30%) [2]
Myalgia/Myopathy (10–30%) [2]

Gastrointestinal/Hepatic
Diarrhea (<10%) [2]
Hepatitis [2]
Nausea (<10%)
Vomiting (<10%) [2]

Respiratory
Influenza [2]

Local
Infusion-site erythema (<5%)
Infusion-site pain (<5%)

Other
Adverse effects [14]
Death [13]
Multiorgan failure [3]
Viscerotropic disease [20]

ZAFIRLUKAST

Trade name: Accolate (AstraZeneca)
Indications: Asthma
Class: Leukotriene receptor antagonist
Half-life: 10 hours
Clinically important, potentially hazardous interactions with: aminophylline, aspirin, carvedilol, CYP2C9 substrates, CYP3A4 substrates, erythromycin, high protein foods, interferon alfa, primidone, vitamin K antagonists, warfarin
Pregnancy category: B
Important contra-indications noted in the prescribing guidelines for: nursing mothers; pediatric patients
Note: Contra-indicated in patients with hepatic impairment including hepatic cirrhosis.

Skin
Churg-Strauss syndrome [6]

Central Nervous System
Fever (2%)
Headache (13%)
Pain (generalized) (2%)
Vertigo (dizziness) (2%)

Neuromuscular/Skeletal
Asthenia (fatigue) (2%)
Back pain (2%)
Myalgia/Myopathy (2%)

Gastrointestinal/Hepatic
Abdominal pain (2%)
Diarrhea (3%)
Nausea (3%)
Vomiting (2%)

Respiratory
Cough [2]

Other
Infection (4%)

ZALCITABINE

Synonyms: dideoxycytidine; ddC
Trade name: Hivid (Roche)
Indications: Advanced HIV infection
Class: Antiretroviral, Nucleoside analog reverse transcriptase inhibitor
Half-life: 2.9 hours
Clinically important, potentially hazardous interactions with: none known
Pregnancy category: C
Important contra-indications noted in the prescribing guidelines for: the elderly; nursing mothers; pediatric patients

Skin
Edema [3]
Exanthems [9]
Pruritus (3–5%)
Rash (2–11%) [2]
Urticaria (3%)

Mucosal
Aphthous stomatitis [6]
Oral lesions (40–73%) [3]
Oral ulceration (3–64%) [4]
Stomatitis (3%)

Central Nervous System
Neurotoxicity [2]

Neuromuscular/Skeletal
Myalgia/Myopathy (<6%)

Other
Side effects [2]

ZALEPLON

Trade name: Sonata (Wyeth)
Indications: Insomnia
Class: Hypnotic, non-benzodiazepine
Half-life: 1 hour
Clinically important, potentially hazardous interactions with: alcohol, cimetidine, erythromycin, imipramine, ketoconazole, promethazine, rifampin, rifapentine, thioridazine
Pregnancy category: C
Important contra-indications noted in the prescribing guidelines for: nursing mothers; pediatric patients

Cardiovascular
Tachycardia [2]

Central Nervous System
Amnesia (2–4%)
Anorexia (<2%)
Confusion [2]
Depersonalization (<2%)
Hallucinations [3]
Headache (30–42%) [3]
Hypoesthesia (<2%)
Paresthesias (3%)
Parosmia (<2%)
Slurred speech [2]
Somnambulism [2]
Somnolence (drowsiness) (5–6%) [4]
Tremor (2%)
Vertigo (dizziness) (7–9%) [4]

Neuromuscular/Skeletal
Asthenia (fatigue) (5–7%)
Ataxia [2]

Gastrointestinal/Hepatic
Abdominal pain (6%)
Nausea (6–8%)
Vomiting [2]

Genitourinary
Dysmenorrhea (3–4%)

Otic
Hyperacusis (<2%)

Ocular
Ocular pain (3–4%)

Other
Adverse effects [2]
Viscerotropic disease [2]

ZANAMIVIR

Trade name: Relenza (GSK)
Indications: Influenza A and B
Class: Antiviral, Neuraminidase inhibitor
Half-life: 2.5–5.1 hours
Clinically important, potentially hazardous interactions with: live attenuated influenza vaccine

Pregnancy category: C
Important contra-indications noted in the prescribing guidelines for: nursing mothers

Skin
Urticaria (<2%)

Mucosal
Nasal discomfort (12%)

Central Nervous System
Anorexia (4%)
Chills (5–9%)
Fever (5–9%)
Headache (13–24%) [2]
Vertigo (dizziness) (<2%)

Neuromuscular/Skeletal
Arthralgia (<2%)
Asthenia (fatigue) (5–8%)
Bone or joint pain (6%)
Myalgia/Myopathy (<8%)

Gastrointestinal/Hepatic
Abdominal pain (<2%)
Diarrhea (3%) [2]
Nausea (3%) [2]

Respiratory
Bronchitis (2%)
Bronchospasm [3]
Cough (7–17%)
Respiratory failure [2]
Sinusitis (2%)
Upper respiratory tract infection (3–13%)
[2]

Endocrine/Metabolic
Appetite decreased (4%)
Appetite increased (4%)

Other
Infection (2%)

ZICONOTIDE

Trade name: Prialt (Jazz)
Indications: Analgesic, severe chronic pain
Class: Neuronal calcium channel blocker
Half-life: 4.6 hours
Clinically important, potentially hazardous interactions with: CNS depressants
Pregnancy category: C
Important contra-indications noted in the prescribing guidelines for: the elderly; nursing mothers; pediatric patients
Note: Ziconotide is a synthetic analog of a substance isolated from the venom of carnivorous oceanic snails that sting their prey with a cocktail of neurotoxins injected through a harpoon-like tube. Ziconotide is 100 to 1,000 times more powerful than morphine.
Warning: NEUROPSYCHIATRIC ADVERSE REACTIONS

Skin
Cellulitis (~2%)
Diaphoresis (5%)
Ecchymoses (~2%)
Edema (~2%)
Pruritus (7%)
Xerosis (~2%)

Mucosal
Xerostomia (~2%)

Cardiovascular
Atrial fibrillation (~2%)
Chest pain (~2%)
Hypertension (~2%)
Hypotension (~2%)
Tachycardia (~2%)

Central Nervous System
Amnesia (8%)
Anorexia (6%)
Anxiety (8%)
Chills (~2%)
Confusion (15%) [5]
Depression (~2%)
Dysarthria (7%)
Dysesthesia (7%)
Dysgeusia (taste perversion) (5%)
Fever (5%)
Hallucinations [3]
Headache (13%)
Hyperesthesia (~2%)
Insomnia (6%)
Pain (11%)
Paresthesias (7%)
Rigors (7%)
Seizures (<2%)
Somnolence (drowsiness) (17%) [3]
Suicidal ideation (<2%)
Tremor (7%)
Twitching (~2%)
Vertigo (dizziness) (47%) [8]

Neuromuscular/Skeletal
Arthralgia (~2%)
Asthenia (fatigue) (18%)
Ataxia (14%)
Back pain (~2%)
Muscle spasm (6%)
Myalgia/Myopathy (~2%)
Rhabdomyolysis (<2%)

Gastrointestinal/Hepatic
Abdominal pain (~2%)
Diarrhea (18%)
Nausea (40%) [3]
Vomiting (16%) [2]

Respiratory
Flu-like syndrome (~2%)
Sinusitis (5%)

Genitourinary
Urinary retention (9%) [3]

Otic
Tinnitus (~2%)

Ocular
Diplopia (~2%)
Nystagmus (8%) [2]
Periorbital edema (~2%)
Photophobia (~2%)
Vision blurred (12%) [2]
Visual disturbances (10%)

Other
Adverse effects [3]
Infection (~2%)

ZIDOVUDINE

Synonyms: azidothymidine; AZT
Trade names: Combivir (ViiV), Retrovir (ViiV), Trizivir (ViiV)
Indications: HIV infection
Class: Antiretroviral, Nucleoside analog reverse transcriptase inhibitor
Half-life: 0.5–3 hours
Clinically important, potentially hazardous interactions with: atovaquone, bone marrow suppressives, clarithromycin, darunavir, diclofenac, doxorubicin, fluconazole, ganciclovir, indinavir, interferon alfa, interferon beta, lopinavir, meloxicam, methadone, NSAIDs, PEG-interferon, phenytoin, probenecid, pyrimethamine, ribavirin, rifampin, rifapentine, stavudine, tipranavir, valproic acid
Pregnancy category: C
Important contra-indications noted in the prescribing guidelines for: the elderly; nursing mothers
Note: Combivir is zidovudine and lamivudine; Trizivir is zidovudine, abacavir and lamivudine.
Warning: HEMATOLOGICAL TOXICITY, MYOPATHY, LACTIC ACIDOSIS AND SEVERE HEPATOMEGALY, and EXACERBATIONS OF HEPATITIS B

Skin
Acneform eruption (<5%)
Bromhidrosis (<5%)
Diaphoresis (5–19%)
Edema of lip (<5%)
Erythema multiforme [2]
Exanthems (<5%) [6]
Lipoatrophy [2]
Lipodystrophy [2]
Pigmentation [10]
Pruritus [4]
Rash (17%) [8]
Stevens-Johnson syndrome [4]
Toxic epidermal necrolysis [3]
Urticaria (<5%) [2]
Vasculitis [2]

Hair
Alopecia [2]
Hypertrichosis (eyelashes) [2]

Nails
Nail pigmentation [27]

Mucosal
Oral lichenoid eruption [2]
Oral pigmentation [7]
Oral ulceration (<5%)
Tongue edema (<5%)
Tongue pigmentation [4]

Central Nervous System
Dysgeusia (taste perversion) (5–19%) [2]
Headache [3]
Paresthesias (<8%)

Neuromuscular/Skeletal
Asthenia (fatigue) [3]
Myalgia/Myopathy [5]

Gastrointestinal/Hepatic
Abdominal pain [3]
Diarrhea [2]
Hepatotoxicity [2]
Nausea [3]

Pancreatitis [3]
Vomiting [2]

Endocrine/Metabolic
Acidosis [6]

Hematologic
Anemia [13]
Neutropenia [3]

Other
Adverse effects [9]
Teratogenicity [2]

ZILEUTON

Trade name: Zyflo (AbbVie)
Indications: Asthma
Class: Leukotriene receptor antagonist
Half-life: 2.5 hours
**Clinically important, potentially hazardous
interactions with:** anisindione, anticoagulants,
astemizole, dicumarol, methylergonovine,
pimozide, propranolol, warfarin
Pregnancy category: C
**Important contra-indications noted in the
prescribing guidelines for:** nursing mothers;
pediatric patients

Neuromuscular/Skeletal
Myalgia/Myopathy (3%)

ZINC

Trade name: Cold-Eeze (The Quigley Corp)
Indications: Supplement to intravenous solutions
given for total parenteral nutrition (TPN)
Class: Food supplement, Trace element
Half-life: N/A
**Clinically important, potentially hazardous
interactions with:** chlorothiazide,
chlortetracycline, chlorthalidone, ciprofloxacin,
cisplatin, deferoxamine, demeclocycline,
doxycycline, eltrombopag, ethambutol, ferrous
sulfate, gatifloxacin, gemifloxacin,
hydrochlorothiazide, indapamide, levofloxacin,
lymecycline, metolozone, minocycline,
moxifloxacin, norfloxacin, ofloxacin,
oxytetracycline, propofol, tetracycline, valproic
acid
Pregnancy category: C
Note: Zinc is found in meats, seafood, dairy
products, legumes, nuts, whole grains. Zinc oxide
and zinc sulfate are used to fortify wheat
products.

Skin
Churg-Strauss syndrome [2]
Dermatitis [4]

Mucosal
Oral mucosal irritation [2]

Central Nervous System
Anosmia [2]
Dysgeusia (taste perversion) [5]

ZIPRASIDONE

Trade name: Geodon (Pfizer)
Indications: Schizophrenia, bipolar I disorder
Class: Antipsychotic
Half-life: 7 hours
**Clinically important, potentially hazardous
interactions with:** acetylcholinesterase
inhibitors, alcohol, alfuzosin, amitriptyline,
amoxapine, amphetamines, antifungals, arsenic,
artemether/lumefantrine, asenapine, astemizole,
carbamazepine, chloroquine, ciprofloxacin,
citalopram, CNS depressants, conivaptan,
dasatinib, degarelix, dolasetron, dopamine
agonists, dopamine agonists, dronedarone, food,
gadobutrol, ketoconazole, lapatinib, levodopa,
levofloxacin, lithium, methylphenidate,
metoclopramide, moxifloxacin, nilotinib,
pazopanib, pimavanserin, pimozide, QT
prolonging agents, quinagolide, quinine,
ranolazine, St John's wort, telavancin,
telithromycin, tetrabenazine, thioridazine,
voriconazole, vorinostat
Pregnancy category: C
**Important contra-indications noted in the
prescribing guidelines for:** the elderly; nursing
mothers; pediatric patients
Note: Ziprasidone should be avoided in patients
with congenital long QT syndrome or a history of
cardiac arrhythmias.
Warning: INCREASED MORTALITY IN
ELDERLY PATIENTS WITH DEMENTIA-
RELATED PSYCHOSIS

Skin
Angioedema [2]
Diaphoresis (2%)
DRESS syndrome [2]
Fungal dermatitis (2%)
Furunculosis (2%)
Lupus erythematosus [2]
Rash (4%)
Urticaria (5%)

Mucosal
Rectal hemorrhage (2%)
Sialorrhea (4%)
Tongue edema (3%)
Xerostomia (<5%)

Cardiovascular
Bradycardia (2%)
Chest pain (3%)
Hypertension (2–3%)
Postural hypotension (5%)
QT prolongation [22]
Tachycardia (2%) [2]
Torsades de pointes [6]

Central Nervous System
Agitation (2%) [3]
Akathisia (2–10%) [5]
Anorexia (2%)
Anxiety (2–5%) [2]
Depression [2]
Dyskinesia (<10%) [2]
Extrapyramidal symptoms (2–31%) [5]
Headache (3–18%) [3]
Hyperesthesia (<2%)
Hypokinesia (<5%)
Insomnia (3%) [5]
Mania [2]

Neuroleptic malignant syndrome [6]
Paralysis (<10%)
Paresthesias (<2%)
Sedation [4]
Somnolence (drowsiness) (8–31%) [10]
Speech disorder (2%)
Tardive dyskinesia [5]
Tremor (<10%) [2]
Twitching (<10%)
Vertigo (dizziness) (3–16%) [2]

Neuromuscular/Skeletal
Asthenia (fatigue) (2–6%) [2]
Dystonia (<10%) [6]
Hypertonia (<10%)
Myalgia/Myopathy (2%)
Rhabdomyolysis [2]

Gastrointestinal/Hepatic
Abdominal pain (<2%)
Constipation (2–9%)
Diarrhea (3–5%)
Dyspepsia (<8%)
Dysphagia (2%)
Nausea (4–12%) [2]
Vomiting (3–5%)

Respiratory
Cough (increased) (3%)
Dyspnea (2%)
Pharyngitis (3%)
Respiratory tract infection (8%)
Rhinitis (<4%)
Upper respiratory tract infection (8%)

Endocrine/Metabolic
Diabetes mellitus [2]
Galactorrhea [3]
Weight gain [7]

Genitourinary
Dysmenorrhea (2%)
Priapism [4]

Ocular
Abnormal vision (3–6%)

Local
Infusion-site pain (7–9%)

Other
Adverse effects [8]
Death [2]

ZOFENOPRIL

See: www.drugeruptiondata.com/drug/id/1312

ZOLEDRONATE

Synonym: zoledronic acid
Trade names: Aclasta (Novartis), Reclast
(Novartis), Zometa (Novartis)
Indications: Hypercalcemia of malignancy,
Paget's disease, osteoporosis
Class: Bisphosphonate
Half-life: 7 days
**Clinically important, potentially hazardous
interactions with:** aminoglycosides,
bisphosphonates, loop diuretics, nephrotoxics

Pregnancy category: D
Important contra-indications noted in the prescribing guidelines for: the elderly; nursing mothers; pediatric patients

Skin
Candidiasis (12%)
Dermatitis (11%)
Dermatomyositis [3]
Edema [3]
Neoplasms (malignant / aggrevated) (20%)
Peripheral edema (5–21%)
Rash [3]

Hair
Alopecia (12%)

Mucosal
Mucositis (5–10%)
Stomatitis (8%)

Cardiovascular
Atrial fibrillation [3]
Chest pain (5–10%)
Hypotension (11%)

Central Nervous System
Agitation (13%)
Anorexia (9–22%)
Anxiety (11–14%)
Chills [2]
Confusion (7–13%)
Depression (14%)
Fever (32–44%) [20]
Headache (5–19%) [4]
Hypoesthesia (12%)
Insomnia (15–16%)
Paresthesias (15%)
Rigors (11%)
Seizures [2]
Somnolence (drowsiness) (5–10%)
Vertigo (dizziness) (18%)

Neuromuscular/Skeletal
Arthralgia (5–10%) [9]
Asthenia (fatigue) (5–39%) [11]
Back pain (15%)
Bone or joint pain (12–55%) [15]
Fractures [4]
Myalgia/Myopathy (23%) [7]
Osteonecrosis [52]
Pain in extremities (14%)

Gastrointestinal/Hepatic
Abdominal pain (14–16%)
Constipation (27–31%) [3]
Diarrhea (17–24%) [2]
Dyspepsia (10%)
Dysphagia (5–10%)
Hepatotoxicity [3]
Nausea (29–46%) [12]
Vomiting (14–32%) [2]

Respiratory
Cough (12–22%)
Dyspnea (22–27%)
Flu-like syndrome [8]
Pharyngolaryngeal pain (8%)
Upper respiratory tract infection (10%)

Endocrine/Metabolic
Appetite decreased (13%)
Creatine phosphokinase increased [2]
Dehydration (5–14%)
Hyperparathyroidism [2]
Hypocalcemia (5–10%) [25]

Hypokalemia (12%)
Hypomagnesemia (11%)
Hypophosphatemia (13%) [3]
Weight loss (16%)

Genitourinary
Urinary tract infection (12–14%)

Renal
Fanconi syndrome [2]
Nephrotoxicity [14]
Renal failure [4]
Renal function abnormal [2]

Hematologic
Anemia (22–33%) [8]
Granulocytopenia (5–10%)
Neutropenia (12%)
Pancytopenia (5–10%)
Thrombocytopenia (5–10%)

Ocular
Ocular adverse effects [2]
Ocular inflammation [3]
Scleritis [2]
Uveitis [10]

Other
Adverse effects [6]
Infection (5–10%)

ZOLMITRIPTAN

Trade name: Zomig (AstraZeneca)
Indications: Migraine attacks
Class: 5-HT1 agonist, Serotonin receptor agonist, Triptan
Half-life: 3 hours
Clinically important, potentially hazardous interactions with: cimetidine, ciprofloxacin, dihydroergotamine, ergot-containing drugs, fluoxetine, fluvoxamine, isocarboxazid, levofloxacin, MAO inhibitors, methysergide, moclobemide, moxifloxacin, naratriptan, norfloxacin, ofloxacin, oral contraceptives, phenelzine, propranolol, rizatriptan, sertraline, sibutramine, SNRIs, SSRIs, St John's wort, sumatriptan, tranylcypromine
Pregnancy category: C
Important contra-indications noted in the prescribing guidelines for: nursing mothers; pediatric patients

Skin
Diaphoresis (2–3%)
Hot flashes (>10%)

Mucosal
Xerostomia (3–5%)

Cardiovascular
Chest pain (2–4%)
Myocardial infarction [4]

Central Nervous System
Dysgeusia (taste perversion) [4]
Headache [2]
Neurotoxicity [2]
Paresthesias (5–9%) [5]
Somnolence (drowsiness) (5–8%)
Vertigo (dizziness) (2–10%) [2]
Warm feeling (5–7%)

Neuromuscular/Skeletal
Jaw pain (4–10%)

Myalgia/Myopathy (2%) [2]
Neck pain (4–10%)

Gastrointestinal/Hepatic
Dyspepsia (<3%)
Dysphagia (<2%)
Nausea (4–9%)

Renal
Nephrotoxicity [2]

Other
Adverse effects [6]

ZOLPIDEM

Trade name: Ambien (Sanofi-Aventis)
Indications: Insomnia
Class: Hypnotic, non-benzodiazepine
Half-life: 2.6 hours
Clinically important, potentially hazardous interactions with: alcohol, antihistamines, azatadine, azelastine, brompheniramine, buclizine, chlorpheniramine, chlorpromazine, cimetidine, clemastine, cobicistat/elvitegravir/ emtricitabine/tenofovir alafenamide, cobicistat/ elvitegravir/emtricitabine/tenofovir disoproxil, dexchlorpheniramine, erythromycin, imipramine, ketoconazole, meclizine, pizotifen, ramelteon, rifampin, rifapentine, ritonavir, telaprevir, voriconazole
Pregnancy category: C
Important contra-indications noted in the prescribing guidelines for: nursing mothers; pediatric patients

Skin
Rash (2%)

Mucosal
Xerostomia (3%) [3]

Cardiovascular
Palpitation (2%)
Tachycardia [2]
Torsades de pointes [2]

Central Nervous System
Amnesia [16]
Anxiety [2]
Compulsions [2]
Confusion [3]
Delirium [5]
Depression (2%)
Dysgeusia (taste perversion) [4]
Gait instability [3]
Hallucinations [13]
Headache (7%) [11]
Nightmares [2]
Seizures [7]
Sleep related disorder [19]
Slurred speech [2]
Somnambulism [16]
Somnolence (drowsiness) (2–8%) [10]
Vertigo (dizziness) (<5%) [12]

Neuromuscular/Skeletal
Asthenia (fatigue) (3%) [4]
Ataxia [3]
Back pain (3%)
Fractures [2]
Myalgia/Myopathy (7%)

Gastrointestinal/Hepatic
Abdominal pain (2%)
Constipation (2%)
Diarrhea (<3%)
Hepatotoxicity [2]
Nausea [5]
Vomiting [2]

Respiratory
Flu-like syndrome (2%)
Pharyngitis (3%)
Sinusitis (4%)

Ocular
Hallucinations, visual [8]

Other
Adverse effects [8]
Allergic reactions (4%)

ZONISAMIDE

Trade name: Zonegran (Concordia)
Indications: Epilepsy
Class: Anticonvulsant, Antiepileptic, sulfonamide
Half-life: 63 hours
Clinically important, potentially hazardous interactions with: caffeine, metformin
Pregnancy category: C
Important contra-indications noted in the prescribing guidelines for: nursing mothers; pediatric patients
Note: Zonisamide is a sulfonamide and can be absorbed systemically. Sulfonamides can produce severe, possibly fatal, reactions such as toxic epidermal necrolysis and Stevens-Johnson syndrome.

Skin
DRESS syndrome [3]
Ecchymoses (2%)
Hypersensitivity [4]
Oligohydrosis [8]
Purpura (2%)
Rash (3%) [6]
Stevens-Johnson syndrome [3]

Mucosal
Xerostomia (2%)

Central Nervous System
Agitation (9%) [4]
Anorexia (13%) [9]
Anxiety (3%)
Cognitive impairment (6%) [4]
Confusion (6%)
Depression (6%) [4]
Dysgeusia (taste perversion) (2%)
Fever [2]
Headache (10%) [7]
Insomnia (6%)
Irritability (9%) [4]
Mania [2]
Nervousness (2%)
Neuroleptic malignant syndrome [2]
Paresthesias (4%)
Psychosis [3]
Restless legs syndrome [3]

Schizophrenia (2%)
Somnolence (drowsiness) (17%) [22]
Speech disorder (2–5%)
Suicidal ideation [2]
Vertigo (dizziness) (13%) [18]

Neuromuscular/Skeletal
Asthenia (fatigue) (7–8%) [9]
Ataxia (6%) [3]

Gastrointestinal/Hepatic
Abdominal pain (6%)
Constipation (2%)
Diarrhea (5%)
Dyspepsia (3%)
Nausea (9%) [2]
Vomiting [2]

Respiratory
Flu-like syndrome (4%)
Pneumonitis [2]
Rhinitis (2%)

Endocrine/Metabolic
Appetite decreased [7]
Weight loss (3%) [20]

Renal
Nephrolithiasis [4]
Nephrotoxicity [2]

Ocular
Diplopia (6%) [2]
Nystagmus (4%)

Other
Adverse effects [12]
Side effects [4]
Teratogenicity [2]

ZOSTER VACCINE

Trade name: Zostavax (Oka/Merck)
Indications: To reduce the risk of developing herpes zoster (in people over 60)
Class: Vaccine
Half-life: N/A
Clinically important, potentially hazardous interactions with: none known
Pregnancy category: C

Skin
Herpes zoster [7]
Rash [2]

Central Nervous System
Fever (<2%)
Headache [4]

Respiratory
Flu-like syndrome (<2%)

Local
Injection-site edema [2]
Injection-site erythema [2]
Injection-site pain [2]
Injection-site reactions [8]

Other
Adverse effects [2]
Death [2]

ZOTAROLIMUS

Trade names: Endeavor (Medtronic), ZoMaxx Drug-Eluting Coronary Stent (AbbVie)
Indications: Ischemic heart disease, restenosis
Class: Angiogenesis inhibitor, Macrolide immunosuppressant (derivative of sirolimus), mTOR inhibitor
Half-life: 33–36 hours
Clinically important, potentially hazardous interactions with: ketoconazole, sirolimus
Pregnancy category: C
Important contra-indications noted in the prescribing guidelines for: nursing mothers; pediatric patients

Skin
Rash (<6%)
Xerosis (<13%)

Cardiovascular
Cardiotoxicity [4]
Myocardial infarction [3]
Subacute thrombosis [2]

Central Nervous System
Headache (4–13%)
Pain (13–63%)

Gastrointestinal/Hepatic
Abdominal pain (<6%)
Diarrhea (<6%)

Genitourinary
Hematuria (<13%)

Local
Application-site reactions (13–63%)
Injection-site reactions (13–38%)

ZUCLOPENTHIXOL

See: www.drugeruptiondata.com/drug/id/1344

ZUCLOPENTHIXOL ACETATE

See: www.drugeruptiondata.com/drug/id/1273

ZUCLOPENTHIXOL DECANOATE

See: www.drugeruptiondata.com/drug/id/1272

ZUCLOPENTHIXOL DIHYDROCHLORIDE

See: www.drugeruptiondata.com/drug/id/1274

DESCRIPTIONS OF IMPORTANT REACTIONS

Acanthosis nigricans

Acanthosis nigricans (AN) is a process characterized by a soft, velvety, brown or grayish-black thickening of the skin that is symmetrically distributed over the axillae, neck, inguinal areas and other body folds.

While most cases of AN are seen in obese and prepubertal children, it can occur as a marker for various endocrinopathies as well as in female patients with elevated testosterone levels, irregular menses, and hirsutism.

It is frequently a concomitant of an underlying malignant condition, principally an adenocarcinoma of the intestinal tract.

Acneform lesions

Acneform eruptions are inflammatory follicular reactions that resemble acne vulgaris and that are manifested clinically as papules or pustules. They are monomorphic reactions, have a monomorphic appearance, and are found primarily on the upper parts of the body. Unlike acne vulgaris, there are rarely comedones present. Consider a drug-induced acneform eruption if:

- The onset is sudden
- There is a worsening of existing acne lesions
- The extent is considerable from the outset
- The appearance is monomorphic
- The localization is unusual for acne as, for example, when the distal extremities are involved
- The patient's age is unusual for regular acne
- There is an exposure to a potentially responsible drug.

The most common drugs responsible for acneform eruptions are: ACTH, androgenic hormones, anticonvulsants (hydantoin derivatives, phenobarbital, trimethadione), corticosteroids, danazol, disulfiram, halogens (bromides, chlorides, iodides), lithium, oral contraceptives, tuberculostatics (ethionamide, isoniazid, rifampin), vitamins B_2, B_6 and B_{12}.

Acute febrile neutrophilic dermatosis

Acute febrile neutrophilic dermatosis is a disorder that appears more frequently in females and has several characteristic features.

The lesions - tender, erythematous or purple, annular plaques or nodules - appear suddenly and are most prominent on the face, neck and upper extremities. Pain and fever often accompany the eruption.

While the cause is unknown, about 15% of the patients have some type of myeloproliferative disorder, primarily leukemias.

Drugs commonly reported to cause Sweet's syndrome are clofazimine, co-trimoxazole, furosemide, granulocyte-colony stimulating factor and minocycline.

Acute generalized exanthematous pustulosis

Arising on the face or intertriginous areas, acute generalized exanthematous pustulosis (AGEP) is characterized by a rapidly evolving, widespread, scarlatiniform eruption covered with hundreds of small superficial pustules.

Often accompanied by a high fever, AGEP is most frequently associated with acetaminophen, carbamazepine, penicillin and macrolide antibiotics, and usually occurs within 24 hours of the drug exposure.

Ageusia

Ageusia is the loss of taste functions of the tongue, essentially the inability to detect sweet, sour, bitter, or salty substances, and umami (the taste of monosodium glutamate).

Atorvastatin, captopril, enalapril, indomethacin, and paroxetine are some of the drugs that can occasion ageusia.

Alopecia

Many drugs have been reported to occasion hair loss. Commonly appearing as a diffuse alopecia, it affects women more frequently than men and is limited in most instances to the scalp. Axillary and pubic hairs are rarely affected except with anticoagulants.

The hair loss from cytostatic agents, which is dose-dependent and begins about 2 weeks after the onset of therapy, is a result of the interruption of the anagen (growing) cycle of hair. With other drugs the hair loss does not begin until 2–5 months after the medication has been begun. With cholesterol-lowering drugs, diffuse alopecia is a result of interference with normal keratinization.

The scalp is normal and the drug-induced alopecia is almost always reversible within 1–3 months after the therapy has been discontinued. The regrown hair is frequently depigmented and occasionally more curly

The most frequent offenders are cytostatic agents and anticoagulants, but hair loss can occur with a variety of common drugs, including hormones, anticonvulsants, amantadine, amiodarone, captopril, cholesterol-lowering drugs, cimetidine, colchicine, etretinate, isotretinoin, ketoconazole, heavy metals, lithium, penicillamine, valproic acid, and propranolol.

Angioedema

Angioedema is a term applied to a variant of urticaria in which the subcutaneous tissues, rather than the dermis, are mainly involved.

Also known as Quincke's edema, giant urticaria, and angioneurotic edema, this acute, evanescent, skin-colored, circumscribed edema usually affects the most distensible tissues: the lips, eyelids, earlobes, and genitalia. It can also affect the mucous membranes of the tongue, mouth, and larynx.

Symptoms of angioedema, frequently unilateral, asymmetrical and non-pruritic, last for an hour or two but can persist for 2–5 days.

The etiological factors associated with angioedema are as varied as that of urticaria (see separate entry).

Anosmia

Anosmia, or odor blindness, is the total absence of the sense of smell. It can be either temporary or permanent.

Some of the drugs that can cause anosmia are ciprofloxacin, doxycycline, enalapril, paroxetine and sparfloxacin.

Aphthous stomatitis

Aphthous stomatitis – also known as canker sores – is a common disease of the oral mucous membranes.

Arising as tiny, discrete or grouped, papules or vesicles, these painful lesions develop into small (2–5 mm in diameter), round, shallow ulcerations having a grayish, yellow base surrounded by a thin red border.

Located predominantly over the labial and buccal mucosae, these aphthae heal without scarring in 10–14 days. Recurrences are common.

Baboon syndrome (SDRIFE)

Baboon syndrome or symmetric drug-related intertriginous and flexural exanthema (SDRIFE) is an unusual presentation of a drug eruption with a characteristic intertriginous distribution pattern. Several drugs have been implicated, notably mercury, nickel, heparin, aminophylline, pseudoephedrine, terbinafine, IVIG, various antibiotics (amoxicillin, ampicillin), and food additives.

Originally described as a type of systemic contact dermatitis characterized by a pruritic exanthems involving the buttocks and major flexures – groins and axillae, some investigators believe that this entity is a form of recall phenomenon. In children, it is important in the differential diagnosis of viral exanthems.

Black tongue (lingua villosa nigra)

Black hairy tongue (BHT) represents a benign hyperplasia of the filiform papillae of the anterior two-thirds of the tongue.

These papillary elongations, usually associated with black, brown, or yellow pigmentation attributed to the overgrowth of pigment-producing bacteria, may be as long as 2 cm.

Occurring only in adults, BHT has been associated with the administration of oral antibiotics, poor dental hygiene, and excessive smoking.

Bullous dermatitis

Bullous and vesicular drug eruptions are diseases in which blisters and vesicles occur as a complication of the administration of drugs. Blisters are a well-known manifestation of cutaneous reactions to drugs.

In many types of drug reactions, bullae and vesicles may be found in addition to other manifestations. Bullae are usually noted in: erythema multiforme; Stevens–Johnson syndrome; toxic epidermal necrolysis; fixed eruptions when very intense; urticaria; vasculitis; porphyria cutanea tarda; and phototoxic reactions (from furosemide and nalidixic acid). Tense, thick-walled bullae can be seen in bromoderma and iododerma as well as in barbiturate overdosage.

Common drugs that cause bullous eruptions and bullous pemphigoid are: nadalol, penicillamine, piroxicam, psoralens, rifampin, clonidine, furosemide, diclofenac, mefenamic acid, and bleomycin.

DRESS syndrome

The DRESS syndrome is an acronym for Drug Rash with Eosinophilia and Systemic Symptoms. It is also known as the Drug-Induced Pseudolymphoma and Drug Hypersensitivity Syndrome.

The symptoms of DRESS syndrome usually begin 1 to 8 weeks after exposure to the offending drug. Common causes include carbamazepine, phenobarbital, phenytoin, terbinafine, and valproic acid.

Erythema multiforme

Erythema multiforme is a relatively common, acute, self-limited, inflammatory reaction pattern that is often associated with a preceding herpes simplex or mycoplasma infection. Other causes are associated with connective tissue disease, physical agents, X-ray therapy, pregnancy and internal malignancies, to mention a few. In 50% of the cases, no cause can be found. In a recent prospective study of erythema multiforme, only 10% were drug related.

The eruption rapidly occurs over a period of 12 to 24 hours. In about half the cases there are prodromal symptoms of an upper respiratory infection accompanied by fever, malaise, and varying degrees of muscular and joint pains.

Clinically, bluish-red, well-demarcated, macular, papular, or urticarial lesions, as well as the classical 'iris' or 'target lesions', sometimes with central vesicles, bullae, or purpura, are distributed preferentially over the distal extremities, especially over the dorsa of the hands and extensor aspects of the forearms. Lesions tend to spread peripherally and may involve the palms and trunk as well as the mucous membranes of the mouth and genitalia. Central healing and overlapping lesions often lead to arciform, annular and gyrate patterns. Lesions appear over the course of a week or 10 days and resolve over the next two weeks.

The following drugs have been most often associated with erythema multiforme: allopurinol, barbiturates, carbamazepine, estrogens/progestins, gold, lamotrigine, NSAIDs, penicillamine, phenytoin, sulfonamides, tetracycline, tolbutamide and valproic acid.

Erythema nodosum

Erythema nodosum is a cutaneous reaction pattern characterized by erythematous, tender or painful subcutaneous nodules commonly distributed over the anterior aspect of the lower legs, and occasionally elsewhere.

More common in young women, erythema nodosum is often associated with increased estrogen levels as occurs during pregnancy and with the ingestion of oral contraceptives. It is also an occasional manifestation of streptococcal infection, sarcoidosis, secondary syphilis, tuberculosis, certain deep fungal infections, Hodgkin's disease, leukemia, ulcerative colitis, and radiation therapy and is often preceded by fever, fatigue, arthralgia, vomiting, and diarrhea.

The incidence of erythema nodosum due to drugs is low and it is impossible to distinguish clinically between erythema nodosum due to drugs and that caused by other factors.

Some of the drugs that are known to occasion erythema nodosum are: antibiotics, estrogens, amiodarone, gold, NSAIDs, oral contraceptives, sulfonamides, and opiates.

Exanthems

Exanthems, commonly resembling viral rashes, represent the most common type of cutaneous drug eruption. Described as maculopapular or morbilliform eruptions, these flat, barely raised, erythematous patches, from one to several millimeters in diameter, are usually bilateral and symmetrical. They commonly begin on the head and neck or upper torso and progress downward to the limbs. They may present or develop into confluent areas and may be accompanied by pruritus and a mild fever.

The exanthems caused by drugs can be classified as:

• Morbilliform eruptions: fingernail-sized erythematous patches
• Scarlatiniform eruptions: punctate, pinpoint, or pinhead-sized lesions in erythematous areas that have a tendency to coalesce. Circumoral pallor and the subsequent appearance of scaling may also be noted.

Maculopapular drug eruptions usually fade with desquamation and, occasionally, postinflammatory hyperpigmentation, in about 2 weeks. They invariably recur on rechallenge.

Exanthems often have a sudden onset during the first 2 weeks of administration, except in cases of semisynthetic penicillin administration, when the exanthems frequently develop after the first 2 weeks following the initial dose.

The drugs most commonly associated with exanthems are: amoxicillin, ampicillin, bleomycin, captopril, carbamazepine, chlorpromazine, co-trimoxazole, gold, nalidixic acid, naproxen, phenytoin, penicillamine, and piroxicam.

Exfoliative dermatitis

Exfoliative dermatitis is a rare but serious reaction pattern that is characterized by erythema, pruritus and scaling over the entire body (erythroderma).

Drug-induced exfoliative dermatitis usually begins a few weeks or longer following the administration of a culpable drug. Beginning as erythematous, edematous patches, often on the face, it spreads to involve the entire integument. The skin becomes swollen and scarlet and may ooze a straw-colored fluid; this is followed in a few days by desquamation.

High fever, severe malaise and chills, along with enlargement of lymph nodes, often coexist with the cutaneous changes.

One of the most dangerous of all reaction patterns, exfoliative dermatitis can be accompanied by any or all of the following: hypothermia, fluid and electrolyte loss, cardiac failure, and gastrointestinal hemorrhage. Death may supervene if the drug is continued after the onset of the eruption. Secondary infection often complicates the course of the disease. Once the active dermatitis has receded, hyperpigmentation as well as loss of hair and nails may ensue.

The following drugs, among others, can bring about exfoliative dermatitis: barbiturates, captopril, carbamazepine, cimetidine, furosemide, gold, isoniazid, lithium, nitrofurantoin, NSAIDs, penicillamine, phenytoin, pyrazolons, quinidine, streptomycin, sulfonamides, and thiazides.

Fixed eruption

A fixed eruption is an unusual hypersensitivity reaction characterized by one or more well-demarcated erythematous plaques that recur at the same cutaneous (or mucosal) site or sites each time exposure to the offending agent occurs. The sizes of the lesions vary from a few millimeters to as much as 20 centimeters in diameter. Almost any drug that is ingested, injected, inhaled, or inserted into the body can trigger this skin reaction.

The eruption typically begins as a sharply marginated, solitary edematous papule or plaque – occasionally surmounted by a large bulla – which usually develops 30 minutes to 8 hours following the administration of a drug. If the offending agent is not promptly eliminated, the inflammation intensifies, producing a dusky red, violaceous or brown patch that may crust, desquamate, or blister within 7 to 10 days. The lesions are rarely pruritic. Favored sites are the hands, feet, face, and genitalia – especially the glans penis.

The reason for the specific localization of the skin lesions in a fixed drug eruption is unknown. The offending drug cannot be detected at the skin site. Certain drugs cause a fixed eruption at specific sites, for example, tetracycline and ampicillin often elicit a fixed eruption on the penis, whereas aspirin usually causes skin lesions on the face, limbs and trunk.

Common causes of fixed eruptions are: ampicillin, aspirin, barbiturates, dapsone, metronidazole, NSAIDs, oral contraceptives, phenolphthalein, phenytoin, quinine, sulfonamides, and tetracyclines.

Gingival hyperplasia/hypertrophy

Gingival hyperplasia, a common, undesirable, non-allergic drug reaction begins as a diffuse swelling of the interdental papillae.

Particularly prevalent with phenytoin therapy, gingival hyperplasia begins about 3 months after the onset of therapy, and occurs in 30 to 70% of patients receiving it. The severity of the reaction is dose-dependent and children and young adults are more frequently affected. The most severe cases are noted in young women.

In many cases, gingival hyperplasia is accompanied by painful and bleeding gums. There is often superimposed secondary bacterial gingivitis. This can be so extensive that the teeth of the maxilla and mandible are completely overgrown.

While it is characteristically a side effect of hydantoin derivatives, it may occur during the administration of phenobarbital, nifedipine, diltiazem and other medications.

Hand-foot syndrome

Hand-foot syndrome (also known as acral erythema, palmar-plantar erythrodysesthesia, palmoplantar erythrodysesthesia, palmar-plantar erythema, and Bergdorf's reaction) is a syndrome that is characterized by well-demarcated painful erythema, edema, numbness and desquamation over the palms and soles that may develop following treatment with a variety of chemotherapeutic agents including bleomycin, cisplatin, cyclophosphamide, hydroxyurea, idarubicin, methotrexate, sorafenib, sunitinib, and others. Tenderness involving the skin overlying the fingers and toes, followed by bulla formation and subsequent desquamation, often supervenes.

This side effect results when a small amount of the culpable drug leaks out of the blood vessels, damaging tissues. This reaction predominates over the palms and soles, where eccrine glands are more numerous, and also as a result of the increased friction and heat that extremities are exposed to through daily activities.

Lichenoid (lichen planus-like) eruptions

Lichenoid eruptions are so called because of their resemblance to lichen planus, a papulosquamous disorder that characteristically presents as multiple, discrete, violaceous, flat-topped papules, often polygonal in shape and which are extremely pruritic.

Not infrequently, lichenoid lesions appear weeks or months following exposure to the responsible drug. As a rule, the symptoms begin to recede a few weeks following the discontinuation of the drug.

Common drug causes of lichenoid eruptions are: antimalarials, beta-blockers, chlorpropamide, furosemide, gold, methyldopa, phenothiazines, quinidine, thiazides, and tolazamide.

Lupus erythematosus

A reaction, clinically and pathologically resembling idiopathic systemic lupus erythematosus (SLE), has been reported in association with a large variety of drugs. There is some evidence that drug-induced SLE, invariably accompanied by a positive ANA reaction with 90% having antihistone antibodies, may have a genetically determined basis. These symptoms of SLE, a relatively benign form of lupus, recede within days or weeks following the discontinuation of the responsible drug. Skin lesions occur in about 20% of cases. Drugs cause fewer than 8% of all cases of SLE.

The following drugs have been commonly associated with inducing, aggravating or unmasking SLE: beta-blockers, carbamazepine, chlorpromazine, estrogens, griseofulvin, hydralazine, isoniazid (INH), lithium, methyldopa, minoxidil, oral contraceptives, penicillamine, phenytoin (diphenylhydantoin), procainamide, propylthiouracil, quinidine, and testosterone.

Onycholysis

Onycholysis, the painless separation of the nail plate from the nail bed, is one of the most common nail disorders.

The unattached portion, which is white and opaque, usually begins at the free margin and proceeds proximally, causing part or most of the nail plate to become separated. The attached, healthy portion of the nail, by contrast, is pink and translucent.

Paresthesias

Paresthesias are abnormal neurological sensations such as burning, prickling, numbness, pruritus, formication, or tingling, often described as 'pins and needles' or of a limb being 'asleep'. It is a symptom of partial damage to a peripheral nerve, as occurs from a head or spinal injury, lack of blood supply to a nerve, or in many cases medications.

Paresthesias can affect various parts of the body; hands, fingers, and feet are common sites but all areas are possibilities.

Scores of generic drugs have been reported to occasion paresthesias including alprazolam, allopurinol, buspirone, celecoxib, ciprofloxacin, cyclosporine, enalapril, glipizine and many others.

Pemphigus vulgaris

Pemphigus vulgaris (PV) is a rare, serious, acute or chronic, blistering disease involving the skin and mucous membranes.

Characterized by thin-walled, easily ruptured, flaccid bullae that are seen to arise on normal or erythematous skin and over mucous membranes, the lesions of PV appear initially in the mouth (in about 60% of the cases) and then spread, after weeks or months, to involve the axillae and groin, scalp, face and neck. The lesions may become generalized.

Because of their fragile roofs, the bullae rupture leaving painful erosions and crusts may develop principally over the scalp.

Peyronie's disease

First described in 1743 by the French surgeon, Francois de la Peyronie, Peyronie's disease is a rare, benign connective tissue disorder involving the growth of fibrous plaques in the soft tissue of the penis. Beginning as a localized inflammation, it often develops into a hardened scar. Affecting as many as 1% of men, it may cause deformity, pain, cord-like lesions, or abnormal curvature of the penis when erect.

It has been associated with several drugs, including all the adrenergic blocking agents (beta-blockers), methotrexate, colchicine and others.

Photosensitivity

A photosensitive reaction is a chemically induced change in the skin that makes an individual unusually sensitive to electromagnetic radiation (light). On absorbing light of a specific wavelength, an oral, injected or topical drug may be chemically altered to produce a reaction ranging from macules and papules, vesicles and bullae, edema, urticaria, or an acute eczematous reaction.

Any eruption that is prominent on the face, the dorsa of the hands, the 'V' of the neck, and the presternal area should suggest an adverse reaction to light. The distribution is the key to the diagnosis.

Initially the eruption, which consists of erythema, edema, blisters, weeping and desquamation, involves the forehead, rims of the ears, the nose, the malar eminences and cheeks, the sides and back of the neck, the extensor surfaces of the forearms and the dorsa of the hands. These reactions commonly spare the shaded areas: those under the chin, under the nose, behind the ears and inside the fold of the upper eyelids. There is usually a sharp cut-off at the site of jewelry and at clothing margins. All light-exposed areas need not be affected equally.

There are two main types of photosensitive reactions: the phototoxic and the photoallergic reaction.

Phototoxic reactions, the most common type of drug-induced photo-sensitivity, resemble an exaggerated sunburn and occur within 5 to 20 hours after the skin has been exposed to a photosensitizing substance and light of the proper wavelength and intensity. It is not a form of allergy – prior sensitization is not required – and, theoretically, could occur in anyone given enough drug and light. Phototoxic reactions are dose-dependent both for drug and sunlight. Patients with phototoxicity reactions are commonly sensitive to ultraviolet A (UVA radiation), the so-called 'tanning rays' at 320–400 nm. Phototoxic reactions may cause onycholysis, as the nailbed is particularly susceptible because of its lack of melanin protection.

Patients with a true photoallergy (the interaction of drug, light and the immune system), a less common form of drug-induced photosensitivity, are often sensitive to UVB radiation, the so-called 'burning rays' at 290–320 nm. Photoallergic reactions, unlike phototoxic responses, represent an immunologic change and require a latent period of from 24 to 48 hours during which sensitization occurs. They are not dose-related.

If the photosensitizer acts internally, it is a photodrug reaction; if it acts externally, it is photocontact dermatitis.

Drugs that are likely to cause phototoxic reactions are: amiodarone, nalidixic acid, various NSAIDs, phenothiazines (especially chlorpromazine), and tetracyclines (particularly demeclocycline).

Photoallergic reactions may occur as a result of exposure to systemically-administered drugs such as griseofulvin, NSAIDs, phenothiazines, quinidine, sulfonamides, sulfonylureas, and thiazide diuretics as well as to external agents such as para-aminobenzoic acid (found in sunscreens), bithionol (used in soaps and cosmetics), paraphenylenediamine, and others.

Pigmentation

Drug-induced pigmentation on the skin, hair, nails, and mucous membranes is a result of either melanin synthesis, increased lipofuscin synthesis, or post-inflammatory pigmentation.

Color changes, which can be localized or widespread, can also be a result of a deposition of bile pigments (jaundice), exogenous metal compounds, and direct deposition of elements such as carotene or quinacrine.

Post-inflammatory pigmentation can follow a variety of drug-induced inflammatory cutaneous reactions; fixed eruptions are known to leave a residual pigmentation that can persist for months.

The following is a partial list of those drugs that can cause various pigmentary changes: anticonvulsants, antimalarials, cytostatics, hormones, metals, tetracyclines, phenothiazine tranquilizers, psoralens and amiodarone.

Pityriasis rosea-like eruption

Pityriasis rosea, commonly mistaken for ringworm, is a unique disorder that usually begins as a single, large, round or oval pinkish patch known as the 'mother' or 'herald' patch. The most common sites for this solitary lesion are the chest, the back, or the abdomen. This is followed in about 2 weeks by a blossoming of small, flat, round or oval, scaly patches of similar color, each with a central collarette scale, usually distributed in a Christmas tree pattern over the trunk and, to a lesser degree, the extremities. This eruption seldom itches and usually limits itself to areas from the neck to the knees.

While the etiology of idiopathic pityriasis rosea is unknown, various medications have been reported to give rise to this disorder. These include: barbiturates, beta-blockers, bismuth, captopril, clonidine, gold, griseofulvin, isotretinoin, labetalol, meprobamate, metronidazole, penicillin, and tripelennamine.

In drug-induced pityriasis rosea, the 'herald patch' is usually absent, and the eruption will often not follow the classic pattern.

Pruritus

Generalized itching, without any visible signs, is one of the least common adverse reactions to drugs. More frequently than not, drug-induced itching – moderate or severe – is fairly generalized.

For most drugs it is not known in what way they elicit pruritus; some drugs can cause itching directly or indirectly through cholestasis. Pruritus may develop by different pathogenetic mechanisms: allergic, pseudoallergic (histamine release), neurogenic, by vasodilatation, cholestatic effect, and others.

A partial list of those drugs that can cause pruritus are as follows: aspirin, NSAIDs, penicillins, sulfonamides, chloroquine, ACE-inhibitors, amiodarone, nicotinic acid derivatives, lithium, bleomycin, tamoxifen, interferons, gold, penicillamine, methoxsalen and isotretinoin.

Pseudolymphoma

Pseudolymphoma is not a specific disease. It is an inflammatory response to various stimuli – known or unknown – that results in a lymphomatous-appearing, but benign, accumulation of inflammatory cells. It may resemble true lymphoma clinically and histologically. Localized, nodular pseudolymphomas typically mimic B-cell lymphoma.

The following drugs, among others, are known to occasion pseudolymphoma: alprazolam, carbamazepine, co-trimoxazole, gold, lamotrigine, lithium, methotrexate, etc.

Pseudoporphyria

Pseudoporphyria is an uncommon, reversible, photoinduced, cutaneous bullous disorder with clinical, histologic and immunofluorescent similarities to porphyria cutanea tarda but without the accompanying biochemical porphyrin abnormalities.

It is commonly seen as localized bullae and skin fragility on sun-exposed skin, often on the dorsum of the hands and fingers. While pseudoporphyria has been linked with numerous causes, including chronic renal failure, dialysis, and ultraviolet radiation, several medications, primarily naproxen and other nonsteroidal inflammatory drugs, have been reported to trigger this reaction pattern. Blue/gray eye color appears to be an independent risk factor for the development of pseudoporphyria.

Psoriasis

Many drugs, as a result of their pharmacological action, have been implicated in the precipitation or exacerbation of psoriasis or psoriasiform eruptions.

Psoriasis is a common, chronic, papulosquamous disorder of unknown etiology with characteristic histopathological features and many biochemical, physiological, and immunological abnormalities.

Drugs that can precipitate psoriasis are, among others, beta-blockers and lithium. Drugs that are reported to aggravate psoriasis are antimalarials, beta-blockers, lithium, NSAIDs, quinidine, and photosensitizing drugs. The effect and extent of these drug-induced psoriatic eruptions are dose-dependent.

Purpura

Purpura, a result of hemorrhage into the skin, can be divided into thrombocytopenic purpura and non-thrombocytopenic purpura (vascular purpura). Both thrombocytopenic and vascular purpura may be due to drugs, and most of the drugs producing purpura may do so by giving rise to vascular damage and thrombocytopenia. In both types of purpura, allergic or toxic (nonallergic) mechanisms may be involved.

Some drugs combine with platelets to form an antigen, stimulating formation of antibody to the platelet–drug combination. Thus, the drug appears to act as a hapten; subsequent antigen–antibody reaction causes platelet destruction leading to thrombocytopenia.

The purpuric lesions are usually more marked over the lower portions of the body, notably the legs and dorsal aspects of the feet in ambulatory patients.

Other drug-induced cutaneous reactions – erythema multiforme, erythema nodosum, fixed eruption, necrotizing vasculitis, and others – can have a prominent purpuric component.

A whole host of drugs can give rise to purpura, the most common being: NSAIDs, thiazide diuretics, phenothiazines, cytostatics, gold, penicillamine, hydantoins, thiouracils, and sulfonamides.

Raynaud's phenomenon

Raynaud's phenomenon is the paroxysmal, cold-induced constriction of small arteries and arterioles of the fingers and, less often, the toes.

Although estimates vary, recent surveys show that Raynaud's phenomenon may affect 5 to 10 percent of the general population in the United States. Occurring more frequently in women, Raynaud's phenomenon is characterized by blanching, pallor, and cyanosis. In severe cases, secondary changes may occur: thinning and ridging of the nails, telangiectases of the nail folds, and, in the later stages, sclerosis and atrophy of the digits.

Rhabdomyolysis

Rhabdomyolysis is the breakdown of muscle fibers, the result of skeletal muscle injury, that leads to the release of potentially toxic intracellular contents into the plasma. The causes are diverse: muscle trauma from vigorous exercise, electrolyte imbalance, extensive thermal burns, crush injuries, infections, various toxins and drugs, and a host of other factors.

Rhabdomyolysis can result from direct muscle injury by myotoxic drugs such as cocaine, heroin and alcohol. About 10–40% of patients with rhabdomyolysis develop acute renal failure.

The classic triad of symptoms of rhabdomyolysis is muscle pain, weakness and dark urine. Most frequently, the involved muscle groups are those of the back and lower calves. The primary diagnostic indicator of this syndrome is significantly elevated serum creatine phosphokinase.

Some of the drugs that have been reported to cause rhabdomyolysis are salicylates, amphotericin, quinine, statin drugs, SSRIs, theophylline, and amphetamines.

Stevens-Johnson syndrome

The Stevens-Johnson syndrome (erythema multiforme major), a severe and occasionally fatal variety of erythema multiforme, has an abrupt onset and is accompanied by any or all of the following: fever, myalgia, malaise, headache, arthralgia, ocular involvement, with occasional bullae and erosions covering less than 10% of the body surface. Painful stomatitis is an early and conspicuous symptom. Hemorrhagic bullae may appear over the lips, mouth and genital mucous membranes. Patients are often acutely ill with high fever. The course from eruption to the healing of the lesions may extend up to six weeks.

The following drugs have been most often associated with Stevens-Johnson syndrome: allopurinol, barbiturates, carbamazepine, estrogens/progestins, gold, lamotrigine, NSAIDs, penicillamine, phenytoin, sulfonamides, tetracycline, tolbutamide, and valproic acid.

Tinnitus

Tinnitus (from the Latin word to tinkle or ring like a bell) is the perception of sound—ringing, buzzing, hissing, humming, whistling, whining, roaring, or ticking, clicking, banging, beeping, pulsating—in the human ear, when none exists. It has also been described as a 'whooshing' sound, like wind or waves, 'crickets' or 'tree frogs' or 'locusts.' To some it's a chirping, clanging, sizzling, rumbling, or a dreadful shrieking noise. And it can be like rushing water, breaking glass or chain saws running. Nearly 40 million Americans suffer from this disorder.

There are more than 200 drugs listed in the Litt's Drug Eruption & Reaction Database that have been reported to trigger tinnitus, the more common being aspirin, quinine, aminoglycoside antibiotics, cytotoxic drugs, diuretics, and NSAIDs.

Toxic epidermal necrolysis (TEN)

Also known as Lyell's syndrome, toxic epidermal necrolysis is a rare, serious, acute exfoliative, bullous eruption of the skin and mucous membranes that usually develops as a reaction to diverse drugs. TEN can also be a result of a bacterial or viral infection and can develop after radiation therapy or vaccinations.

In the drug-induced form of TEN, a morbilliform eruption accompanied by large red, tender areas of the skin will develop shortly after the drug has been administered. This progresses rapidly to blistering, and a widespread exfoliation of the epidermis develops dramatically over a very short period accompanied by high fever. The hairy parts of the body are usually spared. The mucous membranes and eyes are often involved.

The clinical picture resembles an extensive second-degree burn; the patient is acutely ill. Fatigue, vomiting, diarrhea and angina are prodromal symptoms. In a few hours the condition becomes grave.

TEN is a medical emergency and unless the offending agent is discontinued immediately, the outcome may be fatal in the course of a few days.

Drugs that are the most common cause of TEN are: allopurinol, ampicillin, amoxicillin, carbamazepine, NSAIDs, phenobarbital, pentamidine, phenytoin (diphenylhydantoin), pyrazolons, and sulfonamides.

Urticaria

Urticaria induced by drugs is, after exanthems, the second most common type of drug reaction. Urticaria, or hives, is a vascular reaction of the skin characterized by pruritic, erythematous wheals. These welts – or wheals – caused by localized edema, can vary in size from one millimeter in diameter to large palm-sized swellings, favor the covered areas (trunk, buttocks, chest), and are, more often than not, generalized. Urticaria usually develops within 36 hours following the administration of the responsible drug. Individual lesions rarely persist for more than 24 hours.

Urticaria may be the only symptom of drug sensitivity, or it may be a concomitant or followed by the manifestations of serum sickness. Urticaria may be accompanied by angioedema of the lips or eyelids. It may, on rare occasions, progress to anaphylactoid reactions or to anaphylaxis.

The following are the most common causes of drug-induced urticaria: antibiotics, notably penicillin (more commonly following parenteral administration than by ingestion), barbiturates, captopril, levamisole, NSAIDs, quinine, rifampin, sulfonamides, thiopental, and vancomycin.

Vasculitis

Drug-induced cutaneous necrotizing vasculitis, a clinicopathologic process characterized by inflammation and necrosis of blood vessels, often presents with a variety of small, palpable purpuric lesions most frequently distributed over the lower extremities: urticaria-like lesions, small ulcerations, and occasional hemorrhagic vesicles and pustules. The basic process involves an immunologically mediated response to antigens that result in vessel wall damage.

Beginning as small macules and papules, they ultimately eventuate into purpuric lesions and, in the more severe cases, into hemorrhagic blisters and frank ulcerations. A polymorphonuclear infiltrate and fibrinoid changes in the small dermal vessels characterize the vasculitic reaction.

Drugs that are commonly associated with vasculitis are: ACE-inhibitors, amiodarone, ampicillin, cimetidine, coumadin, furosemide, hydantoins, hydralazine, NSAIDs, pyrazolons, quinidine, sulfonamides, thiazides, and thiouracils.

Vertigo

Vertigo, a specific type of dizziness, is a feeling of unsteadiness. It is the sensation of spinning or swaying while actually remaining stationary with respect to the surroundings. It is a result of either motion sickness, a viral infection of the organs of balance, low blood sugar, or medications. It is a symptom of multiple sclerosis, carbon monoxide poisoning, and Meniere's disease.

Vertigo is one of the most common health problems in adults. According to the National Institutes of Health, about 40% of people in the United States experience vertigo at least once during their lifetime. Prevalence is higher in women and increases with age.

Classes of drugs that have been reported to trigger vertigo include, aminoglycoside antibiotics, antihypertensives, diuretics, vasodilators, phenothiazines, tranquilizers, antidepressants, anticonvulsants, hypnotics, analgesics, alcohol, caffeine, and tobacco.

Xerostomia

Xerostomia is a dryness of the oral cavity that makes speaking, chewing and swallowing difficult. Some people also experience changes in taste and salivary gland enlargement. Lack of saliva may predispose one to oral infection, such as candidiasis, and increase the risk of dental caries.

Resulting from a partial or complete absence of saliva production, xerostomia can be caused by more than 400 generic drugs.

DRUGS THAT CAUSE IMPORTANT REACTIONS

Acanthosis nigricans
Amprenavir
Azathioprine
Diethylstilbestrol
Estrogens
Fusidic Acid
Heroin
Insulin
Mechlorethamine
Methsuximide
Methyltestosterone
Niacin
Niacinamide
Oral Contraceptives
Palifermin
Prednisolone
Prednisone
Somatropin
Thioridazine
Tryptophan

Acneform lesions
Acamprosate
Acyclovir
Adalimumab
Adapalene
Afatinib
Alosetron
Alprazolam
Aminolevulinic Acid
Androstenedione
Aprepitant
Aripiprazole
Atorvastatin
Azathioprine
Basiliximab
Bedaquiline
Belatacept
Betamethasone
Bevacizumab
Bexarotene
Bosutinib
Brimonidine
Budesonide
Bupropion
Buserelin
Buspirone
Cabergoline
Capecitabine
Carbamazepine
Ceritinib
Cetirizine
Cetuximab
Chloral Hydrate
Chlorotrianisene
Cidofovir
Ciprofloxacin
Cisplatin
Clobetasol
Clofazimine
Clomipramine
Cobimetinib
Crofelemer
Cyanocobalamin
Cyclophosphamide

Cyclosporine
Dabrafenib
Daclizumab
Dactinomycin
Danazol
Dantrolene
Dapsone
Dasatinib
Deflazacort
Demeclocycline
Dexamethasone
Dexlansoprazole
Diazepam
Diltiazem
Disulfiram
Doxycycline
Duloxetine
Durvalumab
Efalizumab
Eflornithine
Epoetin Alfa
Erlotinib
Erythromycin
Escitalopram
Esmolol
Esomeprazole
Estazolam
Estramustine
Estrogens
Eszopiclone
Etanercept
Ethionamide
Everolimus
Famotidine
Felbamate
Fenoprofen
Finasteride
Fluconazole
Fluorides
Fluorouracil
Fluoxetine
Fluoxymesterone
Fluvoxamine
Folic Acid
Follitropin Alfa/Beta
Fosphenytoin
Gabapentin
Ganciclovir
Gefitinib
Gemcitabine
Gestrinone
Glatiramer
Gold & Gold Compounds
Goserelin
Granulocyte Colony-
    Stimulating Factor (G-CSF)
Grepafloxacin
Halothane
Heroin
Histrelin
Hyaluronic Acid
Hydroquinone
Imatinib
Infliximab

Interferon Alfa
Interferon Beta
Ipilimumab
Irinotecan
Isoniazid
Isotretinoin
Ivacaftor
Ixazomib
Lamotrigine
Lansoprazole
Lapatinib
Leflunomide
Lenalidomide
Letrozole
Leucovorin
Levonorgestrel
Lisdexamfetamine
Lithium
Lopinavir
Maprotiline
MDMA
Medroxyprogesterone
Mephenytoin
Mesalamine
Methotrexate
Methoxsalen
Methyltestosterone
Minoxidil
Mometasone
Mycophenolate
Nabumetone
Nadolol
Nafarelin
Naltrexone
Nandrolone
Naratriptan
Necitumumab
Nefazodone
Nicotine
Nilotinib
Nimodipine
Nisoldipine
Nitrofurantoin
Nivolumab
Nizatidine
Olsalazine
Oral Contraceptives
Osimertinib
Oxcarbazepine
Paclitaxel
Panitumumab
Panobinostat
Pantoprazole
Paroxetine Hydrochloride
Pentostatin
Phenobarbital
Phenylbutazone
Phenytoin
Pimecrolimus
Ponatinib
Potassium Iodide
Prednisolone
Prednisone
Progestins

Propafenone
Propranolol
Propylthiouracil
Psoralens
Pyrazinamide
Pyridoxine
Quinidine
Quinine
Ramipril
Riboflavin
Rifampin
Rifapentine
Risperidone
Ritonavir
Rufinamide
Ruxolitinib
Saquinavir
Sertraline
Sibutramine
Simvastatin
Sirolimus
Smallpox Vaccine
Sodium Oxybate
Sorafenib
Sparfloxacin
Stanozolol
Sunitinib
Tacrine
Temsirolimus
Teriflunomide
Testosterone
Tetracycline
Tiagabine
Tibolone
Tizanidine
Topiramate
Trametinib
Trastuzumab
Tretinoin
Trioxsalen
Triptorelin
Ulipristal
Valdecoxib
Vandetanib
Vemurafenib
Venlafaxine
Verapamil
Vinblastine
Vinorelbine
Vorinostat
Zalcitabine
Zaleplon
Zidovudine
Zolpidem
Zonisamide

Acute febrile neutrophilic dermatosis
Abacavir
Aceclofenac
Aldesleukin
Allopurinol
Amoxapine
Azacitidine
Azathioprine

BCG Vaccine
Bortezomib
Celecoxib
Chloroquine
Ciprofloxacin
Citalopram
Clindamycin
Clofazimine
Clozapine
Co-Trimoxazole
Cytarabine
Dasatinib
Diazepam
Doxycycline
Esomeprazole
Furosemide
Glucagon
Granulocyte Colony-
   Stimulating Factor (G-CSF)
Hydralazine
Imatinib
Infliximab
Influenza Vaccine
Ipilimumab
Isotretinoin
Ixazomib
Lenalidomide
Minocycline
Mitoxantrone
Nilotinib
Nitrofurantoin
Nivolumab
Norfloxacin
Ofloxacin
Omeprazole
Oral Contraceptives
Pandemic Influenza Vaccine
   (HINI)
PEG-Interferon
Perphenazine
Phenylbutazone
Pneumococcal Vaccine
Propylthiouracil
Quinupristin/Dalfopristin
Ribavirin
Sulfamethoxazole
Sulfasalazine
Ticagrelor
Tretinoin
Verapamil
Vorinostat

Acute generalized
exanthematous pustulosis
Acarbose
Acetaminophen
Acetazolamide
Aldesleukin
Allopurinol
Amoxapine
Amoxicillin
Amphotericin B
Ampicillin
Aspirin
Atovaquone/Proguanil
Azathioprine
Azithromycin
Bacampicillin
Bendamustine
Benznidazole
Bupropion
Carbamazepine

Carbimazole
Cefaclor
Cefazolin
Cefepime
Cefotaxime
Ceftazidime
Ceftriaxone
Cefuroxime
Celecoxib
Cephalexin
Cephradine
Cetirizine
Chloramphenicol
Chloroquine
Chlorzoxazone
Ciprofloxacin
Clindamycin
Clopidogrel
Cloxacillin
Clozapine
Co-Trimoxazole
Codeine
Cytarabine
Dalteparin
Dapsone
Daptomycin
Dexamethasone
Dextromethorphan
Dihydrocodeine
Diltiazem
Diphenhydramine
Docetaxel
Doripenem
Doxycycline
Enzalutamide
Epoetin Alfa
Erlotinib
Ertapenem
Erythromycin
Etanercept
Etodolac
Famotidine
Fenofibrate
Fexofenadine
Finasteride
Flucloxacillin
Fluconazole
Furosemide
Galantamine
Gefitinib
Hydrochlorothiazide
Hydroxychloroquine
Hydroxyzine
Ibuprofen
Icodextrin
Imatinib
Imipenem/Cilastatin
Immune Globulin IV
Infliximab
Influenza Vaccine
Iodixanol
Iohexol
Ioversol
Isoniazid
Isotretinoin
Itraconazole
Ketoconazole
Lamivudine
Lamotrigine
Lansoprazole
Levetiracetam

Levofloxacin
Lincomycin
Lindane
Lopinavir
Meloxicam
Meropenem
Metamizole
Methimazole
Methoxsalen
Methylphenidate
Methylprednisolone
Metronidazole
Mexiletine
Midodrine
Mifepristone
Minocycline
Morphine
Moxifloxacin
Naltrexone
Nifedipine
Nimesulide
Nivolumab
Nystatin
Olanzapine
Omeprazole
Pemetrexed
Phenobarbital
Phenytoin
Piperacillin/Tazobactam
Piroxicam
Prednisolone
Pristinamycin
Progestins
Propafenone
Propoxyphene
Pseudoephedrine
Pyrazinamide
Pyrimethamine
Quetiapine
Quinidine
Ranibizumab
Ranitidine
Ranolazine
Rifabutin
Rifampin
Ritodrine
Rivaroxaban
Sertraline
Simvastatin
Sorafenib
Streptomycin
Sulfamethoxazole
Sulfasalazine
Teicoplanin
Telavancin
Terazosin
Terbinafine
Tetrazepam
Thalidomide
Thallium
Ticlopidine
Tigecycline
Tocilizumab
Valdecoxib
Valproic Acid
Vancomycin
Varenicline
Vemurafenib
Zidovudine

Ageusia
Acarbose

Aspirin
Atorvastatin
Azelastine
Betaxolol
Candesartan
Captopril
Carbamazepine
Cetirizine
Chlorhexidine
Clindamycin
Clopidogrel
Cocaine
Cyclobenzaprine
Doxorubicin
Enalapril
Eslicarbazepine
Etidronate
Fluoxetine
Fluvoxamine
Fosinopril
Grepafloxacin
Hydroxychloroquine
Indomethacin
Interferon Alfa
Isotretinoin
Losartan
Methimazole
Nefazodone
Nitroglycerin
Paroxetine Hydrochloride
Penicillamine
Phenylbutazone
Phenytoin
Propofol
Propylthiouracil
Ramipril
Rifabutin
Rifaximin
Rimantadine
Ritonavir
Rivastigmine
Sonidegib
Sulindac
Terbinafine
Tiagabine
Tiopronin
Topiramate
Valrubicin
Venlafaxine
Vismodegib
Voriconazole
Zalcitabine

Alopecia
Abemaciclib
Acetohexamide
Acitretin
Acyclovir
Adalimumab
Ado-Trastuzumab Emtansine
Afatinib
Aflibercept
Albendazole
Aldesleukin
Alectinib
Alitretinoin
Allopurinol
Altretamine
Amantadine
Amiloride
Aminolevulinic Acid
Aminosalicylate Sodium

Amiodarone
Amitriptyline
Amlodipine
Amoxapine
Anagrelide
Anastrozole
Androstenedione
Anidulafungin
Aprepitant
Arsenic
Aspirin
Astemizole
Atenolol
Atorvastatin
Atovaquone/Proguanil
Atropine Sulfate
Axitinib
Azathioprine
Belatacept
Belinostat
Bendamustine
Benznidazole
Betamethasone
Betaxolol
Bevacizumab
Bexarotene
Bezafibrate
Bicalutamide
Bismuth
Bleomycin
Botulinum Toxin (A & B)
Brentuximab Vedotin
Brinzolamide
Bromocriptine
Budesonide
Bupropion
Buspirone
Busulfan
Cabazitaxel
Cabergoline
Cabozantinib
Calcipotriol
Capecitabine
Captopril
Carbamazepine
Carboplatin
Carmustine
Carvedilol
Celecoxib
Certolizumab
Cetirizine
Cetuximab
Cevimeline
Chlorambucil
Chloramphenicol
Chlordiazepoxide
Chlorpropamide
Cidofovir
Cimetidine
Cisplatin
Citalopram
Clarithromycin
Clofibrate
Clomiphene
Clomipramine
Clonazepam
Clonidine
Cobimetinib
Colchicine
Crizotinib
Cyclophosphamide

Cyclosporine
Cytarabine
Dabrafenib
Dacarbazine
Daclatasvir
Daclizumab
Dactinomycin
Dalteparin
Danazol
Dasatinib
Daunorubicin
Decitabine
Deferasirox
Deflazacort
Degarelix
Delavirdine
Desipramine
Dexamethasone
Diazoxide
Diclofenac
Dicumarol
Didanosine
Diethylpropion
Diflunisal
Diltiazem
Dimethyl Fumarate
Docetaxel
Donepezil
Doxazosin
Doxepin
Doxorubicin
Duloxetine
Eculizumab
Efavirenz
Eflornithine
Eltrombopag
Enalapril
Enoxaparin
Entecavir
Epinephrine
Epirubicin
Epoetin Alfa
Eribulin
Erlotinib
Erythromycin
Escitalopram
Eslicarbazepine
Estramustine
Estrogens
Eszopiclone
Etanercept
Ethambutol
Ethionamide
Etoposide
Everolimus
Evolocumab
Exemestane
Febuxostat
Fenofibrate
Fenoprofen
Fingolimod
Flecainide
Fluconazole
Fludarabine
Fluorouracil
Fluoxetine
Fluoxymesterone
Flurbiprofen
Fluvoxamine
Foscarnet
Fulvestrant

Gabapentin
Gadodiamide
Ganciclovir
Gefitinib
Gemcitabine
Gentamicin
Glatiramer
Gold & Gold Compounds
Goserelin
Granisetron
Granulocyte Colony-
    Stimulating Factor (G-CSF)
Grepafloxacin
Haloperidol
Halothane
Heparin
Hepatitis B Vaccine
Human Papillomavirus Vaccine
    (Bivalent)
Hydroxychloroquine
Hydroxyurea
Hyoscyamine
Ibandronate
Ibritumomab
Ibuprofen
Idarubicin
Ifosfamide
Imatinib
Imipramine
Imiquimod
Immune Globulin IV
Indinavir
Indomethacin
Infliximab
Interferon Alfa
Interferon Beta
Ipilimumab
Ipratropium
Irinotecan
Isavuconazonium Sulfate
Isoniazid
Isotretinoin
Itraconazole
Ixabepilone
Ixazomib
Ketoconazole
Ketoprofen
Ketorolac
Labetalol
Lamivudine
Lamotrigine
Lanreotide
Lansoprazole
Lapatinib
Leflunomide
Lenvatinib
Letrozole
Leucovorin
Leuprolide
Levamisole
Levobetaxolol
Levobunolol
Levodopa
Levothyroxine
Liothyronine
Lisinopril
Lithium
Lomustine
Lopinavir
Loratadine
Losartan

Lovastatin
Maprotiline
Mebendazole
Mechlorethamine
Meclofenamate
Medroxyprogesterone
Mefloquine
Meloxicam
Melphalan
Memantine
Mercaptopurine
Mesalamine
Metformin
Methimazole
Methotrexate
Methyltestosterone
Methysergide
Metoprolol
Mexiletine
Minocycline
Minoxidil
Mirtazapine
Mitomycin
Mitotane
Mitoxantrone
Mizoribine
Moexipril
Mycophenolate
Nabumetone
Nadolol
Nalidixic Acid
Naltrexone
Naproxen
Naratriptan
Nefazodone
Neratinib
Nifedipine
Nilotinib
Nimodipine
Nintedanib
Nisoldipine
Nitisinone
Nitrofurantoin
Nivolumab
Nortriptyline
Octreotide
Olanzapine
Olaparib
Olaratumab
Omacetaxine
Omalizumab
Omeprazole
Oral Contraceptives
Oxaliplatin
Oxerutins
Paclitaxel
Palbociclib
Panitumumab
Panobinostat
Pantoprazole
Paricalcitol
Paroxetine Hydrochloride
Pasireotide
Pazopanib
PEG-Interferon
Pegvisomant
Pembrolizumab
Pemetrexed
Penicillamine
Pentosan
Pentostatin

Peplomycin
Pergolide
Pertuzumab
Phentermine
Phenytoin
Piroxicam
Pramipexole
Prazosin
Prednisolone
Prednisone
Procarbazine
Propafenone
Propranolol
Propylthiouracil
Protriptyline
Pyridostigmine
Quetiapine
Quinacrine
Quinapril
Quinidine
Rabeprazole
Raltitrexed
Ramipril
Regorafenib
Ribavirin
Ribociclib
Riluzole
Risperidone
Ritonavir
Rituximab
Rivastigmine
Rofecoxib
Ropinirole
Rucaparib
Selenium
Sertraline
Sodium Oxybate
Sonidegib
Sorafenib
Sotalol
Sparfloxacin
Spinosad
Spironolactone
Strontium Ranelate
Sulfasalazine
Sulfisoxazole
Sulindac
Sunitinib
Tacrine
Tacrolimus
Tamoxifen
Tegafur/Gimeracil/Oteracil
Temozolomide
Temsirolimus
Teniposide
Terbinafine
Terfenadine
Teriflunomide
Testosterone
Thalidomide
Thallium
Thioguanine
Thiotepa
Tiagabine
Timolol
Tinzaparin
Tiopronin
Tizanidine
Tocainide
Tolcapone
Topiramate

Topotecan
Trabectedin
Trametinib
Trastuzumab
Trazodone
Trifluridine & Tipiracil
Trimethadione
Trimipramine
Triptorelin
Ursodiol
Valdecoxib
Valproic Acid
Vandetanib
Vasopressin
Vemurafenib
Venlafaxine
Verapamil
Vinblastine
Vincristine
Vinorelbine
Vismodegib
Vitamin A
Voriconazole
Vorinostat
Warfarin
Zaleplon
Zidovudine
Ziprasidone
Zoledronate
Zonisamide
Zoster Vaccine

Angioedema

Acetaminophen
Acetylcysteine
Acitretin
Acyclovir
Adalimumab
Albendazole
Aldesleukin
Alefacept
Alemtuzumab
Alendronate
Aliskiren
Allopurinol
Alogliptin
Alprazolam
Alteplase
Aminoglutethimide
Aminosalicylate Sodium
Amiodarone
Amitriptyline
Amlodipine
Amodiaquine
Amoxicillin
Ampicillin
Ampicillin/Sulbactam
Anidulafungin
Anthrax Vaccine
Ascorbic Acid
Asenapine
Asparaginase
Aspartame
Aspirin
Atorvastatin
Atracurium
Azatadine
Azathioprine
Azithromycin
Aztreonam
Benazepril
Benznidazole

Bevacizumab
Bezafibrate
Bismuth
Bleomycin
Brivaracetam
Brompheniramine
Budesonide
Bupropion
Butabarbital
Canagliflozin
Candesartan
Captopril
Carbamazepine
Carisoprodol
Carvedilol
Cefaclor
Cefadroxil
Cefixime
Cefoxitin
Cefprozil
Ceftazidime
Ceftriaxone
Cefuroxime
Celecoxib
Cephalexin
Certolizumab
Cetirizine
Chloral Hydrate
Chlorambucil
Chloramphenicol
Chlordiazepoxide
Chloroquine
Chlorpheniramine
Chlorpromazine
Chlorpropamide
Chlorthalidone
Chlorzoxazone
Cilazapril
Cimetidine
Cinoxacin
Ciprofloxacin
Cisplatin
Clarithromycin
Clemastine
Clonazepam
Clonidine
Clopidogrel
Cloxacillin
Clozapine
Co-Trimoxazole
Cocaine
Codeine
Cromolyn
Cyanocobalamin
Cyclamate
Cyclobenzaprine
Cyclophosphamide
Cyclosporine
Cyproheptadine
Dacarbazine
Danazol
Darunavir
Dasabuvir/Ombitasvir/
   Paritaprevir/Ritonavir
Daunorubicin
Deferoxamine
Deflazacort
Delavirdine
Desipramine
Dexchlorpheniramine
Diazepam

Diclofenac
Dicumarol
Diethylstilbestrol
Diflunisal
Dihydrocodeine
Diltiazem
Dimenhydrinate
Diphenhydramine
Dipyridamole
Disulfiram
Dofetilide
Doxazosin
Doxorubicin
Doxycycline
Dronedarone
Droperidol
Dutasteride
Efalizumab
Enalapril
Enoxaparin
Epoetin Alfa
Erythromycin
Esomeprazole
Estramustine
Estrogens
Etanercept
Ethambutol
Etidronate
Etodolac
Etomidate
Etoricoxib
Everolimus
Ezetimibe
Famotidine
Febuxostat
Felodipine
Fenoprofen
Fentanyl
Fluconazole
Fluorouracil
Fluoxetine
Fluphenazine
Flurbiprofen
Fluvoxamine
Fosinopril
Fulvestrant
Glatiramer
Glucagon
Gold & Gold Compounds
Griseofulvin
Haloperidol
Halothane
Heparin
Hepatitis B Vaccine
Heroin
Histrelin
Hyaluronic Acid
Hydralazine
Hydrochlorothiazide
Hydrocortisone
Hydromorphone
Hydroxychloroquine
Hydroxyzine
Ibritumomab
Ibuprofen
Icatibant
Iloperidone
Imidapril
Imiglucerase
Imipenem/Cilastatin
Imipramine

Imiquimod
Indapamide
Indomethacin
Infliximab
Insulin
Interferon Alfa
Iodixanol
Iothalamate
Irbesartan
Isoniazid
Isotretinoin
Itraconazole
Ivacaftor
Ivermectin
Ixekizumab
Ketoconazole
Ketoprofen
Ketorolac
Labetalol
Lacosamide
Lamivudine
Lamotrigine
Ledipasvir & Sofosbuvir
Lepirudin
Levamisole
Levofloxacin
Levothyroxine
Lidocaine
Linezolid
Lisinopril
Lithium
Lixisenatide
Loratadine
Losartan
Lurasidone
MDMA
Mebendazole
Mebeverine
Mechlorethamine
Meclizine
Meclofenamate
Mefenamic Acid
Meloxicam
Melphalan
Meperidine
Mephenytoin
Mephobarbital
Mepivacaine
Meprobamate
Mesna
Metformin
Methohexital
Methotrexate
Methylphenidate
Metoclopramide
Metoprolol
Metronidazole
Miconazole
Midazolam
Minocycline
Mirtazapine
Mitotane
Moexipril
Montelukast
Nabumetone
Nalidixic Acid
Naloxone
Naproxen
Neomycin
Nevirapine
Nicardipine

Nifedipine
Nimesulide
Nitrofurantoin
Ofloxacin
Olanzapine
Olmesartan
Omalizumab
Omeprazole
Oral Contraceptives
Oritavancin
Oxaliplatin
Oxaprozin
Paclitaxel
Pamidronate
Panitumumab
Pantoprazole
Paroxetine Hydrochloride
PEG-Interferon
Pegaptanib
Pegaspargase
Penicillin G
Penicillin V
Pentagastrin
Pentobarbital
Pentoxifylline
Perflutren
Perindopril
Phenelzine
Phenobarbital
Phenolphthalein
Phenylbutazone
Phenytoin
Pioglitazone
Piroxicam
Potassium Iodide
Prasugrel
Praziquantel
Prazosin
Prilocaine
Primaquine
Pristinamycin
Procainamide
Procarbazine
Progestins
Promethazine
Propafenone
Propofol
Propranolol
Propylthiouracil
Protamine Sulfate
Pseudoephedrine
Pyrimethamine
Quinapril
Quinestrol
Quinidine
Quinine
Ramipril
Ranitidine
Riboflavin
Rifampin
Risperidone
Rituximab
Rofecoxib
Ropinirole
Sacubitril/Valsartan
Saxagliptin
Secobarbital
Sertraline
Sirolimus
Sitagliptin
Sorafenib

Sparfloxacin
Streptokinase
Streptomycin
Sulfadoxine
Sulfamethoxazole
Sulfasalazine
Sulfisoxazole
Sulindac
Sumatriptan
Tacrolimus
Tartrazine
Telithromycin
Telmisartan
Tenecteplase
Terbinafine
Terfenadine
Teriflunomide
Tetracycline
Thiamine
Thiopental
Thioridazine
Thiotepa
Ticlopidine
Tinidazole
Tiopronin
Tiotropium
Tocilizumab
Tolmetin
Tositumomab & Iodine[131]
Tosufloxacin
Tramadol
Trandolapril
Trastuzumab
Trazodone
Trifluoperazine
Trimeprazine
Trimetrexate
Tripelennamine
Triprolidine
Triptorelin
Troleandomycin
Trospium
Trovafloxacin
Urokinase
Valsartan
Vancomycin
Vardenafil
Vedolizumab
Venlafaxine
Verapamil
Vildagliptin
Vinblastine
Vincristine
Voriconazole
Vorinostat
Warfarin
Yellow Fever Vaccine
Zalcitabine
Zidovudine
Ziprasidone
Zofenopril

Anosmia
Amikacin
Aspirin
Cocaine
Dorzolamide
Doxycycline
Enalapril
Interferon Alfa
Levodopa
Methazolamide

Methoxsalen
Midodrine
Nifedipine
Propofol
Pyrazinamide
Terbinafine
Uracil/Tegafur
Zinc
Aphthous stomatitis
Afatinib
Aldesleukin
Amodiaquine
Amoxicillin
Anagrelide
Artesunate
Asparaginase
Aspirin
Azathioprine
Azelastine
Aztreonam
Belatacept
Benznidazole
Bupropion
Candesartan
Captopril
Cefaclor
Certolizumab
Cetuximab
Cisplatin
Co-Trimoxazole
Cyclophosphamide
Cyclosporine
Delavirdine
Diclofenac
Docetaxel
Doxepin
Doxorubicin
Epirubicin
Erlotinib
Everolimus
Exemestane
Fenoprofen
Fluorides
Fluorouracil
Fluoxetine
Gold & Gold Compounds
Hepatitis B Vaccine
Imatinib
Imiquimod
Indinavir
Interferon Alfa
Ipilimumab
Ketorolac
Labetalol
Ledipasvir & Sofosbuvir
Lenvatinib
Losartan
Methotrexate
Mycophenolate
Naproxen
Nicorandil
Olanzapine
Omacetaxine
Orlistat
Paclitaxel
Pantoprazole
Paroxetine Hydrochloride
Pemetrexed
Penicillamine
Piroxicam
Prednisone

Pyrimethamine
Rifabutin
Rofecoxib
Sertraline
Siltuximab
Sirolimus
Sorafenib
Sulfadoxine
Sulfamethoxazole
Sulfasalazine
Sulfisoxazole
Tegafur/Gimeracil/Oteracil
Temsirolimus
Tocilizumab
Tosufloxacin
Trametinib
Valsartan
Vedolizumab
Zalcitabine

Baboon syndrome (SDRIFE)
Acetaminophen
Allopurinol
Aminophylline
Amoxicillin
Ampicillin
Aspirin
Betamethasone
Cefadroxil
Cefuroxime
Celecoxib
Cephalexin
Cetuximab
Cimetidine
Cisplatin
Clarithromycin
Cloxacillin
Clozapine
Erythromycin
Everolimus
Fluorouracil
Gemcitabine
Heparin
Hydrochlorothiazide
Hydroxyurea
Immune Globulin IV
Infliximab
Iomeprol
Iopromide
Mesalamine
Mitomycin
Naproxen
Nystatin
Omeprazole
Oral Contraceptives
Oxycodone
Penicillin V
Pseudoephedrine
Ranitidine
Risperidone
Rivastigmine
Roxithromycin
Telmisartan
Terbinafine

Black tongue (lingua villosa nigra)
Amoxicillin
Benztropine
Ceftriaxone
Chloramphenicol
Clarithromycin
Clonazepam

Co-Trimoxazole
Cocaine
Doxycycline
Fluoxetine
Griseofulvin
Lansoprazole
Linezolid
Methyldopa
Minocycline
Nicotine
Nortriptyline
Olanzapine
Oxytetracycline
PEG-Interferon
Ribavirin
Streptomycin
Sulfamethoxazole
Tetracycline
Thiothixene

Bullous dermatitis
Acetazolamide
Acitretin
Afatinib
Aldesleukin
Alemtuzumab
Amifostine
Aminocaproic Acid
Aminophylline
Aminosalicylate Sodium
Amitriptyline
Ampicillin
Anthrax Vaccine
Argatroban
Arsenic
Aspirin
Atropine Sulfate
Bleomycin
Bumetanide
Buspirone
Busulfan
Butabarbital
Butalbital
Captopril
Carbamazepine
Celecoxib
Cetirizine
Cevimeline
Chloral Hydrate
Chloramphenicol
Chlorpromazine
Chlorpropamide
Ciprofloxacin
Clonazepam
Clopidogrel
Co-Trimoxazole
Cocaine
Codeine
Colchicine
Cyanocobalamin
Cyclamate
Cyclosporine
Cytarabine
Dalteparin
Dapsone
Desoximetasone
Dextromethorphan
Diazepam
Diclofenac
Dicumarol
Diethylstilbestrol
Diflunisal

Digoxin
Disulfiram
Enoxaparin
Entacapone
Ephedrine
Erlotinib
Estrogens
Ethambutol
Ethchlorvynol
Felbamate
Fluconazole
Fluorouracil
Fluoxetine
Fluvoxamine
Fondaparinux
Fosphenytoin
Frovatriptan
Furosemide
Ganciclovir
Gemcitabine
Glyburide
Gold & Gold Compounds
Griseofulvin
Heparin
Hydralazine
Hydrochlorothiazide
Hydroxychloroquine
Ibuprofen
Ibutilide
Imipramine
Imiquimod
Indomethacin
Infliximab
Influenza Vaccine
Insulin
Interferon Alfa
Isoniazid
Ivermectin
Ketoprofen
Lamotrigine
Leflunomide
Lindane
Lisinopril
Lithium
Lomefloxacin
Mechlorethamine
Meloxicam
Mephenytoin
Meprobamate
Methicillin
Methotrexate
Methoxsalen
Miconazole
Minoxidil
Mitomycin
Mometasone
Moxifloxacin
Mycophenolate
Nabumetone
Nalidixic Acid
Naproxen
Nifedipine
Norfloxacin
Omeprazole
Oral Contraceptives
Oxacillin
Penicillamine
Pentamidine
Pentobarbital
Pentostatin
Phenobarbital

Phenolphthalein
Phenytoin
Piroxicam
Prednicarbate
Promethazine
Propranolol
Propyphenazone
Pyridoxine
Pyrimethamine
Quinethazone
Reserpine
Rifampin
Risperidone
Ritonavir
Rituximab
Rivastigmine
Rofecoxib
Sertraline
Smallpox Vaccine
Sparfloxacin
Streptomycin
Sulfadoxine
Sulfamethoxazole
Sulfisoxazole
Sunitinib
Temazepam
Tetracycline
Thalidomide
Thiopental
Tinzaparin
Tolbutamide
Tranexamic Acid
Tretinoin
Trioxsalen
Urokinase
Ustekinumab
Valproic Acid
Vancomycin
Vasopressin
Vinblastine
Warfarin
Zalcitabine
Zidovudine
Zolpidem

DRESS syndrome
Abacavir
Acenocoumarol
Acetaminophen
Allopurinol
Amikacin
Amitriptyline
Amoxicillin
Ampicillin
Anakinra
Aspirin
Atenolol
Atorvastatin
Azithromycin
Benznidazole
Boceprevir
Bosentan
Bupropion
Canakinumab
Captopril
Carbamazepine
Cefadroxil
Cefixime
Cefotaxime
Ceftriaxone
Celecoxib
Chlorambucil

Cidofovir
Cilostazol
Ciprofloxacin
Clindamycin
Clomipramine
Clonazepam
Clopidogrel
Co-Trimoxazole
Codeine
Cyclobenzaprine
Cycloserine
Daclatasvir
Dapsone
Darunavir
Dextromethorphan
Diclofenac
Doxycycline
Efalizumab
Efavirenz
Emtricitabine
Erlotinib
Esomeprazole
Ethambutol
Febuxostat
Fenofibrate
Fluoxetine
Hydroxychloroquine
Ibuprofen
Imatinib
Ipilimumab
Isoniazid
Lamotrigine
Leflunomide
Lenalidomide
Leucovorin
Levetiracetam
Linezolid
Lithium
Metamizole
Metformin
Methimazole
Minocycline
Mitoxantrone
Moxifloxacin
Naproxen
Nelfinavir
Nevirapine
Nitrofurantoin
Olanzapine
Oxazepam
Oxcarbazepine
Pandemic Influenza Vaccine
    (HINI)
PEG-Interferon
Penicillin V
Perampanel
Phenobarbital
Phenylbutazone
Phenytoin
Piperacillin/Tazobactam
Piroxicam
Promethazine
Propylthiouracil
Pyrazinamide
Pyrimethamine
Quinine
Raltegravir
Ramipril
Ribavirin
Rifampin
Ritonavir

Rivaroxaban
Sorafenib
Spironolactone
Streptomycin
Strontium Ranelate
Sulfadiazine
Sulfamethoxazole
Sulfasalazine
Teicoplanin
Telaprevir
Tenofovir Disoproxil
Tenoxicam
Terbinafine
Teriflunomide
Thiamine
Tocilizumab
Torsemide
Trimethoprim
Valproic Acid
Vancomycin
Vemurafenib
Ziprasidone
Zonisamide

Erythema multiforme
Acamprosate
Acarbose
Acebutolol
Acetaminophen
Acetazolamide
Adalimumab
Aldesleukin
Alectinib
Alendronate
Allopurinol
Amifostine
Aminosalicylate Sodium
Amiodarone
Amlodipine
Amoxicillin
Amphotericin B
Ampicillin
Anthrax Vaccine
Arsenic
Aspirin
Atovaquone/Proguanil
Atropine Sulfate
Avelumab
Azathioprine
Aztreonam
Benznidazole
Bezafibrate
Bortezomib
Bosutinib
Bumetanide
Bupropion
Busulfan
Butabarbital
Butalbital
Candesartan
Carbamazepine
Carisoprodol
Cefaclor
Cefadroxil
Cefamandole
Cefixime
Cefotaxime
Cefpodoxime
Cefprozil
Ceftazidime
Ceftriaxone
Cefuroxime

Celecoxib
Cephalexin
Cephalothin
Chloral Hydrate
Chlorambucil
Chloramphenicol
Chlordiazepoxide
Chloroquine
Chlorpromazine
Chlorpropamide
Chlorzoxazone
Cimetidine
Ciprofloxacin
Cisplatin
Clindamycin
Clofibrate
Clonazepam
Clozapine
Co-Trimoxazole
Codeine
Collagen (Bovine)
Crizotinib
Cyclobenzaprine
Cyclophosphamide
Danazol
Dapsone
Delavirdine
Desoximetasone
Dexamethasone
Diclofenac
Dicloxacillin
Didanosine
Diflunisal
Dihydrocodeine
Diltiazem
Dimenhydrinate
Docetaxel
Dorzolamide
Doxycycline
Durvalumab
Elotuzumab
Enalapril
Enoxacin
Enoxaparin
Erythromycin
Estrogens
Ethambutol
Ethosuximide
Etodolac
Etoposide
Etoricoxib
Famotidine
Fenbufen
Fenoprofen
Flucloxacillin
Fluconazole
Fluorouracil
Fluoxetine
Flurbiprofen
Fosphenytoin
Furazolidone
Furosemide
Gadoversetamide
Gemfibrozil
Glucagon
Glyburide
Gold & Gold Compounds
Griseofulvin
Hepatitis B Vaccine
Human Papillomavirus (HPV)
    Vaccine

Hyaluronic Acid
Hydrochlorothiazide
Hydroxychloroquine
Hydroxyurea
Hydroxyzine
Ibuprofen
Icodextrin
Imatinib
Imipenem/Cilastatin
Imiquimod
Indapamide
Indomethacin
Infliximab
Interferon Beta
Iomeprol
Ipilimumab
Isoniazid
Isotretinoin
Ixazomib
Ketoprofen
Lamotrigine
Lansoprazole
Leflunomide
Lenalidomide
Levamisole
Levetiracetam
Levofloxacin
Lidocaine
Lithium
Loracarbef
Loratadine
Lorazepam
Maprotiline
Mechlorethamine
Meclofenamate
Mefenamic Acid
Meloxicam
Mephenytoin
Meprobamate
Metamizole
Methenamine
Methicillin
Methotrexate
Methyldopa
Minocycline
Minoxidil
Misoprostol
Mitomycin
Mitotane
Nabumetone
Nalidixic Acid
Naproxen
Neomycin
Nifedipine
Nilotinib
Nitrofurantoin
Nitroglycerin
Nivolumab
Nystatin
Ombitasvir/Paritaprevir/
    Ritonavir
Omeprazole
Oral Contraceptives
Oritavancin
Oxaprozin
Oxazepam
Oxybutynin
Paclitaxel
Pancreatin
Pandemic Influenza Vaccine
    (HINI)

Pantoprazole
Paramethadione
Pembrolizumab
Pemetrexed
Penicillamine
Pentobarbital
Permethrin
Phenobarbital
Phenolphthalein
Phensuximide
Phenylbutazone
Phenytoin
Piroxicam
Pneumococcal Vaccine
Pravastatin
Prednicarbate
Prednisolone
Primidone
Probenecid
Progestins
Promethazine
Propranolol
Pseudoephedrine
Pyrazinamide
Pyrimethamine
Quetiapine
Quinidine
Quinine
Ramipril
Regorafenib
Ribavirin
Rifampin
Ritodrine
Roxatidine
Saquinavir
Scopolamine
Sertraline
Simvastatin
Smallpox Vaccine
Sorafenib
Spironolactone
Streptomycin
Sulfacetamide
Sulfadiazine
Sulfadoxine
Sulfamethoxazole
Sulfasalazine
Sulfisoxazole
Sulindac
Tamsulosin
Telithromycin
Telmisartan
Terbinafine
Tetracycline
Tetrazepam
Thalidomide
Thiabendazole
Thiopental
Thioridazine
Ticlopidine
Tiopronin
Tobramycin
Tocainide
Tolbutamide
Tolcapone
Tolmetin
Trazodone
Trihexyphenidyl
Trimethadione
Valproic Acid
Vancomycin

Vandetanib
Vemurafenib
Verapamil
Vinblastine
Vitamin A
Vitamin E
Voriconazole
Zalcitabine
Zidovudine

Erythema nodosum
Abatacept
Acetaminophen
Acyclovir
Aldesleukin
Amiodarone
Anastrozole
Arsenic
Aspartame
Aspirin
Azathioprine
Benznidazole
Busulfan
Carbamazepine
Carbimazole
Certolizumab
Chlordiazepoxide
Chlorpropamide
Ciprofloxacin
Clomiphene
Co-Trimoxazole
Codeine
Colchicine
Dapsone
Dasatinib
Diclofenac
Disopyramide
Estrogens
Etanercept
Fluoxetine
Furosemide
Glucagon
Gold & Gold Compounds
Granulocyte Colony-
    Stimulating Factor (G-CSF)
Hepatitis B Vaccine
Human Papillomavirus (HPV)
    Vaccine
Hydralazine
Hydroxychloroquine
Ibuprofen
Imatinib
Indomethacin
Interferon Alfa
Isotretinoin
Ixazomib
Levofloxacin
Lidocaine
Meclofenamate
Medroxyprogesterone
Meprobamate
Metamizole
Methyldopa
Minocycline
Montelukast
Naproxen
Nifedipine
Nitrofurantoin
Omeprazole
Oral Contraceptives
Paroxetine Hydrochloride
Penicillamine

Ponatinib
Propylthiouracil
Quinacrine
Smallpox Vaccine
Streptomycin
Sulfamethoxazole
Sulfasalazine
Sulfisoxazole
Terbinafine
Thalidomide
Ticlopidine
Tretinoin
Trimethoprim
Verapamil
Zileuton

Exanthems
Abacavir
Acamprosate
Acebutolol
Acenocoumarol
Acetaminophen
Acetazolamide
Acetohexamide
Acitretin
Acyclovir
Aldesleukin
Allopurinol
Alprazolam
Amantadine
Amcinonide
Amikacin
Amiloride
Aminocaproic Acid
Aminoglutethimide
Aminophylline
Aminosalicylate Sodium
Amiodarone
Amlodipine
Amoxapine
Amoxicillin
Amphotericin B
Ampicillin
Amprenavir
Anastrozole
Anidulafungin
Anistreplase
Anthrax Vaccine
Aprotinin
Arsenic
Aspartame
Aspirin
Astemizole
Atazanavir
Atovaquone
Atovaquone/Proguanil
Azacitidine
Azathioprine
Azelastine
Azithromycin
Aztreonam
Bacampicillin
Baclofen
Benactyzine
Benazepril
Bendamustine
Bendroflumethiazide
Benznidazole
Betamethasone
Bevacizumab
Bexarotene
Bicalutamide

Bismuth
Bleomycin
Bortezomib
Bosentan
Bosutinib
Brompheniramine
Budesonide
Bupropion
Buserelin
Busulfan
Butabarbital
Butalbital
Candesartan
Captopril
Carbamazepine
Carboplatin
Carisoprodol
Carmustine
Carvedilol
Cefaclor
Cefadroxil
Cefamandole
Cefazolin
Cefdinir
Cefepime
Cefoperazone
Cefotaxime
Cefoxitin
Cefpodoxime
Ceftazidime
Ceftriaxone
Cefuroxime
Celecoxib
Cephalexin
Cephalothin
Cephapirin
Cephradine
Ceritinib
Cetirizine
Cetuximab
Cevimeline
Chloral Hydrate
Chlorambucil
Chloramphenicol
Chlordiazepoxide
Chlormezanone
Chloroquine
Chlorothiazide
Chlorpromazine
Chlorpropamide
Cimetidine
Ciprofloxacin
Cisplatin
Citalopram
Cladribine
Clarithromycin
Clemastine
Clindamycin
Clofibrate
Clomiphene
Clonazepam
Clopidogrel
Clorazepate
Cloxacillin
Clozapine
Co-Trimoxazole
Cobimetinib
Codeine
Colchicine
Colestipol
Cyanocobalamin

Cyclamate
Cyclophosphamide
Cycloserine
Cyclosporine
Cyclothiazide
Cyproheptadine
Cytarabine
Dabigatran
Dabrafenib
Dacarbazine
Daclizumab
Dalteparin
Danazol
Dantrolene
Dapsone
Daunorubicin
Deferasirox
Delavirdine
Denosumab
Desipramine
Dexamethasone
Diazepam
Diclofenac
Dicloxacillin
Dicumarol
Dicyclomine
Diethylpropion
Diethylstilbestrol
Diflunisal
Digoxin
Diltiazem
Dimenhydrinate
Diphenhydramine
Dipyridamole
Disopyramide
Disulfiram
Docetaxel
Docusate
Doxazosin
Doxepin
Doxorubicin
Doxycycline
Dronedarone
Durvalumab
Efavirenz
Eletriptan
Elotuzumab
Emtricitabine
Enalapril
Enoxacin
Enoxaparin
Entecavir
Ephedrine
Epoetin Alfa
Eprosartan
Erlotinib
Erythromycin
Esomeprazole
Estramustine
Estrogens
Etanercept
Ethacrynic Acid
Ethambutol
Ethionamide
Ethosuximide
Etodolac
Etoposide
Etoricoxib
Etravirine
Everolimus
Felodipine

Fenofibrate
Fenoprofen
Flecainide
Fluconazole
Flucytosine
Fludarabine
Fluorouracil
Fluoxetine
Flurazepam
Flurbiprofen
Flutamide
Folic Acid
Foscarnet
Fosfomycin
Furazolidone
Furosemide
Gabapentin
Galantamine
Ganciclovir
Gatifloxacin
Gefitinib
Gemcitabine
Gemfibrozil
Gemifloxacin
Gentamicin
Glimepiride
Glipizide
Glucagon
Glyburide
Gold & Gold Compounds
Granulocyte Colony-
    Stimulating Factor (G-CSF)
Grepafloxacin
Griseofulvin
Halothane
Heparin
Heroin
Hydralazine
Hydrochlorothiazide
Hydromorphone
Hydroxychloroquine
Hydroxyurea
Hydroxyzine
Ibrutinib
Ibuprofen
Icodextrin
Idarubicin
Imatinib
Imipenem/Cilastatin
Imipramine
Imiquimod
Indapamide
Indinavir
Indomethacin
Infliximab
Insulin
Interferon Alfa
Iobenguane
Ipilimumab
Irbesartan
Irinotecan
Isocarboxazid
Isoniazid
Isosorbide Dinitrate
Isotretinoin
Isradipine
Itraconazole
Ivermectin
Ixazomib
Ketoconazole
Ketoprofen

Ketorolac
Labetalol
Lamivudine
Lamotrigine
Lapatinib
Lenalidomide
Lenvatinib
Letrozole
Levamisole
Levetiracetam
Levodopa
Levofloxacin
Lidocaine
Lincomycin
Linezolid
Lisinopril
Lithium
Loracarbef
Lovastatin
Maprotiline
Mebendazole
Mechlorethamine
Meclofenamate
Mefenamic Acid
Mefloquine
Meloxicam
Melphalan
Memantine
Mephenytoin
Meprobamate
Mercaptopurine
Meropenem
Mesalamine
Mesna
Metamizole
Methazolamide
Methenamine
Methicillin
Methimazole
Methohexital
Methotrexate
Methoxsalen
Methsuximide
Methyldopa
Methylphenidate
Metoclopramide
Metoprolol
Metronidazole
Mexiletine
Miconazole
Minocycline
Minoxidil
Misoprostol
Mitomycin
Mitotane
Moexipril
Moricizine
Morphine
Nabumetone
Nadolol
Nafarelin
Nafcillin
Nalidixic Acid
Naltrexone
Naproxen
Naratriptan
Nefazodone
Nelfinavir
Neomycin
Nevirapine
Niacin

Nifedipine
Nilotinib
Nimesulide
Nimodipine
Nisoldipine
Nitisinone
Nitrofurantoin
Nivolumab
Norfloxacin
Nystatin
Octreotide
Ofloxacin
Olanzapine
Olmesartan
Olsalazine
Omeprazole
Oral Contraceptives
Oxacillin
Oxaliplatin
Oxaprozin
Oxcarbazepine
Paclitaxel
Paliperidone
Pamidronate
Panobinostat
Pantoprazole
Paromomycin
Paroxetine Hydrochloride
PEG-Interferon
Pembrolizumab
Pemoline
Penbutolol
Penicillamine
Penicillin V
Pentagastrin
Pentamidine
Pentazocine
Pentobarbital
Pentostatin
Perflutren
Perphenazine
Phenazopyridine
Phenobarbital
Phenolphthalein
Phenylbutazone
Phenytoin
Phytonadione
Piperacillin/Tazobactam
Piroxicam
Potassium Iodide
Prazosin
Prednisolone
Primaquine
Primidone
Pristinamycin
Procainamide
Procarbazine
Prochlorperazine
Promazine
Promethazine
Propafenone
Propofol
Propoxyphene
Propranolol
Propylthiouracil
Protamine Sulfate
Pseudoephedrine
Pyrazinamide
Pyrimethamine
Quinacrine
Quinapril

Quinethazone
Quinidine
Quinine
Quinupristin/Dalfopristin
Ramipril
Ranitidine
Rapacuronium
Regorafenib
Repaglinide
Ribavirin
Rifampin
Ritodrine
Ritonavir
Rituximab
Rivastigmine
Rofecoxib
Ropinirole
Rucaparib
Saccharin
Saquinavir
Scopolamine
Sertraline
Simvastatin
Smallpox Vaccine
Sorafenib
Sparfloxacin
Spironolactone
Streptokinase
Streptomycin
Streptozocin
Succimer
Sucralfate
Sulfadiazine
Sulfadoxine
Sulfamethoxazole
Sulfasalazine
Sulfinpyrazone
Sulfisoxazole
Sulindac
Tacrine
Tacrolimus
Tamoxifen
Teicoplanin
Telaprevir
Telmisartan
Temozolomide
Temsirolimus
Terazosin
Terbinafine
Terfenadine
Testosterone
Tetracycline
Tetrazepam
Thalidomide
Thiabendazole
Thiamine
Thimerosal
Thioguanine
Thiopental
Thioridazine
Thiothixene
Tiagabine
Ticarcillin
Ticlopidine
Tinzaparin
Tiopronin
Tipranavir
Tizanidine
Tobramycin
Tocainide
Tolazamide

Tolazoline
Tolbutamide
Tolmetin
Topiramate
Tramadol
Trametinib
Trazodone
Triamcinolone
Trimeprazine
Trimethadione
Trimetrexate
Troleandomycin
Uracil/Tegafur
Valdecoxib
Valproic Acid
Valsartan
Vancomycin
Vardenafil
Vemurafenib
Venlafaxine
Verapamil
Vincristine
Vitamin A
Vorapaxar
Vorinostat
Warfarin
Zalcitabine
Zidovudine
Ziprasidone
Zoledronate
Zonisamide

Exfoliative dermatitis

Acamprosate
Acetaminophen
Acitretin
Afatinib
Aldesleukin
Alitretinoin
Allopurinol
Aminoglutethimide
Aminolevulinic Acid
Aminophylline
Aminosalicylate Sodium
Amiodarone
Amobarbital
Amoxicillin
Amphotericin B
Ampicillin
Arsenic
Aspirin
Avelumab
Azathioprine
Aztreonam
Benzyl Alcohol
Bexarotene
Bismuth
Bosutinib
Bumetanide
Butabarbital
Butalbital
Capecitabine
Captopril
Carbamazepine
Carvedilol
Cefoxitin
Cefpodoxime
Celecoxib
Chlorambucil
Chloroquine
Chlorpropamide
Cimetidine

Ciprofloxacin
Cisplatin
Clofazimine
Clofibrate
Clonazepam
Co-Trimoxazole
Codeine
Cytarabine
Dapsone
Dasatinib
Daunorubicin
Demeclocycline
Desipramine
Dexamethasone
Diazepam
Diclofenac
Dicloxacillin
Diethylstilbestrol
Diflunisal
Diltiazem
Doxorubicin
Efavirenz
Eletriptan
Enalapril
Enoxacin
Ephedrine
Esmolol
Esomeprazole
Estrogens
Ethambutol
Ethosuximide
Fenoprofen
Flecainide
Fluconazole
Flurbiprofen
Fluvoxamine
Fosphenytoin
Furosemide
Gefitinib
Gemcitabine
Gemfibrozil
Gentamicin
Gold & Gold Compounds
Granulocyte Colony-
    Stimulating Factor (G-CSF)
Grepafloxacin
Griseofulvin
Hydroxychloroquine
Ibuprofen
Icodextrin
Idelalisib
Imatinib
Imipramine
Indomethacin
Irinotecan
Isavuconazonium Sulfate
Isoniazid
Isotretinoin
Ixabepilone
Ixazomib
Ketoconazole
Ketoprofen
Ketorolac
Lansoprazole
Lapatinib
Leflunomide
Lenalidomide
Lidocaine
Lisinopril
Lithium
Lomefloxacin

Meclofenamate
Mefenamic Acid
Mefloquine
Mephenytoin
Mephobarbital
Methicillin
Methsuximide
Methylphenidate
Mexiletine
Mezlocillin
Minocycline
Mitomycin
Nalidixic Acid
Nifedipine
Nilotinib
Nisoldipine
Nitisinone
Nitrofurantoin
Nitroglycerin
Nivolumab
Omacetaxine
Ombitasvir/Paritaprevir/
    Ritonavir
Omeprazole
Oxaprozin
Oxcarbazepine
Oxytetracycline
Panitumumab
Pantoprazole
Paramethadione
Pazopanib
Pembrolizumab
Pentobarbital
Pentostatin
Phenobarbital
Phenolphthalein
Phenylbutazone
Phenytoin
Piroxicam
Procarbazine
Propranolol
Propylthiouracil
Pseudoephedrine
Pyrimethamine
Quinacrine
Quinapril
Quinidine
Quinine
Raltitrexed
Rifampin
Risperidone
Rivastigmine
Romidepsin
Secobarbital
Sildenafil
Smallpox Vaccine
Sorafenib
Sparfloxacin
Streptomycin
Strontium Ranelate
Sulfacetamide
Sulfadoxine
Sulfamethoxazole
Sulfasalazine
Sulfisoxazole
Sulindac
Sunitinib
Tacrolimus
Teicoplanin
Terfenadine
Tetracycline

Thalidomide
Tiagabine
Ticlopidine
Tizanidine
Tobramycin
Tocainide
Trazodone
Tretinoin
Trimethadione
Trimethoprim
Trovafloxacin
Vancomycin
Venlafaxine
Verapamil
Vitamin A
Voriconazole
Vorinostat
Zalcitabine
Ziprasidone
Fixed eruption
Aceclofenac
Acetaminophen
Acyclovir
Adalimumab
Albendazole
Alendronate
Allopurinol
Aminosalicylate Sodium
Amitriptyline
Amlexanox
Amodiaquine
Amoxicillin
Amphotericin B
Ampicillin
Arsenic
Aspirin
Atenolol
Atorvastatin
Atropine Sulfate
Azathioprine
Bacampicillin
BCG Vaccine
Bisacodyl
Bismuth
Bisoprolol
Bleomycin
Bucillamine
Butabarbital
Butalbital
Carbamazepine
Carisoprodol
Cefaclor
Cefazolin
Cefixime
Ceftazidime
Ceftriaxone
Celecoxib
Cephalexin
Cetirizine
Chloral Hydrate
Chloramphenicol
Chlordiazepoxide
Chlorhexidine
Chlormezanone
Chloroquine
Chlorothiazide
Chlorpromazine
Chlorpropamide
Cimetidine
Ciprofloxacin
Clarithromycin

Clindamycin
Clioquinol
Clopidogrel
Co-Trimoxazole
Cocaine
Codeine
Colchicine
Cyproterone
Dacarbazine
Danazol
Dapsone
Demeclocycline
Dextromethorphan
Diazepam
Diclofenac
Diflunisal
Dimenhydrinate
Diphenhydramine
Disulfiram
Docetaxel
Doxorubicin
Doxycycline
Ephedrine
Erythromycin
Esomeprazole
Estrogens
Etanercept
Ethchlorvynol
Etodolac
Etoricoxib
Finasteride
Flavoxate
Flecainide
Fluconazole
Flurbiprofen
Foscarnet
Furosemide
Gabapentin
Ganciclovir
Glipizide
Griseofulvin
Guanethidine
Heparin
Heroin
Hydralazine
Hydrochlorothiazide
Hydroxychloroquine
Hydroxyurea
Hydroxyzine
Ibuprofen
Imipramine
Indapamide
Indomethacin
Infliximab
Influenza Vaccine
Iohexol
Iopromide
Isotretinoin
Itraconazole
Ketoconazole
Lamotrigine
Leuprolide
Levamisole
Levocetirizine
Lidocaine
Loperamide
Loratadine
Lorazepam
Meclofenamate
Mefenamic Acid
Meloxicam

Meprobamate
Mesna
Metamizole
Metformin
Methenamine
Methimazole
Methyldopa
Methylphenidate
Metronidazole
Miconazole
Minocycline
Modafinil
Nabumetone
Naproxen
Neomycin
Niacin
Nifedipine
Nimesulide
Nitrofurantoin
Norfloxacin
Nystatin
Ofloxacin
Olanzapine
Olopatadine
Omeprazole
Ondansetron
Oral Contraceptives
Orphenadrine
Oxazepam
Oxcarbazepine
Oxybutynin
Oxytetracycline
Paclitaxel
Papaverine
Paroxetine Hydrochloride
PEG-Interferon
Pentobarbital
Phenobarbital
Phenolphthalein
Phenylbutazone
Phenylephrine
Phenylpropanolamine
Phenytoin
Piperacillin/Tazobactam
Piroxicam
Procarbazine
Prochlorperazine
Promethazine
Propofol
Propranolol
Pseudoephedrine
Pyrazinamide
Pyridoxine
Pyrimethamine
Quinacrine
Quinidine
Quinine
Ranitidine
Ribavirin
Rifampin
Rofecoxib
Ropinirole
Roxithromycin
Rupatadine
Saccharin
Saquinavir
Scopolamine
Sorafenib
Streptomycin
Sulfadiazine
Sulfadoxine

Sulfamethoxazole
Sulfasalazine
Sulfisoxazole
Sulindac
Tadalafil
Tartrazine
Temazepam
Terbinafine
Terfenadine
Tetracycline
Thiabendazole
Thiopental
Ticlopidine
Tinidazole
Tolbutamide
Topiramate
Topotecan
Tosufloxacin
Tranexamic Acid
Triamcinolone
Trifluoperazine
Trimethoprim
Tripelennamine
Triprolidine
Ursodiol
Valproic Acid
Vancomycin
Voriconazole
Zolmitriptan
**Gingival hyperplasia/
hypertrophy**
Amlodipine
Basiliximab
Carbamazepine
Cevimeline
Clarithromycin
Clobazam
Co-Trimoxazole
Cycloserine
Cyclosporine
Diltiazem
Erythromycin
Eslicarbazepine
Everolimus
Felodipine
Fosphenytoin
Isradipine
Ketoconazole
Lamotrigine
Levetiracetam
Levonorgestrel
Lithium
Marihuana
Metoprolol
Mycophenolate
Nicardipine
Nifedipine
Nisoldipine
Oral Contraceptives
Palifermin
Penicillamine
Phenobarbital
Phenytoin
Primidone
Propranolol
Sertraline
Sirolimus
Tacrolimus
Tartrazine
Tiagabine
Topiramate

Valproic Acid
Vemurafenib
Verapamil
Vigabatrin
Voriconazole
Zonisamide
Hand-foot syndrome
Afatinib
Aflibercept
Axitinib
Bevacizumab
Bleomycin
Bosutinib
Brentuximab Vedotin
Cabazitaxel
Cabozantinib
Capecitabine
Carboplatin
Cetuximab
Cisplatin
Clofarabine
Co-Trimoxazole
Cobimetinib
Cyclophosphamide
Cytarabine
Dabrafenib
Dasatinib
Daunorubicin
Docetaxel
Doxorubicin
Epirubicin
Erlotinib
Etoposide
Everolimus
Fluorouracil
Gefitinib
Gemcitabine
Hydroxyurea
Ibandronate
Idarubicin
Imatinib
Infliximab
Interferon Alfa
Ipilimumab
Irinotecan
Ixabepilone
Ketoconazole
Lapatinib
Lenvatinib
Letrozole
Leucovorin
Mercaptopurine
Mesalamine
Methotrexate
Mitomycin
Neratinib
Nintedanib
Olaparib
Oxaliplatin
Paclitaxel
Palifermin
Panitumumab
Pazopanib
PEG-Interferon
Phenytoin
Regorafenib
Rucaparib
Sorafenib
Sunitinib
Tegafur/Gimeracil/Oteracil
Temozolomide

Temsirolimus
Trabectedin
Trametinib
Trastuzumab
Uracil/Tegafur
Valproic Acid
Vandetanib
Varenicline
Vemurafenib
Vincristine
Vinorelbine
Vorinostat
Lichenoid (lichen planus-like) eruptions
Acebutolol
Acyclovir
Adalimumab
Alendronate
Allopurinol
Aminosalicylate Sodium
Amoxicillin
Anakinra
Aspirin
Atenolol
Azathioprine
BCG Vaccine
Captopril
Carbamazepine
Carvedilol
Ceftriaxone
Chloral Hydrate
Chloroquine
Chlorothiazide
Chlorpromazine
Chlorpropamide
Cinnarizine
Clopidogrel
Co-Trimoxazole
Colchicine
Cycloserine
Cyclosporine
Dactinomycin
Demeclocycline
Diazoxide
Diflunisal
Diltiazem
Dorzolamide
Enalapril
Etanercept
Ethambutol
Fluoxymesterone
Flurbiprofen
Fluvastatin
Furosemide
Glimepiride
Glyburide
Gold & Gold Compounds
Granulocyte Colony-
   Stimulating Factor (G-CSF)
Griseofulvin
Hepatitis B Vaccine
Hydrochlorothiazide
Hydroxychloroquine
Hydroxyurea
Ibuprofen
Imatinib
Imiquimod
Immune Globulin IV
Indomethacin
Infliximab
Interferon Alfa

Irbesartan
Isoniazid
Isotretinoin
Ketoconazole
Labetalol
Lansoprazole
Leflunomide
Levamisole
Lisinopril
Lorazepam
Lovastatin
Mercaptopurine
Mesalamine
Metformin
Methamphetamine
Methyldopa
Methyltestosterone
Metoprolol
Nadolol
Naproxen
Nebivolol
Nelfinavir
Nifedipine
Nivolumab
Obinutuzumab
Olanzapine
Omeprazole
Oral Contraceptives
Orlistat
Pantoprazole
PEG-Interferon
Pembrolizumab
Penicillamine
Phenytoin
Pindolol
Piroxicam
Pneumococcal Vaccine
Pravastatin
Propranolol
Propylthiouracil
Pyrimethamine
Quinacrine
Quinidine
Quinine
Ranitidine
Ribavirin
Rifampin
Risperidone
Roxatidine
Salsalate
Sildenafil
Simeprevir
Simvastatin
Sofosbuvir
Solifenacin
Sotalol
Sparfloxacin
Spironolactone
Streptomycin
Sulfadoxine
Sulfamethoxazole
Sulindac
Temazepam
Tenofovir Disoproxil
Terazosin
Terbinafine
Testosterone
Tetracycline
Thimerosal
Thioridazine
Timolol

Tiopronin
Tiotropium
Tolazamide
Tolbutamide
Torsemide
Trichlormethiazide
Tripelennamine
Triprolidine
Ursodiol
Venlafaxine
Zidovudine
Lupus erythematosus
Acebutolol
Acetazolamide
Adalimumab
Albuterol
Aldesleukin
Allopurinol
Aminoglutethimide
Aminosalicylate Sodium
Amiodarone
Amitriptyline
Anastrozole
Anthrax Vaccine
Atenolol
Atorvastatin
Betaxolol
Bevacizumab
Bortezomib
Bupropion
Butabarbital
Butalbital
Capecitabine
Captopril
Carbamazepine
Carbimazole
Cefepime
Cefuroxime
Celecoxib
Celiprolol
Chlorambucil
Chlordiazepoxide
Chlorothiazide
Chlorpromazine
Chlorpropamide
Chlorthalidone
Cilazapril
Cimetidine
Cinnarizine
Citalopram
Clobazam
Clofibrate
Clonidine
Clozapine
Co-Trimoxazole
Cyclophosphamide
Cyclosporine
Cysteamine
Danazol
Dapsone
Dasatinib
Denosumab
Diethylstilbestrol
Diltiazem
Disopyramide
Docetaxel
Domperidone
Doxazosin
Doxorubicin
Doxycycline
Efalizumab

Enalapril
Esomeprazole
Estrogens
Etanercept
Ethambutol
Ethionamide
Ethosuximide
Fluorouracil
Fluoxymesterone
Fluphenazine
Flutamide
Fluvastatin
Fosphenytoin
Furosemide
Gemcitabine
Gold & Gold Compounds
Golimumab
Granulocyte Colony-
　　Stimulating Factor (G-CSF)
Griseofulvin
Hepatitis B Vaccine
Human Papillomavirus (HPV)
　　Vaccine
Hydralazine
Hydrochlorothiazide
Hydroxyurea
Ibandronate
Ibuprofen
Imipramine
Imiquimod
Immune Globulin IV
Immune Globulin SC
Infliximab
Interferon Alfa
Interferon Beta
Isoniazid
Labetalol
Lamotrigine
Lansoprazole
Leflunomide
Letrozole
Leuprolide
Levodopa
Lidocaine
Lisinopril
Lithium
Lovastatin
Mephenytoin
Meprobamate
Mercaptopurine
Mesalamine
Methimazole
Methoxsalen
Methsuximide
Methyldopa
Methyltestosterone
Methysergide
Metoprolol
Mexiletine
Minocycline
Minoxidil
Mitotane
Nafcillin
Nalidixic Acid
Naproxen
Nifedipine
Nitrofurantoin
Olsalazine
Omeprazole
Oral Contraceptives
Paclitaxel

Pantoprazole
PEG-Interferon
Pembrolizumab
Penicillamine
Pentobarbital
Perphenazine
Phenelzine
Phenobarbital
Phenolphthalein
Phenylbutazone
Phenytoin
Pindolol
Piroxicam
Potassium Iodide
Pravastatin
Prazosin
Prednicarbate
Primidone
Procainamide
Promethazine
Propafenone
Propranolol
Propylthiouracil
Psoralens
Quinidine
Quinine
Ranitidine
Reserpine
Ribavirin
Rifabutin
Rifampin
Rituximab
Sertraline
Simvastatin
Smallpox Vaccine
Somatropin
Spironolactone
Streptomycin
Sulfadiazine
Sulfamethoxazole
Sulfasalazine
Sulfisoxazole
Tamoxifen
Terbinafine
Terfenadine
Testosterone
Tetracycline
Thioridazine
Ticlopidine
Timolol
Tiopronin
Tiotropium
Tocainide
Triamterene
Trichlormethiazide
Trientine
Trimethadione
Trimethoprim
Trioxsalen
Uracil/Tegafur
Valproic Acid
Vancomycin
Verapamil
Vitamin E
Voriconazole
Zafirlukast
Zinc
Ziprasidone
Zonisamide
Onycholysis
　　Acitretin

Adalimumab
Allopurinol
Bleomycin
Capecitabine
Captopril
Clofazimine
Dabrafenib
Docetaxel
Doxorubicin
Estrogens
Etoposide
Gold & Gold Compounds
Hydroxyurea
Ibuprofen
Irinotecan
Isotretinoin
Ketoprofen
Methotrexate
Mitoxantrone
Mycophenolate
Nintedanib
Nitrofurantoin
Oral Contraceptives
Paclitaxel
Pemetrexed
Propranolol
Roxithromycin
Tasonermin
Tetracycline
Valproic Acid
Vemurafenib
Paresthesias
　　Acamprosate
　　Acetazolamide
　　Acitretin
　　Acyclovir
　　Adalimumab
　　Adenosine
　　Afamelanotide
　　Agalsidase
　　Alitretinoin
　　Allopurinol
　　Almotriptan
　　Alprazolam
　　Altretamine
　　Amikacin
　　Amiloride
　　Amiodarone
　　Amlodipine
　　Amoxapine
　　Amphotericin B
　　Amprenavir
　　Anagrelide
　　Apraclonidine
　　Arbutamine
　　Arformoterol
　　Aripiprazole
　　Arsenic
　　Artemether/Lumefantrine
　　Articaine
　　Aspirin
　　Astemizole
　　Atorvastatin
　　Avanafil
　　Azatadine
　　Azithromycin
　　Baclofen
　　Basiliximab
　　Bedaquiline
　　Benazepril
　　Benznidazole

Benzthiazide
Bepridil
Betaxolol
Bicalutamide
Blinatumomab
Bortezomib
Brivaracetam
Bromocriptine
Brompheniramine
Bupivacaine
Bupropion
Buspirone
Cabergoline
Cabozantinib
Calcitonin
Candesartan
Capecitabine
Captopril
Carbamazepine
Carboplatin
Carfilzomib
Carisoprodol
Carteolol
Carvedilol
Caspofungin
Ceftazidime
Ceftibuten
Ceftizoxime
Ceftolozane & Tazobactam
Celecoxib
Cephapirin
Ceritinib
Cetirizine
Cevimeline
Chloramphenicol
Chlorothiazide
Chlorpheniramine
Chlorthalidone
Cidofovir
Cilostazol
Cinacalcet
Cinoxacin
Ciprofloxacin
Cisplatin
Citalopram
Clemastine
Clonazepam
Clopidogrel
Clozapine
Coagulation Factor IX
　　(Recombinant)
Colistin
Copanlisib
Crisaborole
Cyclamate
Cyclobenzaprine
Cyclophosphamide
Cyclosporine
Cyproheptadine
Dalfampridine
Daptomycin
Dasatinib
Delafloxacin
Delavirdine
Demeclocycline
Denileukin
Desvenlafaxine
Dexamethasone
Dexchlorpheniramine
Dichlorphenamide
Diclofenac

Diflunisal
Dihydroergotamine
Diltiazem
Dimenhydrinate
Diphenhydramine
Dipyridamole
Dirithromycin
Disopyramide
Dobutamine
Docetaxel
Dofetilide
Dolutegravir
Donepezil
Doxycycline
Duloxetine
Efavirenz
Eflornithine
Eletriptan
Eltrombopag
Emtricitabine
Enalapril
Enoxacin
Entecavir
Enzalutamide
Epirubicin
Epoetin Alfa
Epoprostenol
Eprosartan
Ergotamine
Ertapenem
Escitalopram
Esmolol
Esomeprazole
Estazolam
Eszopiclone
Etanercept
Etelcalcetide
Ethoxzolamide
Etravirine
Evolocumab
Exemestane
Ezetimibe
Ezogabine
Famciclovir
Famotidine
Febuxostat
Felbamate
Felodipine
Fentanyl
Ferric Gluconate
Ferumoxsil
Ferumoxytol
Fingolimod
Flecainide
Fluconazole
Flucytosine
Fludarabine
Flumazenil
Fluorouracil
Fluoxetine
Flurbiprofen
Flutamide
Fosamprenavir
Foscarnet
Fosfomycin
Fosinopril
Fosphenytoin
Frovatriptan
Fulvestrant
Gabapentin
Gadobenate

Gadobutrol
Gadodiamide
Gadofosveset
Gadopentetate
Gadoteridol
Gadoversetamide
Gadoxetate
Galantamine
Ganciclovir
Gatifloxacin
Gemcitabine
Gemfibrozil
Gentamicin
Glatiramer
Glipizide
Glucarpidase
Glyburide
Grepafloxacin
Griseofulvin
Guanadrel
Guanethidine
Guanfacine
Halofantrine
Histrelin
Human Papillomavirus Vaccine
  (Bivalent)
Hydrocodone
Hydroflumethiazide
Imatinib
Imipenem/Cilastatin
Indapamide
Indinavir
Indomethacin
Infliximab
Insulin
Interferon Alfa
Interferon Beta
Iodixanol
Iohexol
Iopromide
Ioversol
Ipilimumab
Ipratropium
Irbesartan
Isavuconazonium Sulfate
Isoniazid
Isradipine
Ixazomib
Ketoconazole
Ketoprofen
Ketorolac
Labetalol
Lamivudine
Lamotrigine
Lansoprazole
Laronidase
Leflunomide
Leucovorin
Leuprolide
Levalbuterol
Levamisole
Levetiracetam
Levobupivacaine
Levofloxacin
Levomilnacipran
Lidocaine
Lisinopril
Lomefloxacin
Loratadine
Lorcainide
Losartan

Lovastatin
Lubiprostone
Maraviroc
MDMA
Meclizine
Meclofenamate
Medroxyprogesterone
Mefloquine
Meloxicam
Menadione
Methazolamide
Methimazole
Methyclothiazide
Methyldopa
Metoclopramide
Metolazone
Metronidazole
Mexiletine
Midodrine
Miglustat
Milnacipran
Miltefosine
Minocycline
Mirtazapine
Mitomycin
Modafinil
Moricizine
Moxifloxacin
Nabumetone
Nadolol
Nafarelin
Naproxen
Naratriptan
Nebivolol
Nefazodone
Nelarabine
Nelfinavir
Nesiritide
Nevirapine
Niacin
Niacinamide
Nicardipine
Nifedipine
Nilotinib
Nilutamide
Nisoldipine
Nitrofurantoin
Nivolumab
Nizatidine
Nusinersen
Ofloxacin
Omacetaxine
Omalizumab
Omeprazole
Ondansetron
Oseltamivir
Oxaliplatin
Oxilan
Oxprenolol
Oxycodone
Oxytetracycline
Paclitaxel
Palifermin
Pandemic Influenza Vaccine
  (HINI)
Pantoprazole
Paricalcitol
Paroxetine Hydrochloride
Pegaspargase
Pegvisomant
Pembrolizumab

Pentamidine
Pentostatin
Pentoxifylline
Perampanel
Perflutren
Pergolide
Perindopril
Phentermine
Phenytoin
Pindolol
Pirbuterol
Piroxicam
Pizotifen
Plasma (Human) Blood
  Product
Posaconazole
Pramipexole
Pravastatin
Prazosin
Prednicarbate
Pregabalin
Prilocaine
Procarbazine
Promethazine
Propafenone
Propylthiouracil
Pyridoxine
Quetiapine
Quinapril
Quinupristin/Dalfopristin
Rabeprazole
Ramipril
Ranolazine
Rasagiline
Rasburicase
Reboxetine
Repaglinide
Rifabutin
Rifampin
Riluzole
Rimantadine
Risedronate
Risperidone
Ritonavir
Rivaroxaban
Rivastigmine
Rizatriptan
Rofecoxib
Romiplostim
Ropinirole
Ropivacaine
Rosuvastatin
Rotigotine
Saquinavir
Sertraline
Sibutramine
Sildenafil
Siltuximab
Sincalide
Sipuleucel-T
Sirolimus
Smallpox Vaccine
Sodium Oxybate
Somatropin
Sotalol
Sparfloxacin
Stavudine
Streptomycin
Succimer
Sufentanil
Sugammadex

Sulfasalazine
Sulindac
Sumatriptan
Tacrine
Tacrolimus
Tadalafil
Taliglucerase
Tartrazine
Tegafur/Gimeracil/Oteracil
Telaprevir
Telbivudine
Telithromycin
Telmisartan
Temozolomide
Terazosin
Terfenadine
Teriflunomide
Teriparatide
Tesamorelin
Testosterone
Tetrabenazine
Tetracycline
Thalidomide
Thallium
Thiamine
Thyrotropin Alfa
Tiagabine
Tibolone
Tiludronate
Timolol
Tinidazole
Tiotropium
Tizanidine
Tobramycin
Tocainide
Tofacitinib
Tolcapone
Tolterodine
Topiramate
Topotecan
Torsemide
Trabectedin
Tramadol
Trandolapril
Trastuzumab
Travoprost
Trazodone
Tretinoin
Triazolam
Trihexyphenidyl
Trimeprazine
Tripelennamine
Triprolidine
Triptorelin
Trovafloxacin
Unoprostone
Valacyclovir
Valdecoxib
Valganciclovir
Valproic Acid
Valsartan
Vardenafil
Venlafaxine
Verapamil
Vernakalant
Vilazodone
Vinblastine
Vincristine
Vinorelbine
Voriconazole
Zaleplon

Ziconotide
Zidovudine
Zileuton
Ziprasidone
Zoledronate
Zolmitriptan
Zolpidem
Zonisamide
Zuclopenthixol

Pemphigus vulgaris
Acetaminophen
Acetazolamide
Aldesleukin
Amoxicillin
Ampicillin
Aspirin
Atorvastatin
Avelumab
Benazepril
Bucillamine
Captopril
Carbamazepine
Carbimazole
Cefaclor
Cefadroxil
Cefazolin
Cefixime
Ceftazidime
Ceftriaxone
Cefuroxime
Cephalexin
Chloroquine
Cilazapril
Clonidine
Cocaine
Cyclophosphamide
Diclofenac
Enalapril
Epinephrine
Famotidine
Fludarabine
Fosinopril
Glyburide
Gold & Gold Compounds
Haloperidol
Hepatitis B Vaccine
Heroin
Hydroxychloroquine
Ibuprofen
Imiquimod
Influenza Vaccine
Ingenol Mebutate
Interferon Alfa
Interferon Beta
Isotretinoin
Ketoprofen
Latanoprost
Levamisole
Levodopa
Meprobamate
Metamizole
Metformin
Methoxsalen
Moexipril
Montelukast
Mycophenolate
Nifedipine
Nivolumab
Omeprazole
Pembrolizumab
Penicillamine

Phenobarbital
Phenylbutazone
Phenytoin
Piroxicam
Propranolol
Psoralens
Quinapril
Ramipril
Rifampin
Rituximab
Secukinumab
Spironolactone
Timolol
Tiopronin
Tocilizumab
Trandolapril
Trioxsalen
Typhoid Vaccine

Peyronie's disease
Acebutolol
Betaxolol
Carvedilol
Labetalol
Methotrexate
Metoprolol
Nadolol
Papaverine
Pindolol
Propranolol
Ropinirole
Timolol

Photosensitivity
Acamprosate
Aceclofenac
Acetohexamide
Acetylcysteine
Acitretin
Acyclovir
Aldesleukin
Alectinib
Allopurinol
Almotriptan
Alprazolam
Amantadine
Amiloride
Aminolevulinic Acid
Aminosalicylate Sodium
Amiodarone
Amitriptyline
Amoxapine
Anagrelide
Arsenic
Astemizole
Atorvastatin
Atropine Sulfate
Azatadine
Azathioprine
Azithromycin
Benazepril
Bendroflumethiazide
Benztropine
Bezafibrate
Bicalutamide
Brompheniramine
Bumetanide
Bupropion
Butabarbital
Butalbital
Calcipotriol
Canagliflozin
Candesartan

Capecitabine
Captopril
Carbamazepine
Carisoprodol
Carvedilol
Cefazolin
Ceftazidime
Celecoxib
Cetirizine
Cevimeline
Chlorambucil
Chlordiazepoxide
Chlorhexidine
Chloroquine
Chlorothiazide
Chlorpheniramine
Chlorpromazine
Chlorpropamide
Chlortetracycline
Chlorthalidone
Ciprofloxacin
Clemastine
Clofazimine
Clofibrate
Clomipramine
Clopidogrel
Clorazepate
Clozapine
Co-Trimoxazole
Cobimetinib
Colchicine
Crizotinib
Cyclamate
Cyproheptadine
Dabrafenib
Dacarbazine
Danazol
Dapsone
Dasatinib
Demeclocycline
Desipramine
Desoximetasone
Dexamethasone
Dexchlorpheniramine
Diazoxide
Diclofenac
Diflunisal
Diltiazem
Dimenhydrinate
Diphenhydramine
Disopyramide
Docetaxel
Doxepin
Doxycycline
Dronedarone
Duloxetine
Eculizumab
Efavirenz
Enalapril
Enoxacin
Epoetin Alfa
Erlotinib
Esomeprazole
Estrogens
Eszopiclone
Ethambutol
Ethionamide
Etodolac
Febuxostat
Felbamate
Fenofibrate

Flucytosine
Fluorouracil
Fluoxetine
Flurbiprofen
Flutamide
Fluvoxamine
Fosinopril
Furazolidone
Furosemide
Ganciclovir
Gatifloxacin
Gemifloxacin
Gentamicin
Glimepiride
Glipizide
Glyburide
Glycopyrrolate
Gold & Gold Compounds
Grepafloxacin
Griseofulvin
Haloperidol
Heroin
Hydralazine
Hydrochlorothiazide
Hydroflumethiazide
Hydroxychloroquine
Hydroxyurea
Hydroxyzine
Hyoscyamine
Ibuprofen
Imatinib
Imipramine
Indapamide
Indomethacin
Interferon Alfa
Interferon Beta
Irbesartan
Irinotecan
Isocarboxazid
Isoniazid
Isotretinoin
Itraconazole
Kanamycin
Ketoconazole
Ketoprofen
Ketorolac
Lamotrigine
Levofloxacin
Lisinopril
Lomefloxacin
Loratadine
Losartan
Loxapine
Maprotiline
Meclizine
Meclofenamate
Meloxicam
Meprobamate
Mercaptopurine
Mesalamine
Mesoridazine
Metformin
Methenamine
Methotrexate
Methoxsalen
Methyclothiazide
Methyldopa
Methylphenidate
Metolazone
Midostaurin
Minocycline

Minoxidil
Mitomycin
Moexipril
Molindone
Moxifloxacin
Nabumetone
Nalidixic Acid
Naproxen
Naratriptan
Nefazodone
Nifedipine
Nimesulide
Nivolumab
Norfloxacin
Nortriptyline
Ofloxacin
Olanzapine
Olmesartan
Omalizumab
Ombitasvir/Paritaprevir/
   Ritonavir
Oral Contraceptives
Oxaprozin
Oxerutins
Oxytetracycline
Paclitaxel
Pantoprazole
Paroxetine Hydrochloride
PEG-Interferon
Pentobarbital
Pentosan
Pentostatin
Phenelzine
Phenobarbital
Phenytoin
Pilocarpine
Pimozide
Pirfenidone
Piroxicam
Polythiazide
Porfimer
Pravastatin
Procainamide
Prochlorperazine
Procyclidine
Promazine
Promethazine
Propranolol
Propylthiouracil
Protriptyline
Psoralens
Pyrazinamide
Pyridoxine
Pyrimethamine
Quetiapine
Quinacrine
Quinapril
Quinethazone
Quinidine
Quinine
Rabeprazole
Ramipril
Ranitidine
Regorafenib
Ribavirin
Rifaximin
Risperidone
Ritonavir
Ropinirole
Rucaparib
Saccharin

Saquinavir
Scopolamine
Sertraline
Sildenafil
Simeprevir
Simvastatin
Sitagliptin
Smallpox Vaccine
Sotalol
Sparfloxacin
Streptomycin
Sulfadiazine
Sulfadoxine
Sulfamethoxazole
Sulfasalazine
Sulfisoxazole
Sulindac
Sumatriptan
Tacrolimus
Tartrazine
Tegafur/Gimeracil/Oteracil
Telmisartan
Terfenadine
Tetracycline
Thimerosal
Thioguanine
Thioridazine
Thiothixene
Tiagabine
Tiopronin
Tiotropium
Tocilizumab
Tolazamide
Tolbutamide
Tolmetin
Topiramate
Torsemide
Trametinib
Tranylcypromine
Trastuzumab
Trazodone
Tretinoin
Triamterene
Triazolam
Trichlormethiazide
Trifluoperazine
Trihexyphenidyl
Trimeprazine
Trimethadione
Trimipramine
Trioxsalen
Tripelennamine
Triprolidine
Trovafloxacin
Uracil/Tegafur
Valdecoxib
Valproic Acid
Valsartan
Vandetanib
Vardenafil
Vemurafenib
Venlafaxine
Verapamil
Verteporfin
Vinblastine
Voriconazole
Xipamide
Zalcitabine
Zaleplon
Ziprasidone
Zolmitriptan

Zolpidem
Pigmentation
Acitretin
Adapalene
Afamelanotide
Alitretinoin
Amantadine
Amifostine
Aminolevulinic Acid
Amiodarone
Amitriptyline
Amlodipine
Amoxicillin
Apomorphine
Arformoterol
Arsenic
Asfotase Alfa
Azacitidine
Azathioprine
Benznidazole
Betaxolol
Bevacizumab
Bimatoprost
Bismuth
Bleomycin
Bortezomib
Bupropion
Busulfan
Cabozantinib
Calcipotriol
Capecitabine
Captopril
Carboplatin
Carmustine
Ceftriaxone
Cetirizine
Cevimeline
Chlorhexidine
Chloroquine
Chlorotrianisene
Chlorpromazine
Cidofovir
Ciprofloxacin
Cisplatin
Citalopram
Clobetasol
Clofazimine
Clomipramine
Clonazepam
Clonidine
Clozapine
Co-Trimoxazole
Cobicistat/Elvitegravir/
   Emtricitabine/Tenofovir
   Disoproxil
Colistin
Collagen (Bovine)
Cyclophosphamide
Dactinomycin
Dapsone
Dasatinib
Daunorubicin
Deferasirox
Degarelix
Deoxycholic Acid
Desipramine
Dexamethasone
Diazepam
Dicumarol
Diethylstilbestrol
Diltiazem

Docetaxel
Donepezil
Doxorubicin
Doxycycline
Eletriptan
Elotuzumab
Eltrombopag
Emtricitabine
Enoxacin
Epirubicin
Erythromycin
Esmolol
Estradiol
Estramustine
Estrogens
Eszopiclone
Etoposide
Ezogabine
Fentanyl
Finasteride
Fluconazole
Fluorouracil
Fluoxetine
Fluphenazine
Fluvoxamine
Foscarnet
Ganciclovir
Gefitinib
Glyburide
Gold & Gold Compounds
Goserelin
Grepafloxacin
Griseofulvin
Halobetasol
Haloperidol
Heroin
Human Papillomavirus (HPV)
    Vaccine
Hyaluronic Acid
Hydrochlorothiazide
Hydroquinone
Hydroxychloroquine
Hydroxyurea
Idarubicin
Ifosfamide
Imatinib
Imipramine
Imiquimod
Indapamide
Indinavir
Insulin
Interferon Alfa
Ipilimumab
Irinotecan
Isotretinoin
Ixabepilone
Ixazomib
Ketoconazole
Ketoprofen
Labetalol
Lamivudine
Lapatinib
Latanoprost
Leflunomide
Lenalidomide
Leuprolide
Levobupivacaine
Levodopa
Levofloxacin
Levonorgestrel
Levothyroxine

Lidocaine
Linezolid
Lithium
Lomefloxacin
Loxapine
Mechlorethamine
Medroxyprogesterone
Mephenytoin
Mercaptopurine
Mesoridazine
Methamphetamine
Methotrexate
Methoxsalen
Methyldopa
Methysergide
Metoclopramide
Minocycline
Minoxidil
Mirtazapine
Mitomycin
Mitotane
Molindone
Naratriptan
Niacin
Nicotine
Nifedipine
Nisoldipine
Nitazoxanide
Nitisinone
Nivolumab
Olanzapine
Omacetaxine
Omeprazole
Oral Contraceptives
Orphenadrine
Oxytetracycline
Paclitaxel
Palifermin
Panitumumab
Pantoprazole
Paromomycin
Paroxetine Hydrochloride
Pazopanib
PEG-Interferon
Pemetrexed
Pentazocine
Pentostatin
Perphenazine
Phenazopyridine
Phenobarbital
Phenolphthalein
Phenytoin
Pimozide
Polidocanol
Porfimer
Prilocaine
Procarbazine
Prochlorperazine
Promazine
Propofol
Propranolol
Psoralens
Pyridoxine
Pyrimethamine
Quinacrine
Quinestrol
Quinidine
Quinine
Rabeprazole
Regorafenib
Ribavirin

Rifabutin
Rifapentine
Risperidone
Ropinirole
Ruxolitinib
Saquinavir
Sertraline
Sildenafil
Siltuximab
Smallpox Vaccine
Sorafenib
Sparfloxacin
Spironolactone
Stanozolol
Sulfadiazine
Sulfasalazine
Sunitinib
Tacrolimus
Tafluprost
Tamoxifen
Tegafur/Gimeracil/Oteracil
Telithromycin
Telmisartan
Terbinafine
Tetracycline
Thioridazine
Thiotepa
Thiothixene
Tiagabine
Tigecycline
Tinidazole
Tolcapone
Topiramate
Trastuzumab
Travoprost
Tretinoin
Triamcinolone
Trifluoperazine
Trioxsalen
Triptorelin
Unoprostone
Uracil/Tegafur
Vandetanib
Venlafaxine
Verapamil
Vinblastine
Vincristine
Vinorelbine
Vitamin A
Voriconazole
Warfarin
Zidovudine
Zinc

Pityriasis rosea-like eruption
Acetaminophen
Acyclovir
Allopurinol
Ampicillin
Arsenic
Asenapine
Aspirin
Atenolol
BCG Vaccine
Bismuth
Captopril
Clonidine
Clozapine
Codeine
Everolimus
Gold & Gold Compounds
Hydrochlorothiazide

Imatinib
Isotretinoin
Ketotifen
Lamotrigine
Lisinopril
Meprobamate
Metronidazole
Mitomycin
Naproxen
Nimesulide
Nortriptyline
Omeprazole
Pneumococcal Vaccine
Terbinafine
Tiopronin
Tripelennamine
Pruritus
Abacavir
Abatacept
Abciximab
Acamprosate
Acebutolol
Acetaminophen
Acetohexamide
Acetylcysteine
Acitretin
Acyclovir
Adalimumab
Adapalene
Adefovir
Ado-Trastuzumab Emtansine
Afatinib
Albendazole
Albuterol
Alcaftadine
Aldesleukin
Alefacept
Alemtuzumab
Alendronate
Alfentanil
Alglucerase
Alitretinoin
Allopurinol
Almotriptan
Alogliptin
Alpha-Lipoic Acid
Alprazolam
Alprostadil
Altretamine
Alvimopan
Amantadine
Amcinonide
Amikacin
Amiloride
Aminoglutethimide
Aminolevulinic Acid
Aminophylline
Aminosalicylate Sodium
Amiodarone
Amitriptyline
Amlodipine
Amodiaquine
Amoxapine
Amoxicillin
Amphotericin B
Ampicillin
Anagrelide
Anastrozole
Anidulafungin
Anthrax Vaccine

Anti-Thymocyte
  Immunoglobulin (Rabbit)
Apomorphine
Apraclonidine
Aprepitant
Arsenic
Artemether/Lumefantrine
Artesunate
Asfotase Alfa
Asparaginase
Aspartame
Aspirin
Astemizole
Atazanavir
Atenolol
Atezolizumab
Atomoxetine
Atorvastatin
Atovaquone
Atovaquone/Proguanil
Atracurium
Avelumab
Axitinib
Azacitidine
Azathioprine
Azithromycin
Aztreonam
Bacampicillin
Bacitracin
Baclofen
Basiliximab
Becaplermin
Bedaquiline
Belinostat
Benazepril
Bendamustine
Bendroflumethiazide
Benzalkonium
Benznidazole
Benzyl Alcohol
Besifloxacin
Betamethasone
Betaxolol
Bevacizumab
Bexarotene
Bezafibrate
Bicalutamide
Bimatoprost
Bismuth
Bleomycin
Boceprevir
Bortezomib
Bosentan
Bosutinib
Botulinum Toxin (A & B)
Brentuximab Vedotin
Brimonidine
Brinzolamide
Brodalumab
Bromfenac
Budesonide
Bumetanide
Bupivacaine
Buprenorphine
Bupropion
Buspirone
Butorphanol
Cabergoline
Calcipotriol
Calcium Hydroxylapatite
Canagliflozin

Capecitabine
Captopril
Carbamazepine
Carbetocin
Carboplatin
Carisoprodol
Carmustine
Carvedilol
Caspofungin
Cefaclor
Cefadroxil
Cefamandole
Cefazolin
Cefdinir
Cefditoren
Cefepime
Cefixime
Cefmetazole
Cefonicid
Cefoperazone
Cefotaxime
Cefotetan
Cefoxitin
Cefpodoxime
Cefprozil
Ceftaroline Fosamil
Ceftazidime
Ceftibuten
Ceftizoxime
Ceftobiprole
Ceftolozane & Tazobactam
Ceftriaxone
Cefuroxime
Celecoxib
Cephalexin
Cephalothin
Cephapirin
Cephradine
Certolizumab
Cetirizine
Cetrorelix
Cetuximab
Cevimeline
Chloral Hydrate
Chlorambucil
Chloramphenicol
Chlordiazepoxide
Chlorhexidine
Chlormezanone
Chloroquine
Chlorothiazide
Chlorpheniramine
Chlorpromazine
Chlorpropamide
Cholestyramine
Ciclopirox
Cidofovir
Cimetidine
Cinoxacin
Ciprofloxacin
Cisplatin
Citalopram
Cladribine
Clarithromycin
Clindamycin
Clobetasol
Clofarabine
Clofazimine
Clofibrate
Clomiphene
Clomipramine

Clonidine
Clopidogrel
Clotrimazole
Cloxacillin
Clozapine
Co-Trimoxazole
Coagulation Factor IX
  (Recombinant)
Cobimetinib
Codeine
Colchicine
Collagen (Bovine)
Conivaptan
Cromolyn
Cyanocobalamin
Cyclamate
Cyclobenzaprine
Cyclophosphamide
Cyclosporine
Cytarabine
Dabrafenib
Dacarbazine
Daclatasvir
Daclizumab
Dactinomycin
Dalbavancin
Dalteparin
Danaparoid
Danazol
Dapsone
Daptomycin
Darbepoetin Alfa
Darifenacin
Darunavir
Dasabuvir/Ombitasvir/
  Paritaprevir/Ritonavir
Dasatinib
Daunorubicin
Decitabine
Deferasirox
Deferoxamine
Defibrotide
Delafloxacin
Delavirdine
Demeclocycline
Denileukin
Denosumab
Deoxycholic Acid
Desipramine
Desonide
Desoximetasone
Dexamethasone
Dexlansoprazole
Diatrizoate
Diazepam
Diclofenac
Dicloxacillin
Dicumarol
Dicyclomine
Didanosine
Diethylpropion
Diethylstilbestrol
Diflunisal
Difluprednate
Digoxin
Dihydrocodeine
Dihydrotachysterol
Diltiazem
Dimethyl Fumarate
Diphenhydramine
Diphenoxylate

Dipyridamole
Dirithromycin
Disopyramide
Dobutamine
Docetaxel
Dolasetron
Dolutegravir
Donepezil
Doripenem
Dorzolamide
Doxapram
Doxazosin
Doxepin
Doxercalciferol
Doxorubicin
Doxycycline
Dronedarone
Droperidol
Duloxetine
Dupilumab
Durvalumab
Ecallantide
Econazole
Eculizumab
Efavirenz
Eflornithine
Eletriptan
Emtricitabine
Enalapril
Enfuvirtide
Enoxacin
Enoxaparin
Enzalutamide
Epinastine
Epinephrine
Epirubicin
Epoetin Alfa
Epoprostenol
Eprosartan
Ergocalciferol
Erlotinib
Ertapenem
Erythromycin
Escitalopram
Esomeprazole
Estazolam
Estramustine
Estrogens
Eszopiclone
Etanercept
Etelcalcetide
Ethambutol
Etidronate
Etodolac
Everolimus
Evolocumab
Exemestane
Exenatide
Ezetimibe
Factor VIII - von Willebrand
  Factor
Famciclovir
Famotidine
Febuxostat
Felbamate
Felodipine
Fenofibrate
Fenoprofen
Fentanyl
Ferric Gluconate
Ferumoxytol

Fidaxomicin
Finafloxacin
Finasteride
Fingolimod
Flecainide
Fluconazole
Fludarabine
Fluocinonide
Fluorides
Fluorouracil
Fluoxetine
Fluphenazine
Flurbiprofen
Fluticasone Propionate
Folic Acid
Follitropin Alfa/Beta
Fondaparinux
Formoterol
Fosamprenavir
Foscarnet
Fosfomycin
Fosinopril
Fosphenytoin
Frovatriptan
Fulvestrant
Furazolidone
Furosemide
Gabapentin
Gadobenate
Gadobutrol
Gadodiamide
Gadofosveset
Gadopentetate
Gadoteridol
Gadoversetamide
Gadoxetate
Ganciclovir
Gatifloxacin
Gefitinib
Gemcitabine
Gemfibrozil
Gemifloxacin
Gemtuzumab
Gentamicin
Glatiramer
Glecaprevir & Pibrentasvir
Gliclazide
Glimepiride
Glipizide
Glucosamine
Glyburide
Glycopyrrolate
Gold & Gold Compounds
Golimumab
Goserelin
Granulocyte Colony-
    Stimulating Factor (G-CSF)
Grepafloxacin
Griseofulvin
Guanabenz
Guanfacine
Guselkumab
Halcinonide
Halobetasol
Halofantrine
Halometasone
Haloperidol
Heparin
Heroin
Histrelin

Human Papillomavirus (HPV)
    Vaccine
Human Papillomavirus Vaccine
    (Bivalent)
Hyaluronic Acid
Hydralazine
Hydrochlorothiazide
Hydrocodone
Hydrocortisone
Hydromorphone
Hydroquinone
Hydroxychloroquine
Hydroxyurea
Ibandronate
Ibritumomab
Ibuprofen
Icatibant
Icodextrin
Idursulfase
Imatinib
Imidapril
Imiglucerase
Imipenem/Cilastatin
Imipramine
Imiquimod
Immune Globulin IV
Immune Globulin SC
Indapamide
Indinavir
Indomethacin
Infliximab
Ingenol Mebutate
Insulin
Insulin Glulisine
Interferon Alfa
Iobenguane
Iodixanol
Iohexol
Iomeprol
Iopromide
Ioversol
Ipilimumab
Ipratropium
Irbesartan
Irinotecan
Isavuconazonium Sulfate
Isocarboxazid
Isoniazid
Isosorbide Mononitrate
Isotretinoin
Isradipine
Itraconazole
Ivermectin
Ixabepilone
Ixazomib
Ixekizumab
Japanese Encephalitis Vaccine
Kanamycin
Ketamine
Ketoconazole
Ketoprofen
Ketorolac
Ketotifen
Labetalol
Lacosamide
Lamivudine
Lamotrigine
Lanreotide
Lansoprazole
Lapatinib
Latanoprost

Ledipasvir & Sofosbuvir
Leflunomide
Lenalidomide
Lepirudin
Letrozole
Leucovorin
Leuprolide
Levalbuterol
Levamisole
Levetiracetam
Levobunolol
Levobupivacaine
Levofloxacin
Levomilnacipran
Levothyroxine
Lidocaine
Lifitegrast
Linagliptin
Lincomycin
Lindane
Linezolid
Liraglutide
Lisinopril
Lithium
Lixisenatide
Lodoxamide
Lomefloxacin
Loracarbef
Loratadine
Losartan
Lovastatin
Loxapine
Luliconazole
Lurasidone
Mafenide
Maraviroc
Mebendazole
Mechlorethamine
Meclofenamate
Medroxyprogesterone
Mefenamic Acid
Mefloquine
Meloxicam
Melphalan
Memantine
Meperidine
Mephenytoin
Mepivacaine
Mepolizumab
Meprobamate
Meropenem
Mesalamine
Mesna
Metamizole
Metformin
Methadone
Methenamine
Methimazole
Methotrexate
Methoxsalen
Methyl salicylate
Methyldopa
Methylprednisolone
Metolazone
Metoprolol
Metronidazole
Mexiletine
Micafungin
Miconazole
Midazolam
Midodrine

Mifepristone
Milnacipran
Miltefosine
Minocycline
Minoxidil
Mirabegron
Mitomycin
Mitotane
Modafinil
Moexipril
Molindone
Mometasone
Moricizine
Morphine
Moxifloxacin
Mupirocin
Muromonab-CD3
Mycophenolate
Nabumetone
Nadolol
Nafarelin
Nalbuphine
Nalidixic Acid
Nalmefene
Naloxone
Naltrexone
Naproxen
Naratriptan
Natalizumab
Necitumumab
Nefazodone
Nelfinavir
Neostigmine
Nepafenac
Nesiritide
Nevirapine
Niacin
Niacinamide
Nicotine
Nifedipine
Nilotinib
Nilutamide
Nimesulide
Nimodipine
Nintedanib
Nisoldipine
Nitazoxanide
Nitisinone
Nitrofurantoin
Nitrofurazone
Nitroglycerin
Nivolumab
Nizatidine
Norfloxacin
Nystatin
Obeticholic Acid
Octreotide
Ofatumumab
Ofloxacin
Olanzapine
Olaparib
Olsalazine
Omacetaxine
Omalizumab
Ombitasvir/Paritaprevir/
    Ritonavir
Omeprazole
Ondansetron
Oral Contraceptives
Oritavancin
Osimertinib

Oxacillin
Oxaliplatin
Oxaprozin
Oxerutins
Oxilan
Oxybutynin
Oxycodone
Oxymetazoline
Oxymorphone
Oxytetracycline
Paclitaxel
Palifermin
Paliperidone
Palonosetron
Pancrelipase
Panitumumab
Pantoprazole
Papaverine
Paricalcitol
Paromomycin
Paroxetine Hydrochloride
Paroxetine Mesylate
Pasireotide
Pazopanib
PEG-Interferon
Pegaspargase
Pegvisomant
Pembrolizumab
Pemetrexed
Penicillamine
Penicillin V
Pentagastrin
Pentamidine
Pentazocine
Pentosan
Pentostatin
Pentoxifylline
Perflutren
Perindopril
Permethrin
Pertuzumab
Phenelzine
Phenobarbital
Phenolphthalein
Phenytoin
Pimecrolimus
Pindolol
Pirfenidone
Piroxicam
Plasma (Human) Blood
    Product
Pneumococcal Vaccine
Podophyllotoxin
Polidocanol
Pomalidomide
Posaconazole
Pralatrexate
Pramipexole
Pravastatin
Praziquantel
Prazosin
Prednicarbate
Prednisolone
Prednisone
Pregabalin
Prilocaine
Primaquine
Pristinamycin
Probenecid
Procainamide
Procarbazine

Prochlorperazine
Propafenone
Propofol
Propranolol
Propylthiouracil
Protriptyline
Psoralens
Pyrazinamide
Pyrimethamine
Quazepam
Quinacrine
Quinapril
Quinethazone
Quinidine
Quinine
Quinupristin/Dalfopristin
Rabeprazole
Raltegravir
Raltitrexed
Ramipril
Ranibizumab
Ranitidine
Rasburicase
Regorafenib
Remifentanil
Repaglinide
Retapamulin
Ribavirin
Ribociclib
Rifampin
Rifapentine
Rifaximin
Risedronate
Risperidone
Ritonavir
Rituximab
Rivaroxaban
Rivastigmine
Rizatriptan
Rocuronium
Rofecoxib
Romidepsin
Ropinirole
Ropivacaine
Rosuvastatin
Rotigotine
Rucaparib
Rufinamide
Saccharin
Sacubitril/Valsartan
Salmeterol
Saquinavir
Sarilumab
Saxagliptin
Scopolamine
Secukinumab
Sertaconazole
Sertraline
Sevelamer
Sevoflurane
Sibutramine
Sildenafil
Siltuximab
Simeprevir
Simvastatin
Sirolimus
Smallpox Vaccine
Sodium Iodide I-131
Sodium Oxybate
Sofosbuvir
Sonidegib

Sorafenib
Sotalol
Sparfloxacin
Spectinomycin
Spinosad
Spironolactone
Streptokinase
Streptomycin
Streptozocin
Succimer
Succinylcholine
Sucralfate
Sufentanil
Sugammadex
Sulfadiazine
Sulfadoxine
Sulfamethoxazole
Sulfasalazine
Sulfisoxazole
Sulindac
Sumatriptan
Sunitinib
Tacrine
Tacrolimus
Tadalafil
Tafluprost
Taliglucerase
Tamoxifen
Tartrazine
Tazarotene
Tedizolid
Tegafur/Gimeracil/Oteracil
Tegaserod
Teicoplanin
Telaprevir
Telavancin
Telbivudine
Telithromycin
Telmisartan
Temozolomide
Temsirolimus
Terazosin
Terbinafine
Terbutaline
Terconazole
Teriflunomide
Tesamorelin
Testosterone
Tetracycline
Thalidomide
Thiabendazole
Thiamine
Thioguanine
Thiopental
Thiotepa
Thyrotropin Alfa
Tiagabine
Tibolone
Ticlopidine
Tigecycline
Tiludronate
Timolol
Tinidazole
Tinzaparin
Tiopronin
Tipranavir
Tizanidine
Tobramycin
Tocainide
Tocilizumab
Tofacitinib

Tolazamide
Tolbutamide
Tolcapone
Tolmetin
Tolterodine
Tolvaptan
Topiramate
Tositumomab & Iodine[131]
Tosufloxacin
Tramadol
Trametinib
Trandolapril
Tranexamic Acid
Trastuzumab
Travoprost
Trazodone
Treprostinil
Tretinoin
Triamcinolone
Triazolam
Trimeprazine
Trimethadione
Trimethoprim
Trimetrexate
Trioxsalen
Triprolidine
Triptorelin
Troleandomycin
Trovafloxacin
Typhoid Vaccine
Ulipristal
Unoprostone
Ursodiol
Ustekinumab
Valdecoxib
Valganciclovir
Valproic Acid
Valrubicin
Valsartan
Vancomycin
Vandetanib
Vardenafil
Varenicline
Varicella Vaccine
Vedolizumab
Vemurafenib
Venlafaxine
Verapamil
Vernakalant
Vincristine
Vitamin A
Voriconazole
Vorinostat
Vortioxetine
Warfarin
Zalcitabine
Zaleplon
Ziconotide
Zidovudine
Zileuton
Zolmitriptan
Zolpidem
Zonisamide
Zoster Vaccine
Zuclopenthixol
Pseudolymphoma
Adalimumab
Aldesleukin
Allopurinol
Alprazolam
Amitriptyline

Amlodipine
Aspirin
Atenolol
Bromocriptine
Captopril
Carbamazepine
Cefixime
Cefuroxime
Chlorpromazine
Cimetidine
Clarithromycin
Clonazepam
Clonidine
Co-Trimoxazole
Cyclosporine
Dapsone
Desipramine
Diclofenac
Diflunisal
Diltiazem
Doxepin
Estrogens
Etanercept
Ethosuximide
Ethotoin
Fluorouracil
Fluoxetine
Fosinopril
Furosemide
Gemcitabine
Gemfibrozil
Glatiramer
Gold & Gold Compounds
Hepatitis A Vaccine
Hepatitis B Vaccine
Hydrochlorothiazide
Ibuprofen
Imatinib
Indomethacin
Infliximab
Interferon Alfa
Ketoprofen
Lamotrigine
Leucovorin
Lisinopril
Lithium
Lorazepam
Losartan
Lovastatin
Methotrexate
Methylphenidate
Metoprolol
Mexiletine
Nabumetone
Naproxen
Nitrofurantoin
Nizatidine
Oxaliplatin
Oxaprozin
Perphenazine
Phenobarbital
Phenytoin
Procainamide
Ranitidine
Sulfamethoxazole
Sulfasalazine
Sulindac
Tamoxifen
Terfenadine
Thioridazine
Valproic Acid

Valsartan
Zoledronate

Pseudoporphyria

Acitretin
Amiodarone
Ampicillin
Ampicillin/Sulbactam
Aspirin
Bumetanide
Carisoprodol
Cefepime
Celecoxib
Chlorthalidone
Ciprofloxacin
Cyclosporine
Diclofenac
Diflunisal
Fluorouracil
Flutamide
Hydrochlorothiazide
Ibuprofen
Imatinib
Indomethacin
Isotretinoin
Ketoprofen
Mefenamic Acid
Metformin
Nabumetone
Nalidixic Acid
Naproxen
Oral Contraceptives
Oxaprozin
Piroxicam
Pyridoxine
Quinidine
Rofecoxib
Tetracycline
Torsemide
Triamterene
Voriconazole

Psoriasis

Abatacept
Acebutolol
Aceclofenac
Acetazolamide
Acitretin
Adalimumab
Aldesleukin
Aminoglutethimide
Amiodarone
Amoxicillin
Ampicillin
Anakinra
Apremilast
Arsenic
Aspirin
Atenolol
Avelumab
BCG Vaccine
Betamethasone
Bisoprolol
Bupropion
Calcipotriol
Candesartan
Captopril
Carbamazepine
Carvedilol
Certolizumab
Cetuximab
Chlorambucil
Chloroquine

Chlorthalidone
Cimetidine
Clarithromycin
Clonidine
Clopidogrel
Co-Trimoxazole
Cyclosporine
Dabrafenib
Daclizumab
Diclofenac
Digoxin
Diltiazem
Dipyridamole
Docetaxel
Donepezil
Doxorubicin
Doxycycline
Durvalumab
Efalizumab
Eletriptan
Enalapril
Esmolol
Etanercept
Fexofenadine
Flecainide
Fluorouracil
Fluoxetine
Fluoxymesterone
Foscarnet
Gemfibrozil
Glyburide
Gold & Gold Compounds
Golimumab
Granulocyte Colony-
    Stimulating Factor (G-CSF)
Human Papillomavirus (HPV)
    Vaccine
Hydroxychloroquine
Hydroxyurea
Ibuprofen
Imatinib
Imiquimod
Indomethacin
Infliximab
Interferon Alfa
Interferon Beta
Ketoprofen
Labetalol
Lapatinib
Letrozole
Levamisole
Levetiracetam
Levobetaxolol
Lisinopril
Lithium
Losartan
MDMA
Meclofenamate
Mefloquine
Meloxicam
Mesalamine
Methicillin
Methotrexate
Methyltestosterone
Metipranolol
Metoprolol
Modafinil
Morphine
Mycophenolate
Nadolol
Nilotinib

Nivolumab
Olanzapine
Ombitasvir/Paritaprevir/
    Ritonavir
Omeprazole
Oral Contraceptives
Oxprenolol
Paroxetine Hydrochloride
PEG-Interferon
Pembrolizumab
Penicillamine
Pentostatin
Perindopril
Phenylbutazone
Pindolol
Potassium Iodide
Prednisolone
Primaquine
Propafenone
Propranolol
Quinacrine
Quinidine
Rabeprazole
Ramipril
Ranitidine
Ribavirin
Risperidone
Ritonavir
Rituximab
Rivastigmine
Rofecoxib
Ropinirole
Saquinavir
Secukinumab
Sertraline
Siltuximab
Sitagliptin
Sorafenib
Sotalol
Sulfamethoxazole
Sulfasalazine
Sulfisoxazole
Tacrine
Tazarotene
Telmisartan
Terbinafine
Terfenadine
Teriflunomide
Testosterone
Tetracycline
Thalidomide
Thioguanine
Tiagabine
Timolol
Tocilizumab
Tofacitinib
Trazodone
Urapidil
Ustekinumab
Valdecoxib
Vedolizumab
Venlafaxine
Voriconazole

Purpura

Acenocoumarol
Acetaminophen
Acetazolamide
Acitretin
Adalimumab
Aldesleukin
Alemtuzumab

Allopurinol
Alteplase
Aminocaproic Acid
Aminoglutethimide
Aminolevulinic Acid
Aminosalicylate Sodium
Amiodarone
Amitriptyline
Amlodipine
Amphotericin B
Ampicillin
Anastrozole
Anti-Thymocyte Globulin
    (Equine)
Arsenic
Artemether/Lumefantrine
Aspartame
Aspirin
Azacitidine
Aztreonam
Bendamustine
Beta-Carotene
Betaxolol
Bevacizumab
Bortezomib
Botulinum Toxin (A & B)
Buspirone
Busulfan
Butabarbital
Butalbital
Capecitabine
Captopril
Carbamazepine
Carbenicillin
Carteolol
Carvedilol
Cefaclor
Cefoxitin
Celecoxib
Cephalothin
Cetirizine
Chloral Hydrate
Chlorambucil
Chloramphenicol
Chlordiazepoxide
Chlorothiazide
Chlorpromazine
Chlorpropamide
Chlorthalidone
Cilostazol
Cinacalcet
Ciprofloxacin
Citalopram
Cladribine
Clarithromycin
Clidinium
Clofibrate
Clomiphene
Clomipramine
Clonazepam
Clopidogrel
Clozapine
Co-Trimoxazole
Cocaine
Codeine
Cycloserine
Cyclosporine
Cytarabine
Dabigatran
Danazol
Dapsone

Deferiprone
Delavirdine
Desipramine
Diazepam
Diclofenac
Dicumarol
Diethylpropion
Diethylstilbestrol
Digoxin
Diltiazem
Diphenhydramine
Dipyridamole
Disopyramide
Disulfiram
Donepezil
Doxazosin
Doxepin
Doxorubicin
Doxycycline
Drotrecogin Alfa
Duloxetine
Enalapril
Enoxacin
Enoxaparin
Entacapone
Ephedrine
Eprosartan
Erlotinib
Escitalopram
Estazolam
Estramustine
Estrogens
Etanercept
Ethacrynic Acid
Ethambutol
Ethchlorvynol
Ethionamide
Ethosuximide
Ethotoin
Famotidine
Febuxostat
Felodipine
Fenoprofen
Fentanyl
Flucloxacillin
Fluconazole
Fluoxetine
Fluvoxamine
Fondaparinux
Frovatriptan
Furosemide
Gabapentin
Galantamine
Gefitinib
Gentamicin
Glatiramer
Glipizide
Glyburide
Gold & Gold Compounds
Griseofulvin
Guanfacine
Heparin
Hepatitis B Vaccine
Heroin
Histrelin
Hyaluronic Acid
Hydralazine
Hydrochlorothiazide
Hydrocortisone
Hydroxyurea
Hydroxyzine

Ibritumomab
Ibuprofen
Imatinib
Imipramine
Indomethacin
Infliximab
Influenza Vaccine
Insulin
Interferon Alfa
Interferon Beta
Iohexol
Ipodate
Isoniazid
Isotretinoin
Itraconazole
Ketoconazole
Ketoprofen
Ketorolac
Labetalol
Lamotrigine
Leflunomide
Lenalidomide
Leuprolide
Levamisole
Levobupivacaine
Levodopa
Levofloxacin
Lidocaine
Lincomycin
Lindane
Linezolid
Lisinopril
Lithium
Lomefloxacin
Loratadine
Losartan
Lovastatin
Maprotiline
Measles, Mumps & Rubella
    (MMR) Virus Vaccine
Mecasermin
Mechlorethamine
Meclofenamate
Medroxyprogesterone
Mefloquine
Meloxicam
Meningococcal Groups C & Y
    & Haemophilus B Tetanus
    Toxoid Conjugate Vaccine
Mephenytoin
Meprobamate
Metformin
Methimazole
Methoxsalen
Methyldopa
Methylphenidate
Metoclopramide
Metolazone
Miconazole
Minocycline
Mirabegron
Mitomycin
Mitoxantrone
Montelukast
Nalidixic Acid
Naproxen
Naratriptan
Natalizumab
Nifedipine
Nimesulide
Nitrofurantoin

Nitroglycerin
Octreotide
Olanzapine
Omacetaxine
Oral Contraceptives
Oxaliplatin
Oxcarbazepine
Oxytetracycline
Pandemic Influenza Vaccine
    (HINI)
Paroxetine Hydrochloride
Pegaspargase
Penicillamine
Pentagastrin
Pentobarbital
Pentosan
Pentostatin
Perindopril
Phenobarbital
Phensuximide
Phenytoin
Pirbuterol
Piroxicam
Plicamycin
Pravastatin
Prednisone
Prilocaine
Procainamide
Prochlorperazine
Promethazine
Propafenone
Propranolol
Propylthiouracil
Pyrimethamine
Quinidine
Quinine
Ramipril
Ranitidine
Rapacuronium
Rifampin
Rifapentine
Risperidone
Rituximab
Rivastigmine
Ropinirole
Rosuvastatin
Rotigotine
Ruxolitinib
Sertraline
Sildenafil
Simvastatin
Sirolimus
Smallpox Vaccine
Streptokinase
Streptomycin
Sulfadoxine
Sulfamethoxazole
Sulfasalazine
Sulfisoxazole
Sulindac
Tacrine
Tacrolimus
Tadalafil
Tamoxifen
Tartrazine
Teicoplanin
Tetracycline
Thalidomide
Thiamine
Thiopental
Ticlopidine

Tinzaparin
Tizanidine
Tolbutamide
Tolmetin
Topiramate
Topotecan
Torsemide
Tosufloxacin
Trichlormethiazide
Trimethadione
Tripelennamine
Valacyclovir
Valproic Acid
Vancomycin
Varicella Vaccine
Vasopressin
Verapamil
Voriconazole
Warfarin
Zolpidem
Zonisamide

Raynaud's phenomenon
Acebutolol
Amphotericin B
Aripiprazole
Arsenic
Atenolol
Bisoprolol
Bleomycin
Bromocriptine
Carboplatin
Carteolol
Cisplatin
Clonidine
Cocaine
Cyclosporine
Dextroamphetamine
Dopamine
Doxorubicin
Estrogens
Ethosuximide
Fluoxetine
Gemcitabine
Gemfibrozil
Hepatitis B Vaccine
Human Papillomavirus (HPV)
    Vaccine
Hydroxyurea
Iloprost
Interferon Alfa
Interferon Beta
Isotretinoin
Labetalol
Lamotrigine
Leflunomide
Methotrexate
Methylphenidate
Metoprolol
Minocycline
Nadolol
Octreotide
Phentermine
Pindolol
Propofol
Propranolol
Quinine
Ribavirin
Rofecoxib
Sotalol
Spironolactone
Sulfasalazine

Sulindac
Sumatriptan
Tegafur/Gimeracil/Oteracil
Tegaserod
Telmisartan
Thiothixene
Timolol
Uracil/Tegafur
Vinblastine
Vincristine
Zolmitriptan

Rhabdomyolysis
Abacavir
Abiraterone
Acetaminophen
Aldesleukin
Allopurinol
Alprazolam
Aminocaproic Acid
Aminophylline
Amiodarone
Amisulpride
Amitriptyline
Amlodipine
Amobarbital
Amoxicillin
Amphotericin B
Aprobarbital
Aspirin
Atorvastatin
Atropine Sulfate
Azacitidine
Azathioprine
Azithromycin
Baclofen
Benztropine
Bezafibrate
Buprenorphine
Bupropion
Butabarbital
Butalbital
Carbamazepine
Chlorpromazine
Cholestyramine
Ciprofibrate
Ciprofloxacin
Cisplatin
Citalopram
Clarithromycin
Clofibrate
Clopidogrel
Clozapine
Co-Trimoxazole
Cobicistat/Elvitegravir/
    Emtricitabine/Tenofovir
    Disoproxil
Cocaine
Colchicine
Colistin
Cyclosporine
Cytarabine
Dacarbazine
Danazol
Daptomycin
Dasatinib
Deferasirox
Delavirdine
Desipramine
Dexketoprofen
Dextroamphetamine
Diatrizoate

Diazepam
Diclofenac
Didanosine
Digoxin
Diltiazem
Diphenhydramine
Distigmine
Dolutegravir
Domperidone
Doxepin
Droperidol
Enflurane
Enoxacin
Epinephrine
Erlotinib
Erythromycin
Esomeprazole
Fenbufen
Fenofibrate
Fluconazole
Fluorouracil
Fluoxetine
Fluphenazine
Fluprednisolone
Fluvastatin
Fusidic Acid
Gabapentin
Gatifloxacin
Gemcitabine
Gemfibrozil
Haloperidol
Halothane
Heroin
Hydroxychloroquine
Ibuprofen
Imatinib
Infliximab
Influenza Vaccine
Interferon Alfa
Interferon Beta
Ipilimumab
Isoflurane
Isoniazid
Isotretinoin
Itraconazole
Ketoconazole
Labetalol
Lamivudine
Lamotrigine
Leflunomide
Lenalidomide
Leuprolide
Levetiracetam
Levodopa
Levofloxacin
Levomepromazine
Lindane
Linezolid
Lithium
Lorazepam
Lovastatin
Loxapine
Lurasidone
Maraviroc
MDMA
Meloxicam
Melphalan
Mephobarbital
Meprobamate
Metformin
Methadone

Methamphetamine
Methohexital
Metoprolol
Minocycline
Mirtazapine
Mizoribine
Molindone
Morphine
Moxifloxacin
Naltrexone
Naproxen
Nefazodone
Nelarabine
Nelfinavir
Nitrazepam
Nivolumab
Norfloxacin
Ofloxacin
Olanzapine
Omeprazole
Paclitaxel
Palbociclib
Paliperidone
Pancuronium
Pantoprazole
PEG-Interferon
Pembrolizumab
Pemetrexed
Pemoline
Pentamidine
Pentobarbital
Perphenazine
Phendimetrazine
Phenelzine
Phenobarbital
Phenylpropanolamine
Phenytoin
Pioglitazone
Pravastatin
Pregabalin
Primidone
Propofol
Protamine Sulfate
Protriptyline
Pyrazinamide
Quetiapine
Quinacrine
Quinine
Rabeprazole
Raltegravir
Ranolazine
Ribavirin
Risperidone
Ritodrine
Ritonavir
Rosuvastatin
Secobarbital
Sertraline
Sevoflurane
Sildenafil
Simeprevir
Simvastatin
Sirolimus
Sitagliptin
Sonidegib
Sotalol
Stanozolol
Streptokinase
Streptomycin
Succinylcholine
Sulfamethoxazole

Sulfasalazine
Sulpiride
Sunitinib
Tacrolimus
Tasonermin
Tenecteplase
Tenofovir Disoproxil
Terbinafine
Terbutaline
Teriflunomide
Terlipressin
Thiopental
Ticagrelor
Tolcapone
Tolvaptan
Trabectedin
Trametinib
Trandolapril
Tranylcypromine
Trifluoperazine
Trimethoprim
Trospium
Valproic Acid
Vasopressin
Venlafaxine
Verapamil
Vinblastine
Warfarin
Ziconotide
Ziprasidone

Stevens-Johnson syndrome
Abacavir
Aceclofenac
Acetaminophen
Acetazolamide
Acyclovir
Adalimumab
Adefovir
Afatinib
Albendazole
Albuterol
Aldesleukin
Allopurinol
Alogliptin
Amifostine
Aminophylline
Amiodarone
Amlodipine
Amobarbital
Amoxicillin
Ampicillin
Amprenavir
Anthrax Vaccine
Aripiprazole
Arsenic
Aspirin
Astemizole
Atovaquone
Atovaquone/Proguanil
Atropine Sulfate
Azathioprine
Azithromycin
Bendamustine
Benznidazole
Bezafibrate
Bleomycin
Bromfenac
Bupropion
Butabarbital
Butalbital
Capecitabine

Captopril
Carbamazepine
Carvedilol
Cefaclor
Cefadroxil
Cefamandole
Cefazolin
Cefdinir
Cefepime
Cefixime
Cefmetazole
Cefonicid
Cefoperazone
Cefotaxime
Cefotetan
Cefoxitin
Cefpodoxime
Cefprozil
Ceftazidime
Ceftibuten
Ceftizoxime
Ceftriaxone
Cefuroxime
Celecoxib
Cephalexin
Cephalothin
Cephapirin
Cephradine
Cetuximab
Chloramphenicol
Chlordiazepoxide
Chlormezanone
Chloroquine
Chlorpropamide
Cimetidine
Ciprofloxacin
Cisplatin
Clarithromycin
Clindamycin
Clobazam
Clofibrate
Clopidogrel
Cloxacillin
Clozapine
Co-Trimoxazole
Cocaine
Cyclophosphamide
Cycloserine
Dapsone
Darunavir
Delavirdine
Dexamethasone
Diclofenac
Dicloxacillin
Didanosine
Diflunisal
Diltiazem
Dimenhydrinate
Dipyridamole
Docetaxel
Doxycycline
Duloxetine
Efavirenz
Enalapril
Enoxacin
Erythromycin
Ethambutol
Ethosuximide
Etodolac
Etoposide
Etoricoxib

Felbamate
Fenbufen
Fenoprofen
Fexofenadine
Flucloxacillin
Fluconazole
Fluoxetine
Flurbiprofen
Furosemide
Gabapentin
Galantamine
Gemcitabine
Glipizide
Griseofulvin
Heparin
Human Papillomavirus (HPV)
    Vaccine
Hydrochlorothiazide
Hydroxychloroquine
Ibuprofen
Imatinib
Immune Globulin IV
Indapamide
Indinavir
Indomethacin
Infliximab
Iohexol
Ipilimumab
Isoniazid
Itraconazole
Ivermectin
Ixazomib
Ketoprofen
Ketorolac
Lacosamide
Lamivudine
Lamotrigine
Lansoprazole
Leflunomide
Lenalidomide
Levamisole
Levetiracetam
Levofloxacin
Lidocaine
Lincomycin
Lomefloxacin
Loracarbef
Lorazepam
Lovastatin
Lymecycline
Maprotiline
Mebendazole
Mechlorethamine
Meclofenamate
Mefenamic Acid
Mefloquine
Meloxicam
Mephenytoin
Mephobarbital
Meprobamate
Metamizole
Methazolamide
Methimazole
Methotrexate
Methsuximide
Methyldopa
Methylprednisolone
Metronidazole
Mexiletine
Miltefosine
Minocycline

Minoxidil
Mizoribine
Modafinil
Nabumetone
Naproxen
Nevirapine
Nifedipine
Nimesulide
Nitrofurantoin
Nivolumab
Norfloxacin
Nystatin
Ofloxacin
Omeprazole
Oral Contraceptives
Oxacillin
Oxaprozin
Oxcarbazepine
Paclitaxel
Pantoprazole
PEG-Interferon
Pembrolizumab
Pentamidine
Pentobarbital
Peplomycin
Phenobarbital
Phenolphthalein
Phenylbutazone
Phenytoin
Piroxicam
Prednisolone
Pristinamycin
Promethazine
Propranolol
Pyrimethamine
Quinine
Raltegravir
Ramipril
Ranitidine
Regorafenib
Ribavirin
Rifampin
Risedronate
Rituximab
Rofecoxib
Secobarbital
Sertraline
Sibutramine
Sitagliptin
Smallpox Vaccine
Sorafenib
Stavudine
Streptomycin
Strontium Ranelate
Sulfacetamide
Sulfadiazine
Sulfadoxine
Sulfamethoxazole
Sulfasalazine
Sulfisoxazole
Sulindac
Tamoxifen
Tegafur/Gimeracil/Oteracil
Teicoplanin
Telaprevir
Temozolomide
Tenofovir Disoproxil
Terbinafine
Teriflunomide
Tetracycline
Tetrazepam

Thalidomide
Thiabendazole
Thiopental
Ticlopidine
Tigecycline
Tiludronate
Tocainide
Tolmetin
Torsemide
Trimethadione
Trimethoprim
Trovafloxacin
Valdecoxib
Valproic Acid
Vancomycin
Vandetanib
Varicella Vaccine
Vemurafenib
Venlafaxine
Verapamil
Vitamin A
Voriconazole
Zidovudine
Zoledronate
Zonisamide

Tinnitus
Acamprosate
Acetaminophen
Acetazolamide
Acitretin
Adalimumab
Almotriptan
Amikacin
Amitriptyline
Anagrelide
Aprepitant
Arsenic
Artemether/Lumefantrine
Artesunate
Aspirin
Atorvastatin
Azithromycin
Bedaquiline
Betaxolol
Bismuth
Bleomycin
Bortezomib
Botulinum Toxin (A & B)
Bupropion
Carbimazole
Carboplatin
Carvedilol
Cefpodoxime
Chlorambucil
Chloramphenicol
Chloroquine
Chlorpromazine
Cilostazol
Ciprofloxacin
Cisplatin
Citalopram
Clarithromycin
Clindamycin
Clomipramine
Colistin
Cyclobenzaprine
Cycloserine
Cyclosporine
Dasatinib
Daunorubicin
Deferoxamine

Degarelix
Delafloxacin
Desvenlafaxine
Dexamethasone
Dexlansoprazole
Doxepin
Doxycycline
Dronabinol
Duloxetine
Eletriptan
Elotuzumab
Eprosartan
Erlotinib
Erythromycin
Escitalopram
Eslicarbazepine
Esomeprazole
Eszopiclone
Etanercept
Ethambutol
Etoposide
Febuxostat
Frovatriptan
Gadodiamide
Gadoteridol
Gadoversetamide
Gentamicin
Glatiramer
Halofantrine
Hepatitis B Vaccine
Hydroxychloroquine
Ibuprofen
Imipramine
Indomethacin
Interferon Alfa
Isavuconazonium Sulfate
Isoniazid
Kanamycin
Ketorolac
Lapatinib
Lenalidomide
Levobetaxolol
Levofloxacin
Lidocaine
Mefloquine
Meloxicam
Mesalamine
Methyl salicylate
Metronidazole
Minocycline
Moexipril
Moxifloxacin
Muromonab-CD3
Nabumetone
Nadolol
Naproxen
Nitroprusside
Omacetaxine
Pamidronate
Paromomycin
PEG-Interferon
Perflutren
Phenelzine
Piroxicam
Propylthiouracil
Quinine
Rabeprazole
Ranitidine
Ranolazine
Ribavirin
Rifaximin

Rivastigmine
Ropivacaine
Rotigotine
Ruxolitinib
Salsalate
Sertraline
Sildenafil
Sirolimus
Sodium Oxybate
Sorafenib
Sumatriptan
Tacrolimus
Tadalafil
Teicoplanin
Tetracycline
Tiagabine
Tobramycin
Tramadol
Triptorelin
Valdecoxib
Valproic Acid
Vancomycin
Vardenafil
Venlafaxine
Vigabatrin
Vinblastine
Vincristine
Voriconazole
Zaleplon
Ziconotide
Ziprasidone
Zolpidem
Zonisamide

Toxic epidermal necrolysis (TEN)
Abacavir
Aceclofenac
Acetaminophen
Acetazolamide
Adefovir
Aldesleukin
Alfuzosin
Allopurinol
Alprostadil
Amifostine
Aminosalicylate Sodium
Amiodarone
Amlodipine
Amobarbital
Amoxapine
Amoxicillin
Ampicillin
Anthrax Vaccine
Arsenic
Asparaginase
Aspirin
Atorvastatin
Atovaquone
Azathioprine
Aztreonam
BCG Vaccine
Bendamustine
Benznidazole
Bezafibrate
Bucillamine
Busulfan
Butabarbital
Butalbital
Captopril
Carbamazepine
Carbenicillin

Caspofungin
Cefaclor
Cefamandole
Cefazolin
Cefixime
Cefotaxime
Cefoxitin
Ceftazidime
Ceftriaxone
Cefuroxime
Celecoxib
Cephalexin
Cephalothin
Cephradine
Cetuximab
Chlorambucil
Chloramphenicol
Chlormezanone
Chloroquine
Chlorpromazine
Chlorpropamide
Chlorthalidone
Cilostazol
Cimetidine
Ciprofloxacin
Cisplatin
Cladribine
Clarithromycin
Clindamycin
Clobazam
Co-Trimoxazole
Codeine
Colchicine
Cyclophosphamide
Cyclosporine
Cytarabine
Dapsone
Darunavir
Deflazacort
Demeclocycline
Denileukin
Dexamethasone
Dextroamphetamine
Diatrizoate
Diclofenac
Diflunisal
Diltiazem
Diphenhydramine
Dipyridamole
Disulfiram
Docetaxel
Dorzolamide
Doxycycline
Dronedarone
Efavirenz
Enalapril
Enoxacin
Ephedrine
Erythromycin
Eslicarbazepine
Ethambutol
Etidronate
Etodolac
Etoricoxib
Famotidine
Felbamate
Fenbufen
Fenofibrate
Fenoprofen
Fexofenadine
Flucloxacillin

Fluconazole
Fludarabine
Fluoxetine
Fluphenazine
Flurazepam
Flurbiprofen
Fluvoxamine
Foscarnet
Furosemide
Gefitinib
Gemcitabine
Gemeprost
Gentamicin
Gold & Gold Compounds
Grepafloxacin
Griseofulvin
Heparin
Heroin
Hydralazine
Hydrochlorothiazide
Hydroxychloroquine
Ibandronate
Ibuprofen
Imatinib
Imipenem/Cilastatin
Immune Globulin IV
Indapamide
Indomethacin
Infliximab
Iohexol
Ipilimumab
Isoniazid
Isotretinoin
Ivermectin
Ketoprofen
Ketorolac
Lacosamide
Lamivudine
Lamotrigine
Lansoprazole
Latanoprost
Leflunomide
Lenalidomide
Letrozole
Levetiracetam
Levofloxacin
Lincomycin
Lomefloxacin
Lomustine
Meclofenamate
Mefenamic Acid
Mefloquine
Meloxicam
Meperidine
Mephenytoin
Meprobamate
Mercaptopurine
Meropenem
Mesna
Metamizole
Methamphetamine
Methazolamide
Methimazole
Methotrexate
Metolazone
Metronidazole
Minocycline
Minoxidil
Moxifloxacin
Mupirocin
Nabumetone

Nalidixic Acid
Naproxen
Neomycin
Nevirapine
Nifedipine
Nitrofurantoin
Nivolumab
Norfloxacin
Ofloxacin
Omeprazole
Ondansetron
Oseltamivir
Oxaprozin
Oxazepam
Oxcarbazepine
Pantoprazole
Papaverine
PEG-Interferon
Pemetrexed
Penicillamine
Penicillin V
Pentamidine
Pentazocine
Pentobarbital
Phenobarbital
Phenolphthalein
Phenylbutazone
Phenytoin
Piroxicam
Plicamycin
Prednisolone
Primidone
Pristinamycin
Procarbazine
Prochlorperazine
Promethazine
Propranolol
Propylthiouracil
Pyridoxine
Pyrimethamine
Quinidine
Quinine
Ranitidine
Regorafenib
Reserpine
Ribavirin
Rifampin
Rifaximin
Ritodrine
Rituximab
Rofecoxib
Smallpox Vaccine
Stavudine
Streptomycin
Streptozocin
Strontium Ranelate
Sulfacetamide
Sulfadiazine
Sulfadoxine
Sulfamethoxazole
Sulfasalazine
Sulfisoxazole
Sulindac
Tegafur/Gimeracil/Oteracil
Telaprevir
Temozolomide
Terbinafine
Terconazole
Teriflunomide
Tetracycline
Tetrazepam

Thalidomide
Thiabendazole
Thiopental
Thioridazine
Timolol
Tolbutamide
Tolmetin
Trimethoprim
Trovafloxacin
Valdecoxib
Valproic Acid
Vancomycin
Vemurafenib
Vinorelbine
Voriconazole
Warfarin
Zidovudine
Zonisamide

Urticaria
Abatacept
Acamprosate
Acarbose
Acebutolol
Aceclofenac
Acetaminophen
Acetohexamide
Acetylcysteine
Acyclovir
Adalimumab
Albendazole
Albiglutide
Albuterol
Alclometasone
Aldesleukin
Alefacept
Alemtuzumab
Alendronate
Alfentanil
Alglucerase
Alglucosidase Alfa
Alirocumab
Allopurinol
Alpha-Lipoic Acid
Alprazolam
Alprostadil
Alteplase
Amcinonide
Aminolevulinic Acid
Aminophylline
Aminosalicylate Sodium
Amiodarone
Amlodipine
Amobarbital
Amodiaquine
Amoxapine
Amoxicillin
Amphotericin B
Ampicillin
Anagrelide
Anakinra
Anidulafungin
Anistreplase
Anthrax Vaccine
Anti-Thymocyte Globulin
   (Equine)
Aprepitant
Arsenic
Artemether/Lumefantrine
Artesunate
Asfotase Alfa
Asparaginase

Asparaginase *Erwinia*
   chrysanthemi
Aspartame
Aspirin
Astemizole
Atenolol
Atorvastatin
Atovaquone/Proguanil
Atracurium
Atropine Sulfate
Azacitidine
Azathioprine
Azithromycin
Aztreonam
Bacitracin
BCG Vaccine
Benazepril
Benznidazole
Bepotastine
Betamethasone
Bezafibrate
Bismuth
Bosutinib
Brinzolamide
Bumetanide
Bupropion
Buspirone
Busulfan
Butorphanol
Calcipotriol
Calcitonin
Canagliflozin
Captopril
Carbamazepine
Carbenicillin
Carboplatin
Carisoprodol
Caspofungin
Cefaclor
Cefadroxil
Cefamandole
Cefazolin
Cefdinir
Cefditoren
Cefepime
Cefixime
Cefmetazole
Cefonicid
Cefoperazone
Cefotaxime
Cefotetan
Cefpodoxime
Cefprozil
Ceftaroline Fosamil
Ceftazidime
Ceftibuten
Ceftizoxime
Ceftolozane & Tazobactam
Ceftriaxone
Cefuroxime
Celecoxib
Cephalexin
Cephalothin
Cephapirin
Cephradine
Certolizumab
Cetirizine
Chloral Hydrate
Chlorambucil
Chloramphenicol
Chlordiazepoxide

Chlorhexidine
Chloroquine
Chlorothiazide
Chlorpromazine
Chlorpropamide
Chlorthalidone
Chlorzoxazone
Cidofovir
Cilostazol
Cimetidine
Cinoxacin
Ciprofloxacin
Cisplatin
Clarithromycin
Clemastine
Clindamycin
Clioquinol
Clofibrate
Clomiphene
Clomipramine
Clonidine
Clopidogrel
Clorazepate
Cloxacillin
Clozapine
Co-Trimoxazole
Coagulation Factor IX
  (Recombinant)
Cocaine
Codeine
Colchicine
Colestipol
Crisaborole
Cromolyn
Cyanocobalamin
Cyclamate
Cyclobenzaprine
Cyclophosphamide
Cycloserine
Cyclosporine
Cysteamine
Cytarabine
Dacarbazine
Daclizumab
Dalbavancin
Dapagliflozin
Dapsone
Darunavir
Dasatinib
Daunorubicin
Decitabine
Deferasirox
Deferoxamine
Deflazacort
Degarelix
Delafloxacin
Delavirdine
Deoxycholic Acid
Desipramine
Desloratadine
Dexamethasone
Dexlansoprazole
Dextroamphetamine
Diazepam
Diclofenac
Dicloxacillin
Dicumarol
Diethylstilbestrol
Diflunisal
Digoxin
Dihydrocodeine

Diltiazem
Dimenhydrinate
Dimethyl Fumarate
Dinutuximab
Diphenoxylate
Dipyridamole
Dirithromycin
Disulfiram
Docetaxel
Donepezil
Doxacurium
Doxazosin
Doxorubicin
Doxycycline
Efalizumab
Efavirenz
Eletriptan
Emtricitabine
Enalapril
Enfuvirtide
Enoxacin
Enoxaparin
Ephedrine
Ertapenem
Erythromycin
Esomeprazole
Estazolam
Estrogens
Eszopiclone
Etanercept
Etelcalcetide
Ethambutol
Ethionamide
Ethosuximide
Etodolac
Etoricoxib
Evolocumab
Exenatide
Famotidine
Febuxostat
Felbamate
Felodipine
Fenofibrate
Fenoprofen
Fentanyl
Ferumoxytol
Fexofenadine
Finasteride
Flecainide
Flucloxacillin
Flumazenil
Fluorides
Fluoxetine
Flurbiprofen
Fluvoxamine
Folic Acid
Foscarnet
Fosinopril
Fulvestrant
Furazolidone
Furosemide
Gadobenate
Gadodiamide
Gadopentetate
Gadoteridol
Gadoversetamide
Ganciclovir
Gefitinib
Gemfibrozil
Gemifloxacin
Gentamicin

Glatiramer
Glimepiride
Glipizide
Glucagon
Glyburide
Gold & Gold Compounds
Golimumab
Granulocyte Colony-
  Stimulating Factor (G-CSF)
Grepafloxacin
Griseofulvin
Halothane
Heparin
Hepatitis B Vaccine
Heroin
Histrelin
Human Papillomavirus Vaccine
  (Bivalent)
Hydrochlorothiazide
Hydrocodone
Hydrocortisone
Hydromorphone
Hydroxychloroquine
Hydroxyzine
Ibritumomab
Ibuprofen
Idarubicin
Idursulfase
Imatinib
Imiglucerase
Imipenem/Cilastatin
Imipramine
Immune Globulin IV
Indapamide
Indinavir
Indomethacin
Infliximab
Insulin
Insulin Glulisine
Interferon Alfa
Interferon Beta
Iodixanol
Iohexol
Iomeprol
Iopromide
Ioversol
Ipilimumab
Ipratropium
Irbesartan
Isavuconazonium Sulfate
Isoniazid
Isotretinoin
Isradipine
Itraconazole
Ivacaftor
Ivermectin
Ixazomib
Ixekizumab
Japanese Encephalitis Vaccine
Ketamine
Ketoconazole
Ketoprofen
Ketorolac
Labetalol
Lamivudine
Lamotrigine
Lansoprazole
Leflunomide
Lenalidomide
Lepirudin
Lesinurad

Leucovorin
Leuprolide
Levamisole
Levetiracetam
Levocetirizine
Levofloxacin
Levomilnacipran
Levonorgestrel
Levothyroxine
Lidocaine
Linaclotide
Linagliptin
Lincomycin
Lindane
Linezolid
Liothyronine
Liraglutide
Lisinopril
Lithium
Lixisenatide
Lomefloxacin
Loracarbef
Loratadine
Losartan
Lubiprostone
Maprotiline
Measles, Mumps & Rubella
  (MMR) Virus Vaccine
Mebeverine
Mechlorethamine
Meclofenamate
Medroxyprogesterone
Mefenamic Acid
Mefloquine
Meloxicam
Melphalan
Memantine
Meperidine
Mephenytoin
Meprobamate
Mercaptopurine
Meropenem
Mesna
Metamizole
Metformin
Methadone
Methamphetamine
Methazolamide
Methimazole
Methohexital
Methotrexate
Methoxsalen
Methsuximide
Methyldopa
Methylphenidate
Methylprednisolone
Metoclopramide
Metolazone
Metronidazole
Mexiletine
Micafungin
Miconazole
Midazolam
Miltefosine
Minocycline
Mirabegron
Mitomycin
Mitotane
Mivacurium
Moexipril
Montelukast

Moricizine
Moxifloxacin
Mycophenolate
Nabumetone
Nafarelin
Nalbuphine
Nalidixic Acid
Naloxone
Naproxen
Naratriptan
Nefazodone
Nelfinavir
Neomycin
Neostigmine
Nevirapine
Niacin
Nicardipine
Nifedipine
Nilotinib
Nimesulide
Nisoldipine
Nitrofurantoin
Nitroglycerin
Nivolumab
Nizatidine
Norfloxacin
Obeticholic Acid
Octreotide
Ofatumumab
Ofloxacin
Olanzapine
Olsalazine
Omalizumab
Ombitasvir/Paritaprevir/
    Ritonavir
Omeprazole
Ondansetron
Oral Contraceptives
Oritavancin
Oxacillin
Oxaliplatin
Oxaprozin
Oxerutins
Oxilan
Oxprenolol
Oxycodone
Oxymorphone
Paclitaxel
Pantoprazole
Pantothenic Acid
Paroxetine Hydrochloride
PEG-Interferon
Pegaptanib
Pegaspargase
Pemetrexed
Penicillamine
Penicillin G
Penicillin V
Pentamidine
Pentosan
Pentostatin
Perflutren
Permethrin
Perphenazine
Phenobarbital
Phenolphthalein
Phenylbutazone
Phenytoin
Phytonadione
Pilocarpine
Pipecuronium

Piroxicam
Pitavastatin
Pizotifen
Plasma (Human) Blood
    Product
Pneumococcal Vaccine
Polidocanol
Pomalidomide
Porfimer
Potassium Iodide
Praziquantel
Prazosin
Prednicarbate
Prednisolone
Prednisone
Prilocaine
Primaquine
Primidone
Pristinamycin
Probenecid
Procainamide
Procarbazine
Progestins
Promethazine
Propafenone
Propofol
Propoxyphene
Propranolol
Propylthiouracil
Propyphenazone
Protamine Sulfate
Psoralens
Quinacrine
Quinapril
Quinestrol
Quinidine
Quinine
Quinupristin/Dalfopristin
Rabeprazole
Ramipril
Ranitidine
Rapacuronium
Remifentanil
Ribavirin
Riboflavin
Rifampin
Rifapentine
Rifaximin
Risedronate
Risperidone
Ritonavir
Rituximab
Rivaroxaban
Rivastigmine
Rofecoxib
Ropinirole
Roxithromycin
Rupatadine
Saccharin
Salmeterol
Salsalate
Saquinavir
Sebelipase Alfa
Secretin
Secukinumab
Sertraline
Sildenafil
Simvastatin
Smallpox Vaccine
Sodium Oxybate
Sorafenib

Sparfloxacin
Spectinomycin
Spironolactone
Streptokinase
Streptomycin
Sufentanil
Sulfadiazine
Sulfamethoxazole
Sulfasalazine
Sulfisoxazole
Sulindac
Sulpiride
Sumatriptan
Tacrine
Tacrolimus
Tartrazine
Tedizolid
Teicoplanin
Telithromycin
Telmisartan
Tenecteplase
Teniposide
Tenofovir Disoproxil
Terbinafine
Terfenadine
Teriflunomide
Tesamorelin
Tetracycline
Thalidomide
Thiabendazole
Thimerosal
Thiopental
Thiotepa
Thyrotropin Alfa
Tiagabine
Ticlopidine
Tigecycline
Tinidazole
Tinzaparin
Tirofiban
Tizanidine
Tocilizumab
Tolazamide
Tolbutamide
Tolcapone
Tolmetin
Topiramate
Torsemide
Tosufloxacin
Tramadol
Trazodone
Triamcinolone
Trimethadione
Trimethoprim
Tripelennamine
Troleandomycin
Trovafloxacin
Urofollitropin
Valdecoxib
Valsartan
Vancomycin
Vardenafil
Varicella Vaccine
Vasopressin
Vedolizumab
Velaglucerase Alfa
Venlafaxine
Verapamil
Voriconazole
Warfarin
Yellow Fever Vaccine

Zalcitabine
Zaleplon
Zanamivir
Zidovudine
Ziprasidone
Zolmitriptan
Zolpidem
Zonisamide

Vasculitis
Abatacept
Acebutolol
Aceclofenac
Acenocoumarol
Acetaminophen
Acyclovir
Adalimumab
Ado-Trastuzumab Emtansine
Aldesleukin
Alemtuzumab
Allopurinol
Aminosalicylate Sodium
Amiodarone
Amitriptyline
Amlodipine
Amoxapine
Amoxicillin
Amphotericin B
Ampicillin
Anastrozole
Anistreplase
Anthrax Vaccine
Asparaginase
Aspartame
Aspirin
Atenolol
Atorvastatin
Azacitidine
Azatadine
Azathioprine
Azithromycin
BCG Vaccine
Bendamustine
Bevacizumab
Bexarotene
Blinatumomab
Bortezomib
Bosentan
Bromocriptine
Busulfan
Captopril
Carbamazepine
Carbimazole
Carvedilol
Caspofungin
Celecoxib
Certolizumab
Cevimeline
Chloramphenicol
Chlordiazepoxide
Chloroquine
Chlorothiazide
Chlorpromazine
Chlorpropamide
Chlorthalidone
Chlorzoxazone
Cimetidine
Cinacalcet
Ciprofloxacin
Citalopram
Cladribine
Clarithromycin

Clindamycin
Clorazepate
Clozapine
Co-Trimoxazole
Cocaine
Colchicine
Cromolyn
Cyclophosphamide
Cyclosporine
Cyproheptadine
Cytarabine
Daclizumab
Delavirdine
Diazepam
Diclofenac
Didanosine
Diflunisal
Digoxin
Diltiazem
Diphenhydramine
Disulfiram
Doxycycline
Dronedarone
Efavirenz
Enalapril
Enfuvirtide
Ephedrine
Epirubicin
Erlotinib
Erythromycin
Estrogens
Etanercept
Ethacrynic Acid
Etodolac
Etoposide
Everolimus
Exemestane
Ezetimibe
Famciclovir
Famotidine
Fenbufen
Flucloxacillin
Fluorouracil
Fluoxetine
Flurbiprofen
Fluticasone Propionate
Furosemide
Gabapentin
Gefitinib
Gemcitabine
Gemfibrozil
Gentamicin
Glatiramer
Glimepiride
Glucagon
Glyburide
Gold & Gold Compounds
Golimumab
Granulocyte Colony-
    Stimulating Factor (G-CSF)
Griseofulvin
Guanethidine
Heparin
Hepatitis B Vaccine
Heroin
Hydralazine
Hydrochlorothiazide
Hydroxychloroquine
Hydroxyurea
Ibuprofen
Icodextrin

Imatinib
Imipenem/Cilastatin
Imipramine
Imiquimod
Immune Globulin IV
Indapamide
Indinavir
Indomethacin
Infliximab
Influenza Vaccine
Insulin
Insulin Aspart
Interferon Alfa
Interferon Beta
Interferon Gamma
Ipilimumab
Isoniazid
Isotretinoin
Itraconazole
Ixazomib
Ketoconazole
Ketorolac
Leflunomide
Leuprolide
Levamisole
Levetiracetam
Levofloxacin
Lisinopril
Lithium
Maprotiline
MDMA
Meclofenamate
Mefenamic Acid
Mefloquine
Meloxicam
Melphalan
Meperidine
Meprobamate
Mercaptopurine
Mesalamine
Metformin
Methimazole
Methocarbamol
Methotrexate
Methoxsalen
Methyldopa
Methylphenidate
Metolazone
Minocycline
Mitotane
Nabumetone
Naproxen
Nelfinavir
Nicotine
Nifedipine
Nimesulide
Nizatidine
Ofloxacin
Olanzapine
Omeprazole
Oxacillin
Oxaliplatin
Pantoprazole
Paroxetine Hydrochloride
PEG-Interferon
Pembrolizumab
Pemetrexed
Penicillamine
Penicillin V
Pergolide
Phenobarbital

Phenylbutazone
Phenytoin
Phytonadione
Piroxicam
Potassium Iodide
Pramipexole
Pregabalin
Procainamide
Propylthiouracil
Psoralens
Pyridoxine
Quinapril
Quinidine
Quinine
Ramipril
Ranitidine
Ribavirin
Rifampin
Risedronate
Ritodrine
Rituximab
Rivastigmine
Rofecoxib
Simvastatin
Sirolimus
Sofosbuvir
Sorafenib
Sotalol
Spironolactone
Streptokinase
Streptomycin
Sulfadiazine
Sulfamethoxazole
Sulfasalazine
Sulfisoxazole
Sulindac
Tacrolimus
Tamoxifen
Tartrazine
Telithromycin
Telmisartan
Terbutaline
Tetracycline
Thalidomide
Thiamine
Thioridazine
Ticlopidine
Tinidazole
Tocainide
Tocilizumab
Torsemide
Trazodone
Tretinoin
Trichlormethiazide
Trimethadione
Trioxsalen
Triptorelin
Ustekinumab
Valproic Acid
Vancomycin
Vemurafenib
Verapamil
Vinorelbine
Warfarin
Zafirlukast
Zidovudine

Vertigo
Abacavir
Abaloparatide
Abarelix
Abatacept

Abemaciclib
Abiraterone
Acamprosate
Acebutolol
Aceclofenac
Acetaminophen
Acetohexamide
Acitretin
Adalimumab
Adenosine
Ado-Trastuzumab Emtansine
Afatinib
Aflibercept
Agalsidase
Albendazole
Albiglutide
Aldesleukin
Alectinib
Alefacept
Alemtuzumab
Alfuzosin
Alirocumab
Aliskiren
Allopurinol
Almotriptan
Alogliptin
Alosetron
Alpha-Lipoic Acid
Alprazolam
Alprostadil
Amantadine
Amiloride
Amiodarone
Amisulpride
Amitriptyline
Amlodipine
Amodiaquine
Amoxapine
Amoxicillin
Anagrelide
Anidulafungin
Anti-Thymocyte
    Immunoglobulin (Rabbit)
Antihemophilic Factor
Apixaban
Apomorphine
Apremilast
Aprepitant
Arformoterol
Aripiprazole
Armodafinil
Arsenic
Artemether/Lumefantrine
Artesunate
Articaine
Asenapine
Atazanavir
Atenolol
Atomoxetine
Atorvastatin
Atovaquone/Proguanil
Avanafil
Avelumab
Axitinib
Azacitidine
Azathioprine
Azilsartan
Azithromycin
Baclofen
Basiliximab
Bedaquiline

Belatacept
Belinostat
Benazepril
Bendamustine
Benznidazole
Benzphetamine
Bepridil
Betaxolol
Bezafibrate
Biperiden
Bismuth
Bisoprolol
Bleomycin
Blinatumomab
Bortezomib
Bosentan
Bosutinib
Botulinum Toxin (A & B)
Brentuximab Vedotin
Brexpiprazole
Brinzolamide
Brivaracetam
Brodalumab
Bromocriptine
Bupivacaine
Buprenorphine
Bupropion
Butorphanol
C1-Esterase Inhibitor
Cabazitaxel
Cabergoline
Cabozantinib
Canagliflozin
Canakinumab
Candesartan
Capecitabine
Carbamazepine
Carbetocin
Carboplatin
Carfilzomib
Cariprazine
Carisoprodol
Carvedilol
Caspofungin
Cefditoren
Cefepime
Cefpodoxime
Ceftaroline Fosamil
Ceftazidime & Avibactam
Ceftolozane & Tazobactam
Ceftriaxone
Cefuroxime
Celecoxib
Celiprolol
Certolizumab
Cevimeline
Chloroquine
Chlorpromazine
Chlorthalidone
Chlorzoxazone
Cholera Vaccine
Choline Fenofibrate
Cilazapril
Cilostazol
Cinacalcet
Cinnarizine
Ciprofloxacin
Cisplatin
Citalopram
Clevidipine
Clobazam

Clofarabine
Clofazimine
Clomipramine
Clonidine
Clozapine
Co-Trimoxazole
Coagulation Factor IX
    (Recombinant)
Cobicistat/Elvitegravir/
    Emtricitabine/Tenofovir
    Disoproxil
Codeine
Colesevelam
Crizotinib
Crofelemer
Cyclobenzaprine
Cycloserine
Cyclosporine
Cysteamine
Cytarabine
Dabigatran
Daclizumab
Dalbavancin
Dalfampridine
Dantrolene
Dapagliflozin
Dapsone
Daptomycin
Darbepoetin Alfa
Darifenacin
Dasatinib
Daunorubicin
Decitabine
Deferasirox
Deflazacort
Degarelix
Delafloxacin
Denileukin
Denosumab
Desvenlafaxine
Deutetrabenazine
Dexamethasone
Dexketoprofen
Dextroamphetamine
Dextromethorphan
Diatrizoate
Diazepam
Diazoxide
Diclofenac
Dicyclomine
Diethylpropion
Dihydrocodeine
Dihydroergotamine
Diltiazem
Diphenhydramine
Dipyridamole
Disopyramide
Disulfiram
Docetaxel
Dofetilide
Dolasetron
Dolutegravir
Donepezil
Doxazosin
Doxepin
Doxercalciferol
Doxorubicin
Doxycycline
Dronabinol
Dronedarone
Droxidopa

Duloxetine
Dutasteride
Eculizumab
Edaravone
Edrophonium
Efavirenz
Eflornithine
Eletriptan
Eliglustat
Elotuzumab
Eluxadoline
Empagliflozin
Emtricitabine
Enalapril
Entacapone
Entecavir
Enzalutamide
Eplerenone
Epoetin Alfa
Eprosartan
Eribulin
Escitalopram
Eslicarbazepine
Esomeprazole
Estramustine
Eszopiclone
Etanercept
Etravirine
Everolimus
Evolocumab
Exenatide
Ezetimibe
Ezogabine
Factor VIII - von Willebrand
    Factor
Famotidine
Febuxostat
Felbamate
Fentanyl
Ferric Gluconate
Ferumoxytol
Fesoterodine
Finasteride
Fingolimod
Flecainide
Flibanserin
Flumazenil
Fluorouracil
Fluoxetine
Fluphenazine
Flurbiprofen
Fluticasone Furoate
Fluticasone Propionate
Fluvoxamine
Follitropin Alfa/Beta
Fomepizole
Fomivirsen
Formoterol
Fosfomycin
Fosphenytoin
Frovatriptan
Fulvestrant
Furazolidone
Gabapentin
Gadobenate
Gadobutrol
Gadodiamide
Gadofosveset
Gadopentetate
Gadoteridol
Gadoversetamide

Gadoxetate
Galantamine
Gatifloxacin
Gefitinib
Gemifloxacin
Gentamicin
Glatiramer
Gliclazide
Glimepiride
Glipizide
Glycopyrrolate
Golimumab
Goserelin
Granisetron
Granulocyte Colony-
    Stimulating Factor (G-CSF)
Guanabenz
Guanadrel
Guanethidine
Guanfacine
Halofantrine
Haloperidol
Human Papillomavirus (HPV)
    Vaccine
Human Papillomavirus Vaccine
    (Bivalent)
Hydrochlorothiazide
Hydrocodone
Hydromorphone
Hydroxychloroquine
Ibandronate
Ibritumomab
Ibrutinib
Icatibant
Icodextrin
Idebenone
Iloperidone
Iloprost
Imatinib
Imidapril
Imiglucerase
Imipramine
Imiquimod
Immune Globulin IV
Indapamide
Indinavir
Indoramin
Infliximab
Influenza Vaccine
Insulin
Insulin Detemir
Interferon Alfa
Interferon Beta
Iobenguane
Iodixanol
Iohexol
Iomeprol
Iopromide
Ioversol
Ipilimumab
Irinotecan
Isavuconazonium Sulfate
Isocarboxazid
Isosorbide Mononitrate
Isradipine
Itraconazole
Ivabradine
Ivacaftor
Ivermectin
Ixabepilone
Japanese Encephalitis Vaccine

Kanamycin
Ketamine
Ketoconazole
Ketorolac
Lacosamide
Lamivudine
Lamotrigine
Lansoprazole
Lapatinib
Latanoprost
Ledipasvir & Sofosbuvir
Leflunomide
Lenalidomide
Lenvatinib
Lesinurad
Letrozole
Levetiracetam
Levodopa
Levofloxacin
Levomepromazine
Levomilnacipran
Levonorgestrel
Lidocaine
Linagliptin
Linezolid
Liothyronine
Liraglutide
Lisdexamfetamine
Lisinopril
Lithium
Lixisenatide
Lomitapide
Lopinavir
Loratadine
Lorazepam
Lorcainide
Lorcaserin
Losartan
Lovastatin
Loxapine
Lubiprostone
Lumiracoxib
Lurasidone
Maraviroc
Mazindol
MDMA
Mebendazole
Mefloquine
Meloxicam
Memantine
Meperidine
Mepolizumab
Meptazinol
Mesalamine
Metamizole
Metaxalone
Metformin
Methocarbamol
Methotrexate
Methoxyflurane
Methylnaltrexone
Methylphenidate
Methylprednisolone
Metronidazole
Micafungin
Midazolam
Midostaurin
Mifepristone
Miglustat
Milnacipran
Miltefosine

Minocycline
Minoxidil
Mirabegron
Mirtazapine
Mivacurium
Mizoribine
Moclobemide
Modafinil
Moexipril
Montelukast
Morphine
Moxifloxacin
Moxonidine
Mupirocin
Muromonab-CD3
Mycophenolate
Nabilone
Nabumetone
Nadolol
Nalbuphine
Nalmefene
Naloxegol
Naltrexone
Naproxen
Naratriptan
Nateglinide
Nebivolol
Nefazodone
Nelarabine
Nelfinavir
Nesiritide
Netupitant & Palonosetron
Niacin
Nicorandil
Nifedipine
Nilotinib
Nilutamide
Niraparib
Nisoldipine
Nitazoxanide
Nivolumab
Nizatidine
Norfloxacin
Nortriptyline
Obeticholic Acid
Octreotide
Ofloxacin
Olanzapine
Olmesartan
Olodaterol
Omacetaxine
Omalizumab
Ombitasvir/Paritaprevir/
    Ritonavir
Omeprazole
Ondansetron
Oral Contraceptives
Oritavancin
Orlistat
Oxaliplatin
Oxcarbazepine
Oxerutins
Oxilan
Oxprenolol
Oxybutynin
Oxycodone
Oxymorphone
Paclitaxel
Palbociclib
Paliperidone
Palonosetron

Pancrelipase
Pandemic Influenza Vaccine
    (HINI)
Panitumumab
Panobinostat
Pantoprazole
Paricalcitol
Paroxetine Hydrochloride
Paroxetine Mesylate
Pasireotide
PEG-Interferon
Pegaptanib
Pegaspargase
Peginesatide
Pegloticase
Pegvisomant
Pembrolizumab
Pemetrexed
Pentamidine
Pentazocine
Perampanel
Perflutren
Pergolide
Perindopril
Pertuzumab
Phendimetrazine
Phenelzine
Phenobarbital
Phenoxybenzamine
Phentermine
Pilocarpine
Pioglitazone
Piracetam
Pirfenidone
Piroxicam
Pizotifen
Pomalidomide
Ponatinib
Posaconazole
Pramipexole
Pramlintide
Pranlukast
Prasugrel
Pravastatin
Praziquantel
Prazosin
Prednicarbate
Prednisolone
Pregabalin
Prenylamine
Promazine
Promethazine
Propafenone
Propoxyphene
Propranolol
Pseudoephedrine
Pyrimethamine
Quetiapine
Quinagolide
Quinapril
Quinidine
Quinine
Rabeprazole
Radium-223 Dichloride
Raltegravir
Ramelteon
Ramipril
Ranolazine
Rasagiline
Reboxetine
Regadenoson

Remifentanil
Repaglinide
Ribavirin
Rifabutin
Rifampin
Rifapentine
Rifaximin
Rilpivirine
Riluzole
Rimantadine
Rimonabant
Riociguat
Risedronate
Risperidone
Ritonavir
Rituximab
Rivaroxaban
Rivastigmine
Rizatriptan
Rofecoxib
Roflumilast
Rolapitant
Romiplostim
Ropinirole
Ropivacaine
Rosuvastatin
Rotigotine
Roxatidine
Rucaparib
Rufinamide
Rupatadine
Ruxolitinib
Sacubitril/Valsartan
Safinamide
Salmeterol
Saxagliptin
Scopolamine
Secnidazole
Selegiline
Selenium
Selexipag
Sertraline
Sibutramine
Sildenafil
Silodosin
Simvastatin
Sincalide
Sipuleucel-T
Sitaxentan
Sodium Oxybate
Sofosbuvir
Solifenacin
Sonidegib
Sorafenib
Spectinomycin
Streptomycin
Strontium Ranelate
Sucralfate
Sugammadex
Sulfadoxine
Sulfasalazine
Sumatriptan
Sunitinib
Suvorexant
Tacrine
Tacrolimus
Tadalafil
Taliglucerase
Talimogene Laherparepvec
Tamoxifen
Tamsulosin

Tapentadol
Tedizolid
Tegafur/Gimeracil/Oteracil
Tegaserod
Teicoplanin
Telavancin
Telbivudine
Telithromycin
Telmisartan
Temozolomide
Tenofovir Disoproxil
Terazosin
Terbutaline
Teriparatide
Tetrabenazine
Tetracaine & Oxymetazoline
Thalidomide
Thiabendazole
Thioridazine
Thyrotropin Alfa
Tiagabine
Tianeptine
Ticagrelor
Tigecycline
Tiludronate
Timolol
Tinidazole
Tiotropium
Tipranavir
Tizanidine
Tocainide
Tocilizumab
Tofacitinib
Tolcapone
Tolterodine
Tolvaptan
Topiramate
Toremifene
Torsemide
Tositumomab & Iodine[131]
Tosufloxacin
Trabectedin
Tramadol
Trametinib
Trandolapril
Tranylcypromine
Trastuzumab
Trazodone
Treprostinil
Trimipramine
Triptorelin
Troglitazone
Trospium
Trovafloxacin
Typhoid Vaccine
Ulipristal
Unoprostone
Urapidil
Ursodiol
Ustekinumab
Valbenazine
Valproic Acid
Valrubicin
Valsartan
Vancomycin
Vardenafil
Varenicline
Varicella Vaccine
Velaglucerase Alfa
Venlafaxine
Verapamil

Verteporfin
Vigabatrin
Vilazodone
Vildagliptin
Vismodegib
Voriconazole
Vorinostat
Vortioxetine
Warfarin
Zafirlukast
Zaleplon
Zanamivir
Ziconotide
Zidovudine
Ziprasidone
Zofenopril
Zoledronate
Zolmitriptan
Zolpidem
Zonisamide
Zoster Vaccine
Zuclopenthixol

Xerostomia

Abemaciclib
Acamprosate
Acebutolol
Acetaminophen
Acetazolamide
Acitretin
Aclidinium
Ado-Trastuzumab Emtansine
Afatinib
Aflibercept
Albendazole
Albuterol
Aldesleukin
Almotriptan
Alprazolam
Alprostadil
Amantadine
Amifostine
Amiloride
Amisulpride
Amitriptyline
Amlodipine
Amoxapine
Amoxicillin
Apraclonidine
Aprepitant
Arbutamine
Aripiprazole
Armodafinil
Arsenic
Asenapine
Astemizole
Atomoxetine
Atropine Sulfate
Azatadine
Azelastine
Baclofen
Balsalazide
Bendamustine
Bendroflumethiazide
Benzphetamine
Benztropine
Bepridil
Betaxolol
Bexarotene
Bicalutamide
Bisacodyl
Bismuth

Bisoprolol
Botulinum Toxin (A & B)
Brexpiprazole
Brimonidine
Brinzolamide
Bromocriptine
Brompheniramine
Bumetanide
Buprenorphine
Bupropion
Buspirone
Butorphanol
Cabergoline
Canagliflozin
Captopril
Cariprazine
Carisoprodol
Carvedilol
Cefditoren
Cefixime
Ceftibuten
Celecoxib
Cetirizine
Cetuximab
Cevimeline
Chlordiazepoxide
Chlormezanone
Chlorpheniramine
Chlorpromazine
Ciprofloxacin
Cisplatin
Citalopram
Clarithromycin
Clemastine
Clindamycin
Clomipramine
Clonazepam
Clonidine
Clorazepate
Clozapine
Codeine
Conivaptan
Crofelemer
Cromolyn
Cyclobenzaprine
Cyproheptadine
Dapagliflozin
Darifenacin
Dasatinib
Daunorubicin
Degarelix
Delavirdine
Desipramine
Desloratadine
Desvenlafaxine
Deutetrabenazine
Dexamethasone
Dexchlorpheniramine
Dexketoprofen
Dexlansoprazole
Dexmedetomidine
Dexmethylphenidate
Dextroamphetamine
Diazepam
Diclofenac
Dicyclomine
Didanosine
Diethylpropion
Diflunisal
Dihydrocodeine
Dihydroergotamine

Diltiazem
Dimenhydrinate
Diphenhydramine
Diphenoxylate
Dirithromycin
Disopyramide
Domperidone
Donepezil
Doxazosin
Doxepin
Dronabinol
Duloxetine
Dutasteride
Efavirenz
Eletriptan
Eltrombopag
Enalapril
Enfuvirtide
Enoxacin
Entacapone
Ephedrine
Epinephrine
Eprosartan
Eribulin
Escitalopram
Eslicarbazepine
Esmolol
Estazolam
Eszopiclone
Etravirine
Everolimus
Exemestane
Ezogabine
Famotidine
Felbamate
Felodipine
Fenoprofen
Fentanyl
Fesoterodine
Flavoxate
Flecainide
Flibanserin
Fluconazole
Flumazenil
Fluorides
Fluoxetine
Fluphenazine
Flurazepam
Flurbiprofen
Fluvoxamine
Formoterol
Fosfomycin
Fosinopril
Fosphenytoin
Frovatriptan
Furosemide
Gabapentin
Gadobenate
Gadodiamide
Gadopentetate
Gadoteridol
Gadoversetamide
Gadoxetate
Ganciclovir
Gemifloxacin
Glatiramer
Glycopyrrolate
Goserelin
Granisetron
Grepafloxacin
Griseofulvin

Guanabenz	Midodrine	Pentoxifylline	Sucralfate
Guanadrel	Mifepristone	Perflutren	Sugammadex
Guanethidine	Miglustat	Pergolide	Sulfamethoxazole
Guanfacine	Milnacipran	Perindopril	Sulfasalazine
Haloperidol	Minocycline	Phendimetrazine	Sulindac
Hydrocodone	Mirabegron	Phenelzine	Sulpiride
Hydromorphone	Mirtazapine	Phenobarbital	Sumatriptan
Hydroxyzine	Mizolastine	Phenoxybenzamine	Sunitinib
Hyoscyamine	Modafinil	Phentermine	Suvorexant
Ibuprofen	Moexipril	Pilocarpine	Tacrine
Iloperidone	Molindone	Pimozide	Tadalafil
Imatinib	Moricizine	Pirfenidone	Tamoxifen
Imipramine	Morphine	Piroxicam	Tamsulosin
Indapamide	Moxifloxacin	Pizotifen	Tapentadol
Indinavir	Moxisylyte	Posaconazole	Tasimelteon
Insulin	Moxonidine	Pramipexole	Tedizolid
Interferon Alfa	Mupirocin	Prazepam	Telithromycin
Ioversol	Nabilone	Prazosin	Telmisartan
Ipilimumab	Nabumetone	Pregabalin	Temazepam
Ipratropium	Nadolol	Prochlorperazine	Terazosin
Isocarboxazid	Nalbuphine	Procyclidine	Terbutaline
Isoetharine	Nalmefene	Promethazine	Terfenadine
Isoproterenol	Naloxone	Propafenone	Thalidomide
Isotretinoin	Naltrexone	Propantheline	Thiabendazole
Isradipine	Naproxen	Propofol	Thioguanine
Itraconazole	Nedocromil	Propoxyphene	Thioridazine
Ketoprofen	Nefazodone	Propranolol	Thiothixene
Ketorolac	Neostigmine	Protriptyline	Tiagabine
Ketotifen	Neratinib	Pseudoephedrine	Tianeptine
Lamivudine	Nevirapine	Pyridostigmine	Tigecycline
Lamotrigine	Nicardipine	Pyrimethamine	Tiludronate
Lansoprazole	Nicotine	Quazepam	Timolol
Leflunomide	Nifedipine	Quetiapine	Tinidazole
Lenalidomide	Nilotinib	Quinapril	Tiotropium
Lenvatinib	Nilutamide	Rabeprazole	Tizanidine
Letrozole	Niraparib	Raltitrexed	Tocainide
Levocetirizine	Nisoldipine	Ramipril	Tolcapone
Levodopa	Nitrofurantoin	Ranolazine	Tolterodine
Levofloxacin	Nitroglycerin	Rasagiline	Tolvaptan
Levomilnacipran	Nivolumab	Reboxetine	Topiramate
Lisdexamfetamine	Nizatidine	Regadenoson	Toremifene
Lisinopril	Norfloxacin	Regorafenib	Tosufloxacin
Lithium	Nortriptyline	Remifentanil	Tramadol
Lomefloxacin	Ofloxacin	Reserpine	Trametinib
Loperamide	Olanzapine	Rifaximin	Trandolapril
Loratadine	Olaparib	Riluzole	Tranylcypromine
Lorazepam	Omacetaxine	Rimantadine	Trazodone
Lorcaserin	Omeprazole	Risperidone	Tretinoin
Losartan	Ondansetron	Ritonavir	Triamcinolone
Lovastatin	Orlistat	Rivaroxaban	Triamterene
Loxapine	Oxaliplatin	Rivastigmine	Triazolam
Lubiprostone	Oxazepam	Rizatriptan	Trihexyphenidyl
Maprotiline	Oxcarbazepine	Rofecoxib	Trimeprazine
Marihuana	Oxprenolol	Ropinirole	Trimipramine
Mazindol	Oxybutynin	Rotigotine	Tripelennamine
MDMA	Oxycodone	Rucaparib	Triprolidine
Meclizine	Oxymorphone	Rupatadine	Trospium
Meloxicam	Oxytocin	Salmeterol	Trovafloxacin
Meperidine	Paliperidone	Saquinavir	Tryptophan
Mesalamine	Palonosetron	Scopolamine	Ulipristal
Metamizole	Panobinostat	Selegiline	Umeclidinium
Methadone	Pantoprazole	Sertindole	Unoprostone
Methamphetamine	Papaverine	Sertraline	Valbenazine
Methantheline	Paricalcitol	Sevoflurane	Valdecoxib
Methazolamide	Paromomycin	Sibutramine	Valproic Acid
Methyldopa	Paroxetine Hydrochloride	Sildenafil	Valsartan
Methylphenidate	PEG-Interferon	Solifenacin	Vardenafil
Metoclopramide	Pembrolizumab	Sorafenib	Varenicline
Metolazone	Pemetrexed	Sotalol	Vemurafenib
Metronidazole	Pentamidine	Sparfloxacin	Venlafaxine
Mexiletine	Pentazocine	Spironolactone	Verapamil

Vilazodone	Vortioxetine	Zidovudine	Zonisamide
Vitamin A	Zalcitabine	Ziprasidone	Zuclopenthixol
Voriconazole	Zaleplon	Zolmitriptan	
Vorinostat	Ziconotide	Zolpidem	

Main Classes of Drugs

5-HT1 agonist
Almotriptan
Eletriptan
Frovatriptan
Naratriptan
Rizatriptan
Sumatriptan
Zolmitriptan

5-HT3 antagonist
Alosetron
Dolasetron
Granisetron
Ondansetron
Palonosetron

ACE inhibitor
Benazepril
Captopril
Cilazapril
Enalapril
Fosinopril
Imidapril
Lisinopril
Moexipril
Perindopril
Quinapril
Ramipril
Trandolapril
Zofenopril

Adrenergic alpha-receptor agonist
Clonidine
Dexmedetomidine
Dopamine
Ephedrine
Guanabenz
Guanadrel
Guanethidine
Guanfacine
Methyldopa
Midodrine
Mirtazapine
Phenylephrine
Phenylpropanolamine
Polythiazide
Pseudoephedrine

Adrenergic alpha-receptor antagonist
Alfuzosin
Doxazosin
Phenoxybenzamine
Phentolamine
Prazosin
Silodosin
Tamsulosin
Terazosin
Urapidil

Adrenergic alpha2-receptor agonist
Apraclonidine
Brimonidine
Tizanidine

Adrenergic beta-receptor agonist
Arbutamine
Dobutamine
Isoetharine
Isoproterenol
Isoxsuprine
Metoprolol

Adrenergic beta-receptor antagonist
Betaxolol
Carteolol
Carvedilol
Esmolol
Labetalol
Levobetaxolol
Levobunolol
Metipranolol
Nadolol
Nebivolol
Penbutolol
Pindolol
Timolol

Alkylating agent
Altretamine
Bendamustine
Busulfan
Carboplatin
Carmustine
Chlorambucil
Cisplatin
Cyclophosphamide
Dacarbazine
Estramustine
Ifosfamide
Lomustine
Mechlorethamine
Melphalan
Mitomycin
Oxaliplatin
Procarbazine
Streptozocin
Temozolomide
Thiotepa

Amphetamine
Benzphetamine
Dextroamphetamine
Diethylpropion
MDMA
Methamphetamine
Methylphenidate
Pemoline
Phendimetrazine
Phentermine
Prenylamine

Analeptic
Doxapram
Modafinil

Analgesic
narcotic
Dextromethorphan

non-narcotic
Acetaminophen
non-opioid
Ketorolac
opioid
Alfentanil
Dihydrocodeine
Fentanyl
Meptazinol
Tapentadol
urinary
Pentosan
Phenazopyridine

Anesthetic
Alfentanil
Edrophonium
Fentanyl
Ketamine
general
Chloral Hydrate
Propofol
Sodium Oxybate
Sufentanil
inhalation
Desflurane
Enflurane
Halothane
Isoflurane
Methoxyflurane
Sevoflurane
local
Articaine
Bupivacaine
Cocaine
Levobupivacaine
Lidocaine
Mepivacaine
Ropivacaine
Tetracaine & Oxymetazoline

Angiotensin II receptor antagonist (blocker)
Azilsartan
Candesartan
Eprosartan
Irbesartan
Losartan
Olmesartan
Telmisartan
Valsartan

Anti-inflammatory
Amlexanox
Amodiaquine
Clofazimine
Colchicine
Fluprednisolone
Roflumilast

Antiarrhythmic
class Ia
Disopyramide
Procainamide
Quinidine

class Ib
Lidocaine
Mexiletine
Phenytoin
Tocainide
class Ic
Flecainide
Lorcainide
Moricizine
Propafenone
class II
Acebutolol
Atenolol
Esmolol
Labetalol
Metoprolol
Nadolol
Propranolol
Sotalol
class III
Amiodarone
Bretylium
Dofetilide
Dronedarone
Ibutilide
Sotalol
Vernakalant
class IV
Adenosine
Amlodipine
Bepridil
Digoxin
Diltiazem
Verapamil

Antibiotic
Doripenem
Ertapenem
Imipenem/Cilastatin
Meropenem
Meropenem & Vaborbactam
aminoglycoside
Amikacin
Gentamicin
Kanamycin
Neomycin
Paromomycin
Streptomycin
Tobramycin
anthracycline
Bleomycin
Dactinomycin
Daunorubicin
Doxorubicin
Epirubicin
Idarubicin
Mitomycin
Mitoxantrone
Peplomycin
Valrubicin
beta-lactam
Ampicillin/Sulbactam
Aztreonam
Ceftazidime & Avibactam

Ceftolozane & Tazobactam
Flucloxacillin
fluoroquinolone
Besifloxacin
Ciprofloxacin
Delafloxacin
Enoxacin
Finafloxacin
Gatifloxacin
Gemifloxacin
Levofloxacin
Lomefloxacin
Moxifloxacin
Norfloxacin
Ofloxacin
Sparfloxacin
Tosufloxacin
glycopeptide
Daptomycin
Teicoplanin
Vancomycin
imidazole
Clotrimazole
Ketoconazole
Mebendazole
Miconazole
Sertaconazole
Thiabendazole
lincosamide
Clindamycin
Clindamycin/Tretinoin
Lincomycin
macrolide
Azithromycin
Clarithromycin
Dirithromycin
Erythromycin
Fidaxomicin
Roxithromycin
Telithromycin
Troleandomycin
nitrofuran
Furazolidone
Nitrofurazone
nitroimidazole
Benznidazole
Metronidazole
Secnidazole
Tinidazole
oxazolidinone
Linezolid
Tedizolid
penicillin
Amoxicillin
Ampicillin
Ampicillin/Sulbactam
Bacampicillin
Carbenicillin
Cloxacillin
Dicloxacillin
Methicillin
Mezlocillin
Nafcillin
Oxacillin
Penicillin G
Penicillin V
Piperacillin
Ticarcillin
quinolone
Cinoxacin
Grepafloxacin

Nalidixic Acid
Trovafloxacin
rifamycin
Rifabutin
Rifampin
Rifapentine
Rifaximin
streptogramin
Pristinamycin
Quinupristin/Dalfopristin
sulfonamide
Co-Trimoxazole
Sulfacetamide
Sulfadiazine
Sulfadoxine
Sulfamethoxazole
Sulfisoxazole
tetracycline
Chlortetracycline
Demeclocycline
Doxycycline
Lymecycline
Minocycline
Oxytetracycline
Tetracycline
Tigecycline
topical
Mupirocin
Retapamulin
triazole
Fluconazole
Itraconazole
Posaconazole
Terconazole
Voriconazole
miscellaneous
Aminosalicylate Sodium
Bacitracin
Capreomycin
Ceftriaxone
Chloramphenicol
Cycloserine
Dapsone
Ethionamide
Fosfomycin
Isoniazid
Methenamine
Nitrofurantoin
Plicamycin
Pyrazinamide
Quinacrine
Spectinomycin
Tigecycline
Trimethoprim

Anticonvulsant
Brivaracetam
Carbamazepine
Ezogabine
Felbamate
Gabapentin
Lacosamide
Lamotrigine
Levetiracetam
Mephenytoin
Oxcarbazepine
Perampanel
Phenacemide
Phenobarbital
Phensuximide
Phenytoin

Pregabalin
Primidone
Tetrazepam
Tiagabine
Topiramate
Valproic Acid
Vigabatrin
Zonisamide
antiepileptic
Brivaracetam
Clobazam
Eslicarbazepine
Lacosamide
Lamotrigine
Perampanel
Rufinamide
Vigabatrin
hydantoin
Ethotoin
Fosphenytoin
Mephenytoin
Phenytoin
oxazolidinedione
Paramethadione
Trimethadione
succinimide
Ethosuximide
Methsuximide

Antidepressant
Bupropion
Citalopram
Desvenlafaxine
Duloxetine
Escitalopram
Fluoxetine
Fluvoxamine
Isocarboxazid
Levomilnacipran
Milnacipran
Moclobemide
Nefazodone
Paroxetine Hydrochloride
Phenelzine
Reboxetine
Selegiline
Sertraline
Tianeptine
Tranylcypromine
Tryptophan
Venlafaxine
Vilazodone
Vortioxetine
tetracyclic
Maprotiline
Mianserin
Mirtazapine
tricyclic
Amitriptyline
Amoxapine
Clomipramine
Desipramine
Doxepin
Imipramine
Nortriptyline
Protriptyline
Trazodone
Trimipramine

Antiemetic
Aprepitant
Chlorpromazine

Dexamethasone
Dimenhydrinate
Diphenhydramine
Domperidone
Dronabinol
Droperidol
Granisetron
Haloperidol
Marihuana
Meclizine
Metoclopramide
Nabilone
Ondansetron
Palonosetron
Perphenazine
Prochlorperazine
Rolapitant
Scopolamine
Trimethobenzamide

Antifungal
Amphotericin B
Caspofungin
Ciclopirox
Clioquinol
Econazole
Efinaconazole
Griseofulvin
Micafungin
Nystatin
Terbinafine
azole
Clotrimazole
Fluconazole
Isavuconazonium Sulfate
Itraconazole
Ketoconazole
Luliconazole
Miconazole
Posaconazole
Voriconazole
oxaborole
Tavaborole

Antimalarial
Amodiaquine
Artemether/Lumefantrine
Artesunate
Atovaquone
Atovaquone/Proguanil
Chloroquine
Halofantrine
Hydroxychloroquine
Mefloquine
Primaquine
Pyrimethamine
Quinacrine
Quinidine
Quinine
Sulfadoxine

Antimycobacterial
Bedaquiline
Clofazimine
Dapsone
Ethambutol
Flucytosine
Isoniazid
Potassium Iodide
echinocandin
Anidulafungin

Antineoplastic

Anastrozole
Arsenic
Asparaginase
Asparaginase *Erwinia chrysanthemi*
Azacitidine
Bexarotene
Cabazitaxel
Capecitabine
Carboplatin
Cetuximab
Cisplatin
Cladribine
Cytarabine
Dacarbazine
Dasatinib
Decitabine
Denileukin
Docetaxel
Eribulin
Erlotinib
Everolimus
Floxuridine
Fludarabine
Fluorouracil
Gefitinib
Gemcitabine
Gemtuzumab
Hydroxyurea
Ibritumomab
Imatinib
Irinotecan
Ixabepilone
Lapatinib
Levamisole
Mercaptopurine
Mitotane
Mitoxantrone
Nelarabine
Nilotinib
Nilutamide
Oxaliplatin
Paclitaxel
Panitumumab
Pazopanib
Pegaspargase
Pentostatin
Porfimer
Raltitrexed
Sorafenib
Streptozocin
Sunitinib
Tegafur/Gimeracil/Oteracil
Temozolomide
Temsirolimus
Teniposide
Testolactone
Thioguanine
Topotecan
Tositumomab & Iodine[131]
Trabectedin
Trastuzumab
Tretinoin
Trifluridine & Tipiracil
Vorinostat

Antiplatelet

Abciximab
Aspirin
Cangrelor
Cilostazol
Clopidogrel
Dipyridamole
Eptifibatide
Ticagrelor
Tirofiban

CPTP

Cangrelor
Ticagrelor

thienopyridine

Clopidogrel
Prasugrel
Ticlopidine

Antiprotozoal

Atovaquone
Chloroquine
Hydroxychloroquine
Mefloquine
Nitazoxanide
Pentamidine
Primaquine
Pyrimethamine
Quinidine
Quinine

Antipsychotic

Amisulpride
Aripiprazole
Asenapine
Brexpiprazole
Carbamazepine
Cariprazine
Chlorpromazine
Clozapine
Droperidol
Fluphenazine
Haloperidol
Iloperidone
Levomepromazine
Lithium
Lurasidone
Mesoridazine
Molindone
Olanzapine
Paliperidone
Perphenazine
Pimavanserin
Pimozide
Prochlorperazine
Promazine
Quetiapine
Risperidone
Sertindole
Thioridazine
Thiothixene
Trifluoperazine
Trimeprazine
Valproic Acid
Ziprasidone
Zuclopenthixol
Zuclopenthixol Acetate
Zuclopenthixol Decanoate
Zuclopenthixol Dihydrochloride

tricyclic

Loxapine

Antiretroviral

Adefovir
Amprenavir
Atazanavir
Cobicistat/Elvitegravir/ Emtricitabine/Tenofovir Alafenamide
Cobicistat/Elvitegravir/ Emtricitabine/Tenofovir Disoproxil
Darunavir
Delavirdine
Didanosine
Dolutegravir
Efavirenz
Emtricitabine
Enfuvirtide
Fosamprenavir
Hydroxyurea
Indinavir
Lamivudine
Lopinavir
Maraviroc
Nelfinavir
Nevirapine
Raltegravir
Rilpivirine
Ritonavir
Saquinavir
Stavudine
Tenofovir Disoproxil
Zalcitabine
Zidovudine

Antiviral

Acyclovir
Amantadine
Cytarabine
Entecavir
Famciclovir
Foscarnet
Ganciclovir
Imiquimod
Oseltamivir
Penciclovir
Peramivir
Podophyllotoxin
Rimantadine
Tenofovir Alafenamide
Trifluridine
Valacyclovir
Valganciclovir
Zanamivir

nucleoside analog

Ribavirin
Vidarabine

nucleotide analog

Cidofovir

topical

Acyclovir
Docosanol

Anxiolytic

Buspirone
Chlormezanone
Meprobamate
Tetrazepam

Barbiturate

Amobarbital
Aprobarbital
Butabarbital
Butalbital
Mephobarbital
Methohexital
Pentobarbital
Phenobarbital
Primidone
Secobarbital
Thiopental

Benzodiazepine

Alprazolam
Chlordiazepoxide
Clobazam
Clonazepam
Clorazepate
Diazepam
Estazolam
Flurazepam
Lorazepam
Midazolam
Nitrazepam
Oxazepam
Prazepam
Quazepam
Temazepam
Tetrazepam
Triazolam

Bisphosphonate

Alendronate
Etidronate
Ibandronate
Pamidronate
Risedronate
Tiludronate
Zoledronate

Calcium channel blocker

Amlodipine
Bepridil
Clevidipine
Diltiazem
Felodipine
Isradipine
Nicardipine
Nifedipine
Nimodipine
Nisoldipine
Prenylamine
Verapamil

Carbonic anhydrase inhibitor

Acetazolamide
Brinzolamide
Dichlorphenamide
Dorzolamide
Ethoxzolamide
Methazolamide

CB1 Cannabinoid receptor antagonist

Rimonabant

Central muscle relaxant

Carisoprodol
Chlormezanone
Chlorzoxazone
Cyclobenzaprine
Meprobamate
Metaxalone
Methocarbamol
Orphenadrine

Cephalosporin
1st generation

Cefadroxil
Cefazolin
Cephalexin

Cephalothin
Cephapirin
Cephradine
2nd generation
Cefaclor
Cefamandole
Cefmetazole
Cefonicid
Cefotetan
Cefoxitin
Cefprozil
Cefuroxime
Loracarbef
3rd generation
Cefdinir
Cefditoren
Cefixime
Cefoperazone
Cefotaxime
Cefpodoxime
Ceftazidime
Ceftazidime & Avibactam
Ceftibuten
Ceftizoxime
Ceftriaxone
4th generation
Cefepime
5th generation
Ceftaroline Fosamil
Ceftobiprole
Ceftolozane & Tazobactam

Cholinesterase inhibitor
Donepezil
Edrophonium
Galantamine
Neostigmine
Physostigmine
Rivastigmine
Succinylcholine
Tacrine

CNS stimulant
Cocaine
Dexmethylphenidate
Dextroamphetamine
Lisdexamfetamine
Modafinil

Corticosteroid
Alclometasone
Amcinonide
Beclomethasone
Betamethasone
Budesonide
Ciclesonide
Clobetasol
Cortisone
Deflazacort
Desonide
Desoximetasone
Dexamethasone
Difluprednate
Fludrocortisone
Flumetasone
Flunisolide
Fluocinolone
Fluocinonide
Fluprednisolone
Fluticasone Furoate
Fluticasone Propionate
Halcinonide

Halobetasol
Halometasone
Hydrocortisone
Loteprednol
Methylprednisolone
Mometasone
Prednicarbate
Prednisolone
Prednisone
Tixocortol
Triamcinolone
antagonist
Mifepristone
Misoprostol

COX-2 inhibitor
Celecoxib
Etodolac
Etoricoxib
Meloxicam
Nimesulide
Rofecoxib
Valdecoxib

CYP3A4 inhibitor
Amiodarone
Aprepitant
Boceprevir
Chloramphenicol
Cimetidine
Ciprofloxacin
Clarithromycin
Conivaptan
Dasabuvir/Ombitasvir/
    Paritaprevir/Ritonavir
Delavirdine
Diltiazem
Erythromycin
Fluconazole
Fluvoxamine
Imatinib
Indinavir
Itraconazole
Ketoconazole
Mifepristone
Nefazodone
Nelfinavir
Norfloxacin
Ombitasvir/Paritaprevir/
    Ritonavir
Ritonavir
Saquinavir
Telaprevir
Telithromycin
Verapamil
Voriconazole

Dermal filler
Azficel-T
Calcium Hydroxylapatite

**Disease-modifying
antirheumatic drug
(DMARD)**
Abatacept
Adalimumab
Azathioprine
Bucillamine
Certolizumab
Chloroquine
Cyclosporine
Etanercept
Gold & Gold Compounds

Golimumab
Hydroxychloroquine
Infliximab
Leflunomide
Methotrexate
Minocycline
Penicillamine
Rituximab
Sulfasalazine
Tocilizumab

Diuretic
Acetazolamide
Brinzolamide
Dorzolamide
Eplerenone
Isosorbide
Methazolamide
Spironolactone
loop
Bumetanide
Ethacrynic Acid
Furosemide
Torsemide
potassium-sparing
Amiloride
Triamterene
thiazide
Bendroflumethiazide
Benzthiazide
Chlorothiazide
Chlorthalidone
Cyclothiazide
Hydrochlorothiazide
Hydroflumethiazide
Indapamide
Methyclothiazide
Metolazone
Polythiazide
Quinethazone
Trichlormethiazide

Dopamine receptor agonist
Apomorphine
Bromocriptine
Cabergoline
Dopexamine
Fenoldopam
Pergolide
Pramipexole
Quinagolide
Ropinirole
Rotigotine

**Dopamine receptor
antagonist**
Amisulpride
Domperidone
Metoclopramide
Sulpiride

**Endothelin receptor (ETR)
antagonist**
Ambrisentan
Bosentan
Macitentan
Sitaxentan

**Epidermal growth factor
receptor (EGFR) inhibitor**
Cetuximab
Erlotinib
Gefitinib

Lapatinib
Necitumumab
Nilotinib
Panitumumab
Pazopanib
Sorafenib
Sunitinib

Eugeroic
Armodafinil

Fibrinolytic
Alteplase
Anistreplase
Reteplase
Streptokinase
Tenecteplase
Urokinase

**Gonadotropin-releasing
hormone (GnRH)
agonist**
Buserelin
Goserelin
Histrelin
Leuprolide
Nafarelin
Triptorelin
antagonist
Abarelix
Cetrorelix
Degarelix
Ganirelix

Histamine
H1 receptor antagonist
Alcaftadine
Astemizole
Azatadine
Azelastine
Bepotastine
Brompheniramine
Buclizine
Carbinoxamine
Cetirizine
Chlorpheniramine
Cinnarizine
Clemastine
Cyproheptadine
Desloratadine
Dexchlorpheniramine
Diphenhydramine
Epinastine
Fexofenadine
Hydroxyzine
Ketotifen
Levocetirizine
Loratadine
Meclizine
Mizolastine
Olopatadine
Phenindamine
Promethazine
Pyrilamine
Rupatadine
Terfenadine
Trimeprazine
Tripelennamine
Triprolidine
H2 receptor antagonist
Cimetidine
Famotidine
Nizatidine

Ranitidine
Roxatidine

Histone deacetylase (HDAC) inhibitor
Belinostat
Panobinostat
Romidepsin
Vorinostat

HMG-CoA reductase inhibitor
Atorvastatin
Fluvastatin
Lovastatin
Pravastatin
Rosuvastatin
Simvastatin

Hormone
Estradiol
Levonorgestrel
Oral Contraceptives
Sincalide
polypeptide
Glucagon
Insulin
Insulin Aspart
Mecasermin
Nesiritide
Secretin

Immunomodulator
Aldesleukin
Efalizumab
Glatiramer
Imiquimod
Immune Globulin IV
Immune Globulin SC
Interferon Alfa
Interferon Beta
Interferon Gamma
Lenalidomide
Levamisole
Natalizumab
Palivizumab
PEG-Interferon
Pimecrolimus
Pomalidomide
Sinecatechins

Immunosuppressant
Alefacept
Alemtuzumab
Anti-Thymocyte Globulin
(Equine)
Anti-Thymocyte
Immunoglobulin (Rabbit)
Azathioprine
Belatacept
Belimumab
Cyclosporine
Daclizumab
Everolimus
Fingolimod
Mizoribine
Muromonab-CD3
Mycophenolate
Pirfenidone
Rituximab
Sirolimus
Tacrolimus
Thalidomide

Mast cell stabilizer
Cromolyn
Lodoxamide
Nedocromil
Pemirolast

Monoamine oxidase (MAO) inhibitor
Isocarboxazid
Phenelzine
Tranylcypromine

mTOR inhibitor
Everolimus
Temsirolimus
Zotarolimus

Muscarinic antagonist
Amitriptyline
Amoxapine
Atropine Sulfate
Benactyzine
Benztropine
Biperiden
Chlorpheniramine
Chlorpromazine
Cinnarizine
Clidinium
Clomipramine
Darifenacin
Dicyclomine
Diphenhydramine
Disopyramide
Doxepin
Fesoterodine
Flavoxate
Glycopyrrolate
Hydroxyzine
Hyoscyamine
Imipramine
Ipratropium
Maprotiline
Mepenzolate
Olanzapine
Orphenadrine
Oxybutynin
Phenelzine
Prochlorperazine
Procyclidine
Propantheline
Scopolamine
Solifenacin
Tiotropium
Tolterodine
Trihexyphenidyl
Trospium
Umeclidinium

Muscarinic cholinergic agonist
Bethanechol
Carbachol
Cevimeline
Methantheline
Pilocarpine

Non-depolarizing neuromuscular blocker
Atracurium
Cisatracurium
Doxacurium
Pancuronium
Pipecuronium
Rapacuronium

Rocuronium
Vecuronium

Non-nucleoside reverse transcriptase inhibitor
Delavirdine
Efavirenz
Emtricitabine/Rilpivirine/
Tenofovir Alafenamide
Etravirine
Nevirapine
Rilpivirine

Non-steroidal anti-inflammatory (NSAID)
Aceclofenac
Acemetacin
Aspirin
Benzydamine
Bromfenac
Celecoxib
Dexibuprofen
Dexketoprofen
Diclofenac
Diflunisal
Etodolac
Etoricoxib
Fenbufen
Fenoprofen
Flurbiprofen
Ibuprofen
Indomethacin
Ketoprofen
Ketorolac
Meclofenamate
Mefenamic Acid
Meloxicam
Metamizole
Methyl salicylate
Nabumetone
Naproxen
Nepafenac
Nimesulide
Oxaprozin
Phenylbutazone
Piroxicam
Pranoprofen
Rofecoxib
Salsalate
Sulindac
Tenoxicam
Tolmetin
Valdecoxib

Nucleoside analog reverse transcriptase inhibitor
Abacavir
Cobicistat/Elvitegravir/
Emtricitabine/Tenofovir
Alafenamide
Cobicistat/Elvitegravir/
Emtricitabine/Tenofovir
Disoproxil
Didanosine
Emtricitabine
Emtricitabine/Rilpivirine/
Tenofovir Alafenamide
Lamivudine
Stavudine
Telbivudine
Tenofovir Disoproxil
Zalcitabine

Zidovudine

Oligonucleotide
Defibrotide

Opiate agonist
Codeine
Heroin
Hydrocodone
Hydromorphone
Loperamide
Meperidine
Methadone
Morphine
Nalbuphine
Oxycodone
Oxymorphone
Pentazocine
Propoxyphene
Sufentanil
Tramadol

Phosphodiesterase inhibitor
Apremilast
Avanafil
Cilostazol
Inamrinone
Milrinone
Roflumilast
Sildenafil
Tadalafil
Vardenafil

Programmed death receptor-1 (PD-1) inhibitor
Nivolumab
Pembrolizumab

Prostaglandin
Alprostadil
Dinoprostone
Iloprost
Treprostinil
Unoprostone

Prostaglandin analog
Bimatoprost
Gemeprost
Latanoprost
Tafluprost
Travoprost

Proton pump inhibitor (PPI)
Dexlansoprazole
Esomeprazole
Lansoprazole
Omeprazole
Pantoprazole
Rabeprazole

Retinoid
Acitretin
Adapalene
Alitretinoin
Bexarotene
Clindamycin/Tretinoin
Isotretinoin
Tretinoin

Selective estrogen receptor modulator (SERM)
Chlorotrianisene
Clomiphene
Ospemifene
Raloxifene

Tamoxifen
Tibolone
Toremifene

Selective serotonin reuptake inhibitor (SSRI)
Citalopram
Escitalopram
Fluoxetine
Fluvoxamine
Paroxetine Hydrochloride
Paroxetine Mesylate
Sertraline

Serotonin
Buspirone
Sibutramine
serotonin receptor agonist
Almotriptan
Eletriptan
Frovatriptan
Lorcaserin
Rizatriptan
Sumatriptan
Vortioxetine
Zolmitriptan
serotonin receptor antagonist
Naratriptan
Vortioxetine
serotonin reuptake inhibitor
Duloxetine
Trazodone
Vortioxetine
serotonin type 3 receptor antagonist
Alosetron
Dolasetron
Granisetron
Netupitant & Palonosetron
Ondansetron
Palonosetron
serotonin type 4 receptor agonist
Tegaserod
serotonin-norepinephrine reuptake inhibitor
Desvenlafaxine

Levomilnacipran
Venlafaxine
Vilazodone

Statin
Atorvastatin
Fluvastatin
Lovastatin
Pitavastatin
Pravastatin
Rosuvastatin
Simvastatin

Sulfonylurea
Acetohexamide
Chlorpropamide
Gliclazide
Glimepiride
Glipizide
Glyburide
Tolazamide
Tolazoline
Tolbutamide

Topoisomerase 1 inhibitor
Irinotecan
Topotecan

Topoisomerase 2 inhibitor
Etoposide
Teniposide

Trace element
Arsenic
Selenium
Zinc

Tyrosine kinase inhibitor
Afatinib
Axitinib
Bosutinib
Brigatinib
Cabozantinib
Ceritinib
Crizotinib
Dasatinib
Erlotinib
Gefitinib
Imatinib

Lapatinib
Leflunomide
Lenvatinib
Nilotinib
Nintedanib
Pazopanib
Ponatinib
Regorafenib
Sorafenib
Sunitinib
Vandetanib

Vaccine
Anthrax Vaccine
BCG Vaccine
Cholera Vaccine
Diphtheria Antitoxin
Hemophilus B Vaccine
Hepatitis A Vaccine
Hepatitis B Vaccine
Human Papillomavirus (HPV) Vaccine
Human Papillomavirus Vaccine (Bivalent)
Inactivated Polio Vaccine
Influenza Vaccine
Japanese Encephalitis Vaccine
Measles, Mumps & Rubella (MMR) Virus Vaccine
Meningococcal Group B Vaccine
Meningococcal Groups C & Y & Haemophilus B Tetanus Toxoid Conjugate Vaccine
Pandemic Influenza Vaccine (H1N1)
Pneumococcal Vaccine
Sipuleucel-T
Smallpox Vaccine
Typhoid Vaccine
Varicella Vaccine
Yellow Fever Vaccine
Zoster Vaccine

Vasodilator
Ambrisentan
Amyl Nitrite
Benazepril

Bosentan
Captopril
Cilazapril
Diazoxide
Enalapril
Fosinopril
Hydralazine
Iloprost
Isosorbide Dinitrate
Isosorbide Mononitrate
Minoxidil
Nesiritide
Nitroglycerin
Nitroprusside
Prenylamine
Quinapril
Ramipril
Trandolapril
peripheral
Cilostazol
Papaverine
Pentoxifylline

Vitamin
Ascorbic Acid
Beta-Carotene
Cyanocobalamin
Ergocalciferol
Folic Acid
Niacin
Niacinamide
Pantothenic Acid
Phytonadione
Pyridoxine
Riboflavin
Thiamine
Vitamin A
Vitamin E

Vitamin D receptor agonist
Dihydrotachysterol
Doxercalciferol
Paricalcitol

Xanthine alkaloid
Aminophylline
Pentoxifylline

CLASSES OF DRUGS THAT CAN CAUSE IMPORTANT INTERACTIONS

ARBs
Angiotensin II receptor antagonists (blockers)
- Candesartan
- Eprosartan
- Irbesartan
- Losartan
- Olmesartan
- Telmisartan
- Valsartan

Anticholinergics
- Amoxapine
- Atropine
- Benztropine
- Biperiden
- Chlorpheniramine
- Clomipramine
- Cyproheptadine
- Desipramine
- Dicyclomine
- Digoxin
- Diphenhydramine
- Disopyramide
- Furosemide
- Glycopyrrolate
- Hyoscyamine
- Oxybutynin
- Propantheline
- Tiotropium
- Tolterodine

Anticoagulants
- Acenocoumarol
- Apixaban
- Aspirin
- Clopidogrel
- Dabigatran
- Dalteparin
- Fondaparinux
- Phenindione
- Rivarobaxan
- Ticlopidine
- Urokinase
- Warfarin

CYP 3A4 inhibitors
- Amiodarone
- Anastrozole
- Azithromycin
- Cimetidine
- Clarithromycin
- Cyclosporine
- Danazol
- Delavirdine
- Dexamethasone
- Diltiazem
- Dirithromycin
- Disulfiram
- Entacapone
- Erythromycin
- Fluconazole
- Fluoxetine
- Fluvoxamine
- Grapefruit juice
- Indinavir
- Isoniazid
- Ketoconazole
- Metronidazole
- Mibefradil
- Nefazodone
- Nelfinavir
- Nevirapine
- Norfloxacin
- Omeprazole
- Paroxetine
- Propoxyphene
- Quinidine
- Quinine
- Ranitidine
- Ritonavir
- Saquinavir
- Sertindole
- Sertraline
- Troglitazone
- Troleandomycin
- Valproic acid

MAOIs
Monamine Oxidase Inhibitors
- Amitriptyline
- Amoxapine
- Atomoxetine
- Benzphetamine
- Brompheniramine
- Bupropion
- Chlorpheniramine
- Citalopram
- Clomipramine
- Cocaine
- Cyclobenzaprine
- Desipramine
- Desvenlafaxine
- Dextroamphetamine
- Dextromethorphan
- Doxepine
- Duloxetine
- Ephedrine
- Escitalopram
- Fentanyl
- Fluoxetine
- Fluvoxamine
- Imipramine
- Ketamine
- Lisdexamfetamine
- Maprotiline
- Mazindol
- MDMA ("Ecstasy")
- Meperidine
- Methadone
- Methamphetamine
- Methylphenidate
- Milnacipran
- Nefazodone
- Nortriptyline
- Paroxetine
- Pemoline
- Phencyclidine
- Phendimetrazine
- Pheniramine
- Phentermine
- Phenylephrine
- Phenylalanine
- Propoxyphene
- Protripyline
- Pseudoephedrine
- Reboxetine
- Sertraline
- Sibutramine
- Tramadol
- Trazodone
- Trimipramine
- Tryptophan
- Venlafaxine

NSAIDs*
Non Steroidal Anti-Inflammatory Drugs
- Aspirin
- Celecoxib
- Diclofenac
- Diflunisal
- Etodolac
- Fenoprofen
- Flurbiprofen
- Ibuprofen
- Indomethacin
- Ketoprofen
- Magnesium salicylate
- Meclofenamate sodium
- Mefenamic acid
- Meloxicam
- Nabumetone
- Naproxen
- Oxaprozin
- Piroxicam
- Rofecoxib
- Salsalate
- Sodium salicylate
- Sulindac
- Tolmetin
- Valdecoxib

Statins
HMG-CoA reductase inhibitors
- Atorvastatin
- Fluvastatin
- Lovastatin
- Pitavastatin
- Pravastatin
- Rosuvastatin
- Simvastatin

---

* Note that acetaminophen (Paracetamol; Tylenol) is not on this list; unlike other common analgesics such as aspirin and ibuprofen, it has no anti-inflammatory properties, and so it is not a member of the class of drugs known as non-steroidal anti-inflammatory drugs. Acetaminophen relieves pain in mild arthritis but has no effect on the underlying inflammation, redness and swelling of the joint. It belongs to a class of drugs called analgesics (pain relievers) and antipyretics (fever reducers) and is thought to relieve pain by elevating the pain threshold (that is, by requiring a greater amount of pain to develop before it is felt). It reduces fever through its action on the heat-regulating center of the brain; specifically, it tells the center to lower the body's temperature when the temperature is elevated.

CLASS REACTIONS*

ACE INHIBITORS

	B	C	E	F	L	P	Q	R	T	Z	=
SKIN											
Anaphylaxis		[1]	[1]		•	[1]		•			✓
Angioedema	[8]	[45] (15%)	[73]	[3]	[43] (70%)	[6]	[9]	[11]	[3]	[1]	✓✓
Bullous dermatitis		[1]			[1]						
Bullous pemphigoid		[2]	[2]								
Dermatitis		[3]		[1]				[1]			
Diaphoresis	[1]		[1]	•	•	•	[3]	[2]			✓
DRESS syndrome		[2]						[1]			
Edema			[1]	•		•	[4]	[1]	•		✓
Erythema		[1]	[1]		•	•		[1]			✓
Erythema multiforme			•					•			
Erythroderma		[2]	[1]	[1]							
Exanthems	[1]	[19] (10%)	[9]		[4]		[1]	[1]			✓
Exfoliative dermatitis		[4]	•		[2]		•				
Facial edema					[1]	•	[1]				
Jaundice		[1]						[1]			
Kaposi's sarcoma		[2]			[2]		[1]				
Lichen planus pemphigoides		[2]						[3]			
Lichenoid eruption		[12]	[2]		[2]						
Linear IgA	[1]	[5]									
Lupus erythematosus		[8]	[2]		[1]						
Mycosis fungoides		[2]	[1]								
Palmar–plantar pustulosis		[1]				[1]					
Pemphigus	[1]	[23]	[10]	[1]			[1]	[1]	•		✓

B Benazepril; **C** Captopril; **E** Enalapril; **F** Fosinopril; **L** Lisinopril; **P** Perindopril; **Q** Quinapril; **R** Ramipril; **T** Trandolapril; **Z** Zofenopril

These tables concentrate on skin, hair, nails and mucosal reactions.

* The following conventions are followed in these tables:

•	reaction noted (package inserts)
[3]	number of published reports of a reaction
(8%)	highest incidence that has ever been noted or reported
?	20 reports or over or an incidence of 20% or over recorded for this reaction for a minority of drugs in the class
✓	at least half the drugs in the class selection have this reaction noted or reported
✓✓	all drugs in the class selection have this reaction noted or reported
Note:	reactions noted or reported for only one drug in a class selection have been excluded

	B	C	E	F	L	P	Q	R	T	Z	=
Pemphigus foliaceus	[1]	[2]	[2]	[1]	[2]	[1]	[1]	[1]	[1]		✓
Peripheral edema	[3]		[2]		[1]	[3]	[3]				✓
Photosensitivity	•	[3]	[2]	•	•		[2]	[2]			✓
Pityriasis rosea		[6]			[2]						
Pruritus	[1]	[8] (10%)	[3]	[1]	•	(<10%)	[7]	[3]	•		✓
Pseudolymphoma		[2]		[1]	[1]						
Psoriasis		[8]	[3]		[1]	•		[1]			✓
Purpura		[1]	[1]		[2]	•		•			✓
Rash	[1]	[12] (4–7%)	[5]	[1]	[5]	[1] (<10%)	[5]	[4]	•	•	✓✓
Stevens–Johnson syndrome		[1]	•					[1]			
Toxic epidermal necrolysis		[3]	•								
Urticaria	[1]	[9] (7%)	[5]	•	[2]		•	•			✓
Vasculitis		[7]	[2]		[1]		•	[1]			✓
Xerosis		[1]				•					
HAIR											
Alopecia		[4]	[1]		[1]		•	(<10%)			✓
NAILS											
Nail dystrophy		[2]	[1]								
MUCOSAL											
Burning mouth syndrome		[1]	[1]		[1]						
Glossitis		[3]	•								
Glossopyrosis		[1]	[1]								
Oral burn		[1]	[1]								
Oral ulceration		[4]	[2]								
Sialorrhea		[1]						•			
Tongue edema			[2]		[2]	[2]					
Xerostomia		[1]	•	•	•	•	•	•	•		✓

B Benazepril; C Captopril; E Enalapril; F Fosinopril; L Lisinopril; P Perindopril; Q Quinapril; R Ramipril; T Trandolapril; Z Zofenopril

ANTIARRHYTHMICS

	A	Di	Dr	F	I	L	Pn	Pf	Pr	Q	S	=
SKIN												
Acneform eruption								•	[2]	[2]		
AGEP								[1]		[2]		
Anaphylaxis	[2]		[2]			[7]			[1]			
Angioedema	[2]					[3]	[1]	[1]	[2]	•		✓
Bullous dermatitis					[1]				[1]			
Dermatitis		•	(5%) [1]			[27]	[1] (6%)		[2]	[4]		✓
Diaphoresis	[2]			•	[1]	[1]		•			•	✓
Eczema			(5%) [1]			[3]			[2]			
Edema	(<10%)	•		•		[2]		•			(5%)	✓
Erythema			(5%)			[3]		[1]	[1]			
Erythema multiforme	[1]					[2]			[1]	[1]		
Erythema nodosum	[2]	[1]				[1]						
Exanthems	[5]	[1] (<5%)	[1]	[1]		[2]	[5] (8%)	[1]	[4]	[6] (17%)		✓
Exfoliative dermatitis	[1]			•		[2]			[1]	[5]		
Fixed eruption				[1]		[2]			[1]	[2]		
Hypersensitivity	[1]		[1]			[9]	[2]			[1]		
Leukocytoclastic vasculitis									[1]		[1]	
Lichen planus							[1]			[7]		
Lichenoid eruption									[3]	[6]	[1]	
Lupus erythematosus	[5] (5%)	[3]				[1]	[175] (15–20%)	[3]	[2]	[35]		✓
Necrosis	[1]								[3]			
Photosensitivity	[41] (10–75%)	[1]	[1]				[1]		[1]	[21]	•	✓
Phototoxicity	[3]		[1]						[1]	[1]		
Pigmentation	[68] (<10%)					[1]				[3]		?
Pruritus	[2] (<5%)	•	(5%) [1]	•		[3]	•	•	[1]	[3]	(<10%)	✓
Psoriasis	[2]			[2]				[2]	[21]	[5]	[3]	✓
Purpura	[1]	[1]				[1]	[3]	•	[1]	[13]		✓
Rash	[1]	•	[8] (<10%)	•		•	•	•	[2] (<10%)	(<10%)	•	✓

A Amiodarone; **Di** Disopyramide; **Dr** Dronedarone; **F** Flecainide; **I** Ibutilide; **L** Lidocaine; **Pn** Procainamide; **Pf** Propafenone; **Pr** Propranolol; **Q** Quinidine; **S** Sotalol

	A	Di	Dr	F	I	L	Pn	Pf	Pr	Q	S	=
Raynaud's phenomenon									[3] (59%)		•	?
Sjögren's syndrome							[1]			[1]		
Stevens–Johnson syndrome	•			[1]					[2]			
Toxic epidermal necrolysis	[2]		[1]						[1]	[2]		
Toxicity	[5]	[1]	[1]			[3]		[1]				
Urticaria	[1]		•			[5]	[1] (<5%)	[1]	[3]	[1]		✓
Vasculitis	[6]		[1]				[5]			[5]	[1]	
HAIR												
Alopecia	[5]			•				•	[6]	[1]	•	✓
MUCOSAL												
Oral lesions		[1] (40%)						[1] (>5%)				?
Oral mucosal eruption							[1]			[2]		
Oral ulceration		[1]				[1]			[1]			
Sialorrhea	(<10%)							[1]				
Xerostomia		[2] (40%)		•				•	[1]		•	?

A Amiodarone; **Di** Disopyramide; **Dr** Dronedarone; **F** Flecainide; **I** Ibutilide; **L** Lidocaine; **Pn** Procainamide; **Pf** Propafenone; **Pr** Propranolol; **Q** Quinidine; **S** Sotalol

ANTIBIOTICS, MACROLIDE

	A	C	E	=
SKIN				
AGEP	[3]		[2]	✓
Anaphylaxis	[2]	[2]	[2]	✓✓
Angioedema	[1]	[1]	[1]	✓✓
Dermatitis	[1]		[4]	✓
Exanthems	[3]	[2]	[4] (<5%)	✓✓
Fixed eruption		[3]	[6]	✓
Hypersensitivity	[3]	[3]	[3] (<10%)	✓✓
Jarisch–Herxheimer reaction	[2]		[1]	✓
Pruritus	[3]	[1]		✓
Pustules	[1]		[1]	✓
Rash	[6] (2–10%)	[2]	[3]	✓✓
SDRIFE		[1]	[2]	✓
Stevens-Johnson syndrome	[6]	[1]	[7]	✓✓
Toxic epidermal necrolysis		[4]	[7]	✓
Toxicity	[1]	[1]		✓
Urticaria	[2]	[1]	[4]	✓✓
Vasculitis	[1]	[3]	[1]	✓✓
HAIR				
Alopecia		[1]	[1]	✓
MUCOSAL				
Gingival hyperplasia/hypertrophy		[1]	[1]	✓

A Azithromycin; **C** Clarithromycin; **E** Erythromycin

ANTICONVULSANTS

	B	C	G	La	Le	O	Phb	Phy	Ti	To	V	Z	=
SKIN													
Acne keloid		[1]						[2]					
Acneform eruption		[1]	•	[1]		•	[1]	[8]	•	•		•	✓
AGEP		[5]		[1]	[1]		[1]	[5]			[1]		✓
Angioedema	•	[5]		[1] (<10%)			•	[2]					
Anticonvulsant hypersensitivity syndrome		[19]	[2]	[17]		[1]	[10]	[10]			[6]		✓
Bullae		[1]					[1]						
Bullous dermatitis		[4]		[1]			[5]	[1]			[1]		
Bullous pemphigoid			[2]		[1]								
Dermatitis		[7]					[1]		•	•			
Diaphoresis		(<10%)		•		•	[1]		•	•	[1]	•	✓
DRESS syndrome		[48] (77%)		[17] (11%)	[7]	[6]	[13] (6%)	[32] (68%)			[9]	[3]	✓
Ecchymoses				•	•	•			(<6%)		[4] (<5%)	•	✓
Eczema		[2]		•					•	•		•	
Edema			[5]		[1]	•	[1]		•	•	[3]	•	✓
Epidermolysis bullosa		[1]						[1]					
Erythema		[1]		[2] (~10%)	[2]								
Erythema multiforme		[16]		[4]	[2]		[7]	[11]			[3]		✓
Erythroderma		[12]			[1]		[2] (16%)	[9] (6%)			[3]		
Exanthems		[35] (17%)	[2]	[18] (20%)	[1]	[4]	[13] (70%)	[22] (71%)	•	[1]	[3] (14%)	•	✓
Exfoliative dermatitis		[24]				[1]	[6]	[15]	•				?
Facial edema		[2]	•	•					•	[1]	•	•	✓
Fixed eruption		[10]		[1]		[1]	[9]	[5]		[2]	[1]		✓
Furunculosis									•		(<5%)		
Granuloma annulare					[1]					[1]			
Hand–foot syndrome								[1]			[1]		
Hot flashes			[1]	(<10%)		•				(<10%)			
Hyperhidrosis				[1]		•							
Hypersensitivity	•	[71]	[1]	[29] (<10%)		[6]	[12]	[47] (23%)			[5]	[4]	✓

B Brivaracetam; **C** Carbamazepine; **G** Gabapentin; **La** Lamotrigine; **Le** Levetiracetam; **O** Oxcarbazepine; **Phb** Phenobarbital; **Phy** Phenytoin; **Ti** Tiagabine; **To** Topiramate; **V** Valproic Acid; **Z** Zonisamide

	B	C	G	La	Le	O	Phb	Phy	Ti	To	V	Z	=
Leukocytoclastic vasculitis			[1]		[1]								
Lichen planus		[2]						[1]					
Lichenoid eruption		[8]						[1]					
Linear IgA		[1]						[8]					
Lupus erythematosus		[35]		[4]			[2]	[19]			[5]	[1]	✓
Lymphadenopathy		[1]		[1]		•			•		•		
Lymphoma		[2]						[6]					
Lymphoproliferative disease		[5]						[1]					
Mycosis fungoides		[3]			[1]	[1]		[7]					
Neoplasms								[1]	•				
Oligohydrosis										[1]		[8]	
Pemphigus		[3]					[1]	[2]					
Peripheral edema		[1]	[12] (8%)				[1]	[1]	•		(<5%)	•	✓
Petechiae		[1]		•					•		[1] (<5%)	•	
Photosensitivity		[9]		[2]			[1]	[1]	•	•	[1]		✓
Pigmentation							[1]	[4]	•	•			
Pruritus		[7]	[1]	[3]	[1]		[1]	[5]	•	[3]	[1] (>5%)	[1] (2–6%)	✓
Pseudolymphoma		[17]		[1]			[1]	[31]			[2]		?
Psoriasis		[1]			[1]				•				
Purpura		[8]	[1]	[1]		•	[2]	[4]		•	[2]	•	✓
Pustules		[5]					[1]	[3]				•	
Rash		[30] (12%)	[2]	[53] (12–22%)	[5]	[11] (9%)	[4]	[13] (17%)	[2] (5%)	[3] (6%)	[7] (>5%)	[6] (7%)	✓
Scleroderma								[1]			[1]		
Sjögren's syndrome				[1]			[1]	[1]			[1]		
Stevens-Johnson syndrome		[98] (68%)	[2]	[49] (30%)	[3]	[10]	[21] (15%)	[58] (68%)			[11]	[3]	✓
Toxic epidermal necrolysis		[88] (68%)		[51] (13%)	[2]	[4]	[26] (13%)	[65] (68%)			[7]	[1]	✓
Toxicity		[2]	[1]					[1]					
Toxicoderma		[1]					[1]						
Urticaria		[14] (7%)		[1]	[2]		[1]	[5]	•	[1]		[1]	✓
Vasculitis		[7]	[1]		[1]		[1]	[11]			[3]		✓
Vesiculobullous eruption									•			•	

B Brivaracetam; **C** Carbamazepine; **G** Gabapentin; **La** Lamotrigine; **Le** Levetiracetam; **O** Oxcarbazepine; **Phb** Phenobarbital; **Phy** Phenytoin; **Ti** Tiagabine; **To** Topiramate; **V** Valproic Acid; **Z** Zonisamide

	B	C	G	La	Le	O	Phb	Phy	Ti	To	V	Z	=
Xerosis				•					•	[1]		[1]	
HAIR													
Alopecia		[7] (~6%)	[2]	[2]				[3]	•	[2]	[22] (<10%)	•	✓
Hirsutism		[1] (25%)		•				[8] (13%)	•		[2] (60%)	•	✓
Poliosis							[1]				[1]		
NAILS													
Nail changes								[2]		•			
Nail hypoplasia		[1]					[2]	[3]					
Nail pigmentation								[1]			[2]		
Onychomadesis		[1]									[1]		
MUCOSAL													
Epistaxis						•			•				
Gingival hyperplasia/hypertrophy		[1]		•	[1]		[4] (16%)	[57] (16–94%)	•	[2]	[8] (42%)	•	✓
Gingivitis			•	•	•				•	•		•	✓
Glossitis									•	(<5%)	•		
Halitosis									•	[1]			
Mucocutaneous eruption		[4]						[2]					
Mucocutaneous lymph node syndrome		[2]						[1]					
Oral ulceration		[2]		[1]	[1]			[1]	•		•		✓
Rectal hemorrhage						•			•		•		
Sialorrhea				•					•	[1] (4–5%)			
Stomatitis				•					•	•	(<5%)	•	
Ulcerative stomatitis									•		•		
Xerostomia			[1] (5%)	(6%)		•	[1]		[1]	[5] (16%)	[2] (<5%)	•	✓

B Brivaracetam; **C** Carbamazepine; **G** Gabapentin; **La** Lamotrigine; **Le** Levetiracetam; **O** Oxcarbazepine; **Phb** Phenobarbital; **Phy** Phenytoin; **Ti** Tiagabine; **To** Topiramate; **V** Valproic Acid; **Z** Zonisamide

Litt's Drug Eruption & Reaction Manual © 2018 by Taylor & Francis Group, LLC

ANTIDEPRESSANTS, TRICYCLIC

	Ami	Amo	C	I	N	T	=
SKIN							
Angioedema	[1]			[1]			
Bullous dermatitis	[1]			[1]			
Dermatitis	[1]		[1]				
Diaphoresis	[1] (<10%)	(<10%)	[2] (43%)	[8] (25%)	(<10%)	[1] (<10%)	✓✓
DRESS syndrome	[2]			[1]			
Edema	[1]	(<10%)	•	[1]			✓
Exanthems		[2]		[6] (6%)			
Fixed eruption	[1]			[1]			
Hypersensitivity	[1]		[2]				
Lichen planus	[1]			[1]			
Lupus erythematosus	[1]			[1]			
Photosensitivity	[3]	•	[3]	[3]	[2]	•	✓✓
Pigmentation	[4]		[1]	[13]			✓
Pruritus	[3]	[1]	[1] (6%)	[6]			✓
Purpura	[2]		•	[3]			✓
Rash		(<10%)	(8%)				
Urticaria		•	[1]	[6]			✓
Vasculitis	[1]	[1]		[1]			✓
HAIR							
Alopecia	[1]	•	•	[2]	•	•	✓✓
Alopecia areata			[1]	[1]			
MUCOSAL							
Stomatitis	[1]			[2]			
Xerostomia	[16] (79%)	[1] (14%)	[6] (84%)	[16] (21%)	[9] (<10%)	[2] (<10%)	✓✓

Ami Amitriptyline; **Amo** Amoxapine; **C** Clomipramine; **I** Imipramine; **N** Nortriptyline; **T** Trimipramine;

ANTIHISTAMINES (HI)

	Ce	Chl	Des	Dy	Fex	H	Lev	Lor	O	P	=
SKIN											
AGEP	[1]			[1]	[1]	[3]					
Anaphylaxis	[2]	[1]		[4]		[2]		•		[1]	✓
Angioedema	•	(<10%)		[1]		[3]		[1]		•	✓
Bullous dermatitis	•									•	
Dermatitis	•	[4] (<10%)		[4]		[1]	[1]	•		[3]	✓
Desquamation	[1]					[1]					
Diaphoresis	•							•			
Eczema				[2]						[1]	
Edema				•		•					
Erythema multiforme						[2]		•		[2]	
Exanthems	[1]			[1]		[3]				[1]	
Fixed eruption	[6]			[4]		[3]	[3]	[3]	[1]	[1]	✓
Hypersensitivity						[1]				[1]	
Palmar erythema	[1]					[1]					
Photosensitivity	•	(<10%)		[3]		•		•		[12]	✓
Phototoxicity	•			[1]		[1]				[1]	
Pruritus	[1]	[1]		[2]				[1]			
Purpura	•			[1]		[1]		•		[2]	✓
Rash	•			•		•		[1]		[1]	✓
Stevens-Johnson syndrome					[1]					[1]	
Toxic epidermal necrolysis				[3]	[1]					[2]	
Toxicity				[2]		[1]					
Urticaria	[9]		[2]		[3]	[4]	[1]	[4]		[3]	✓
Xerosis	•							•			
HAIR											
Alopecia	•							•			
MUCOSAL											
Oral ulceration			[1]							[1]	
Sialorrhea	•							•			
Stomatitis	•							•			
Xerostomia	[2] (6%)	(<10%)	[5]	[1] (<10%)		[4] (12%)	•	[9]		[2] (<10%)	✓

Ce Cetirizine; **Chl** Chlorpheniramine; **Des** Desloratadine; **Dy** Diphenhydramine; **Fex** Fexofenadine; **H** Hydroxyzine; **Lev** Levocetirizine; **Lor** Loratadine; **O** Olopatadine; **P** Promethazine

ANTIMALARIALS

	Amo	A/L	Art	A/P	C	H	M	P	Quc	Qud	Qun	S	=
SKIN													
Acneform eruption										[2]	[2]		
AGEP				[1]	[1]	[22] (25%)		[1]		[2]			?
Anaphylaxis						[1]	[2]	•					
Angioedema	[1]				[1]	•		[2]		•	•	[1]	✓
Bullous dermatitis						[2]		[2]				[1]	
Dermatitis		[1]			[2]	[1]		•		[4]	[6]		✓
DRESS syndrome						[2]		[2]		[1]			
Erythema								[2]	[1]			[1]	
Erythema annulare centrifugum					[2]	[3]							
Erythema multiforme				[2]	•	[2]		[4]		[1]	[2]	[3]	✓
Erythema nodosum						[1]			[1]				
Erythroderma					[3]	[3]							
Exanthems					[1]	[3] (<5%)	[4] (<5%)	[1] (30%)	[3]	[3] (80%)	[6] (17%)	[3] (<5%)	[1]	✓
Exfoliative dermatitis					[4]	[3]	[1]	[2]	[3] (8%)	[5]	[2]	[3]	✓
Fixed eruption	[1]				•	•		[3]	[3]	[2]	[12]	[2]	✓
Hypersensitivity		[1]						[1]		[1]	[1]	(>10%)	
Lichen planus						[1]				[7]	[3]		
Lichenoid eruption					[6]	[4]		[2]	[6] (12%)	[6]	[3]		✓
Livedo reticularis										[6]	[3]		
Lupus erythematosus										[35]	[1]		?
Lymphoproliferative disease						[1]		[1]		[1]			
Ochronosis										[2]		[1]	
Pemphigus					[1]	[1]							
Photosensitivity					[8]	[6]		[3] (<10%)	[1]	[21]	[19]	[2] (>10%)	✓
Phototoxicity					[1]	[1]	[3]			[1]			
Pigmentation					[15]	[19] (<10%)		[5]	[9]	[3]	[6]		✓
Pruritus	[3]	[2]	[3]	(<10%)	[36] (47%)	[13] (47%)	[2] (4–10%)	[2]	•	[3]	[1]	[2]	✓✓
Psoriasis					[18]	[13]	[2]		[1]	[5]			

Amo Amodiaquine; **A/L** Artemether/Lumefantrine; **Art** Artesunate; **A/P** Atovaquone/Proguanil; **C** Chloroquine; **H** Hydroxychloroquine; **M** Mefloquine; **P** Pyrimethamine; **Quc** Quinacrine; **Qud** Quinidine; **Qun** Quinine; **S** Sulfadoxine

	Amo	A/L	Art	A/P	C	H	M	P	Quc	Qud	Qun	S	=
Purpura		[1]					[1]	[1]		[13]	[13]	[1]	✓
Pustules		[1]			[1]	[1]		[1]		[1]			
Rash		[6] (11%)			[1]	[4] (<10%)	[1] (<10%)	•	[1]	(<10%)	[1]	•	✓
Stevens-Johnson syndrome			[1]		[4]	[1]	[2]	[25] (<10%)			[2]	[24] (<10%)	✓
Thrombocytopenic purpura						[2]					[8]		
Toxic epidermal necrolysis					[5]	[3]	[2]	[15]		[2]	[3]	[17]	✓
Toxicity					[2]	[1]							
Urticaria	[1]	[2]	[1]	[1]	[4]	[2]	[1]		[1]	[1]	[2]		✓
Vasculitis						[1]	[3]			[5]	[5]		
HAIR													
Alopecia				[1]		[2]	•		[2] (80%)	[1]			?
Hair pigmentation					[10]	[8] (<10%)	•						
NAILS													
Discoloration					[1]	[1]							
Nail pigmentation					[2]	[3]			[2]				
MUCOSAL													
Aphthous stomatitis	[1]		[1]					[1]			[1]		
Gingival pigmentation					[1]	[1]							
Glossitis								•				•	
Oral edema			[1]					[1]			[1]		
Oral mucosal eruption										[2]	[1]		
Oral pigmentation					[12]	[7]			[4]	[1]			
Oral ulceration				[3] (6%)	[1]						[1]		
Stomatitis					•	[2]				'	[1]		

Amo Amodiaquine; A/L Artemether/Lumefantrine; Art Artesunate; A/P Atovaquone/Proguanil; C Chloroquine; H Hydroxychloroquine; M Mefloquine; P Pyrimethamine; Quc Quinacrine; Qud Quinidine; Qun Quinine; S Sulfadoxine

ANTIPSYCHOTICS

	Ap	As	Chl	Clo	H	L	O	Pal	Per	Q	R	Z	=
SKIN													
Acneform eruption	[I]										•		
AGEP				[I]			[I]			[I]			
Anaphylaxis			[I]				[I]	•					
Angioedema		[I]	[I]	[2]	[I]	•	[2]				[6]	[2]	✓
Bullous dermatitis			[I]								•		
Candidiasis							•			•			
Dermatitis			[I]	•	•		[I]						
Diaphoresis				[4] (31%)	[2]		•			(<10%)	•	[I]	✓
DRESS syndrome							[I]					[2]	
Ecchymoses							•					•	
Eczema				•			•	[I]			[I]	•	
Edema				•			[3]	•		[I]	[3]		
Erythema multiforme			•	•						[I]			
Exanthems			[8] (13%)	[2]			•	[I]	[2]			•	✓
Exfoliative dermatitis											•	•	
Facial edema			[I]				•			•		•	
Fixed eruption		•					[I]						
Furunculosis											•	•	
Hypersensitivity		[I]					[2]						
Lichenoid eruption			[I]				[I]				•		
Lupus erythematosus			[12]	[4]					[4]			[2]	
Peripheral edema		[I]					[5] (<10%)	[4]		[5]	[4] (16%)	•	✓
Photosensitivity			[22] (<10%)	[I]	[3]		•			•	[2] (<10%)	•	✓
Pigmentation			[16]		•		[I]		•		•		
Pityriasis rosea		[I]		[2]									
Pruritus			[2] (<10%)	•	•	•	•		[I]		•		✓
Pseudolymphoma			[I]						[I]				
Psoriasis							[2]				•		
Purpura			[6]	•			(<10%)				•		
Pustules			[I]				[I]						

Ap Aripiprazole; **As** Asenapine; **Chl** Chlorpromazine; **Clo** Clozapine; **H** Haloperidol; **L** Lurasidone; **O** Olanzapine; **Pal** Paliperidone; **Per** Perphenazine; **Q** Quetiapine; **R** Risperidone; **Z** Ziprasidone;

	Ap	As	Chl	Clo	H	L	O	Pal	Per	Q	R	Z	=
Rash	[2] (7%)		(<10%)	[2]	•	•	[2]	[1]	(<10%)	•	[1]	•	✓
SDRIFE				[1]							[1]		
Seborrhea							•				•		
Seborrheic dermatitis			[4]		[2]								
Stevens-Johnson syndrome	[1]			[1]									
Sweet's syndrome				[1]					[1]				
Ulcerations							•				•		
Urticaria			[4]	•			•		[1]		[2]	[1] (5%)	✓
Vasculitis			[3]	•			[1]						
Vesiculobullous eruption							•					•	
Xerosis							•			•	•		
HAIR													
Alopecia					[1]		[3]			[1]	[2]	•	
Alopecia areata			[1]	[2]									
MUCOSAL													
Epistaxis							(<10%)				[1]	•	
Gingival bleeding											[1]	•	
Gingivitis							•			[1]	•	[1]	
Glossitis							•				•		
Glossodynia		[1]		•									
Nasal congestion								•			[1]		
Oral ulceration							•				•		
Sialorrhea	[5] (4–11%)	[1]		[75] (30–80%)	[1]	•	[4]	[2] (<6%)		[3]	[11] (13%)	•	✓
Stomatitis							•				•	•	
Tongue edema							•	•		•	•	•	
Tongue pigmentation							•				•		
Xerostomia	[7] (15%)	[1]	[1] (<10%)	[3] (6%)	[4] (21%)		[11] (19%)	[1]		[22] (31%)	[7] (18%)	[1] (<5%)	✓

Ap Aripiprazole; **As** Asenapine; **Chl** Chlorpromazine; **Clo** Clozapine; **H** Haloperidol; **L** Lurasidone; **O** Olanzapine; **Pal** Paliperidone; **Per** Perphenazine; **Q** Quetiapine; **R** Risperidone; **Z** Ziprasidone;

BENZODIAZEPINES

	A	Cln	Clo	D	L	M	O	=
SKIN								
Acneform eruption	[1]			[1]				
Anaphylaxis				[1]		[1]		
Angioedema	[1]	[1]		[1]		[1]		✓
Bullous dermatitis		[2]		[1]				
Dermatitis	[5]	(<10%)	(<10%)	[3] (<10%)	(<10%)		(<10%)	✓
Diaphoresis	(16%)	[1] (>10%)	(>10%)	(>10%)	(>10%)		(>10%)	✓
DRESS syndrome		[1]					[1]	
Edema	(5%)					[2]		
Erythema multiforme		[1]			[1]		[1]	
Exanthems	[1]	[1]	[1]	[6]				✓
Exfoliative dermatitis		[1]		[2]				
Fixed eruption				[2]	[1]		[1]	
Peripheral edema				[1]		•		
Photosensitivity	[4]		[1]					
Pruritus	[2] (<10%)			[1]		[3]		
Pseudolymphoma	[1]	[2]			[2]			
Purpura		[1]		[4]				
Rash	[4] (11%)	(>10%)	(>10%)	[2] (>10%)	(>10%)	•	(>10%)	✓✓
Urticaria			[1]	[1]		[2]		
Vasculitis			[1]	[1]				
MUCOSAL								
Sialopenia	(33%)	(>10%)	(>10%)		(>10%)		(>10%)	✓
Sialorrhea	•	(<10%)	(<10%)		[1]	•	(<10%)	✓
Xerostomia	[6] (15%)	[1] (>10%)	(>10%)	(>10%)	(>10%)		(>10%)	✓

A Alprazolam; **Cln** Clonazepam; **Clo** Clorazepate; **D** Diazepam; **L** Lorazepam; **M** Midazolam; **O** Oxazepam

BETA BLOCKERS

	A	B	C	N	P	S	=
SKIN							
Anaphylaxis	[2]				[1]		
Cold extremities		[1]			[6] (36%)		?
Dermatitis	[1]			[1]	[2]		✓
Diaphoresis		•	[1]			•	✓
Edema		[1]				(5%)	
Fixed eruption	[1]	[1]			[1]		✓
Leukocytoclastic vasculitis					[1]	[1]	
Lichenoid eruption	[1]			[1]	[3]	[1]	✓
Lupus erythematosus	[2]		[1]		[2]		✓
Necrosis	[3]				[3]		
Peripheral edema		(<10%)		•			
Photosensitivity					[1]	•	
Pruritus	(<5%)				[1]	(<10%)	✓
Psoriasis	[7]	[1]			[21]	[3]	✓
Rash	[1]	(<10%)		•	[2] (<10%)	•	✓
Raynaud's phenomenon	[2]	(<10%)			[3] (59%)	•	✓
Urticaria	[2]				[3]		
Vasculitis	[1]					[1]	
HAIR							
Alopecia	[1]				[6]	•	✓
MUCOSAL							
Xerostomia		•			[1]	•	✓

A Atenolol; **B** Bisoprolol; **C** Celiprolol; **N** Nebivolol; **P** Propranolol; **S** Sotalol

BIOLOGICS

	Ald	Alm	Be	Bo	C	D	E	G	Ib	In	Ip	L	P	R	=
SKIN															
Acne keloid			[1]				[2]								
Acneform eruption			[6] (83%)		[62] (97%)	[2] (<10%)	[27] (73–80%)	[32] (66–85%)	[2]	•	[1]	[1]	[18] (81%)		✓
AGEP	[1]						[1]	[1]	[7]						
Anaphylaxis		•			[5] (13%)		[1] (30%)	[1]				[1]	[1]	[7]	✓
Angioedema	[2]	•	[1]							[3]			[1]	[4] (11%)	
Bullae	[1]					[1]									
Bullous dermatitis	[1]	•					[1]			[4]				[1]	
Bullous pemphigoid	[1]						[1]								
Burning				[1]	[1]										
Carcinoma		[2]							[1]						
Cellulitis		•	[1]									(5%)		[1]	
Dermatitis	[2]		[1]	[1]	[4] (80%)	[1] (<10%)	[4] (30%)			[1] (6%)	[12] (12%)	[1]		[2]	✓
Dermatomyositis									[1]	[1]	[2]				
Desquamation	[1]		[1] (8%)		[3] (89%)		[1]	[2] (39%)					[3] (13%)		?
Diaphoresis									(13%)	[1]			[2] (15%)		
DRESS syndrome							[2]		[3]			[1]	[2]		
Ecchymoses				[1] (16%)								[1] (16%)			
Eczema					[1]	(<10%)	[1]	[1]		[6] (39%)	[1]		[2]		✓
Edema	[3] (47%)		[1] (15%)	(23%)		[6] (38%)	[1]		[35] (80%)	[2] (15%)		[1] (10%)	[1] (15%)	[1]	✓
Embolia cutis medicamentosa (Nicolau syndrome)				[1]						[1]					
Erythema	[5] (41%)	[1]	[1]	[2]	[3] (14%)	[2]	(18%)	[1]	[5] (<10%)	[2]	[3]	(5%)	[5] (65%)	[2] (16%)	✓✓
Erythema multiforme	[1]		[1] (16%)						[2]		[1]	[1] (16%)			
Erythema nodosum	[3]					•			[1]	[1]					
Erythroderma	[4] (>5%)								[3]						
Exanthems	[5]		[1]	[1] (16%)	[5]		[3] (8%)	[3] (21%)	[9]	[3]	[5] (20%)	[3] (16%)		[1]	✓

Ald Aldesleukin; **Alm** Alemtuzumab; **Be** Bevacizumab; **Bo** Bortezomib; **C** Cetuximab; **D** Dasatinib; **E** Erlotinib; **G** Gefitinib; **Ib** Imatinib; **In** Interferon Alfa; **Ip** Ipilimumab; **L** Lenalidomide; **P** Panitumumab; **R** Rituximab

	Ald	Alm	Be	Bo	C	D	E	G	Ib	In	Ip	L	P	R	=
Exfoliative dermatitis	[1] (18%)					[1]		[1]	[4]			[1]	[2] (25%)		?
Facial edema		•					[1]		[3] (<10%)					[1]	
Fissures					[4] (14%)		[1]						[4] (21%)		?
Folliculitis			[2]		[13] (83%)		[9] (11%)	[4]	[1]		[1] (7%)	[2]	[3]		✓
Graft-versus-host reaction	[1]						[1]		[1]		[1] (14%)	[2] (43%)			?
Granulomas		[1]								[1]	[3]				
Hand–foot syndrome			[12] (57%)		[5] (6%)	[1]	[3] (30–60%)	[2]	[3]	[1] (10%)	[1]		[3] (23%)		✓
Hematoma		•	[1]		[1]										
Herpes		[2] (16%)				(<10%)									
Herpes simplex		[2] (6%)								[2]				[2]	
Herpes zoster		[3] (9%)		[13] (10–15%)										[7]	
Hyperhidrosis			[1] (8%)			[1] (<10%)			[1]			[2] (11%)			
Hypersensitivity			[1] (7%)		[8]	•				[1]	[1]			[5]	
Kaposi's sarcoma	[1]									[2]				[3]	
Keratoses										[1]	[1]				
Lesions										[1]	[1] (8%)				
Lichen planus										[5]	[8]				
Linear IgA	[4]									[3]					
Livedo reticularis								[1]		[2]					
Lupus erythematosus	[1]		[1]	[1]		[1]				[17]				[1]	
Lupus syndrome			[1]							[2]	[1]			[1]	
Lymphoma		[2]												[1]	
Malignancies										[1]		[6]			
Malignant lymphoma		•								[1]					
Necrolysis								[1]	[1]						
Necrosis	[2]		[2]				[1]			[6]				[1]	
Neutrophilic eccrine hidradenitis					[1]				[3]						

Ald Aldesleukin; **Alm** Alemtuzumab; **Be** Bevacizumab; **Bo** Bortezomib; **C** Cetuximab; **D** Dasatinib; **E** Erlotinib; **G** Gefitinib; **Ib** Imatinib; **In** Interferon Alfa; **Ip** Ipilimumab; **L** Lenalidomide; **P** Panitumumab; **R** Rituximab

	Ald	Alm	Be	Bo	C	D	E	G	Ib	In	Ip	L	P	R	=
Panniculitis						[4]			[3]						
Papulopustular eruption					[7] (83%)		[9] (29%)	[3] (21%)					[4] (21–41%)		?
Pemphigus	[2]									[2]				[1]	
Peripheral edema	(28%)	(13%)	[1] (8%)	[5] (83%)	[1] (40%)	[3] (44%)		•	[5] (75%)			[4] (83%)	[1] (12%)	[1] (14%)	✓
Petechiae	•								[1] (<10%)						
Photosensitivity	[1]				[1]	[1]			[3] (<10%)	[2]					
Pigmentation			[1] (>10%)	[1] (16%)		[1]		[1]	[12] (60%)	[3] (21%)	[1] (23%)	[2] (16%)	[1]		✓
Pityriasis rubra pilaris			[1]						[1]						
Pruritus	[7] (24%)	(14–24%)	[1] (91%)	[1] (11%)	[9] (40%)	[4] (14%)	[8] (21%)	[5] (61%)	[3] (10%)	[4] (30%)	[22] (65%)	[3] (42%)	[9] (91%)	[8] (14%)	✓✓
Pseudolymphoma	[1]								[3]	[1]					
Psoriasis	[4] (>5%)				[1]				[3]	[22]				[4]	?
Purpura	[1]	(8%)	[1]	[2]			[3]	[1]	[1]	[2]		[1]		[1]	✓
Pustules					[1]			[1]					[1]		
Pyoderma gangrenosum								[1]	[1]	[1]		[1]		[3]	
Radiation recall dermatitis			[1]		[2]		[1]			[1]					
Rash	[2] (42%)	[5] (13–40%)	[16] (91%)	[9] (67%)	[47] (89%)	[10] (34%)	[112] (80%)	[63] (66–85%)	[26] (69%)	[5] (11%)	[28] (83%)	[16] (36%)	[30] (91%)	[12] (58%)	✓✓
Rosacea					[1]		[2]		[1]	[1]	[1]				
Sarcoidosis	[1]									[47]	[4]			[2]	?
Scleroderma	[2]									[1]					
Sclerosis	[1]									[1]					
Seborrheic dermatitis	[1]						[1]			[2]					
Serum sickness												[1] (8%)	[21] (<20%)		?
Sjögren's syndrome										[4]	[1]				
Skin reactions				[1]			[1]								
Squamous cell carcinoma		[1]						[1]	[2]	[1] (7%)					
Stevens-Johnson syndrome	[1]				[1]				[13]	[3]		[5]		[5]	
Sweet's syndrome	[1]			[7]		[1]			[3]		[1]	[3]			

Ald Aldesleukin; **Alm** Alemtuzumab; **Be** Bevacizumab; **Bo** Bortezomib; **C** Cetuximab; **D** Dasatinib; **E** Erlotinib; **G** Gefitinib; **Ib** Imatinib; **In** Interferon Alfa; **Ip** Ipilimumab; **L** Lenalidomide; **P** Panitumumab; **R** Rituximab

	Ald	Alm	Be	Bo	C	D	E	G	Ib	In	Ip	L	P	R	=
Telangiectasia					[1]		[1]		[1]	[1]			[1]		
Thrombocytopenic purpura		[10]	[1]							[2]	[1]				
Toxic epidermal necrolysis	[2]				[2]			[1]	[1]		[3]	[1]		[3]	✓
Toxicity	[6]	[1]	[9] (16%)	[4] (38%)	[18] (63%)	[7] (36%)	[9] (84%)	[10] (68%)	[9] (30–44%)	[4]	[3] (35%)	[6] (75%)	[26] (95%)	[3] (12%)	✓✓
Transient acantholytic dermatosis					[1]						[2]				
Tumor lysis syndrome				[2] (17%)		[1] (<5%)					[1]	[3] (<5%)		[3] (21%)	?
Tumors												[5] (11%)		[1] (11%)	
Ulcerations			[3]	[1]	[1]	[1]		[2]		[1]	[1]				✓
Urticaria	[3]	[2] (16–30%)				[1] (<10%)		[1]	[3]	[3]	[2]	[1]		[5] (8%)	✓
Vasculitis	[1]	[1]	[1]	[4]			[1]	[1]	[2]	[7]	[1]			[4]	✓
Vitiligo	[3]									[9]	[3]				
Xerosis	(15%)		[1] (>10%)	[1] (16%)	[14] (49%)	[1] (<10%)	[12] (56%)	[12] (53%)	[2] (<10%)	[1] (>10%)	[1] (13%)	[2] (16%)	[12] (62%)		✓
HAIR															
Abnormal hair growth					[2]							[1]			
Alopecia	[2] (10%)		[5] (43%)		(5%)	[3] (<10%)	[10] (14%)	[6]	[2] (10–15%)	[16] (48%)	[3] (19%)		[3] (54%)	[1]	✓
Hair changes					[3]		[4] (20%)						[2] (9%)		?
Hair pigmentation						[2]				[3] (18%)					
Hirsutism							[1]			[1]					
Hypertrichosis					[3]		[4]	[2]		[3]					
NAILS															
Nail changes					[1] (21%)		[3] (25%)	[1] (17%)					[2] (9–29%)		?
Nail disorder					[2]	[1]			[1]						
Nail pigmentation								[1]	[1]						
Paronychia			[1]		[15] (14%)		[11] (15%)	[13] (14–32%)					[13] (85%)		?
Pyogenic granuloma					[1]		[1]	[2]					[1]		

Ald Aldesleukin; **Alm** Alemtuzumab; **Be** Bevacizumab; **Bo** Bortezomib; **C** Cetuximab; **D** Dasatinib; **E** Erlotinib; **G** Gefitinib; **Ib** Imatinib; **In** Interferon Alfa; **Ip** Ipilimumab; **L** Lenalidomide; **P** Panitumumab; **R** Rituximab

MUCOSAL

	Ald	Alm	Be	Bo	C	D	E	G	Ib	In	Ip	L	P	R	=
MUCOSAL															
Aphthous stomatitis	[1] (5%)				[1]		[1]		[1]	[2]	[1]				
Epistaxis			[5] (17%)					[1]		[1] (17%)		(15%)	[1]		
Mucocutaneous eruption					[1]				[1]					[2]	
Mucosal inflammation			[2] (59%)				[1] (18%)			[1]			(6%)		?
Mucositis			[11] (75%)	[2] (45%)	[10] (>10%)	[1] (16%)	[10] (21%)	[4] (6–17%)	[2] (15%)		[1]		[4] (75%)		✓
Oral lichenoid eruption									[3]	[1]					
Oral mucositis					[2] (82%)			[1] (33%)							?
Oral pigmentation									[3]	[1]					
Oral ulceration	[1]		[2] (18%)	[1]	[1]		[1]	[1]	[3] (15%)						✓
Oropharyngeal pain										[1]				[1]	
Perianal fistula			[1] (67%)								[1]				?
Rectal hemorrhage				[1]		[1]									
Stomatitis	[1] (22%)	[1] (14%)	[8] (75%)	[1] (43%)	[3] (25%)	[1]	[10] (26%)	[7] (6–17%)		[1] (30%)			[4] (100%)	[2] (69%)	✓
Xerostomia	[1]				(11%)	[1] (33%)			[1] (44%)	[4] (41%)	[1]	(7%)			✓

Ald Aldesleukin; **Alm** Alemtuzumab; **Be** Bevacizumab; **Bo** Bortezomib; **C** Cetuximab; **D** Dasatinib; **E** Erlotinib; **G** Gefitinib; **Ib** Imatinib; **In** Interferon Alfa; **Ip** Ipilimumab; **L** Lenalidomide; **P** Panitumumab; **R** Rituximab

BISPHOSPHONATES

	A	E	I	P	R	Z	=
SKIN							
Angioedema	[2]	•		•			✓
Candidiasis				(6%)		(12%)	
Eczema	[1] (13%)				[1]		
Edema				•		[3]	
Exanthems				[1]		[1]	
Hypersensitivity	[3] (19%)	•		•	[1]		✓
Peripheral edema	[1]				(8%)	(5–21%)	✓
Pruritus	[1]	[1]	[1] (4–5%)		•		✓
Rash	[5]	•	[1]	[1]	[1] (8%)	[3] (6%)	✓✓
Stevens-Johnson syndrome					[1]	[1]	
Toxic epidermal necrolysis		[1]	[1]				
Urticaria	[1]				[1]		
HAIR							
Alopecia			[1]			[1] (12%)	
MUCOSAL							
Stomatitis	[1]			•		(8%)	✓

A Alendronate; **E** Etidronate; **I** Ibandronate; **P** Pamidronate; **R** Risedronate; **Z** Zoledronate

Litt's Drug Eruption & Reaction Manual © 2018 by Taylor & Francis Group, LLC

CALCIUM CHANNEL BLOCKERS

	A	D	F	I	Nic	Nif	Nis	V	=
SKIN									
Acneform eruption		[1]					•	[1]	
AGEP		[21]				[3]			?
Anaphylaxis					[1]	[1]			
Angioedema	[6] (6%)	[3]	[1]		[1]	[2]		[3]	✓
Dermatitis	(<10%)	[1]				[1]			
Diaphoresis	•	[2]	[1]	•		[2]	•	[2]	✓
Ecchymoses		•					•	[1]	
Eczema	[1]	[1]							
Edema	[20] (5–14%)	[4] (<10%)	[1]	[6] (7%)	•	[3]	[1]	[1]	✓✓
Erythema		[2]	•			[2]			
Erythema multiforme	[2]	[11] (31%)				[5]		[4]	✓
Erythema nodosum						[2]		[1]	
Exanthems	[2]	[17] (31%)	[2]	[1]		[9]	[1]	[8]	✓
Exfoliative dermatitis		[6]				[5]	•	[2]	✓
Facial edema			•			•	•		
Hyperkeratosis		[1]						[2]	
Hypersensitivity	[1]	[2]							
Lichenoid eruption		[1]				[3]			
Linear IgA	[1]							[1]	
Lupus erythematosus		[5]				[3]		[2]	
Peripheral edema	[44] (34%)	[1] (5–8%)	[6] (22%)		[2] (7%)	[12] (6%)	[6] (22%)	[1] (<10%)	✓
Petechiae	[1]	•					•		
Photosensitivity		[11]				[5]		[4]	
Pigmentation	[2]	[10]					•		
Pruritus	[3]	[6]	•	[1] (6%)		[3]	•	[6]	✓
Pseudolymphoma	[1]	[1]							
Purpura	[1]	[3]	[1]			[3]		[1]	✓
Pustules		[2]					•		
Rash	(<10%)	[4]	•	•	[3]	[2]	•	[2]	✓✓

A Amlodipine; **D** Diltiazem; **F** Felodipine; **I** Isradipine; **Nic** Nicardipine; **Nif** Nifedipine; **Nis** Nisoldipine; **V** Verapamil

	A	D	F	I	Nic	Nif	Nis	V	=
Stevens-Johnson syndrome	[1]	[4]				[3]		[5]	✓
Telangiectasia	[5]		[2]			[2]			
Toxic epidermal necrolysis	[2]	[4]				[2]			
Toxicity	[2]	[2]						[1]	
Ulcerations						[1]	•		
Urticaria	[1]	[5]	[1]	•	[3]	[7]	•	[5]	✓✓
Vasculitis	[2]	[6]				[4]		[2]	✓
Xerosis	•						•		
HAIR									
Alopecia	•	[2]				[4]	•	[5]	✓
Hair pigmentation						[1]		[1]	
NAILS									
Nail dystrophy		[1]				[1]		[1]	
MUCOSAL									
Gingival hyperplasia/hypertrophy	[30] (31%)	[10] (74%)	[5] (2–10%)	[1]	[2]	[75] (75%)	•	[10] (19%)	✓✓
Oral ulceration		[1]					•	[1]	
Xerostomia	[1]	[2]	[1]	•	•	•	•	•	✓✓

A Amlodipine; **D** Diltiazem; **F** Felodipine; **I** Isradipine; **Nic** Nicardipine; **Nif** Nifedipine; **Nis** Nisoldipine; **V** Verapamil

CEPHALOSPORINS

	Cdxl	Cclor	Ctan	Coxm	Cnir	Cixm	Ctxm	Czim	Caxn	Cpm	CF	Cple	=
SKIN													
AGEP		[2]		[2]			[1]	[1]	[4]	[1]			✓
Anaphylaxis	[1]	[4]	[3]	[7]		[1]	[1]	[3]	[15]		•		✓
Angioedema	[1]	•		•		•		•	[3]				✓
Candidiasis			•		•			•	[3] (5%)	•			
Dermatitis		[1]							[2]				
DRESS syndrome	[1]					[1]	[4]		[2]				
Erythema	[1]			[1]								(9%)	
Erythema multiforme	•	[6]		•		[1] (13%)	[2]	[1]	[1]				✓
Exanthems	[1]	[9]		[2] (6%)	•		[3]	[1]	[7] (6%)	•			✓
Fixed eruption		[2]				[1]			[1]				
Hypersensitivity			[1]	[4]		[1]	[2]	[1]	[4]	[2]	[2]	[1]	✓
Jarisch–Herxheimer reaction				[1]					[1]				
Lupus erythematosus				[1]					[2]				
Pemphigus	[1]			[1]		[1]			[1]				
Pemphigus erythematodes				[1]				[2]					
Pruritus	[1]	[4]	•	•	•	[1]	[3]	[3]	[2]	[3]	[7]	[1] (9%)	✓✓
Pseudolymphoma				[1]		[1]							
Pustules		[1]		[1]									
Rash	•	[2] (12%)	[2]	[1]	•	[2]	[3]	[5]	[5]	[12] (51%)	[9] (10%)	[1]	✓✓
SDRIFE	[1]			[1]									
Serum sickness	•	[7]											
Serum sickness-like reaction		[23]	•	[2]	•	[1]			[2]				✓
Stevens-Johnson syndrome	•	[1]	•	•	•	[1]	[1]	•	[1]	[1]			✓
Toxic epidermal necrolysis		[1]		[2]		•	[1]	[1]	[1]				✓
Urticaria	[2]	[5]	•	[2]	•	[2] (13%)	•	•	[4]	[1]	•		✓
MUCOSAL													
Glossitis	[1]								[2]				
Oral candidiasis				[1]					[1]	•			
Oral mucosal eruption	[1]								[1]				

1st generation: **Cdxl** Cefadroxil; 2nd generation: **Cclor** Cefaclor, **Ctan** Cefotetan, **Coxm** Cefuroxime; 3rd generation: **Cnir** Cefdinir, **Cixm** Cefixime, **Ctxm** Cefotaxime, **Czim** Ceftazidime, **Caxn** Ceftriaxone; 4th generation: **Cpm** Cefepime; 5th generation: **CF** Ceftaroline Fosamil; **Cple** Ceftobiprole

DISEASE-MODIFYING ANTIRHEUMATIC DRUGS (DMARDS)

	Ab	Ad	Az	Ce	Cy	E	G	H	I	M	P	R	S	=
SKIN														
Abscess		[1]				[2]			[4]	[2]				
Acneform eruption		[3]	[2]		[7] (13%)	[1]			[6]	[1] (67%)				?
AGEP			[2]			[1]		[22] (25%)	[2]				[3]	?
Anaphylaxis		[1]	[1]		[8]	[2]		[1]	[10]	[9] (<10%)		[7]	[4]	✓
Angioedema		[3]	[2]	•	[1]	[1]		•	[2] (11%)	[1]		[4] (11%)	[3]	✓
Angioma					[1]					[1]				
Atrophy								[1]			[1]			
Basal cell carcinoma	[3]		[2]		[4]		[1]		[1]	[1]				
Bullous dermatitis					[1]			[2]	[1]	[4]	[3]	[1]		
Bullous pemphigoid		[1]				[1]					[6]		[3]	
Burning					[1]					[1]				
Candidiasis		[1]			[2] (16%)				[4] (5%)	[1]				
Carcinoma		[2]	[3]			[2]				[2]				
Cellulitis	[1]	[2] (<5%)				[2]			[5]	[1]		[1]		
Churg-Strauss syndrome			[1]		[1]									
Cicatricial pemphigoid			[1]								[2]			
Cyst					[5]						[1]			
Dermatitis		[1]	[4]	•		[3]		[1]	[4]	[2]	[4]	[2]	[2]	✓
Dermatomyositis		[5]				[4]		[1]		[14]				
Diaphoresis											[2] (15%)	[1]		
DRESS syndrome								[2]				[31] (7%)		?
Ecchymoses								[1]	[1]	[1]				
Eccrine squamous syringometaplasia					[1]					[1]				
Eczema	[2] (15%)	[2]							[5] (19–30%)				[1]	?
Edema					[1] (5–14%)				[3]	[2]		[1]	[1]	
Erysipelas	[1]	(<5%)												

Ab Abatacept; **Ad** Adalimumab; **Az** Azathioprine; **Ce** Certolizumab; **Cy** Cyclosporine; **E** Etanercept; **G** Golimumab; **H** Hydroxychloroquine; **I** Infliximab; **M** Methotrexate; **P** Penicillamine; **R** Rituximab; **S** Sulfasalazine

	Ab	Ad	Az	Ce	Cy	E	G	H	I	M	P	R	S	=
Erythema		[1]	[1]		[1]				[1]	[1] (7%)		[2] (16%)		
Erythema annulare centrifugum								[3]				[1]		
Erythema multiforme		[1]	[2]					[2]	[2]	[4]	(<5%)		[8]	✓
Erythema nodosum	[1]		[4]	[1]		[1]		[1]		[1]			[2]	✓
Erythroderma								[3]		[2]			[1]	
Exanthems			[10] (5%)		[1]	[2]		[4] (<5%)	[4]	[5] (15%)	[8]	[1]	[23] (23%)	✓
Exfoliative dermatitis			[1]					[3]					[5]	
Facial edema	[1]				[1]				[1]	[1]	[1]	[1]	[1]	✓
Fixed eruption		[1]	[1]			[1]		•	[1]				[7]	
Folliculitis					[8]	[1]			[2]	[2]				
Fungal dermatitis			[1] (42%)		[1]									?
Furunculosis	[1]	[1]							[1]					
Granuloma annulare						[1]			[1]					
Granulomas		[1]				[2]			[1]					
Granulomatous reaction		[5]				[5]			[1]		[1]			
Hand–foot syndrome									[2] (31%)	[3]				?
Henoch–Schönlein purpura		[2]				[3]			[1]					
Herpes		[1]			[1]				[2]					
Herpes simplex	[3] (>5%)	[1]	[3] (35%)		[4]	[1]			[4] (10%)	[2]		[2]		✓
Herpes zoster	[3]	[10]	[8] (27%)	[3]	[2]	[5]			[11]	[7]		[7]		✓
Hidradenitis		[2]			[1]	[2]			[1]			[1]		
Hyperkeratosis					[1]		[1]							
Hypersensitivity	[2]	[3]	[28]	•	[2]	[1]			[11] (11%)	[4]	[3]	[5]	[21] (9%)	✓
Kaposi's sarcoma		[1]	[14]		[5]				[1]			[3]		
Keratoacanthoma			[1]		[1]				[1]					
Leprosy		[1]				[2]			[1]					
Lesions		[2]							[1]					
Leukocytoclastic vasculitis		[1]					[1]		[2]					
Lichen planus						[2]		[1]	[2]		[4]		[3]	
Lichenoid eruption		[5]	[1]		[1]	[3]		[4]	[3]		[7]			✓
Linear IgA					[2]				[1]					

Ab Abatacept; **Ad** Adalimumab; **Az** Azathioprine; **Ce** Certolizumab; **Cy** Cyclosporine; **E** Etanercept; **G** Golimumab; **H** Hydroxychloroquine; **I** Infliximab; **M** Methotrexate; **P** Penicillamine; **R** Rituximab; **S** Sulfasalazine

	Ab	Ad	Az	Ce	Cy	E	G	H	I	M	P	R	S	=
Lupus erythematosus		[16]			[1]	[25]	[3]		[35] (59%)		[43]	[1]	[34]	✓
Lupus syndrome		[3]		[1]		[3]			[11]		[1]	[1]		
Lymphadenopathy		[1]							[1]	[1]				
Lymphoma		[8]	[1]		[12]	[3]	[1]		[9]	[5]		[1]		✓
Lymphomatoid papulosis		[1]			[1]									
Lymphoproliferative disease			[4]		[2]	[1]		[1]	[1]			[1]		
Malignancies	[10] (23%)	[4]	[1]		[2] (8%)	[3]	[5]		[2]	[1]				✓
Melanoma		[6]			[1]	[2]	[1]		[1]	[1]				
Molluscum contagiosum		[1]							[2]	[2]				
Morphea		[1]				[1]					[2]			
Necrosis										[6]		[1]	[1]	
Necrotizing fasciitis					[1]	[1]			[1]	[1]				
Neoplasms		[2]	[2]	[2]	[1]	[2]			[2]	[2]		[1]		✓
Neutrophilic dermatosis	[1]	[1]	[4] (76%)											?
Nevi			[3]			[1]			[2]					
Nodular eruption					[1]	[3]				[15]				
Non-Hodgkin's lymphoma		[1]	[1]							[2]				
Palmar–plantar pustulosis									[3]			[1]		
Pemphigus								[1]			[75]	[1]		?
Pemphigus foliaceus			[1]							[16]				
Peripheral edema	[1]	(<5%)			[3] (10%)	[1]			[1]		(<10%)	[1] (14%)		✓
Photoallergic reaction								[1]				[1]		
Photosensitivity		[1]						[6]		[9] (5%)			[4] (10%)	
Phototoxicity								[3]		[1]				
Pigmentation			[1] (37%)					[19] (<10%)	(<10%)				[3]	?
Pityriasis lichenoides chronica		[1]				[1]			[2]					
Porokeratosis			[4]		[1]	[1]								
Pruritus	•	[6]	[1]	[1]	[2] (12%)	[2] (14%)		[13] (47%)	[8] (20%)	[1] (<5%)	[2] (44–50%)	[8] (14%)	[8] (10%)	✓
Pseudolymphoma		[1]			[6]	[1]			[2]	[10]			[2]	

Ab Abatacept; **Ad** Adalimumab; **Az** Azathioprine; **Ce** Certolizumab; **Cy** Cyclosporine; **E** Etanercept; **G** Golimumab; **H** Hydroxychloroquine; **I** Infliximab; **M** Methotrexate; **P** Penicillamine; **R** Rituximab; **S** Sulfasalazine

	Ab	Ad	Az	Ce	Cy	E	G	H	I	M	P	R	S	=
Psoriasis	[13]	[39]		[6]	[2]	[19]	[2]	[13]	[56] (19%)		[4]	[4]	[1]	✓
Purpura					[4]						[5]	[1]	[1]	
Pustules		[1]				[2]		[1]	[5]				[2]	
Pyoderma gangrenosum		[1]	[1]			[1]			[1]			[3]		
Rash	[6] (23%)	[4] (12%)	[10] (<10%)	[2] (5%)	[1] (7-12%)	[7] (15%)	[3]	[4] (<10%)	[13] (25%)	[11] (5%)	[6] (44-50%)	[12] (58%)	[19] (>10%)	✓✓
Raynaud's phenomenon					[2]					[1]			[3]	
Rosacea		[1]				[1]			[1]					
Sarcoidosis		[8]				[10]			[5]	[1]		[2]	[1]	
Scabies			[5]			[1]				[1]				
Scleroderma		[1]	[1]								[7]			
Serum sickness				•					[2]			[21] (<20%)	[1]	?
Serum sickness-like reaction				•					[5]		[1]	[5] (<17%)		
Sjögren's syndrome	[4]										[1]			
Skin cancer		[1]							[1]					
Squamous cell carcinoma	[5]	[5]	[11]		[12]	[4]	[1]		[1]	[2]				✓
Stevens-Johnson syndrome		[2]	[1]					[1]	[1]	[4]		[5]	[9]	✓
Striae					[1]					[1] (9%)				
Sweet's syndrome			[12]							[1]			[1]	
Thrombocytopenic purpura		[1]			[5]			[2]						
Tinea		[1]	[3]											
Toxic epidermal necrolysis			[1]		[1]			[3]	[2]	[8]	[2]	[3]	[13] (<10%)	✓
Toxicity		[1]	[3] (6%)	[1]	[2]		[1]	[1]	[2] (75%)	[9] (10%)		[3] (12%)		✓
Tumors		[1]	[8] (14%)	[1]	[1]							[1] (11%)		
Ulcerations			[1]		•				[1]	[12]				
Urticaria	[1]	[3]	[5]	•	[2]	[2]		[2]	[6] (17%)	[4]	[2] (44-50%)	[5] (8%)	[11] (<5%)	✓
Vasculitis	[2]	[9] (13%)	[5]	•	[3]	[23] (25%)	[1]	[1]	[18] (63%)	[9] (>10%)	[7]	[4]	[4]	✓✓
Vesiculation		[1]								[1]	[1]			
Vitiligo		[2]			[1]				[4]					

Ab Abatacept; Ad Adalimumab; Az Azathioprine; Ce Certolizumab; Cy Cyclosporine; E Etanercept; G Golimumab; H Hydroxychloroquine;
I Infliximab; M Methotrexate; P Penicillamine; R Rituximab; S Sulfasalazine

	Ab	Ad	Az	Ce	Cy	E	G	H	I	M	P	R	S	=
Xerosis	[1]										[1]		[1]	
HAIR														
Alopecia		[5]	[9] (54%)	[1]	[2]	[5] (20%)		[2]	[6]	[25] (10%)	[3]	[1]	[6]	✓
Alopecia areata		[7]			[6]	[1]	[1]		[3]					
Follicular mucinosis		[1]							[1]					
Hair pigmentation								[8] (<10%)		[1]				
Hirsutism					[10]						[2]			
NAILS														
Discoloration			[1]					[1]						
Leukonychia (Mees' lines)					[2]					[1]	[1]			
Nail pigmentation								[3]		[2]	[4]			
Onychocryptosis		[1]			[1]			[1]						
Onycholysis		[1]								[1]				
Onychomycosis			[2] (5%)						[1] (33%)	[1]				?
Pyogenic granuloma					[1]	[1]								
MUCOSAL														
Aphthous stomatitis			•	•	[2] (9%)					[2]	[2]		[1]	
Cheilitis					[1] (10%)					[1]			[1]	
Gingival hyperplasia/hypertrophy					[157] (86%)						[1]			?
Gingivitis					•	[1] (7%)				(>10%)			[1]	
Glossitis					[1]					(10%)	[1]			
Mucocutaneous reactions						[1]				[2]	[1]	[2]	[2] (6%)	
Mucosal ulceration			[1]							[1]				
Oral candidiasis									[1]	[1] (11%)	[1]			
Oral mucositis			[1]						[1]	[6]				
Oral ulceration			[2]		[2]	[1]				[11] (61%)	[5]		[3]	?
Oropharyngeal pain						[1] (9%)						[1]		
Stomatitis	[3] (24%)		[1]		(5–7%)			[2]		[18] (43%)	[6]	[2] (69%)	[1] (<10%)	✓

Ab Abatacept; **Ad** Adalimumab; **Az** Azathioprine; **Ce** Certolizumab; **Cy** Cyclosporine; **E** Etanercept; **G** Golimumab; **H** Hydroxychloroquine; **I** Infliximab; **M** Methotrexate; **P** Penicillamine; **R** Rituximab; **S** Sulfasalazine

DPP-4 INHIBITORS

	Alog	Lina	Saxa	Sita	=
SKIN					
Anaphylaxis	[1]			[1]	✓
Angioedema	[1]		[1]	[3]	✓
Edema			[1]	[3]	✓
Hypersensitivity	[2]	[1]	[1]		✓
Peripheral edema	[1]	[1] (10%)	•		✓
Pruritus	[2]	[1]	[1]		✓
Rash	[1]		[1]	[2]	✓
Stevens-Johnson syndrome	[1]			[1]	✓

Alog Alogliptin; **Lina** Linagliptin; **Saxa** Saxagliptin; **Sita** Sitagliptin

EGFR INHIBITORS

	C	E	G	L	Nec	Nil	P	Sor	Sun	=
SKIN										
Acneform eruption	[62] (97%)	[27] (73–80%)	[32] (66–85%)	[4] (90%)	[1] (23–43%)	[1] (<10%)	[18] (81%)	[6] (<10%)	[1] (<10%)	✓✓
AGEP		[1]	[1]					[2]		
Anaphylaxis	[5] (13%)	[1] (30%)	[1]				[1]			?
Angioedema							[1]	[1]		
Bullous dermatitis		[1]							[1] (7%)	
Dermatitis	[4] (80%)	[4] (30%)				(<10%)				?
Desquamation	[3] (89%)	[1]	[2] (39%)				[3] (13%)	[9] (50%)		✓
DRESS syndrome		[2]						[1]		
Eczema	[1]	[1]	[1]			(<10%)	[2]	[2]		✓
Edema		[1]		[1] (29%)		[3]	[1] (15%)	[3] (11%)	[6] (32%)	✓
Erythema	[3] (14%)	(18%)	[1]	[1]		[2] (<10%)	[5] (65%)	[4] (19%)	[6] (7%)	✓
Erythema multiforme						[1]		[11] (17%)		
Exanthems	[5]	[3] (8%)	[3] (21%)	[2]		[2]		[3]		✓
Exfoliative dermatitis		[1]		[1] (14%)		[1]	[2] (25%)	[1] (<10%)	[1] (10%)	✓
Facial edema		[1]				•		[1]	[3] (24%)	?
Fissures	[4] (14%)	[1]			[1] (22%)		[4] (21%)			?
Folliculitis	[13] (83%)	[9] (11%)	[4]	[1]		(<10%)	[3]	[3]		✓
Hand–foot syndrome	[5] (6%)	[3] (30–60%)	[2]	[9] (76%)			[3] (23%)	[113] (89%)	[68] (45–65%)	✓
Hematoma	[1]					(<10%)				
Hypersensitivity	[8]				[1]			[2]		
Jaundice				[1] (35%)		•		[1]	[1]	?
Keratosis pilaris		[1]				[1]		[2]		
Necrosis		[1]							[1]	
Nevi						[1]		[3]	[2]	
Papulopustular eruption	[7] (83%)	[9] (29%)	[3] (21%)				[4] (21–41%)			?

C Cetuximab; **E** Erlotinib; **G** Gefitinib; **L** Lapatinib; **Nec** Necitumumab; **Nil** Nilotinib; **P** Panitumumab; **Sor** Sorafenib; **Sun** Sunitinib

Litt's Drug Eruption & Reaction Manual © 2018 by Taylor & Francis Group, LLC

	C	E	G	L	Nec	Nil	P	Sor	Sun	=
Peripheral edema	[1] (40%)		•			[1] (44%)	[1] (12%)		[1] (17%)	✓
Pigmentation			[1]	[1] (18%)			[1]	[2]	[14] (38%)	✓
Pruritus	[9] (40%)	[8] (21%)	[5] (61%)	[3] (33%)	[2] (60%)	[13] (21%)	[9] (91%)	[10] (21%)	[3] (<10%)	✓✓
Psoriasis	[1]			[1]		[1]		[2]		
Purpura		[3]	[1]							
Pustules	[1]		[1]				[1]			
Pyoderma gangrenosum			[1]						[8]	
Radiation recall dermatitis	[2]	[1]						[3]	[1]	
Rash	[47] (89%)	[112] (80%)	[63] (66–85%)	[25] (55%)	[9] (76–81%)	[16] (56%)	[30] (91%)	[51] (30–75%)	[17] (14–38%)	✓✓
Rosacea	[1]	[2]				[1]				
Seborrheic dermatitis		[1]						[2]	[1]	
Skin reactions		[1]						[1]		
Squamous cell carcinoma			[1]			[1]		[8]		
Stevens-Johnson syndrome	[1]							[2]		
Telangiectasia	[1]	[1]					[1]			
Toxic epidermal necrolysis	[2]		[1]							
Toxicity	[18] (63%)	[9] (84%)	[10] (68%)	[6] (46%)	[2] (8%)	[7]	[26] (95%)	[16] (75%)	[24] (67%)	✓✓
Ulcerations	[1]		[2]						[1]	
Urticaria			[1]			(<10%)		•		
Vasculitis		[1]	[1]					[1]		
Xerosis	[14] (49%)	[12] (56%)	[12] (53%)	[1] (29%)	[2] (67%)	[2] (13–17%)	[12] (62%)	[6] (14%)	[3] (17%)	✓✓
HAIR										
Alopecia	(5%)	[10] (14%)	[6]	[2] (33%)		[4] (<10%)	[3] (54%)	[26] (67%)	[5] (5–12%)	✓
Hair changes	[3]	[4] (20%)					[2] (9%)	[1] (26%)		?
Hair pigmentation								[2]	[8] (38%)	?
Hypertrichosis	[3]	[4]	[2]							
NAILS										
Nail changes	[1] (21%)	[3] (25%)	[1] (17%)				[2] (9–29%)			?

C Cetuximab; **E** Erlotinib; **G** Gefitinib; **L** Lapatinib; **Nec** Necitumumab; **Nil** Nilotinib; **P** Panitumumab; **Sor** Sorafenib; **Sun** Sunitinib

	C	E	G	L	Nec	Nil	P	Sor	Sun	=
Nail disorder	[2]			[1] (10%)					[1] (<10%)	
Paronychia	[15] (14%)	[11] (15%)	[13] (14–32%)	[3] (27%)			[13] (85%)			✓
Pyogenic granuloma	[1]	[1]	[2]				[1]			
Splinter hemorrhage								[4] (70%)	[2]	?
Subungual hemorrhage								[2]	[4]	
MUCOSAL										
Aphthous stomatitis	[1]	[1]					[1]			
Cheilitis				[1] (14%)			[1]			
Epistaxis			[1]				[1]	[2] (11%)	[2] (13%)	
Glossodynia								(<10%)	[1] (15%)	
Mucosal inflammation		[1] (18%)		[1] (15%)			(6%)		[4] (54%)	?
Mucositis	[10]	[10] (21%)	[4] (6–17%)	[2] (11–35%)			[4] (75%)	[12] (28%)	[18] (~60%)	✓
Oral mucositis	[2] (82%)		[1] (33%)						[1] (20%)	?
Oral ulceration	[1]	[1]	[1]			•		[1] (5%)		✓
Oropharyngeal pain					•			[1] (10%)		
Stomatitis	[3] (25%)	[10] (26%)	[7] (6–17%)	[1] (41%)	(11%)	•	[4] (100%)	[13] (28%)	[17] (60%)	✓✓
Xerostomia	(11%)					[1] (11%)		[1] (<10%)	[2] (~60%)	?

C Cetuximab; **E** Erlotinib; **G** Gefitinib; **L** Lapatinib; **Nec** Necitumumab; **Nil** Nilotinib; **P** Panitumumab; **Sor** Sorafenib; **Sun** Sunitinib

FLUOROQUINOLONES

	B	C	L	M	N	=
SKIN						
AGEP		[4]	[1]	[2]		✓
Anaphylaxis		[15]	[6]	[5]		✓
Angioedema		[8]	[1]			
Bullous dermatitis		[1]		[2]	[1]	✓
Candidiasis		[2]	•	•		✓
Diaphoresis		[5]	[1]	•	•	✓
DRESS syndrome		[1]		[1]		
Edema		•	[1]			
Erythema			[2]		[1]	
Erythema multiforme		[5]	[1]			
Erythema nodosum		[1]	[1]			
Exanthems		[4]	[2]		[2]	✓
Fixed eruption		[13]			[3]	
Hypersensitivity	[1]	[5]	[5]	[6]		✓
Peripheral edema		[1]		[1]		
Photosensitivity		[19]	[3]	[5]	[1]	✓
Phototoxicity		[5]	[5]		[4]	✓
Pigmentation		[1]	[1]			
Pruritus		[11]	[3]	[3]	[1]	✓
Purpura		[4]	[2]			
Radiation recall dermatitis		[1]	[2]			
Rash		[13] (<10%)	[2]	[4]	•	✓
Stevens-Johnson syndrome		[9]	[2]		[1]	✓
Sweet's syndrome		[1]			[1]	
Thrombocytopenic purpura		[1]		[2]		
Toxic epidermal necrolysis		[11]	[5]	[2]	[2]	✓
Toxicity		[3]	[1]			
Urticaria		[9]	[1]	[3]	[1]	✓
Vasculitis		[11]	[3]			
Xerosis		[1]	[1]	•		✓

B Besifloxacin; **C** Ciprofloxacin; **L** Levofloxacin; **M** Moxifloxacin; **N** Norfloxacin

	B	C	L	M	N	=
MUCOSAL						
Stomatitis		[4]		[1]		
Xerostomia		[3]	[1]	[1]	•	✓

NON-STEROIDAL ANTI-INFLAMMATORY DRUGS (NSAIDs)

	A	C	D	E	F	Ib	In	Ktp	Ktl	Mx	Np	O	P	S	=
SKIN															
AGEP	[1]	[7]		[1]		[5] (50%)				[1]			[2]		?
Anaphylaxis	[8] (<10%)	[8]	[16] (48%)		[1]	[5] (25%)	•	[4]	[3]	[1]	[2]	•	•	[4]	✓
Angioedema	[32] (22%)	[9]	[2]	[1]	[1]	[8]	[2]	[1]	[1]	[3]	[5]	•	[3]	•	✓✓
Bullous dermatitis	[4]	[1]	[2]			[3]	[2]	[1] (29%)		•	[5]		[1]		✓
Bullous pemphigoid	[1]	[1]	[1]			[2]									
Churg-Strauss syndrome	[1]						[1]								
Dermatitis		[2] (14%)	[10]		[1]	[5]	[5]	[29]	•				[5]	[1]	✓
Dermatitis herpetiformis	[1]		[2]		[1]	[1]	[2]								
Dermatomyositis	[1]		[1]												
Diaphoresis		•	•			[1]	•	[1]	[2] (<10%)		[3]	•	[1]		✓
DRESS syndrome	[1]	[1]	[1]			[4]					[4]		[1]		
Ecchymoses						[1]	•		•	[1]	(3–9%)	•	•	•	✓
Eczema			•		•	[1]	[1]	[3]		[1]					
Edema		[5] (6%)			(3–9%)	[1]	[1] (6%)		(<10%)	[1] (6%)	[1] (<9%)	•	•		✓
Embolia cutis medicamentosa (Nicolau syndrome)			[16]			[2]		[1]					[1]		
Erythema		[2] (14%)	[4]					[4] (21%)	[1]	[2]	[1]		[1]	[1]	✓
Erythema multiforme	[9]	[3]	[6]	•	•	[11] (13%)	[1]	[1]		[1]	[2]	[1]	[12]	[8]	✓
Erythema nodosum	[9]		•			[1] (<5%)	[1]				[1]				
Erythroderma	[2]												[2]		
Exanthems	[11] (18%)	[7] (49%)	[6] (<5%)	[2]	[3]	[9]	[7] (11%)	[3]	[1]	[1]	[9] (14%)	[1]	[8] (>5%)	[9] (<5%)	✓✓
Excoriations						[1] (6%)		[1]							
Exfoliative dermatitis	[1]	[1]	[1]		•	[1]	[1]	•	•			•	[1]	•	✓
Facial edema		[1]	[1]	[2]				•		[1]					
Fixed eruption	[22]	[2]	[4] (18%)	[2]	[2]	[15]	[2]			[1]	[25] (24%)		[15]	[5]	✓

A Aspirin; **C** Celecoxib; **D** Diclofenac; **E** Etodolac; **F** Flurbiprofen; **Ib** Ibuprofen; **In** Indomethacin; **Ktp** Ketoprofen; **Ktl** Ketorolac; **Mx** Meloxicam; **Np** Naproxen; **O** Oxaprozin; **P** Piroxicam; **S** Sulindac

	A	C	D	E	F	Ib	In	Ktp	Ktl	Mx	Np	O	P	S	=
Hematoma	[1]								[2]	[3]					
Henoch–Schönlein purpura						[1]				[1]					
Herpes simplex	[1]	•									[1]				
Herpes zoster		•				[1]									
Hot flashes		•			•	•	•	•		•	[1]		•	•	✓
Hypersensitivity	[5]	[8]	[5]		[4]	[5]	[1]		[2]	[2] (5%)	[2]		[1]	•	✓
Jaundice		[1]			[1]					•				[1]	
Lichen planus							[1]				[3]			[1]	
Lichenoid eruption	[2]										[3]		[5]		
Linear IgA			[6]					[1]			[1]	[1]	[3]		
Lupus erythematosus		[1]				[5]					[2]		[1]		
Pemphigus	[1]		[1]			[1]		[1]					[3]		
Peripheral edema	[1]	[2]	[1]	[1]		[2] (5%)	•			[1]	[1]		[1]		✓
Petechiae							•						•		
Photoallergic reaction		[1]	[1]					[2]							
Photosensitivity		•	[4]	[1]	•	[6]	[1]	[35] (11%)	•	•	[16]	•	[40]	[2]	✓
Phototoxicity											[1]	[1]			
Pityriasis rosea	[3]										[1]				
Pruritus	[6] (>5%)	[6]	[6] (<10%)	[7] (<10%)	[1] (<5%)	[5] (<5%)	[3] (<10%)	[4] (<10%)	[1] (<10%)	[3]	[5] (17%)	(<10%)	[6] (<10%)	[5] (<10%)	✓✓
Pseudolymphoma	[1]		[1]			[1]	[1]	[1]			[1]	[1]		[1]	✓
Psoriasis	[3]		[1]			[2]	[7]	[1]		[1]					
Purpura	[8]	[1]	[2]			[1]	[5]	[1]	[1] (<10%)	•	[4]		[2]	[2]	✓
Purpura fulminans			[2]						[1]						
Pustules		[1]									[2]				
Rash	(<10%)	[11] (40%)	[4] (>10%)	[5]	•	[2] (>10%)	[1] (>10%)	[1] (>10%)	[1] (<10%)	[3]	[2] (3–9%)	[2] (>10%)	[1]	(>10%)	✓✓
SDRIFE	[1]	[1]									[1]				
Serum sickness												•	•	[1]	
Serum sickness-like reaction						[1]	[1]				[1]				
Stevens-Johnson syndrome	[6]	[2]	[5]	•	•	[10] (17%)	•	•		•	[1]	[1]	[2]	[5]	✓✓
Toxic epidermal necrolysis	[9]	[5]	[4]	•	[1]	[8] (6%)	[6]	[1]	•	[1]	[5]	[4]	[12]	[13]	✓✓

A Aspirin; **C** Celecoxib; **D** Diclofenac; **E** Etodolac; **F** Flurbiprofen; **Ib** Ibuprofen; **In** Indomethacin; **Ktp** Ketoprofen; **Ktl** Ketorolac; **Mx** Meloxicam; **Np** Naproxen; **O** Oxaprozin; **P** Piroxicam; **S** Sulindac

	A	C	D	E	F	Ib	In	Ktp	Ktl	Mx	Np	O	P	S	=
Urticaria	[72] (83%)	[11]	[7]	•	•	[10] (>10%)	[7]	[6]	[1]	[4]	[6] (<5%)	•	[7]	[4]	✓✓
Vasculitis	[2]	[4]	[3]	[2]	[1]	[8]	[5]		[1]	•	[9]		[3]	•	✓
Vesiculobullous eruption						[2]					[1]				
Wound complications						[1]			[1]						
Xerosis		•	[3]						[1]				[1]		
HAIR															
Alopecia	[1]	[3]	•		•	[2]	•	[1]	•	•	[3]		[3]	•	✓
NAILS															
Nail changes		•			•	[1]									
Onycholysis						[1]		[1]							
MUCOSAL															
Aphthous stomatitis	[3]		[1]						[1]		[1]		[4]		
Epistaxis	[1]								•	[1]					
Glossitis									•					•	
Oral lesions						[1]	[2] (7%)	[1]							
Oral lichenoid eruption					[2]	[1]	[1]							[1]	
Oral mucosal eruption	[3]													[2]	
Oral mucosal fixed eruption											[1]		[1]		
Oral ulceration	[4]		[1]			[1]	[4]				[1]		[1]		
Rectal hemorrhage									•	[1]					
Rectal mucosal ulceration	[1]													[1]	
Stomatitis		[4] (8%)	•					•	(<10%)		•	•	•	[2]	✓
Tongue edema			[1]				[1]		•						
Ulcerative stomatitis							[1]			•					
Xerostomia		•	[2] (26%)		•	•		[1]	[2]	•	[2]		[1]	[2]	✓

A Aspirin; **C** Celecoxib; **D** Diclofenac; **E** Etodolac; **F** Flurbiprofen; **Ib** Ibuprofen; **In** Indomethacin; **Ktp** Ketoprofen; **Ktl** Ketorolac; **Mx** Meloxicam; **Np** Naproxen; **O** Oxaprozin; **P** Piroxicam; **S** Sulindac

PROTON PUMP INHIBITORS (PPI)

	D	E	L	O	P	R	=
SKIN							
Acneform eruption	•	•	•		•		✓
AGEP			[1]	[2]			
Anaphylaxis	•	[1]	[6]	[7]	[7]		✓
Angioedema		•		[5]	•		✓
Candidiasis		•	•				
Dermatitis	•	•	[1]	[1]	•		✓
Diaphoresis		•	[1]	[1]	[1]	•	✓
Ecchymoses					•	•	
Eczema		[1]		[2]	[1] (9%)		✓
Edema		•	[1]	[2] (<10%)	•		✓
Erythema	•			[1]			
Erythema multiforme			[2]	[1]	•		✓
Erythroderma			[1]	[2]			
Exanthems		•		[1]	•		✓
Exfoliative dermatitis		[1]	[1]	[3]			✓
Facial edema			[2]	[1]	[1]	•	✓
Fixed eruption		[2]		[1]			
Fungal dermatitis		•			•		
Herpes zoster	•				•	•	
Hypersensitivity			[3]	[2]	[1]	[1]	✓
Lichenoid eruption			[1]	[2]	[1]		✓
Lupus erythematosus		[2]	[3]	[5]	[3]		✓
Peripheral edema		•	[2]	[2]	[2]	•	✓
Photosensitivity		[1]			[1]	•	✓
Pigmentation				[1]		•	
Pruritus	•	•	[1] (3–10%)	[8] (<10%)	[1]	[2]	✓✓
Pruritus ani et vulvae		•	[1]				
Psoriasis				[1]		•	
Rash	•	[1]	(3–10%)	[6]	[3] (9%)	[2]	✓✓
Stevens-Johnson syndrome			[1]	•	•		✓

D Dexlansoprazole; **E** Esomeprazole; **L** Lansoprazole; **O** Omeprazole; **P** Pantoprazole; **R** Rabeprazole

	D	E	L	O	P	R	=
Sweet's syndrome		[1]		[1]			
Toxic epidermal necrolysis			[4]	[5]	•		✓
Urticaria	•	[1]	[3]	[9] (<10%)	[2]	•	✓✓
Vasculitis				[2]	[1]		
Xerosis		[1]		[2]	•	•	✓
HAIR							
Alopecia			[1]	[2]	•	•	✓
MUCOSAL							
Gingivitis					•	•	
Glossitis			[1]		•	•	✓
Oral candidiasis	•			[3]	•		✓
Stomatitis			[2]	[1]	•	•	✓
Tongue edema		•			[1]		
Xerostomia	•		•	[2] (<10%)	•	•	✓

D Dexlansoprazole; **E** Esomeprazole; **L** Lansoprazole; **O** Omeprazole; **P** Pantoprazole; **R** Rabeprazole

STATINS

	A	F	L	Pi	Pr	R	S	=
SKIN								
Acneform eruption	•						[1] (36%)	?
Dermatomyositis	[4]	[1]	[1]		[2]		[5]	✓
Diaphoresis	•						[1]	
Ecchymoses	•					•		
Eczema	•				[2]		[4] (5%)	
Edema	•		[1] (6%)		•		[1]	✓
Eosinophilic fasciitis	[1]						[2]	
Erythema multiforme					[1]		[2]	
Exanthems			[3] (5%)				[1]	
Herpes zoster	[1]	[1]	[1]		[1]	[1]	[1]	✓
Hypersensitivity			[1]	•			[1]	
Jaundice	[2]						[1]	
Lichenoid eruption		[1]	[1]		[2]		[1]	✓
Lupus erythematosus	[2]	[2]	[4]		[1]		[5]	✓
Peripheral edema		·				•	[2] (50%)	?
Petechiae	•						[1]	
Photosensitivity	•				[1]		[7]	
Pruritus	[1]		[2] (5%)		[2]	•	[3]	✓
Purpura			[1]		[1]		[3]	
Radiation recall dermatitis						[1]	[1]	
Rash	[2]	•	[3] (5%)	•	[7] (5–7%)	•	[4] (<10%)	✓✓
Toxicity	[2]					[1]	[1]	
Urticaria	[1]			•			[1]	
Vasculitis	[1]						[2]	
HAIR								
Alopecia	[1]		•					
MUCOSAL								
Cheilitis	•						[1]	
Stomatitis	•						[2] (64%)	?

A Atorvastatin; **F** Fluvastatin; **L** Lovastatin; **Pi** Pitavastatin; **Pr** Pravastatin; **R** Rosuvastatin; **S** Simvastatin

TNF INHIBITORS

	A	C	E	G	I	=
SKIN						
Abscess	[1]		[2]		[4]	✓
Acneform eruption	[3]		[1]		[6]	✓
AGEP			[1]		[2]	
Anaphylaxis	[1]		[2]		[10]	✓
Angioedema	[3]	•	[1]		[2] (11%)	✓
Basal cell carcinoma				[1]	[1]	
Bullous pemphigoid	[1]		[1]			
Candidiasis	[1]				[4] (5%)	
Carcinoma	[2]		[2]			
Cellulitis	[2] (<5%)		[2]		[5]	✓
Dermatitis	[1]	•	[3]		[4]	✓
Dermatomyositis	[5]		[4]			
Eczema	[2]				[5] (19–30%)	?
Erythema	[1]				[1]	
Erythema multiforme	[1]				[2]	
Erythema nodosum		[1]	[1]			
Exanthems			[2]		[4]	
Fixed eruption	[1]		[1]		[1]	✓
Folliculitis			[1]		[2]	
Granuloma annulare			[1]		[1]	
Granulomas	[1]		[2]		[1]	✓
Granulomatous reaction	[5]		[5]		[1]	✓
Henoch–Schönlein purpura	[2]		[3]		[1]	✓
Herpes	[1]				[2]	
Herpes simplex	[1]		[1]		[4] (10%)	✓
Herpes zoster	[10]	[3]	[5]		[11]	✓
Hidradenitis	[2]		[2]		[1]	✓
Hypersensitivity	[3]	•	[1]		[11] (11%)	✓
Kaposi's sarcoma	[1]				[1]	

A Adalimumab; **C** Certolizumab; **E** Etanercept; **G** Golimumab; **I** Infliximab

	A	C	E	G	I	=
Leprosy	[1]		[2]		[1]	✓
Lesions	[2]				[1]	
Leukocytoclastic vasculitis	[1]			[1]	[2]	✓
Lichen planus			[2]		[2]	
Lichenoid eruption	[5]		[3]		[3]	✓
Lupus erythematosus	[16]		[25]	[3]	[35] (59%)	✓
Lupus syndrome	[3]	[1]	[3]		[11]	✓
Lymphadenopathy	[1]				[1]	
Lymphoma	[8]		[3]	[1]	[9]	✓
Lymphoproliferative disease			[1]		[1]	
Malignancies	[4]		[3]	[5]	[2]	✓
Melanoma	[6]		[2]	[1]	[1]	✓
Molluscum contagiosum	[1]				[2]	
Morphea	[1]		[1]			
Necrotizing fasciitis			[1]		[1]	
Neoplasms	[2]	[2]	[2]		[2]	✓
Nevi			[1]		[2]	
Peripheral edema	(<5%)		[1]		[1]	✓
Pityriasis lichenoides chronica	[1]		[1]		[2]	✓
Pruritus	[6]	[1]	[2] (14%)		[8] (20%)	✓
Pseudolymphoma	[1]		[1]		[2]	✓
Psoriasis	[39]	[6]	[19]	[2]	[56] (19%)	✓✓
Pustules	[1]		[2]		[5]	✓
Pyoderma gangrenosum	[1]		[1]		[1]	✓
Rash	[4] (12%)	[2] (5%)	[7] (15%)	[3]	[13] (25%)	✓✓
Rosacea	[1]		[1]		[1]	✓
Sarcoidosis	[8]		[10]		[5]	✓
Serum sickness		•			[2]	
Skin cancer	[1]				[1]	
Squamous cell carcinoma	[5]		[4]	[1]	[1]	✓

A Adalimumab; **C** Certolizumab; **E** Etanercept; **G** Golimumab; **I** Infliximab

	A	C	E	G	I	=
Stevens-Johnson syndrome	[2]				[1]	
Toxicity	[1]	[1]		[1]	[2] (75%)	✓
Tumors	[1]	[1]				
Urticaria	[3]	•	[2]		[6] (17%)	✓
Vasculitis	[9] (13%)	•	[23] (25%)	[1]	[18] (63%)	✓✓
Vitiligo	[2]				[4]	
HAIR						
Alopecia	[5]	[1]	[5] (20%)		[6]	✓
Alopecia areata	[7]		[1]	[1]	[3]	✓
Follicular mucinosis	[1]				[1]	

A Adalimumab; **C** Certolizumab; **E** Etanercept; **G** Golimumab; **I** Infliximab

TYROSINE-KINASE INHIBITORS

	Aft	Axt	Cbo	Crz	Dsa	Erl	Gft	Imt	Lpt	Lnv	Nlo	Nnt	Srf	Snt	Vnd	=
SKIN																
Acneform eruption	[25] (92%)				[2] (<10%)	[27] (73–80%)	[32] (66–85%)	[2]	[4] (90%)		[1] (<10%)		[6] (<10%)	[1] (<10%)	[4] (35%)	✓
AGEP						[1]	[1]	[7]					[2]			
Anaphylaxis						[1] (30%)	[1]									
Bullous dermatitis	•					[1]								[1] (7%)		
Cyst				[1]									[1]			
Dermatitis	[1] (21%)				[1] (<10%)	[4] (30%)					(<10%)				[1]	?
Desquamation						[1]	[2] (39%)						[9] (50%)			?
Diaphoresis								(13%)					[1] (6%)			
DRESS syndrome						[2]		[3]					[1]			
Eczema					(<10%)	[1]	[1]				(<10%)		[2]			
Edema				[11] (23–55%)	[6] (38%)	[1]		[35] (80%)	[1] (29%)		[3]		[3] (11%)	[6] (32%)		✓
Erythema		[1]	(11%)		[2]	(18%)	[1]	[5] (<10%)	[1]		[2] (<10%)		[4] (19%)	[6] (7%)		✓
Erythema multiforme				[1]				[2]			[1]		[11] (17%)		[1]	
Erythema nodosum					•			[1]								
Exanthems						[3] (8%)	[3] (21%)	[9]	[1]	(21%)	[2]		[3]			?
Exfoliative dermatitis	•					[1]		[1]	[4]	[1] (14%)		[1]		[1] (<10%)	[1] (10%)	✓
Facial edema						[1]		[3] (<10%)			•		[1]	[3] (24%)		?
Fissures	[2] (12%)					[1]										
Folliculitis	[1]					[9] (11%)	[4]	[1]	[1]		(<10%)		[3]		[5] (49%)	✓
Graft-versus-host reaction						[1]		[1]								
Hand–foot syndrome	[2] (10%)	[15] (64%)	[17] (50%)		[1]	[3] (30–60%)	[2]	[3]	[9] (76%)	[2] (47%)		[2]	[113] (89%)	[68] (45–65%)	[4] (36%)	✓
Herpes						(<10%)					•					
Hyperhidrosis					[1] (<10%)			[1]			(<10%)	[1] (12%)				

Aft Afatinib; **Axt** Axitinib; **Cbo** Cabozantinib; **Crz** Crizotinib; **Dsa** Dasatinib; **Erl** Erlotinib; **Gft** Gefitinib; **Imt** Imatinib; **Lpt** Lapatinib; **Lnv** Lenvatinib; **Nlo** Nilotinib; **Nnt** Nintedanib; **Srf** Sorafenib; **Snt** Sunitinib; **Vnd** Vandetanib

	Aft	Axt	Cbo	Crz	Dsa	Erl	Gft	Imt	Lpt	Lnv	Nlo	Nnt	Srf	Snt	Vnd	=
Hyperkeratosis			(7%)							(7%)			[4]			
Hypersensitivity					•								[2]			
Hypomelanosis								[5]						[1]		
Jaundice			(25%)						[1] (35%)		•		[1]	[1]		?
Keratosis pilaris						[1]					[1]		[2]			
Lesions								[1]						[2] (38%)		?
Leukocytoclastic vasculitis	[1]							[1]								
Lichen planus								[5]			[1]					
Necrolysis							[1]	[1]								
Necrosis						[1]								[1]		
Nevi											[1]		[3]	[2]		
Palmar–plantar hyperkeratosis								[1]						[1]		
Panniculitis					[4]			[3]								
Papulopustular eruption						[9] (29%)	[3] (21%)								[1]	?
Peripheral edema				[6] (28%)	[3] (44%)		•	[5] (75%)		[3] (37%)	[1] (44%)			[1] (17%)		?
Photosensitivity				[2]	[1]	[1]		[3] (<10%)						[8] (23%)		?
Phototoxicity													[1]		[3]	
Pigmentation					[1]		[1]	[12] (60%)	[1] (18%)				[2]	[14] (38%)	[6]	✓
Pityriasis rubra pilaris								[1]					[1]			
Pruritus	[2] (13%)	[1] (8%)			[4] (14%)	[8] (21%)	[5] (61%)	[3] (10%)	[3] (33%)		[13] (21%)	[1] (19%)	[10] (21%)	[3] (<10%)	[2] (11%)	✓
Psoriasis								[3]	[1]		[1]		[2]			
Purpura						[3]	[1]	[1]								
Pyoderma gangrenosum							[1]	[1]						[8]		
Radiation recall dermatitis						[1]							[3]	[1]		
Rash	[49] (92%)	[3] (14%)	[1] (30%)	[4] (16%)	[10] (34%)	[112] (80%)	[63] (66–85%)	[26] (69%)	[25] (55%)	[1] (23%)	[16] (56%)	[4] (41%)	[51] (30–75%)	[17] (14–38%)	[34] (67%)	✓✓
Rosacea						[2]		[1]			[1]					
Seborrheic dermatitis						[1]							[2]	[1]		
Skin reactions						[1]							[1]			

Aft Afatinib; **Axt** Axitinib; **Cbo** Cabozantinib; **Crz** Crizotinib; **Dsa** Dasatinib; **Erl** Erlotinib; **Gft** Gefitinib; **Imt** Imatinib; **Lpt** Lapatinib; **Lnv** Lenvatinib; **Nlo** Nilotinib; **Nnt** Nintedanib; **Srf** Sorafenib; **Snt** Sunitinib; **Vnd** Vandetanib

	Aft	Axt	Cbo	Crz	Dsa	Erl	Gft	Imt	Lpt	Lnv	Nlo	Nnt	Srf	Snt	Vnd	=
Squamous cell carcinoma							[1]	[2]			[1]		[8]			
Stevens-Johnson syndrome	[1]							[13]					[2]		[2]	
Sweet's syndrome					[1]			[3]			[3]					
Telangiectasia						[1]		[1]								
Toxic epidermal necrolysis							[1]	[1]								
Toxicity	[3]		[2]		[7] (36%)	[9] (84%)	[10] (68%)	[9] (30–44%)	[6] (46%)	[2]	[7]		[16] (75%)	[24] (67%)	[9] (48–50%)	✓
Ulcerations						[1]		[2]						[1]		
Urticaria					[1] (<10%)		[1]	[3]			(<10%)		•			
Vasculitis						[1]	[1]	[2]					[1]			
Wound complications			[1]										[1]		[1]	
Xerosis	[6] (15%)	(10%)	[1] (23%)		[1] (<10%)	[12] (56%)	[12] (53%)	[2] (<10%)	[1] (29%)	[1] (20%)	[2] (13–17%)		[6] (14%)	[3] (17%)	[3] (15%)	✓
HAIR																
Alopecia	[1] (7%)	[2] (6%)	(16%)	[1] (7%)	[3] (<10%)	[10] (14%)	[6]	[2] (10–15%)	[2] (33%)	(12%)	[4] (<10%)	[2] (71%)	[26] (67%)	[5] (5–12%)	[1]	✓✓
Hair changes			(34%)			[4] (20%)							[1] (26%)		[2]	?
Hair pigmentation			[2] (34%)		[2]								[2]	[8] (38%)		?
Hypertrichosis						[4]	[2]									
NAILS																
Nail changes	[2] (16%)					[3] (25%)	[1] (17%)									?
Nail disorder					[1]			[1]	[1] (10%)					[1] (<10%)		
Nail pigmentation							[1]	[1]								
Paronychia	[10] (33–85%)					[11] (15%)	[13] (14–32%)		[3] (27%)					[5] (7%)		?
Pyogenic granuloma						[1]	[2]									
Splinter hemorrhage													[4] (70%)	[2]	[2]	?
Subungual hemorrhage													[2]	[4]		

Aft Afatinib; **Axt** Axitinib; **Cbo** Cabozantinib; **Crz** Crizotinib; **Dsa** Dasatinib; **Erl** Erlotinib; **Gft** Gefitinib; **Imt** Imatinib; **Lpt** Lapatinib; **Lnv** Lenvatinib; **Nlo** Nilotinib; **Nnt** Nintedanib; **Srf** Sorafenib; **Snt** Sunitinib; **Vnd** Vandetanib

	Aft	Axt	Cbo	Crz	Dsa	Erl	Gft	Imt	Lpt	Lnv	Nlo	Nnt	Srf	Snt	Vnd	=
MUCOSAL																
Aphthous stomatitis	•					[1]		[1]		(41%)			[1]			?
Cheilitis	[1] (7%)							[1]	[1] (14%)				[1]			
Epistaxis	[3] (17%)	[1] (8%)					[1]			[1] (24%)		[2]	[2] (11%)	[2] (13%)		?
Glossodynia		[1]								(25%)			(<10%)	[1] (15%)		?
Mucocutaneous eruption					[1]			[1]			[1]					
Mucosal inflammation	[7] (69%)	[2] (15%)	[2] (23%)			[1] (18%)			[1] (15%)	[1] (50%)				[4] (54%)	[1] (27%)	✓
Mucositis	[10] (50–90%)	[1] (30%)	[1]		[1] (16%)	[10] (21%)	[4] (6–17%)	[2] (15%)	[2] (11–35%)				[12] (28%)	[18] (~60%)	[2] (14%)	✓
Oral mucositis		[1]					[1] (33%)							[1] (20%)		?
Oral ulceration						[1]	[1]	[3] (15%)		(41%)	•		[1] (5%)			
Oropharyngeal pain								[1]		(25%)			[1] (10%)			?
Rhinorrhea	(11%)												•			
Stomatitis	[19] (50–90%)	[1] (15%)	(51%)	[1] (11%)	[1]	[10] (26%)	[7] (6–17%)		[1] (41%)	[3] (47%)	•	[1]	[13] (28%)	[17] (60%)	[2] (33%)	✓
Xerostomia	[1] (20%)				[1] (33%)			[1] (44%)		(17%)	[1] (11%)		[1] (<10%)	[2] (~60%)		?

Aft Afatinib; **Axt** Axitinib; **Cbo** Cabozantinib; **Crz** Crizotinib; **Dsa** Dasatinib; **Erl** Erlotinib; **Gft** Gefitinib; **Imt** Imatinib; **Lpt** Lapatinib; **Lnv** Lenvatinib; **Nlo** Nilotinib; **Nnt** Nintedanib; **Srf** Sorafenib; **Snt** Sunitinib; **Vnd** Vandetanib

CONCORDANCE OF SYNONYMS AND TRADE NAMES WITH GENERIC NAMES

Synonym/Trade name	Generic	Synonym/Trade name	Generic
13-cis-retinoic acid	isotretinoin	Acnamino	minocycline
3,4-methylenedioxymethamphetamine	MDMA	Acnavit	tretinoin
3TC	lamivudine	Acon	vitamin A
4-aminopyridine	dalfampridine	Act-3	ibuprofen
4-demethoxydaunorubicin	idarubicin	*ACT*	dactinomycin
4-DMDR	idarubicin	Acta	tretinoin
5-aminosalicylic acid	mesalamine	Actacode	codeine
5-ASA	mesalamine	Actemra	tocilizumab
5-aza-2'-deoxycytidine	decitabine	ActHIB	Hemophilus B vaccine
5-fluorouracil	fluorouracil	Actigall	ursodiol
6-mercaptopurine	mercaptopurine	Actilyse	alteplase
6-MP	mercaptopurine	Actimmune	interferon gamma
		actinomycin-D	dactinomycin

A

Synonym/Trade name	Generic	Synonym/Trade name	Generic
		Actiprofen	ibuprofen
A-Acido	tretinoin	Actiq	fentanyl
A-Gram	amoxicillin	Activacin	alteplase
Abaprim	trimethoprim	Activase	alteplase
Abbocillin	penicillin V	Actonel	risedronate
Abelcet	amphotericin B	Actos	pioglitazone
Aberal	tretinoin	Acuitel	quinapril
Aberela	tretinoin	Acular	ketorolac
Abetol	labetalol	Acupril	quinapril
Abilify	aripiprazole	*ACV*	acyclovir
Abilitat	aripiprazole	Acyclo-V	acyclovir
Abraxane	paclitaxel	*acycloguanosine*	acyclovir
Abrifam	rifampin	Acyvir	acyclovir
Abstral	fentanyl	Aczone	dapsone
Ac-De	dactinomycin	Adalat	nifedipine
Acaren	vitamin A	Adalate	nifedipine
Accolate	zafirlukast	Adant	hyaluronic acid
AccuNeb	albuterol	Adapin	doxepin
Accupril	quinapril	Adaquin	quinine
Accuprin	quinapril	Adasuve	loxapine
Accupro	quinapril	Adcetris	brentuximab vedotin
Accuretic	hydrochlorothiazide, quinapril	Adcirca	tadalafil
Accutane	isotretinoin	Adderall	dextroamphetamine
Acenor-M	fosinopril	Addyi	flibanserin
Acenorm	captopril	Adempas	riociguat
Aceon	perindopril	Adenic	adenosine
Acepril	captopril	Adeno-Jec	adenosine
Acerbon	lisinopril	Adenocard	adenosine
Acertil	perindopril	Adenocur	adenosine
Acetazolam	acetazolamide	Adenoject	adenosine
acetylsalicylic acid	aspirin	Adenoscan	adenosine
Acfol	folic acid	Adiblastine	doxorubicin
aciclovir	acyclovir	Adipex-P	phentermine
Acid A Vit	tretinoin	Adipine	nifedipine
Acidulated phosphate fluoride	fluorides	Adlyxin	lixisenatide
Acifur	acyclovir	Adocor	captopril
Acimox	amoxicillin	Adofen	fluoxetine
Aciphex	rabeprazole	Adoxa	doxycycline
Aclasta	zoledronate	Adrecar	adenosine
Aclinda	clindamycin	Adrenaclick	epinephrine

Adrenalin	epinephrine	Alfotax	cefotaxime
adrenaline	epinephrine	Algocetil	sulindac
Adriablastine	doxorubicin	Alimta	pemetrexed
Adriacin	doxorubicin	Alinia	nitazoxanide
Adriamycin	doxorubicin	Aliqopa	copanlisib
Adriblatina	doxorubicin	Alka-Seltzer	aspirin
Adsorbocarbine	pilocarpine	Alkeran	melphalan
Adumbran	oxazepam	*all-trans-retinoic acid*	tretinoin
Adursall	ursodiol	Allegra-D	pseudoephedrine
Advantan	methylprednisolone	Allegra	fexofenadine
Advicor	lovastatin, niacin	Allegron	nortriptyline
Advil	ibuprofen	Aller-Chlor	chlorpheniramine
Aerolate	aminophylline	Allerdryl	diphenhydramine
Aerovent	aldesleukin	Allerglobuline	immune globulin IV
Afaxin	vitamin A	Allermax	diphenhydramine
Afinitor	everolimus	Allermin	diphenhydramine
Aflodac	sulindac	Alli	orlistat
Aflorix	miconazole	Allo 300	allopurinol
Afluria	influenza vaccine	Allo-Puren	allopurinol
Afstyla	antihemophilic factor	Alloprin	allopurinol
Aggrenox	aspirin, dipyridamole	Allvoran	diclofenac
Agilect	rasagiline	Almarytm	flecainide
Agisolvan	acetylcysteine	Almatol	spironolactone
Agrippal	influenza vaccine	Almodan	amoxicillin
AH3 N	hydroxyzine	Almogran	almotriptan
Airol	tretinoin	Aloid	miconazole
AK-Chlor	chloramphenicol	Alopexy	minoxidil
Ak-Zol	acetazolamide	Alora	estradiol
Akarpine	pilocarpine	Aloxi	palonosetron
Akatinol	memantine	*alpha tocopherol*	vitamin E
Aknemin	minocycline	Alphagan P	brimonidine
Aknemycin Plus	tretinoin	Alphapress	hydralazine
AKTob Ophthalmic	tobramycin	Alprim	trimethoprim
Akynzeo	netupitant & palonosetron	Alprox	alprazolam
AL-R	chlorpheniramine	Alquingel	tretinoin
Alapril	lisinopril	Alrheumat	ketoprofen
Alavert	loratadine	Alrheumun	ketoprofen
Albenza	albendazole	Alsuma	sumatriptan
Albiotic	lincomycin	Altace	ramipril
Alcloxidine	chlorhexidine	Alten	tretinoin
Alcomicinx	gentamicin	Alti-Diltiazem	diltiazem
Aldactazide	hydrochlorothiazide, spironolactone	Alti-Doxepin	doxepin
Aldactone	spironolactone	Alti-Ipratropium	ipratropium
Aldara	imiquimod	Alti-Minocycline	minocycline
Aldoclor	methyldopa	Alti-MPA	medroxyprogesterone
Aldocumar	warfarin	Alti-Trazodone	trazodone
Aldomet	methyldopa	Altocor	lovastatin
Aldopur	spironolactone	Altoprev	lovastatin
Aldoril	hydrochlorothiazide, methyldopa	Alunbrig	brigatinib
Alecensa	alectinib	Aluvira	lopinavir
Alendronic acid	alendronate	Alveolex	acetylcysteine
Alepsal	phenobarbital	Amaryl	glimepiride
Alercet	cetirizine	Ambi	hydroquinone
Alerid	cetirizine	Ambien	zolpidem
Alertec	modafinil	AmBisome	amphotericin B
Alesse	oral contraceptives	Amdepin	amlodipine
Aleve	naproxen	Ameluz	aminolevulinic acid
Alexan	cytarabine	*amethopterin*	methotrexate
Alfadil	doxazosin	Ametycine	mitomycin
Alfatil	cefaclor	Amfipen	ampicillin
Alferon N	interferon alfa	Amias	candesartan

Amicacina	amikacin	Antabus	disulfiram
Amicasil	amikacin	Antabuse	disulfiram
Amikacin sulfate	amikacin	Antagonil	nicardipine
Amikal	amiloride	Antaxone	naltrexone
Amikan	amikacin	*antegren*	natalizumab
Amineurin	amitriptyline	Anten	doxepin
Aminophyllin	aminophylline	Antepsin	sucralfate
Amipress	labetalol	Antiflog	piroxicam
Amisalen	procainamide	Antilak	etodolac
Amitiza	lubiprostone	Antilirium	physostigmine
Amjevita	adalimumab	Antipressan	atenolol
Amlodin	amlodipine	Antra	omeprazole
Amlogard	amlodipine	Antrex	leucovorin
Amlopin	amlodipine	Apacef	cefotetan
Amlor	amlodipine	*APAP*	acetaminophen
Amnesteem	isotretinoin	Apatef	cefotetan
Amodex	amoxicillin	Apdormin	hydralazine
Amodopa	methyldopa	Apekumarol	dicumarol
Amoxan	amoxapine	Aphtiria	lindane
Amoxapine	amoxapine	Apidra	insulin glulisine
Amoxil	amoxicillin	APO-Alpraz	alprazolam
amoxycillin	amoxicillin	Apo-Amoxi	amoxicillin
Amphocin	amphotericin B	Apo-Atenol	atenolol
Amphotec	amphotericin B	Apo-Bisoprolol	bisoprolol
Ampicin	ampicillin	Apo-Bromocriptine	bromocriptine
Amprace	enalapril	Apo-Buspirone	buspirone
Ampyra	dalfampridine	APO-Capto	captopril
Amrix	cyclobenzaprine	Apo-Carbamazepine	carbamazepine
Amterene	triamterene	Apo-Cefaclor	cefaclor
Amuno	indomethacin	Apo-Cephalex	cephalexin
Amycil	mebendazole	Apo-Cimetidine	cimetidine
Anacin-3	acetaminophen	Apo-Clomipramine	clomipramine
Anacin	aspirin	Apo-Diclo	diclofenac
Anacobin	cyanocobalamin	Apo-Doxy	doxycycline
Anafranil Retard	clomipramine	Apo-Enalapril	enalapril
Anafranil	clomipramine	Apo-Ethambutol	ethambutol
Anamantle HC	lidocaine	Apo-Famotidine	famotidine
Anamorph	morphine	Apo-Fenofibrate	fenofibrate
Anaprox	naproxen	Apo-Fluoxetine	fluoxetine
Anaspaz	hyoscyamine	Apo-Fluphenazine	fluphenazine
Anatensol	fluphenazine	Apo-Flurbiprofen	flurbiprofen
Anaxanil	hydroxyzine	Apo-Fluvoxamine	fluvoxamine
Anco	ibuprofen	Apo-Folic	folic acid
Andro LA	testosterone	Apo-Furosemide	furosemide
Androcur	cyproterone	Apo-Gain	minoxidil
Androderm	testosterone	Apo-Hydro	hydrochlorothiazide
AndroGel	testosterone	Apo-Imipramine	imipramine
Android	methyltestosterone	Apo-Indomethacin	indomethacin
Andronaq	testosterone	Apo-ISDN	isosorbide dinitrate
Androral	methyltestosterone	Apo-Lorazepam	lorazepam
Andrumin	dimenhydrinate	Apo-Lovastatin	lovastatin
Anectine	succinylcholine	Apo-Metformin	metformin
Aneol	ketoprofen	Apo-Metronidazole	metronidazole
Anergan	promethazine	Apo-Minocycline	minocycline
Anestacon	lidocaine	Apo-Nadolol	nadolol
Angilol	propranolol	Apo-Nicotinamide	niacin
Angiomax	bivalirudin	Apo-Nifed	nifedipine
Angioverin	papaverine	Apo-Nortriptyline	nortriptyline
Anitrim	co-trimoxazole	Apo-Oxazepam	oxazepam
Ansaid	flurbiprofen	Apo-Pen	penicillin V
Ansail	buspirone	Apo-Pentoxifylline	pentoxifylline

Apo-Perphenazine	perphenazine	Arythmol	propafenone
Apo-Piroxicam	piroxicam	Arzerra	ofatumumab
Apo-Propranolol	propranolol	ASA	aspirin
Apo-Ranitidine	ranitidine	Asacol	mesalamine
Apo-Selegiline	selegiline	Asacolitin	mesalamine
Apo-Sulfatrim	co-trimoxazole	Asclera	polidocanol
APO-Sulin	sulindac	Ascriptin	aspirin
Apo-Tamox	tamoxifen	Asendis	amoxapine
Apo-Temazepam	temazepam	Aside	etoposide
Apo-Tetra	tetracycline	Asig	quinapril
Apo-Trimip	trimipramine	Asmaven	albuterol
APO-Verap	verapamil	Aspergum	aspirin
Apocard	flecainide	Aspro	aspirin
Aponal	doxepin	ASS	aspirin
Apranax	naproxen	Assival	diazepam
Apresazide	hydralazine	AsthmaHaler	epinephrine
Apresolin	hydralazine	Astramorph	morphine
Apresoline	hydralazine	Atabrine	quinacrine
Aprical	nifedipine	Atacand HCT	hydrochlorothiazide
Aprovel	irbesartan	Atacand	candesartan
Apsifen	ibuprofen	Ataline	terbutaline
Apsolol	propranolol	Atarax	hydroxyzine
Aptiom	eslicarbazepine	AteHexal	atenolol
Aptivus	tipranavir	Atelvia	risedronate
Aquachloral	chloral hydrate	Atem	aldesleukin
Aquamid	hyaluronic acid	Atendol	atenolol
Aquamycetin	chloramphenicol	Atisuril	allopurinol, salsalate
Aquarius	ketoconazole	Ativan	lorazepam
Aquasol A	vitamin A	Atosil	promethazine
Aquasol E	vitamin E	ATP	adenosine
ara-C	cytarabine	ATRA	tretinoin
Arabitin	cytarabine	Atragen	tretinoin
Arace	cytarabine	Atrenta	artesunate
Aracytine	cytarabine	Atreol	carbamazepine
Aragest 5	medroxyprogesterone	Atridox	doxycycline
Aralen	chloroquine	Atripla	efavirenz, emtricitabine, tenofovir disoproxil
Aranesp	darbepoetin alfa	Atronase	aldesleukin
Aratac	amiodarone	Atropine Martinet	atropine sulfate
Arcapta Neohaler	indacaterol	Atropt	atropine sulfate
Aredia	pamidronate	Atrovent	ipratropium
Arestin	minocycline	Atruline	sertraline
Argesic-SA	salsalate	Aubagio	teriflunomide
Aricept Evess	donepezil	Audazol	omeprazole
Aricept	donepezil	Augmentin	amoxicillin
Arimidex	anastrozole	Austedo	deutetrabenazine
Aristada	aripiprazole	Autologen	collagen (bovine)
Arixtra	fondaparinux	Auvi-Q	epinephrine
Aromasin	exemestane	Avage	tazarotene
Arovit	vitamin A	Avalide	hydrochlorothiazide, irbesartan
Arpamyl LP	verapamil	Avandamet	metformin, rosiglitazone
Arsacol	ursodiol	Avandaryl	glimepiride, rosiglitazone
Artal	pentoxifylline	Avandia	rosiglitazone
Artamin	penicillamine	Avapro	irbesartan
Artecoll	collagen (bovine)	Avastin	bevacizumab
Artha-G	salsalate	Avaxim	hepatitis A vaccine
Arthaxan	nabumetone	Avelox	moxifloxacin
Arthro-Aid	glucosamine	Aventyl	nortriptyline
Arthrocine	sulindac	Aviane	oral contraceptives
Arthrotec	diclofenac, misoprostol	Avinza	morphine
Artifar	carisoprodol	Avipur	vitamin A
ARTZ	hyaluronic acid	Avirax	acyclovir

Avita	tretinoin	Basaglar	insulin glargine
Avitcid	tretinoin	Basoquin	amodiaquine
Avitene	collagen (bovine)	Batrizol	co-trimoxazole
Avitin	vitamin A	Bavencio	avelumab
Avitoin	tretinoin	Baxan	cefadroxil
Avloclor	chloroquine	Baxdela	delafloxacin
Avlosulfon	dapsone	Baxo	piroxicam
Avodart	dutasteride	Baygam	immune globulin IV
Avonex	interferon beta	Baymycard	nisoldipine
Avycaz	ceftazidime & avibactam	BB	clindamycin
Axerol	vitamin A	Beatryl	fentanyl
Axert	almotriptan	Becenun	carmustine
Axoban	ranitidine	Beconase AQ	beclomethasone
Aygestin	progestins	Begrivac	influenza vaccine
Azamedac	azathioprine	Behapront	phentermine
Azamune	azathioprine	Beleodaq	belinostat
Azantac	ranitidine	Belladenal	atropine sulfate
Azasan	azathioprine	Bellafill	collagen (bovine)
AzaSite	azithromycin	Bellergal-S	atropine sulfate
Azatrilem	azathioprine	Beloc-Zoc	metoprolol
Azenil	azithromycin	Belsomra	suvorexant
azidothymidine	zidovudine	Belviq	lorcaserin
Azilect	rasagiline	Benadryl	diphenhydramine, pseudoephedrine
Azitrocin	azithromycin	Benahist	diphenhydramine
Azitromax	azithromycin	Benaxima	cefotaxime
Azol	danazol	Benaxona	ceftriaxone
Azopt	brinzolamide	Bencid	probenecid
AZT	zidovudine	Benecid	probenecid
Azucimet	cimetidine	Benhex Cream	lindane
Azulfidine	sulfasalazine	Benicar	olmesartan
Azupamil	verapamil	Benuryl	probenecid
Azupentat	pentoxifylline	Benylin	dextromethorphan, diphenhydramine
Azutranquil	oxazepam	Benzaclin	clindamycin
Azzalure	botulinum toxin (A & B)	Benzamin	cyclobenzaprine
		Benzylpenicillin	penicillin G
		Beriglobulin	immune globulin IV

B

Bacille Calmette-Guerin	BCG vaccine	Berkatens	verapamil
Baclofen	baclofen	Berlthyrox	levothyroxine
Baclon	baclofen	Berubigen	cyanocobalamin
Baclosal	baclofen	Bespar	buspirone
Bacomine	hydrocodone	Besponsa	inotuzumab ozogamicin
Bactelan	co-trimoxazole	Beta-Adalat	atenolol
Bactin	trimethoprim	Beta-Cardone	sotalol
Bactocill	oxacillin	Betades	sotalol
Bactocin	ofloxacin	Betaferon	interferon beta
Bactoscrub	chlorhexidine	Betaloc	metoprolol
BactoShield	chlorhexidine	Betanis	mirabegron
Bactrim	co-trimoxazole, sulfamethoxazole, trimethoprim	Betapace	sotalol
Baklofen	baclofen	Betasept	chlorhexidine
BAL5788	ceftobiprole	Betaseron	interferon beta
Balcoran	vancomycin	Betazok	metoprolol
Balminil	dextromethorphan, pseudoephedrine	Betolvex	cyanocobalamin
Ban-Tuss HC	hydrocodone	Betoptic [Ophthalmic]	betaxolol
Banophen	diphenhydramine	Betoptic S	betaxolol
Bantenol	mebendazole	Betoptima	betaxolol
Baraclude	entecavir	Bevyxxa	betrixaban
Barazan	norfloxacin	Bex	aspirin
Barbilixir	phenobarbital	Bexsero	meningococcal group B vaccine
Barbita	phenobarbital	*BG-12*	dimethyl fumarate
Barbital	phenobarbital	Bi-Profenid	ketoprofen
Barclyd	clonidine	Biaxin HP	clarithromycin

Biaxin	clarithromycin	Bronkaid	epinephrine
Bicide	lindane	Bronkodyl	aminophylline
Biclin	amikacin	Brothine	terbutaline
BiCNU	carmustine	Brovana	arformoterol
Bidocef	cefadroxil	Brufen	ibuprofen
Biklin	amikacin	Bucaril	terbutaline
Biliepar	ursodiol	Bufigen	nalbuphine
Bilim	tamoxifen	Busetal	disulfiram
Biltricide	praziquantel	Busirone	buspirone
Bimaran	trazodone	BuSpar	buspirone
Binocrit	epoetin alfa	Bustab	buspirone
Binosto	alendronate	Butaline	terbutaline
Binotal	ampicillin	Butibel	atropine sulfate
Bio E	vitamin E	Bydureon	exenatide
Bio-Well	lindane	Byetta	exenatide
Biocet	cephalexin	Bystolic	nebivolol
Biocoryl	procainamide	Byvalson	nebivolol, valsartan
Biofanal	nystatin		
Biosint	cefotaxime	**C**	
BioThrax	anthrax vaccine	Caduet	amlodipine, atorvastatin
Biozolene	fluconazole	Calamine	zinc
Biron	buspirone	Calan	verapamil
Bismatrol	bismuth	Calcicard	diltiazem
Bismuth Iodoform Paraffin Paste (BIPP)	bismuth	*calcidiol*	calcifediol
Bismuth subcitrate	bismuth	Calcidrine	codeine
Bismuth subgallate	bismuth	Calcilat	nifedipine
Bismuth sucralfate	bismuth	Calcilean	heparin
Bleminol	allopurinol	Calcimar	calcitonin
Blenoxane	bleomycin	Calciparin	heparin
bleo	bleomycin	*calcipotriene*	calcipotriol
Bleocin	bleomycin	Calm-X	dimenhydrinate
Bleomycine	bleomycin	Caltine	calcitonin
Bleomycinum	bleomycin	Calypsol	ketamine
Blephamide	prednisolone	Cambia	diclofenac
Blincyto	blinatumomab	Camochin	amodiaquine
BLM	bleomycin	Camoquin	amodiaquine
Blocan	cimetidine	Camoquinal	amodiaquine
Bobsule	hydroxyzine	Campath	alemtuzumab
Bocouture	botulinum toxin (A & B)	Camptosar	irinotecan
Bolutol	gemfibrozil	Canasa	mesalamine
Bondronat	ibandronate	Cancidas	caspofungin
Boniva	ibandronate	Candio-Hermal	nystatin
Bonnox	promethazine	*cannabis*	marihuana
Bonzol	danazol	Caplenal	allopurinol
Botox	botulinum toxin (A & B)	Capoten	captopril
Brek	loperamide	Capozide	captopril, hydrochlorothiazide
Brethine	terbutaline	Caprelsa	vandetanib
Brevibloc	esmolol	Caprilon	tranexamic acid
Brevicon	oral contraceptives	Caprin	aspirin, heparin
Bricanyl	terbutaline	Captolane	captopril
Bridion	sugammadex	Captoril	captopril
Brilinta	ticagrelor	Carac	fluorouracil
Brisdelle	paroxetine mesylate	Carace	lisinopril
Bristopen	oxacillin	Carafate	sucralfate
Britiazem	diltiazem	Carbatrol	carbamazepine
Briviact	brivaracetam	Carbex	selegiline
Brocadopa	levodopa	*carbidopa*	levodopa
Bromed	bromocriptine	Carbolith	lithium
Bromfed	pseudoephedrine	Carbometyx	cabozantinib
Broncho-Spray	albuterol	Carboplat	carboplatin
Bronitin	epinephrine	Carbosap	anthrax vaccine

Carbosin	carboplatin	Ceporex	cephalexin
Carcinil	leuprolide	Ceporexine	cephalexin
Cardem	celiprolol	Ceptaz	ceftazidime
Cardene	nicardipine	Cerdelga	eliglustat
Cardicor	bisoprolol	Cerepax	temazepam
Cardigox	digoxin	Certican	everolimus
Cardine	quinidine	Cerubidine	daunorubicin
Cardiosteril	dopamine	Cervarix	human papillomavirus vaccine (bivalent)
Cardizem	diltiazem	Cervidel	dinoprostone
Cardol	sotalol	Cerviprime	dinoprostone
Cardoxan	doxazosin	Cerviprost	dinoprostone
Cardoxin	dipyridamole	Cesamet	nabilone
Cardular	doxazosin	Cetrine	cetirizine
Cardura	doxazosin	Cetrotide	cetrorelix
Carisoma	carisoprodol	Cezin	cetirizine
Carmubris	carmustine	Champix	varenicline
Cartia-XT	diltiazem	Chantix	varenicline
Casodex	bicalutamide	Chemet	succimer
Cassadan	alprazolam	Cheracol-D	dextromethorphan
Cataflam	diclofenac	Cheracol	codeine
Catapres	clonidine	Chibro-Atropine	atropine sulfate
Catapresan	clonidine	Chibroxin	norfloxacin
Caved-S	bismuth	Chibroxine	norfloxacin
Caverject	alprostadil	Chibroxol	norfloxacin
CDDP	cisplatin	Chinine	quinine
Cebenicol	chloramphenicol	Chitosamine	glucosamine
Cebutid	flurbiprofen	Chlo-Amine	chlorpheniramine
CEC 500	cefaclor	Chlor-Pro	chlorpheniramine
Ceclor	cefaclor	Chlor-Trimeton	chlorpheniramine
Cedocard	isosorbide dinitrate	Chlor-Tripolon	chlorpheniramine
Cedrox	cefadroxil	Chloractil	chlorpromazine
Cefabiocin	cefaclor	Chloraldurat	chloral hydrate
cefalexin	cephalexin	Chlorate	chlorpheniramine
Cefamox	cefadroxil	Chlorazin	chlorpromazine
Cefaxim	cefotaxime	Chlorhexamed	chlorhexidine
Cefaxona	ceftriaxone	Chloroptic	chloramphenicol
Cefaxone	ceftriaxone	chlorphenamine	chlorpheniramine
Ceforal	cephalexin	Chlorpromanyl	chlorpromazine
Cefotan	cefotetan	Chlorquin	chloroquine
Cefotax	cefotaxime	Chol-Less	cholestyramine
Cefspan	cefixime	Cholacid	ursodiol
Ceftazim	ceftazidime	Cholbam	cholic acid
Ceftenon	cefotetan	Choledyl	aminophylline
Ceftin	cefuroxime	Cholestagel	colesevelam
Cefuril	cefuroxime	Cholit-Ursan	ursodiol
Celebrex	celecoxib	Cholofalk	ursodiol
Celectol	celiprolol	Chronovera	verapamil
Celexa	citalopram	Cialis	tadalafil
Celipres	celiprolol	Cibacalcine	calcitonin
Celipro	celiprolol	Cibace	benazepril
CellCept	mycophenolate	Cibacen	benazepril
Cellmusin	estramustine	Cibacene	benazepril
Celol	celiprolol	Ciclosporin	cyclosporine
Celsentri	maraviroc	Cidomycin	gentamicin
Celupan	naltrexone	Ciflox	ciprofloxacin
Celvapan	pandemic influenza vaccine (H1N1)	Cillimicina	lincomycin
Cemidon	isoniazid	Cillimycin	lincomycin
Centedrin	methylphenidate	Ciloxan Ophthalmic	ciprofloxacin
Cepan	cefotetan	Cimedine	cimetidine
Cepazine	cefuroxime	Cimehexal	cimetidine
Cephoral	cefixime	Cimogal	ciprofloxacin

Cimzia	certolizumab	Colazal	balsalazide
Cin-Quin	quinidine	Colazide	balsalazide
Cinqair	reslizumab	ColBenemid	colchicine
Ciplox	ciprofloxacin	Colchiquim	colchicine
Cipramil	citalopram	Colcrys	colchicine
Cipro	ciprofloxacin	Cold-Eeze	zinc
Ciprobay Uro	ciprofloxacin	Coledos	ursodiol
Cipromycin	ciprofloxacin	Colestrol	cholestyramine
Ciproxin	ciprofloxacin	Colgout	colchicine
Cisplatyl	cisplatin	Colo-Fresh	bismuth
Cisticid	praziquantel	Colo-Pleon	sulfasalazine
Citanest	prilocaine	Combivent	albuterol, ipratropium
Citax	immune globulin IV	Combivir	lamivudine, zidovudine
Citosulfan	busulfan	Cometriq	cabozantinib
Citrec	leucovorin	Compazine	prochlorperazine
citrovorum factor	leucovorin	Complera	emtricitabine, tenofovir disoproxil
Ciuk	cimetidine	Compoz	diphenhydramine
Civeran	loratadine	Comtan	entacapone
Clacine	clarithromycin	Comtess	entacapone
Claforan	cefotaxime	Comvax	Hemophilus B vaccine, hepatitis B vaccine,
Clamoxyl	amoxicillin		influenza vaccine
Claragine	aspirin	Concerta	methylphenidate
Claratyne	loratadine	Concor	bisoprolol
Claravis	isotretinoin	Consolan	nabumetone
Clarinex	desloratadine	Consupren	cyclosporine
Clarith	clarithromycin	Contalgin	morphine
Claritin-D	loratadine	Contergan	thalidomide
Claritin	loratadine	Contigen	collagen (bovine)
Claritine	loratadine	Contramal	tramadol
Clarus	isotretinoin	Contrave	naltrexone
Classen	mercaptopurine	Convon	terbutaline
Clasynar	calcitonin	Copaxone	glatiramer
Claversal	mesalamine	Copegus	ribavirin
Cleocin-T	clindamycin	copolymer-1	glatiramer
Cleocin	clindamycin	Coracten	nifedipine
Cleridium	dipyridamole	Coradur	isosorbide dinitrate
Clexane	enoxaparin	Corax	chlordiazepoxide
Climara	estradiol	Corbionax	amiodarone
Clindacin	clindamycin	Cordarex	amiodarone
Clindagel	clindamycin	Cordarone X	amiodarone
Clindets	clindamycin	Cordarone	amiodarone
Clinofem	medroxyprogesterone	Cordes VAS	tretinoin
Clinoril	sulindac	Cordiax	celiprolol
Cloben	cyclobenzaprine	Cordilox	verapamil
Clofen	baclofen	Coreg	carvedilol
Clofranil	clomipramine	Corflene	flecainide
Clonex	clonazepam	Corgard	nadolol
Clont	metronidazole	Coric	lisinopril
Clopress	clomipramine	Coricidin D	aspirin
Closerin	cycloserine	Corifam	rifampin
Closerina	cycloserine	Corlanor	ivabradine
Closin	promethazine	Corogal	nifedipine
Clothia	hydrochlorothiazide	Coronarine	dipyridamole
Clozaril	clozapine	Corophyllin	aminophylline
club drug	MDMA	Corotrend	nifedipine
Coartem	artemether/lumefantrine	Coroxin	dipyridamole
Cobex	cyanocobalamin	Corsodyl	chlorhexidine
Cobutolin	albuterol	Cortastat	dexamethasone
Codamine	hydrocodone	Cortone	cortisone
Codicept	codeine	Cortosporin	neomycin
Codiforton	codeine	Corvert	ibutilide

Corzide	nadolol	D-Zol	danazol
Cosentyx	secukinumab	*D4T*	stavudine
Cosmegen Lyovac	dactinomycin	Dacatic	dacarbazine
Cosmegen	dactinomycin	Dacogen	decitabine
Cosopt	dorzolamide	Dagan	nicardipine
Cotellic	cobimetinib	Daipres	clonidine
Cotempla	methylphenidate	Daklinza	daclatasvir
Cotrim	co-trimoxazole	Daktarin	miconazole
Coumadin	warfarin	Dalacin C	clindamycin
Coumadine	warfarin	Dalacin	clindamycin
Covera-HS	verapamil	Dalacine	clindamycin
Coversum	perindopril	Daliresp	roflumilast
Coversyl	perindopril	Dalisol	folic acid
Cozaar	losartan	Danocrine	danazol
CPM	cyclophosphamide	Danol	danazol
Cranoc	fluvastatin	Dantamacrin	dantrolene
Crasnitin	asparaginase	Dantrium	dantrolene
Cresemba	isavuconazonium sulfate	Dantrolen	dantrolene
Crestor	rosuvastatin	Daonil	glyburide
Crixivan	indinavir	Dapa-tabs	indapamide
Cryocriptina	bromocriptine	Dapatum D25	fluphenazine
Cryodoxin	sulfadoxine	Dapotum D	fluphenazine
Cryptaz	nitazoxanide	Dapson-Fatol	dapsone
Crystamine	cyanocobalamin	Dapson	dapsone
Crystapen	penicillin G	Daraprim	pyrimethamine
Crysti-12	cyanocobalamin	Darvocet-N	acetaminophen
CsA	cyclosporine	Darvon Compound	aspirin
CTX	cyclophosphamide	Darzalex	daratumumab
Cubicin	daptomycin	*daunomycin*	daunorubicin
Curantyl N	dipyridamole	DaunoXome	daunorubicin
Curretab	progestins	Davedax	reboxetine
Cuvitru	immune globulin sc	Davesol	lindane
Cuvposa	glycopyrrolate	Davitamon E	vitamin E
CyA	cyclosporine	Daxas	roflumilast
Cyanoject	cyanocobalamin	Daypro	oxaprozin
Cyben	cyclobenzaprine	Daytrana	methylphenidate
Cycloblastin	cyclophosphamide	Dazamide	acetazolamide
Cyclomen	danazol	DDAVP	desmopressin
Cyclomycin	cycloserine	*ddC*	zalcitabine
Cyclorine	cycloserine	De-Nol	bismuth
Cyclostin	cyclophosphamide	Deca-Durabolin	nandrolone
Cycosin	cycloserine	Decadron	dexamethasone
Cyklokapron	tranexamic acid	Decentan	perphenazine
Cymbalta	duloxetine	Deconsal	pseudoephedrine
Cynomel	liothyronine	Decrelip	gemfibrozil
Cyomin	cyanocobalamin	Dedralen	doxazosin
Cyramza	ramucirumab	Defanyl	amoxapine
Cystrin	oxybutynin	Defiltran	acetazolamide
CYT	cyclophosphamide	Defirin	desmopressin
Cytamen	cyanocobalamin	Defitelio	defibrotide
Cytarbel	cytarabine	Deflam	oxaprozin
Cytomel	liothyronine	Dehydrobenzperidol	droperidol
Cytosar-U	cytarabine	Delatest	testosterone
Cytosar	cytarabine	Delatestryl	testosterone
Cytospaz	hyoscyamine	Delice	lindane
Cytotec	misoprostol	Delsym	dextromethorphan
Cytoxan	cyclophosphamide	Delta-Cortef	prednisolone
		Delta-Lutin	progestins
		Deltasone	prednisone

D

D-Amp	ampicillin	Deltazen	diltiazem
D-Penamine	penicillamine	Delursan	ursodiol

Demadex	torsemide	Diaformin	metformin
Demerol	meperidine	Dialar	diazepam
Demolox	amoxapine	Diamox	acetazolamide
Demulen	oral contraceptives	Diapax	diazepam
Denan	simvastatin	Diar-Aid	loperamide
Densul	methyldopa	Diarr-Eze	loperamide
Dentipatch	lidocaine	Diarrol	triamterene
Denzapine	clozapine	Diarstop-L	loperamide
Depacon	valproic acid	Diastat	diazepam
Depade	naltrexone	Diatracin	vancomycin
Depakene	valproic acid	Diazemuls	diazepam
Depakote	valproic acid	Diazid	isoniazid
Depen	penicillamine	Dibloc	carvedilol
Depo-Provera	medroxyprogesterone	Diblocin	doxazosin
DepoCyt	cytarabine	Dibrondrin	diphenhydramine
Deprax	trazodone	DIC	dacarbazine
deprenyl	selegiline	Dichlotride	hydrochlorothiazide
Derm A	tretinoin	Dicolmax	diclofenac
DermaDeep	hyaluronic acid	Dicumarol	dicumarol
DermaFlex	lidocaine	Dicumol	dicumarol
Dermairol	tretinoin	dideoxycytidine	zalcitabine
DermaLive	hyaluronic acid	Didronate	etidronate
Dermalogen	collagen (bovine)	Didronel	etidronate
Dermojuventus	tretinoin	Differin	adapalene
Desconex	loxapine	Diflucan	fluconazole
Descovy	emtricitabine, tenofovir alafenamide	Diformin	metformin
Deseril	methysergide	Difosfen	etidronate
Desernil	methysergide	Digacin	digoxin
Deserril	methysergide	Digoxine	digoxin
Deseryl	methysergide	Dilacor XR	diltiazem
Desferal	deferoxamine	Dilanorm	celiprolol
Desferin	deferoxamine	Dilantin	phenytoin
Desirel	trazodone	Dilatrate-SR	isosorbide dinitrate
Desmospray	desmopressin	Dilatrend	carvedilol
Desocol	ursodiol	Dilaudid-HP	hydromorphone
Desogen	oral contraceptives	Dilaudid	hydromorphone
Desoxil	ursodiol	Dilocaine	lidocaine
Desoxyn	methamphetamine	Dilrene	diltiazem
Destolit	ursodiol	Diltahexal	diltiazem
Desyrel	trazodone	Diltia-XT	diltiazem
Detensol	propranolol	Dimetabs	dimenhydrinate
Deticene	dacarbazine	dimethyl (E) butenedioate	dimethyl fumarate
Detimedac	dacarbazine	Diminex	phentermine
Detrol	tolterodine	Dimitone	carvedilol
Detulin	vitamin E	Dimodan	disopyramide
Deurcil	ursodiol	Dinol	etidronate
Devrom	bismuth	Diocarpine	pilocarpine
Dexacine	neomycin	Diochloram	chloramphenicol
Dexambutol	ethambutol	Diogent	gentamicin
Dexamphetamine	dextroamphetamine	Dionephrine	phenylephrine
Dexamphetamini	dextroamphetamine	Diotame	bismuth
Dexedrine	dextroamphetamine	Diovan HCT	hydrochlorothiazide, valsartan
Dexilant	dexlansoprazole	Diovan	valsartan
Dexo	ursodiol	Diphenylan	phenytoin
Dexone	dexamethasone	diphenylhydantoin	phenytoin
Dextrostat	dextroamphetamine	Diphos	etidronate
DHC-Continus	dihydrocodeine	Dipridacot	dipyridamole
Di-Hydran	phenytoin	Diprivan	propofol
Diabeta	glyburide	Diram	spironolactone
Diabex	metformin	Dirythmin SA	disopyramide
diacetylmorphine	heroin	Disalgesic	salsalate

Discoid	furosemide	DTIC-Dome	dacarbazine
Disonorm	disopyramide	DTIC	dacarbazine
Disprin	aspirin	Duboisine	hyoscyamine
Distaclor	cefaclor	Ducene	diazepam
Distamine	penicillamine	Duexis	famotidine
Distaval	thalidomide	Dulera	formoterol
Distocide	praziquantel	Dumirox	fluvoxamine
Ditropan	oxybutynin	Dumyrox	fluvoxamine
Diu-Melsin	hydrochlorothiazide	Dunate	artesunate
Diuchlor H	hydrochlorothiazide	Duoneb	albuterol, ipratropium
Diuramid	acetazolamide	Duopa	levodopa
Diuteren	triamterene	Dupixent	dupilumab
divalproex	valproic acid	Dura-Vent	phenylephrine
Divigel	estradiol	Duracef	cefadroxil
Dixarit	clonidine	Duraclon	clonidine
Dizac	diazepam	Duragesic	fentanyl
DMSA	succimer	Duralith	lithium
DNR	daunorubicin	Duralutin	progestins
Dobetin	cyanocobalamin	Durametacin	indomethacin
Doblexan	piroxicam	Duramorph	morphine
Dolac	ketorolac	Duraperidol	haloperidol
Dolantin	meperidine	Duraprox	oxaprozin
Dolce	vitamin A	Durater	famotidine
Dolestan	diphenhydramine	Duratest	testosterone
Dolestine	meperidine	Duratuss	hydrocodone
Dolophine	methadone	Durazepam	oxazepam
Dolosal	meperidine	Durazolam	lorazepam
Dom-Baclofen	baclofen	Durbis	disopyramide
Dom-Fluoxetine	fluoxetine	Duricef	cefadroxil
Domical	amitriptyline	Durlaza	aspirin
Doneurin	doxepin	Duzallo	allopurinol, lesinurad
Donnagel	atropine sulfate	Dyazide	hydrochlorothiazide, triamterene
Donnamar	hyoscyamine	Dyloject	diclofenac
Donnatal	atropine sulfate	Dymenalgit	naproxen
Donnazyme	atropine sulfate	Dyna-Hex	chlorhexidine
Dopaflex	levodopa	Dynacil	fosinopril
Dopamet	methyldopa	Dynacin	minocycline
Dopamin AWD	dopamine	Dynacirc SRO	isradipine
Dopamin	dopamine	DynaCirc	isradipine
Doparl	levodopa	Dynatra	dopamine
Dopastat	dopamine	Dyrenium	triamterene
Dormicum	midazolam	Dysman	mefenamic acid
Doryx	doxycycline	Dyspamet	cimetidine
Dostinex	cabergoline	Dysport	botulinum toxin (A & B)
Dovonex	calcipotriol	Dytac	triamterene
Doxil	doxorubicin		
Doximed	doxycycline	**E**	
Doxy-100	doxycycline	E Perle	vitamin E
Doxycin	doxycycline	E-Mycin	erythromycin
Doxytec	doxycycline	E-Pam	diazepam
Dozic	haloperidol	E-Vitamin Succinate	vitamin E
DPH	phenytoin	E102	tartrazine
Dramamine	dimenhydrinate	*E*	MDMA
Dridase	oxybutynin	Ebixa	memantine
Drogenil	flutamide	Ebufac	ibuprofen
Droleptan	droperidol	Ecalta	anidulafungin
Droperidol	droperidol	Ecomucyl	acetylcysteine
Droxia	hydroxyurea	Economycin	tetracycline
Droxine	levothyroxine	Ecotrin	aspirin
Dryptal	furosemide	Ecridoxan	etodolac
Dryvax	smallpox vaccine	*ecstasy*	MDMA

Ectaprim	co-trimoxazole	Enapren	enalapril
Ectasule	ephedrine	Enarmon	methyltestosterone
ED-SPAZ	hyoscyamine	Enbrel	etanercept
Edenol	furosemide	Encore	acetylcysteine
Edex	alprostadil	Endeavor	zotarolimus
Edisylate	prochlorperazine	Endep	amitriptyline
Edolan	etodolac	Endobulin	immune globulin IV
Edronax	reboxetine	Endocodone	oxycodone
EES	erythromycin	Endoxan	cyclophosphamide
Efedron	ephedrine	Endoxana	cyclophosphamide
Eferox	levothyroxine	Ener-B	cyanocobalamin
Effexor XL	venlafaxine	Engerix B	hepatitis B vaccine
Effexor	venlafaxine	Entex HC	hydrocodone
Effient	prasugrel	Entex	pseudoephedrine
Efracea	doxycycline	Entresto	sacubitril/valsartan
Efudex	fluorouracil	Entumin	clozapine
Efudix	fluorouracil	Entumine	clozapine
Efurix	fluorouracil	Entyvio	vedolizumab
Egacene Durettes	hyoscyamine	Envarsus XR	tacrolimus
Egazil	hyoscyamine	Epanutin	phenytoin
ELA-Max	lidocaine	Epaxal	hepatitis A vaccine
Elavil	amitriptyline	Epclusa	sofosbuvir & velpatasvir
Eldeprine	selegiline	Ephedsol	ephedrine
Eldepryl	selegiline	Ephynal	vitamin E
Elderin	etodolac	Epi E-Z Pen	epinephrine
Eldopal	levodopa	Epi-Aberel	tretinoin
Elentol	lindane	Epiduo	adapalene
Elepsia XR	levetiracetam	Epifrin	epinephrine
Elestrin	estradiol	Epimorph	morphine
Elidel	pimecrolimus	Epipen	epinephrine
Eligard	leuprolide	Epitol	carbamazepine
Eliquis	apixaban	Epivir	lamivudine
Elisor	pravastatin	EPO	epoetin alfa
Elixophyllin	aminophylline	Epogen	epoetin alfa
Ellence	epirubicin	Epoxitin	epoetin alfa
Elobact	cefuroxime	Eppy	epinephrine
Eloctate	antihemophilic factor	Eppystabil	epinephrine
Elorgan	pentoxifylline	Eprex	epoetin alfa
Eloxatin	oxaliplatin	Eprolin	vitamin E
Elspar	asparaginase	Eptadone	methadone
Eltor 120	pseudoephedrine	Epzicom	abacavir, lamivudine
Eltroxin	levothyroxine	Equagesic	aspirin
EMB	ethambutol	Equibar	methyldopa
Embolin	dicumarol	Eramycin	erythromycin
Emcor	bisoprolol	Eraxis	anidulafungin
Emcyt	estramustine	Erbaprelina	pyrimethamine
Emend	aprepitant	Erbitux	cetuximab
Emeset	ondansetron	Ercar	carboplatin
Emeside	ethosuximide	Ercoquin	hydroxychloroquine
Emflaza	deflazacort	Erelzi	etanercept
EMLA	lidocaine	Ergomar	ergotamine
Emorhalt	tranexamic acid	Ergometrine	ergometrine
Empirin	aspirin	Ergostat	ergotamine
Empliciti	elotuzumab	Erivedge	vismodegib
Emquin	chloroquine	Ery-Ped	erythromycin
Emsam	selegiline	Ery-Tab	erythromycin
Emselex	darifenacin	Eryc	erythromycin
Emtriva	emtricitabine	Erypar	erythromycin
Enablex	darifenacin	Erypo	epoetin alfa
Enaladil	enalapril	Erythrocin	erythromycin
Enantone	leuprolide	*erythropoiesis stimulating protein*	darbepoetin alfa

erythropoietin	epoetin alfa	Famodil	famotidine
Eryzole	erythromycin	Famoxal	famotidine
Esbriet	pirfenidone	Famvir	famciclovir
Esclim	estradiol	Fanapt	iloperidone
eserine	physostigmine	Fansidar	pyrimethamine, sulfadoxine
Esidrex	hydrochlorothiazide	Fareston	toremifene
Eskalith	lithium	Farmablastina	doxorubicin
Esmino	chlorpromazine	Farmagard	nadolol
Esperal	disulfiram	Farxiga	dapagliflozin
Estazor	ursodiol	Farydak	panobinostat
Esteprim	co-trimoxazole	Faverin	fluvoxamine
Estrace	estradiol	Favoxil	fluvoxamine
Estraderm	estradiol	FazaClo	clozapine
Estratest	methyltestosterone	FD&C yellow No.5	tartrazine
Estring	estradiol	Felden	piroxicam
Estrogel	estradiol	Feldene	piroxicam
Estrostep	oral contraceptives	Femara	letrozole
Etapiam	ethambutol	Fempatch	estradiol
Ethymal	ethosuximide	Fenac	diclofenac
Etibi	ethambutol	Fentanest	fentanyl
Etopos	etoposide	Fentazin	perphenazine
Etosid	etoposide	Fenytoin	phenytoin
Etrafon	perphenazine	Feraheme	ferumoxytol
Eucrisa	crisaborole	Ferndex	dextroamphetamine
Eudigox	digoxin	Ferriprox	deferiprone
Eudyna	tretinoin	Fetzima	levomilnacipran
Euflex	flutamide	Fevarin	fluvoxamine
Euflexxa	hyaluronic acid	Fexmid	cyclobenzaprine
Euglucan	glyburide	Fibrel	collagen (bovine)
Euglucon	glyburide	Fibrocit	gemfibrozil
Euhypnos	temazepam	Fiorinal	aspirin
Eulexin	flutamide	*fisalamine*	mesalamine
Eulexine	flutamide	Fisamox	amoxicillin
Eupen	amoxicillin	Fixime	cefixime
Euphyllin	aminophylline	Flagyl	metronidazole
Evamist	estradiol	Flanax	naproxen
Evista	raloxifene	Flavoquin	amodiaquine
Evitocor	atenolol	Flecaine	flecainide
Evomela	melphalan	Flector Patch	diclofenac
Evotaz	atazanavir	Flexeril	cyclobenzaprine
Evoxac	cevimeline	Flexiban	cyclobenzaprine
Evra	oral contraceptives	Flexitec	cyclobenzaprine
Evzio	naloxone	Flexyx	flucloxacillin
Exacyl	tranexamic acid	Flobasin	ofloxacin
Exalgo	hydromorphone	Flodine	folic acid
Excedrin	acetaminophen, aspirin	Flolan	epoprostenol
Exelon	rivastigmine	Flomax	tamsulosin
Exforge	amlodipine, valsartan	Flopen	flucloxacillin
Exidine Scrub	chlorhexidine	Florazole	metronidazole
Exjade	deferasirox	Florid	miconazole
Exocine	ofloxacin	Florocycline	tetracycline
Exodus	nicotine	Floxan	ofloxacin
Exomuc	acetylcysteine	Floxapen	flucloxacillin
Extavia	interferon beta	Floxil	ofloxacin
Eylea	aflibercept	Floxin	ofloxacin
Ezetrol	ezetimibe	Floxstat	ofloxacin
		Fluad	influenza vaccine

F

		Fluarix	influenza vaccine
Fabior	tazarotene	Flucazol	fluconazole
Fabrol	acetylcysteine	Flucinom	flutamide
Falciquin	artesunate	Fluclox	flucloxacillin

Fluctin	fluoxetine	Funcort	miconazole
Fluctine	fluoxetine	Fungarest	ketoconazole
Fludac	fluoxetine	Fungata	fluconazole
Fludara	fludarabine	Fungilin	amphotericin B
Fludecate	fluphenazine	Fungizone	amphotericin B
Fludex	indapamide	Fungoid Tincture	miconazole
Fluimucil	acetylcysteine	Fungoral	ketoconazole
Flukacide	praziquantel	Furadantin	nitrofurantoin
Fluken	flutamide	Furadantina	nitrofurantoin
Flukezol	fluconazole	Furadoine	nitrofurantoin
Flulem	flutamide	Furalan	nitrofurantoin
FluMist	influenza vaccine	Furan	nitrofurantoin
Fluorophosphate	fluorides	Furobactina	nitrofurantoin
Fluoroplex	fluorouracil	Furorese	furosemide
Fluorouracil Injection, USP	fluorouracil	Furoside	furosemide
Fluoxac	fluoxetine	Fusid	furosemide
Fluoxeren	fluoxetine	Fuzeon	enfuvirtide
Flurix	influenza vaccine	Fycompa	perampanel
Flurofen	flurbiprofen		
Flurozin	flurbiprofen	**G**	
Fluviral	influenza vaccine	G-Well	lindane
Fluxil	fluoxetine	GAB	lindane
Fluzone	fluconazole, influenza vaccine	Gabbroral	paromomycin
Focalin	dexmethylphenidate	Gabitril	tiagabine
Focetria	pandemic influenza vaccine (H1N1)	Gablofen	baclofen
folacin	folic acid	Gabrilen Retard	ketoprofen
folate	folic acid	Gabroral	paromomycin
Folina	folic acid	Galecin	clindamycin
folinic acid	leucovorin	Galedol	diclofenac
Folinsyre	folic acid	Galmax	ursodiol
Folitab	folic acid	Galzin	zinc
Folsan	folic acid	Gamabenceno	lindane
Fontex	fluoxetine	Gamafine	immune globulin IV
Foradil	formoterol	Gamastan	immune globulin IV
Formula-Q	quinine	Gambex	lindane
Forsteo	teriparatide	Gamene	lindane
Fortamet	metformin	Gamikal	amikacin
Fortaz	ceftazidime	Gamimune	immune globulin IV
Forteo	teriparatide	Gamma 16	immune globulin IV
Fortesta	testosterone	*gamma benzene hexachloride*	lindane
Fortipine	nifedipine	Gammabulin	immune globulin IV
Fortum	ceftazidime	Gammagard	immune globulin IV
Forvade	cidofovir	Gammalin	lindane
Fosalan	alendronate	Gammar PIV	immune globulin IV
Fosamax	alendronate	Gammer-IV	immune globulin IV
Fosinorm	fosinopril	Gammonayiv	immune globulin IV
Foxsalepsin	carbamazepine	Gamunex	immune globulin IV
Fozitec	fosinopril	Ganor	famotidine
Fragmin	dalteparin	Garamycin	gentamicin
Fragmine	dalteparin	Garatec	gentamicin
Fraurs	ursodiol	Gardasil	human papillomavirus (HPV) vaccine
Frenal	pimozide	Gardenal	phenobarbital
Froben	flurbiprofen	Gastro	famotidine
Froxal	cefuroxime	Gastrodyn	glycopyrrolate
Frusid	furosemide	Gastroloc	omeprazole
Fugerel	flutamide	Gastrosed	hyoscyamine
Fulcin	griseofulvin	Gattex	teduglutide
Fulvicin	griseofulvin	Gazyva	obinutuzumab
Fulvina P/G	griseofulvin	GBH	lindane
Fulyzaq	crofelemer	Geangin	verapamil
Fumaderm	dimethyl fumarate	Gelnique	oxybutynin

Gelprin	aspirin
Geluprane	acetaminophen
Gemicina	neomycin
Gemlipid	gemfibrozil
Gemzar	gemcitabine
Gen-Baclofen	baclofen
Gen-Fibro	gemfibrozil
Gen-Metformin	metformin
Gen-XENE	clorazepate
Genabid	papaverine
Genahist	diphenhydramine
Genin	quinine
Genoptic	gentamicin
Genora	oral contraceptives
Genoxal	cyclophosphamide
Genpril	ibuprofen
Gentacidin	gentamicin
Gentalline	gentamicin
Gentalol	gentamicin
Genvoya	cobicistat/elvitegravir/emtricitabine/tenofovir alafenamide
Geodon	ziprasidone
Geroxalen	methoxsalen
Gestapuran	medroxyprogesterone
Gesterol 50	progestins
Gevilon Uno	gemfibrozil
Gilenya	fingolimod
Gilex	doxepin
Gilotrif	afatinib
Glatopa	glatiramer
Gleevec	imatinib
Gliadel Wafer	carmustine
glibenclamide	glyburide
Glibenese	glipizide
Glimel	glyburide
Glioten	enalapril
Glipid	glipizide
Glivec	imatinib
Glucagon Emergency Kit	glucagon
Glucal	glyburide
Glucobay	acarbose
Glucomet	metformin
Glucophage	metformin
Glucosamine sulfate	glucosamine
Glucotrol	glipizide
Glucovance	glyburide, metformin
Gluquine	quinidine
glybenclamide	glyburide
glyceryl trinitrate	nitroglycerin
glycopyrronium bromide	glycopyrrolate
Glyde	glipizide
Glynase	glyburide
Glypressin	terlipressin
Glyxambi	empagliflozin, linagliptin
GoNitro	nitroglycerin
Goodnight	promethazine
Gopten	trandolapril
Goutnil	colchicine
Gralise	gabapentin
grass	marihuana
Green-Alpha	interferon alfa

Grifulvin V	griseofulvin
Gris-PEG	griseofulvin
Grisefuline	griseofulvin
Griseostatin	griseofulvin
Grisovin	griseofulvin
Guiatuss AC	codeine
Gynodiol	estradiol

H

Habitrol Patch	nicotine
Haemiton	clonidine
Haemopressin	terlipressin
Hairgaine	minoxidil
Halaven	eribulin
Haldol	haloperidol
Halfprin	aspirin
Haloper	haloperidol
Halotussin	codeine
Haltran	ibuprofen
Hamarin	allopurinol
Harkoseride	lacosamide
Harvoni	ledipasvir & sofosbuvir
hashish	marihuana
Havrix	hepatitis A vaccine
Heitrin	terazosin
Helidac	bismuth, tetracycline
Heliopar	chloroquine
Helminzole	mebendazole
Heloxatin	oxaliplatin
Hemangeol	propranolol
Hemi-Daonil	glyburide
Hemovas	pentoxifylline
Henexal	furosemide
Hep-Flush	heparin
Hep-Lock	heparin
Hepalean	heparin
Heparin-Leo	heparin
Heparine	heparin
Hepsera	adefovir
Herceptin	trastuzumab
Herklin	lindane
Heroin	heroin
Herpefug	acyclovir
Hetlioz	tasimelteon
hexachlorocyclohexane	lindane
Hexadrol	dexamethasone
Hexicid	lindane
Hexit	lindane
Hexol	chlorhexidine
Hibiclens	chlorhexidine
Hibident	chlorhexidine
Hibidil	chlorhexidine
Hibiscrub	chlorhexidine
Hibistat	chlorhexidine
Hibitane	chlorhexidine
HibMenCY	meningococcal groups C & Y & Haemophilus B tetanus toxoid conjugate vaccine
HibTITER	Hemophilus B vaccine
Histantil	promethazine
Hitrin	terazosin
Hivid	zalcitabine

Hizentra	immune globulin sc	Imitrex	sumatriptan
Holoxan	ifosfamide	Imlygic	talimogene laherparepvec
Horizant	gabapentin	Imodium	loperamide
HPV4	human papillomavirus (HPV) vaccine	Imossel	loperamide
Huberplex	chlordiazepoxide	Imovane	eszopiclone
Humagel	paromomycin	Imovax	influenza vaccine
Humatin	paromomycin	Implanta	cyclosporine
Humira	adalimumab	Impril	imipramine
Hyalgan	hyaluronic acid	Imuprin	azathioprine
hyaluronidase	hyaluronic acid	Imuran	azathioprine
Hybloc	labetalol	Imurek	azathioprine
Hycamtin	topotecan	Imurel	azathioprine
Hyco	hyoscyamine	Inapsin	droperidol
Hycosol SI	hyoscyamine	Inapsine	droperidol
Hycotuss	hydrocodone	Incivek	telaprevir
Hydeltrasol	prednisolone	Incruse	umeclidinium
Hydopa	methyldopa	Inderal LA	propranolol
Hydrea	hydroxyurea	Inderal	propranolol
Hydrogen fluoride [HF]	fluorides	Inderide	hydrochlorothiazide
Hydromet	hydrocodone	Indochron	indomethacin
Hydrosaluric	hydrochlorothiazide	Indocin	indomethacin
HydroStat IR	hydromorphone	Indolar SR	indomethacin
hydroxycarbamide	hydroxyurea	indometacin	indomethacin
hydroxydaunomycin	doxorubicin	Indotec	indomethacin
Hylaform	hyaluronic acid	Inegy	simvastatin
Hylan G-F 20	hyaluronic acid	INF	interferon alfa
Hylutin	progestins	Infergen	interferon alfa
Hynorex Retard	lithium	Inflamase	prednisolone
Hyospaz	hyoscyamine	Inflectra	infliximab
Hypolar	nifedipine	Inflexal V	influenza vaccine
Hysingla ER	hydrocodone	Influsome	influenza vaccine
Hytrin	terazosin	Infumorph	morphine
Hytrine	terazosin	Infurin	nitrofurantoin
Hytrinex	terazosin	Ingrezza	valbenazine
Hyzaar	hydrochlorothiazide, losartan	INH	isoniazid
		Inhibitron	omeprazole

I

		Inlyta	axitinib
IB-Stat	hyoscyamine	Innofem	estradiol
ibandronic acid	ibandronate	Innohep	tinzaparin
Ibrance	palbociclib	Innopran XL	propranolol
Idamycin	idarubicin	Innovace	enalapril
Idhifa	enasidenib	Insomnal	diphenhydramine
Idotrim	trimethoprim	Integrex	reboxetine
Ifex	ifosfamide	Integrilin	eptifibatide
IFN	interferon alfa	Intelence	etravirine
Ifoxan	ifosfamide	Intercon	oral contraceptives
IG Gamma	immune globulin IV	Interglobin	immune globulin IV
IGIM	immune globulin IV	interleukin-2	aldesleukin
IGIV	immune globulin IV	Intrarosa	prasterone
Iktorivil	clonazepam	Intron A	interferon alfa
IL-2	aldesleukin	Introna	interferon alfa
Ilaris	canakinumab	Introne	interferon alfa
Ilosone	erythromycin	Intropin	dopamine
Ilotycin	erythromycin	Invanz	ertapenem
Imbrilon	indomethacin	Invega	paliperidone
Imbruvica	ibrutinib	Invirase	saquinavir
Imdur	isosorbide mononitrate	Invivac	influenza vaccine
Imfinzi	durvalumab	Invokamet	canagliflozin, metformin
Imidol	imipramine	Invokana	canagliflozin
Imigran	sumatriptan	Ionamin	phentermine
Imipramin	imipramine	Iopidine	apraclonidine

Ipamix	indapamide
Ipolab	labetalol
Ipral	trimethoprim
Ipratropium Steri-Neb	ipratropium
Iquix	levofloxacin
Iremofar	hydroxyzine
Irenor	reboxetine
Iressa	gefitinib
Isavuconazole	isavuconazonium sulfate
Isentress	raltegravir
Ismipur	mercaptopurine
Ismo	isosorbide mononitrate
Ismotic	isosorbide
Isobac	co-trimoxazole
Isoptin	verapamil
Isoptine	verapamil
Isopto Atropine	atropine sulfate
Isopto Eserine	physostigmine
Isopto Pilocarpine	pilocarpine
Isopto-Epinal	epinephrine
Isopto	atropine sulfate
Isordil	isosorbide dinitrate
Isorythm	disopyramide
Isotamine	isoniazid
Isotrex	isotretinoin
Isox	itraconazole
Isozid	isoniazid
Istin	amlodipine
Istodax	romidepsin
Istubol	tamoxifen
Italnik	ciprofloxacin
Itranax	itraconazole
Itrin	terazosin
IV Globulin-S	immune globulin IV
Iveegam	immune globulin IV
IVIG	immune globulin IV
Ixiaro	Japanese encepahlitis vaccine
Izba	travoprost

J

Jacutin	lindane
Jadelle	levonorgestrel
Jadenu	deferasirox
Jalyn	dutasteride, tamsulosin
Janumet	metformin, sitagliptin
Januvia	sitagliptin
Jardiance	empagliflozin
Jenamicin	gentamicin
Jetrea	ocriplasmin
Jezil	gemfibrozil
Jodatum	potassium iodide
Jodid	potassium iodide
Jublia	efinaconazole
Jumex	selegiline
Jurnista	hydromorphone
Juvederm	hyaluronic acid
Juxtapid	lomitapide

K

Kabikinase	streptokinase

Kadcyla	ado-trastuzumab emtansine
Kadian	morphine
Kalcide	praziquantel
Kaletra	lopinavir, ritonavir
Kalium	potassium iodide
Kallmiren	buspirone
Kalma	alprazolam
Kalten	atenolol
Kaluril	amiloride
Kalydeco	ivacaftor
Kanamicina	kanamycin
Kanamycine	kanamycin
Kanamytrex	kanamycin
Kanbine	amikacin
Kanescin	kanamycin
Kannasyn	kanamycin
Kantrex	kanamycin
Kanuma	sebelipase alfa
Kaywan	phytonadione
Kcentra	prothrombin complex concentrate (human)
Keduril	ketoprofen
Kefarol	cephalexin
Keflex	cephalexin
Kefolor	cefaclor
Keftab	cephalexin
Kelac	ketorolac
Kelatin	penicillamine
Kenaprol	metoprolol
Kengreal	cangrelor
Kenzoflex	ciprofloxacin
Kepivance	palifermin
Keppra	levetiracetam
Kerlon	betaxolol
Kerlone	betaxolol
Kerydin	tavaborole
Kessar	tamoxifen
Ketalar	ketamine
Ketalin	ketamine
Ketanest	ketamine
Ketoderm	ketoconazole
Ketoisidin	ketoconazole
Ketolar	ketamine
Ketonic	ketorolac
Kevadon	thalidomide
Kevzara	sarilumab
Keytruda	pembrolizumab
Khedezla	desvenlafaxine
KI	potassium iodide
Kidrolase	asparaginase
Kie	potassium iodide
Kildane	lindane
Kineret	anakinra
Kinidin	quinidine
Kisqali	ribociclib
Klacid	clarithromycin
Klaricid	clarithromycin
Klexane	enoxaparin
Klonopin	clonazepam
Kloramfenicol	chloramphenicol
Klozapol	clozapine
Kodapan	carbamazepine

Koffex	dextromethorphan	Lenal	temazepam
Kolkicin	colchicine	Lencid	lindane
Konakion	phytonadione	Lenoxin	digoxin
Konicine	colchicine	Lentizol	amitriptyline
Korec	quinapril	Lentorsil	ursodiol
Korlym	mifepristone	Lenvima	lenvatinib
Kovaltry	antihemophilic factor	Leponex	clozapine
Kovanaze	tetracaine & oxymetazoline	Leptanal	fentanyl
KP-E	dinoprostone	Leptopsique	perphenazine
Kredex	carvedilol	Lescol	fluvastatin
Krenosin	adenosine	Letairis	ambrisentan
Krenosine	adenosine	Leucovorin	leucovorin
Kripton	bromocriptine	Leukerin	mercaptopurine
Krystexxa	pegloticase	Leukosulfan	busulfan
Kwell	lindane	Leunase	asparaginase
Kwildane	lindane	Leuprorelin	leuprolide
Kybella	deoxycholic acid	Leustatin	cladribine
Kyleena	levonorgestrel	Levanxene	temazepam
Kyprolis	carfilzomib	Levaquin	levofloxacin
		Levate	amitriptyline
		Levbid	hyoscyamine

L

L-asparaginase	asparaginase	Levemir	insulin detemir
L-Cysteine	acetylcysteine	Levitra	vardenafil
L-deprenyl	selegiline	Levlen	oral contraceptives
L-dopa	levodopa	Levlite	oral contraceptives
L-DOPS	droxidopa	Levo-T	levothyroxine
L-Gent	gentamicin	Levodopa-Woelm	levodopa
L-Polamidon	methadone	Levora	oral contraceptives
L-thyroxine sodium	levothyroxine	Levothyroid	levothyroxine
Labrocol	labetalol	Levothyrox	levothyroxine
Ladogal	danazol	Levoxyl	levothyroxine
Lagaquin	chloroquine	Levsin/SL	hyoscyamine
lambrolizumab	pembrolizumab	Levsin	hyoscyamine
Lamictal	lamotrigine	Levsinex	hyoscyamine
Lamisil	terbinafine	Levulan Kerastick	aminolevulinic acid
Lamocot	diphenoxylate	Lexapro	escitalopram
Landsen	clonazepam	Lexin	carbamazepine
Lanicor	digoxin	Lexinor	norfloxacin
Lanoxin	digoxin	Lexiva	fosamprenavir
Lantarel	methotrexate	Lexpec	folic acid
Lantus	insulin glargine	Lexxel	enalapril
Lapole	flurbiprofen	Lialda	mesalamine
Laraflex	naproxen	Libritabs	chlordiazepoxide
Larapam	piroxicam	Librium	chlordiazepoxide
Largactil	chlorpromazine	Lidaprim	trimethoprim
Lariam	mefloquine	Lidifen	ibuprofen
Laricam	mefloquine	Lidodan	lidocaine
Laroferon	interferon alfa	Lidoderm	lidocaine
Laroxyl	amitriptyline	Lidoject-2	lidocaine
Lartruvo	olaratumab	Lifaton B$_{12}$	cyanocobalamin
Lasilix	furosemide	lignocaine	lidocaine
Lasix	furosemide	Likudin M	griseofulvin
Laspar	asparaginase	Limbitrol	amitriptyline, chlordiazepoxide
Lastet	etoposide	Lin-Amnox	amoxicillin
Latisse	bimatoprost	Lincocin	lincomycin
Latuda	lurasidone	Lincocine	lincomycin
Laubeel	lorazepam	Linzess	linaclotide
Lebic	baclofen	Liocarpina	pilocarpine
Lederfolin	leucovorin	Lioresal	baclofen
Ledertrexate	methotrexate	Lipex	simvastatin
Ledoxina	cyclophosphamide	Lipitor	atorvastatin

Liponorm	simvastatin
Lipostat	pravastatin
Liptruzet	atorvastatin, ezetimibe
Lipur	gemfibrozil
Liquemin	heparin
Liquiprin	acetaminophen
Liroken	diclofenac
Lisino	loratadine
Lismol	cholestyramine
Litalir	hydroxyurea
Litanin	ursodiol
Lithicarb	lithium
Lithizine	lithium
Lithobid	lithium
Lithonate	lithium
Lithotabs	lithium
Litocure	ursodiol
Litoff	ursodiol
Litursol	ursodiol
Livalo	pitavastatin
Lo/Ovral	oral contraceptives
Locion-V	lindane
Locol	fluvastatin
Lodales	simvastatin
Lodimol	dipyridamole
Lodine	etodolac
Lodosyn	carbidopa
Loestrin	oral contraceptives
Lofene	atropine sulfate, diphenoxylate
Logastric	omeprazole
Logen	atropine sulfate, diphenoxylate
Lomaira	phentermine
Lomanate	atropine sulfate, diphenoxylate
Lomarin	dimenhydrinate
Lomir SRO	isradipine
Lomir	isradipine
Lomotil	atropine sulfate, diphenoxylate
Lomper	mebendazole
Lonazep	clonazepam
Lonine	etodolac
Loniten	minoxidil
Lonolox	minoxidil
Lonoten	minoxidil
Lonox	diphenoxylate
Lonsurf	trifluridine & tipiracil
Lop-Dia	loperamide
Loperhoe	loperamide
Lopid	gemfibrozil
Lopirin	captopril
Lopressor	hydrochlorothiazide, metoprolol
Lopril	captopril
Lorastine	loratadine
Lorcet	acetaminophen
Lorexane	lindane
Lortab	hydrocodone
Losec	omeprazole
Lotensin HCT	benazepril, hydrochlorothiazide
Lotensin	benazepril, hydrochlorothiazide
Lotrel	amlodipine, benazepril
Lovalip	lovastatin
Lovenox	enoxaparin

Low-Quel	diphenoxylate
Loxapac	loxapine
Loxen	nicardipine
Loxitane	loxapine
Lozapin	clozapine
Lozide	indapamide
Lozol	indapamide
Lucassin	terlipressin
Lucentis	ranibizumab
Lucrin	leuprolide
Lugol's solution	potassium iodide
Lukadin	amikacin
Lumigan	bimatoprost
Luminal	phenobarbital
Luminaletten	phenobarbital
Lunelle	medroxyprogesterone, oral contraceptives
Lunesta	eszopiclone
Lupron Depot-Ped	leuprolide
Lupron	leuprolide
Lustra	hydroquinone
Luvox	fluvoxamine
Luzu	luliconazole
Lyeton	ursodiol
Lynparza	olaparib
Lyovac	dactinomycin
Lyple	alprostadil
Lyrica	pregabalin
Lyrinel	oxybutynin
Lysalgo	mefenamic acid
Lysatec rt-PA	alteplase
Lyxumia	lixisenatide

M

M-KYA	quinine
M-M-R II	measles, mumps & rubella (MMR) virus vaccine
Maalox Anti-Diarrheal	loperamide
Maalox	loperamide
MabCampath	alemtuzumab
Mablin	busulfan
MabThera	rituximab
Macladin	clarithromycin
Macrobid	nitrofurantoin
Macrodantin	nitrofurantoin
Macugen	pegaptanib
Malarivon	chloroquine
Malarone	atovaquone/proguanil
Malocide	pyrimethamine, sulfadoxine
Maloprim	dapsone
Mamofen	tamoxifen
Mapap	acetaminophen
Marax	ephedrine, hydroxyzine
Marcillin	ampicillin
Mareen	doxepin
Marevan	warfarin
marijuana	marihuana
Marinol	dronabinol
Marmine	dimenhydrinate
Marthritic	salsalate
Masmoran	hydroxyzine
Maveral	fluvoxamine
Mavik	trandolapril

Mavyret	glecaprevir & pibrentasvir	Metrolotion	metronidazole
Maxalt	rizatriptan	Metrolyl	metronidazole
Maxcef	cefepime	Mevacor	lovastatin
Maxidone	hydrocodone	Meval	diazepam
Maxiphed	pseudoephedrine	Mevinacor	lovastatin
Maxipime	cefepime	Mevinolin	lovastatin
Maxitrol	neomycin	Miacalcic	calcitonin
Maxtrex	methotrexate	Miacalcin	calcitonin
Maxzide	hydrochlorothiazide, triamterene	Miacin	amikacin
Mazepine	carbamazepine	Miaquin	amodiaquine
Measurin	aspirin	Micardis	hydrochlorothiazide, telmisartan
Mebensole	mebendazole	Micotef	miconazole
Med-Glibe	glyburide	Micronase	glyburide
Medamor	amiloride	Micronor	progestins
Medianox	chloral hydrate	Microzide	hydrochlorothiazide
MedihalerEpi	epinephrine	Midamor	amiloride
Medilium	chlordiazepoxide	Midol 220	ibuprofen
Medimet	methyldopa	Midoride	amiloride
Medipren	ibuprofen	Mifeprex	mifepristone
Medispaz	hyoscyamine	Miglucan	glyburide
Medrol	methylprednisolone	Mindiab	glipizide
Mefac	mefenamic acid	Mindol	mebendazole
Mefic	mefenamic acid	Minidiab	glipizide
Megace	progestins	Miniprostin E(2)	dinoprostone
Megacillin	penicillin G	Minirin	desmopressin
Mekinist	trametinib	Minitran	nitroglycerin
Meladinine	methoxsalen	Minobese-Forte	phentermine
Melizide	glipizide	Minocin	minocycline
Menabol	stanozolol	Minoclir 50	minocycline
Menhibrix	meningococcal groups C & Y & Haemophilus B tetanus toxoid conjugate vaccine	Minodiab	glipizide
		Minogalen	minocycline
Menostar	estradiol	Minomycin	minocycline
mepacrine	quinacrine	Minoximen	minoxidil
Mephaquin	mefloquine	Minprog	alprostadil
Mephaquine	mefloquine	Minurin	desmopressin
Mephenon	methadone	Miocarpine	pilocarpine
Mephyton	phytonadione	Miracol	miconazole
Merabis	spironolactone	Mirapex	pramipexole
Merlit	lorazepam	Mircette	oral contraceptives
Meronem	meropenem	Mirena	levonorgestrel
Merrem IV	meropenem	Mirvaso	brimonidine
mesalazine	mesalamine	Misulban	busulfan
Mesasal	mesalamine	*mitomycin-C*	mitomycin
Mestacine	minocycline	Mitomycin	mitomycin
Mestatin	nystatin	Mitomycine	mitomycin
Mestinon	pyridostigmine	Mitoxana	ifosfamide
Metadate CD	methylphenidate	Mitran	chlordiazepoxide
Metadon	methadone	Mobic	meloxicam
Metaglip	glipizide, metformin	Mobilin	sulindac
Metandren	methyltestosterone	Modamide	amiloride
Metex	methotrexate	Modecate	fluphenazine
Metforal	metformin	Modicon	oral contraceptives
Methadose	methadone	Moditen	fluphenazine
Methipox	sulfadoxine	Moduretic	amiloride, hydrochlorothiazide
Methoprim	trimethoprim	Molelant	cefotaxime
Methylin	methylphenidate	Molipaxin	trazodone
methylmorphine	codeine	*molly*	MDMA
Meticorten	prednisone	Monazole-7	miconazole
Metomin	metformin	Monistat	miconazole
Metrocream	metronidazole	Mono-Gesic	salsalate
MetroGel	metronidazole	Monocor	bisoprolol

Monodox	doxycycline
Monoflam	diclofenac
Monofluorophosphate [MFP]	fluorides
Monoket	isosorbide mononitrate
Mononate	artesunate
Monopril	fosinopril
Monotrim	trimethoprim
Mopral	omeprazole
Morcomine	hydrocodone
Moronal	nystatin
Morphabond	morphine
Morphine-HP	morphine
MOS	morphine
Moscontin	morphine
Motiax	famotidine
Motifene	diclofenac
Motrin	ibuprofen
Movantik	naloxegol
Movergan	selegiline
Moxacef	cefadroxil
Moxeza	moxifloxacin
MS Contin	morphine
MS-IR	morphine
MS/S	morphine
MSIR Oral	morphine
MST Continus	morphine
MTC	mitomycin
MTX	methotrexate
Mucofillin	acetylcysteine
Mucolit	acetylcysteine
Mucolitico	acetylcysteine
Mucoloid	acetylcysteine
Mucomiste	acetylcysteine
Mucomyst-10	acetylcysteine
Mucomyst	acetylcysteine
Mucosil-10	acetylcysteine
Multaq	dronedarone
Multipax	hydroxyzine
Multum	chlordiazepoxide
Murelax	oxazepam
Muse	alprostadil
Mustargen	mechlorethamine
Mustine Hydrochloride Boots	mechlorethamine
mustine	mechlorethamine
Mutamycin	mitomycin
Myambutol	ethambutol
Mycamine	micafungin
Myciguent	neomycin
Mycobax	BCG vaccine
Mycobutin	rifabutin
Mycol	metoprolol
Mycology-II	nystatin
mycophenolate mofetil, mycophenolate sodium	mycophenolate
Mycostatin	nystatin
Mydayis	dextroamphetamine
Myfortic	mycophenolate
Mylanta AR	famotidine
Myleran	busulfan
Mylocel	hydroxyurea
Mynocine	minocycline
Myobloc	botulinum toxin (A & B)

Myolax	carisoprodol
Myrbetriq	mirabegron

N

N-acetyl-glucosamine (NAG)	glucosamine
N-acetylcysteine	acetylcysteine
Nabuser	nabumetone
NAC	acetylcysteine
Nadic	nadolol
Nalcryn SP	nalbuphine
Nalorex	naltrexone
Nalpin	naloxone
Namenda	memantine
Naplin	indapamide
Naprelan	naproxen
Naprogesic	naproxen
Napron X	naproxen
Naprosyn	naproxen
Naprosyne	naproxen
Narcan	naloxone
Narcanti	naloxone
Narcotan	naloxone
Narilet	aldesleukin
Narol	buspirone
Nascobal	cyanocobalamin
Natesto	testosterone
Natrilix	indapamide
Nauseatol	dimenhydrinate
Nausicalm	dimenhydrinate
Navelbine	vinorelbine
Naxen	naproxen
Nazoltec	ketoconazole
Nebilet	nebivolol
NebuPent	pentamidine
Necon	oral contraceptives
NEE	oral contraceptives
Nelova	oral contraceptives
Nemasol	mebendazole
Nemexin	naltrexone
Neo-Synephrine	phenylephrine
Neomicina	neomycin
Neomycine Diamant	neomycin
Neopap	acetaminophen
Neoral	cyclosporine
Neosar	cyclophosphamide
Neosporin	neomycin
Neosulf	neomycin
Neotigason	acitretin
NEPA	netupitant & palonosetron
Nephronex	nitrofurantoin
Nergadan	lovastatin
Nerlynx	neratinib
Nesina	alogliptin
Neupro	rotigotine
Neurap	pimozide
Neurobloc	botulinum toxin (A & B)
Neurontin	gabapentin
Neurosine	buspirone
Nexavar	sorafenib
Nexiclon	clonidine
Nexium	esomeprazole

Nia-Bid	niacin	Norfenon	propafenone
Niac	niacin	Norgesic	aspirin
Niacels	niacin	Norinyl	oral contraceptives
Niacinamide	niacinamide	Noritate	metronidazole
Niacor	niacin	Noritren	nortriptyline
Niaspan	niacin	Norlutate	progestins
Nicabate	nicotine	Norlutin	progestins
Nicardal	nicardipine	Normison	temazepam
Nico-Vert	dimenhydrinate	Normorytmin	propafenone
Nicobid	niacin	Normozide	labetalol
Nicobion	niacin	Noroxin	norfloxacin
Nicodel	nicardipine	Norpace	disopyramide
Nicoderm	nicotine	Norphyl	aminophylline
Nicolan	nicotine	Norplant	levonorgestrel
Nicorette Plus	nicotine	Norpress	nortriptyline
Nicorette	nicotine	Northera	droxidopa
Nicotibine	isoniazid	Nortrilen	nortriptyline
nicotinamide	niacinamide	Norvas	amlodipine
Nicotinell-TTS	nicotine	Norvasc	amlodipine
Nicotinex	niacin	Norvir	ritonavir
nicotinic acid	niacin	Noten	atenolol
Nicotrans	nicotine	Novahistine DH	codeine
Nicotrol	nicotine	Novahistine	phenylephrine
Nicovital	niacin	Novamin	prochlorperazine
Nicozid	isoniazid	Novamoxin	amoxicillin
Nida Gel	metronidazole	Novantrone	mitoxantrone
Nifecor	nifedipine	Novapen-VK	penicillin V
Nifedipress	nifedipine	Novasen	aspirin
Nikofrenon	nicotine	Novazam	diazepam
Ninlaro	ixazomib	Novitropan	oxybutynin
Niotal	zolpidem	Novo-Atenol	atenolol
Nirulid	amiloride	Novo-AZT	zidovudine
Nistaquim	nystatin	Novo-Chlorpromazine	chlorpromazine
Nitro-Dur	nitroglycerin	Novo-Cycloprine	cyclobenzaprine
NitroBid	nitroglycerin	Novo-Digoxin	digoxin
Nitrocap	nitroglycerin	Novo-Dipiradol	dipyridamole
Nitrocine	nitroglycerin	Novo-Doxepin	doxepin
Nitrodur	nitroglycerin	Novo-Doxylin	doxycycline
nitrogen mustard	mechlorethamine	Novo-Flutamide	flutamide
Nitroglin	nitroglycerin	Novo-Furan	nitrofurantoin
nitroglycerol	nitroglycerin	Novo-Hylazin	hydralazine
Nitrolingual	nitroglycerin	Novo-Ipramide	ipratropium
Nitromist	nitroglycerin	Novo-Keto	ketoprofen
Nitronal	nitroglycerin	Novo-Lexin	cephalexin
Nitrospan	nitroglycerin	Novo-Medrone	medroxyprogesterone
Nitrostat	nitroglycerin	Novo-Metformin	metformin
Nitrumon	carmustine	Novo-Naprox	naproxen
Nivemycin	neomycin	Novo-Pramine	imipramine
Nizoral	ketoconazole	Novo-Purol	allopurinol
Nobegyl	salsalate	Novo-Seleginine	selegiline
Nocbin	disulfiram	Novo-Semide	furosemide
Noctec	chloral hydrate	Novo-Spiroton	spironolactone
Noctiva	desmopressin	Novo-Sundac	sulindac
Nodine	ketorolac	Novo-Zolamide	acetazolamide
Nolvadex	tamoxifen	Novochlorhydrate	chloral hydrate
Nor-QD	progestins	Novocimetine	cimetidine
Norboral	glyburide	Novoclopate	clorazepate
Norco	hydrocodone	Novofen	tamoxifen
Nordette	oral contraceptives	NovoLog	insulin aspart
Norebox	reboxetine	Novomit	prochlorperazine
Norethin	oral contraceptives	Novopen-G	penicillin G

Novopoxide	chlordiazepoxide
NovoRapid	insulin aspart
Novotriptyn	amitriptyline
Novoxapam	oxazepam
Noxafil	posaconazole
NTG	nitroglycerin
Nu-Alprax	alprazolam
Nu-Amoxi	amoxicillin
Nu-Atenol	atenolol
Nu-Baclo	baclofen
Nu-Buspirone	buspirone
Nu-Capto	captopril
Nu-Cimet	cimetidine
Nu-Clonidine	clonidine
Nu-Diclo	diclofenac
Nu-Diltiaz	diltiazem
Nu-Doxycycline	doxycycline
Nu-Famotidine	famotidine
Nu-Flurprofen	flurbiprofen
Nu-Gemfibrozil	gemfibrozil
Nu-Hydral	hydralazine
Nu-Indo	indomethacin
Nu-Loraz	lorazepam
Nu-Medopa	methyldopa
Nu-Naprox	naproxen
Nu-Nifed	nifedipine
Nu-Pirox	piroxicam
Nu-Ranit	ranitidine
Nu-Temazepam	temazepam
Nu-Verap	verapamil
Nubain SP	nalbuphine
Nubain	nalbuphine
Nucala	mepolizumab
Nucofed	codeine
Nucynta ER	tapentadol
Nucynta	tapentadol
Nulev	hyoscyamine
Nulojix	belatacept
Nuplazid	pimavanserin
Nuprin	ibuprofen
Nuvigil	armodafinil
Nyaderm	nystatin
Nystacid	nystatin
Nystan	nystatin
Nystex	nystatin
Nytol	diphenhydramine

O

Ocaliva	obeticholic acid
Ocrevus	ocrelizumab
Octagam	immune globulin IV
Octocaine	lidocaine
Octostim	desmopressin
Ocuflox	ofloxacin
Ocumycin	gentamicin
Ocusert Pilo	pilocarpine
Odefsey	emtricitabine/rilpivirine/tenofovir alafenamide
Odomzo	sonidegib
Odrik	trandolapril
Ofev	nintedanib
Ofirmev	acetaminophen

Oflocet	ofloxacin
Oflocin	ofloxacin
Oforta	fludarabine
Oftalmotrisol-T	tobramycin
Oleomycetin	chloramphenicol
Oleptro	trazodone
Olmetec	olmesartan
Olysio	simeprevir
Omed	omeprazole
Omnicef	cefdinir
OmniHIB	Hemophilus B vaccine
OMS Oral	morphine
Onbrez Breezhaler	indacaterol
Oncaspar	pegaspargase
Onco-Carbide	hydroxyurea
Oncocarbin	carboplatin
Oncoden	ondansetron
oncovin	vincristine
Onglyza	saxagliptin
Onicit	palonosetron
Onivyde	irinotecan
Onmel	itraconazole
Onzetra Xsail	sumatriptan
Opana	oxymorphone
Opdivo	nivolumab
Ophthochlor	chloramphenicol
Opistan	meperidine
Opizone	naltrexone
Opsumit	macitentan
Optenyl	papaverine
Optipres	betaxolol
Optovit-E	vitamin E
Oracea	doxycycline
Oracefal	cefadroxil
Oramorph SR	morphine
Oranor	norfloxacin
Oranyst	nystatin
Orap	pimozide
Oravig	miconazole
Orbactiv	oritavancin
Orencia	abatacept
Orientomycin	cycloserine
Oritaxim	cefotaxime
Orkambi	lumacaftor/ivacaftor
Ormazine	chlorpromazine
Ornade	chlorpheniramine
Ornidyl	eflornithine
Oroken	cefixime
Ortho Tri-Cyclen	oral contraceptives
Ortho-Cept	oral contraceptives
Ortho-Cyclen	oral contraceptives
Ortho-Novum	oral contraceptives
Orthovisc	hyaluronic acid
Orudis	ketoprofen
Oruvail	ketoprofen
Osiren	spironolactone
Ospen	penicillin V
Ospexin	cephalexin
Osphena	ospemifene
Osteum	etidronate
Otarex	hydroxyzine

Otezla	apremilast	Paveral	codeine
Otrexup	methotrexate	Paxene	paclitaxel
Otrivine	xylometazoline	Paxil CR	paroxetine hydrochloride
Ovcon	oral contraceptives	Paxil	paroxetine hydrochloride
Ovral	oral contraceptives	Paxistil	hydroxyzine
Ovrette	progestins	Paxtibi	nortriptyline
Oxiklorin	hydroxychloroquine	PCC	prothrombin complex concentrate (human)
Oxpam	oxazepam	PCE	erythromycin
Oxsoralen	methoxsalen, psoralens	PCV	pneumococcal vaccine
Oxsoralon	methoxsalen	Pedi-Dri	nystatin
Oxtellar XR	oxcarbazepine	Pediapred	prednisolone
Oxyban	oxybutynin	Pediatrix	hepatitis B vaccine
Oxybutyn	oxybutynin	Pediazole	erythromycin
OxyContin	oxycodone	PedivaxHIB	Hemophilus B vaccine
Oxydess	dextroamphetamine	Pegasys	PEG-interferon
OxyIR	oxycodone	PegIntron	PEG-interferon
Oxytrol	oxybutynin	Penbeta	penicillin V
Ozoken	omeprazole	Penbritin	ampicillin
Ozurdex	dexamethasone	Pendramine	penicillamine
		Pennsaid	diclofenac
		Penstabil	ampicillin

P

		Pentacarinat	pentamidine
Pacerone	amiodarone	Pentaglobin	immune globulin IV
Pacifen	baclofen	Pentam 300	pentamidine
Paclimer	paclitaxel	Pentamycetin	chloramphenicol
Palaron	aminophylline	Pentasa SR	mesalamine
Palexia	tapentadol	Pentasa	mesalamine
Palladone	hydromorphone	Pentazine	promethazine
Palmitate A	vitamin A	Pentoxi	pentoxifylline
Palux	alprostadil	Pentoxil	pentoxifylline
Pameion	papaverine	Pepcid	famotidine
Pamelor	nortriptyline	Pepcidine	famotidine
Pamid	indapamide	Pepdul	famotidine
Pamprin	ibuprofen	Pepeom Amide	niacin
Panadol	acetaminophen	Peptard	hyoscyamine
Panbesy	phentermine	Peptaron	ursodiol
Panbesyl	phentermine	Pepto-Bismol	bismuth
Pandemrix	pandemic influenza vaccine (H1N1)	Peptol	cimetidine
Panglobulin	immune globulin IV	Peratsin	perphenazine
Panoral	cefaclor	Percocet	acetaminophen, oxycodone
Panretin	alitretinoin	Percogesic	acetaminophen
Pantelmin	mebendazole	Perforomist	formoterol
Panuric	probenecid	Peridex	chlorhexidine
Papaverine 60	papaverine	Peridol	haloperidol
Papaverini	papaverine	PerioChip	chlorhexidine
paracetamol	acetaminophen	Periogard	chlorhexidine
Paraplatin	carboplatin	Periostat	doxycycline
Paraplatine	carboplatin	Perlane	hyaluronic acid
Parilac	bromocriptine	Perlutex	medroxyprogesterone
Parizac	omeprazole	Perphenan	perphenazine
Parkemed	mefenamic acid	Persantin	dipyridamole
Parlodel	bromocriptine	Persantine	dipyridamole
Parsabiv	etelcalcetide	Pertussin	dextromethorphan
Parvolex	acetylcysteine	Petar	ketamine
Pasmex	hyoscyamine	pethidine	meperidine
Pasotomin	prochlorperazine	Petidin	meperidine
Pataday	olopatadine	Petnidan	ethosuximide
Patanol	olopatadine	Pexal	pentoxifylline
Pavabid	papaverine	PGE	alprostadil
Pavagen	papaverine	Phenaemal	phenobarbital
Pavased	papaverine	Phenaphen	acetaminophen
Pavatine	papaverine		

Phenazine	promethazine	Pradaxa	dabigatran
Phenergan	promethazine	Praluent	alirocumab
Phenetron	chlorpheniramine	Prandin E2	dinoprostone
Phenhydan	phenytoin	Pravachol	pravastatin
phenobarbitone	phenobarbital	Pravasin	pravastatin
Phenoxymethylpenicillin	penicillin V	Pravasine	pravastatin
phenylethylmalonylurea	phenobarbital	Pravidel	bromocriptine
Phenytek	phenytoin	Praxbind	idarucizumab
phenytoin sodium	phenytoin	Praxiten	oxazepam
Pheryl-E	vitamin E	Prazite	praziquantel
Phyllocontin	aminophylline	Pre-Par	ritodrine
Phyllotemp	aminophylline	Precaptil	captopril
Phytomenadione	phytonadione	Precose	acarbose
Picato	ingenol mebutate	Pred-G	gentamicin
Pidilat	nifedipine	Prefrin Liquifilm	phenylephrine
Pilo Grin	pilocarpine	Prelone	prednisolone
Pilogel	pilocarpine	Premphase	medroxyprogesterone
Pilopine	pilocarpine	Prempro	medroxyprogesterone
Pilopt	pilocarpine	Prepidil	dinoprostone
Pimodac	pimozide	Pres	enalapril
Pink Bismuth	bismuth	Prescal	isradipine
Pirimecidan	pyrimethamine	Presinol	methyldopa
Pitocin	oxytocin	Presoken	diltiazem
Pitressin	vasopressin	Presolol	labetalol
Placil	clomipramine	Prestalia	amlodipine, perindopril
Plan B	levonorgestrel	Pretz-D	ephedrine
Planphylline	aminophylline	Prevacid	lansoprazole
Planum	temazepam	Prevalite	cholestyramine
Plaquenil	hydroxychloroquine	Preveon	adefovir
Plaquinol	hydroxychloroquine	Prevnar	pneumococcal vaccine
Plasmotrim	artesunate	Prevpac	amoxicillin
Plasticin	cisplatin	Prexum	perindopril
Platiblastin	cisplatin	Prezcobix	darunavir
Platinex	cisplatin	Prezista	darunavir
Platinol-AQ	cisplatin	Priadel	lithium
Platinol	cisplatin	Prialt	ziconotide
Platistil	cisplatin	Pridemon	tranexamic acid
Plavix	clopidogrel	Prilosec	omeprazole
Plegridy	interferon beta	Primacor	milrinone
Pletal	cilostazol	Primafen	cefotaxime
Plurimen	selegiline	Primatene Mist	epinephrine
PMS-Baclofen	baclofen	Primatene	epinephrine
PMS-Cholestyramine	cholestyramine	Primiprost	dinoprostone
PMS-Isoniazid	isoniazid	Primonil	imipramine
PMS-Lindane	lindane	Primosept	trimethoprim
PncOMP	pneumococcal vaccine	Primsol	trimethoprim
Pneumovax II	pneumococcal vaccine	Principen	ampicillin
Pnu-Immune	pneumococcal vaccine	Princol	lincomycin
Polinal	methyldopa	Prinil	lisinopril
Poly-Pred	neomycin	Prinivil	lisinopril
Polygam S/D	immune globulin IV	Prinzide	hydrochlorothiazide, lisinopril
Polygris	griseofulvin	Pristiq	desvenlafaxine
Polytrim	trimethoprim	Pro-Amox	amoxicillin
Pomalyst	pomalidomide	Pro-Ampi	ampicillin
Ponstan	mefenamic acid	Pro-Cure	finasteride
Ponstel	mefenamic acid	Pro-Depo	progestins
Ponstyl	mefenamic acid	Pro-Trin	co-trimoxazole
Portrazza	necitumumab	Probalan	probenecid
pot	marihuana	Probuphine	buprenorphine
Potiga	ezogabine	Procan SR	procainamide
PPV	pneumococcal vaccine	Procan	procainamide

Procanbid	procainamide
Procardia	nifedipine
Procid	probenecid
Procoralan	ivabradine
Procren Depot	leuprolide
Procrin	leuprolide
Procrit	epoetin alfa
Procytox	cyclophosphamide
Prodac	nabumetone
Prodopa	methyldopa
Prodox	progestins
Profen	ibuprofen
Proflex	ibuprofen
Progestaject	progestins
Progevera	medroxyprogesterone
Prograf	tacrolimus
ProHIBIT	Hemophilus B vaccine
Prolaken	metoprolol
Proleukin	aldesleukin
Prolex-D	phenylephrine
Prolex-DH	hydrocodone
Prolia	denosumab
Prolift	reboxetine
Prolixin	fluphenazine
Promacta	eltrombopag
Prometh-50	promethazine
Promine	procainamide
Pronestyl	procainamide
Propachem	hydrocodone
Propaphenin	chlorpromazine
Propecia	finasteride
Propess	dinoprostone
Prorazin	prochlorperazine
Proscar 5	finasteride
Proscar	finasteride
prostaglandin E₁	alprostadil
Prostaphlin	oxacillin
Prostarmon	dinoprostone
Prostigmin	neostigmine
Prostin E2	dinoprostone
Prostin VR	alprostadil, dinoprostone
Prostin	dinoprostone
Prostine VR	alprostadil
Prostine	dinoprostone
Prostivas	alprostadil
Prothiazine	promethazine
Protium	pantoprazole
Protogen	dapsone
Protonix	pantoprazole
Protopam	pralidoxime
Protopic	tacrolimus
Proventil	albuterol
Provera	medroxyprogesterone, progestins
Provigil	modafinil
Prozac	fluoxetine
Prozin	chlorpromazine
Pryleugan	imipramine
Psicofar	chlordiazepoxide
Pulmicort Turbuhaler	budesonide
Punktyl	lorazepam
Puri-Nethol	mercaptopurine

Purinethol	mercaptopurine
Purinol	allopurinol
Puvasoralen	methoxsalen
Pyknolepsinum	ethosuximide
Pyoredol	phenytoin
Pyrethia	promethazine

Q

Q-Vel	quinine
Qnasl	beclomethasone
Qsymia	phentermine, topiramate
Qtern	dapagliflozin, saxagliptin
Qualaquin	quinine
Quantalan	cholestyramine
Qudexy	topiramate
Quellada	lindane
Quensyl	hydroxychloroquine
Querto	carvedilol
Questran Lite	cholestyramine
Questran	cholestyramine
Quibron	aminophylline
Quiess	hydroxyzine
Quinalan	quinidine
Quinate	quinidine
Quinazil	quinapril
Quini Durules	quinidine
Quinoctal	quinine
Quinora	quinidine
Quinsan	quinine
Quinsul	quinine
Quintasa	mesalamine
Quiphile	quinine
Quixin	levofloxacin
Qvar	beclomethasone

R

Ra-223 dichloride	radium-223 dichloride
Radicava	edaravone
Radiesse	calcium hydroxylapatite
Ralovera	medroxyprogesterone
Ralozam	alprazolam
Ramicin	rifampin
Randikan	kanamycin
Ranexa	ranolazine
Raniben	ranitidine
Raniplex	ranitidine
Ranisen	ranitidine
Ranvil	nicardipine
Rapaflo	silodosin
Rapamune	sirolimus
rapamycin	sirolimus
Rapivab	peramivir
Rasuvo	methotrexate
Rayaldee	calcifediol
Razadyne	galantamine
Reactine	cetirizine
Rebetol	ribavirin
Rebetron	interferon alfa, ribavirin
Rebif	interferon beta
Reclast	zoledronate

Recombivax HB	hepatitis B vaccine	Rhythmin	procainamide
Rectiv	nitroglycerin	Ride	amiloride
Redisol	cyanocobalamin	Ridene	nicardipine
Redusa	phentermine	Rifadin	rifampin
Refobacin	gentamicin	Rifaldin	rifampin
Refolinin	leucovorin	Rifamate	isoniazid
Refusal	disulfiram	Rifamed	rifampin
Regaine	minoxidil	rifampicin	rifampin
Regitin	phentolamine	Rifater	isoniazid
Regitine	phentolamine	Rilatine	methylphenidate
Regonol	pyridostigmine	Rimactane	rifampin
Relafen	nabumetone	Rimpin	rifampin
Relenza	zanamivir	Rimycin	rifampin
Relief	tretinoin	Rinatec	ipratropium
Relif	nabumetone	Riomet	metformin
Relifex	nabumetone	Risperdal Consta	risperidone
Relpax	eletriptan	Risperdal	risperidone
Remeron	mirtazapine	Ritalin	methylphenidate
Remethan	diclofenac	Ritmocamid	procainamide
Remicade	infliximab	Ritmolol	metoprolol
Reminyl	galantamine	Rituxan	rituximab
Renflexis	infliximab	Rivotril	clonazepam
Renitec	enalapril	RMS	morphine
Reniten	enalapril	Roaccutan	isotretinoin
Renova	tretinoin	Roaccutane	isotretinoin
Repatha	evolocumab	Roacutan	isotretinoin
Reposans-10	chlordiazepoxide	Roacuttan	isotretinoin
Requip	ropinirole	Robaxisal	aspirin
Rescufolin	leucovorin	Robidrine	pseudoephedrine
Rescuvolin	leucovorin	Robimycin	erythromycin
Resmin	diphenhydramine	Robinul	glycopyrrolate
Respirol	terbutaline	Robitussin AC	codeine
Respontin	ipratropium	Robitussin-CF	pseudoephedrine
Restasis	cyclosporine	Robitussin	dextromethorphan
Restoril	temazepam	Rocefin	ceftriaxone
Restylane Fine Lines	hyaluronic acid	Rocephalin	ceftriaxone
retigabine	ezogabine	Rocephin	ceftriaxone
Retin-A Micro	tretinoin	Roceron-A	interferon alfa
Retinoic Acid	tretinoin	Rofact	rifampin
Retinova	tretinoin	Roferon-A	interferon alfa
Retrovir	zidovudine	Rogaine	minoxidil
Revapole	mebendazole	Rogal	piroxicam
Revatio	sildenafil	Rogitene	phentolamine
ReVia	naltrexone	Rogitine	phentolamine
Revimine	dopamine	Rotarix	rotavirus vaccine
Reviten	triamterene	RotaTeq	rotavirus vaccine
Revlimid	lenalidomide	Roubac	co-trimoxazole
Revolade	eltrombopag	Rovacor	lovastatin
Revonto	dantrolene	Rowasa	mesalamine
Rexulti	brexpiprazole	Roxanol	morphine
Reyataz	atazanavir	Roxicodone	oxycodone
Rezine	hydroxyzine	Rozerem	ramelteon
rFVIIIFc	antihemophilic factor	Rtsun	artesunate
Rheumatrex	methotrexate	Ru-Tuss	hydrocodone
Rhinocort	budesonide	Rubesol-1000	cyanocobalamin
Rhodacine	indomethacin	Rubex	doxorubicin
Rhodis	ketoprofen	rubidomycin	daunorubicin
Rhofade	oxymetazoline	Rubifen	methylphenidate
Rhonal	aspirin	Rubraca	rucaparib
Rhotrimine	trimipramine	Rubramin	cyanocobalamin
Rhovail	ketoprofen	Rufen	ibuprofen

Ryanodex	dantrolene	Selectin	pravastatin
Rybix ODT	tramadol	Selectol	celiprolol
Rydapt	midostaurin	Selektine	pravastatin
Rydene	nicardipine	Selipran	pravastatin
Rynatan	phenylephrine	Seloken-Zok	metoprolol
Rynatuss	ephedrine	Selozok	metoprolol
Rytary	levodopa	Selzentry	maraviroc
Rythmex	propafenone	Sendoxan	cyclophosphamide
Rythmol	propafenone	Septra	co-trimoxazole, sulfamethoxazole, trimethoprim
Rytmonorm	propafenone	Ser-Ap-Es	hydralazine
Ryzodeg	insulin aspart, insulin degludec	Serax	oxazepam

S

		Serenace	haloperidol
		Serepax	oxazepam
S-1	tegafur/gimeracil/oteracil	Serocryptin	bromocriptine
S-2	epinephrine	Seromycin	cycloserine
Sabril	vigabatrin	Seroquel	quetiapine
Sacbexyl	lindane	Seroxat	paroxetine hydrochloride
Saccharin	saccharin	Serozide	etoposide
Saflutan	tafluprost	Sesamol	flucloxacillin
Salagen	pilocarpine	Setamine	hyoscyamine
salazopyrin	sulfasalazine	Sevredol	morphine
Salbulin	albuterol	Sideril	trazodone
salbutamol	albuterol	Sigacefal	cefaclor
Salflex	salsalate	Sigafam	famotidine
Salgesic	salsalate	Silenor	doxepin
salicylazosulfapyridine	sulfasalazine	Silgard	human papillomavirus (HPV) vaccine
Salina	salsalate	Silicofluoride	fluorides
Salisulf	sulfasalazine	Siliq	brodalumab
Salmagne	labetalol	Simatin	ethosuximide
Salofalk	mesalamine	Simcor	niacin, simvastatin
Sandimmun	cyclosporine	Simovil	simvastatin
Sandimmune	cyclosporine	Simplene	epinephrine
Sandoglobulin	immune globulin IV	Simponi	golimumab
Sandoglobulina	immune globulin IV	Simulect	basiliximab
Sandoglobuline	immune globulin IV	Sinaplin	ampicillin
Sandostatin	octreotide	Sinemet	levodopa
Sandostatina	octreotide	Singulair	montelukast
Sandostatine	octreotide	Sinomin	sulfamethoxazole
Sanoma	carisoprodol	Sinosid	paromomycin
Sansert	methysergide	Sinquan	doxepin
Saphris	asenapine	Sintodian	droperidol
Sarafem	fluoxetine	Sinutab	acetaminophen
Sarconyl	lindane	Siran	acetylcysteine
Saridine	sulfasalazine	Sirdalud	tizanidine
Saroten	amitriptyline	Sirtal	carbamazepine
SAS-500	sulfasalazine	Sirturo	bedaquiline
Savaysa	edoxaban	Sitavig	acyclovir
Savella	milnacipran	Sivastin	simvastatin
Savlon	chlorhexidine	Sivextro	tedizolid
Saxenda	liraglutide	Sizopin	clozapine
Scabecid	lindane	Skelaxin	metaxalone
Scabene	lindane	Sklice	ivermectin
Scabex	lindane	Slo-Bid	aminophylline
Scabi	lindane	Slo-Niacin	niacin
Scabisan	lindane	SMX-TMP	co-trimoxazole
SCIG	immune globulin sc	SMZ-TMP	co-trimoxazole
Sebomin	minocycline	Sno Pilo	pilocarpine
Sebvio	telbivudine	Sobelin	clindamycin
Sedanazin	gentamicin	Sodium fluoride [NaF]	fluorides
Sediat	diphenhydramine	Sodium monofluorophosphate	fluorides
Seebri Neohaler	glycopyrrolate	Sodol	carisoprodol

Solage	tretinoin	Starlix	nateglinide
Solaraze Gel	diclofenac	Statex	morphine
Solcodein	codeine	Steclin	tetracycline
Solesorin	hydralazine	SteiVAA	tretinoin
Solfoton	phenobarbital	Stelara	ustekinumab
Solgol	nadolol	Stella	prochlorperazine
Soliqua	insulin glargine, lixisenatide	Stemetil	prochlorperazine
Soliris	eculizumab	Stendra	avanafil
Solis	diazepam	Stieva-A	tretinoin
Solium	chlordiazepoxide	Stilnoct	zolpidem
Solodyn	minocycline	Stilnox	zolpidem
Solosec	secnidazole	Stimate	desmopressin
Solpurin	probenecid	Stiolto Respimat	olodaterol, tiotropium
Solu-Medrol	methylprednisolone	Stomedine	cimetidine
Solutrat	ursodiol	Stopit	loperamide
Solvex	reboxetine	Storzine	pilocarpine
Soma Compound	aspirin	Strattera	atomoxetine
Soma	carisoprodol	Strensiq	asfotase alfa
Somadril	carisoprodol	Streptase	streptokinase
Somatuline Autogel	lanreotide	Streptomycin	streptomycin
Somatuline Depot	lanreotide	Stribild	cobicistat/elvitegravir/emtricitabine/tenofovir
Somatuline LA	lanreotide		disoproxil
Somavert	pegvisomant	Striverdi Respimat	olodaterol
Sominex 2	diphenhydramine	Stromba	stanozolol
Somnox	chloral hydrate	Stromectol	ivermectin
Somophyllin	aminophylline	Strumazol	methimazole
Sonata	zaleplon	Stubit	nicotine
Soolantra	ivermectin	Sublimaze	fentanyl
Sopamycetin	chloramphenicol	Suboxone	buprenorphine, naloxone
Sorbitrate	isosorbide dinitrate	Subutex	buprenorphine
Soriatane	acitretin	Sucrabest	sucralfate
Soridol	carisoprodol	Sucrets	dextromethorphan
Sorine	sotalol	Sudafed	pseudoephedrine
Sostril	ranitidine	Sular	nisoldipine
Sotacor	sotalol	Sulcrate	sucralfate
Sotahexal	sotalol	Sulene	sulindac
Sotalex	sotalol	*sulfamethoxazole-trimethoprim*	co-trimoxazole
Sotilen	piroxicam	Sulfatrim	co-trimoxazole
Sotret	isotretinoin	Sulfazine	sulfasalazine
Sovaldi	sofosbuvir	Sulfona	dapsone
Spectro Gram	chlorhexidine	Sulfur hexafluoride [SF6]	fluorides
Spersacarpine	pilocarpine	Sulic	sulindac
Spinax	baclofen	Sulmidine	clonidine
Spinraza	nusinersen	Suloril	sulindac
Spiriva	tiotropium	Suloton	triamterene
Spiroctan	spironolactone	Sumacef	cefadroxil
Spirosine	cefotaxime	Sumavel DosePro	sumatriptan
Splenda	sucralose	Sumontil	trimipramine
Sporacid	itraconazole	Sumycin	tetracycline
Sporal	itraconazole	Supartz	hyaluronic acid
Sporanox	itraconazole	Supeudol	oxycodone
Sprycel	dasatinib	Suppress	dextromethorphan
SSKI	potassium iodide	Supradol	naproxen
Stable	hydralazine	Supran	cefixime
Stalevo	entacapone, levodopa	Suprax	cefixime
Stamaril	yellow fever vaccine	Suprenza	phentermine
Stambutol	ethambutol	Supressin	doxazosin
Stangyl	trimipramine	Suretin	tazarotene
Stannous fluoride [SF]	fluorides	Surmontil	trimipramine
Stapenor	oxacillin	Sustiva	efavirenz
Staril	fosinopril	Sutent	sunitinib

suxamethonium	succinylcholine
Sweet'N Low	saccharin
Sylatron	PEG-interferon
Symbicort	budesonide, formoterol
Symbol	misoprostol
Symbyax	fluoxetine, olanzapine
Symjepi	epinephrine
Symproic	naldemedine
Syn-Minocycline	minocycline
Syn-Nadolol	nadolol
Synagis	palivizumab
Syndros	dronabinol
Synflex	naproxen
Synjardy	empagliflozin, metformin
Synribo	omacetaxine
Synthroid	levothyroxine
Syntocinon	oxytocin
Syraprim	trimethoprim
Syscor	nisoldipine
Sytobex	cyanocobalamin

T

T-20	enfuvirtide
T-DM1	ado-trastuzumab emtansine
T-VEC	talimogene laherparepvec
T₃ sodium	liothyronine
T₃	liothyronine
T₄	levothyroxine
Tabalom	ibuprofen
Tabco	flecainide
Tabrin	ofloxacin
Tacex	ceftriaxone
Tachydaron	amiodarone
Tadol	tramadol
Tafil	alprazolam
Tafinlar	dabrafenib
Taflutan	tafluprost
Tagal	ceftazidime
Tagamet	cimetidine
Tagrisso	osimertinib
Taks	diclofenac
Taloken	ceftazidime
Taltz	ixekizumab
Talwin Compound	aspirin
Talwin-NX	naloxone
Tamaxin	tamoxifen
Tambocor	flecainide
Tamiflu	oseltamivir, pandemic influenza vaccine (H1N1)
Tamofen	tamoxifen
Tamoxan	tamoxifen
Tanzeum	albiglutide
Tapazole	methimazole
Tapros	leuprolide
Taravid	ofloxacin
Tarceva	erlotinib
Targiniq	naloxone, oxycodone
Targocid	teicoplanin
Targretin	bexarotene
Tarka	trandolapril, verapamil
Taro-Ampicillin Trihydrate	ampicillin
Taro-Atenol	atenolol

Tasigna	nilotinib
Taucor	lovastatin
Tavanic	levofloxacin
Tavor	lorazepam
Taxagon	trazodone
Taxol	paclitaxel
Taxotere	docetaxel
Taxus	tamoxifen
Tazicef	ceftazidime
Tazorac	tazarotene
Tecentriq	atezolizumab
Tecfidera	dimethyl fumarate
Technivie	ombitasvir/paritaprevir/ritonavir
Tecoplanin	teicoplanin
Tecprazin	praziquantel
Teczem	diltiazem, enalapril
Tedolan	etodolac
Tefamin	aminophylline
Teflaro	ceftaroline fosamil
Teflin	tetracycline
Tega-Cert	dimenhydrinate
Tega-Vert	dimenhydrinate
Tegretol XR	carbamazepine
Tegretol	carbamazepine
Teichomycin-A2	teicoplanin
Tekamlo	amlodipine
Tekturna HCT	hydrochlorothiazide
Telachlor	chlorpheniramine
Teldrin	chlorpheniramine
Teline	tetracycline
Temazepam	temazepam
Tementil	prochlorperazine
Temesta	lorazepam
Temgesic	buprenorphine
Temodar	temozolomide
Tenif	atenolol, nifedipine
Teniken	praziquantel
Tenolin	atenolol
Tenoret 50	atenolol
Tenoretic	atenolol
Tenormin	atenolol
Tenormine	atenolol
Tensin	spironolactone
Tensipine MR	nifedipine
Tensopril	lisinopril
Teralithe	lithium
Teril	carbamazepine
Terlipressin	terlipressin
Ternalax	tizanidine
Ternelin	tizanidine
Tertroxin	liothyronine
Tesavel	sitagliptin
Testandro	testosterone
Testim	testosterone
Testoderm	testosterone
Teston	methyltestosterone
Testopel	testosterone
Testotonic 'B'	methyltestosterone
Testovis	methyltestosterone
Testred	methyltestosterone
Tetradin	disulfiram

tetrahydrocannabinol	dronabinol	Tramal	tramadol
Tetramig	tetracycline	Tramed	tramadol
Teveten HCT	hydrochlorothiazide	Tramol	tramadol
Teveten	eprosartan	Trandate	labetalol
Texate	methotrexate	Transderm-Nitro	nitroglycerin
Teysuno	tegafur/gimeracil/oteracil	Transene	clorazepate
Thacapzol	methimazole	Transtec	buprenorphine
Thalomid	thalidomide	Tranxal	clorazepate
THC	dronabinol	Tranxen	clorazepate
Theo-Dur	aminophylline	Tranxene	clorazepate
theophylline ethylenediamine	aminophylline	Tranxilen	clorazepate
Thevier	levothyroxine	Tranxilium	clorazepate
Thiamazol	methimazole	Trasamlon	tranexamic acid
thiamazole	methimazole	Travatan Z	travoprost
Thinex	lindane	Travatan	travoprost
Thioprine	azathioprine	Travel Tabs	dimenhydrinate
Thorazine	chlorpromazine	Trazalon	trazodone
Thyroid-Block	potassium iodide	Tremfya	guselkumab
Thyronine	liothyronine	Trendar	ibuprofen
Thyrozol	methimazole	Trental	pentoxifylline
tiabendazole	thiabendazole	Tresiba	insulin degludec
Tiamate	diltiazem	Trexan	naltrexone
Tiazac	diltiazem	Tri-Levlen	oral contraceptives
Tibinide	isoniazid	Tri-Norinyl	oral contraceptives
TICE BCG	BCG vaccine	Triadapin	doxepin
Tidocol	mesalamine	Triaken	ceftriaxone
Tiempe	trimethoprim	Triaminic DM	dextromethorphan
Tifomycine	chloramphenicol	Triaminic	chlorpheniramine
Tilazem	diltiazem	Trian	triamterene
Tildiem	diltiazem	Triasox	thiabendazole
Timonil	carbamazepine	Triavil	perphenazine
Titus	lorazepam	Tricodein	codeine
Tivicay	dolutegravir	Tricor	fenofibrate
TMP-SMX	co-trimoxazole	Tridil	nitroglycerin
TMP-SMZ	co-trimoxazole	Tridol	tramadol
TOBI	tobramycin	Triflucan	fluconazole
Tobra	tobramycin	Trijodthyronin BC N	liothyronine
TobraDex	tobramycin	Trikacide	metronidazole
Tobrex	tobramycin	Trilafon	perphenazine
Tofranil	imipramine	Trileptal	oxcarbazepine
Tolak	fluorouracil	Trilifan Retard	perphenazine
Toloxim	mebendazole	Trimopan	trimethoprim
Topadol	ketorolac	Trimox	amoxicillin
Topamax	topiramate	Trimzol	co-trimoxazole
Topicort	desoximetasone	Trinalin	pseudoephedrine
Topicycline	tetracycline	Trintellix (formerly Brintellix)	vortioxetine
Toprol XL	metoprolol	Triomin	perphenazine
Toradol	ketorolac	Triostat	liothyronine
Torem	torsemide	Triphasil	oral contraceptives
Toremonil	hydroxychloroquine	Triprim	trimethoprim
Torental	pentoxifylline	Triptone	dimenhydrinate
Torisel	temsirolimus	Trisoralen	psoralens
Torolac	ketorolac	Trisulfa	co-trimoxazole
Torvin	ketorolac	Tritace	ramipril
Totacillin	ampicillin	Triumeq	abacavir, dolutegravir, lamivudine
Totapen	ampicillin	Trivora	oral contraceptives
Toviaz	fesoterodine	Triz	cetirizine
tPA	alteplase	Trizivir	abacavir, lamivudine, zidovudine
Tracleer	bosentan	Trobalt	ezogabine
Tradjenta	linagliptin	Trocal	dextromethorphan
Tradol	tramadol	Trokendi XR	topiramate

Tronoxal	ifosfamide	Urdox	ursodiol
Tropax	oxybutynin	Urem	ibuprofen
Tropium	chlordiazepoxide	Urex	furosemide
Tropyn Z	atropine sulfate	Urief	silodosin
Troxyca	naltrexone, oxycodone	Urised	atropine sulfate, hyoscyamine
Trulance	plecanatide	Uritol	furosemide
Trulicity	dulaglutide	Uro-cephoral	cefixime
Trumenba	meningococcal group B vaccine	Urobak	sulfamethoxazole
Truphylline	aminophylline	Urocid	probenecid
Trusopt	dorzolamide	Urofuran	nitrofurantoin
Truvada	emtricitabine, tenofovir disoproxil	Uromax	oxybutynin
Tryptanol	amitriptyline	Uroxatral	alfuzosin
Tryptizol	amitriptyline	Urozide	hydrochlorothiazide
TS-1	tegafur/gimeracil/oteracil	Urso 250	ursodiol
Tussar-2	codeine	Urso Forte	ursodiol
Tussgen	hydrocodone	Urso Heumann	ursodiol
Tussi-12D	phenylephrine	Urso Vinas	ursodiol
Tussi-Organidin	codeine	Ursochol	ursodiol
Tussionex	hydrocodone	*ursodeoxycholic acid*	ursodiol
Tussogest	hydrocodone	Ursofal	ursodiol
Twinrix	hepatitis B vaccine	Ursofalk	ursodiol
Tykerb	lapatinib	Ursoflor	ursodiol
Tylenol	acetaminophen	Ursogal	ursodiol
Tylox	oxycodone	Ursolac	ursodiol
Tymlos	abaloparatide	Ursolism	ursodiol
Typherix	typhoid vaccine	Ursolvan	ursodiol
Typhim Vi	typhoid vaccine	Urson	ursodiol
Tysabri	natalizumab	Ursoproge	ursodiol
Tyzeka	telbivudine	Ursosan	ursodiol
		Ursotan	ursodiol
		USCA	ursodiol

U

UDC Hexal	ursodiol	Utibron Neohaler	glycopyrrolate, indacaterol
UDC	ursodiol	Utinor	norfloxacin
UDCA	ursodiol	Utradol	etodolac
Udrik	trandolapril		

V

Uducil	cytarabine		
Ulcar	sucralfate	V-cillin K	penicillin V
Ulcedine	cimetidine	Vabomere	meropenem & vaborbactam
Ulcogant	sucralfate	Vacanyl	terbutaline
Ulcol	sulfasalazine	Vagifem	estradiol
Ulcyte	sucralfate	Valadol	acetaminophen
Uloric	febuxostat	Valcyte	valganciclovir
Ulsen	omeprazole	Valdrene	diphenhydramine
Ultra-MOP	methoxsalen	Valium	diazepam
Ultracet	tramadol	Valni XL	nifedipine
Ultram	tramadol	Valodex	tamoxifen
Umbradol	salsalate	*valproate sodium*	valproic acid
Umine	phentermine	Valtrex	valacyclovir
Unasyn	ampicillin/sulbactam	Valturna	valsartan
Unat	torsemide	Vamate	hydroxyzine
Uniflox	ciprofloxacin	Vanatrip	amitriptyline
Unimazole	methimazole	Vanceril	beclomethasone
Unimetone	nabumetone	Vancocin	vancomycin
Uniparin	heparin	Vancotil	loperamide
Uniretic	hydrochlorothiazide	Vandazole	metronidazole
Unithroid	levothyroxine	Vaniqa	eflornithine
Unitrim	trimethoprim	Vanmicina	vancomycin
Unituxin	dinutuximab	Vanquish	aspirin
Unizuric	allopurinol	Vaprisol	conivaptan
Uptravi	selexipag	Vaqta	hepatitis A vaccine
Urbal	sucralfate	Varilrix	varicella vaccine

Variquel	terlipressin
Varithena	polidocanol
Varivax	varicella vaccine
Varsan	lindane
Varubi	rolapitant
Vascal	isradipine
Vaseretic	enalapril, hydrochlorothiazide
Vasopril	fosinopril
Vasostrict	vasopressin
Vasotec	enalapril
Vaxchora	cholera vaccine
Vaxigrip	influenza vaccine
Veclam	clarithromycin
Vectibix	panitumumab
Velban	vinblastine
Velbe	vinblastine
Velcade	bortezomib
Veletri	epoprostenol
Velodan	loratadine
Velsar	vinblastine
Velsay	naproxen
Veltassa	patiromer
Vemlidy	tenofovir alafenamide
Venclexta	venetoclax
Venoglobulin	immune globulin IV
Ventolin	albuterol
Ventoline	albuterol
VePesid	etoposide
Vepeside	etoposide
Veraken	verapamil
Verelan	verapamil
Vermicol	mebendazole
Vermox	mebendazole
Versed	midazolam
Vertab	dimenhydrinate
Vertigon	prochlorperazine
Verzenio	abemaciclib
Vesanoid	tretinoin
Vesicare	solifenacin
Vestra	reboxetine
Vfend	voriconazole
Viadur	leuprolide
Viaflex	heparin
Viagra	sildenafil
Viberzi	eluxadoline
Vibra-Tabs	doxycycline
Vibramycin-D	doxycycline
Vicapan N	cyanocobalamin
Vicard	terazosin
Vicks Formula 44	dextromethorphan
Vicks Vatronol	ephedrine
Vicodin	acetaminophen, hydrocodone
Vicoprofen	hydrocodone, ibuprofen
Victoza	liraglutide
Victrelis	boceprevir
Vidaza	azacitidine
Videx	didanosine
Vidopen	ampicillin
Viekira Pak	ombitasvir/paritaprevir/ritonavir
Viekira XR	dasabuvir/ombitasvir/paritaprevir/ritonavir
Viekirax	ombitasvir/paritaprevir/ritonavir

Viibryd	vilazodone
Vimizim	elosulfase alfa
Vimpat	lacosamide
Vincasar	vincristine
Viracept	nelfinavir
Viramid	ribavirin
Viramune	nevirapine
Virazid	ribavirin
Virazole	ribavirin
Viread	tenofovir disoproxil
Virilon	methyltestosterone
Virlix	cetirizine
Viromone	methyltestosterone
Vistabel	botulinum toxin (A & B)
Vistacarpin	pilocarpine
Vistaril	hydroxyzine
Vistide	cidofovir
Visudyne	verteporfin
Vita Plus E	vitamin E
Vita-E	vitamin E
Vitak	phytonadione
Vitamin B$_{12}$	cyanocobalamin
vitamin B$_3$	niacin, niacinamide
vitamin B$_9$	folic acid
vitamin K$_1$	phytonadione
Vitamin K	phytonadione
Vitatropine	atropine sulfate
Vitec	vitamin E
Vitrase	hyaluronic acid
Vivaglobin	immune globulin sc
Vivatec	lisinopril
Vivelle-Dot	estradiol
Vivelle	estradiol
Vividyl	nortriptyline
Vivitrex	naltrexone
Vivitrol	naltrexone
Vivol	diazepam
Vivotif	typhoid vaccine
Vogan	vitamin A
Volibris	ambrisentan
Volmax	albuterol
Voltaren	diclofenac
Voltarene	diclofenac
Voltarol	diclofenac
Vomacur	dimenhydrinate
Vomex A	dimenhydrinate
Vomisen	dimenhydrinate
Vonum	indomethacin
Vosevi	sofosbuvir/velpatasvir/voxilaprevir
Vozet	levocetirizine
VP-TEC	etoposide
Vraylar	cariprazine
Vytorin	ezetimibe, simvastatin
Vyvanse	lisdexamfetamine

W

Waran	warfarin
Warfilone	warfarin
Waytrax	ceftazidime
Wehamine	dimenhydrinate
Welchol	colesevelam

Wellbutrin	bupropion	Zantic	ranitidine
Welldorm	chloral hydrate	Zantryl	phentermine
Wigrettes	ergotamine	Zapex	oxazepam
Winobanin	danazol	Zaponex	clozapine
Winstrol	stanozolol	Zariviz	cefotaxime
Wintrocin	erythromycin	Zarondan	ethosuximide
Wyamicin S	erythromycin	Zarontin	ethosuximide

X

X	MDMA	Zavedos	idarubicin
Xadago	safinamide	Zebeta	bisoprolol
Xalatan	latanoprost	Zebinix	eslicarbazepine
Xalkori	crizotinib	Zecuity	sumatriptan
Xanax	alprazolam	Zedolac	etodolac
Xanef	enalapril	Zefone	ceftriaxone
Xarelto	rivaroxaban	Zeftera	ceftobiprole
Xatral	alfuzosin	Zejula	niraparib
Xelevia	sitagliptin	Zelapar	selegiline
Xeljanz	tofacitinib	Zelboraf	vemurafenib
Xeloda	capecitabine	Zenapax	daclizumab
Xenical	orlistat	Zentropil	phenytoin
Xeomin	botulinum toxin (A & B)	Zeos	loratadine
Xermelo	telotristat ethyl	Zepatier	elbasvir & grazoprevir
Xgeva	denosumab	Zerbaxa	ceftolozane & tazobactam
Xifaxan	rifaximin	Zerit	stavudine
Xifaxanta	rifaximin	Zestoretic	hydrochlorothiazide, lisinopril
Xigduo XR	dapagliflozin, metformin	Zestril	lisinopril
Xiidra	lifitegrast	Zetia	ezetimibe
Xofigo	radium-223 dichloride	Zeto	azithromycin
Xolair	omalizumab	Ziac	bisoprolol, hydrochlorothiazide
Xomolix	droperidol	Ziagen	abacavir
Xozal	levocetirizine	Zicam	zinc
Xtampza ER	oxycodone	Zimovane	eszopiclone
Xtandi	enzalutamide	Zinacef	cefuroxime
Xtoro	finafloxacin	Zinacet	cefuroxime
Xultophy	insulin degludec, liraglutide	Zinat	cefuroxime
Xusal	levocetirizine	Zinbryta	daclizumab
xylocaine	lidocaine	Zinnat	cefuroxime
Xylocard	lidocaine	Zinplava	bezlotoxumab
Xyzal	levocetirizine	Zioptan	tafluprost

Y

		Zipan	tramadol
		Zipsor	diclofenac
		Zirtin	cetirizine
Yamatetan	cefotetan	Zithromax	azithromycin
Yasmin	oral contraceptives	Zitromax	azithromycin
Yaz	oral contraceptives	*ziv-aflibercept*	aflibercept
Yectamid	amikacin	Zmax	azithromycin
Yentreve	duloxetine	Zocor	simvastatin
Yervoy	ipilimumab	Zocord	simvastatin
YF-VAX	yellow fever vaccine	Zofran	ondansetron
Yosprala	aspirin, omeprazole	Zofron	ondansetron
Yuma	hydroxychloroquine	Zohydro ER	hydrocodone
Yurelax	cyclobenzaprine	Zoldan-A	danazol
		Zole	miconazole

Z

		zoledronic acid	zoledronate
		Zolinza	vorinostat
		Zoloft	sertraline
Zaltrap	aflibercept	ZoMaxx Drug-Eluting Coronary Stent	zotarolimus
Zanaflex	tizanidine	Zometa	zoledronate
Zanosar	streptozocin	Zomig	zolmitriptan
Zantab	ranitidine	Zonegran	zonisamide
Zantac-C	ranitidine	Zontivity	vorapaxar
Zantac	ranitidine	Zorac	tazarotene

Zorbenal-G	tetracycline	Zyclir	acyclovir
Zoref	cefuroxime	Zydelig	idelalisib
Zoroxin	norfloxacin	Zyderm	collagen (bovine)
Zortress	everolimus	Zydone	hydrocodone
Zorvolex	diclofenac	Zyflo	zileuton
Zostavax	zoster vaccine	Zyloprim	allopurinol
Zosyn	piperacillin/tazobactam	Zyloric	allopurinol
Zovia	oral contraceptives	Zymerol	cimetidine
Zovirax	acyclovir	Zynox	naloxone
Zumalin	lincomycin	Zyplast	collagen (bovine)
Zunden	piroxicam	Zyprexa Relprevv	olanzapine
Zuplenz	ondansetron	Zyprexa	olanzapine
Zurampic	lesinurad	Zyrtec	cetirizine
Zyban	bupropion	Zytiga	abiraterone
Zyclara	imiquimod	Zyvox	linezolid

This information is intended for
personal use only and is not an
endorsement or referral.
Please consult your physician
with specific questions.